Advanced Practice Nursing

An Integrative Approach

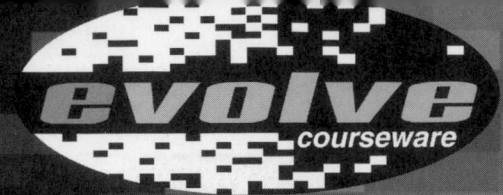

The Latest *Evolution* in Learning.

Evolve provides online access to free learning resources and activities designed specifically for the textbook you are using in your class.
The resources will provide you with information that enhances the material covered in the book and much more.

Visit the Web address listed below to start your learning evolution today!

▶▶ LOGIN: *http://evolve.elsevier.com/Hamric/*

Evolve Student Learning Resources for Hamric, Spross, and Hanson's *Advanced Practice Nursing: An Integrative Approach*, third edition offers:

- **WebLinks**
  An invaluable resource that lets you link to hundreds of websites chosen to supplement each chapter of the book. The WebLinks are regularly updated so that you will have access to the most cutting-edge information in the field.

Evolve Instructor Resources for Hamric, Spross, and Hanson's *Advanced Practice Nursing: An Integrative Approach*, third edition offers the following features:

- **"Things to Think About" Discussion Questions**
  includes discussion topics and questions for each chapter

- **PowerPoint Lecture Slides**
  includes highlighted points from each chapter and all of the tables and boxes presented in the text

- **Electronic Image Collection**
  includes all of the illustrations from the text

- **WebLinks**
  includes all websites cited in the text and other related websites

Think outside the book... EVOLVE.

Advanced Practice Nursing
An Integrative Approach
Third Edition

ANN B. HAMRIC, PhD, RN, FAAN
Associate Professor
University of Virginia School of Nursing
Charlottesville, Virginia

JUDITH A. SPROSS, PhD, RN, AOCN, FAAN
Associate Professor
University of Southern Maine
College of Nursing and Health Professions
Portland, Maine

CHARLENE M. HANSON, EdD, RN, CS, FNP, FAAN
Professor Emerita
Georgia Southern University
Statesboro, Georgia

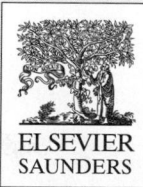

ELSEVIER
SAUNDERS

ELSEVIER
SAUNDERS

11830 Westline Industrial Drive
St. Louis, Missouri 63146

ADVANCED PRACTICE NURSING: AN INTEGRATIVE APPROACH
Copyright © 2005, 2000, 1996 by Elsevier Inc.

Previous editions copyrighted 2000, 1996

Library of Congress Cataloging-in-Publication Data

Hamric, Ann B.
    Advanced practice nursing: an integrative approach/Ann Hamric, Judith Spross,
Charlene Hanson.—3rd ed.
        p.; cm.
    Rev. ed. of: Advanced nursing practice, 2nd ed. c2000.
    Includes bibliographical references and index.
    ISBN-13: 978-0-7216-0330-8   ISBN-10: 0-7216-0330-0
        1. Nurse practitioners. 2. Midwives. 3. Nurse anesthetists. I. Spross, Judith A. II.
Hanson, Charlene M. III. Hamric, Ann B. Advanced nursing practice. IV. Title.
    [DNLM: 1. Specialties, Nursing—methods. 2. Nurse Anesthetists. 3. Nurse Clinicians.
4. Nurse Midwives. 5. Nurse Practitioners. WY 101 H232a 2000]
RT82.8H355 2005
610.73—dc22

2004046662

Executive Publisher: Barbara Nelson Cullen
Developmental Editor: Adrienne Simon
Publishing Services Manager: Deborah. L. Vogel
Designer: Amy Buxton

ISBN-13: 978-0-7216-0330-8
ISBN-10: 0-7216-0330-0

Printed in United States of America

Last digit is the print number: 9 8 7 6 5

CONTRIBUTORS

Ann Reid Anderson, MSN, RNC, ANP
Nurse Practitioner
Medical College of Virginia
Virginia Commonwealth University Health System
Richmond, Virginia
Chapter 13: The Primary Care Nurse Practitioner

Anne-Marie Barron, PhD, RN, CS
Assistant Professor
Department of Nursing
School for Health Studies
Simmons College
Boston, Massachusetts

Psychiatric Clinical Nurse Specialist
Oncology/Bone Marrow Transplant Unit
Massachusetts General Hospital
Boston, Massachusetts
Chapter 7: Consultation

Jeri L. Bigbee, PhD, RN, CS, FNP, FAAN
Orvis Endowed Professor
Orvis School of Nursing
University of Nevada
Reno, Nevada
*Chapter 1: History and Evolution of Advanced Practice
    Nursing*

Sarah Jo Brown, PhD, RN
Research Consultant
Practice-Research Integrations
Norwich, Vermont
Chapter 5: Direct Clinical Practice

Karen A. Brykczynski, DNSc, RN, FNP
Associate Professor
University of Texas Medical Branch School of Nursing
Galveston, Texas
*Chapter 4: Role Development of the Advanced Practice
    Nurse*

Paula A. Caron, ARNP, MS, AOCN
Advanced Practice Nurse
Norris Cotton Cancer Center
Dartmouth-Hitchcock Medical Center
Lebanon, New Hampshire
*Chapter 15: The Blended Role of the Clinical Nurse Specialist
    and the Nurse Practitioner*

Judith A. DePalma, PhD, RN
Associate Professor
Slippery Rock University
Slippery Rock, Pennsylvania

President
J. A. DePalma Consulting
Pittsburgh, Pennsylvania
Chapter 8: Research

Margaret W. Dorroh, MN, CNM, FNP-C
Certified Nurse-Midwife and Family Nurse Practitioner
The Family Health and Birth Center
Rincon, Georgia
Chapter 16: The Certified Nurse-Midwife

Susan E. D. Doughty, RNC, MSN, WHNP
Owner
New England WomenCenter
South Portland, Maine
Chapter 21: Marketing and Contracting Considerations

Margaret Faut-Callahan, DNSc, CRNA, FAAN
Professor and Chair, Adult Health Nursing
Director, Nurse Anesthesia Program
Rush University College of Nursing
Chicago, Illinois
Chapter 17: The Certified Registered Nurse Anesthetist

Jane Guttendorf, RN, MSN, CRNP, APRN-BC
Acute Care Nurse Practitioner
Cardiothoracic Intensive Care Unit
University of Pittsburgh Medical Center
Pittsburgh, Pennsylvania
Chapter 14: The Acute Care Nurse Practitioner

Ann B. Hamric, PhD, RN, FAAN
Associate Professor
University of Virginia School of Nursing
Charlottesville, Virginia
Chapter 3: A Definition of Advanced Practice Nursing
Chapter 11: Ethical Decision Making
Chapter 15: The Blended Role of the Clinical Nurse Specialist
and the Nurse Practitioner
Chapter 19: Evolving and Innovative Opportunities for
Advanced Practice Nursing

Charlene M. Hanson, EdD, RN, CS, FNP, FAAN
Professor Emerita
Georgia Southern University
Statesboro, Georgia
Chapter 9: Clinical and Professional Leadership
Chapter 10: Collaboration
Chapter 20: Business Planning and Reimbursement
Mechanisms
Chapter 22: Understanding Regulatory, Legal, and
Credentialing Requirements

Donna R. Hodnicki, PhD, APRN, BC, FNP, FAAN
Professor and MSN Program Director
Georgia Southern University
Statesboro, Georgia
Chapter 21: Marketing and Contracting Considerations

Marilyn Hravnak, PhD, RN, CRNP-BC, CCRN, FCCM
Assistant Professor
Acute Care Nurse Practitioner Program
University of Pittsburgh
School of Nursing
Pittsburgh, Pennsylvania
Chapter 14: The Acute Care Nurse Practitioner

Gail L. Ingersoll, EdD, RN, FAAN, FNAP
Professor, Nursing
Director, Clinical Nursing Research
University of Rochester Medical Center
Rochester, New York
Chapter 25: Outcome Evaluation and Performance
Improvement

Jean Johnson, PhD, RN, FAAN
Associate Dean and Professor
George Washington University
School of Medicine and Health Sciences
Washington, District of Columbia
Chapter 23: Health Policy Issues in Changing Environments

Arlene W. Keeling, PhD, RN
Professor
Director, The Center for Nursing Historical Inquiry
Director, Acute Care Nurse Practitioner Program
University of Virginia School of Nursing
Charlottesville, Virginia
Chapter 1: History and Evolution of Advanced Practice
Nursing

Maureen A. Kelley, PhD, CNM, FACNM
Clinical Associate Professor
Chair, Family and Community Nursing
Emory University
Nell Hodgson Woodruff School of Nursing
Atlanta, Georgia
Chapter 16: The Certified Nurse-Midwife

Christina C. King, MSN, APRN-BC
Clinical Nurse Specialist
Capital Health – University of Alberta Hospital
Edmonton, Alberta
Chapter 20: Business Planning and Reimbursement
Mechanisms

Ruth M. Kleinpell, PhD, RN-CS, FAAN, CCRN
Associate Professor, Adult Health Nursing
Rush University College of Nursing
Chicago, Illinois
Chapter 14: The Acute Care Nurse Practitioner

Mary D. Knudtson, MSN, FNP
Clinical Professor
Director of FNP Program
Department of Family Medicine
University of California, Irvine
Irvine, California
Chapter 24: Strengthening Advanced Nursing Practice in Organizational Structures and Cultures

Michael J. Kremer, DNSc, CRNA, FAAN
Associate Professor, Adult Health Nursing
Co-Director, Rush University Simulation Labs
Assistant Director, Nurse Anesthesia Program
Rush University College of Nursing
Chicago, Illinois
Chapter 17: The Certified Registered Nurse Anesthetist

Marjorie Thomas Lawson, PhD, RN, FNP
Associate Professor
College of Nursing and Health Professions
University of Southern Maine
Portland, Maine
Chapter 2: Conceptualizations of Advanced Practice Nursing

Kathy S. Magdic, MSN, RN, APRN, BS
Instructor and Coordinator, Acute Care Nurse Practitioner Program
University of Pittsburgh School of Nursing
Pittsburgh, Pennsylvania
Manager, Cardiopulmonary Clinical Emphasis
University of Pittsburgh Medical Center Cardiac Pavilion Service
Pittsburgh, Pennsylvania
Chapter 14: The Acute Care Nurse Practitioner

Vicky A. Mahn-DiNicola, MS, RN
Vice President, Clinical Decision Support Services
ACS MIDAS+
Tucson, Arizona
Adjunct Clinical Instructor
University of Arizona College of Nursing
Tucson, Arizona
Chapter 18: The Advanced Practice Nurse Case Manager
Chapter 25: Outcome Evaluation and Performance Improvement

Deborah B. McGuire, PhD, RN, FAAN
Professor and Coordinator, Oncology Specialty
University of Maryland
School of Nursing
Baltimore, Maryland
Chapter 8: Research

Brenda M. Nevidjon, MSN, RN
Associate Clinical Professor
Chief, Division of Health Care Leadership, Education, and Management
Duke University School of Nursing
Durham, North Carolina
Chapter 24: Strengthening Advanced Nursing Practice in Organizational Structures and Cultures

L. Gregory Pawlson, MD, MPH
Clinical Professor of Medicine and Health Care Sciences
George Washington University
School of Medicine and Health Sciences
Washington, District of Columbia
Adjunct Professor
George Washington University
School of Public Health
Washington, District of Columbia
Executive Vice President
National Committee for Quality Assurance
Washington, District of Columbia
Chapter 23: Health Policy Issues in Changing Environments

Juanita Reigle, MSN, RN, ACNP-CS
Associate Professor of Nursing
University of Virginia School of Nursing
Charlottesville, Virginia
Chapter 11: Ethical Decision Making

Jeanne Salyer, PhD, RN
Associate Professor, Adult Health Nursing
Virginia Commonwealth University
Richmond, Virginia
Chapter 19: Evolving and Innovative Opportunities for Advanced Practice Nursing

Karen Skalla, MSN, ARNP, AOCN
Nurse Practitioner, Hematology/Oncology
Dartmouth-Hitchcock Medical Center and Valley Regional
    Hospital
Lebanon, New Hampshire

Instructor in Medicine, Hematology/Oncology
Dartmouth Medical School
Hanover, New Hampshire
*Chapter 15: The Blended Role of the Clinical Nurse Specialist
    and the Nurse Practitioner*

Patricia S. A. Sparacino MS, RN, FAAN
Coordinator of Clinical Practice
Clinical Nurse Specialist
UCSF Home Health Care
San Francisco, California

Clinical Professor
UCSF School of Nursing
University of California, San Francisco
San Francisco, California
Chapter 12: The Clinical Nurse Specialist

Judith A. Spross, PhD, RN, AOCN, FAAN
Associate Professor
University of Southern Maine
College of Nursing and Health Professions
Portland, Maine
Chapter 2: Conceptualizations of Advanced Practice Nursing
Chapter 6: Expert Coaching and Guidance
Chapter 9: Clinical and Professional Leadership
Chapter 10: Collaboration

Patricia A. White MS, APRN, BC
Assistant Professor
Department of Nursing
School for Health Studies
Simmons College
Boston, Massachusetts

Adult Nurse Practitioner
Hingham-Weymouth Family Medical Associates
North Weymouth, Massachusetts
Chapter 7: Consultation

Donna J. Zazworsky, MS, RN, CCM, FAAN
Adjunct Clinical Assistant Professor
University of Arizona College of Nursing
Tucson, Arizona

Director, Community Nursing and Outreach
St. Elizabeth of Hungary Clinic
Tucson, Arizona

Managing Partner
Case Manager Solutions, LLC
Tucson, Arizona
Chapter 18: The Advanced Practice Nurse Case Manager

REVIEWERS

Connie Gleim Bareford, PhD, RN, CS
Director, Graduate Program in Nursing
William Paterson University of New Jersey
Wayne, New Jersey

Toni O. Barnett, PhD, FNP-C, AANP, ANCC
Director, Family Nurse Practitioner Program
North Georgia College and State University
Department of Nursing
Dahlonega, Georgia

Nancey E. M. France, PhD, RN
Coordinator, Master's of Science in Nursing Program and
    Research
Murray State University
College of Science, Department of Nursing
Murray, Kentucky

Brenda L. Hage, MSN, CRNP
Assistant Professor, Nursing
College Misericordia
Division of Health Sciences
Department of Nursing
Dallas, Pennsylvania

Marcia Murphy, MS, RN, CS-ANP
Assistant Professor
Rush University College of Nursing
Chicago, Illinois

The environment within which nurses and, more specifically, advanced practice nurses (APNs) are educated and practice has become more complex since the events of September 11, 2001 and the war in Iraq. These are troubled times economically and in health care. However, advanced nursing practice has continued to develop and flourish as evidence accumulates that the advanced practice of nursing is good for patients/consumers. Continuing concerns regarding cost containment have sustained a focus on evidence-based practice. Despite calls for more cooperation among providers (IOM, 2001)*, market and social forces continue to foster competition among providers, notably physicians and APNs. Increased health-care regulations in the wake of reports of medical errors, privacy concerns, and research lapses have complicated practice for all providers, including APNs. All of these developments have heightened the need for clarity about advanced practice nursing and promulgation of standards to ensure the competence of all APN providers.

At the same time, the United States has experienced one of the most serious nursing shortages in its history. Despite efforts to recruit men into nursing, most nurses are women. While the shortage is attributed, in part, to a wider range of career choices for women, those within and outside the profession recognize that for many nurses, working conditions are often inhospitable, characterized by limited autonomy, a lack of interdisciplinary collaboration, and a lack of recognition of the impact of nursing care on patient outcomes and resource utilization. Clinically, expanding populations of elderly persons and those with chronic diseases, an increasing volume of information (guidelines, research), new technologies, and other innovations have increased the complexity of care delivery and clinical decision making. The nursing profession is responding to these changes by using media campaigns and other strategies to enhance the public image of nursing and recruit new nurses into the profession. Innovative education and practice strategies are also being implemented to ensure that the United States will have sufficient nurses who are prepared to address the challenges of 21st century health care.

There are signs that some of these trends are creating favorable conditions for APNs. Physician-dominated primary care is being reexamined, and the time is right for primary and specialty care provided by APNs to flourish. The clinical nurse specialist (CNS) role is experiencing a resurgence as hospitals recognize the need for strong mentoring of nursing staff. Acute care nurse practitioners (ACNPs) and blended roles are finding strong markets as changes continue within institutional structures. Interestingly, APN programs, particularly for NPs, have stayed stable although issues of quality, faculty preparation and practice, and standardization continue to be serious concerns. All of these changes have required a major revision of this book.

PURPOSE

Our goal remains to describe an integrated understanding of advanced practice nursing that will provide clarity and structure for students, practicing APNs, and the profession at

---

*Institute of Medicine. (2001). Crossing the quality chasm: A new health system for the 21st century. Washington, DC: National Academies Press.

large. We have thoroughly updated this edition with state-of-the-science information to ensure that APNs can proactively manage the environments in which they practice so that advanced practice nursing not only survives but also thrives in the system's ongoing turbulence.

We believe that this third edition defines and strengthens our understanding of advanced practice nursing—its definition, competencies, roles, and the issues facing APNs—with more clarity and authority than our earlier efforts. There is now a clearer understanding of all APN roles, both established and evolving, that are valuable in achieving the goals of various care delivery systems. There are clear signs of progress toward a unified understanding of advanced practice nursing, though much remains to be done.

This edition also updates the opportunities for advanced practice that can be envisioned in a future health-care system where APNs and all nurses participate more fully, visibly, and equitably with their medical colleagues and others. We have approached this revision with openness to these potential opportunities and have focused much of this text on strategies to assist APNs to take advantage of the uncertainty and complexity of the health-care environment and to set the stage for the exploration of new roles for advanced practice nursing.

UNDERLYING PREMISES

This book is grounded in the conviction that advanced practice nursing must have a definable and describable core that provides a framework for standardizing the profession's understanding of this level of practice. At the same time, the core must be flexible enough to accommodate the differing roles necessary to enact the varied practices of all APNs. As new roles evolve, this advanced practice core becomes ever more important. Several premises underlie this conviction:

- For certain patient populations, APNs are the best providers for delivering quality care at a reasonable cost.
- A uniform definition of advanced nursing practice and standards for educating and credentialing that are consistent across APN groups are essential for continued legitimacy of APN roles and regulatory parity with other providers. In the absence of a consistent definition, the instability of the health-care system and increased competition among providers pose a threat to the legitimacy of all APNs as providers; such threats may lead to the loss of hard-won legal and regulatory battles.
- A consistent definition of core competencies for APNs is essential in order to standardize APN education and regulation and to evaluate outcomes of APN care across roles. It is also imperative that APNs practice these competencies in order to demonstrate the value-added component they bring to care delivery, so that advanced practice nursing is not confused with physician substitution.
- A consistent definition is essential for interdisciplinary teamwork. Administrators and other providers must be able to rely on a core set of role expectations to design and implement cost-effective health-care delivery systems that fully utilize all APN roles.
- We remain convinced that advanced practice nursing is good for patients, but a higher level of standardization must be attained for the larger health-care establishment to agree with this claim.

ORGANIZATION

As with our previous work, this third edition of *Advanced Practice Nursing: An Integrative Approach* has been extensively updated and revised to reflect current literature and trends. We have retitled this edition to *Advanced Practice Nursing* in line with common terminology, though we continue to use the term interchangeably with *advanced nursing practice*.

There are a number of major revisions in this latest edition. In Part I, "Historical and Developmental Aspects of Advanced Practice Nursing," Chapter 1 has been reframed into an exciting decade-by-decade history of advanced practice nursing which clearly shows the origins of advanced practice and the tremendous strides APNs have made over time. Chapter 2 adds newer conceptual work including new models and commentary to direct a much-needed common language for advanced practice nursing. An important addition is an outline of future directions and recommendations to help foster a professional consensus on advanced practice. In Part II, "Competencies of Advanced Practice Nursing," the seven core competencies are examined. The chapters describing the competencies of research and ethical decision making have been extensively revised and updated to reflect current APN practice. Chapter 8 strengthens the current emphasis on evidence-based practice in discussing the research competency of the APN and clearly describes a model for teaching, learning, and implementing evidence-based concepts for outcomes evaluation. Chapter 11 proposes a more complete description of the ethical decision-making competency, including ethical issues affecting current APN practices.

The chapters in Part III, "Advanced Practice Roles: The Operational Definitions of Advanced Practice Nursing," have been revised to reflect the current practices of each APN role. Each chapter explicitly incorporates the core competencies and demonstrates how these competencies are played out in specific APN roles. Features unique to each APN role are also described, and a variety of exemplars are used to help students understand how to implement the particular APN role. Chapters describing the three newest APN roles—acute care nurse practitioner (ACNP), the blended CNS/NP, and the APN case manager—have been extensively reworked to reflect their current state of practice. The blended CNS/NP role chapter clarifies this evolving practice through a model that incorporates key CNS and NP competencies as well as features unique to the blended role. In the face of the proposed new non-APN role of the Clinical Nurse Leader, Chapter 18 offers a clear description of the APN case manager role and demonstrates the need for APN case management leadership. An important new chapter in this edition, Chapter 19, explores opportunities for new and evolving APN roles and clarifies important distinctions among specialty practice, subspecialty practice, and advanced nursing practice. This provocative chapter opens new vistas for APNs and at the same time presents a standardized framework for assessing the potential of evolving roles and specialties to become a new APN role.

Part IV, "Critical Elements in Managing Advanced Nursing Practice Environments," continues to explore key environmental factors affecting APN practice. Again, each chapter has been substantially updated. Chapter 23, which is about health policy, has been expanded to include a new section on legal issues. Chapter 24 has been revised to consider the critical issue of administrative support for APNs from both acute care and primary care perspectives. Chapter 25 is essentially a new chapter in this edition. It focuses on a thorough review of existing APN outcome research and gives strategies for individual APNs to demonstrate their impact on clinical outcomes and performance enhancements.

AUDIENCE

This book is intended for graduate students, practicing APNs in all roles, educators, administrators, and leaders in the nursing profession. For students in any APN graduate program, the book provides a comprehensive resource useful throughout their program of study. Initial clarity and understanding about the definition and competencies of advanced practice nursing can guide students as they enter their clinical coursework. We strongly recommend the book's use early in the program of study, in theory, in policy, and in APN role courses. The text is a valuable tool for use throughout clinical courses as students see the various APN roles and related competencies in action and as they begin practicing their chosen APN role. Students nearing graduation in role transition or capstone courses will appreciate the role development chapter, the in-depth information about implementing evidence-based practice, and the content in Part IV that explores business practices and environmental issues that they must be prepared to manage in the workplace.

For practicing APNs, the book updates both theoretical and practical content to guide role implementation. Individuals interested in strengthening or changing their roles will find many strategies for accomplishing these changes. The exploration of current issues in the health-care environment makes the book particularly useful to practicing clinicians who face issues within a marketplace that changes daily. The interdisciplinary, collaborative focus in many chapters may be useful to clinicians and educators in other fields. For example, interdisciplinary teams could benefit from discussions of such chapters as expert coaching and guidance, collaboration, ethical decision-making skills and health-care policy.

For educators, the book will serve as a comprehensive curricular resource in preparing APNs for practice. It also serves as a guide to standardize core education for advanced practice. An exciting new feature for faculty is the new Instructor's Resource that accompanies the text. It includes over 1,500 PowerPoint lecture slides presented by chapter including key text, tables, and boxes. There is also an electronic Image Collection with all of the images from the text, "Things to Think About" discussion topics and questions for each chapter, and WebLinks to all websites cited in the text. It is available both on the Evolve website (http://evolve.elsevier.com/Hamric/) and on CD-ROM. Extensive current references and additional reading lists can assist educators to design relevant courses on all the facets of advanced nursing practice. Nursing administrators will appreciate the descriptions of various APN roles and the strategies for justifying and supporting APN positions.

For nursing leaders, educators, and practicing clinicians alike, this book is a clarion call to reach greater consensus regarding our understanding of and preparation for advanced nursing practice and the roles APNs assume so that we speak with increasing authority and consistency to policymakers, to those in other disciplines, and to one another. Clarity regarding advanced practice nursing is a professional imperative.

APPROACH

We have sought to describe advanced practice nursing at its best, as it is being enacted by APNs throughout the country. There is still much work to be done: not all APN students are educated to practice with the competencies described here; faculty are aging and there are insufficient numbers of new faculty to replace them; too many nurses are in advanced nursing practice roles without the necessary credentials or competencies, so that true advanced practice is not demonstrated; and there is still too much "alphabet soup" in role titles (for example, the APN case manager is variously called outcomes manager, clinical outcomes consultant, disease management specialist, and so on).

Roles are continuing to evolve as nursing matures in its understanding and enactment of advanced practice, but advanced practice nursing must be distinct, recognizable, and describable if it is to continue to flourish. It will be clear to the reader that the diverse roles described in Part 3, while they share the core criteria and competencies of advanced practice nursing, are different and distinct from one another in their role enactment. This should be a cause for celebration, as nursing recognizes its strength and range in meeting patient/client needs.

Creating this new edition has once again been a challenging undertaking. We are grateful for the hard work of our contributors who substantially revised their chapters to portray a cutting-edge understanding of advanced practice nursing. We are privileged to participate with them in shaping this ever-changing area of nursing practice. Advanced nursing practice is a relatively young idea in the profession's evolution. We continue to be impressed by how complex it is to integrate and incorporate the perspectives of all APN specialties. Not all groups have addressed the core concept of advanced practice or the competencies of APNs in a complete or consistent manner. The literature from the various advanced practice specialty groups remains unfortunately separated, and clinicians and educators tend to read and cite only their own group's literature. One of the major contributions of this third edition is the effort to solidify our conceptualization of advanced practice nursing and to struggle with the complexities of new and evolving APN roles. Adopting this integrative approach, as challenging as it continues to be, has in our view immeasurably enriched this work.

We challenge readers to examine and apply the ideas put forth in this book, thereby adding to the evidence about the importance and quality of advanced nursing practice. As a critical component of present and future health care delivery systems, APNs are and must continue to be active participants in solving some of the pressing problems in health care delivery. We remain convinced that advanced practice nursing is essential to improving the health and well-being of the citizens of this nation and that increasing numbers of competent, well-prepared APNs will be needed as this century unfolds.

Ann B. Hamric
Judith A. Spross
Charlene M. Hanson

CONTENTS

PART I

Historical and Developmental Aspects of Advanced Practice Nursing

CHAPTER 1

The History of Advanced Practice Nursing in the United States

ARLENE W. KEELING • JERI L. BIGBEE

INTRODUCTION

For an understanding of the challenges facing advanced practice nursing today and to determine a path for the future, looking to the past is essential. This chapter presents some highlights of the history of advanced practice nursing in the United States from the late 19th century to the present. It examines four established and one emerging advanced practice roles—certified registered nurse anesthetists (CRNAs), certified nurse-midwives (CNMs), clinical nurse specialists (CNSs), nurse practitioners (NPs), and advanced practice nurse case managers (APNCMs)—in the context of the social, political, and economic environment of each decade and within the context of the history of medicine and advances in technology and science. Legal issues and issues related to gender and healthcare manpower are considered. The chapter's focus is the history of advanced practice in nursing, rather than the history of specialization in nursing, although the two are often intertwined. The roles profiled in this chapter are referred to as *advanced practice nursing roles*, although the terminology and understanding of advanced practice nursing were not used during much of the 20th century.

Although the development of advanced practice nursing has been complex, the trends that emerge are clear: (1) development was arduous and involved interprofessional and intraprofessional conflicts, as well as legal battles over acceptance of the various roles and the advance practice nurse's (APN's) scope of practice; (2) societal forces including wars, advances in science and technology, federal government funding and legislation, economic conditions, gender issues, and the women's movement played a significant part in the history of advanced practice nursing; and (3) organizational efforts, certification at the national level, and the move toward graduate education as a requirement for advanced practice were critical to the credibility of APNs' roles. Historical events relating directly to the development of advanced practice nursing are described. The reader is encouraged to consult the references of this chapter for further information.

The use of the term *specialist* in nursing can be traced to the turn of the 20th century, when it was used to designate a nurse who had completed a postgraduate course in a clinical specialty area or who had extensive experience and expertise in a particular clinical practice area. With the introduction of the NP role during the 1960s and 1970s, the terms *expanded role* and *extended role* were used, implying a horizontal movement to encompass expertise from medicine and other disciplines. The more contemporary term, *advanced practice*, which began to be seen in the 1980s, reflects a more vertical or hierarchical movement encompassing graduate education within nursing, rather than a simple expansion of expertise by development of knowledge and skills used by other disciplines. Since the 1980s, state nursing practice acts have increasingly adopted the term *advanced practice nurses* (APNs) to delineate CRNAs, CNMs, CNSs, and NPs. This regulatory influence served to unite the advanced practice specialty roles conceptually and legislatively, thereby promoting collaboration and cohesion among APNs.

PRE-1930s: THE ROOTS OF ADVANCED PRACTICE NURSING

The history of advanced practice nursing can be traced to the 19th century when two key events converged. The conflict between states' rights and the federal union came to a head, resulting in the American Civil War (1861 to 1865), and the medical profession discovered that chloroform could be used as an anesthetic agent during surgery. The intersection of these two factors would lead to the birth of professional nursing in the United States and to the roots of specialty practice in nurse anesthesia.

The Roots of Nurse Anesthesia

The specialty of nurse anesthesia emerged directly from the pre-professional work of women in the Civil War. There were no professional nurses in the United States when the first shots were fired on Fort Sumter in 1861. With the call to arms, thousands of women from both the North and the South volunteered to care for wounded and dying soldiers. They did so in makeshift hospitals created from hastily converted churches and warehouses or in their homes. Besides the lay volunteers, Catholic sisters served as nurses. Part of their work included assisting in surgery, particularly with the administration of chloroform. According to one author, on June 5, 1863, Mother Francis took four sisters "especially trained in the care of surgical cases" to Cincinnati where the nuns "often assisted in giving the anesthetic" (Jolly, 1927, p. 119). That same year, religious sisters administered anesthesia at West Pennsylvania Hospital in Pittsburgh (Jolly, 1927).

The creation of training schools for nurses was also a direct outcome of the war. Influenced by the decrease in mortality and morbidity rates that resulted from the women's nursing efforts during the Civil War, prominent physicians and members of the U.S. Sanitary Commission (a volunteer organization that sought to improve sanitary conditions and medical treatment in the Union army), lobbied for formal training[1] for nurses afterward. Moreover, Florence Nightingale's training school for nurses at St Thomas' Hospital in England was gaining international acclaim. Modeled according to Nightingale's recommendations, in 1873 the first schools of nursing opened in New York City; Boston; and New Haven, Connecticut. Soon thereafter, most hospitals were staffed by student nurses. In fact, very few graduate nurses were employed in hospitals. One exception to this trend was the employment of graduate nurses as nurse anesthetists. These nurse anesthetists were readily accepted by surgeons, who valued the fact that, unlike the disinterested medical students who had formerly assisted with anesthesia, nurse anesthetists concentrated on administering the anesthesia rather than observing the surgery. Moreover, they used a "gentle touch" during the process (Olsen, 1940). One of the first nurse anesthetists in the United States was Alice Magaw, who worked with the Mayo family surgeons at their clinic in Rochester, Minnesota. Commonly referred to as the *mother of anesthesia*, Magaw (1900) wrote that the responsibility for administering anesthesia should be given to nurses rather than physicians in training. According to her:

No anesthetizer can learn to be a surgeon at the same time he is administering an anesthetic, but many doctors think they will let the anesthetic take care of itself, especially in giving ether, and learn what they can at this time. When finally the attention is attracted to the patient, the result is that artificial respiration and drugs are resorted to . . . we think a well qualified, especially trained nurse for this purpose, can get better results, as her interests are undivided. (p. 153)

Magaw was one of the first specialty nurses to document and publish the outcomes of her practice. In an article published in the *St. Paul's Medical Journal* in 1900, she reports her "Observations on 1092 Cases of Anesthesia from January 1, 1899 to January 1, 1900":

In that time, we administered an anesthetic 1,092 times; ether alone 674 times; chloroform 245 times; ether and chloroform combined, 173 times. I can report that out of this number, 1,092 cases, we have not had an accident; we have not had occasion to use artificial respiration once; nor one case of ether pneumonia; neither have we had any serious renal results. Tongue forceps were used but once, the operation was on the jaw and it was quite necessary. (p. 306)

---

[1]The word *training* was commonly used to describe nursing education in this era.

During her tenure at the Mayo Hospital, Magaw helped separate hospital-based anesthesia services from the traditional nursing service administrative structures, on the basis of the assertion that anesthesia was a specialized field requiring advanced education beyond the credentials of graduate nurses (Thatcher, 1953). This decision to separate nurse anesthetists from the established nursing structure at the Mayo Hospital would set the stage for the continued division between nurse anesthesia and mainstream nursing for many years to follow.

The Roots of Nurse-Midwifery

Like the origins of nurse anesthesia, the origins of nurse-midwifery in America can be traced to the pre-professional work of women. Throughout the 18th and 19th centuries, lay midwives, rather than professional nurses or physicians, assisted women in childbirth. Midwives, who were brought to the United States with the slave trade in 1619 and who later came with waves of European immigration, were respected and rewarded community members in early Native American, colonial, and pioneer communities. Typically employed by European immigrants who lived in culturally isolated ethnic communities in urban areas of the Northeast, these untrained "old country midwives" would lose respect later in the century as "scientific," hospital-based deliveries became the norm. Meanwhile, women in isolated communities throughout the country, particularly in rural settings, continued to employ midwives for deliveries well into the 20th century. In fact, providing care for the poor and underserved would become a hallmark of APN practice in general.

The Roots of Clinical Nurse Specialization: Psychiatric Nursing

The roots of the clinical nurse specialist role are also embedded in the second half of the 19th century. Recognized as the first clinical specialty in nursing, psychiatric nursing had its origins in the reform movement initiated earlier in the century by Quakers at the York Retreat in England. These reformers challenged the brutal treatment of the insane and advocated "moral treatment," emphasizing gentler methods of social control in a domestic setting (D'Antonio, 1991, p. 411).

The first American training program for psychiatric nurses was founded in 1880 at McLean Hospital in Massachusetts (Critchley, 1985). According to Linda Richards, an 1873 graduate of The New England Hospital School of Nursing, from the outset, the McLean Hospital maintained high standards and demonstrated "the value of trained nursing for the many persons afflicted with mental disease"(Richards, 1911, p. 109). During a time when nursing's role in the care of the mentally ill was essentially custodial, Linda Richards served as superintendent of nurses at the Taunton Insane Hospital for 4 years, beginning in 1899. She subsequently organized a nursing school for the preparation of psychiatric nurses at the Worcester Hospital for the Insane and finally went to the Michigan Insane Hospital in Kalamazoo where she remained until 1909 (Richards, 1911). Because of this work, Richards is credited with founding the specialty of psychiatric nursing.

The Roots of the Concepts of Nurse Practitioners and Case Management

Although the term *nurse practitioner* did not emerge until the 1960s and the phrase *case management* was not coined until the 1980s, their origins also date to the late 1800s.

During this period of social reform, nurses played a major role in the development of case management models while they provided primary care for poverty-stricken immigrants in New York City. In 1893, Lillian Wald, a young graduate nurse from the New York Training School for Nurses, established the Henry Street Settlement (HSS) House in the lower east side of Manhattan. Its purpose was to address the needs of poor immigrants, many of whom who lived in overcrowded, rat-infested tenements. For several decades the HSS visiting nurses, like other district nurses, would manage large caseloads of patients (Wald, 1922). The needs of this disadvantaged community were limitless. According to one HSS nurse:

There were nursing infants, many of them with the summer bowel complaint that sent infant mortality soaring during the hot months; there were children with measles, not quarantined; there were children with opthalmia, a contagious eye disease; there were children scarred with vermin bites; there were adults with typhoid; there was a case of puerperal septicemia, lying on a vermin-infested bed without sheets or pillow cases; a family consisting of a pregnant mother, a crippled child and two others living on dry bread . . . ; a young girl dying of tuberculosis amid the very conditions that had produced the disease . . . (Duffus, 1938, p. 43)

In addition to making home visits and providing basic primary care, the HSS nurses also established a nurses' dispensary in one room of the settlement house, where "simple complaints and emergencies not requiring referral elsewhere were treated" (Buhler-Wilkerson, 2001, p. 107). As their clientele expanded, however, the HHS nurses became an economic threat to Manhattan physicians. According to nurse historian Karen Buhler-Wilkerson (2001):

As the number of ambulatory visits grew, the settlement risked attracting the unwelcome attention of the increasingly disagreeable "uptown docs." The New York Medical Society's recent success in attaching a clause to the Nursing Registration Bill prohibiting nurses from practicing medicine gave the society a new opportunity to disrupt the settlement's neighborly activities. While initially the first aid rooms went unnoticed, by 1904 . . . Lavinia Dock [a colleague of Lillian Wald] wrote to Wald about doctors' concerns that nurses were carrying ointments and even giving pills outside the strict control of physicians. (p. 110)

As is apparent in this scenario, from early in the century there is evidence of interprofessional conflicts with medicine as nurses began to expand their scope of practice. On the other hand, there is also evidence of emerging collaboration between the professions, as physicians and nurses worked out solutions to the boundary problems. In this case, the HSS nurses, with the endorsement of the local medical society, established "standing orders" (Buhler-Wilkerson, 2001, p. 110) for emergency medications and treatments. What is clear, even in these early years, is that nurses were considered "good enough" to care for the poor, whereas physicians would care for the middle class and the rich.

Turn of the 20th Century

As immigrants continued to flood into the cities and towns of the Northeast, problems of excessive crowding, tenement house dwelling, and the spread of infectious diseases intensified. Coinciding with the trend toward urbanization and industrialization, medicine was establishing itself as a respectable and economically viable profession, one that was dominated by men. At the same time, the nursing profession made significant progress, particularly in the area of licensure. In 1903, state licensure registration for nurses was initiated in North Carolina, New Jersey, New York, and Virginia. Licensure was a first step in regulating the profession of nursing at the state level. Moreover, it was crucial to the upgrading of nursing education because it determined what requirements a nurse must meet before she would be eligible for licensure. Licensure would set the stage for nursing to move from a trade occupation to a profession.

The "Specialties," circa 1900s

The use of the term *specialist* in nursing can be traced to the turn of the 20th century when hospitals offered postgraduate courses in a variety of specialty areas including anesthesia, tuberculosis, operating room, laboratory, and dietetics. In the first issue of the *American Journal of Nursing (AJN)*, Katherine Dewitt (1900) describes the role and the specialist's need for continuing education in an article titled "Specialties in Nursing" as follows:

Those who devote themselves to one branch of nursing often do so because of the keen interest they feel in it. The specialist can and should reach greater perfection in her sphere when she gives her entire time to it. Her studies should be continued in that direction, she should try constantly to keep up with the rapid advances in medical science. . . . The nurse who is a specialist can often supplement the doctor's work to a great extent. The surgeon or obstetrician who has a patient in the country can often leave the aftercare of a case in the hands of a nurse who is familiar with his mode of treatment. (p. 16)

1910s: The Impact of the Progressive Era and World War I

In the 1910s, dramatic events on the national scene and continued problems in the United States had a direct effect on the profession's growth. In 1912, the National Organization for Public Health Nursing (NOPHN) was established. That same year, Lillian Wald spearheaded the creation of the Children's Bureau, a federal organization whose early studies of infant and maternal mortality rates led to the conclusion that a substantial number of maternal and infant deaths could be prevented by adequate prenatal care. Meanwhile, the women's campaign for the right to vote was at its height. Later in the decade in 1917, two significant events coincided: an influenza epidemic swept the country and the United States entered World War I. Both events would challenge the nursing profession and promote greater autonomy in nursing practice.

Midwifery, circa 1910s

Negative attitudes toward traditional midwives peaked in the 1910s, resulting in heated debates surrounding issues of midwife licensing and control. Despite resistance from the medical profession, several states passed laws granting legal recognition to midwives as increasing awareness of the social problems of the poor continued to create a demand for their services in underserved areas. In 1911, Bellevue Hospital established a school of midwifery, "specifically designed to aid the forty thousand New York women who were being assisted in delivery by untrained women" (Donahue, 1996, p. 309).The history does not indicate whether this school was for the training of lay or nurse midwives. Most likely, it was for lay midwives because the term *nurse-midwife* was not introduced until 1914 when Frederick Taussig, MD, spoke at the annual meeting of the NOPHN in St. Louis.

He proposed that the creation of "nurse-midwives" might solve the "midwife question" and suggested that nurse-midwifery schools be established to train graduate nurses (Taussig, 1914). Later in the decade, the Children's Bureau called for efforts to instruct pregnant women in nutrition and recommended that public health nurses teach principles of hygiene and prenatal care to "granny midwives" (Rooks, 1997). A landmark in the history of nurse-midwifery was the establishment of the Maternity Center Association (MCA), a nonprofit voluntary health-care agency that remains a leader in the field today. The MCA was established in 1918 in response to a study conducted by the New York City health commissioner that indicated the need for comprehensive prenatal care. It served as the central organization for a network of community-based maternity centers throughout the city. Overall, this was a decade of continued progress for nurse-midwives.

Red Cross Rural Nursing Service, circa 1910s

In 1910, Lillian Wald proposed the formation of a rural public health service, which was established in 1912 as the Red Cross Rural Nursing Service. (Later, it would be known as the Town and Country Nursing Service.) In many communities, the Red Cross Rural nurse was the only health-care provider other than lay midwives. These rural nurses provided traditional community nursing services, including home care, maternal-child health care in homes and schools, detection and management of infectious diseases, and sanitation and immunization programs. They did so in an independent practice environment that required well-developed skills in community intervention and patient management. This innovative model for health-care delivery contributed to the eventual establishment of official public health departments in counties nationwide (Bigbee & Crowder, 1985) and laid the foundation for autonomous nursing practice.

Nurse Anesthesia, circa 1910s

During the 1910s, nurse anesthetists faced practice barriers, as well as new opportunities. Early in the decade, the medical profession began to question the right of nurses to administer anesthesia, claiming that these nurses were practicing medicine without a license. In 1911, the New York State Medical Society unsuccessfully declared that the administration of an anesthetic by a nurse violated state law (Thatcher, 1953). A year later, the Ohio State Medical Board passed a resolution specifying that only physicians could administer anesthesia. Despite this resolution, nurse anesthetist Agatha Hodgins established The Lakeside Hospital School of Anesthesia in Cleveland, Ohio, in 1915, culminating in a lawsuit brought against the Lakeside Hospital program by the state medical society. This lawsuit was unsuccessful and resulted in an amendment to the Ohio Medical Practice Act, protecting the practice of nurse anesthesia. However, medical opposition to the practice of nurse anesthesia continued. In a landmark decision, the Kentucky appellate court, in the case of *Frank v. South* (1917), ruled that anesthesia provided by nurse anesthetist Margaret Hatfield did not constitute the practice of medicine if it was given under the orders and supervision of a licensed physician (Dr. Louis Frank). The significance of this decision lay in the fact that the courts declared nurse anesthesia legal but "subordinate" to the medical profession, a decision that would have lasting implications for the specialty and for advanced practice nursing in general.

Later in the decade, opportunities for CRNAs increased when the United States entered World War I. By October 1917, 1,100 nurses had been deployed to Britain and

France. The realities of the front were gruesome: shrapnel created devastating wounds, and mustard gas destroyed lungs and caused profound burns (Beeber, 1990). The resulting need for pain relief and anesthesia care for the wounded soldiers created an immediate demand for nurse anesthetists' knowledge and skills.

Concurrent with the war effort, scientific investigation into new methods of administering anesthesia began. At the well-established Lakeside Hospital anesthesia program in Cleveland (one of five postgraduate schools of nurse anesthesia in the country), nurse anesthetist Agatha Hodgins and her physician colleague George W. Crile experimented with combined nitrous oxide–oxygen administration. They also investigated the use of morphine and scopolamine as adjuncts to anesthesia.

Overall, while World War I and scientific advances in clinical anesthesia greatly enhanced the visibility and public enthusiasm for nurse anesthetists,[2] some physicians continued to claim that nurse anesthetists' work was an encroachment on medical practice. In fact, legal battles between physicians and nurse anesthetists would continue well into the century.

1920s: The Roaring Twenties

In 1920, Congress passed the Nineteenth Amendment to the United States Constitution, granting women the right to vote. That same year, Congress also approved a bill that provided nurses military rank (Dock & Stewart, 1920). Both acts of Congress helped open the decade of the Roaring Twenties, a time in which the new-found freedom for women was reflected in their shortened hairstyles, rising hemlines, and use of cigarettes and cosmetics. The decade also saw an increase in acceptance of the scientific basis of medicine and increased use of hospitals, especially for surgery (Howell, 1996). Of particular importance, in 1921 Congress passed the Shephard Towner Maternity and Infant Protection Act, providing health-care services to mothers and children throughout the nation.

During this decade, the nursing profession undertook a study on nursing education supported by the Rockefeller Foundation. The Goldmark Report, published in 1923, advocated the establishment of collegiate schools of nursing rather than hospital-based diploma programs (Goldmark, 1923). Championed mainly by a group of nursing faculty at Columbia's Teachers College, the report provided a significant opportunity for nursing to become professionalized through collegiate education. Hoping the Goldmark Report would gain for nursing the status the Flexner Report (1910)[3] had gained for medicine, the Columbia nursing faculty group, led by Adelaide Nutting, strongly supported collegiate programs at Yale University and Case Western Reserve University and pressed other colleagues to take advantage of the opportunity. However, hospital administrators and physicians largely ignored the report, arguing that the plan was not practical (Baer, 2001). In the end, although some collegiate programs were established, strong support never materialized for university education for nurses, and the majority of aspiring nurses continued to be trained in diploma schools. In essence, organized nursing's response to the Goldmark Report may be considered a "missed opportunity" in the history of advanced practice nursing.

---

[2]Nurse anesthetist Sophie Winton, who provided anesthesia care to soldiers in France, received the Crox de Guerre in recognition of her service (Faut-Callahan & Kremer, 1996).
[3]The Flexner Report ended medical apprenticeship training in the United States, and medical education became university based after this study (Flexner, 1910).

Nurse Anesthetists, circa 1920s

Although the decade of the 1920s was one of continued progress for some nurse anesthetists, it was also a decade in which resistance to their role grew behind the scenes. In 1922 nurse anesthetist Alice M. Hunt responded to a request by Samuel Harvey, a Yale professor of surgery, to "send me a nurse anesthetist" (Thatcher, 1953, p. 101) by accepting the offer herself. The offer included her appointment as an instructor of anesthesia with university rank at the Yale Medical School, a significant and prestigious appointment for a nurse. However, not all nurse anesthetists had this kind of opportunity. In fact, during the 1920s, many nurse anesthetists struggled to find practice opportunities as more physicians began to choose anesthesia as their medical specialty. Female physicians were among the first to specialize in the role of anesthetists because the low pay and status of anesthesia practice made it unattractive to many male physicians. These women were active in the establishment of the Association of Anesthetists of the United States and Canada in the early 1920s (Bankert, 1989). Unfortunately, although they shared a great deal with nurse anesthetists in terms of sex discrimination and stereotyping, the early women anesthesiologists were actively opposed to nurse anesthetists, probably because they saw CRNAs as competitors for their jobs.

Nurse-Midwifery, circa 1920s

During the 1920s, societal class differences and the public's growing acceptance of hospitals and scientific medicine resulted in a declining use of lay midwives for deliveries. In fact, many upper and middle class urban white women began to use obstetricians to deliver their babies in hospital delivery rooms (Rinker, 2000). In contrast, poor urban European immigrants continued to employ midwives to deliver their babies at home. Likewise, in rural southern states such as Mississippi, where half the population was black, the majority of women (80% of African American and 8% of white women) continued to rely on African American "granny midwives" to deliver their babies (Smith, 1994). The same pattern seen at the turn of the century continued: physician-assisted, hospital births were associated with patients of higher socioeconomic status. Midwives could attend the poor.

The Frontier Nursing Service: A New Model for Nurse-Midwifery

In 1925 Mary Breckinridge, a 1910 graduate of St. Luke's Training School in New York City and a British-trained nurse-midwife (Donahue, 1996), founded the Frontier Nursing Service (FNS), which firmly established the specialty of nurse-midwifery in the United States. In an economically depressed rural mountain area of Leslie County, Kentucky, Breckinridge established a network of clinics to serve the Appalachian community. Originally, Breckinridge staffed the FNS with British nurse-midwives and American public health nurses whom she had sent to England for midwifery training (Rooks, 1997; Breckinridge, 1981). Because there were few roads in the mountainous region, the nurses traveled by horseback to attend births, carrying their supplies in saddlebags. One FNS nurse, Vanda Summers (1938), described how the bags also contained a list of standing orders, or *Medical Routines*, by which a physician committee supervised their practice:

The whole of the district work of the FNS in the Kentucky mountains is done with the aid of two pairs of saddle-bags. . . . The "midwifery" saddle-bags weigh about 42 pounds when packed. . . . In these bags we have everything needed for a home delivery. . . . In one of the pockets we carry our *Medical Routines* which tells us what we may—and may not—do. A very treasured possession! (pp. 1183-1184)

The FNS nurses maintained outstanding patient data from the outset. Reflecting on her work in later years, Breckinridge (1981) notes that "trained statisticians were to come later, through a grant from the Carnegie Corporation, but from the start we had records and report sheets and kept them carefully" (p. 166). When findings were analyzed by the Metropolitan Life Insurance Company in 1951, they indicated that 8,596 births had been attended, with 6,533 occurring in homes, since 1925. More important, the FNS maternal mortality rate of 1.2 per 1000 was significantly lower than the national average of 3.4 per 1000 during the same period (Varney, 1987). Besides caring for patients, the FNS nurses formally organized the Kentucky State Association of Midwives in 1928. Later, this organization would become known as The American Association of Nurse-Midwives (AANM) and would play a key role in the progress of this advanced practice specialty. Meanwhile, the FNS nurses' documentation of the outcomes of their care would serve to advance the FNS cause.

Settlement Nurses Provide Case Management Services, circa 1920s

Influenced by both the 1921 Shephard Towner Act that increased federal funding for maternal-child care and the phenomenal increase in demand for their services, the HSS visiting nurses expanded their services to 18 nursing centers throughout New York City during the 1920s. "By 1926, the service cared for over 49,000 patients and made nearly 347,000 home visits" (Buhler-Wilkerson, 2001, p. 111). In effect, these nurses served as case managers and precursors of primary care NPs, because they not only provided direct patient care but also coordinated social services for their patients. One nurse, writing in 1925, reported that because of nurses' sympathetic interest and the provision of direct care, "families seem less reluctant to admit their needs to the nurse than perhaps to any other person" (Hunt, 1925, p. 137). Although it would be more than 50 years later that the CNM role would be described in the nursing literature, case management was a reality of visiting nursing in the early years of the 20th century.

1930s-1950s: THE EMERGENCE OF ADVANCED PRACTICE NURSING IN THE UNITED STATES

By the time President Franklin Roosevelt took the oath of office in March 1933, the United States was mired in an economic depression that affected the entire industrialized world. Over the next 6 years, Roosevelt's social programs under the New Deal would dramatically affect U.S. citizens. Rural rehabilitation programs, including health-care programs sponsored by the Farm Security Administration (FSA), would be particularly important for poverty-stricken farmers and their families.

In addition, the Depression would change the hospital workforce. During these fiscally stringent times, many private hospitals were forced to close their schools of nursing, and hospitals without student labor began to employ graduate nurses to staff their wards. Soon, increasing numbers of unemployed private duty nurses began to turn to hospitals for secure employment, giving up the autonomy of private duty nursing to work in physician-dominated hospital bureaucracies. This change marked a major shift in the nursing workforce during which the majority of nurses became hospital employees rather than independent practitioners. With the shift, nurses also forfeited the freedom to bill for their services. The change would have profound implications for APNs later in the century as nursing services were first considered as part of the room rate and later "bundled" under physician services.

Nurse Anesthetists, circa 1930s

Despite the turmoil of the Depression years, Lakeside Hospital nurse anesthetist Agatha Hodgins established the American Association of Nurse Anesthetists (AANA) in 1931 and served as the organization's first president. At the first meeting of the association, the group voted to affiliate with the American Nurses Association (ANA). However, the AANA was rebuffed, probably because the ANA was afraid to assume legal responsibility for a group that could be charged with practicing medicine without a license (Thatcher, 1953).

The ANA's fears were not unfounded. During the 1930s, legal challenges to the practice of nurse anesthesia continued. In California, the Los Angeles County Medical Association sued nurse anesthetist Dagmar Nelson in 1934 for practicing medicine without a license. Nelson won. In response, William Chalmers-Frances, MD, filed another suit against Nelson in 1936, which again resulted in a judgment for Nelson (*Chalmers-Frances v. Nelson*, 1936). In 1938, the judgment was appealed to the California Supreme Court, which again ruled in favor of Nelson, stating that she was not practicing medicine because she was supervised by the operating surgeon. The case became famous. In fact, with this decision, the courts established legal precedent: the practice of nurse anesthesia was legal and within the scope of nursing practice, *as long as it was done under the guidance of a supervising physician.*

Nurse-Midwifery, circa 1930s

During the decade of the Great Depression, nurse-midwifery also made significant strides. In 1930, a group of MCA board members, including Mary Breckinridge, incorporated as the Association for the Promotion and Standardization of Midwifery, and in 1931, opened the Lobenstine Clinic in New York City, the nation's second nurse-midwifery service. Its purpose was to prepare public health nurses, not to deliver babies, but to teach and supervise traditional midwives and nurses with limited obstetrical training. The school set high standards. In fact, most of its first class of six students were college graduates (Rooks, 1997).

In 1939, the entry of Britain into World War II proved to be the catalyst for the establishment of another school for nurse-midwifery in the United States. That year, the Kentucky FNS faced a crisis because many of their British nurse-midwives returned to England to work. To deal with this shortage of qualified nurse-midwives, Breckinridge established the Frontier Graduate School of Midwifery, specifically to train American nurses (Buck, 1940).[4] Key to the midwives' success was the fact that they were not posing a threat to private obstetricians. The Lobenstine Clinic prepared public health

---

[4]This program was for nurses who already had a degree in nursing (i.e., registered nurses) but was not a *graduate program* in the modern sense of the term.

nurses to care for the urban poor, and the FNS delivered babies in the backwoods of Kentucky.

The Emergence of "Primary Care Practitioners," circa 1930s

In addition to providing midwifery services, the FNS nurses in Leslie County, Kentucky, informally modeled what would become, in the 1960s, the primary care NP role. In fact, during the 1930s, the FNS continued the work Breckinridge had started in 1928, providing most of the primary health care needed by people living in rural Appalachia. Working out of eight centers that covered about 78 square miles in remote mountainous regions, the FNS nurses had considerable autonomy in decision making. In reality, they made diagnoses and treated patients, dispensing both herbs and medicines (including morphine) with permission of their medical advisory committee (FNS, 1936).Working from standing orders written by the FNS medical advisory committee, the nurses also dispensed aspirin, ipecac, cascara, and castor oil at their own discretion (FNS, 1936).

Besides the FNS nurses, other nurses working among the poor in rural areas in the Depression also had unprecedented autonomy in their scope of practice. In particular, the FSA nurses "were given unusual latitude in their clinical roles" (Grey, 1999, p. 94) in migrant health programs in the western region of the United States. According to historian Michael Grey (1999), who chronicled the history of rural health programs during the Great Depression:

With the verbal approval of the camp doctor, they [FSA nurses] could write prescriptions and dispense drugs from the clinic formulary. . . . They staffed well baby clinics, coordinated immunization programs . . . decided whether a sick migrant required referral to a physician . . . and provided emergency care. (p. 94)

Like the FNS nurses, FSA nurses practiced according to standing orders issued by the FSA medical offices and approved by local physicians. As Dr. H. Daniels recalled in a 1984 interview, "Nurses functioned pretty autonomously. They were able to do a lot of what NPs do after a lot of training, but these nurses did it through experience" (Grey, 1999, p. 96). Essential to this practice autonomy for both the FNS and FSA nurses, however, was the tacit requirement that the patients be poor and have little access to physician-provided medical care.

Clinical Specialization in Psychiatry, circa 1930s

The 1930s also witnessed growth in the area of psychiatry. In this period Harry Stack Sullivan's classic writings and the work of Sigmund Freud changed psychiatric nursing dramatically. The emphasis on interpersonal interaction with patients and milieu treatment supported the movement of nurses into a more direct role in the psychiatric care of hospitalized patients. Scientific advances in the field, including the use of insulin and chemotherapies, required nurses to assume an increasingly active role in patient treatment.

1940s: World War II Challenges the Nation and the Profession

During the 1940s, the rise of medical specialization and the increase in technology and scientific knowledge further influenced the trend toward specialization in the profession and the expansion of nurses' responsibilities. However, the effect of these factors did not compare with the impact of World War II on the profession. The demands of the battle-front, scientific discoveries made as a result of experiments to protect soldiers from chemical warfare, and the shortage of nurses on the home front would all create opportunities for the nursing profession.

As in other wars, the demands of the battlefield forced nurses to assume responsibilities that went beyond their usual scope of practice. One example of this expansion of the nurse's role and practice autonomy is evidenced in a 1943 *AJN* article on flight nursing, an emerging nursing specialty:

Once in the air, the nurse is in complete charge of the patients, assisted by a trained staff sergeant. . . . She may have to readjust splints, administer sedatives or stimulants, arrest sudden hemorrhage, treat shock, administer oxygen. . . . She will be responsible for handling any emergency and for doing anything a doctor would have to do, except operate. (White, 1943, p. 344)

It was simple: if a physician was unavailable or too busy with other cases, the nurse's role could expand from "caring" to "curing." In contrast, if a physician was readily available, the nurse was expected to practice within the traditional "caring" boundaries of the profession (Lynaugh & Fairman, 1992; Reverby, 1987).

Scientific discoveries made as a result of experiments related to chemical warfare also provided opportunities for the expansion of nursing practice, particularly for what would later become the specialty of oncology nursing. It was during World War II that the United States military's investigations of nitrogen mustard[5] led to the significant scientific discovery that the agent had substantial activity against lymphocytes. This discovery promoted further study of agents that could effectively kill rapidly spreading cancer cells. In fact, the discovery would herald the beginning of the "era of cytotoxic chemotherapy" (Friereich, 1984), a landmark event that would presage major changes in clinical oncology and cancer nursing.

In addition to the demands of the battlefront and the scientific discoveries of the era, the nursing shortages that occurred after the United States entered the war on December 7, 1941, led to federal legislation that would ultimately benefit the profession. Reacting to the nursing shortage, Congress passed the Bolton Act, forming the Cadet Nurse Corps. The bill, sponsored by Congresswoman Frances Payne Bolton and signed into law by President Roosevelt in 1943, subsidized the nursing education of 179,000 students and provided funds to graduate nurses for advanced education to increase the number of nursing instructors (Spalding, 1943). The Bolton Act not only ensured an adequate supply of nurses for both military and civilian hospitals but also had positive effects on nursing education. Federal funding, paid directly to schools, facilitated the separation of nursing education from nursing service. Moreover, Cadet Nurse Corps funds were also allocated for postgraduate study in certificate programs such as those preparing CRNAs or in programs in administration and education. By the time the program ended, "more than 3 million dollars had been spent for postgraduate study for more than 10,000 registered nurses throughout the country" (U.S. Federal Security Agency, 1950, p. 61).

---

[5]Although gas warfare was not used in World War II, a stock of mustard gas canisters was held in the Italian port of Bari. An accident involving leakage of one of these canisters rekindled interest begun in World War I about the myelosuppressive effect of nitrogen mustard (Baguley, 2002).

Nurse Anesthetists, circa 1940s

The specialty of medical anesthesia made significant progress during the war. In fact, World War II is often hailed as "a juncture in the growth of anesthesiology as a medical specialty in the United States" (Waisel, 2001, p. 907). Just before the war, in 1939, the first written examination for board certification was given for anesthesiologists, but the specialty practice of medical anesthesiology still sought legitimacy. By the 1940s, demands for anesthetists, advances in the types of anesthesia available, and continuing education in the field stimulated physicians' interest in the specialty. The medical journal *Anesthesiology*, established in 1940, further strengthened medicine's claim to anesthesia practice. In particular, according to physicians, the use of the new drug sodium pentothal required specialized knowledge of physiology and pharmacology and underscored the emerging view that only physicians could provide anesthesia. In fact, the administration of anesthesia was becoming more complex, and anesthesiologists demonstrated their expertise not only in administering sodium pentothal but also in performing endotracheal intubation and regional blocks (Waisel, 2001). All of these factors increased medicine's hold on the specialty.

Meanwhile, there were shortages of anesthetists on the battlefields. Despite these shortages, the U.S. military would not grant nurse anesthetists a specific designation within the military. Notwithstanding efforts by the AANA in lobbying the military to provide CRNAs with special status, experienced nurse anesthetists who volunteered for duty were required to accept general nurse status. However, CRNAs could be promoted within nursing as administrators and educators. In the Army Nurse Corps, for example, nurse anesthetists were sometimes advanced to the rank of chief nurse and served as administrators or instructors in addition to administering anesthesia. Later, when shortages became severe, the Army Nurse Corps trained staff nurses as anesthetists. Overall, the war years represented a time of growth in the knowledge base for the anesthesia specialty and an expansion in responsibilities for individual CRNAs meeting the demands of the battlefront. Paradoxically, this was also a period in which organized medicine increased its claim over the field of anesthesiology.

After the war, the specialty of nurse anesthesia continued to make progress. Probably in response to the advances made during the war, the AANA instituted mandatory certification for CRNAs in 1945. This formal credentialing of CRNAs preceded credentialing of nurses in the other specialties and marked a significant milestone in the history of advanced practice, because it specified the requirements a nurse had to meet to practice in this area of specialization.

Nurse-Midwives, circa 1940s

While the United States was at war, nurse-midwives continued their work on the home front. Key to their development in the 1940s was the establishment of a formal organization of practicing nurse-midwives, the AANM, which incorporated in 1941 under the leadership of Mary Breckinridge, its first president. By July 1942, the AANM had a "membership of 71 graduate nurses" who had specialty training in midwifery (News Here and There, 1942, p. 832). Three years later, in 1944, the National Organization of Public Health Nurses established a section for nurse-midwives[6]

---

[6]Expanded preparation for nurse-midwives also influenced the practice of lay midwives. As the CNMs gained knowledge, they began to share it with the lay midwives. During this decade minority nurses were also encouraged to become CNMs, albeit in segregated institutions. On March 13, 1942, "the first class of three Negro nurse midwives graduated from the midwifery school operated at the Tuskegee Institute under the auspices of the Macon County Health Department" (Negro Nurse-Midwives, 1942, p. 705).

within their organization. This group prepared a roster of all midwives in the country and defined their practice, making it clear that nurse-midwives would continue to practice under physician authority, an idea that was first implemented by Breckinridge in 1928.

In the FNS , the medical advisory board continued to supervise the nurses' work in a revised edition of *Medical Routines* (FNS, 1948). The introduction to the 1948 version explicitly stated that FNS nurses are to work only within the guidelines provided:

The routines set forth in this book are the orders given by the physicians of the medical advisory committee of the FNS for the use of nurses in the service. They must be followed exactly. No other medications or treatments may be used. . . . In a grave emergency you may act according to your own judgment, but must report the case in full to the Medical Director. (FNS, 1948, p. 3)

Psychiatric Nursing, circa 1940s

Because of an increased public awareness of psychiatric problems in returning soldiers, (Critchley, 1985), World War II would also affect the specialty of psychiatric nursing. During the 1940s, new treatments were introduced for the care of the mentally ill, including the widespread use of electroshock therapy. The new treatments would require nurses who had specialized knowledge and training to assist with the procedures used to implement them. According to a 1942 *AJN* article, "Only the nurse skilled in her profession and with additional psychiatric background has a place in mental hospitals today" (Schindler, 1942, p. 861). By 1943, three postgraduate programs in psychiatric nursing had been established. In 1946, after Congress passed the National Mental Health Act designating psychiatric nursing as a core discipline in mental health, federal funding for graduate and undergraduate educational programs and research became available; and programs in psychiatric-mental health were included in schools of nursing throughout the United States. Psychiatric nursing knowledge was now widely accepted as essential content in the nursing curriculum. Psychiatric nursing was also becoming established as a graduate level specialty, one that would lead the way for clinical nurse specialization in the next decade.

1950s: The Growth of Hospitals, Scientific Nursing, and the GI Bill

In the period after World War II, optimism about the possibilities of research and scientific knowledge permeated the United States. Advances in medical science and technology were promoted and celebrated in the popular culture. In the immediate post-war period, Americans were impressed by specialists, turning to Dr. Benjamin Spock for advice on childcare and to Norman Vincent Peale for spiritual guidance. Without a doubt, specialization and a scientific approach to medical care had captured America's interest.

Nevertheless, science and medical specialization were only two of the many factors that set the stage for dramatic changes that would take place in health care in the 1950s. Another important factor was economic, as federally funded hospital construction reshaped the setting in which physicians and nurses practiced. In 1946, the federal government passed the Hospital Survey and Construction Act, known as *the Hill Burton Act*, which provided large-scale funding to modernize aging hospitals and build new ones. These modern hospitals eliminated the large open wards in which nurses could easily observe patients. Instead, the renovated hospitals had long halls with numerous private and semiprivate rooms. Although they were pleasing to middle-class patients who demanded privacy, the new hospital spaces, along with the increasing severity of illness in patients and the national nursing shortage, changed the way in which care was given. The sickest patients required observation and grouping in one place, soon to be labeled the *intensive care unit* (ICU) (Fairman & Lynaugh, 1998). Caring for patients in the ICU required specialized knowledge and skills, a trend that clearly contributed to an increase in specialization in nursing.

In addition to funding new hospitals, the federal government also supported nurse education in the postwar years. Nurses returning from World War II were eligible to pursue advanced education under the GI Bill, and many took advantage of the opportunity to return to school. Prompted by the Brown Report of 1948, the National League of Nursing Education (NLNE) established a committee that catalogued all nursing programs, including those leading to a master's degree, in a 1949 issue of *AJN* (Donahue, 1996). Governmental support during this decade and thereafter proved to be critically important to the evolution of graduate education for nurses.

Nurse Anesthetists, circa 1950s

During the 1950s, the growth of nurse anesthesia was affected by the increasing dominance of organized medicine in the specialty. By this time, increasing numbers of male physicians were choosing this specialty and women physicians' leadership in the field declined. However, nurse anesthetists held their ground. In 1952, the American Association of Nurse Anesthetists established an accreditation program to monitor the quality of nurse anesthetist education. Meanwhile, the United States was once again at war, this time with Korea, and once again, war provided a setting in which opportunities abounded for nurse anesthetists, particularly for men. By the end of the decade, the army had established nurse anesthesia educational programs, including one at Walter Reed General Hospital, which graduated its first class in 1961. This class consisted of only men. Soon after, the Letterman General Hospital School of Anesthesia in San Francisco also graduated an all-male class. This significant movement of men into a nursing specialty has been unparalleled in any of the other specialties.

Nurse-Midwives, circa 1950s

Numerous factors increased the demand for obstetrical care during the 1950s, not the least of which was the high post-war birth rate. In the 1950s, most urban mothers were delivered of their babies in hospitals where scientific methods, including the use of scopolamine during labor and general anesthesia during delivery, were the norm. Meanwhile, women in rural areas, especially in the South, continued to rely on "granny midwives" or CNMs to deliver their babies. Practice, educational, and organizational efforts in nurse-midwifery also continued. During this period, nurse-midwives attempted to establish hospital-based practices, and in 1955 Columbia Presbyterian Sloan Hospital opened its doors to nurse-midwives. Concomitantly, Columbia University established a graduate program in maternal nursing, the first to provide midwifery education in an academic medical center. A cooperative program involving Columbia University's Department of Nursing and School of Public Health and Administrative Medicine, the obstetrics and gynecology departments of Presbyterian-

Sloan Hospital and Kings County Hospital, and the MCA led to a master of science degree in nursing and a nurse-midwifery certificate (Rooks, 1997). Soon afterward, educational programs for nurse-midwives increased in number, and by 1956, there were three certificate programs and two master's degree programs in the United States. Given the conservative mood of the country in this decade and the increasing emphasis on the scientific management for labor and delivery, it is surprising that nurse-midwives fared as well as they did. Overall, they not only held their ground but also made some progress in establishing programs at the graduate level. It is noteworthy that they were among the first specialties to advocate graduate education, a significant move toward advanced practice status.

Psychiatric Clinical Nurse Specialists, circa 1950s

Psychiatric nursing blossomed as a specialty in the 1950s. In 1954, Hildegarde E. Peplau, professor of psychiatric nursing, established the first master's program in psychiatric nursing in the United States at Rutgers University in New Jersey. Considered the first CNS educational program, this program and the growth of specialty knowledge in psychiatric nursing that ensued provided support for psychiatric nurses to begin exploring new leadership roles in the care of patients with mental illness in both inpatient and outpatient settings. Scholarship in psychiatric nursing also flourished. Among the most significant publications were the writings of Peplau, who proposed the first conceptual framework for psychiatric nursing, *Interpersonal Relations in Nursing, a Conceptual Frame of Reference for Psychodynamic Nursing* (1952), providing theory-based practice for the specialty. Clearly, the link between academia and specialization was becoming stronger. The specialty of psychiatric nursing was leading the way, with midwifery not far behind.

American Nurses Association Defines Nursing Practice, circa 1950s

The seminal work of nurse scholar Virginia Henderson on scientifically based patient-centered care laid the foundation for changes in advanced practice nursing that would occur in the second half of the 20th century. Influenced by both Henderson and Peplau, innovative nurses like France Reiter at New York Medical College initiated a clinical nurse graduate curriculum designed to provide nurses with an intellectual clinical component based on a liberal arts education, in effect, supporting a broader role for nurses (Fairman, 2001). However, although academic nursing was making strides toward establishing specialty education and expanding the nurse specialist's scope of practice, the ANA developed a model definition of nursing that would unduly restrict nursing practice for the next several decades. The definition, prepared in 1955 and adopted by many states, reads as follows:

The practice of professional nursing means the performance for compensation of any act in the observation, care and counsel of the ill . . . or in the maintenance of health or prevention of illness . . . or the administration of medications and treatments as prescribed by a licensed physician. . . . The foregoing shall not be deemed to include acts of diagnosis or prescription of therapeutic or corrective measures. (ANA, 1955, p. 1474)

Although the ANA may simply have been seeking clarity in defining the discipline's boundaries, its exclusion of the acts of diagnosis and prescription stifled the development of advanced practice nursing. Discussing the impact of the ANA's restrictions on diagnosis and prescription, law professor Barbara Safriet (1992) argued: "Even at the time the ANA's model definition was issued . . . it was unduly restrictive when measured by then current nursing practice" (p. 417). Nurses had been assessing patients for more than 50 years and continued to do so in this period. According to historian Bonnie Bullough (1984), "The fascinating thing about the disclaimer [regarding diagnosis and prescription] is that it was made not by the American Medical Association, but the American Nurses Association. . . . In effect, organized nursing surrendered without any battle over boundaries" (p. 374). The ANA's 1955 definition of nursing would restrict the expansion of scope of practice for advanced practice nursing for the remainder of the 20th century, as the profession struggled with the dichotomy of "care versus cure" and the legalities of "medical" versus "nursing" diagnosis. The definition reversed years of hard-won gains in expanding the scope of nursing practice.

1960s: INNOVATION AND GROWTH IN ADVANCED PRACTICE NURSING

The federal legislation of the Great Society, the national problems of heart disease and stroke, and the war in Vietnam set the stage for innovation and growth in advanced practice nursing during the 1960s. In 1964 Congress passed the Nurse Training Act (Title VIII of the Public Health Service Act), specifically funding nursing education. The Nurse Training Act provided a comprehensive financial package for student grants and loans, as well as for the construction of nursing schools and faculty recruitment and development. A year later, in his 1965 inaugural address, President Lyndon Johnson outlined his plans for the Great Society, proposing a massive legislative agenda that included Medicare and Medicaid programs (under Title XVIII of the Social Security Act), providing millions of Americans with health-care benefits. In addition, the agenda included funding for regional medical programs to coordinate state and local efforts to combat cancer, heart disease, and stroke.

Of particular importance to the future of education for advanced practice nursing, the ANA published its "First Position on Education for Nursing" in 1965, calling for nursing education for professional practice to take place in colleges and universities (ANA, 1965). Had that position been enacted formally, it would have united the profession on the issue of nurse preparation. As it was, the position paper incited much debate on the issue of preparation for "entry into practice" but did little else. What became very clear was that although collegiate education in nursing was here to stay, it would not be the only entry route into the nursing profession. However, the foundation was laid for nurses to seek postbaccalaureate education in master's programs. Furthermore, the funds allocated by the 1964 Nurse Training Act were available to pay their tuition fees.

Nurse Anesthetists, circa 1960s

As was the case in wars of other eras, the war in Vietnam provided nurses with opportunities to stretch the boundaries of the discipline as they treated thousands of casualties in evacuation hospitals and aboard hospital ships. Not surprisingly, nurse anesthetists in particular played an active role in the Vietnam War, providing vital services in the prompt surgical treatment of the wounded. According to one account:

The nurse anesthetist suddenly became a part of a new concept in the treatment of the severely wounded. The Dust-Off helicopter brings medical aid to severely wounded casualties who formerly would have died before or perhaps during evacuation. . . . Very often it is a nurse anesthetist who first is available to intubate a casualty, and by so doing may avoid the need for tracheostomy. (Jenicek, 1967, p. 348)

However, opportunity was not without cost. Of the 10 nurses killed in Vietnam, two were male nurse anesthetists (Bankert, 1989).

Nurse-Midwives, circa 1960s

During the 1960s, progress for nurse-midwives was mixed. Some advances were made in defining their role when, in 1962, the ACNM established the definitions of the nurse-midwife and nurse-midwifery. These definitions clearly emphasized that the role was an "extension" of nursing practice (ACNM, 1962). However, the states were slow to grant statutory recognition to CNMs. In fact, as late as 1963, only Kentucky, New Mexico, and New York City had legally sanctioned CNM practice (Rooks, 1997). That same year, only 11% of CNMs who responded to a national survey reported that they were practicing midwifery. This proportion increased to 23% by 1967. However, about one in four of these CNMs were practicing overseas through church and international health organizations. Within the United States, the proportion of CNMs actually practicing midwifery was highest in areas with strong educational programs—again, New Mexico, Kentucky, and New York City, where they cared primarily for indigent women (ACNM, 1968). Once again, the trend is clear: as long as CNMs cared for underserved populations and proved no economic threat to physicians, they could practice unopposed.

Clinical Nurse Specialists, circa 1960s

The 1960s are most often noted as the decade in which clinical nurse specialization took its modern form. Nurse educator Hildegarde Peplau (1965) contended that development of areas of specialization is preceded by three social forces: (1) an increase in specialty-related information, (2) new technological advances, and (3) a response to public need and interest. All of these forces clearly helped shape the development of the psychiatric CNS role in the 1960s. The expansion of that role in outpatient mental health was greatly enhanced by the Community Mental Health Centers Act of 1963, as well as the growing interest in child and adolescent mental health care.

After the enactment of the 1964 Nurse Training Act, an abundance of CNS master's programs were created. These new clinically focused graduate programs were instrumental in developing and defining the role of the CNS. In a 1966 AJN article, nurse educator Frances Reiter, who had first used the term *nurse clinician* in 1943 to describe a nurse with advanced "curative" knowledge and clinical competence committed to providing the highest quality of direct patient care, expounded on her view, noting that graduate education represented an efficient means of preparing these specialized practitioners (Reiter, 1966). She proved to be correct, and graduates of these early programs, convincing hospital administrators to create CNS jobs, pioneered the role. "Through their successes, CNSs were hired, job descriptions were created and CNSs moved into the mainstream of hospital employees" (Fulton, 2002, p. 167). One of the new clinical specialty areas to emerge in the 1960s was cardiology. With the establishment of the Bethany Hospital Coronary Care Unit (CCU) in Kansas City in 1962, the concept of specialization in the care of the acutely ill patient with heart disease was conceived. Expansion of the role soon followed as nurses identified specialty knowledge for CCU nurses and added a new dimension to their previous role (Pinneo, 1967). As CCUs proliferated across the country with the support of federally funded regional medical programs, nurses and physicians acquired more knowledge about the diagnosis and treatment of cardiac arrhythmias. Together, they discussed clinical questions and negotiated responsibilities (Lynaugh & Fairman, 1992). In doing so, CCU nurses expanded their scope of practice. When nurses diagnosed arrhythmias, administered intravenous medications, and defibrillated patients who had lethal ventricular fibrillation, they blurred the invisible boundary separating the disciplines of nursing and medicine. They were diagnosing and treating, and in fact "curing," in dramatic life-saving moments. Moreover, they challenged the very definition of nursing that had been published by the ANA only a few years earlier (Keeling, 2004). What they did not do, however, was to differentiate specialization from advanced practice nursing. That differentiation would come later as master's programs were developed to prepare cardiovascular CNSs.

Although creation of the CCU may have caused confusion about "specialization" and "advanced practice," it unleashed a new era for nurses. The changes that occurred in the clinical setting of the CCU helped establish collegial relationships between nurses and physicians that would be important for CNSs and NPs in the decades to follow. Collaborative practice became the norm in intensive and coronary care units. "Most importantly, nurses and physicians learned to trust each other as they practiced in their own areas of expertise" (Lynaugh & Fairman, 1992, p. 24). Furthermore, nurses began to form new specialty organizations. By 1969, a large group of nurses who specialized in the care of patients with heart disease formed the American Association of Cardiovascular Nurses, later renamed the American Association of Critical-Care Nurses to reflect its inclusiveness (Lynaugh & Fairman, 1992).

In all, the decade was one of unprecedented growth in both the number and variety of ICUs and the latitude and scope of practice for nurses in these areas. What was necessary now was to move preparation for specialty nursing from the informal realm of in-service education to the formal setting of graduate school.

Nurse Practitioners, circa 1960s

Although the NP role had been modeled informally in the FNS in the 1930s, it was during the 1960s that the role was first formally described and implemented in primary care, originating in part as a response to a shortage of primary care physicians. As the trend toward medical specialization drew increasing numbers of physicians away from primary care, many areas of the country were designated *underserved* with respect to numbers of primary care providers. In fact, "report after report issued by the AMA and the Association of American Medical Colleges, although applauding the high level of expertise and technology found in U.S. hospitals and medical schools, decried the shortage of physicians in poor rural and urban areas" (Fairman, 2002, p. 163). At the same time, consumers across the nation were demanding accessible, affordable, and sensitive health care, while healthcare delivery costs were increasing at an annual rate of 10% to 14% (Jonas, 1981).

Pediatric Nurse Practitioners

The landmark event marking the birth of the modern NP role was the establishment of the first pediatric NP (PNP) program by Loretta Ford, RN, and Henry Silver, MD, at the University of Colorado in 1965. This demonstration project, funded by the Commonwealth Foundation, was designed to prepare professional nurses to provide comprehensive well-child care and to manage common childhood health problems. The 4-month program, which certified registered nurses (RNs) as PNPs without requiring master's preparation, emphasized health promotion and the inclusion of the family. Ford (1991) saw the development of the PNP as a reclaiming of the nurse's role in well-child care, which was lost in the 1930s when the American Academy of Pediatrics claimed that well-child care was the domain of pediatricians rather than public health nurses.

A study evaluating the project demonstrated that PNPs were highly competent in assessing and managing 75% of well and ill children in community health settings. In addition, PNPs increased the number of patients served in private pediatric practice by 33% (Ford & Silver, 1967). Like early nurse-midwife and nurse anesthetist data, these positive findings demonstrated support for this APN role.

Despite this major advance for NP practice, there was significant intraprofessional controversy over NP education. As was the case with nurse anesthesia and nurse-midwifery, early NP education did not develop within the mainstream of nursing education. Instead, certificate programs based on the Colorado project rapidly came into existence. According to Ford (1991), some of these programs shifted the emphasis of PNP preparation from a nursing to a medical model. As a result, one of the major areas of controversy in academia was over the fact that NPs made "medical" diagnoses and wrote prescriptions for medications, essentially stepping over the invisible medical boundary into the realm of "curing." Because of this, some nurse educators and other nurse leaders questioned whether the NP role could be conceptualized as being within the discipline of nursing, a profession that had historically been "ordered to care" (Reverby, 1987). While nursing professors debated the educational preparation of NPs (Rogers, 1972), the NP role attracted considerable attention from professional groups and policymakers. Health policy groups, such as the National Advisory Commission on Health Manpower, issued statements in support of the NP concept (Moxley, 1968). At the grass-roots level, nurse practitioners were employed and accepted. Educators continued to argue over whether to accept the NP role as an advanced practice nursing role and prepare NPs in master's programs, but "the horse was out of the barn" with regard to the idea of the role itself. Ford herself conceptualized the role as firmly rooted within nursing's domain, noting later in her life that the idea "thrived because the foundation of the nurse practitioner was deeply rooted in the enduring values and goals of professional nursing" (Ford, 1991, p. 287).

Physician Assistants

If nurses in academe were upset about NPs, they were even more reactive to the role of the physician assistant (PA) when it was introduced at Duke University in North Carolina in 1965 by Eugene Stead, MD. In fact, organized nursing was opposed to the idea of the PA from the beginning (Ballweg, 1994). According to Christman (1998), "The idea of having an NP program for medical surgical nursing at Duke, modeled after the PNP program established at Colorado, collapsed because the National League for Nursing (NLN) refused to accredit a program in which physicians would teach much of the curriculum.

Moreover, some of the prominent nurses at Duke did not support the idea" (p. 56). Frustrated by organized nursing's refusal to collaborate to create this new medical-surgical NP, the physicians who conceived of the idea concluded that "nurse leaders were very antagonistic to innovation and change" (Christman, 1998, p. 56). Meanwhile, Duke had recently had experience with training firefighters, excorpsmen, and other noncollege graduates to resolve personnel shortages in the clinical services of Duke University Hospital. The school proceeded with plans to open a PA program. The 2-year training program defied established concepts of medical education and accepted some applicants who had no prior college education but who had practical experience under battlefield conditions. Moreover, it provided for sharing the knowledge base formerly "owned" by medicine, but mandated that the PA would work under the license of a preceptor-physician (Ballweg, 1994). Relationships between PAs and NPs, at least at the academic level, continued to be fraught with tension as more programs developed. At the clinical level, PAs and NPs began to work together.

Nurse Case Managers, circa 1960s

Changes that occurred in social policies for health-care delivery in the early 1960s also fostered the development of the nurse case manager role. In 1962, the President's Commission on Mental Retardation recommended the use of a "program coordinator" to help individuals with chronic mental illness and developmental disabilities stay in the community rather than be cared for in institutions. Community mental health nurses fulfilled many of these roles, ensuring availability of services. Moreover, they expedited the delivery and responsiveness of care (Tahan, 1998). The 1965 Medicare Bill reinforced the concept of case management by including reimbursement to the elderly for the costs of home health-care services. Despite this federal support, the case management role would remain "on the back burner" for several decades.

1970s: ADVANCED PRACTICE NURSING BECOMES ESTABLISHED

The 1970s ushered in a period of rapid growth and development in advanced practice nursing, a decade in which it would not only gain momentum but would also become firmly established. However, the term *advanced* was most often used to describe advanced education and study in the writings of this period (e.g., see Georgopoulos and Christman, 1970), rather than the current concept of advanced practice nursing.

According to historians Lynaugh and Brush (1996): "What was historically unique . . . was the emerging [public] consensus that nursing, the largest single health-care group, should expand its scope of practice to provide direct services to patients, including services previously considered solely in the physician's domain" (p. 38). In fact, in 1971, this new view of nursing was documented in a report to Elliot Richardson, the Secretary of Health, Education, and Welfare titled *Extending the Scope of Nursing Practice*. The report called for nurses in primary, acute, and long-term care to expand their responsibilities to collect medical data and make clinical decisions about patients (Lynaugh & Brush, 1996). Recognizing the need for leadership, the ANA Congress of Nursing Practice published educational standards, described the NP and CNS roles, and attempted to define the expanding scope of nursing practice (ANA Congress for Nursing Practice, 1974). However, considerable conflict developed within the nursing profession as nurses themselves struggled to identify the boundaries of the discipline and the scope of advanced practice nursing. These changes took place within the context of the women's movement, the *Roe v. Wade* Supreme Court decision legalizing abortion, growing public disillusion with government, widespread resistance to continuing the war in Vietnam, an awareness and concern about environmental issues, and increasing federal legislation to provide health care to the handicapped and disabled.

Certified Nurse-Midwives, circa 1970s

The renewed public interest in natural childbirth that stemmed from the women's movement was particularly beneficial to the practice of nurse-midwifery in the 1970s. In fact, the demand for nurse-midwifery services increased dramatically in this decade. In addition, sociopolitical developments including the increased employment of CNMs in federally funded health-care projects, the official recognition of CNMs by the American College of Obstetricians and Gynecologists in 1971, and the increased birth rate resulting from baby boomers reaching adulthood coupled with inadequate numbers of obstetricians fostered the rapid growth of CNM practice (Varney, 1987). In 1971 only 37% of CNMs who responded to an ACNM survey were employed in clinical midwifery practice. By 1977, this percentage increased to 51%. Not surprisingly, the majority practiced in the rural, underserved areas of the Southwest and Southeast, including Appalachia.

Even at the national level, there was support for nurse-midwives. In 1971, the ACNM, the American College of Obstetricians and Gynecologists, and the Nurses' Association of the American College of Obstetricians and Gynecologists issued a joint statement supporting the development and employment of nurse-midwives in obstetrical teams directed by a physician. The joint statement, which was critical to the evolution of nurse-midwifery, reflected some resolution of the interprofessional tension that existed through much of the 20th century. However, it did not provide for autonomy for CNMs. The statement made clear the fact that the medical profession would retain supervisory authority over the practice of nurse-midwifery. By 1978, the ACNM revised its definitions of CNM practice and its philosophy, emphasizing the distinct midwifery and nursing origins of the role (ACNM, 1978a, 1978b). This conceptualization of nurse-midwifery as the combination of two disciplines, nursing and midwifery, was unique among the advanced practice nursing specialties. It served to align nurse-midwives with nonnurse midwives, thereby broadening their organizational and political base. Nonetheless, the conceptualization created some distance from other APN specialties that conceptualized the advanced practice role as based solely within the discipline of nursing. This distinction would continue to isolate CNMs from mainstream APNs for the next several decades as they persisted in aligning with nonnurses.

Nurse Anesthetists, circa 1970s

The 1970s proved to be a difficult decade for nurse anesthetists. In 1972, years after the inception of nurse anesthesia as a specialty role, only four state practice acts specifically mentioned them. Nevertheless, some progress was made in interprofessional relations that year. After years of negotiation, in 1972, the AANA and the American Society of Anesthesiologists (ASA) issued a "Joint Statement on Anesthesia Practice," promoting the concept of the anesthesia team. However, a few years later, in 1976, the ASA Board of Directors voted to withdraw support from the 1972 statement, endorsing one that explicitly supported physician control and leadership over CRNA practice (Bankert, 1989).

During the mid-1970s, the number of nurse anesthesia educational programs declined significantly, largely because of the closure of many small certificate programs that did not award a master's degree. Physician pressure, inadequate financial support, limited clinical facilities, and lack of accessible universities with which programs could be affiliated contributed to these closures (Faut-Callahan & Kremer, 1996). However, the new requirement that programs offer a graduate degree was not without benefit for CRNAs. In 1973 the University of Hawaii opened the first master's degree program for nurse anesthesia, making it clear that the role was one of advanced practice.

The economic implications of third-party payment also affected nurse anesthetists. Beginning in 1977, the AANA led a long and complex effort to secure third-party reimbursement under Medicare so that CRNAs could bill for their services. The organization would finally succeed in 1989.

Clinical Nurse Specialists, circa 1970s

The rapid proliferation of programs and jobs for CNSs, as well as the emerging role ambiguity and confusion facing them, defined the 1970s for these APNs. During this decade, psychiatric CNSs continued to provide leadership in the educational and clinical arenas, and federal funding from the Professional Nurse Traineeship Program provided fiscal support to new programs. Meanwhile, several specialty nursing organizations, including the American Association of Critical Care Nurses (AACN) and the Oncology Nursing Society (ONS) were founded. In addition, the ANA's Congress of Nursing Practice operationally defined the role of the CNS, and nursing began to conduct evaluative research on the outcomes of CNS care.

Psychiatric CNSs were particularly visible in the 1970s. Early in the decade, a cadre of graduate-prepared psychiatric CNSs assumed roles as individual, group, family, and milieu therapists and obtained direct third-party reimbursement for their services. Soon after, psychiatric nurses identified minimal educational and clinical criteria for CNSs and established national specialty certification through the ANA (Critchley, 1985).

The specialties of critical care and oncology nursing also received attention during the 1970s. The AACN, established by a small group of concerned nurses at the end of the previous decade, further organized to meet the continuing educational needs of new specialists in the areas of coronary care and intensive care nursing. Only 4 years later, after the first National Cancer Nursing Research Conference sponsored by the ANA and the American Cancer Society (ACS), a group of oncology nurses met to discuss the need for a national organization to support their specialty. Officially incorporated in 1975, the ONS provided a forum for issues related to cancer nursing and supported the growth of advanced practice nursing in this specialty (Oncology Nursing Society, 1994).

By the middle of the decade, the ANA officially recognized the CNS role, operationally defining the CNS as an expert practitioner and a change agent. Of particular significance, the ANA's definition included master's education as a requirement for the CNS (ANA Congress of Nursing Practice, 1974).

As with the other advanced nursing specialties, the development of the CNS role included early evaluation research that served to validate and promote the innovation. Landmark studies by Georgopoulos and colleagues (Georgopoulos & Christman, 1970; Georgopoulos & Jackson, 1970; Georgopoulos & Sana, 1971) evaluated the effect of CNS practice on nursing process and outcomes in inpatient adult health-care settings. These and other evaluative studies (Ayers, 1971; Girouard, 1978; Little & Carnevali, 1967) demonstrated the positive effect of the introduction of the CNS in relation to nursing care improvements and functioning.

Overall, the 1970s can probably be considered the golden age for the CNS. It was a period in which there was unprecedented growth in the health-care field in an era of expanding opportunities for women. Moreover, there was an increasing demand from society to cure illness with high-tech solutions and a willingness on the part of hospital administrators to support specialization in nursing and to hire CNSs, particularly in revenue-producing ICUs.

Nurse Practitioners, circa 1970s

Nurse practitioners also made considerable progress in the 1970s, increasing their visibility within the health-care system, negotiating with physicians to expand their scope of practice, and demonstrating their cost-effectiveness in providing quality care. Nevertheless, it was also a period characterized by intraprofessional conflict as some leaders within the nursing community continued to reject the role. In contrast, state legislatures and the AMA increasingly recognized these expanded roles of RNs, and a group of "pro-NP" nursing faculty, already teaching in NP programs, held their first national meeting in Chapel Hill, North Carolina, in 1974. This meeting would lay the foundation for the formation of the National Organization of Nurse Practitioner Faculties (NONPF).

In the early 1970s, Health, Education, and Welfare Secretary Elliott Richardson established the Committee to Study Extended Roles for Nurses. This group of health-care leaders was charged with evaluating the feasibility of expanding nursing practice (Kalisch & Kalisch, 1986). They concluded that extending the scope of the nurse's role was essential to providing equal access to health care for all Americans. According to a 1971 editorial in *AJN*, "The kind of health care Lillian Wald began preaching and practicing in 1893 is the kind the people of this country are still crying for" (Schutt, 1971, p. 53). The committee urged the establishment of innovative curricular designs in health science centers and increased financial support for nursing education. It also advocated standardizing nursing licensure and national certification and developed a model nurse practice law suitable for national application. In addition, in a report the committee called for further research related to cost-benefit analyses and attitudinal surveys to assess the impact of the new role (U.S. Department of HEW, 1972). This report resulted in increased federal support for training programs for the preparation of several types of NPs including family NPs, adult NPs, and emergency department NPs.

One of the new types of NPs to emerge was the neonatal NP. Originating in the late 1970s in response to a shortage of neonatologists coinciding with restrictions in the total time pediatric residents could devote to neonatal intensive care, the neonatal NP was the forerunner of the acute care NP of the 1990s. These highly skilled, experienced neonatal nurses assumed a wide range of new responsibilities formerly undertaken by pediatric residents, including interhospital transport of critically ill infants and newborn resuscitation (Clancy & Maguire, 1995).

As noted, conflict and discord about the NP role characterized the relationships between NPs and other nurses during this decade. Resistance continued from some members of academia who believed that NPs were not practicing nursing (Ford, 1982). Nurse theorist Martha Rogers, one of the most outspoken opponents of the NP concept, argued that the development of the NP role was a ploy to lure nurses away from nursing to medicine and thereby undermine nursing's unique role in health care (Rogers, 1972). Subsequently, nurse leaders and educators took sides for and against the establishment of educational programs for NPs within mainstream master's programs. Over time, a move toward standardizing NP educational programs at the master's level, initiated by the group of faculty who formed NONPF, would serve to reduce intraprofessional tension.

Despite this resistance, physicians increasingly accepted NPs in individual health-care practices. Working together in local practices, NPs and MDs established collegial relationships, negotiating with each other to construct work boundaries and reach agreement about their collaborative practice. "In the NP-MD dyad, negotiations centered on the NP's right to practice an essential part of traditional medicine: the process or skill set of clinical thinking . . . to perform a physical examination, elicit patient symptoms . . . create a diagnosis, formulate treatment options, prescribe treatment and make decisions about prognosis"(Fairman, 2002, pp. 163-164).The proximity of a supervising physician was thought to be key to effective practice, and "on-site" supervision was the norm. According to early NP Corene Johnson, "Initially, we had to always have a physician on site. . . . I didn't resent that. Actually, I needed the backup"(Fairman, 2002, p. 164).

During the 1970s, one of the most contentious areas of interprofessional conflict involved prescriptive authority for nursing. As one author so aptly notes, "Nursing's efforts to obtain the legal authority to prescribe may be seen as the second chapter in the struggle over the use of the word 'diagnosing' in Nurse Practice Acts" (Hadley, 1989, p. 291). Basically, prescriptive authority was dependent on the authority of NPs to provide treatment. In 1971 Idaho became the first state to recognize diagnosis and treatment as part of the scope of practice of specialty nurses (Idaho Code 54-1413, 1971). However, "As path-breaking as the statute was, it was still rather restrictive in that any acts of diagnosis and treatment had to be authorized by rules and regulations promulgated by the Idaho State Boards of Medicine and Nursing" (Safriet, 1992, p. 445). Moreover, the Drug Enforcement Act required that practitioners wishing to prescribe controlled substances obtain Drug Enforcement Agency (DEA) registration numbers, and only those practitioners with broad prescriptive authority (e.g., physicians and dentists) could obtain these numbers. In spite of these barriers, by the end of the decade, PNPs obtained legal authority to prescribe drugs for infants and children using standing protocols developed by physicians (Ford, 1979).[7]

Nurse Case Managers, circa 1970s

The practice of providing care through case management also made significant progress in the decade of the 1970s. The term *case management* appeared first in social welfare literature in the 1970s but soon emerged in public health nursing journals as well. During this decade case management services became increasingly available, particularly for elderly and disabled people, as mandated by federal legislation. The Allied Services Act of 1972 resulted in a series of demonstration projects creating the role of systems agent. These agents coordinated resources for patients with complex health-care and social services needs because many programs had become so fragmented and complex that it was difficult for patients to seek appropriate services independently. Several long-term demonstration projects that provided case management services funded by both Medicaid and Medicare were established. The Older Americans Act of 1973, which led to the development of the Area Agencies on Aging throughout the country, served as a powerful impetus to

---

[7]Alaska and North Carolina authorized PNPs to write prescriptions in 1975.

the development and dissemination of case management services during the 1970s. These agencies provided comprehensive services for the elderly, allowing them to remain independent as long as possible (Gerber, 1994). To do so, the agencies used case management teams, composed of RNs and social workers, to assess the need for services, implement the care provided, and evaluate outcomes. They also served as brokers to obtain access to appropriate community resources for patients.

Another impetus to the development of the concept of case management was the Education for All Handicapped Children Act of 1975. This legislation brought case management into the nation's school systems, as nurses and social workers collaborated with teachers and administrators to coordinate services. A third impetus was the passage of the Developmental Disabilities Assistance and Bill of Rights Act of 1975. This legislation, stipulating that each mentally disabled person be assigned a program coordinator for comprehensive services after hospital discharge, laid the groundwork for another case management role. Three years later, the President's Commission on Mental Health would recognize case management as the key to integration of services for deinstitutionalized patients (Kersbergen, 1996). Throughout the decade, what is significant is that case management had a team approach. It was becoming a specialty, but not a nursing specialty. Later, this background would become important as the nursing profession strived to carve its niche.

1980s: ADVANCE PRACTICE NURSING MATURES AND EXPANDS

During the 1980s, the ANA provided the leadership APNs would need to continue to mature and for APN roles to become institutionalized in the health-care system. Critical to this support was the ANA's 1980 Social Policy Statement, which declared that "specialization in nursing is now clearly established" (ANA, 1980, p. 22). Despite this gain, the lack of consensus about educational preparation for APNs and the titles to identify them continued to plague the profession. According to nurse educator Grace Sills (1983), "The issue of titles was hotly debated in the nursing literature. Nurse clinician, advanced clinical nurse, nurse practitioner—all such titles had different meaning, differing descriptions of the preparation needed and of the performance expected"(p. 566).

On the positive side, however, during the 1980s the concept of advanced nursing practice began to be defined and used in the literature. In 1983, Harriet Kitzman, an associate professor at the University of Rochester, explored the interrelationships between CNSs and NPs (Kitzman, 1983). She used the term *advanced practice* throughout her discussion, applying the term not only to advanced education but also to CNS and NP practice. She noted, "Recognition for advanced practice competence is already established for both NPs and CNSs through the profession's certification programs . . . advanced nursing practice cannot be setting-bound, because nursing needs are not exclusively setting-restricted" (Kitzman, 1983, pp. 284, 288). Building on Kitzman's ideas, Spross and Hamric (1983) proposed the term *advanced registered nurse practitioner* for a blended CNS/NP model of practice (see Chapter 15). In 1984, an associate professor at the University of Wisconsin–Madison, Joy Calkin, proposed a model for advanced nursing practice, specifically identifying CNSs and NPs with master's degrees as APNs (Calkin, 1984). By the end of the decade, the term was in common use.

The increasing emphasis on cost containment in the 1980s produced legislative and economic changes that affected advanced practice nursing and the health-care delivery system as a whole. In particular, the establishment of a prospective payment system in which diagnosis-related groups (DRGs) were used for hospitalized Medicare recipients in 1983 was a landmark event. This payment system represented an effort to control rising costs and reimbursement to hospitals by shifting reimbursement from "payment for services provided" to "payment by case" (capitation). As a result, hospital administrators put increasing pressure on nurses and physicians to save money by decreasing the length of time patients remained in the hospital. The emphasis on cost containment also heralded budget cuts for hospitals that forced nursing administrators to carefully evaluate the cost-effectiveness of CNSs (then the most commonly employed APNs), resulting in elimination of some of these positions.

Nonetheless, the economic climate was not all negative for nursing. In fact, the need to provide cost-effective, quality care to American citizens prompted the Senate Committee on Appropriations to request a report on the contributions of NPs, CNMs, and PAs in meeting the nation's health-care needs. The report, released in 1986 and titled "Nurse Practitioners, Physician Assistants and Certified Nurse-Midwives," was based on an analysis of numerous studies that assessed quality of care, patient satisfaction, and physician acceptance. It concluded that "within their areas of competence NPs . . . and CNMs provide care whose quality is equivalent to that of care provided by physicians" (Office of Technology Assessment, 1986, p. 5). However, while the Office of Technology Assessment was conducting this study, the AMA House of Delegates, threatened by the possibility of competition from APNs, passed a resolution to "oppose any attempt at empowering non-physicians to become unsupervised primary care providers and be directly reimbursed" (Safriet, 1992, p. 429).

Nurse Anesthetists, circa 1980s

Despite progress on the educational front, interprofessional conflicts with medicine continued. Although the earlier litigation, *Frank et al. v. South* (1917) and *Chalmers-Frances v. Nelson* (1936) provided the critical legal basis of nurse anesthesia practice, tension between physicians and nurse anesthetists continued, particularly in relation to malpractice policies, antitrust issues, and restraint of trade issues. In 1986, *Oltz v. St. Peter's Community Hospital* established the right of CRNAs to sue for anticompetitive damages when anesthesiologists conspired to restrict practice privileges. A second case, *Bhan v. NME Hospitals, Inc.* (1985), established the right of CRNAs to be awarded damages when exclusive contracts were made between hospitals and physician anesthesiologists. Undeniably, CRNAs were winning the legal battles and overcoming barriers to their practice erected by hospital administrators and physicians.

Like other APNs during the 1980s, nurse anesthetists also had to overcome barriers to reimbursement for their service by third-party payors. The chief problem was that nurse anesthetists could not bill for their services and hospitals had to consider them as a cost center rather than as a revenue-generating service, creating reimbursement disincentives for hospitals to use them (Diers, 1991). Overall, the decade was one of legal success for CRNAs and gradual progress in a difficult economic environment.

Nurse-Midwives, circa 1980s

By the 1980s, the public's acceptance of nurse-midwives had grown, and demand for their services had increased. By the middle of 1982, there were almost 2,600 CNMs, the majority located on the East Coast. "Nurse-midwifery had become not only acceptable but also desirable and demanded. Now the problem was that, after years during which nurse-midwives struggled for existence there was nowhere near the supply to meet the demand" (Varney, 1987, p. 31).

Conflict with the medical profession increased as obstetricians perceived a growing threat to their practices. The denial of hospital privileges, attempts to deny third-party reimbursement, and state legislative battles over statutory recognition of CNMs ensued. In particular, the problem of restraint of trade was significant. In 1980 Congress and the Federal Trade Commission conducted a hearing to determine the extent of the restraint-of-trade issues experienced by CNMs. In two cases, one in Tennessee and one in Georgia, the Federal Trade Commission obtained restraint orders against hospitals and insurance companies that attempted to limit the practice of CNMs (Diers, 1991), in essence, assuring CNMs that they could practice. Third-party reimbursement for CNMs was a second issue. It was first approved in 1980 for CNMs working under the Civilian Health and Medical Program of the Uniformed Services (CHAMPUS) for military dependents. Third-party payment for CNMs was also included under Medicaid. Statutory recognition by state legislatures was a third problem that would be addressed in the 1980s. By 1984, all states had recognized nurse-midwifery within state laws or regulations (Varney, 1987).

Throughout this decade, nurse-midwifery was immersed in interprofessional struggles over disciplinary boundaries. The support they received in the Office of Technology Assessment study, as well as backing from the Federal Trade Commission and the state legislatures, was critical to their continued survival.

Clinical Nurse Specialists, circa 1980s

Of particular significance to the maturation of the CNS role during the 1980s was the ANA's Social Policy Statement (1980), which clearly delineated the criteria required to assume the title of CNS. According to that statement:

The specialist in nursing practice is a nurse who, through study and supervised clinical practice at the graduate level (masters or doctorate), has become expert in a defined area of knowledge and practice in a selected clinical area of nursing. . . . Upon completion of a graduate program degree in a university graduate program with an emphasis on clinical specialization, the specialist in nursing practice should meet the criteria for specialty certification through nursing's professional society. (p. 23)

In the early 1980s, nurse executives were eager to hire CNSs and the demand for programs increased. In February 1983, the first meeting of the executive committee of the ANA's Council of Clinical Nurse Specialists provided a forum for CNSs and a general repository for documents and information about the role. By 1984, the NLN had accredited 129 programs for preparation of CNSs (NLN, 1984). However, about that time, concerns related to the future of the CNS role were surfacing in light of the increasing concern with health-care cost containment (Hamric, 1989). Concurrently, some nurse researchers studied the outcomes related to CNS practice. In 1987, for example, McBride et al. demonstrated that nursing practice, particularly in relation to documentation, improved as a result of the introduction of a CNS in an inpatient psychiatric setting. By the late 1980s, many CNSs shifted the focus of their practice away from the clinical area and instead focused on the educational and organizational aspects of the CNS role. This shift was supported by the view that CNSs were too valuable to spend their time on direct patient care (Wolfe, 1984). Meanwhile, others who asserted that the essence of the CNS role was clinical expertise were publishing articles and books on the topic (Hamric & Spross, 1983, 1989; Sparacino, Cooper, & Minarik, 1990). In addition, articles describing the practice of CNSs and consensus reports on this APN role began to appear in critical care, oncology, and other nursing specialty journals. These publications helped lay the groundwork for curriculum development in APN specialties.

Also during the 1980s, the ANA Council of Clinical Nurse Specialists (CCNS) and Council of Primary Health Care Nurse Practitioners (CPHCNP) began to explore together commonalities of the two roles. In 1988, the councils conducted a survey of all NP and CNS graduate programs and identified considerable overlap in curricula. Subsequently, between 1988 and 1990, the two councils discussed a proposal to merge, and in 1991, the new Council of Nurses in Advanced Practice was formed. Unfortunately, it was short-lived because of the restructuring of ANA during the early 1990s. Nevertheless, this merger was a landmark event in the organizational coalescence of advanced practice nursing (ANA, 1991).

Nurse Case Managers, circa 1980s

During the 1980s, a new phase in case management history emerged in which case management was recognized as a specialized nursing role, but not yet an advanced practice specialty. In the late 1980s, Karen Zander developed the acute care nurse case management model at the New England Medical Center hospital in Boston, Massachusetts. Envisioned as an evolution and further development of primary nursing, Zander's model used clinical pathways that focused on prospective planning of nursing care and measurement of outcomes (Zander, 1988). These critical pathways led to the development of multidisciplinary case management tools.

Also in this decade, the ANA set initial educational guidelines for the nurse case manager (NCM) (ANA, 1988; Bower, 1992). The minimum recommended education was a baccalaureate degree in nursing with 3 years of appropriate clinical experience. However, a year after these recommendations were made, Cronin and Maklebust (1989) studied case-managed care at Harper Hospital and found that nurses with bachelor's degrees were frustrated with their inability to case manage effectively while delivering patient care. In contrast, when case managers with master's degrees were employed, improvements were noted for patients and the hospital. These researchers concluded that APNs saved time and money by using early interventions based on in-depth clinical expertise (Cronin & Maklebust, 1989). The move toward requiring the NCM to be an APN was under way.

Nurse Practitioners, circa 1980s

The fight for prescriptive authority for NPs characterized the 1980s. In 1983, only Oregon and Washington granted NPs statutory independent prescriptive authority. Other states granting prescriptive authority to NPs did so with the provision that the NP be directly supervised by a licensed physician. Despite these legal barriers, NP practice increased immeasurably during the 1980s. By 1984, approximately 20,000 graduates of NP programs were employed, for the most part in settings "that the founders envisioned": outpatient clinics, health maintenance organizations, health departments, community health centers, rural clinics, schools, occupational health clinics, and private offices (Kalisch & Kalisch, 1986, p. 715).

During this period, multiple roles for NPs including those of emergency NP, PNP, family NP, and neonatal NP continued to develop, creating competing interests that would affect NPs' ability to speak with one voice on legislative issues. In an attempt to rectify this situation, the ANA established the Primary Health Care Nurse Practitioner Council in the early 1980s. At about the same time, the Alliance of Nurse Practitioners was established as an umbrella organization for all the various NP associations.

Throughout the 1980s, NPs worked tirelessly to convince state legislatures to pass laws and establish reimbursement policies that would support their practice. Interprofessional conflicts with organized medicine, and to a lesser extent with pharmacists, centered on control issues and the degree of independence the NP was allowed. These conflicts intensified as NPs moved beyond the "physician extender" model to a more autonomous one. In a 1980 landmark case, *Sermchief v. Gonzales* (1983), the Missouri medical board charged two women's health-care NPs with practicing medicine without a license (Doyle & Meurer, 1983). The initial ruling was against the NPs, but on appeal, the Missouri Supreme Court overturned the decision, concluding that the scope of practice of APNs may evolve without statutory constraints (Wolff, 1984). In essence, this case provided a model for new state nurse practice acts to address issues related to APN practice with very generalized wording, a change that allowed for expansion in APNs' roles and functions.

1990s: ADVANCED PRACTICE NURSING RESPONDS TO MANAGED CARE

The 1990s continued to be a period of growth and change for advanced practice nursing as the profession responded to regulatory and economic turmoil. The 1990s opened with the United States' war with Iraq, a war in which thousands of American military nurses were deployed to the Persian Gulf. The cost of health care was a constant concern, and by 1992, when William Jefferson Clinton was elected President of the United States, the country was in serious need of health-care reform. Determined to take a proactive stance in the movement, the ANA wrote its *Agenda for Health Care Reform* (1992). The plan focused on restructuring the U.S. health-care system to reduce costs and improve access to care (Keeling, 1997). Although the Clinton administration's efforts for health-care reform failed, radical changes were made by the private sector in which the once dominant "fee for service" insurance plans were overtaken by managed care organizations (Safriet, 1998). The changing marketplace created new challenges for APNs as they struggled not only with restrictive outdated state laws on prescriptive authority but also with "nongovernmental, market-based impediments" to their practices (Safriet, 1998, p. 25). In this environment, APNs continued to expand their roles, their educational programs, and their practice settings. During this decade, at the national Nursing Summit organized by the tri-council organizations in August 1993, representatives of 63 of 66 organizations attending the conference agreed to the criterion of master's education for advanced practice nursing (Cronenwett, 1995).

Nurse Practitioners, circa 1990s

During the 1990s, the number of NPs increased dramatically in response to increasing demand, the national emphasis on primary care, and the concomitant decrease in the number of medical residencies in the subspecialties (a factor spurring growth of acute care

NPs). In 1990, there were 135 master's degree and 40 certificate NP programs. Between 1992 and 1994, the number of institutions offering NP education more than doubled from 78 to 158. In 1994 these institutions offered a total of 384 NP tracks in master's programs throughout the United States. By 1998, the number of institutions offering NP education again doubled, representing a total of 769 distinct NP specialty tracks (National Organization of Nurse Practitioner Faculties [NONPF] 1997; AACN, 1999). The majority of the programs were at the master's or post-master's level. In fact, by 1998, only 12 post-basic RN certificate programs remained in existence. This rapid expansion created concern about the need for so many programs and the quality of the programs. In the end, most nurse educators supported the master's degree as the educational requirement for NP practice, and many used the NONPF guidelines in determining their curricula (NONPF, 1997).

In the mid-1990s, NPs attempted to unify their organizational voice by establishing the American Academy of Nurse Practitioners (AANP). Membership in this organization included national organizational affiliates, state NP organizations, and individuals. Supposedly, the focus of the organization was to address public policy issues that affected all NPs. However, NPs never unified. Throughout this period many were angry about the establishment of the AANP. The Alliance of Nurse Practitioners continued to be active, and the American College of Nurse Practitioners was born. In addition, PNPs formed the National Association of Pediatric Nurse Associates and Practitioners (NAPNAP), and nurses interested in women's' health formed the Association of Women's Health, Obstetric, & Neonatal Nurses (AWHONN). Multiple certification examinations were developed by these various groups, in addition to the ANA's Credentialing Center (ANCC). In fact, dissension about which group should speak for NPs continued throughout the 1990s and into the 21st century.

Like the neonatal NP role of the late 1970s, the adult acute care NP (ACNP) role developed during this decade in response to residency shortages in ICUs, although this time the shortage was due to decreases in the number of residents available to work in the medical subspecialties. In addition, increasingly complicated tertiary care systems lacked coordination of care. Advanced practice nursing responded quickly to this need, creating a role that promoted both quality patient care and nursing's leadership in health-care delivery (Daly, 1997). University of Pennsylvania Professor Anne Keane and Theresa Richmond, RN, MSN, (1993) were among the first to document the emergence of the tertiary NP (TNP), noting:

The TNP is an advanced practice nurse educated at the master's level with both a theoretical and experiential focus on complex patients with specialized health needs. . . . There is precedent for the NP in tertiary care. For example, neonatal nurse practitioners are central to the provision of care in many intensive care nurseries. . . . It is our belief that the TNP can provide clinically expert specialized care in a holistic manner in a system that is often typified by fragmentation, lack of communication among medical specialists and a loss of recognition of the patient and patient's needs as central to the care delivered. (p. 282)

From 1992 to 1995, ACNP tracks in master's programs proliferated across the country.[8] Soon, questions abounded about the content of the curriculum. To resolve these, the

---

[8]The University of Pittsburgh, Case Western Reserve University, the University of Connecticut, The University of Rochester, Rush Presbyterian University, and the University of Pennsylvania were among the first university schools of nursing to embrace the idea and implement programs, most of which were originally at the post-master's level (Daly, 2002).

educators met annually at ACNP consensus conferences, beginning in 1993. The first ACNP certification examination was given in December 1995 by the ANCC, and by 1997, there were 43 tracks nationwide that prepared ACNPs either at the master's or post-master's level (Kleinpell, 1997). In 2002, ACNPs formally merged with the American Academy of Nurse Practitioners (AANP) with the goal of uniting both primary care and acute care NPs under an umbrella organization. By this time, the ACNP role was beginning to be accepted. ACNPs were employed in multiple specialties including cardiology, cardiovascular surgery, neurosurgery, emergency/trauma, internal medicine, and radiology services (Daly, 2002).

Federal legislation regulating narcotics in the Controlled Substances Act (1991 and 1992) would be of major significance to NP progress in implementing prescriptive authority in this decade. As NPs began to gain prescriptive authority for controlled substances in the different states, they required a parallel authority granted by the federal Drug Enforcement Agency (DEA). In 1991, the DEA first responded to this situation by proposing registration for "affiliated practitioners" (56FR 4181). This proposal called for those NPs who had prescriptive authority pursuant to a practice protocol or collaborative practice agreement to be assigned a registration number for controlled substances tied to the number of the physician with whom they worked. This proposal received much criticism specifically related to restricting accessibility to health care and to the legal liability of the prescribers. Because of these criticisms, the proposal was revoked in 1992. Later in the year, in July 1992, the DEA amended its regulations by adding a category of "mid-level providers" (MLPs) who would be issued individual provider DEA numbers as long as they were granted prescriptive authority by the state in which they practiced. The MLP's number would begin with an M for "mid-level provider," rather than an A or B. The MLP provision took effect in 1993, significantly expanding NPs' ability to prescribe.

Nurse Anesthetists, circa 1990s

The 1990s saw significant growth in CRNA educational programs, although many of the programs were very small. As the decade opened, there were 17 master's programs in nurse anesthesia; by 1999, there were 82 (Bigbee & Amidi-Nouri, 2000). As of 1998, all accredited programs in nurse anesthesia were required to be at the master's level; however, they were not uniformly located within schools of nursing. Rather, they were housed in a variety of disciplines, including schools of nursing, medicine, allied health, and basic science. As it had been throughout the century, nurse anesthetist programs continued to be regarded by the profession as "on the fringe." At the turn of the 21st century, however, CRNA programs are becoming increasingly institutionalized in graduate nursing programs.

Nurse-Midwives, circa 1990s

During the 1990s, increasing demand for CNM services resulted in gradual expansion in the scope of nurse-midwifery practice. CNMs began to provide care to women with relatively high-risk pregnancies in collaboration with obstetricians in some of the nations' academic tertiary care centers (Rooks, 1997). During this decade, two practice models emerged: the CNM service model in which CNMs were responsible for the care of a caseload of women determined to be eligible for midwifery care, and the CNM/MD team model. Nurse-midwives made significant progress in establishing laws and regulations needed to support their practice. In fact, over the course of the decade, every state gave statutory recognition to CNMs. Moreover, CNMs were also granted prescriptive privileges and third-party reimbursement (Rooks, 1997, p. 161).

As recently as 1999, nurse-midwifery programs were required to award a minimum of a bachelor's degree (rather than a master's degree) to be eligible for ACNM accreditation. This requirement diverged from the trend among other APN specialties to require graduate preparation. At about the same time, economic conditions created new problems for CNMs. The rapid transition to managed care, as well as an increase in the cost of liability insurance, began to threaten nurse-midwifery practice.

Clinical Nurse Specialists, circa 1990s

The 1990s were also a challenging decade for CNSs, beginning with cutbacks in their employment opportunities because of the financial problems within hospitals and ending with national recognition by the federal government for Medicare reimbursement for their services. In the early 1990s, CNS programs were the most numerous of all the master's nursing programs nationally, serving more than 11,000 students (NLN, 1994). The largest area of specialization was adult health/medical-surgical nursing. However, with the increasing emphasis on primary care in the mid-1990s, the rapid growth of NP programs, the financial challenges faced by hospital administrators, and the introduction of the ACNP role in tertiary care centers, there was a sharp decline in the number of CNS positions in hospitals. Consequently, there was also a sharp decline in the number of nurses interested in pursuing master's degrees for the CNS role.

The 1996 Sample Survey of Registered Nurses also revealed that a significant number (7,802) of CNSs were also prepared as NPs (see Chapter 3). According to that report, these dual-role–prepared APNs were more likely to be employed as NPs rather than as CNSs. By 1996, of the 61,601 CNSs in the United States, only 23% were practicing in CNS-specific positions (U.S. Department of Health and Human Services, 1996). This low percentage may reflect the fact that CNSs accepted different positions as, for example, administrators or staff educators. It may also reflect the decline in the number of CNS positions available because of budget cutbacks. Certification for CNS practice was particularly complicated. In many specialties, nurses were allowed to take examinations for certification if they were clinical experts in the field and had a baccalaureate degree. For example, in oncology, basic certification was available for several years through the ONS. It was not until 1995 that the ONS administered the first certification examination for advanced practice in oncology nursing.

Despite these realities, the decade was not without its positive side for CNSs. The creation of the National Association of Clinical Nurse Specialists (NACNS), established in 1995, represented a major step in the organizational development of this specialty. In 1997, CNSs were specifically identified for Medicare reimbursement eligibility in the Balanced Budget Act (Public Law 105-33) (Safriet, 1998). This law, providing Medicare Part B direct payment to NPs and CNSs, regardless of their geographic area of practice, allowed both CNSs and NPs to be paid 85% of the fee paid to physicians for the same services. Moreover, the law's inclusion and definition of CNSs corrected a previous omission of this group for reimbursement (Safriet, 1998). The possibility of reimbursement for services was an important step in the continuing development of the CNS role because hospital administrators would continue to focus on the cost of having APNs provide patient care.

Nurse Case Managers, circa 1990s

The Case Management Society of America (CMSA), a multidisciplinary organization, was founded in 1990. Throughout the decade, the development of nurse case management accelerated significantly as a result of the rapid proliferation of managed care. In 1985, only 19% of the U.S. population received care through health maintenance organizations, as compared with 56% in 1995 (Fox, 1997). This major shift in health-care financing resulted in a dramatic increase in the use of case managers by both health-care institutions and insurers.

Also, in the 1990s, several nursing leaders contended that case management was best done by APNs (Connors, 1993; Fralic, 1992; Hamric, 1992). In 1996, Mahn and Spross differentiated the basic NCM from the Advanced Practice Nurse Case Manager (APNCM). They proposed that the APNCM was a master's prepared APN who, like an NCM, maintains a direct clinical relationship with patients and families but also assesses the need for system or process improvements (Mahn & Spross, 1996). During the late 1990s, the American Nurses Credentialing Center (ANCC) established the first certification program specifically for NCMs. Eligibility requirements for the ANCC examination included a bachelor's degree in nursing and 2000 hours of experience in nurse case management within the preceding 2 years. These requirements were not consistent with those for advanced practice specialty certification through the ANCC, which required graduate education.

The entry of NCMs into health-care delivery produced a moderate amount of interprofessional and intraprofessional conflict. From the interprofessional perspective, some debate within the case management community focused on which discipline is most appropriate to provide case management services. In addition, some direct care providers, particularly physicians, voiced strident opposition to NCMs' review and decision-making power within institutions and managed care organizations, arguing that NCMs were an inappropriate intrusion in the patient-provider relationship. From the intraprofessional perspective, the major point of contention has centered on the educational and practice preparation necessary for nurses to function as NCMs and APNCMs. Some authors argue that all professional nurses are NCMs (Conti, 1996). Others argue that CNSs or NPs are best prepared to provide case management services (Schroer, 1991; Trinidad, 1993; Wagner & Menke, 1992; Mahn & Spross, 1996). In fact, within the emerging APNCM role, considerable overlap with other APN specialties remained, particularly with CNSs and ACNPs. However, as of 2002, ANA had not yet formally recognized the role of case manager as advanced nursing practice (Murphy-Ende, 2002).

THE 21ST CENTURY: NEW CHALLENGES AND OPPORTUNITIES FOR ADVANCED PRACTICE NURSING

The turn of the 21st century brought new challenges to APNs. Computerized charting, the widespread use of the Internet to access information, an emphasis on evidence-based practice, and an increasing awareness of the global community were just a few of the challenges facing the profession. In addition, public health nursing and the rebuilding of the public health system received increased attention after the September 11, 2001, attacks on the World Trade Center in New York City, as the threat of infectious disease from bioterrorism became a clinical reality.

Today, America is faced with a health-care system at risk of imploding with spiraling costs and increasing percentages of the population that are uninsured or underinsured.

Along with a downturn in the national economy, an increasingly diverse and aging population, military conflicts in Afghanistan and Iraq, and a critical nursing shortage, the health-care system faces significant problems that must be addressed. Legislative battles continue over the scope of APN prescriptive authority, especially for controlled substances. More importantly, current market forces represent more significant barriers than regulatory ones. As Safriet (1998) noted:

No longer is governmental prohibition or restriction the only—or even the principal problem. Now an increase in the competitive chaos of the marketplace has thrown APNs into unfamiliar territory in which private contracting, market-share, and capital requirements may pose potentially serious obstacles. (p. 25)

Full recognition of APNs by insurers and managed care organizations is currently the most important challenge. Legislative efforts to secure third-party reimbursement continue to be critical to the economic survival of advanced practice nursing.

SUMMARY AND CONCLUSIONS: ADVANCED PRACTICE NURSING IN CONTEXT

In a brief analysis of the history of advance practice nursing in the 20th century, several themes emerge: (1) Throughout the century, APNs have been permitted by organized medicine and state legislative bodies to provide care to the underserved poor, particularly in rural areas of the nation. However, when that care competes with physician's reimbursement for their services, there is resistance from organized medicine and resulting interprofessional conflict. (2) Documentation of the outcomes of APN practice continues to be of critical importance to the survival of this level of practice. (3) Organizational efforts, certification at the national level, and the move toward graduate education as a requirement for advanced practice have been critical to the credibility of advanced practice nursing. (4) There has been recurrent intraprofessional and interprofessional resistance to expanding the boundaries of the nursing discipline. (5) Societal forces including wars, the economic climate, and health-care policy have influenced the evolution of advanced practice nursing.

Providing care to people in underserved areas has, by default, been assigned to nursing throughout the 20th century. Moreover, history is clear that the concept of expanding the scope of practice for nurses was inextricably entwined in that assignment. The HSS visiting nurses cared for poor immigrants of the Lower East Side unopposed by physicians until MDs perceived them as a threat. The FNS nurses made diagnoses and treated patients in remote areas of Appalachia with the blessings of the physician committee who supervised them, and the FSA nurses "cured," as best they could, migrant workers in their care. In other instances, if one considers time as place, "after midnight" nurses expanded their scope of practice by defibrillating patients in CCUs across the nation, and army nurses did whatever needed to be done (Keeling, 2004) on the battlefront. Only when APNs threatened physicians' practice and income did organized medicine accuse them of practicing medicine without a license. Moreover, organized nursing itself was responsible for resisting the expansion of the scope of practice of nursing. However, it is also clear that when nurses and physicians focused on providing quality care for their patients, they were capable of working collaboratively and interdependently.

Further analysis of the history of advanced practice nursing demonstrates the importance of evaluative research in documenting the contributions of APNs to the health-care system and patients' well-being. As evidenced by nurse anesthetist Alice Magaw's 1900 publication on outcomes, the early APNs were particularly visionary in their use of data to document their effectiveness. Throughout the century, evaluative research based on measurable outcomes served as a tool for the profession to argue its position to both health-care policymakers and the medical profession (Brooten et al., 1986; Hamric, Lindbak, Jaubert, & Worley, 1998; Mitchell-DiCenso et al., 1996; Shah, Brutlomesso, Sullivan, & Lattanzio, 1997; Wammack, & Mabrey, 1998). As Beck (1995) states in the *University of San Francisco Law Review*, "It is inconsistent for a state medical association to maintain a position that quality health care is their objective . . . [while] . . . disregarding data demonstrating the positive impact of APNs on health care" (p. 15).

The powerful influence of organizational efforts also emerges as a theme. National organization has been key to APN progress. Within the development of each of the advanced nursing specialties, several common features emerge. Strong national organizational leadership has been clearly demonstrated to be of critical importance in enhancing the growth and protection of the specialty. On the basis of the experience of the two oldest specialties, nurse anesthesia and nurse-midwifery, the process of establishing an effective national organization has taken a minimum of 3 decades. Members of the newest advanced practice specialties—NPs, CNSs, and APNCMs—are still dealing with their organizational development. As demonstrated within the specialties of nurse anesthesia and nurse-midwifery, specialty organizations have also historically played a critical role in the credentialing process for individuals within the specialty. The strength, unity, and depth of the organizational development of the two oldest advanced nursing specialties should serve as a model for the younger developing specialties.

An additional theme to emerge is the importance of professional unity regarding the requisite education of APNs. Early in the century, specialty education was considered to be postgraduate; however, that education was commonly post-diploma, not post-baccalaureate, and did not result in a master's degree. These early programs were of variable length and quality. The establishment of credible and stable educational programs has been a crucial step in the evolution of advanced nursing specialties. As educational programs moved from informal, institutionally based models with a strong apprenticeship approach to more formalized graduate education programs, the credibility of the APN role increased. Today, there is emerging consensus that graduate education at the master's level is a requirement for advanced nursing practice.[9] However, not all specialty organizations agree, and this lack of unity is impeding progress in the adoption of this educational criterion. Chief among these is the ACNM's commitment to expanding the pool of available midwives to ensure access to care. This commitment makes it difficult for the organization to advocate master's preparation for all CNMs.

The powerful influence of interprofessional struggles is apparent in all the advanced specialties, with the possible exception of CNSs. The legal battles between nursing and medicine are longstanding, particularly in relation to nurse anesthesia and nurse-midwifery. Most of these tensions revolve around issues of control, autonomy, and economic competition. However, the outcomes of the legal battles have proven to be positive for nursing for the most part and have helped to legitimize APN roles.

Nurse anesthetists, nurse-midwives, and NPs specifically challenged the boundaries between nursing and medical practice. When they did, organized medicine responded, and today, these predictable responses should not be unexpected or underestimated.

---

[9]In contrast to academic programs for NPs, CNMs, and CRNAs, educational preparation for CNSs evolved within master's programs exclusively.

According to Inglis and Kjervik (1993), "It should be noted that organized medicine, largely through lobbying, has played a central role in creating and perpetuating the states' contradictory and constraining provisions of APN practice" (p. 196).

Controversy within the nursing community was also a strong theme as the specialties developed. CRNAs, CNMs, and to some extent NPs and NCMs developed outside of mainstream nursing; whereas from the start, CNSs developed within the mainstream. Nevertheless, each specialty has had to deal with resistance from other nurses. These intraprofessional struggles can be understood within the context of change: each of the APN specialties represented innovations that challenged the status quo of the nursing establishment and the health-care system. Intraprofessional conflict over certification continues today, particularly in relation to certification for CNSs.

Throughout the century, prescriptive authority for advanced practice nursing, inextricably linked to economic and boundary issues between medicine and nursing, has been a particularly volatile legislative issue. Today, in most states, NPs, CNMs, and CRNAs can prescribe drugs with varying degrees of physician involvement and supervision. Although CNSs can prescribe in many states, they have not received the full recognition that has been granted to the other APN groups. Thus despite a great deal of progress in the role of APNs over the last century and the gradual changes in state legislation and third-party reimbursement, APNs have not reached their full potential to fulfill the nation's health-care needs. Barriers to enhancement of prescriptive authority for APNs include (1) exclusive reimbursement patterns, (2) anticompetitive practices and resistance of organized medicine, (3) state regulation and practice acts, and (4) DEA registration laws (Beck, 1995).

Societal forces have clearly influenced the development of advanced nursing practice. Gender issues have affected all the specialties to some degree because of the unique position of nursing as a female-dominated profession. The specialty of nurse anesthesia has been the exception, with large numbers of men entering this field. Within nurse-midwifery, the status of women and women's health were powerful forces in the establishment and development of the specialty. In the second half of the century, CNMs responded to the growing demands of middle-class women for comprehensive, family-focused prenatal care. Throughout the century, CNMs have consistently met the needs of the poor and underserved communities in which physicians chose not to practice. Wars and the relationship of nursing and the military establishment also influenced advanced practice nursing. Overall, war has served as a catalyst to the development of advanced nursing practice, education, and professional organization. Finally, economic changes, particularly in relation to health-care financing, have had a powerful effect on the development of advanced practice nursing. The dramatic growth of managed care systems in the 1990s in particular presented new challenges and opportunities for APNs related to reimbursement, scope of practice, and autonomy (Safriet, 1998). The recent growth of the APNCM role has largely been a result of the economic restructuring of health care in the 1990s.

Throughout the latter half of the 20th century, state regulations influenced the evolution of advanced practice as an increasing number of states mandated a master's degree as a prerequisite for APN licensure. Undoubtedly, as law professor Safriet (1998) has argued, consistency in the definition of advanced practice nursing and in the criteria for licensure as an APN is critical to autonomy in practice.

With unremitting changes in nursing and health care, it is apparent that the advanced nursing practice specialties will continue to evolve and diversify. Current examples of these newly evolving roles include the wound, ostomy, and continence nurse and the genetics APN (see Chapter 19). The beauty of the concept of advanced practice nursing is its inherent flexibility and creativity to quickly adapt to changing health-care needs. As new roles emerge, the history of advanced practice nursing continues to be written. What remains to be seen is whether the profession can unite on issues related to the definition of advanced practice nursing and standardized criteria for education and practice to ensure that APNs are permitted to practice as other professionals. "The past is prologue" (Shakespeare, 2002).

REFERENCES

American Association of Colleges of Nursing. (1999). *Enrollment and graduations in baccalaureate and graduate programs in nursing.* Washington, DC: Author.

American College of Nurse-Midwives. (1962). *Definition of a certified nurse-midwife.* Washington, DC: Author.

American College of Nurse-Midwives. (1968). *Descriptive data, nurse-midwives—U.S.A.* Washington, DC: Author.

American College of Nurse-Midwives. (1978a). *Definition of a certified nurse-midwife.* Washington, DC: Author.

American College of Nurse-Midwives. (1978b). *Philosophy.* Washington, DC: Author.

American Nurses Association. (1955). ANA board approves a definition of nursing practice. *American Journal of Nursing, 5,* 1474.

American Nurses Association. (1965). ANA's first position on education for nursing. *American Journal of Nursing, 65,* 106-111.

American Nurses Association. (1980). *Nursing: A social policy statement.* Kansas City, MO: Author.

American Nurses Association. (1988). *Nursing case management.* Kansas City, MO: Author.

American Nurses Association. (1991, April). *Report of the Congress on Nursing Practice to ANA Board of Directors on the merger of the Council of Clinical Nurse Specialists and the Council of Primary Health Care Nurse Practitioners into the Council of Nurses.* Washington, DC: Author.

American Nurses Association. (1992). *Agenda for health care reform.* Washington, DC: Author.

American Nurses Association Congress for Nursing Practice. (1974). *Definition: Nurse practitioner, nurse clinician and clinical nurse specialist.* Kansas City, MO: American Nurses Association.

Ayers, R. (1971). Effects and development of the role of the clinical nurse specialist. In R. Ayers (Ed.), *The clinical nurse specialist: An experiment in role effectiveness and role development* (pp. 32-49). Duarte, CA: City of Hope National Medical Center.

Baer, E. (2001). Aspirations unattained: The story of the Illinois Training School's search for university status. In E. Baer, P. D'Antonio, S. Rinker , & J. Lynaugh (Ed.), *Enduring issues in American Nursing* (pp. 150-164). New York: Springer.

Baguley, B. (2002). A brief history of cancer chemotherapy. In B. Baguley & D. Kerr (Eds.), *Anticancer drug development* (pp. 1-9). New York: Academic Press.

Ballweg, R. (1994). History of the profession. In R. Ballweg, S. Stolberg, & E. M. Sullivan (Eds.), *Physician assistant* (pp. 1-20). Philadelphia: W. B. Saunders.

Bankert, M. (1989). *Watchful care: A history of America's nurse anesthetists.* New York: Continuum.

Beck, M. (1995). Improving America's health care: Authorizing independent prescriptive privileges for advanced practice nurses. *University of San Francisco's Law Review, 29,* 951.

Beeber, L. S. (1990). To be one of the boys: Aftershocks of the WWI nursing experience. *Advances in Nursing Science, 12,* 32-43.

Bhan v. NME Hospitals, Inc., ct al., 772 F.2d 1467 (9th Cir. 1985).

Bigbee, J., & Amidi-Nouri, A. (2000). History and evolution of advanced nursing practice. In A. B. Hamric, J. A. Spross, & C. M. Hanson (Eds.), *Advanced nursing practice: An integrative approach* (2nd ed., pp. 3-32). Philadelphia: W. B. Saunders.

Bigbee, J., & Crowder, E. (1985). The Red Cross Rural Nursing Service: An innovative model of public health nursing delivery. *Public Health Nursing, 2,* 109-121.

The Bolton Hill. (1943, July). *American Journal of Nursing, 43,* 617.

Bower, K. A. (1992). Case management by nurses. Kansas City, MO: American Nurses Association.

Breckinridge, M. (1981). *Wide neighborhoods: A story of the Frontier Nursing Service.* Lexington: The University Press of Kentucky.

Brooten, D., Kumar, S., Brown, L. P., Butts, P., Finkler, S. A., Bakewell-Sachs, S., Gibbons, A., et al. (1986). A randomized clinical trial of early hospital discharge and home follow-up of very-low-birth-weight infants. *New England Journal of Medicine, 315,* 934-939.

Brown, E. L. (1948). *Nursing for the future.* New York: Russell Sage Foundation.

Buck, D. F. (1940). The nurses on horseback ride on. *American Journal of Nursing, 40,* 993-995.

Buhler-Wilkerson, K. (2001). *No place like home: A history of nursing and home care in the United States.* Baltimore: The Johns Hopkins University Press.

Bullough, B. (1984). The current phase of the development of nurse practice acts. *St. Louis Law Journal, 28,* 365-395.

Calkin, J. D. (1984). A model for advanced nursing practice. *Journal of Nursing Administration, 14,* 24-30.

Chalmers-Frances v. Nelson, 6 Cal.2d 402 (1936).

Christman, L. (1998). Advanced practice nursing: Is the physician's assistant an accident of history or a failure to act? *Nursing Outlook, 46,* 56-59.

Clancy, G. T., & Maguire, D. (1995). Advanced practice nursing in the neonatal intensive care unit. *Critical Care Nursing Clinics of North America, 7,* 71-76.

Connors, H. (1993). Impact of care management modalities on curricula. In K. Kelly & M. Maas (Eds.), *Managing nursing care: Promise and pitfalls* (pp. 190-207). St. Louis, MO: Mosby.

Conti, R. M. (1996). Nurse case manager roles: Implications for practice and education. *Nursing Administration Quarterly, 21,* 67-80.

Critchley, D. L. (1985). Evolution of the role. In D. L. Critchley & J. T. Maurin (Eds.), *The clinical specialist in psychiatric mental health nursing* (pp. 5-22). New York: John Wiley & Sons.

Cronenwett, L. R. (1995). Modeling the future of advanced practice nursing. *Nursing Outlook, 43,* 112-118.

Cronin, C. J., & Maklebust, J. (1989). Case-managed care: Capitalizing on the CNS. *Nursing Management, 20,* 38-47.

Daly, B. (1997). *The acute care nurse practitioner.* New York: Springer.

Daly, B. (2002). ACNP 2002: "Where we've been and where we're going." Original manuscript, keynote address presented at the April 2002 ACNP Consensus Conference, Charlottesville, VA. The Keeling Collection, Center for Nursing Historical Inquiry, UVA.

D'Antonio, P. (1991). Staff needs and patient care: Seclusion and restraint in a nineteenth-century insane asylum. *Transactions and Studies of the College of Physicians of Philadelphia 13*(4), 411-423.

Dewitt, K. (1900). Specialties in nursing. *American Journal of Nursing, 1,* 14-17.

Diers, D. (1991). Nurse-midwives and nurse anesthetists: The cutting edge in specialist practice. In L. H. Aiken & C. M. Fagin (Eds.), *Charting nursing's future: Agenda for the 1990s* (pp. 159-180). New York: J. B. Lippincott.

Dock, L. & Stewart, I. (1920). *A short history of nursing.* New York: Putnam.

Donahue, P. M. (1996). *Nursing, the finest art: An illustrated history.* 2nd ed. St. Louis, MO: Mosby.

Doyle, E., & Meurer, J. (1983). Missouri legislation and litigation: Practicing medicine without a license. *Nurse Practitioner, 8,* 41-44.

Drug Enforcement Agency. (1991). *Definition and exemption of affiliated practitioners,* 56 Fed. Reg. 4181.

Duffus, R. L. (1938). *Lillian Wald: Neighbor and crusader.* New York: The Macmillan Company.

Fairman, J. (1992). Watchful vigilance: Nursing care, technology, and the development of intensive care units. *Nursing Research, 41,* 56-60.

Fairman, J. (2001). Delegated by default or negotiated by need?: Physicians, nurse practitioners, and the process of clinical thinking. In E. Baer, P. D'Antonio, S. Rinker, & J. Lynaugh (Eds.), *Enduring issues in American nursing* (pp. 309-333). New York: Springer.

Fairman, J. (2002). The roots of collaborative practice: Nurse practitioner pioneers' stories. *Nursing History Review, 10,* 159-174.

Fairman, J., & Lynaugh, J.(1998). *Critical care nursing: A history.* Philadelphia: University of Pennsylvania.

Faut-Callahan, M., & Kremer, M. (1996). The certified registered nurse anesthetist. In A. B. Hamric, J. A. Spross, & C. M. Hanson (Eds.), *Advanced nursing practice: An integrative approach* (pp. 421-444). Philadelphia: W. B. Saunders.

Flexner, A. (1910). *Medical Education in the United States and Canada.* New York: Carnegie Foundation.

Ford, L. C. (1970). A nurse for all settings: The nurse practitioner. *Nursing Outlook, 27,* 516-521.

Ford, L. C. (1982). Nurse practitioners: History of a new idea and predictions for the future. In L. H. Aiken (Ed.), *Nursing in the 80s* (pp. 231-248). Philadelphia: J. B. Lippincott.

Ford, L. C. (1991). Advanced nursing practice: Future of the nurse practitioner. In L. H. Aiken & C. M. Fagin (Eds.), *Charting nursing's future: Agenda for the 1990s* (pp. 287-299). New York: J. B. Lippincott.

Ford, L. C., & Silver, H. K. (1967). The expanded role of the nurse in child care. *Nursing Outlook, 15,* 43-45.

Fox, P. D. (1997). An overview of managed care. In P. R. Kongstvedt (Ed.), *Essentials of managed health care* (pp. 3-16). Gaithersburg, MD: Aspen.

Fralic, M. (1992). The nurse case manager: Focus, selection, preparation, and measurement. *Journal of Nursing Administration, 22,* 13-14, 46.

Frank et al. v. South et al., 175 KY. 416-428 (1917).

Friereich, E. (1984). Landmark perspective: Nitrogen mustard therapy. *Journal of the American Medical Association. 251,* 2262-2263.

Frontier Nursing Service. (1948). *Medical routines.* Lexington, KY: University of Kentucky, Frontier Nursing Service Collection.

Fulton, J. S. (2002). Defining our practice [Editorial]. *Clinical Nurse Specialist, 16,* 167-168.

Georgopoulos, B. S., & Christman, L. (1970). The clinical nurse specialist: A role model. *American Journal of Nursing, 70,* 1030-1039.

Georgopoulos, B. S., & Jackson, M. M. (1970). Nursing Kardex behavior in an experimental study of patient units with and without clinical specialists. *Nursing Research, 19,* 196-218.

Georgopoulos, B. S., & Sana, M. (1971). Clinical nursing specialization and intershift report behavior. *American Journal of Nursing, 71,* 538-545.

Gerber, L. S. (1994). Case management models. *Journal of Gerontological Nursing, 20,* 18-24.

Girouard, S. (1978). The role of the clinical nurse specialist as change agent: An experiment in preoperative teaching. *International Journal of Nursing Studies, 15,* 57-65.

Goldmark, J. (1923). *Nursing and nursing education in the United States.* Report of the Committee for the Study of Nursing Education. New York: Garland.

Grey, M. (1999). *New Deal medicine: The rural health programs of the Farm Security Administration.* Baltimore: Johns Hopkins University.

Hadley, E. (1989). Nurses and prescriptive authority: A legal and economic analysis. *American Journal of Law and Medicine, 15,* (213): 245-299.

Hamric, A., Lindbak, S., Jaubert, S., & Worley, D. (1998). Outcomes associated with advanced nursing practice prescriptive authority. *Journal of the American Academy of Nurse Practitioners, 10,* 113-118.

Hamric, A. B. (1989). History and overview of the CNS role. In A. B. Hamric & J. A. Spross (Eds.), *The clinical nurse specialist in theory and practice* (2nd ed., pp. 3-18). Philadelphia: W. B. Saunders.

Hamric, A. B. (1992). Creating our future: Challenges and opportunities for the clinical nurse specialist. *Oncology Nursing Forum, 19*(Suppl. 1), 11-15.

Hamric, A. B., & Spross, J. (Eds.). (1983). *The clinical nurse specialist in theory and practice.* New York: Grune & Stratton.

Hamric, A. B., & Spross, J. A. (Eds.). (1989). *The clinical nurse specialist in theory and practice* (2nd ed.). Philadelphia: W. B. Saunders.

Howell, J. (1996). *Technology in the hospital.* Baltimore: Johns Hopkins University Press.

Hunt, V. E. (1925).With Henry St. Nurses. *American Journal of Nursing, 25,* 136-137.

Idaho Code 54-1413 (1971).

Inglis, A. D., & Kjervik, D.K. (1993). Empowerment of advanced practice nurses: Regulation reform needed to increase access to care. *Journal of Law, Medicine and Ethics, 21*(2), 193-205.

Jenicek, J. (1967). Vietnam—new challenges for the army nurse anesthetist. *Journal of the American Association of Nurse Anesthetists, 67,* 347-352.

Jolly, E. (1927). *Nuns of the battlefield.* Providence, RI: The Providence Visitor Press.

Kalisch, P. A., & Kalisch, B. J. (1986). *The advance of American nursing.* (2nd ed.). Boston: Little, Brown and Company.

Keane, A. & Richmond, T. (1993). Tertiary nurse practitioners. *Image: Journal of Nursing Scholarship, 25,* 281-284.

Keeling, A. (2001). Professional nursing comes of age: 1859-2000. In K. Chitty (Ed.), *Professional nursing: Concepts and challenges* (3rd ed., pp. 1-32). St Louis, MO: Mosby.

Keeling, A. (2004). Blurring the boundaries between medicine and nursing: Coronary care nursing, circa the 1960s. *Nursing History Review, 12,* 139-164.

Kersbergen, A. L. (1996). Case management: A rich history of coordinating care to control costs. *Nursing Outlook, 44,* 169-172.

Kitzman, H. J. (1983). The CNS and the nurse practitioner. In A. B. Hamric & J. A. Spross (Eds.), *The clinical nurse specialist in theory and practice* (pp. 275-290). New York: Grune & Stratton.

Kleinpell, R. M. (1997). Acute care nurse practitioners: Roles and practice profiles. *AACN Clinical Issues, 8,* 156-162.

Linda Richards. (1900). *American Journal of Nursing, 1,* 11-13.

Little, D. E., & Carnevali, D. (1967). Nurse specialist effect on tuberculosis. *Nursing Research, 16,* 321-326.

Lynaugh, J. E., & Brush, B. L. (1996). *American nursing: From hospitals to health systems.* Cambridge, MA: Milbank Memorial Fund and Blackwell Publishers.

Lynaugh, J. E., & Fairman, J. (1992). New nurses, new spaces: A preview of the AACN history study. *American Journal of Critical Nursing, 1*(1), 19-24

Magaw, A. (1900, May). Observations on 1092 cases of anesthesia from January 1, 1899 to January 1, 1900.*St. Paul's Medical Journal,* 306-311.

Mahn, V. A., & Spross, J. A. (1996). Nurse case management as an advanced practice role. In A. B. Hamric, J. A. Spross, & C. M. Hanson (Eds.), *Advanced nursing practice: An integrative approach* (pp. 445-465). Philadelphia: W. B. Saunders.

McBride, A. B., Austin, J. K., Chestnut, E. E., Main, C. S., Richards, B. S., & Roy, B. A. (1987). Evaluation of the impact of the clinical nurse specialist in a state psychiatric hospital. *Archives of Psychiatric Nursing, 1,* 55-61.

Mitchell-DiCenso, A., Guyatt, G., Marrin, M., Goeree, R., Willan, A., Southwell, D., et al. (1996). A controlled trial of nurse practitioners in neonatal intensive care. *Pediatrics, 98,* 1143-1148.

Moxley, J. (1968). The predicament in health manpower. *American Journal of Nursing, 68,* 1489-1492.

Murphy-Ende, K. (2002). Advanced practice nursing: Reflections on the past, issue for the future. *Oncology Nursing Forum, 29,* 106-112.

National League for Nursing. (1984). *Master's education in nursing: Route to opportunities in contemporary nursing, 1984-1985.* New York: Author.

National League for Nursing. (1994). *Graduate Education in Nursing, Advanced Practice Nursing.* New York: Author.

National Organization of Nurse Practitioner Faculties. (1997). *Criteria for evaluation of nurse practitioner programs.* Washington, DC: National Task Force on Quality Nurse Practitioner Education.

Negro nurse-midwives.(1942). *American Journal of Nursing, 42,* 705.

News about nursing: Nursing and national defense: Nurse anesthetists in the Army Nurse Corps. (1942). *American Journal of Nursing, 42,* 451.

News here and there: American Association of Nurse-Midwives.(1942). *American Journal of Nursing, 42,* 832.

Office of Technology Assessment. (1986). *Nurse practitioners, physicians assistants and certified nurse-*

midwives: A policy analysis. Washington DC: US Congress, HCS 37. Washington, DC: Author.

Olsen, G. W. (1940). The nurse anesthetists: Past, present and future. *Bulletin of the American Association of Nurse Anesthetists, 8,* 296-299.

Oltz v. St. Peter's Community Hospital, CV 81-271-H-Res (D. Mont. 1986).

Oncology Nursing Society (1994). *ONS online.* Retrieved February 13, 2004, from http://www.ons.org/xp6/ONS

Peplau, H. E. (1952). *Interpersonal relations in nursing, a conceptual frame of reference for psychodynamic nursing.* New York: Putnam.

Peplau, H. E. (1965). Specialization in professional nursing. *Nursing Science, 3,* 268-287.

Pinneo, R. (1967, February). A new dimension in nursing: Intensive coronary care. Reprint, *American Association of Industrial Nurses Journal.* The Pinneo Collection, Center for Nursing Historical Inquiry, University of Virginia.

Reiter, F. (1966). The nurse-clinician. *American Journal of Nursing, 66,* 274-280.

Reverby, S. M. (1987). *Ordered to care: The dilemma of American nursing, 1850-1945.* New York: Cambridge University Press.

Richards, L. (1911). *Reminiscences of America's first trained nurse.* (Reprint.) Boston: Whitcomb and Barrows.

Rinker, S. (2000). To cultivate a feeling of confidence: The nursing of obstetric patients, 1890-1940. *Nursing History Review, 8,* 117-142.

Rogers, M. E. (1972). Nursing: To be or not to be. *Nursing Outlook, 20,* 42-46.

Rooks, J. (1997). *Midwifery and childbirth in America.* Philadelphia: Temple University Press.

Safriet, B. J. (1992). Health care dollars and regulatory sense: The role of advance practice nursing. *Yale Journal on Regulation, 9,* 417-488.

Safriet, B. J. (1998). Still spending dollars, still searching for sense: Advanced practice nursing in an era of regulatory and economic turmoil. *Advanced Practice Nursing Quarterly, 4,* 24-33.

Schindler, F. (1942). Nursing in electro-shock therapy. *American Journal of Nursing, 42,* 858-861.

Schroer, K. (1991). Case management: Clinical nurse specialist and nurse practitioner, converging roles. *Clinical Nurse Specialist, 5,* 190-194.

Schutt, B. (1971). A prophet honored. *American Journal of Nursing, 71*(1), 53.

Sermchief v. Gonzales, 660 S.W.2d 683 (1983).

Shah, H., Brutlomesso, K., Sullivan, D., & Lattanzio, J. (1997). An evaluation of the role and practices of the acute care nurse practitioner. *AACN Clinical Issues, 8,* 147-155.

Shakespeare, W. (2002). The Tempest. In S. Orgel & A. R. Braunmuller (Eds.), *William Shakespeare 1564-1616: The complete works* (2.1.245-253). New York: Penguin.

Sills, G. M. (1983). The role, function of the clinical nurse specialist. In N.L. Chaska (Ed.), *The nursing profession: A time to speak* (pp. 563-579). New York: McGraw-Hill.

Smith, S. (1994).White nurses, black midwives, and public health in Mississippi, 1920-1950. *Nursing History Review, 2,* 29-49.

Spalding, E. (1943). The Bolton Act provides federal funds for postgraduate programs. *American Journal of Nursing, 43,* 833.

Sparacino, P. (1990). A historical perspective on the development of the CNS role. In P. Sparacino, D. M. Cooper, & P. A. Minarik (Eds.), *The CNS: Implementation and impact* (Chapter 1, pp. 3-10), Norwalk, CT: Appleton and Lange.

Spross, J., & Hamric, A. B. (1983). A model for future clinical specialist practice. In Hamric, A. B., & Spross, J. (Eds.), *The clinical nurse specialist in theory and practice* (pp. 291-306). New York: Grune & Stratton.

Summers, V. (1938). Saddle bag and log cabin technic. *The American Journal of Nursing, 38,* 1183-1189.

Tahan, H. A. (1998). Case management: A heritage more than a century old. *Nursing Case Management, 3,* 55-60.

Thatcher, V. S. (1953). *A history of anesthesia: With emphasis on the nurse specialist.* Philadelphia: J. B. Lippincott.

Trinidad, E. A. (1993). Case management: A model of CNS practice. *Clinical Nurse Specialist, 7,* 221-223.

U.S. Department of Health, Education, & Welfare Secretary's Committee to Study Extended Roles for Nurses. (1972). *Extending the scope of nursing practice: A report of the Secretary's Committee* (pp. 3-6). Washington, DC: U.S. Government Printing Office.

U.S. Department of Health and Human Services. (1996). The registered nurse population March 1996: Findings from the National Sample Survey of Registered Nurses. Washington, DC: Author.

U.S. Federal Security Agency. (1950). *Cadet Nurse Corps and other federal nurse training programs.* Washington, DC: U.S. Government Printing Office.

Varney, H. (1987). *Nurse-midwifery* (2nd ed.). Boston: Blackwell Scientific.

Wagner, J. D., & Menke, E. M. (1992). Case management of homeless families. *Clinical Nurse Specialist, 6,* 65-71.

Waisel, D. (2001). The role of World War II and the European theater of operations in the development of anesthesiology as a physician specialty in the USA. *Anesthesiology, 94,* 907-912.

Wald, L. (1922). The origin and development of Henry Street Settlement. *Text for Broadcasting, The Westinghouse Electric and Manufacturing Co.,* Reel #25, *Lillian Wald Papers,* New York Public Library.

White, R. (1943). Army nurses—in the air! *American Journal of Nursing, 43,* 344.

Wolff, M. A. (1984). Court upholds expanded practice roles for nurses. *Law, Medicine and Health Care, 12,* 26-29.

Wolff, M. A. (1984, February). Court upholds expanded practice roles for nurses. *Law, Medicine and Health Care,* 26-29.

Woodrow, M., & Bell, J. (1971). Clinical specialization: Conflict between reality and theory. *Journal of Nursing Administration, 1,* 23-27.

Zander, K. (1988). Nurse case management: Resolving the DRG paradox. *Nursing Clinics of North America, 23,* 503-520.

CHAPTER 2

Conceptualizations of Advanced Practice Nursing

JUDITH A. SPROSS • MARJORIE THOMAS LAWSON

INTRODUCTION

Fundamental to the sound progress of any practice field is the development of a common language and conceptual framework for communication and for guiding and evaluating practice, education, policy, research, and theory. Although such a foundation is particularly crucial at this stage in the development of advanced practice nursing, a professional consensus on the nature of advanced practice nursing has not been reached. Through a literature review, several types of articles related to model development and advanced practice nursing were identified. These models could be characterized as:

- Curriculum models (e.g., Atkins & Ersser, 2000; Curran & Roberts, 2002; Woods, 1997; Plager, Conger, & Craig, 2003; Williams & Kelly, 1998; Williams et al., 1998)
- Administrative or organizational models (e.g., Whitcomb et al., 2002; Gibbins, Green, Scott, & Watson MacDonell, 2000; Valentine, Antai-Otong, Kupecz, Lynn, & Chaffee, 2000)
- Models that differentiate among advanced practice roles (e.g., Williams & Valdivieso, 1994; Lincoln, 2000)
- Models that differentiate between basic and advanced practice nursing (e.g., Calkin, 1984; Oberle & Allen, 2001)
- Models of the nature of advanced practice nursing (Brown, 1998; Hamric, 1996, 2000, and see Chapter 3)
- Models of role development of advanced practice nurses (APNs) (e.g., Brown & Olshansky, 1997 and see Chapter 5)
- Models that APNs would find useful (e.g., Curley, 1998; Mitchell, Ferketich, & Jennings, 1998; Sidani & Irvine, 1998; Thibodeau & Haukins, 1994)
- Others (e.g., Raudonis & Anderson, 2002, on specialty certification; Styles, 1998, on advanced practice credentialing)

In addition, professional organizations with interests in defining, educating, and accrediting APNs can be viewed as operating from some conceptualization of advanced practice nursing, whether implicit or explicit.

The purpose of this chapter is to lay the foundation for thinking about the concepts underlying advanced practice nursing and to outline future directions and recommendations that may foster a professional consensus on advanced practice nursing. Using published documents from national professional organizations and the literature, the authors focus selectively on the following types of models of APN practice: those promulgated by professional organizations and ones that address a specific APN role; those that aim to explicate the nature of advanced practice nursing; and conceptualizations that are useful for APNs seeking to demonstrate the value-added, distinct character of advanced practice nursing. This review is not exhaustive. For example, in limiting the scope of this chapter, statements on advanced practice nursing by specialty organizations and conceptualizations of advanced practice nursing proposed by authors writing about advanced practice in foreign countries have not been examined—issues we address in the discussion of recommendations and future directions. We invite readers to debate and enlarge upon the models, issues, and thinking put forward in this chapter.

The authors and editors express their gratitude to Margretta Styles and Carolyn Lewis, authors of this chapter in the first and second editions, for their keen insights and clarity of thinking about advanced practice nursing. We also acknowledge Ann Hamric and Charlene Hanson for their contributions in revising the chapter.

THE NATURE, PURPOSES, AND COMPONENTS OF CONCEPTUAL MODELS

What is a conceptual model? What purposes does it serve? What are its components? There are a number of answers to these questions in the nursing literature. Fawcett (2000, 2001) identified a conceptual model as "a set of relatively abstract and general concepts that address the phenomena of central interest to a discipline, the propositions that broadly describe these concepts, and the propositions that state relatively abstract and general relations between two or more of the concepts" (2001, p. 380). In describing nurse-midwifery, Carveth (1987) drew heavily from various expert sources to arrive at a clear, comprehensive, and general explanation of a conceptual model, paraphrased as follows:

A conceptual model is that which orders, clarifies, and systematizes selected components of the phenomenon (e.g., nursing) it serves to depict. The components of conceptual models are concepts and relationships (i.e., concepts in meaningful configuration) serving as building blocks that reflect assumptions about the philosophy, values, and practices of a profession. The model then becomes a tool for interrelating concepts in a way in which the concepts can be better understood and explained.

Conceptual models serve many purposes. Models may help APNs articulate *professional role identity* and *function*, serving as a framework for organizing their beliefs and knowledge about their professional roles and practice, and providing a sound base for further development of knowledge. The Strong Memorial Model, discussed later in the chapter, is such a model. In *clinical practice*, APNs use conceptual models to understand the bigger picture so that holistic, comprehensive care is provided. For example, the authors of Chapter 18 provide an exemplar of an APN case manager who used the concepts from the theory of self-efficacy to assess and intervene with a complex patient. Models may also be used to differentiate among levels of nursing practice (e.g., staff nursing and advanced pratice [as discussed later in Calkin's model]). In research and other scholarly activities, investigators use conceptual models to guide the *conceptualization of research* and *theory development*. An investigator could decide to focus on the study of one concept or examine relationships among selected concepts to elucidate testable theories. For example, research by Fenton (1985) and Brykczynski (1989), described later in this chapter, elucidated new domains of practice for clinical nurse specialists (CNSs) and nurse practitioners (NPs), respectively. In education, faculty use conceptual models to *plan curricula*, identify important concepts and the relationships among them, and make choices about course content and clinical experiences, based on such models. For example, Plager, Conger, and Craig (2003) developed a model that helped their faculty differentiate among APN roles and informed the design of the curricula for NPs and CNSs. Despite the utility and benefits of conceptual models, some difficulties are apparent when the advanced practice nursing literature is examined.

CONCEPTUALIZATIONS OF ADVANCED PRACTICE NURSING: PROBLEMS AND IMPERATIVES

As one reviews the literature, it is clear that there are problems with conceptualizations of advanced practice nursing. In addition, when one examines the clinical and professional issues inherent in advanced practice nursing, imperatives for clarifying advanced practice and arriving at a professional consensus on what it is and what it is not are apparent. Three areas of conceptual confusion or uncertainty in the evolution of advanced practice nursing can be identified.

The first issue is that there is an absence of well-defined and consistently applied terms of reference. A core, stable vocabulary, a *lingua franca*, is needed for definition and model building. The lack of a consistent, stable vocabulary can be seen in the literature. For example, the basic elements or building blocks of conceptual models of advanced practice nursing literature are variously labeled *domains*, *theories*, *roles*, *subroles*, *hallmarks*, *competencies*, *functions*, *activities*, *skills*, and *abilities*. The problem in comparing, refining, or developing models is that these terms are used with no universal meaning or frame of reference; occasionally, no definition is offered at all, or the meaning seems uncertain or inconsistent. Shuler and Davis (1993a), in introducing their nurse practitioner (NP) model, stated that "one of the greatest barriers to using nursing models in practice relates to vocabulary and communication within the models" (p. 11). This instability and inconsistency are evident in the various models cited in this chapter. It is rightly anticipated that conceptual models of the field and its practice change over time. However, the evolution of advanced practice nursing and its comprehension by nurses, policymakers, and others would be enhanced if scholars and practitioners in the field could agree on the use and definition of fundamental terms of reference.

The second issue is that many attempts to articulate models of advanced practice nursing fail to consider extant literature that is directly relevant to such conceptualizing activities. In part, this seems to be due to a lag between the conceptualizing effort and its ultimate publication, as well as the knowledge explosion. For example, some articles reviewed for this chapter with publication dates of 2001 and 2002 cited work from the 1990s; revised publications, though apparently available, were not cited. We note this as a caution to be considered in proposing, evaluating, or refining advanced practice nursing models.

The third issue is a lack of clarity regarding conceptualizations that differentiate between and among levels of clinical practice. There is much to understand about how advanced practice nursing is different from that of experienced nurses and how specialty nursing practiced by APNs is different from that of experienced, non-master's-prepared nurses (Harson & Hamric, 2003). For example, many authors who write about advanced practice nursing cite Benner's model of expert practice (1984) without clearly indicating that the model was derived from the study of nurses who were experts by experience, not APNs. Certainly, Benner's model is relevant to efforts to conceptualize advanced practice nursing as Fenton 's (1985) and Brykczynski's (1989) work, reviewed later in this chapter, demonstrates. Given that clinical practice is the raison d'être for the profession of nursing and is central to advanced practice nursing, models that help the profession differentiate levels of practice are needed.

In addition to these problems, imperatives for reaching a conceptual consensus can be identified in three broad, interrelated areas: policymaking, licensing and credentialing, and in practice. In the policymaking arena, for example, not all APNs are eligible to be reimbursed by insurers, and even those activities that are reimbursable are often billed incident to a physician's care, rendering the work of APNs invisible. Further evidence of the need for consensus is the National Council of State Boards of Nursing (NCSBN)'s proposal for a uniform licensing compact that would standardize criteria for advanced practice nursing licensing (NCSBN, 2002). In practice, little is understood about the impact of APN-physician collaboration on practice or strategies for matching the level of nursing knowledge and skill to the needs of patient populations. These are examples of many professional imperatives for reaching a consensus on the nature and definition of advanced practice nursing. As outlined in Chapters 22 and 23, the profession is at a critical juncture in terms of policymaking: policies are being created today that will have far-reaching effects. Indeed these policies will shape every aspect of APN practice— APN education, APN regulation and credentialing, scopes of APN practice, the populations with whom, and the environments in which, APNs work, compensation for APN activities, and research priorities. To fully appreciate the interrelationships between conceptualizations of advanced practice nursing their effects on APN practice, the reader is encouraged to refer back to Chapter 2 when reading Chapters 12 through 19 in Part III and Chapters 22 and 23 in Part IV.

Some conceptual models, as reviewed in this chapter, are more narrowly focused than others. Some advanced practice models are more homogeneous and some are mixed with respect to the phenomenon studied. Some could be seen as micromodels in terms of the unit of analysis, and others could be seen as meta-models, incorporating a number of conceptual frameworks. Some models explain systems; others explain relationships between systems. All these foci are important, depending on the purposes to be served. However, in the development of conceptual models, the phenomenon to be modeled must be carefully defined. For example, is the model intended to encompass the entire field of advanced practice nursing, or is it confined to distinctive concepts such as collaborative practice between physicians and nurses? When the phenomenon and its related concepts are not clearly delimited, there is the possibility of the model being so inconsistent or mixed or far-reaching as to be confusing or to dilute or lose the impact of the contribution.

As previously stated, assumptions about the philosophy, values, and practices of the profession are reflected in conceptual models. The present discussion of conceptualizations of advanced practice nursing is guided by two assumptions. The first is that the development and strengthening of the field of advanced practice nursing depends on a professional consensus regarding the nature of advanced practice nursing. The second is that advanced practice nursing will reach its full potential to the extent that identified conceptual components are appropriately addressed. Clarification and consensus on conceptualization of the nature of advanced practice nursing will lead to the following *outcomes*:

1. Clear differentiation of advanced practice nursing from other levels of clinical nursing practice
2. Clear differentiation between advanced practice nursing and the clinical practice of other nonnurse providers within a specialty
3. Clear delineation of the similarities and differences among APN roles
4. APN regulation and credentialing that protects the public and ensures equitable treatment of all APNs
5. A maximum social contribution by APNs in health care, including improvement in health outcomes and health-related quality of life
6. The actualization of practitioners of advanced practice nursing

CONCEPTUALIZATIONS OF ADVANCED PRACTICE NURSING

Practice is the central, the clinical work of the field. Practice is the reason for which nursing was created. What are the characteristics of advanced practice nursing? How does it differ from other types of nursing practice, particularly the clinical practice of nurses who are not master's prepared, who are experts by experience and who are often certified in a specialty? What is the scope and purpose of advanced practice nursing? How do APNs' scopes of practice differ from those of other providers offering similar or related services? What knowledge and skills are required? Within what settings does this practice occur? When has a specialty evolved to the point that society needs APNs in a new field? When should health-care systems employ APNs and what types of patients particularly benefit from advanced practice nursing care? For what types of pressing health-care problems are APNs a solution in terms of outcomes, quality of care, and cost-effectiveness?

These and other questions have encouraged scores of writers to describe advanced practice nursing from a variety of perspectives. Specialty organizations, such as the Oncology Nursing Society and the American Association of Critical-Care Nurses have addressed advanced practice nursing. These models and standards are important to students and APNs but are not addressed in this chapter. As students and readers consider their own APN practices, they may want to review both the history of advanced practice nursing (Chapter 1) and evolving advanced practice nursing roles (Chapter 19) to inform their efforts to conceptualize their own practice of advanced nursing.

In the next section, we examine the implicit and explicit conceptualizations of advanced practice nursing promulgated by professional organizations concerned with defining APN practice and with clarifying particular APN roles.

Professional Organizations' Conceptualizations

Although not all of the documents described in this chapter are conceptual models, many include a conceptual framework or reference a conceptual framework. Some of the problems with the absence of a core vocabulary noted previously are apparent as one reads the different approaches taken by organizations, so comparisons are difficult to make because terms of reference and their meanings vary. To help the reader appreciate the challenge of developing a common language to characterize advanced practice, dictionary definitions of terms used in conceptualizations of advanced practice nursing are found in Box 2-1. In spite of differences in terminology, the efforts of the profession to come to grips with a definition of advanced practice nursing are evident in all of these documents. Reflection on and discussion of the various terms used and debate about interpreting them—for example, roles, domains, and competencies—may contribute to clarification of conceptual models and the emergence of a common language. The descriptions of each model in the following sections are necessarily limited. The reader is encouraged to refer to the original documents and publications to more fully understand advanced practice nursing as described by organizations and individual authors. Website addresses for national APN organizations are found in Chapter 22.

BOX 2-1 • DEFINITION OF TERMS

Competent—having requisite or adequate ability or qualities; legally qualified or adequate; having the capacity to function or develop in a particular way; (sufficient)

Competence/Competency—the quality or state of being competent; the knowledge that enables a person to speak and understand a language

Component—a constituent part; ingredient

Domain—a sphere of knowledge, influence or activity

Role—a socially expected behavior pattern usually determined by an individual's status in a particular society

Hallmark—distinguishing characteristic, trait or feature

Sphere—an area or range over or within which someone or something acts, exists, or has influence or significance

Scope—space or opportunity for unhampered motion, activity or thought; extent of treatment, activity, or influence

Standard—something established by authority, custom, or general consent as a model or example; something set up and established by an authority as a rule for the measure of quantity, weight, extent, value or quality

---

From Mish, F.C. (Ed.) (2001). *Merriam-Webster's collegiate dictionary* (10th ed.). Springfield, MA: Merriam-Webster, International.

AMERICAN NURSES ASSOCIATION

In 1995 the American Nurses Association (ANA) published a revision of *Nursing's Social Policy Statement* (ANA, 1980; 1995); the statement included concepts that differentiated advanced practice nursing from basic nursing practice: specialization, expansion, and advancement. In a more recent edition of this statement, the ANA (2003) recognized certified nurse-midwives (CNMs), CNSs, certified registered nurse anesthetists (CRNAs), and NPs as APNs and noted that APNs use both expanded and specialized knowledge and skills in their practices, defining expansion and specialization as follows:

Expansion refers to the acquisition of new practice knowledge and skills, including the knowledge and skills that legitimize role autonomy within areas of practice that may overlap traditional boundaries of medical practice.

Specialization is concentrating or delimiting one's focus to part of the whole field of nursing (such as ambulatory care, pediatric, maternal-child, psychiatric, palliative care, or oncology nursing).

Advanced practice is characterized by the integration of a broad range of theoretical, research-based, and practical knowledge that occurs as part of graduate education. Advanced practice registered nurses are either certified or approved to practice in their expanded, specialized roles. (p. 9)

AMERICAN ASSOCIATION OF COLLEGES OF NURSING

In 1994 the American Association of Colleges of Nursing (AACN) convened a task force to define the essential elements for master's level advanced practice nursing education. A series of regional meetings provided a national forum that led to the development of a consensus-based document. The *Essentials of Master's Education for Advanced Practice Nursing* (AACN, 1996) defined content that should be part of master's level education for all APNs. The organization described a master's level curriculum that has three components: a graduate nursing core, an advanced practice nursing core, and specialty nursing content.

The graduate nursing core includes content for all graduate nursing programs whether in advanced practice, administration, or education (e.g., ethics and theory courses). The advanced practice nursing core includes advanced health/physical assessment, advanced physiology and pathophysiology, and advanced pharmacology. Specialty curricula include content and clinical practica that help students acquire the knowledge and skills essential to a specific advanced practice role.

While not a conceptual model per se, the AACN *Essentials* document addresses concepts and content that are evident in the educational components of the majority of other advanced practice nursing documents that address scopes of practice and education. A recent initiative of AACN, "The Clinical Nurse Leader, Developing a New Nurse," proposes a new clinical nursing role that will require postbaccalaureate education and a new scope of practice (AACN, 2002). How this proposed new role is similar to or different from such APN roles as CNS and APN case manager has not been articulated. Initiatives such as these point to the urgency of conceptualizing advanced practice nursing so that new clinical nursing roles can be adequately distinguished from advanced practice at the bedside, in the boardroom, and in policy arenas.

NATIONAL ORGANIZATION OF NURSE PRACTITIONER FACULTIES

The mission of the National Organization of Nurse Practitioner Faculties (NONPF) is to provide leadership in promoting quality NP education. In 1990 (Price et al., 1992; Zimmer, Brykczynski, Martin, et al., 1990), NONPF published a set of domains and core competencies for nurse practitioners (NPs) based on Benner's (1984) domains of expert nursing practice and the results of Brykczynski's study (1989) of the use of these domains by primary care NPs. These domains and core competencies were intended to serve as a framework for primary care NP curricula. Subsequent work done to validate the NP domains and competencies resulted in revisions, the most recent of which was published in 2002 (NONPF, 2002). In addition, domains and competencies for psychiatric mental health nurse practitioners (PMHNP) have been published—a collaborative effort of "six national organizations whose foci include advanced practice nursing education, psychiatric-mental health practice, and certification for the PMHNP" (NONPF, 2003, p. 1). Each competency within the domains is further described by a list of learning objectives students are expected to meet. The domains used in each of the documents are as follows:

1. Management of patient health/illness status
2. The nurse practitioner-patient relationship
3. The teaching-coaching function
4. Professional role (includes leadership)
5. Managing and negotiating health-care delivery systems
6. Monitoring and ensuring the quality of health-care practice
7. Cultural competence

These domains can be considered an implicit conceptual model, derived from the practice of NPs and empirically validated (NONPF, 2002, 2003). The model is intended to inform curriculum design and regulatory and credentialing mechanisms. These two documents are notable for several reasons: the domains and competencies for NPs were developed collaboratively by stakeholder organizations; a similar collaborative process was used by the group that developed domains and competencies for PMHNPs; and empirical validation has been used to affirm the domains and competencies for each of the two APN roles.

NATIONAL ASSOCIATION OF CLINICAL NURSE SPECIALISTS

The National Association of Clinical Nurse Specialists (NACNS) published a *Statement on Clinical Nurse Specialist Practice and Education* in 1998 and revised it in 2004. While acknowledging the early conceptualization of CNS practice as subroles proposed by Hamric and Spross (1983, 1989), the authors of the NACNS statement believed that this conceptualization failed to differentiate CNS practice from that of other APNs and proposed a new statement to resolve the ambiguity about this particular APN role. Three spheres of influence are posited: patient, nurses and nursing practice, and organization/system, each of which requires a unique set of competencies (NACNS, 2004) (Figure 2-1). In addition, the statement outlines expected outcomes of CNS practice for each sphere. For each sphere, competencies that parallel the nursing process are identified. Thus for each sphere, CNSs have sphere-specific competencies of assessment, diagnosis, intervention, and evaluation. Previous descriptions of CNS subroles informed the delineation of CNS competencies.

Several components of conceptual models are incorporated into the NACNS statement: a definition of nursing on which the definition of a CNS is based, assumptions that inform the model, essential characteristics, description of the spheres of influence and associated competencies, and recommendations for graduate education. A key assumption, which has empirical validation, is that CNSs have an impact on patients, nursing

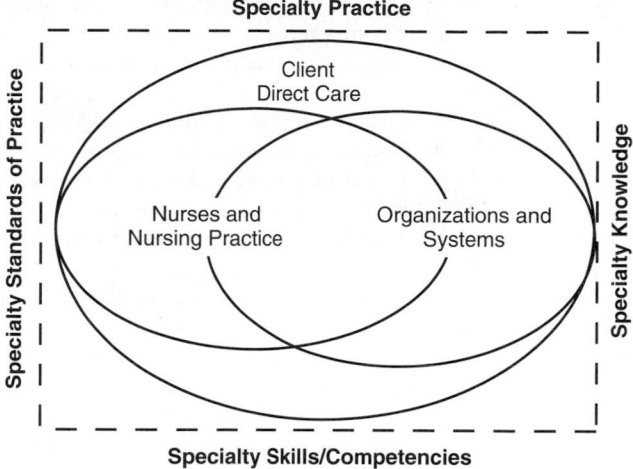

Specialty Practice

Specialty Standards of Practice

Specialty Knowledge

Client
Direct Care

Nurses and
Nursing Practice

Organizations and
Systems

Specialty Skills/Competencies

FIGURE 2-1 • National Association of Clinical Nurse Specialists Model. Clinical nurse specialist practice conceptualized as core competencies in three interacting spheres actualized in specialty practice, and guided by specialty knowledge and specialty standards. (Copyright for this figure belongs to J.S. Fulton, © 2004.)

practice, and institutional outcomes. NACNS has taken a position opposing second licensure for credentialing CNSs as advanced practice nurses (NACNS, 2004). Within the advanced practice community, this is a minority position and, as the reader can appreciate, makes it difficult to reach consensus on a uniform definition of advanced nursing practice.

AMERICAN ASSOCIATION OF NURSE ANESTHETISTS AND AMERICAN COLLEGE OF NURSE-MIDWIVES

Official statements of the American Association of Nurse Anesthetists (AANA) (1996, 2002) and the American College of Nurse Midwives (ACNM) (1997a, 2003) describe the advanced nursing practice models of certified registered nurse anesthetists (CRNA) and certified nurse-midwives (CNMs). These statements include scopes of practice, standards, and other documents that describe CRNA and CNM practices. Although the nature of advanced practice nursing is amplified and clarified by these role-specific documents, the level of conceptualization is different from that usually associated with conceptual models.

The most recent revision of the AANA's *Scope and Standards for Nurse Anesthesia Practice* was published in 2002. In this document, the CRNA's scope of practice is defined. The scope is followed by 10 items that we would characterize as clinical competencies or responsibilities (e.g., managing a patient's airway). These are followed by seven "*additional responsibilities*" (AANA, 2002) that are within the CRNA's scope of practice and which we would characterize as leadership behaviors (e.g., quality assessment). Eleven *standards* and an interpretation for each are also listed. The purposes of the standards are to: (1) provide a guide for evaluating CRNA care, (2) provide a common foundation on which CRNAs can develop a quality practice, (3) help the public understand what they can expect from CRNAs, and (4) support and preserve the basic rights of patients.

The scope of practice for CNMs (and certified midwives [CMs] who are not nurses) is defined in two ACNM documents, *The Core Competencies for Basic Midwifery Practice* (ACNM, 1997a) and *Standards for the Practice of Midwifery* (ACNM, 2003). The first document addresses basic midwifery, and ACNM notes that there is a position statement that addresses expanding midwifery practices beyond the basic core competencies (ACNM, 1997b) (see the ACNM website [www.acnm,org]). The *core competencies* include 16 *hallmarks* of the art and science of midwifery and *components* of midwifery care within which are prescribed competencies. Competencies are defined as the knowledge, skills, and attitudes expected of a new practitioner. The components of midwifery care are identified as follows:

- Professional responsibilities of CNMs and CMs
- Midwifery management process
- Fundamentals (e.g., knowledge such as anatomy and physiology)
- Primary health care of women
- The childbearing family (includes care of childbearing women and newborns)

These components and associated core competencies are said to comprise the foundation on which practice guidelines and curricula are built.

In addition to the competencies, there are eight ACNM standards with interpretive statements that midwives are expected to meet (ACNM, 2003). The standards address such issues as qualifications, safety, patient rights, assessment, documentation, and expansion of midwifery practice. It is important to note that ACNM has issued a statement that is not in support of state-mandated requirements for a master's degree to be licensed as a CNM (ACNM, 1998), a position that conflicts with the standard of graduate education for APNs promoted by most organizations.

SUMMARY/IMPLICATIONS FOR ADVANCED PRACTICE NURSING CONCEPTUALIZATIONS

In conclusion, the organizational models just described enable the reader to understand who engages in advanced practice nursing and in what capacity. Thus, these models primarily address professional role *identity* and *function, curriculum planning,* as well as *clinical practice*—some of the purposes identified on p. 49. The descriptive statements about APN roles—CNS, NP, CNM, CRNA—demonstrate that there are common elements across all APN roles. These elements include a central focus on, and accountability for, patient care; knowledge and skills specific to each APN role; and a concern for patient rights. Table 2-1 was constructed based on the content of official statements of AANA, ACNM, NACNS, and NONPF and illustrates these commonalities. Despite the existence of common elements, some organizations have taken stands that may prevent the profession from reaching a consensus on advanced practice nursing. Even so, these models provide templates against which (1) levels of practice can be distinguished; (2) educational programs can be developed and evaluated; (3) knowledge and behaviors can be measured for certification purposes; (4) practitioners can understand, examine, and improve their own practice; and (5) job descriptions can be developed.

Conceptualizations of the Nature of Advanced Practice Nursing

The APN role-specific models promulgated by professional organizations naturally lead to the following questions: What is common across APN roles? Can an overarching conceptualization of advanced practice nursing be articulated? Some authors have attempted to discern the nature of advanced practice nursing and address these questions. The extent to which they have considered all existing APN roles is not always clear: some authors have only considered the CNS and NP roles.

In this section, the focus is on those frameworks that address the nature of advanced practice nursing. The term *role* is used loosely and variably, sometimes seeming to describe

TABLE 2-1 COMPARISON OF AANA, ACNM, NACNS, AND NONPF STATEMENTS ON PRIMARY CRITERIA AND APN COMPETENCIES*

ORGANIZATION	PRIMARY CRITERIA			COMPETENCIES						
	GRADUATE EDUCATION	CERTIFICATION (IF AVAILABLE)	PRACTICE FOCUSED ON PATIENT/FAMILY	DIRECT CARE	PATIENT & FAMILY GUIDANCE/ COACHING	COLLABORATION	CONSULTATION	RESEARCH	LEADERSHIP	ETHICAL DECISION MAKING
AANA	Y	Y	Y	Y	Y	Y (implied)	Y	Y	Y	Y
ACNM	N	Y	Y	Y	Y	Y	Y	Y	Y	Y
NACNS	Y	Varies†	Y	Y	Y	Y	Y	Y	Y	Y
NONPF	Y		Y	Y	Y	Y	Y	Y	Y	Y

*Each organization's primary statements on the nature of the advanced practice role were used to complete the grid as follows:
AANA (1996, 2002)
ACNM (1997a, 2003)
NACNS (2004)†
NONPF (2002)
†Although NACNS has identified over 40 specialties, CNS certification examinations are not available for all specialties.

functions, such as management or teaching or research or consultation, and sometimes taking a psychological or sociological perspective on developing social roles or selves in relation to environment. Dictionary definitions add to the confusion by using the terms *role, function, occupation,* and *duties* to define one another. For example, *role* is usually used to refer to titles appearing in legal documents, certification programs, or job descriptions. From this perspective, the CNS, NP, CNM, and CRNA designations represent advanced practice roles. From the present review of a number of frameworks, it can be seen that *domain* and *competency* may be the most commonly used concepts in explaining nursing practice and advanced practice nursing. However, meanings are not consistent.

FENTON'S AND BRYKCZYNSKI'S EXPERT PRACTICE DOMAINS OF THE CNS AND NP: BUILDING ON BENNER'S MODEL OF EXPERT PRACTICE

In order to appreciate the contributions of Fenton (1985) and Brykczynski (1989) to the understanding of advanced practice, it is important to highlight some of Benner's key findings about nurses who are experts by experience. Although many authors have used Benner's (1984) seminal work, *From Novice to Expert,* in their conceptualizations of advanced practice nursing, it is important to note that Benner did not study advanced practice nurses; her research described nurses who were experts by experience. In using an interpretive approach to identifying and describing clinical knowledge, Benner defined two key terms as follows (pp. 292-293):

Competency: An interpretively defined area of skilled performance identified and described by its intent, function, and meanings
   Domain: A cluster of competencies that have similar intents, functions, and meanings

Through the analysis of clinical exemplars discussed in interviews, Benner derived a group of competencies. Clustering the competencies resulted in further identification of seven domains of expert nursing practice. Within her lexicon, these domains are a combination of roles, functions, and competencies, although the three have not been precisely differentiated. The seven domains are as follows:

1. The helping role
2. Administering and monitoring therapeutic interventions and regimens
3. Effective management of rapidly changing situations
4. The diagnostic and monitoring function
5. The teaching-coaching function
6. Monitoring and ensuring the quality of health care practices
7. Organizational and work-role competencies (Benner, 1984)

Fenton (1985) and Brykczynski (1989) each independently applied Benner's model of expertise to APNs, examining the practice of CNSs and NPs, respectively. In a later publication, Fenton and Brykczynski (1993) compared their earlier research findings to identify similarities and differences between CNSs and NPs. They used Benner's understanding of the concepts of domains, competencies, roles, and functions. Fenton and Brykczynski verified that nurses in advanced practice were indeed experts, as defined by Benner, and identified some additional domains and competencies as outlined in Figure 2-2. Fenton's research identified an eighth domain for CNSs—that of consultation by the nurse. In her study of NPs, Brykczynski also identified an eighth domain—management of health/illness in ambulatory care settings. Their contributions can be viewed as

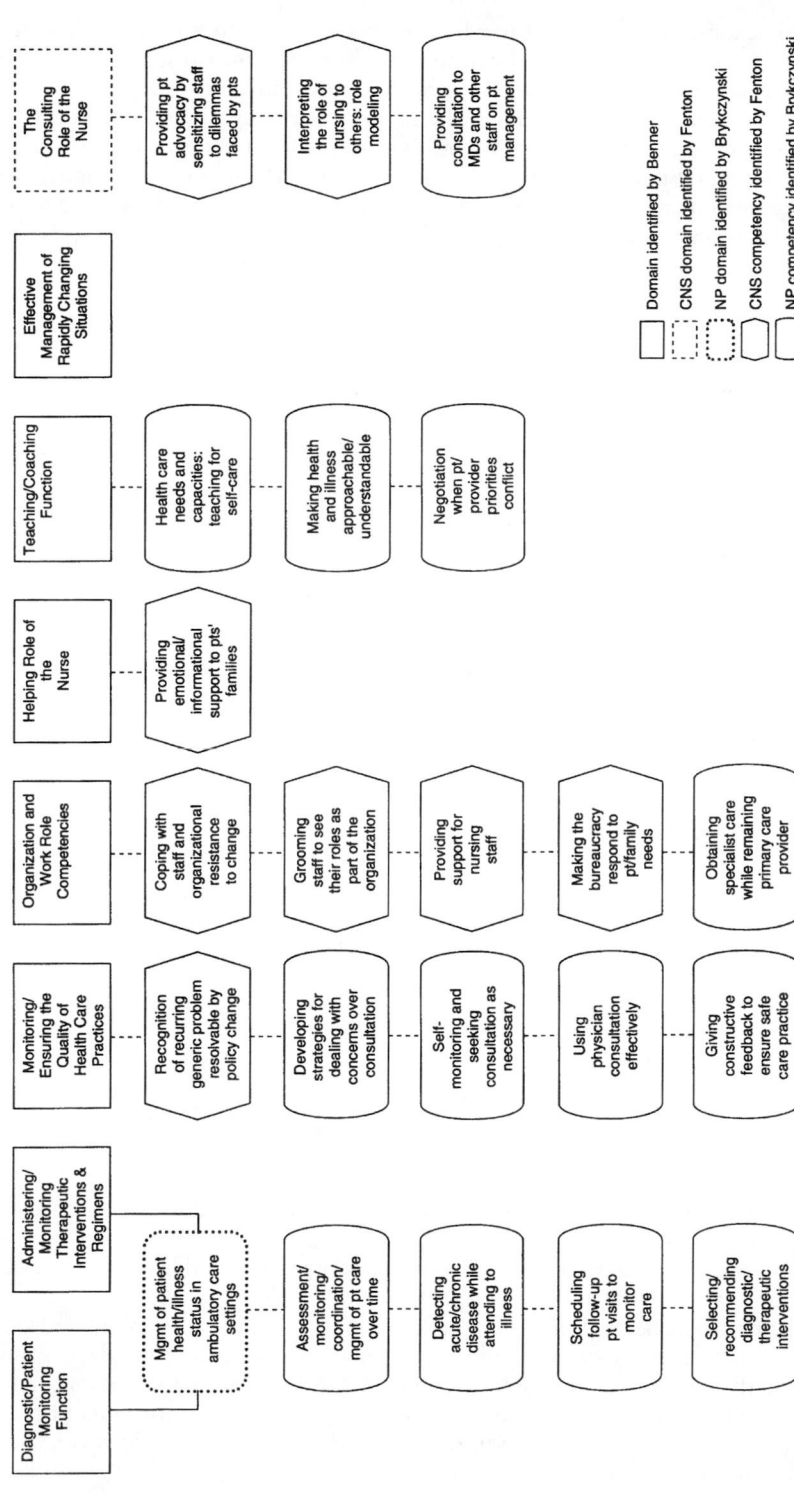

FIGURE 2-2 • Fenton's and Brykczynski's Expert Practice Domains of the Clinical Nurse Specialist (CNS) and Nurse Practitioner (NP). (From Fenton, M. V., & Brykczynski, K. A. [1993]. Qualitative distinctions and similarities in the practice of clinical nurse specialists and nurse practitioners. *Journal of Professional Nursing, 9,* 313-326.)

not only examining the extent to which APNs demonstrate the seven domains found in experts by experience but also beginning to describe how these two advanced practice nursing roles may be different with regard to practice domains.

In considering the applications of the Benner model and the refinements to CNS practice made by Fenton (1985), Spross and Baggerly (1989) made recommendations for further development. With some modification, their recommendations apply to advanced practice nursing in general. Spross and Baggerly (1989) indicated the need for the following: (1) further application of the model to advanced practice nursing, (2) extension of the teaching/coaching domain to educating nurses, (3) comparison of the non-master's-prepared clinician's competencies with the APN's competencies to further elucidate components of expert versus advanced practice, and (4) student experience with ethnographic methods to enable graduates to address Benner's challenge to uncover the knowledge embedded in practice.

CALKIN'S MODEL OF ADVANCED NURSING PRACTICE

Calkin's model (1984) was the first to explicitly distinguish advanced practice nursing as practiced by CNSs and NPs. Calkin developed the model to help nurse administrators determine how to differentiate advanced practice nursing from other levels of clinical practice in personnel policies. She proposed that this could be accomplished by matching (1) patient responses to health problems (as nursing was defined in the ANA 1980 Social Policy Statement) with (2) the skill level and (3) the knowledge level of nursing personnel. In Calkin's model, three curves were overlaid on a normal distribution chart. Calkin depicted the skills and knowledge of novices, experts-by-experience, and APNs in relation to knowledge required in caring for patients whose responses to health-care problems (i.e., health-care needs) ranged from simple and common to complex and complicated (Figure 2-3).

Calkin used the framework to explain how APNs perform under different sets of circumstances: when there is a high degree of unpredictability; when there are new conditions or a new patient population or new sets of problems; and when there are a wide variety of health problems requiring the services of "specialist generalists," as she called them. She defined what APNs do in terms of functions. For example, when patients' health problems elicit a wide range of human responses with continuing and substantial unpredictable elements, the APN should do the following (Calkin, 1984, p. 28):

- Identify and develop interventions for the unusual by providing direct care
- Transmit this knowledge to nurses and, in some settings, to students
- Identify and communicate the need for research or to carry out research related to human responses to these health problems
- Anticipate factors that may lead to the presence of unfamiliar responses
- Provide anticipatory guidance to nurse administrators when the changes in the diagnosis and treatment of these responses may require altered levels or types of resources

A principal advantage to Calkin's model is that the skills, education, and knowledge of the nurses needed are considered based on patient needs. It provides a framework for scholars to use in studying the function of APNs in a variety of work situations, and it should be a useful conceptualization for administrators who must maximize a multilevel nursing workforce and thus need to rationalize the use of APNs. However, the model has been left for others to test.

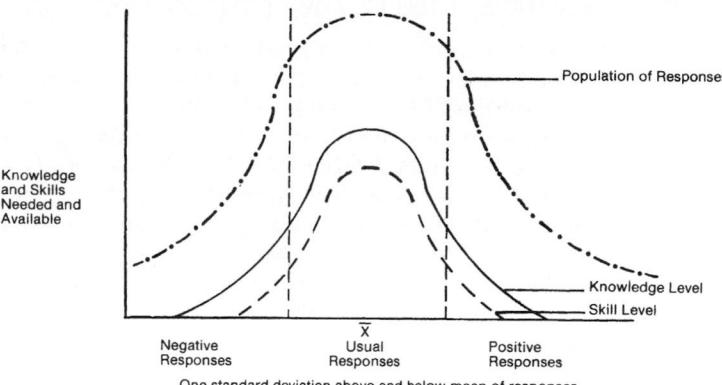

A

Beginning Practitioners

FIGURE 2-3 • Calkin's Model of Advanced Nursing Practice. Patient responses correlated with the knowledge and skill of beginning practitioners, experienced nurses, and advanced practice nurses.(From Calkin, J. D. [1984]. A model for advanced nursing practice. *Journal of Nursing Administration, 14,* 24-30.)

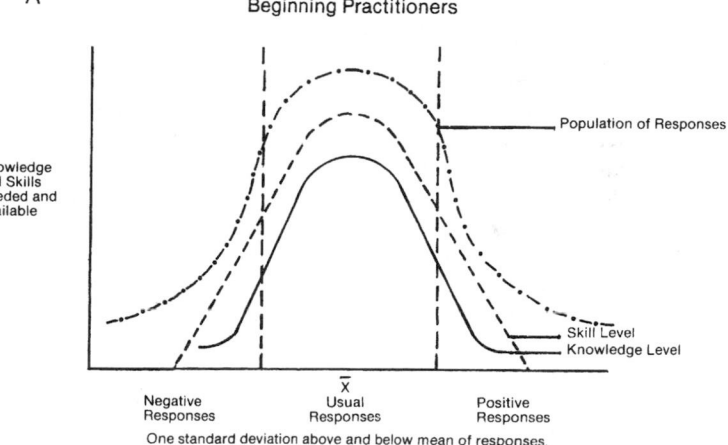

B

Experienced Nurses

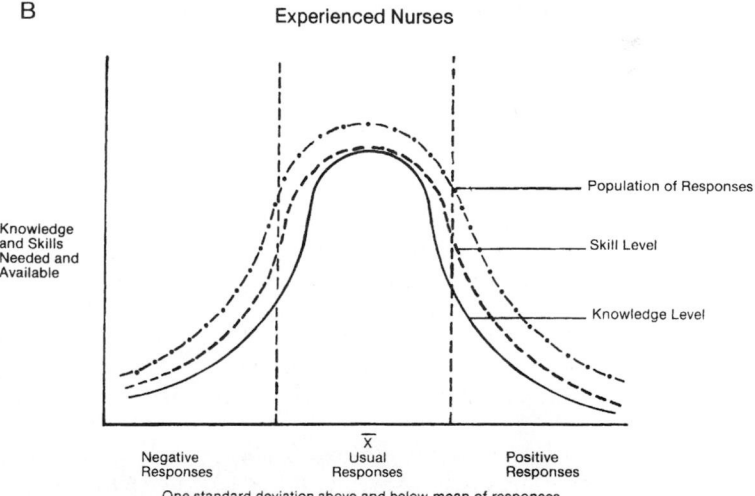

C

Advanced Nurse Practitioners

HAMRIC'S MODEL OF ADVANCED PRACTICE NURSING

One of the earliest efforts to synthesize a model of advanced practice that would apply to all APN roles was developed by Hamric (1996). Hamric, whose early conceptual work was done on the CNS role (Hamric & Spross, 1983, 1989), proposed an integrative understanding of the core of advanced practice nursing, based on literature from all APN specialties. She proposed a conceptual definition of advanced practice nursing and defining characteristics that included primary criteria (graduate education, certification in the specialty, and a focus on clinical practice with patients) and a set of core competencies (direct clinical practice, collaboration, coaching and guidance, research, ethical decision making, consultation, and leadership). This early model was further refined together with Hanson and Spross in 2000 and again in the current edition of this text (see Chapter 3), based on dialogue among the editors of this text. The revised model (Figure 2-4) retains the

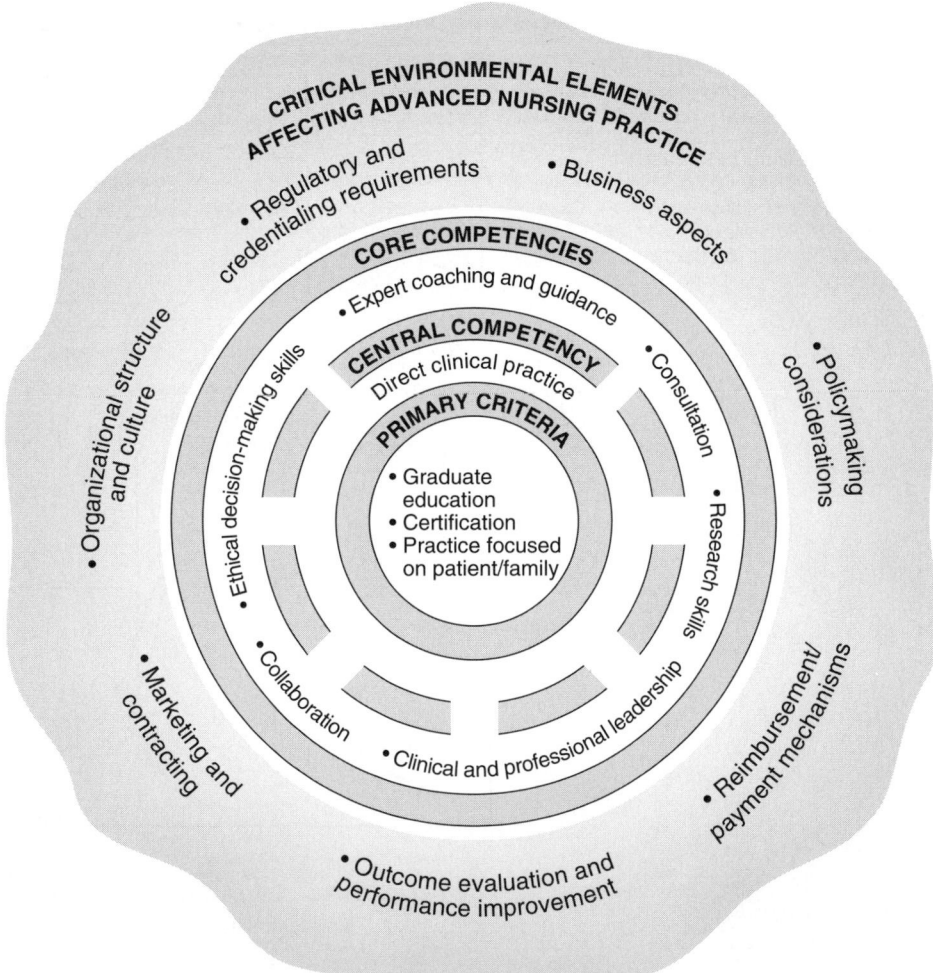

FIGURE 2-4 • Hamric's Model of Advanced Practice Nursing.

primary criteria, proposed direct care as the core competency on which the other advanced practice nursing competencies depend, and adds a variety of contextual factors present in the environments where APNs practice, which must be managed for advanced practice nursing to flourish. These changes highlight the dynamic feature of conceptual models, which are refined over time according to changes in practice, research, and theoretical understanding. This model forms the understanding of advanced practice nursing used throughout this text and provides the book's structure.

Using Hamric's model, some contributors to this text have further elaborated the specific competencies she proposed (Hamric, 2000; see Chapter 3) by describing concepts relevant to the specific competency and depicting them graphically. The competencies include coaching (Spross, Clarke, & Beauregard, 2000; see Chapter 6), consultation (Barron & White, 2000; see Chapter 7), and ethical decision making (Reigle & Boyle, 2000; see Chapter 11).

BROWN'S FRAMEWORK FOR ADVANCED PRACTICE NURSING

Brown (1998) developed a framework for the entire field of advanced practice nursing, including the environments that surround and impact upon practice (see Figure 2-5). She synthesized existing literature to propose a conceptual framework that included 4 main and 17 specific concepts (the specific concepts are in parentheses): *environments* (society, health-care economy, local conditions, nursing, advanced practice community); *role legitimacy* (graduate education, certification, licensure); *advanced practice nursing* (scope, clinical

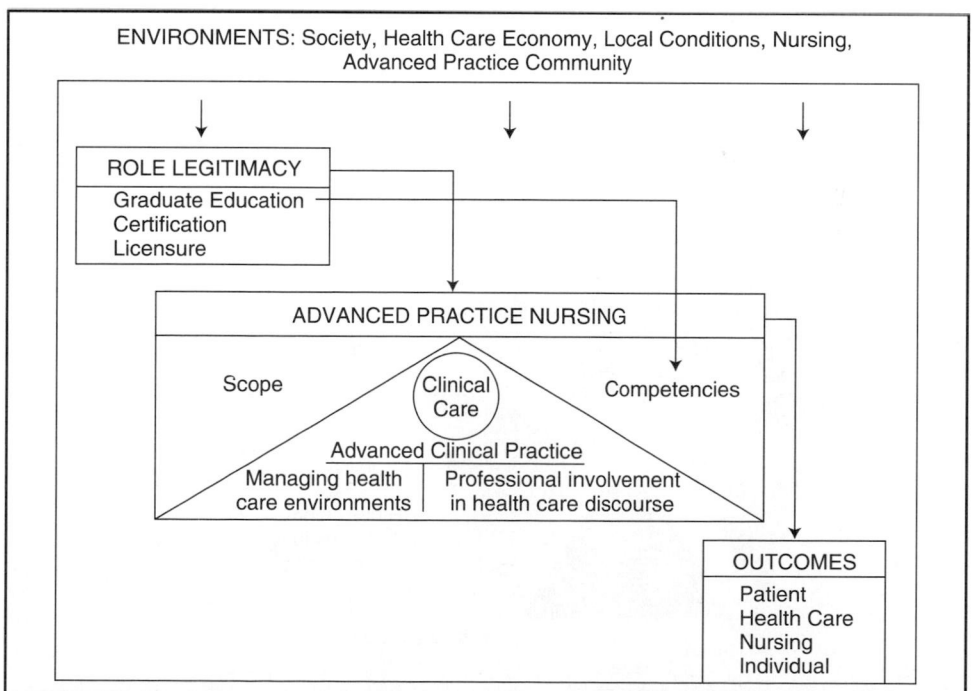

FIGURE 2-5 • Brown's Framework for Advanced Practice Nursing. (From Brown, S. J. [1998]. A framework for advanced practice nursing. *Journal of Professional Nursing, 14,* 157-164.)

care, competencies, managing health-care environments, professional involvement in health-care discourse); and *outcomes* (patient, health-care system, the nursing profession, individual APN outcomes) (Figure 2-5).

The central concept, conceptually and visually, is advanced practice nursing. Brown (1998) proposed a definition of advanced practice nursing: "professional health care activities that (1) focus on clinical services rendered at the nurse-client interface, (2) use a nursing orientation, (3) have a defined but dynamic and evolving scope, and (4) are based on competencies that are acquired through graduate nursing education" (p. 161).

This comprehensive model is one of the few that explicates a conceptual framework as described in the beginning of this chapter. Brown defines the concepts or "building blocks" of the model, articulates assumptions, and proposes linkages among concepts that could be tested. The model is comprehensive in that it addresses both the nature of the practice and the context in which the practice occurs. She notes the importance of a nursing orientation, particularly when APNs perform activities traditionally done by physicians. Brown notes that scope is "defined but dynamic and evolving" (p. 161), an observation that reflects the rapidity with which knowledge accrues and practice changes. The model is sufficiently explicated that it could be used for all of the purposes conceptual models can serve: differentiating practice, designing curricula, and evaluating advanced practice. Like the NONPF model, Brown uses domains and competencies to describe the work of APNs.

STRONG MEMORIAL HOSPITAL'S MODEL OF ADVANCED PRACTICE NURSING

APNs at Strong Memorial Hospital developed a model of advanced practice nursing (Ackerman, Clark, Reed, Van Horn, & Francati, 2000; Ackerman, Norsen, Martin, Wiedrich, & Kitzman, 1996; Mick & Ackerman, 2000). The model (Figure 2-6) evolved from the delineation of the domains and competencies of the acute care NP (ACNP) role,

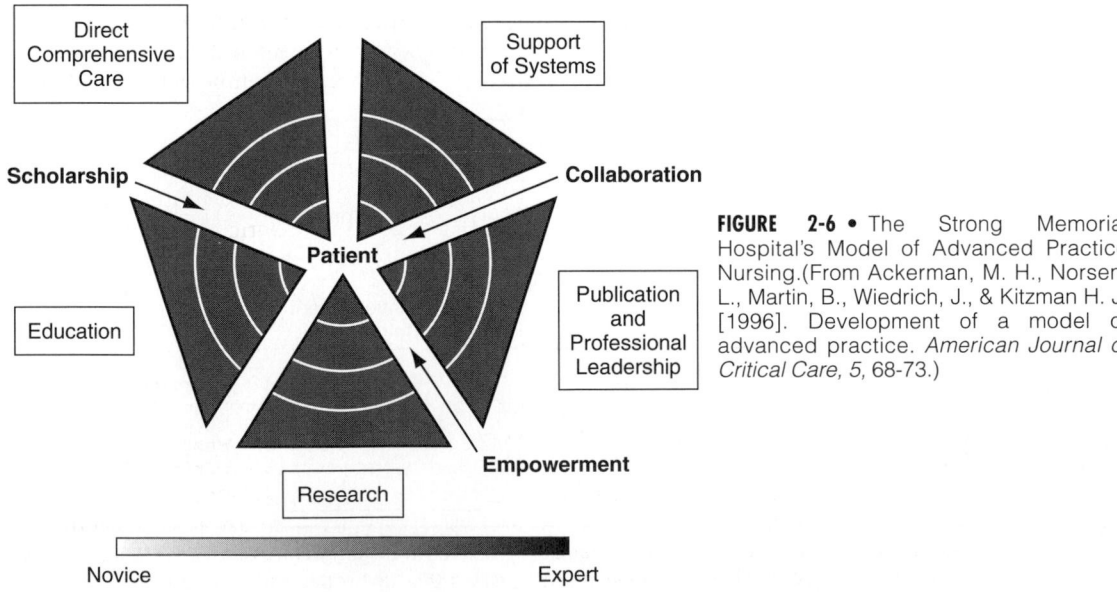

FIGURE   2-6 • The   Strong   Memorial Hospital's Model of Advanced Practice Nursing.(From Ackerman, M. H., Norsen, L., Martin, B., Wiedrich, J., & Kitzman H. J. [1996]. Development of a model of advanced practice. *American Journal of Critical Care, 5,* 68-73.)

conceptualized as a role that "combines the clinical skills of the NP with the systems acumen, educational commitment, and leadership ability of the CNS" (Ackerman et al., 1996, p. 69). There are five domains: direct comprehensive patient care, support of systems, education, research, and publication and professional leadership. All domains have direct and indirect activities associated with them. In addition, there are necessary, unifying threads that influence each domain, which are illustrated as circular and continuous threads in Figure 2-6: collaboration, scholarship, and empowerment (Ackerman et al., 1996). These threads are operationalized in each practice domain. Ackerman et al. (2000) noted that the model is based on an understanding of the role development of APNs—the concept of novice (APN) to expert (APN) is foundational to the Strong Model.

Direct comprehensive care includes a range of assessments and interventions performed by APNs including history taking; physical assessment; requesting and/or performing diagnostic studies; performing invasive procedures; interpreting clinical and laboratory data; prescribing medications and other therapies; and case management of complex, critically ill patients. The support of systems domain includes indirect patient care activities that support the clinical enterprise and serve to improve the quality of care. These activities include consultation, participating or leading strategic planning, quality improvement initiatives, establishing and evaluating standards of practice, precepting students, and promoting APN practice. The education domain includes a variety of activities such as evaluating educational programs; providing formal and informal education to staff; educating patients and families; and identifying and disseminating educational resources. The research domain addresses both the use and conduct of research. The publication and professional leadership domain includes those APN functions involved with disseminating knowledge about the ACNP role, participating in professional organizations as a member or leader, influencing health and public policy, and publishing. APNs are expected to exert influence within and outside of their institution.

The unifying threads of collaboration, scholarship, and empowerment are attributes of advanced practice that exert influence across all five domains and characterize the professional model of nursing practice. Collaboration ensures that the contributions of all caregivers are valued. APNs are expected to create and sustain a culture that supports scholarly inquiry whether it is questioning a common nursing practice or developing and disseminating an innovation. APNs support the empowerment of staff, ensuring that nurses have authority over nursing practice and opportunities to improve practice.

The Strong Model is a parsimonious model that has many similarities with other advanced practice conceptualizations. For example, its domains are consistent with the competencies delineated in the Hamric Model. Unlike the Hamric Model, which posits direct care as the central competency that informs all other advanced nursing practice competencies, in the Strong Model all domains of practice, including direct care, are considered "mutually exclusive of each other and exhaustive of practice behaviors" (Ackerman et al., 1996, p. 69). Like the Synergy Model, discussed later, role development is incorporated within the model (novice to expert). As described in the original article, the Strong Model emerged form consideration of the ACNP as a combined CNS/NP role—this is considered a blended role that is not the same as an ACNP in this textbook (see Chapters 14 and 15)—highlighting our point that work remains to be done on a unifying conceptualization of advanced nursing practice. Even so, we agree with the authors' conclusion that the model may be useful to other APNs and administrators (Ackerman et al., 1996). It is notable that this model was the result of a collaborative effort between practicing APNs and APN faculty members. One could infer that such a model would be useful for guiding clinical practice and planning curricula, two of the purposes of conceptual models outlined earlier in the chapter.

OBERLE AND ALLEN: THE NATURE OF ADVANCED PRACTICE NURSING

For Oberle and Allen (2001), current conceptualizations of advanced practice were limited: particular gaps are the lack of clear distinctions between the expert practice of experienced nurses and the expert practice of APNs, as well as the lack of nursing theories to address such levels of practice. The authors note that although the literature on expert nursing is mostly focused on expertise as it unfolds in the context of relationships, the literature on advanced practice nursing seems to focus more on expertise as "skills acquisition and critical thinking abilities" (p. 148).

According to Oberle and Allen (2001), any conceptualization of advanced practice nursing should be embedded in a conceptual understanding of nursing. To elucidate their model of advanced practice nursing, the authors first propose a conceptualization of nursing practice. They refer to practice as *praxis*, a term that captures the values-oriented, reflective, and creative nature of the work of nurses. They conceive of nursing as a dialectical process between the nurse's knowledge and his or her experiences and relationships with patients. In this process, the nurse considers general and particular knowledge, synthesizes this knowledge, and generates options for care that he or she can offer to the patient. Over time, this dialectical process occurring in relationship with patients contributes to developing expertise.

The conceptualization of advanced practice nursing proposed by Oberle and Allen (2001) is illustrated in Figure 2-7. Box 2-2 defines each of the elements in the model. Oberle and Allen differentiate between experts by experience and APNs as follows: "The inherent difference between expert and advanced practice is that the expert nurse's knowledge base is largely experientially acquired, whereas the APN has a greater store of theoretical knowledge acquired through graduate study" (p. 151).

Although Figure 2-7 is meant to illustrate advanced practice nursing, the elements in the model are the same as those used for the textual description of experts-by-experience; there are not separate illustrations of the two levels of practice. Differences between experts-by-experience and APNs are offered in the text, and Oberle and Allen propose that graduate education is a process in which students have experiences that lead to transformations in self and in practice, a dialectical process that results in "Transformative Practice" (p. 152). Although the notion of transformative practice is provocative and likely to resonate with students and faculty, neither the model nor the text helps the reader understand what this transformative practice is and how it is different from the practice of experts-by-experience. Graduate students could use the article and model as a starting point for considering their own experiences as expert staff nurses and the ways in which graduate education is transforming them.

Oberle and Allen acknowledge that they do not consider the specifics of advanced practice. Neither do they address the environment or contexts of practice in their model, which we consider a limitation of the model. Environment is a significant theoretical concept for nursing in general and for advanced practice nursing in particular. Another limitation of the model is the emphasis on practical experience in nursing. With more and more career changers entering nursing through direct-entry programs that prepare APNs, future conceptualizations of advanced practice nursing will need to take into account how nonnursing experience helps graduate nursing students experience the dialectical process that is at the heart of praxis and helps them develop the practical wisdom that is essential to effective nursing practice. Graduate APN students who do not have nursing experience

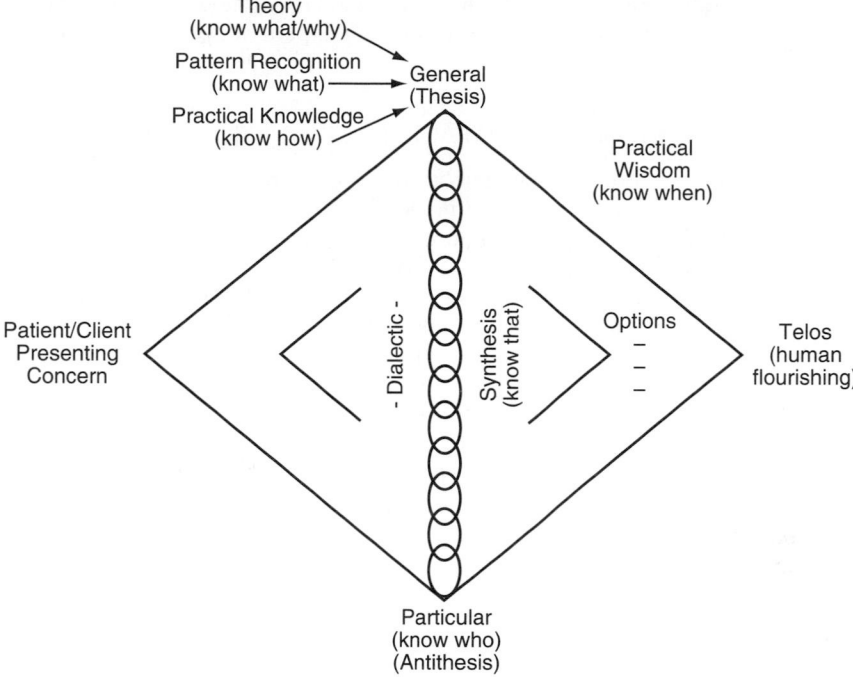

FIGURE 2-7 • Oberle and Allen's Conceptualization of Advanced Practice. (From Oberle, K., & Conceptualization of Allen, M. [2001]. The nature of advanced practice nursing. *Nursing Outlook, 49,* 148-53.)

BOX 2-2 • ELEMENTS OF OBERLE AND ALLEN'S CONCEPTUALIZATION OF ADVANCE PRACTICE

Patient/client presenting concern—problem or potential problem for which an individual needs nursing care.
General and particular knowledge—Nurses move back and forth between global knowledge (such as the features of an illness or the nursing care that usually works for a particular problem) and specific knowledge (specifics about the individual patient or situation).

GENERAL KNOWLEDGE
• Theory—Know what and know why
• Pattern recognition—Know what
• Practical knowledge—Know how

PARTICULAR KNOWLEDGE
• Client's meanings, desired outcomes, and acceptable actions—Know who
Dialectic—The process by which nurses consider general and particular knowledge and synthesize this information to generate options and propose actions to the patient to move the patient toward his or her goals.
Synthesis—Know that [a particular action is called for in a specific situation].
Practical wisdom—Know when [a particular ought to be taken]. The dialectical process and experience with synthesis, informed by praxis, lead to the development of "practical wisdom."

From Oberle, K., & Allen, M. (2001). The nature of advanced practice nursing. *Nursing Outlook, 49,* 148-153.

are encouraged to reflect on and expand on this model, considering how their life and professional experiences account for their experience of transformation and their mastery of advanced practice nursing.

SHULER'S MODEL OF NP PRACTICE: A THEORETICAL FRAMEWORK

Shuler's efforts to integrate both nursing and medical knowledge skills into the NP role led her to develop a conceptual model that would make apparent the unique contribution NPs made to patient care and outcomes. Thus, Shuler purposefully addressed the need for a model that reflects the acquisition of expertise by the NP in two health-care disciplines: nursing and medicine. Shuler's NP practice model (Figure 2-8) is a complex systems model that is holistic and wellness oriented. It is both definitive and detailed in terms of how the NP-patient interaction, patient assessment, intervention, and evaluation should occur (Shuler & Davis, 1993a). Its complexity is likely to overwhelm beginning NP students, and its value for understanding NP practice may not become clear until they have experience as practicing NPs. To simplify the presentation of the model, Table 2-2 outlines key model constructs and related theories, many of which should be familiar to students. Knowing that these familiar concepts are embedded in this very complex model may help readers as they read about and examine Figure 28-8. To fully understand the model, the reader should go back to the original publication; the following discussion highlights selected elements.

Within NP practice, Shuler conceptualizes patient visits as fitting into one of three categories: episodic (Figure 2-8, patient/NP throughput A), comprehensive exam with an existing acute (Figure 2-8, patient/NP throughput B1) or chronic (Figure 2-8, patient/NP throughput B2) problem, or comprehensive exam without an existing health problem (Figure 2-8, patient/NP throughput C). Input categories are similar regardless of the type of visit. Students can see the integration of nursing and medicine in the Inputs box—in addition to information that one would assess in the usual history and physical, the NP incorporates less traditional elements such as spiritual elements. NP characteristics are also viewed as inputs in that NPs' own wellness orientations may exert influence on NP-patient interactions and patient outcomes through role modeling. Throughputs vary somewhat according to the type of visit. A close look at the throughputs indicates that both patient data from the history, physical, and other assessments and NP interventions are identified. The Outputs box could be viewed as outcomes—patient outputs such as reduced complications and adherence to treatment and NP outputs such as adoption of healthy behaviors and identification of professional learning needs.

In addition to integrating nursing and medicine, the model incorporates concepts from a number of disciplines (e.g., psychology). From the figure alone, the reader will appreciate that it is most ambitious; it incorporates multiple theoretical constructs within a systems framework that integrates internal and external environments and input-throughput-output processes. From a review we discerned that the systems model incorporates the following: (1) the four concepts of nursing's metaparadigm (person, health, nursing, and environment), (2) the nursing process, (3) humanistically based assumptions about patients and nurse practitioners, and (4) theoretical concepts underlying practice model constructs. Indeed, the model could be characterized as a network or system of frameworks.

Shuler's model is intended "to impact the NP domain at four levels: theoretical, clinical, educational, and research" (Shuler & Davis, 1993a, p. 17). Clinical application of the Shuler model is intended to ensure demonstration of the NP's combined (i.e., nursing and medicine) role with the proposed benefits for both the practitioner and the patient and to provide a framework by which NP services can be evaluated (Shuler & Davis, 1993b). For example, if NPs purposefully include patients in the assessment, planning, intervention,

TABLE 2-2 MODEL CONSTRUCTS AND UNDERLYING THEORETICAL CONCEPTS INCLUDED IN SHULER'S MODEL OF NURSE PRACTITIONER PRACTICE

MODEL CONSTRUCTS	WHOLISTIC PATIENT NEEDS	NP-PATIENT INTERACTION	SELF-CARE	HEALTH PREVENTION	HEALTH PROMOTION	WELLNESS
Underlying Theoretical Concepts	Basic needs Wellness activities Health/illness Psychological health Family Culture Social support Environmental health Spirituality	Contracting Role modeling Self-care activities Teaching/learning Communication Problem solving Decision making	Wellness activities Preventive health activities Health promotion activities Compliance Problem solving Teaching/learning Contracting Culture Family Social support Environmental health	Primary prevention Secondary prevention Tertiary prevention Preventive health behavior Family Culture Environmental health	Health promotion behavior Wellness Family Culture Environmental health Social support	Self-care activities Wellness activities Disease prevention activities Health promotion activities Family Culture Social support Environmental health Spirituality Contracting Teaching/learning

From Shuler, P. A., & Davis, J. E. (1993). The Shuler nurse practitioner practice model: A theoretical framework for nurse practitioner clinicians, educators, and researchers, Part 1. *Journal of the American Academy of Nurse Practitioners, 5,* 11-18; reprinted with permission.

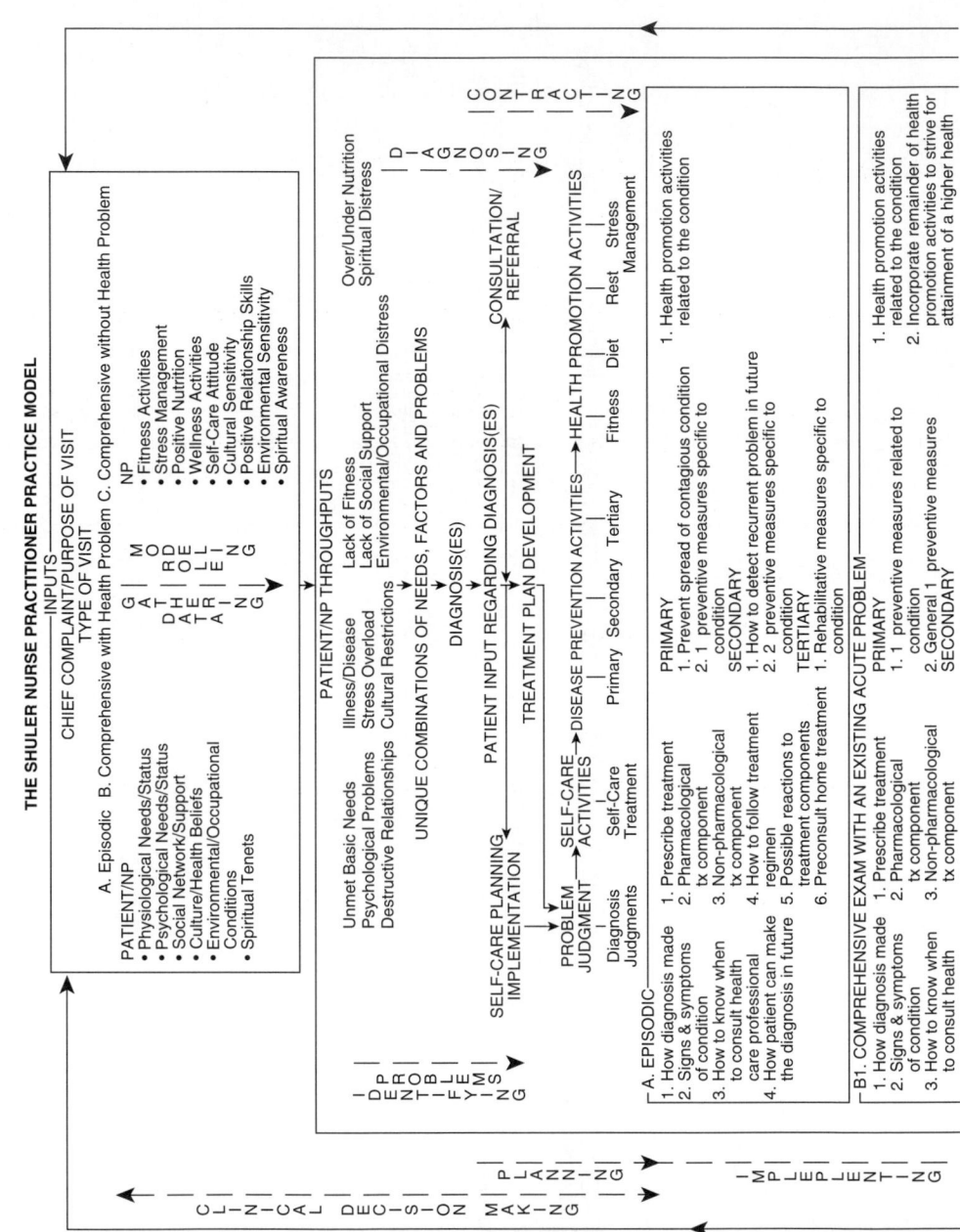

THE SHULER NURSE PRACTITIONER PRACTICE MODEL

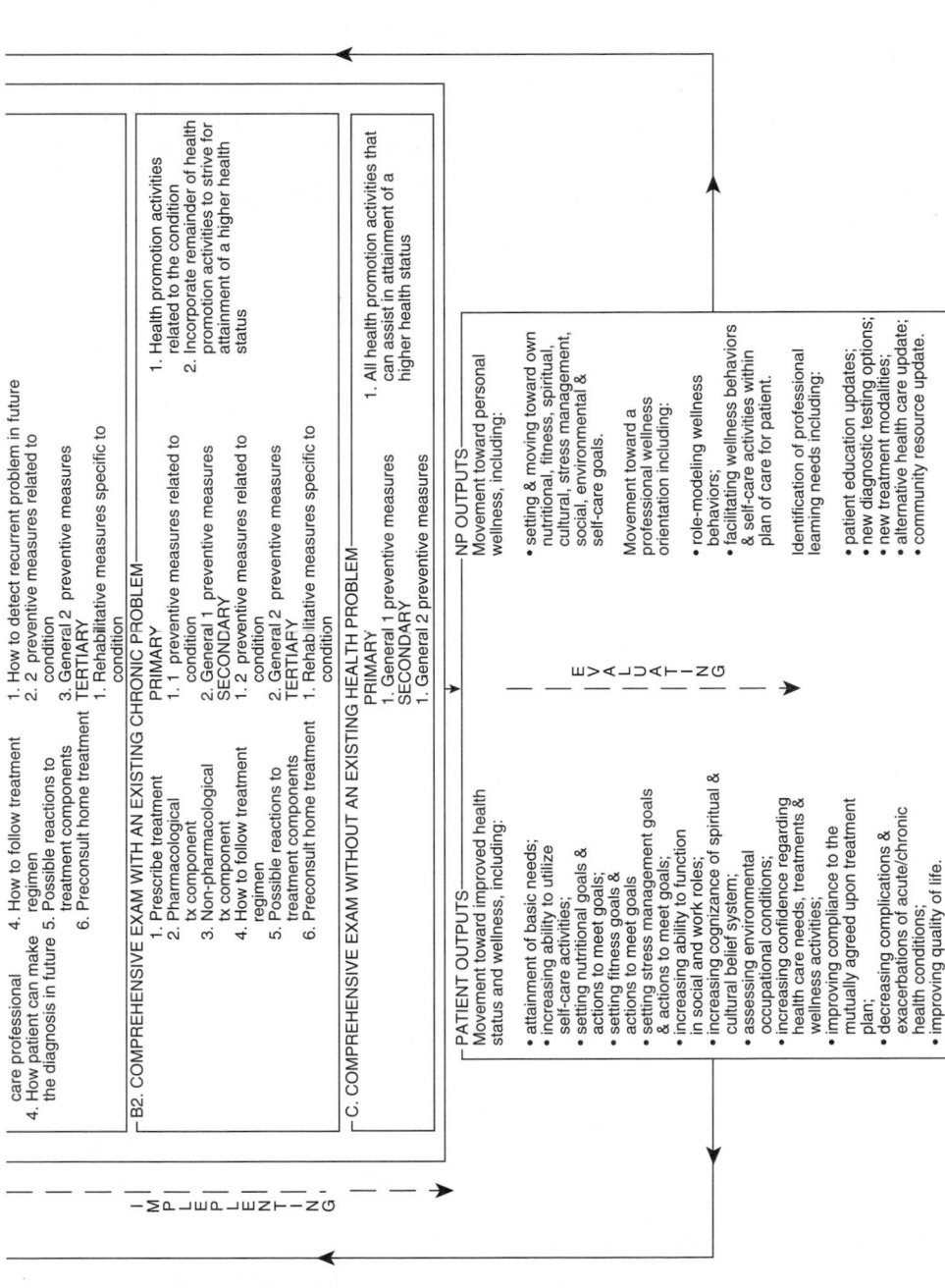

FIGURE 2-8 • The Shuler Nurse Practitioner Practice Model. (From Shuler, P. A., & Davis, J. E. [1993a]. The Shuler nurse practitioner practice model: A theoretical framework for nurse practitioner clinicians, educators, and researchers, Part 1. *Journal of the American Academy of Nurse Practitioners, 5,* 11-18.)

and evaluation processes an improvement in patient adherence to a mutually agreed upon treatment/wellness plan would be anticipated.

Shuler & Davis (1993b) published a template for conducting a visit with guidelines on what types of information should be solicited during a comprehensive exam when there is an existing health problem—the template is 17 pages long! The scope and intent of the model are enormous. Although it is difficult to imagine ready implementation into the busy NP practices of today, Shuler and colleagues have proposed examples of applying the model, which included (1) providing care to patients with an existing health problem seen for a comprehensive exam (Shuler & Davis, 1993b), (2) delivering primary care through school-based health centers (Shuler, 2000), and (3) providing holistic health care to elders (Shuler, Huebscher, & Hallock, 2001). These examples illustrate the model's comprehensiveness and vastness. The ability to use the entire framework in the context of individual patient encounters may prove overwhelming, especially for NP students. Faculty may be able to use the complete model to help NP students see how nursing and medical knowledge and skills come together in this advanced practice role or to demonstrate the complexity of NP practice—the view from the mountaintop, if you will. However, the model may be best utilized when a student or reader isolates and tries to grasp one or two constructs and then visualizes these constructs within the larger whole. For practicing NPs, the model's benefit may lie in providing NPs with a guide on how to promote and retain the nursing focus on care in the context of a combined role that integrates medical knowledge and skills into nursing.

SUMMARY/IMPLICATIONS FOR ADVANCED PRACTICE NURSING CONCEPTUALIZATIONS

When one considers conceptualizations of advanced practice nursing described by professional organizations and individual authors, similarities and differences emerge. Many conceptual models address competencies that APNs must possess. All are in agreement that the direct care of patients is central to APN practice. Some models (e.g., Calkin and Strong Models) address the issue of skill mix as it relates to APNs, an issue of concern to administrators who hire APNs. On the other hand, processes of care such as consultation and collaboration are infrequently addressed. There is a fairly consistent emphasis on outcomes—how does APN practice influence patient and institutional outcomes. However, different models may emphasize different competencies. Some models address concepts such as research, scholarly inquiry, and ethics more explicitly than others. A notable difference is the extent to which the concept of environment as it relates to APN practice is addressed. In the next section we review models that have not necessarily emerged from an APN perspective, but they are ones that APNs may find useful as they develop and evaluate their own practices.

MODELS THAT APNs WILL FIND USEFUL IN THEIR PRACTICE

Other models exist that can contribute to conceptualizing and studying advanced practice nursing. In addition to the ones described in the following sections, conceptual models of APN role development that help students, faculty, and APNs understand how an individual APN's knowledge and practice evolve over time are fully explored in Chapter 4.

Models Useful for Differentiating Levels of Nursing Practice

THE AMERICAN ASSOCIATION OF CRITICAL-CARE NURSES' SYNERGY MODEL

The American Association of Critical-Care Nurses created the Synergy Model (Figure 2-9), and it is in an effort to link nursing practice with patient outcomes (Curley, 1998). Components of the model are patients' characteristics; nurses' competencies; and patient,

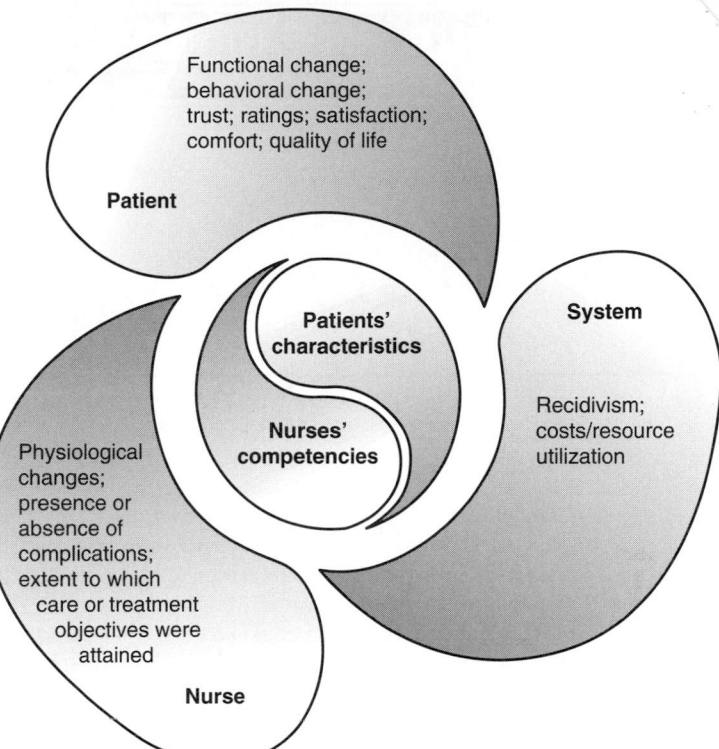

FIGURE 2-9 • The American Association of Critical Care Nurses' Synergy Model. The Synergy Model delineates three levels of outcomes: those derived from the patient, those derived from the nurse, and those derived from the health-care system. (From Curley, M. A. Q. [1998]. Patient-nurse synergy: Optimizing patient's outcomes. *American Journal of Critical Care, 7,* 64-72.)

nurse, and system level outcomes. Patients' capacity for health and their vulnerability to illness are influenced by biological, genetic, psychological, and socioecological determinants. The Synergy Model posits a unique cluster of *personal characteristics* that arise from these determinants and exist along a continuum that parallels health and illness states: stability, complexity, predictability, resiliency, vulnerability, participation in decision making and care, and resource availability (Box 2-3). An important function of the nurse is to ensure the patient's "safe passage" through the health-care situation.

Nursing competencies are derived from the needs of patients and also exist along continua. There are eight nursing competency continua: clinical judgment, advocacy and moral agency, caring practices, facilitation of learning, collaboration, systems thinking, diversity of responsiveness, and clinical inquiry (Box 2-4). The continua for these competencies range from "competent" (level 1) to "expert" (level 5). A discussion of the interpretation of these levels is beyond the scope of this chapter. The reader is referred to the American Association of Critical-Care Nurses website (http://www.aacn.org) and publications (American Association of Critical-Care Nurses [AACN], 2003; Curley, 1998).

Outcomes are conceptualized as being derived from patient, nurse, and/or system. For example, trust of the caregiver and patient satisfaction are patient outcomes that arise or are derived from the patient. Physiological outcomes are derived from the nurse (i.e., the nurse's interventions). System level outcomes are derived from the hospital or insurer (e.g., readmission to the hospital for a preventable complication).

The model is interesting for several reasons. Apparently, certification examinations are based on the conceptualization of levels of competency and represent an effort to ensure

2-3 • THE SYNERGY MODEL: THE SEVEN CONTINUA OF PATIENT CHARACTERISTICS

	1	2	3	4	5
	Minimally resilient				Highly resilient
	Highly vulnerable				Minimally vulnerable
	Minimally stable				Highly stable
	Minimally complex				Highly complex
	Not predictable				Highly predictable
	Few resources available				Many resources available
	No participation in decision making and care				Full participation in decision making and care

Adapted from American Association of Critical-Care Nurses. (2003). *The AACN Synergy Model for patient care.* Retrieved December 7, 2003, from http://www.aacn.org/certcorp/certcorp.nsf/vwdoc/SynModel?opendocument

conceptual coherence between the nature of the practice and how one's knowledge of the practice is tested. Since certification examinations are based on the model, it seems likely that programs preparing APNs in critical care would use the model to structure curricula. APNs have used the model to understand complex cases (e.g., Collopy, 1999; Moloney-Harmon, 1999). Finally, the model could serve as the basis for differentiating among critical care APN roles. For example, one might study ACNPs, CNSs, and APN case managers in critical care to determine whether characteristics and competencies vary across these APN roles or whether differences exist in how these APNs operationalize their advanced practice nursing roles.

Models Useful for Studying Outcomes of Advanced Practice Nursing

APNs, regardless of role, must be prepared to articulate the relationships among their practice, patient outcomes, and resource use. The following models can be used to

BOX 2-4 • THE SYNERGY MODEL: THE EIGHT CONTINUA OF NURSE CHARACTERISTICS/NURSING COMPETENCIES

	1	2	3	4	5
Clinical judgment	*Competent*				*Expert*
Advocacy/Moral agency	*Competent*				*Expert*
Caring practices	*Competent*				*Expert*
Collaboration	*Competent*				*Expert*
Systems thinking	*Competent*				*Expert*
Response to diversity	*Competent*				*Expert*
Clinical inquiry or Innovator/Evaluator	*Competent*				*Expert*
Facilitator of patient and family learning	*Competent*				*Expert*

Adapted from American Association of Critical-Care Nurse. (2003). *The AACN Synergy Model for patient care.* Retrieved December 7, 2003, from http://www.aacn.org/certcorp/certcorp.nsf/vwdoc/SynModel?opendocument

inform the design and conduct of quality improvement projects and research projects aimed at demonstrating the links between advanced practice nursing and outcomes (see Chapter 25).

BROOTEN'S MODEL OF TRANSITIONAL CARE

Brooten used a conceptual framework proposed by Doessel and Marshall (1985). Doessel and Marshall synthesized medical and economic concepts to propose a definition of quality of health care whose key concepts were outcomes, patient satisfaction, and cost. Brooten et al. (1988) integrated these three concepts into their evaluation of outcomes of APN transitional care with different populations such as very low birth weight infants, hospitalized elderly patients, and women who had undergone cesarean deliveries. APN transitional care was defined as "comprehensive discharge planning designed for each patient group plus APN home follow-up through a period of normally expected recovery or stabilization" (Brooten et al., 2002, p. 370). Brooten's model was intended to address outlier patient populations (e.g., those patients who were complex, at high risk for complications, who represented a significant proportion of those whose care was expensive). Across all studies, care was provided by NPs and/or CNSs whose clinical expertise was matched to the needs of the patient population. APN care was associated with improved patient outcomes and reduced costs (see Chapter 25). Research conducted by Brooten and others who have used this model provided empirical support for several elements important to a conceptualization of advanced practice nursing. In a summary of the studies conducted to date, the investigators identified several factors that contribute to APNs' effectiveness: content expertise, interpersonal skills, knowledge of systems, the ability to implement change, and ability to access resources (Brooten, Youngblut, Deatrick, Naylor, & York, 2003). This finding provides empirical support for the importance of the APN competencies of direct care, collaboration, coaching, and leadership/change agent. Two other important findings were the existence of patterns of morbidity within patient populations and an apparent "dose effect" (i.e., outcomes seemed to be related to how much time, how many interactions patients had with APNs, and numbers and types of APN interventions) (Booten et al., 2003). These findings suggest that characteristics of patients and characteristics of APN interventions are likely to be important to any conceptualization of advanced practice nursing. Finally, the fact that this program of research has used both NPs and CNSs to intervene with patients provides support for elucidating a conceptual model that encompasses characteristics, competencies, and other concepts that are common across advanced practice nursing roles.

MITCHELL AND JENNINGS' QUALITY HEALTH OUTCOMES MODEL

For APNs involved in quality improvement, the Quality Health Outcomes Model (QHOM) (Figure 2-10) is particularly relevant. It is interesting that this model builds on Donabedian's (1966) theoretical work on the quality of health care, a model Hamric (1983, 1989) proposed using for evaluating CNS practice. A key premise of Donabedian's theory is that structure, process, and outcome variables influence the quality and outcomes of health care.

Although the QHOM model has not been used to evaluate advanced practice nursing specifically, it is relevant for examining nursing and interdisciplinary practice. From the perspective of knowledge building, it evolved from Donabedian's Structure-Process-Outcome model of quality assurance (Donabedian, 1966; Mitchell, Ferketich, & Jennings, 1998).

One of the challenges in evaluating the quality of nursing care is disentangling or accounting for the influence of other factors such as physician care, staffing levels, or

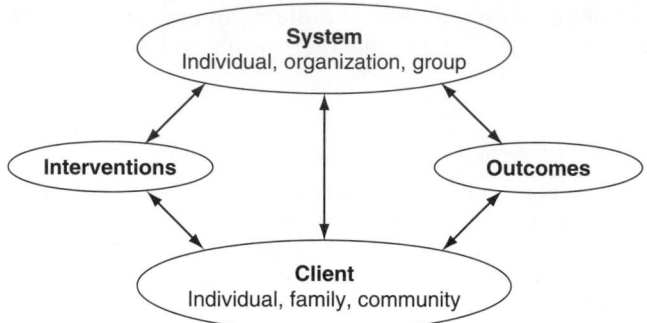

FIGURE 2-10 • Mitchell and Jennings' Quality Health Outcomes Model. This model proposes two-direction relationships among components, with interventions always acting through characteristics of the system and of the patient. (From Mitchell P. H., Ferketich S., & Jennings B. M. [1998]. Quality health outcomes model. American Academy of Nursing Expert Panel on Quality Health Care. *Image: The Journal of Nursing Scholarship, 30,* 43-46.)

availability of resources. By proposing a model that allows for multiple inputs at the level of patient, personnel and system, the authors of the QHOM suggest that using the model will enable evaluators to analyze the contribution of specific variables to patient outcomes. The authors note that the model provides a structure for studying complex relationships among patient, provider, and system level variables so that studies guided by this model might produce results that improve our understanding of patient outcomes. Because the model incorporates organization/system level influences, it can guide studies of system level interventions such as program initiatives or reimbursement changes; results of such studies can be used to influence health policy. In a refinement of this model, Radwin (2002) proposed that client characteristics could be further understood in terms of state and trait, arguing that nursing interventions cannot influence trait variables such as age or gender (which may exert influences on health outcomes) (Figure 2-11).

One can see that this approach to evaluation would allow one to evaluate some of the models of advanced practice nursing previously discussed. For example, concepts in this model parallel the spheres of CNS influence posited by the NACNS (2004). The model incorporates the concept of system or environment, consistent with such models as Brown's Framework for Advanced Practice Nursing and Hamric's model of advanced practice nursing (1996, 2000; see Chapter 3).

SIDANI AND IRVINE'S NURSING ROLE EFFECTIVENESS MODEL FOR STUDYING OUTCOMES OF ACUTE CARE NURSE PRACTITIONERS

The original Nursing Role Effectiveness Model (NREM) model (Irvine, Sidani, & McGilliss Hall, 1995) was developed to "facilitate the identification and investigation of nursing-sensitive outcomes" (Sidani & Irvine, 1998, p. 59). The authors believed that inconsistencies among published findings about outcomes of ACNP practice were due in part to inadequate conceptualization of the practice. NREM (Figure 2-12) provides a framework for evaluating outcomes of acute care nurse practitioner (ACNP) practice. The authors used literature to support the elucidation of concepts and relationships among concepts, enabling them to make propositions about the various relationships and their impact on outcome. Unlike the QHOM model, this framework is linear—no reciprocal influences are posited—and no differentiation is made between patient state and trait characteristics, factors that one might want to consider in using the framework. Although Sidani and Irvine revised the NREM model to examine ACNP practice, we believe all APNs will find it useful for evaluating their practices. APNs can also use both the Quality Health Outcomes Model and NREM to guide quality improvement activities.

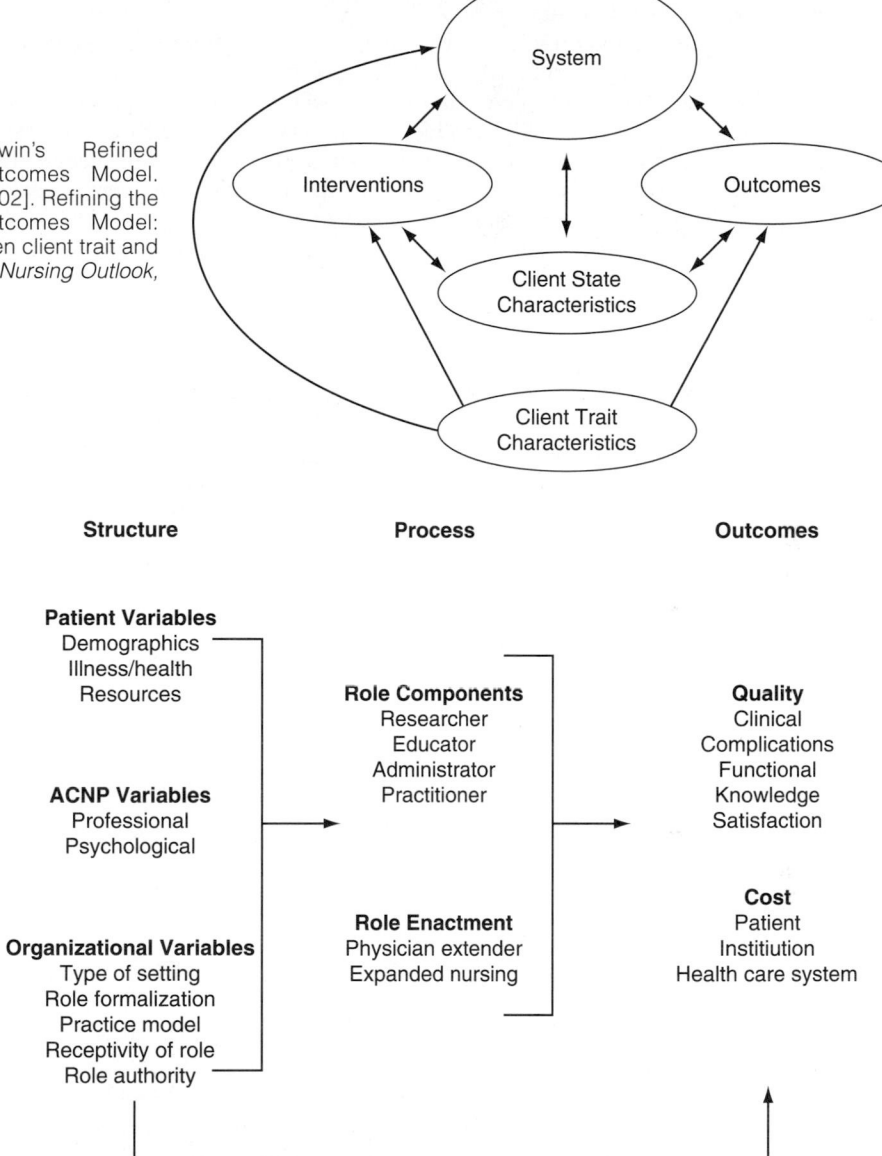

FIGURE 2-11 • Radwin's Refined Quality Health Outcomes Model. (From Radwin, L. [2002]. Refining the Quality Health Outcomes Model: Differentiating between client trait and state characteristics. *Nursing Outlook, 50*[4], 168-169.)

FIGURE 2-12 • Sidani and Irvine's Nursing Role Effectiveness Model (NREM) for acute care nurse practitioners. (From Sidani, S., & Irvine, D. [1998]. A conceptual framework for evaluating the nurse practitioner role in acute care settings. *Journal of Advanced Nursing 30*(1), 58-66.)

Models Useful for Conceptualizing Interdisciplinary Practice

DUNPHY AND WINLAND-BROWN'S CIRCLE OF CARING: A TRANSFORMATIVE MODEL

A central premise of Dunphy and Winland-Brown's model (1998) is that the health-care needs of individuals, families, and communities are not being met in a health-care system that is dominated by medicine and one in which medical language (i.e., the *International*

Classification of Disease Codes [ICD-10-CM]) is the basis for reimbursement. They proposed the Circle of Caring: A Transformative Model in order to foster a more active and visible nursing presence in the health-care system and to explain and promote medical-nursing collaboration. Dunphy and Winland-Brown's transformative model (Figure 2-13) is a synthesized problem-solving approach to advanced practice nursing that builds on both nursing and medical models (Dunphy & Winland-Brown, 1998).

The authors argue that a model such as theirs is needed because nursing and medicine have two very different traditions with the medical model being viewed as primarily reductionistic and nursing being regarded as primarily humanistic. Neither a nursing nor medical model of practice, in isolation or in combination, is seen as providing a structure that allows APNs to be recognized for their day-to-day practice and the positive patient health outcomes that can be attributed to APNs' care. The model's authors viewed the development of *nursing diagnoses* as an attempt to differentiate nursing care from medical care. Though this initiative gave nurses a taxonomy for naming problems that are within the nursing domain to treat, nursing diagnoses are not recognized by current reimbursement systems, even though APNs may use them in the context of their practices. Dunphy and Winland-Brown further noted the challenge facing APNs to identify and cost out the unique characteristics of advanced practice nursing that are associated with improved patient outcomes.

The Circle of Caring model is said to incorporate the strengths of medicine and nursing in a transforming way. The conceptual elements are the *processes* of assessment, planning, intervention, and evaluation with a feedback loop. Each of these processes is greatly

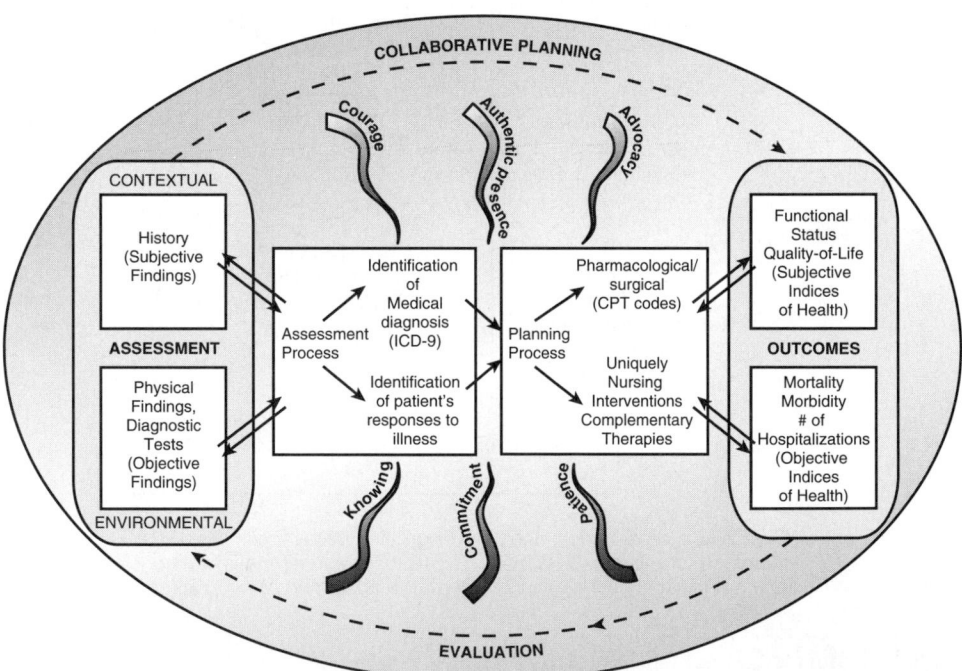

FIGURE 2-13 • Dunphy and Winland-Brown's Circle of Caring Model. (From Dunphy, L. M., & Winland-Brown, J. E. [1998]. The Circle of Caring: A transformative model of advanced practice nursing. *Clinical Excellence for Nurse Practitioners, 2,* 241-247.)

enriched by a multiparadigmatic perspective. By superimposing a nursing-based template on a traditional medical model, the following occurs:

- The assessment and evaluation are contextualized, incorporating subjective and environmental elements into traditional history taking and physical examination.
- The approach to therapeutics is broadened to include holistic approaches to healing and makes nursing care more visible.
- Measured outcomes include patients' perceptions of health and care, not just physiological outcomes, and resource utilization.

The assessment-planning-intervention-evaluation processes in linear configuration are encircled by caring. Caring is actualized through interpersonal interactions with patients and caregivers to which NPs bring patience, courage, advocacy, authentic presence, commitment, and knowing (Dunphy & Winland-Brown, 1998). Contextual definitions of these concepts would add to the understanding of how these processes interact with and affect the caregiving of APNs. The authors suggested that the model promotes the incorporation of the lived experience of the patient into the provider-patient interaction and that the process of caring is prerequisite to APNs providing effective and meaningful care to patients.

The Circle of Caring is seen as an integrated model of caregiving that incorporates the discrete strengths of both nursing and medicine. For NP graduate students this is an important concern. They struggle with integrating their nursing expertise and philosophy with new knowledge and skills that were traditionally viewed as medicine. Though the authors view the concept of caring as a way to bridge "the gap" between advanced practice nursing and medicine and raise awareness, the model provides no clear guidance on how faculty can help students or how students themselves can use the model to bridge the gap.

Several issues remain to be considered. Dunphy and Winland-Brown intended that the model be applied on both the micro level of one-to-one relationships in acute care and the macro level of caring for communities and populations, although the feasibility, desirability, or implementation of the latter are not specifically addressed. How this might be done is not addressed. For example, if one goal of proposing the model is to resolve differences about the diagnostic language used by medicine and nursing to obtain reimbursement, the model offers no specific mechanism for APNs to resolve this issue. Indeed, the model does not seem sufficiently described to understand how it might be used to guide policymaking. The conceptual significance of encircling the four practice processes with the six caring processes is unclear. Practically, one would expect the caring processes, which appear to be attitudes and values, to be integrated throughout each practice step in a value-added collaborative model. Since the model was first proposed, we did not find literature that indicated it has been tested empirically. Such testing would help determine whether the model: (1) is applicable to all advanced practice nursing roles; (2) has the potential to be used in practice at the basic (clinician) level; (3) is viewed by other disciplines as having an interdisciplinary focus that would promote collaboration; and (4) would result in more visibility for NPs and other APNs within the health-care system.

RECOMMENDATIONS AND FUTURE DIRECTIONS

It is understandable that students may feel overwhelmed at the variety of conceptualizations and inconsistency in terminology. The challenge for students is to find a model that works for them—that enables them to understand and evaluate their practices.

Based on this review of models of advanced practice nursing, we have formulated some recommendations for further work on conceptualizing advanced practice in three areas: conceptualizations of advanced practice nursing, consensus building around advanced practice nursing, and research on APN practice and outcomes.

Conceptualizations of Advanced Practice Nursing

We acknowledge that our review of extant models of advanced practice nursing is rather cursory and may be incomplete—it is more a survey or overview than a review of the literature. Although there is some agreement on selected elements of advanced practice, by and large, there is no synthesis of existing work and limited evidence of new conceptualizations building on earlier work. In order to promote a unified conceptualization of advanced practice nursing we suggest the following:

1. A rigorous content analysis of the statements published by professional organizations that describe the advanced practice nursing of recognized APNs (CNMs, CNSs, CRNAs, NPs)
2. A similar content analysis of statements that address advanced nursing practice promulgated by specialty organizations
3. Based on recommendations 1 and 2, a synthesis of results should be generated that can be used to propose a definition of the phenomenon—advanced nursing practice—and related concepts
4. A policy analysis of proposed standards for APN credentialing and licensing that includes a delineation of anticipated policy and patient outcomes of minority stances such as those taken by NACNS and ACNM and proposed strategies for addressing the legitimate concerns of these organizations (such as grandfathering)

The purpose of these activities would be to more clearly identify areas of agreement, to propose a common language (e.g., domains and competencies) for describing advanced practice nursing, propose a prospective process for creating and credentialing APNs in evolving areas of advanced practice nursing, and identify areas that are priorities for negotiation and resolution by stakeholder groups. Now is the time for the focus to shift toward bringing the practice of all APNs, including CNMs and CRNAs, into conceptual unity. This is not to suggest that the practice is identical for all, but that the common elements should be identified and differences noted. Such a comprehensive approach is needed if our profession is to make room for evolving APN roles while making the expertise of APNs prepared 20 years ago available to the public; the latter is particularly important considering the shortage of nurses. The need to move forward with one voice on this issue is urgent if APNs and the nursing profession as a whole are to fulfill their social contract with the individuals, the institutions, and the communities we serve.

Other purposes could be served by a rigorous and comprehensive synthesis of conceptualizations of advanced practice nursing including communicating within and across disciplines; evolving a process for expanding scopes of practice for APNs as knowledge, technology, and other elements of health-care delivery change; and strengthening the political influence of APNs. A unified conceptualization of advanced practice nursing would assist the NCSBN and state Boards of Nursing to address legislative and regulatory issues relative to APN licensing when promulgating new standards or responding to challenges.

Consensus Building Around Advanced Practice Nursing

Although we are aware that historically our profession has had difficulty reaching consensus on issues of importance (see Chapter 1; C.M. Hanson, personal communication, April 12, 2004), we believe a proposal for a collaboratively developed conceptualization of advanced practice nursing is a prerequisite for building consensus among APNs and stakeholder professional organizations. Once such a proposal has been drafted, we recommend the following:

1. Under the auspices of an organization with demonstrated success at bringing diverse groups together, the proposal would be circulated among groups for discussion and input in a town meeting–like setting; such groups should include a diverse representation of APN roles, APN faculty, and others who have a direct interest in how advanced practice nursing is conceptualized.
2. That stakeholder groups agree to a process for using input, identifying those areas on which consensus is needed, and establishing a process and timeline for reaching consensus. For example, the process might be structured such that agreement to move forward as a profession could be elicited with a provision for expressing minority opinions.

Divisiveness after having accomplished so much for APNs will not serve our patients or our profession. We believe this collaborative work is critical to ensuring that patients will continue to benefit from advanced practice nursing.

Research on APN and Outcomes

Research on patient outcomes and cost-effectiveness that leads to increased knowledge about advanced practice nursing is critical (see Chapter 25). The worth of any service depends on the extent to which practice meets the needs and priorities of health-care systems, the public policy arena, and society in general. These needs are, by and large, for appropriate services at a reasonable cost. In addition to research that links advanced practice nursing with outcomes we recommend the following:

1. That promising conceptual models of advanced practice nursing be refined based on research that validates key concepts and tests theoretical propositions associated with such models.
2. That research on APNs is necessary to examine the interpersonal processes they use in the course of providing care to patients and collaborating with colleagues within and across disciplines—across many of the models reviewed in this chapter the APN's skill in communication and collaboration is considered important. Descriptive data on the interpersonal strategies APNs use will enable researchers to examine links between these less tangible aspects of APN care and patient outcomes.
3. That studies be undertaken that examine advanced practice nursing across APN roles. Such studies can identify the extent to which the assumptions that a core set of competencies are used by APNs are valid regardless of role. In addition the activities that differentiate one APN role from another can be identified.
4. When there is a better empirical understanding of the similarities and differences across roles, this knowledge must be packaged and presented to colleagues in other disciplines, policymakers, and the public. Such information is important to

educating physicians, consumers, and policymakers about the meaning and relevance of advanced practice nursing to the health of our society.

For further discussion of research directions relevant to advanced practice nursing, see Chapter 25.

SUMMARY

Conceptual models serve many purposes for the fields they seek to describe. Importantly, they are useful for guiding and evaluating the evolution of advanced practice nursing. Such progress is dependent on the extent to which practice meets the needs and priorities of the society, health-care systems, and the public policy arena. We have identified problems and imperatives related to conceptualizing advanced practice nursing, reviewed a number of models, and made some recommendations for future work on conceptualizing advanced practice nursing that address the problems and imperatives. A unified conceptualization of advanced practice nursing will focus the efforts of the profession on preparing APNs, promulgating policies, and fostering research that can enable the realization of the two goals put forward at the beginning of this chapter: maximizing the social contribution of the advanced practice nursing to the health needs of society and promoting the actualization of APNs.

REFERENCES

Ackerman, M., Clark J., Reed, T., Van Horn, L. & Francati, M. (2000). A nurse-practitioner managed cardiovascular intensive care unit. In J. Hickey, R. Ouimette, & S. Venegoni (Eds.), *Advanced practice nursing: Changing roles and clinical applications* (pp. 470-480). Philadelphia: Lippincott.

Ackerman, M. H., Norsen, L., Martin, B., Wiedrich, J., & Kitzman, H. J. (1996). Development of a model of advanced practice. *American Journal of Critical Care, 5,* 68-73.

American Association of Colleges of Nursing. (1996). *Essentials of master's education for advanced practice nursing.* Washington, DC: Author.

American Association of Colleges and Nursing. (2002). *The clinical nurse leader, developing a new nurse.* Retrieved March 1, 2004, from http://www.aacn.nche.edu/NewNurse/index.htm

American Association of Critical-Care Nurses. (2003). *The AACN Synergy Model for patient care.* Retrieved December 7, 2003, from http://www.aacn.org/certcorp/certcorp.nsf/vwdoc/SynModel?opendocu

American Association of Nurse Anesthetists. (1996). *Scope and standards for nurse anesthesia practice.* Park Ridge, IL: Author.

American Association of Nurse Anesthetists. (2002). *Scope and standards for nurse anesthesia practice.* Retrieved March 1, 2004, from http://www.aana.com/crna/prof/scope.asp

American College of Nurse-Midwives. (1997a). *The core competencies for basic midwifery practice.* Washington, DC: Author.

American College of Nurse-Midwives. (1997b). *Position statement: Expansion of midwifery practice and skills beyond basic core competencies.* Retrieved March 1, 2004, from http://www.midwife.org/prof/display.cfm?id=118

American College of Nurse Midwives. (1998). *State mandated master's degrees: A tip sheet for ACNM legislative contacts Number 18.* Retrieved January 13, 2004, from http://www.acnm.org/legis/display.cfm?id=175

American College of Nurse-Midwives. (2003). *Standards for the practice of midwifery.* Retrieved March 1, 2004, from http://www.acnm.org/prof/display.cfm?id=138

American Nurses Association. (1980). *Nursing: A social policy statement.* Kansas City, MO: Author.

American Nurses Association. (1995). *Nursing's social policy statement.* Washington, DC: Author.

American Nurses Association. (1996). *Scope and standards of advanced practice registered nursing.* Washington, DC: Author.

American Nurses Association. (2003). *Nursing's social policy statement* (2nd ed.). Washington, DC: Author.

Atkins, S., & Ersser, S. (2000). Education for advanced nursing practice: An evolving framework. *International Journal of Nursing Studies, 37,* 523-533.

Barron, A., & White, P. A. (2000). Consultation. In A. B. Hamric, J. A. Spross, & C. M. Hanson (Eds.), *Advanced nursing practice: An integrative approach* (2nd ed., pp. 217-246). Philadelphia: W. B. Saunders.

Benner, P. (1984). *From novice to expert.* Menlo Park, CA: Addison-Wesley.

Benner, P. (1985). The oncology clinical nurse specialist as expert coach. *Oncology Nursing Forum, 12,* 40-44.

Brooten, D., Brown, L., Munro, B., York, R., Cohen, S., Roncoli, M., et al. (1988). Early discharge and specialist transitional care. *Image: Journal of Nursing Scholarship, 20,* 64-68.

Brooten, D., Naylor, M., York, R., Brown, L., Munro, B., Hollingsworth, A., et al. (2002). Lessons learned from testing the quality cost model of advanced practice nursing (APN) transitional care. *Journal of Nursing Scholarship, 34,* 359-375.

Brooten, D., Youngblut, J., Deatrick, J., Naylor, M., & York, R. (2003). Patient problems, advanced practice nurse (APN) interventions, time and contacts among five patient groups. *Journal of Nursing Scholarship, 35*(1), 73-79.

Brown, M. A., & Olshansky, E. F. (1997). From limbo to legitimacy: A theoretical model of the transition to the primary care nurse practitioner role. *Nursing Research, 46,* 46-51.

Brown, S. J. (1998). A framework for advanced practice nursing. *Journal of Professional Nursing, 14,* 157-164.

Brykczynski, K. A. (1989). An interpretive study describing the clinical judgment of nurse practitioners. *Scholarly Inquiry for Nursing Practice, 3,* 75-104.

Calkin, J. D. (1984). A model for advanced nursing practice. *Journal of Nursing Administration, 14,* 24-30.

Carveth, J. A. (1987). Conceptual models in nurse-midwifery. *Journal of Nurse-Midwifery, 32,* 20-25.

Collopy, K. (1999). The Synergy Model in practice: Advanced practice nurses guiding families through system. *Critical Care Nurse 19*(5), 80-85.

Curran, C., & Roberts, W. (2002). Columbia University's competency and evidence-based acute care nurse practitioner program. *Nursing Outlook, 50,* 232-237.

Curley, M. A. Q. (1998). Patient-nurse synergy: Optimizing patient's outcomes. *American Journal of Critical Care, 7,* 64-72.

Doessel, D., & Marshall, J. (1985). A rehabilitation of health outcomes in quality assessment. *Social Science and Medicine, 21*(12), 1319-1328.

Donabedian, A. (1966). Evaluating the quality of medical care. *Milbank Memorial Fund Quarterly, 44*(part 2), 166-206.

Dunphy, L. M., & Winland-Brown, J. E. (1998). The circle of caring: A transformative model of advanced practice nursing. *Clinical Excellence for Nurse Practitioners, 2,* 241-247.

Fawcett, J. (2000). *Analysis and evaluation of contemporary nursing knowledge: Nursing models and theories.* Philadelphia: F. A. Davis.

Fawcett, J. (2001). Integrating conceptual models, theories, research, and practice. In D. Robinson &

C. Kish (Eds.), *Core concepts in advanced practice nursing* (pp. 380-391). St. Louis: Mosby.

Fenton, M. V. (1985). Identifying competencies of clinical nurse specialists. *Journal of Nursing Administration, 15,* 31-37.

Fenton, M. V., & Brykczynski, K. A. (1993). Qualitative distinctions and similarities in the practice of clinical nurse specialists and nurse practitioners. *Journal of Professional Nursing, 9,* 313-326.

Gibbins, S. Green, P., Scott, P., & Watson MacDonell, J. (2000). The role of the clinical nurse specialist/neonatal nurse practitioner in a breastfeeding clinic: A model of advanced practice. *Clinical Nurse Specialist, 14*(2), 56-59.

Hamric, A. B. (1996). A definition of advanced practice nursing. In A. B. Hamric, J. A. Spross, & C. M. Hanson (Eds.), *Advanced nursing practice: An integrative approach* (pp. 25-41). Philadelphia: W. B. Saunders.

Hamric, A. B. (2000). A definition of advanced practice nursing. In A. B. Hamric, J. A. Spross, & C. M. Hanson (Eds.), *Advanced nursing practice: An integrative approach* (2nd ed., pp. 53-74). Philadelphia: W. B. Saunders.

Hamric, A. B., & Spross, J. A. (1983). A model for future clinical specialist practice. In A. B. Hamric & J. A. Spross (Eds.), *The clinical nurse specialist in theory and practice* (pp. 291-306). New York: Grune & Stratton.

Hamric, A. B., & Spross, J. A. (1989). *The clinical nurse specialist in theory and practice* (2nd ed). Philadelphia: W. B. Saunders

Hanson, C. M., & Hamric, A. B. (2003). Reflections on the continuing evolution of advanced practice nursing. *Nursing Outlook, 51*(5), 203-210.

Irvine, D., Sidani, S., & McGillis Hall, L. (1998). Linking outcomes to nurses' roles in health care. *Nursing Economics, 16*(2), 58-64.

Lincoln, P. (2000). Comparing CNS and NP role activities: A replication. *Clinical Nurse Specialist, 14*(6), 269-277.

Mick, D., & Ackerman, M. (2000). Advanced practice nursing role delineation in acute and critical care: Application of the Strong Model of advanced practice. *Heart and Lung, 29*(3), 210-221.

Mitchell, P. H., Ferketich, S., & Jennings, B. M. (1998). Quality health outcomes model. American Academy of Nursing Expert Panel on Quality Health Care. *Image: The Journal of Nursing Scholarship, 30,* 43-46.

Moloney-Harmon, P. (1999). The Synergy Model: Contemporary practice of the clinical nurse specialist. *Critical Care Nurse, 19*(2), 101-104.

National Association of Clinical Nurse Specialists. (1998). *Statement on clinical nurse specialist practice and education.* Glenview, IL: Author.

National Association of Clinical Nurse Specialists. (2004). *Statement on clinical nurse specialist practice and education.* Harrisburg, PA: Author.

National Council of State Boards of Nursing. (2002). *Nurse licensure compact.* Retrieved March 11, 2004, from http://www.ncsbn.org/nlc/aprncompact.asp

National Organization of Nurse Practitioner Faculties (2002). *Nurse practitioner primary care competencies in specialty areas: Adult, family gerontological, pediatric, and women's health.* Retrieved March 6, 2004, from http://www.nonpf.com/-finalaug2002.pdf

National Organization of Nurse Practitioner Faculties (2003). *Psychiatric-mental health nurse practitioner competencies.* Retrieved March 6, 2004, from http://www.nonpf.com/finalcomps03.pdf

Oberle, K., & Allen, M. (2001). The nature of advanced practice nursing. *Nursing Outlook, 49,* 148-153.

Plager, K., Conger, M., & Craig, C. (2003). Education for differentiated role development for NP and CNS practice: One nursing program's approach. *Journal of Nursing Education, 42*(9), 406-416.

Price, M. J., Martin, A. C., Newberry, Y. G., Zimmer, P. A., Brykczynski, K. A., Warren, B. (1992). Developing national guidelines for nurse practitioner education: An overview of the product and the process. *Journal of Nursing Education, 31,* 10-15.

Radwin, L. (2002). Refining the Quality Health Outcomes Model: Differentiating between client trait and state characteristics. *Nursing Outlook, 50*(4), 168-169.

Raudonis, B., & Anderson, C. (2002). A theoretical framework for specialty certification in nursing practice. *Nursing Outlook, 50,* 247-252

Reigle, J., & Boyle, R. J. (2000). Ethical decision-making skills. In A. B. Hamric, J. A. Spross, & C. M. Hanson (Eds.), *Advanced nursing practice: An integrative approach* (2nd ed., pp. 273-295). Philadelphia: W. B. Saunders.

Shuler, P. A. (2000). Evaluating student services provided by school-based health centers: Applying the Shuler Nurse Practitioner Practice model. *Journal of School Health, 70,* 348-352.

Shuler, P. A., & Davis, J. E. (1993a). The Shuler nurse practitioner practice model: A theoretical framework for nurse practitioner clinicians, educators, and researchers, Part 1. *Journal of the American Academy of Nurse Practitioners, 5,* 11-18.

Shuler, P. A., & Davis, J. E. (1993b). The Shuler nurse practitioner practice model: Clinical application, Part 2. *Journal of the American Academy of Nurse Practitioners, 5,* 73-88.

Shuler, P. A., Huebscher, R., & Hallock, J. (2001). Providing wholistic health care for the elderly: Utilization of the Shuler Nurse Practitioner Practice Model. *Journal of the American Academy of Nurse Practitioners, 13,* 297-303.

Sidani, S., & Irvine, D. (1998). A conceptual framework for evaluating the nurse practitioner role in acute care settings. *Journal of Advanced Nursing, 30*(1), 58-66.

Spross, J. A., & Baggerly, J. (1989). Models of advanced nursing practice. In A. B. Hamric & J. A. Spross (Eds.), *The clinical nurse specialist in theory and practice* (2nd ed., pp. 19-40). Philadelphia: W. B. Saunders.

Spross, J. A., Clarke, E. B., & Beauregard, J. (2000). Expert coaching and guidance. In A. B. Hamric, J. A. Spross, & C. M. Hanson (Eds.), *Advanced nursing practice: An integrative approach* (2nd ed., pp. 183-216). Philadelphia: W. B. Saunders.

Styles, M. (1998). An international perspective: APN credentialing. *Advanced Practice Nursing Quarterly, 4* (3), 1-5.

Thibodeau, J. A., & Hawkins, J. W. (1994). Moving toward a nursing model in advanced practice. *Western Journal of Nursing Research, 16,* 205-218.

Valentine, N. Antai-Otong, D., Kupecz, D., Lynn, M., & Chaffee, M. (2000). Advanced practice nursing in the Department of Veterans Affairs: A model for the future. In J. Hickey, R. Ouimette, & S. Venegoni (Eds.), *Advanced practice nursing: Changing roles and clinical applications* (pp. 378-389). Philadelphia: Lippincott.

Walton, M. K., Jakobowski, D. S., & Barnsteiner, J. H. (1993). A collaborative practice model for the clinical nurse specialist. *Journal of Nursing Administration, 23,* 55-59.

Whitcomb, R., Wilson, S., Chang-Dawkins, S., Durand, J., Pitcher, D., Lauzon, C., & Aleman, D. (2002). Advanced practice nursing: Acute care model in progress. *Journal of Nursing Administration, 32*(3), 123-125.

Williams, C. A., & Valdivieso, G. C. (1994). Advanced practice models. A clinical comparison of clinical nurse specialist and nurse practitioner activities. *Clinical Nurse Specialist, 8,* 311-318.

Williams, C., Pesut, D., Boyd, M., Russell, S., Morrow, J., & Head, K. (1998). Toward an integration of competencies for advanced practice mental health nursing. *Journal of the American Psychiatric Nurses Association, 4*(2), 48-56.

Williams, D., & Kelley, M. (1998). Core competency-based education, certification, and practice: the nurse-midwifery model. *Advanced Practice Nursing Quarterly, 4*(3), 63-71.

Woods, L. P. (1997). Conceptualizing advanced nursing practice: curriculum issues to consider in the educational preparation of advanced practice nurses in the UK. *Journal of Advanced Nursing, 25,* 820-828.

Zimmer, P., Brykczynski, K. A., Martin, A. C., et al. (1990). *Advanced nursing practice: Nurse practitioner curriculum guidelines* (Final Report: NONPF Education Committee). Washington, DC: National Organization of Nurse Practitioner Faculties.

CHAPTER 3

A Definition of Advanced Practice Nursing

ANN B. HAMRIC

INTRODUCTION

The advanced practice of nursing builds on the foundation and core values of the nursing discipline. According to the American Nurses Association (ANA) (1995, 2003), contemporary nursing practice has four essential features: (1) inclusion of the full range of human experiences and responses to health and illness without restriction to a problem-focused orientation; (2) practice based on the integration of objective and subjective experience; (3) the ability to apply scientific knowledge to diagnostic and treatment processes; and (4) the ability to provide a caring relationship that facilitates health and healing. These four characteristics are equally essential for advanced practice nursing. Core values that guide nurses in practice include advocating for patients; respecting patient and family values and informed choices; viewing individuals holistically within their environments, communities, and cultural traditions; and maintaining a focus on disease prevention, health restoration, and health promotion (Creasia & Parker, 2001; Leddy, 1998; ANA, 2001). These core professional values also inform the central perspective of advanced practice. As Smith (1995) states, "The core of advanced practice nursing lies within nursing's disciplinary perspective on human-environment and caring interrelationships that facilitate health and healing. This core is delineated specifically in the philosophic and theoretic foundations of nursing" (p. 3).

Advanced practice nursing is a dynamic and evolving entity. Differing interpretations are evident at this stage of its development as compared with those included in the first edition of this text. Despite efforts to standardize the definition of advanced practice (American Association of Colleges of Nursing, 1995; ANA, 1996; National Council of State Boards of Nursing [NCBSN], 1993; Hamric, 1996, 2000), different interpretations of advanced practice, debates about who is and is not an advanced practice nurse (APN), and debates on educational preparation for APNs remain. For advanced practice nursing to achieve its full potential and for new APN roles to evolve, the profession must come to agreement on the key issues of definition, education, and credentialing. In this chapter, the definition of advanced practice nursing (first proposed in 1996 and expanded in 2000) is reiterated, and the scope of practice of APNs is discussed. Various APN roles are differentiated, and key factors in advanced practice nursing environments are identified. The importance of a common and unified understanding of the distinguishing characteristics of advanced practice nursing is emphasized in this chapter and throughout the book.

DISTINGUISHING BETWEEN SPECIALIZATION AND ADVANCED PRACTICE NURSING

Before the definition of advanced practice nursing can be explored, it is important to distinguish between specialization in nursing and advanced practice nursing. Specialization involves concentration in a selected clinical area within the field of nursing. All nurses with extensive experience in a particular area of practice (e.g., pediatric nursing or trauma nursing) are specialized in this sense. As the profession has advanced and responded to changes in health care, specialization and the need for specialty knowledge have increased. Thus there are few nurses who are generalists in the true sense of the word (Kitzman, 1989). Although family nurse practitioners (NPs) have traditionally seen themselves as generalists, they are also specialists in the sense being discussed here because they have specialized in one of the many facets of health care, namely, primary care. As Keeling and Bigbee note in Chapter 1, early specialization involved primarily on-the-job training or hospital-based training courses, and many nurses continue to develop specialty skills through practice experiences and continuing education. Examples of such currently evolving specialties include parish nursing and clinical research nurse coordination. As specialties mature, they may develop graduate-level clinical preparation and incorporate the competencies of advanced practice nursing as the concept is defined in this chapter (Hanson & Hamric, 2003; see Chapter 19). This progression is clearly seen in such APN roles as those of the certified registered nurse anesthetist (CRNA) and the NP.

The nursing profession has responded in a variety of ways to the increasing need for specialization in both clinical and clinical support arenas. The creation of specialty organizations, such as the American Association of Critical-Care Nurses and the Oncology Nursing Society, has been one response. The creation of advanced clinical practice roles—the CRNA and certified nurse-midwife (CNM) roles early in nursing's evolution and the clinical nurse specialist (CNS) and NP roles more recently—has been another response. The development of specialized faculty, such as pediatrics and obstetrics faculty; researchers who focus on particular phenomena, such as nursing ethics or the care of dying patients; and nursing administrators who direct clinical nursing services has been a third response. Nurses in all of these roles can be considered specialists in an area of nursing; some of these roles may involve advanced education in a clinical specialty as well. However, they are not necessarily advanced practice nursing roles. Advanced practice nursing includes specialization but also involves expansion, advancement (ANA, 1995; Cronenwett, 1995), and other characteristics. In *Nursing's Social Policy Statement* (ANA, 1995), these elements are defined as follows:

Expansion refers to the acquisition of new practice knowledge and skills, including the knowledge and skills that legitimize role autonomy within areas of practice that overlap traditional boundaries of medical practice. Advancement involves both specialization and expansion and is characterized by the integration of a broad range of theoretical, research-based, and practical knowledge that occurs as a part of graduate education in nursing. (p. 14)[1]

APNs are further characterized by their autonomy to practice at the edges of the expanding boundaries of nursing, their predominantly self-initiated treatment regimens rather than dependent functions, and the greater complexity of their clinical decision making and skill in managing organizations and environments as compared with basic nursing practice (ANA, 1996).

DEFINING ADVANCED PRACTICE NURSING

As recently as 1996, O'Malley, Cummings, and King wrote, "In most settings, the role of APNs has not been fully understood . . . APNs are still not identified by the public as primary care providers, partially due to misunderstanding of their roles" (p. 63). Significant progress has been made in the public and policy arenas, as exemplified by legislation introduced in Congress—the Medicaid Nursing Incentive Act of 2003—which if passed, will allow Medicaid plans to cover primary care services provided by APNs. However, the concept of advanced practice nursing continues to be defined in various ways in the nursing literature. The *Cumulative Index to Nursing and Allied Health Literature* defines advanced practice broadly as anything beyond the staff nurse role: "The performance of

[1]In the 2003 draft of the ANA's social policy statement, this definition has been reworded slightly, although the characteristics have not changed.

additional acts by registered nurses who have gained added knowledge and skills through post-basic education and clinical experience" (Advanced Nursing Practice, 2003). A definition this broad incorporates many specialized nursing roles, not all of which should be considered advanced practice. For example, some authors have proposed the "health policy analyst" as an advanced practice role (Stimpson & Hanley, 1991). This role contains no direct practice component, focusing as it does on consultation with decision makers regarding health policy. As the ANA (1995) notes, "The term advanced practice is used to refer exclusively to advanced *clinical* practice" (p. 15). In the understanding being developed here, the health policy analyst is a specialized nursing role but not an advanced practice role.

Advanced practice nursing is most often defined as a constellation of four roles: the NP, CNS, CNM, and CRNA (ANA, 1992; Donley, 1995; Ray & Hardin, 1995). For example, a 2003 ANA press release states:

Advanced practice registered nurses (APRNs) are registered nurses (RNs) who have attained advanced education and expertise and specialize in such medical fields as pediatrics, anesthesiology, gerontology, neonatology and mental health. APRNs include nurse practitioners, clinical nurse specialists, certified nurse-midwives and certified registered nurse anesthetists. (ANA, 2003)

Some authors, although they explicitly state that they are addressing advanced practice, discuss only NP and CNS roles (Lindeke, Canedy, & Kay, 1997; Rasch & Frauman, 1996). Others have focused exclusively on the NP role (Hickey, Ouimette, & Venegoni, 1996; Thibodeau & Hawkins, 1994). Snyder and Mirr (1995) define advanced practice nursing as the merged roles of the CNS and NP. These definitions of advanced practice in terms of particular roles limit the concept and deny the reality that nurses practicing in other roles are also APNs. These definitions are also limiting because they do not incorporate evolving APN roles, such as case management. Thus it seems preferable to define advanced practice nursing without reference to particular roles.

A definition should also clarify the critical point that advanced practice nursing involves advanced *nursing* knowledge and skills; it is not a *medical* practice, although APNs perform expanded medical therapeutics in many roles. Throughout nursing's history, nurses have assumed "medical" roles. For example, common nursing tasks such as blood pressure measurement and administration of chemotherapeutic agents were once exclusively performed by physicians. When APNs begin to transfer new skills or interventions into their repertoire, they become nursing skills, informed by the clinical practice values of the profession.

In addition, advanced practice nursing needs to be understood in a conceptually clear fashion that recognizes the core competencies that all APNs share. Conceptual clarity can guide educational curricula to ensure that all APNs learn the core competencies so essential to successful practice.

CORE DEFINITION OF ADVANCED PRACTICE NURSING

As can be seen from this brief review, advanced practice nursing is defined in different and sometimes contradictory ways. A central and agreed-upon definition of advanced practice nursing and clarity regarding its application in various health-care settings are critical to the continued development of advanced practice nursing and to the nursing profession itself.

The definition proposed in this chapter builds on and extends the understanding of advanced practice proposed in the first two editions of this book. In this section a core definition of advanced practice nursing is proposed; the differences among the advanced practice roles are described in the following section. Important assertions of this discussion are as follows:

- Advanced practice nursing is a function of educational and practice preparation *and* a constellation of primary criteria and core competencies.
- Direct clinical practice is the central competency of any APN role.
- All APNs share the same core criteria and competencies, though the actual clinical skill set varies depending on the needs of the patient population.
- Actual practices differ significantly based on the needs of the specialty patient population served and the organizational framework within which the role is performed. Particular APN roles have different "shapes" and include additional competencies specific to them. This is most clearly exemplified in the CRNA and CNM roles, but it is true for all the APN roles. Consequently, it is both necessary and preferable to retain varied job titles that reflect these actual practices, rather than reduce all APNs to one title.

In spite of the need to keep job descriptions and job titles distinct in practice settings, it is critical that the public's confusion about advanced practice be decreased and its acceptance of advanced practice nursing be enhanced. As Safriet (1993, 1998) noted, nursing's future depends on reaching consensus on titles and consistent preparation for title holders. The burden is clearly on the nursing profession and its APNs to be clear, concrete, and consistent about APN titles and their functions in discussions with nursing's larger constituencies: consumers, other health-care professionals, health-care administrators, and health-care policymakers.

Conceptual Definition

Davies and Hughes (1995) note, "The term advanced nursing practice extends beyond roles. It is a way of thinking and viewing the world based on clinical knowledge, rather than a composition of roles" (p. 157). In the ANA's *Scope and Standards of Advanced Practice Registered Nursing* (1996) the central activities of APNs are defined as follows:

Advanced practice registered nurses manifest a high level of expertise in the assessment, diagnosis, and treatment of the complex responses of individuals, families, or communities to actual or potential health problems, prevention of illness and injury, maintenance of wellness, and provision of comfort. The advanced practice registered nurse has a master's or doctoral education concentrating in a specific area of advanced nursing practice, had supervised practice during graduate education, and has ongoing clinical experiences. Advanced practice registered nurses continue to perform many of the same interventions used in basic nursing practice. The difference in this practice relates to a greater depth and breadth of knowledge, a greater degree of synthesis of data, and complexity of skills and interventions. (p. 2)

Integrating this understanding with the ANA's (1995, 2003) components of advanced practice, I conceptualize advanced practice nursing as follows:

Advanced practice nursing is the application of an expanded range of practical, theoretical, and research-based competencies to phenomena experienced by patients within a specialized clinical area of the larger discipline of nursing.[2]

---

[2]The term *patient* is intended to be used interchangeably with *individual* and *client*.

The term *competencies* refers to any area of skillful performance. In this context, competencies encompass any of the activities undertaken as part of delivering advanced nursing care, including assessment, diagnosis, planning, intervention/treatment, and evaluation. Some competencies are processes that APNs use in all dimensions of their practice, such as collaboration and leadership. Through graduate education and practice experiences, APNs expand their capability to provide and direct care. As noted, although certain activities may also be performed by physicians and other health-care professionals, the experiential, theoretical, and philosophical perspectives of nursing make these activities advanced *nursing* practice when they are carried out by an APN. In addition, advanced practice nursing involves highly developed nursing skills, as well as performance of selected medical therapies, as the defining characteristics will clarify. The nursing profession needs to be clear on this point, for *the advanced practice of nursing is not the junior practice of medicine.*

The definition recognizes that not all nursing competencies are research based at this point in nursing's evolution. Theoretical understanding and practice expertise are also key adjuncts to advanced practice. The definition acknowledges the strong experiential component necessary to develop the competencies of advanced practice nursing. Although graduate education in nursing provides a critical foundation for the expanded knowledge and theory base necessary to support advanced practice nursing, in-depth clinical experiences are equally critical. Graduate education and clinical practice experience work synergistically to develop the APN. The definition also emphasizes the patient-focused and specialized nature of advanced practice nursing. Finally, the critical importance of ensuring that any type of advanced practice is grounded within the larger discipline of nursing is made explicit.

Advanced practice nursing is further defined by three primary criteria and seven core competencies, one of them central to the others. This discussion and the chapters in Part II isolate each of these core competencies to clarify them. The reader should recognize that this is only a cognitive device for clarifying the conceptualization of advanced practice nursing used in this book. In reality, these elements are integrated into an APN's practice; they are not separate and distinct features. The concentric circles in Figures 3-1 through 3-3 represent the seamless nature of this interweaving of elements. In addition, the APN's skills function synergistically to produce a whole that is greater than the sum of its parts. The essence of advanced practice nursing is found not only in the primary criteria and competencies demonstrated but also in the synthesis of these elements, along with individual nurse characteristics, into a unified composite practice (Davies & Hughes, 1995) that conforms to the conceptual definition presented earlier.

Primary Criteria

Certain criteria (or qualifications) must be met before a nurse can be considered an APN. Although these baseline criteria are not *sufficient* in and of themselves, they are *necessary* core elements of advanced practice nursing. The three primary criteria for advanced practice are shown in Figure 3-1 and include an earned graduate degree with a concentration in an advanced practice nursing category, professional certification of practice at an advanced level within a given specialty, and a practice that is focused on patients and their families. These criteria are most often the ones used by states to regulate APN practice because they are objective and easily measured.

First, the APN must possess an *earned graduate (master's or doctoral) degree with a concentration in an APN category.* Advanced practice students acquire specialized knowledge and skills through study and supervised practice at either the master's or the doctoral level.

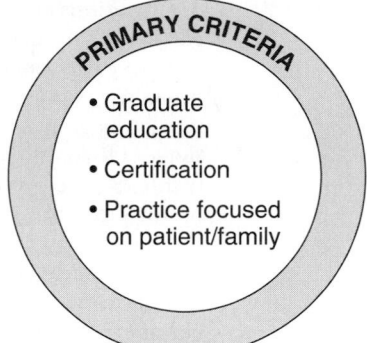

FIGURE 3-1 • Primary criteria of advanced practice nursing.

The content of study includes theories and research findings relevant to the core of a particular advanced nursing specialty. The expansion of practice skills is acquired through clinical experience in addition to faculty-supervised practice (ANA, 1995; American Association of Colleges of Nursing, 1996). As noted previously in the ANA's definition, there is consensus that a master's education in nursing is a requirement for advanced practice nursing, with the exception of the nurse-midwifery specialty. (The issue of educational requirements for nurse-midwifery is explored in depth in Chapter 16; see also Hanson & Hamric, 2003.)

Why is graduate educational preparation necessary for advanced practice nursing? As the knowledge base within specialties has grown, so too has the need for formal education at the graduate level. Some of the differences between basic and advanced nursing practice are apparent in the range and depth of APNs' clinical knowledge; in APNs' ability to anticipate patient responses to health, illness, and nursing interventions; in their ability to analyze clinical situations and explain why a phenomenon has occurred or why a particular intervention has been chosen; and in their skill in assessing and addressing nonclinical variables that influence patient care. Because of the interaction and integration of graduate education in nursing and their extensive clinical experience, APNs are able to exercise a level of discrimination in clinical judgment that is unavailable to other experienced clinicians (Spross & Baggerly, 1989). Professionally, requiring graduate preparation is important to create parity among all APN roles so that all can move forward together in addressing policy-making and regulatory issues. This parity advances the profession's standards and ensures more uniform credentialing mechanisms. Creating a normative educational expectation also enhances nursing's image and credibility with other disciplines. Moves by other health-care providers, such as physical therapists and social workers, to require graduate preparation for practice argue for nursing to have master's-prepared experts to achieve parity with other disciplines. Nursing has a particular need to achieve greater credibility with medicine. Organized medicine has historically been eager to point to nursing's internal differences in APN education as evidence that APNs are inferior providers. Finally, the research skills necessary for evidence-based practice (EBP) and the theory base required for advanced practice nursing mandate education at the graduate level.

Second, APNs must have *professional certification for practice at an advanced level within a clinical specialty.* The continuing growth of specialization has dramatically increased the amount of knowledge and experience required to practice safely in modern health-care settings. National certification examinations have been developed by specialty organizations and are used to determine whether nurses meet standards for practice in a particular clinical specialty. Historically, these examinations tested the specialty knowledge of experienced nurses and not knowledge at the advanced level of practice. Two notable exceptions are the CNM and CRNA certifying examinations (see Chapter 1). As regulatory groups, particularly state boards of nursing, have increasingly used the certification credential to recognize APN providers, the picture has changed and more APN certifications have been developed (see Chapter 22). NPs now have a number of certification options for both primary care and acute care practices. Although the American Nurses Credentialing Center has sponsored CNS certification examinations in medical-surgical and psychiatric areas for years, advanced practice certification examinations in particular specialties such as maternal-child health have been slow to develop. However, the number of examination options for CNSs is increasing. For example, the Oncology Nursing Society began administering an advanced practice certification examination in 1995, and advanced practice certifications for CNSs exist in such specialties as critical care and rehabilitation nursing (see Chapter 19 for additional examples). If no certification examination exists for the advanced practice level of a particular specialty, the APN should be certified at the highest level available, or alternative mechanisms should be developed to ensure competency for APN practice. The ANA and various specialty organizations should continue to develop certification for advanced practice nursing based on graduate education so that all APN certifications will be at the graduate level. Lyon (2002) notes the importance of states including "alternative mechanism" language to allow state boards of nursing to develop alternative ways for CNSs to demonstrate competency during the time when there is no national certification examination available in their specialty (see Lyon & Minarik, 2001, for a full description of one such alternative mechanism). This alternative is essential for CNSs in certain specialties and is being used in a number of states (see Chapters 12 and 22).

Why is it important that national certification at an advanced practice level be a primary criterion for advanced practice nursing? As early as 1980, in the seminal document *Nursing: A Social Policy Statement*, the ANA definitively stated:

[T]he public needs clear evidence that a nurse who claims to be a specialist does indeed have expertise of a particular kind. The profession of nursing has a social obligation to the public to satisfy that need, which it does by means of certification of specialists and by accreditation of the graduate programs that educate specialists in nursing practice. These two methods by which the public is protected against false claims are in accord with the prerogative of self-regulation (within the profession) that society has accorded as a trust to its professions. It is in the absence of such within-profession credentialing that the public turns to the law for its protection. Through credentialing of those nurses who claim competence at an expert level, the nursing profession assures the public that these claims of a higher standard of nursing competence are not false. (ANA, 1980, p. 24)

The NCSBN's recent position paper on the *Regulation of Advanced Practice Nursing* (2002) reiterates that certification is one of the core qualifications for recognition and regulation of APNs. In addition, continuing variability in graduate curricula make sole reliance on graduate education insufficient to protect the public. For example, a recent survey of CNS programs in the United States (Walker et al., 2003) revealed tremendous variability in both program length (varying from 27 to 60 credit hours required) and clinical practice experiences (ranging from 3 to 42 credit hours required). Given this variability, it is difficult to argue (as has the National Association of Clinical Nurse Specialists [NACNS], 2003) that graduate education alone can provide sufficient evidence of competence for regulatory purposes. National certifying examinations provide a consistent standard that each APN must meet to demonstrate beginning competency for an advanced level of practice in his or her specialty. Finally, certification enhances title recognition in the regulatory arena, which promotes the visibility of advanced practice nursing and enhances the public's access to APN services.

Table 3-1 lists numbers of APNs and numbers certified in the United States from 1992 through 2000. Certification percentages have increased for all APN specialty groups, with the exception of CRNAs, who have a consistently high percentage of certified practitioners.

Third, the APN engages in a *practice focused on patients and their families.* To promote clarity about advanced practice nursing, it is critical that the term should be used to describe advanced *clinical* practice (ANA, 1995) and to refer to roles that have direct clinical practice as their central focus. This does not imply that direct practice is the only activity that APNs undertake. APNs also educate others, participate in and conduct research, and serve as consultants (Brown, 1998). However, to be considered an APN role, the patient/family direct practice focus must be primary. As noted earlier, there are other important specialized roles in the profession, notably, education, administration, and research. These roles are valuable and vital to the profession's continued development. They are "critical to the preparation of nurses for practice, the provision of environments that are conducive to nursing practice, and the continued development of the knowledge base that nurses use in practice" (ANA, 1995, p. 15). Some of the nurses in these roles possess advanced practice knowledge and skills as well. However, if they do not have a patient/family-focused clinical practice, they are not considered APNs by this definition.

The central clinical requirement puts some community health nurses in a gray area between advanced nursing practice and specialized practices of program development or consultation. Some APNs in community-based practices take a community view of their practice and consider the community to be their patient or client. Certainly, the broad perspective of the APN encompasses the community and society in which care is provided (Davies & Hughes, 1995); effecting positive outcomes for populations of patients is an important expectation for APNs in general. The National Organization of Nurse Practitioner Faculties (NONPF) has integrated community health concepts into NP education and considers them to be a core competency of NP practice (NONPF, 2000).

However, advanced practice nursing, as it is conceptualized by the profession, is focused on and realized at the level of clinical practice with patients and families. As long as APNs in community health practices maintain a direct clinical practice focused on patients and their families in addition to programmatic or consultative responsibilities, they are APNs by this definition. Community health specialists who do not have a patient-focused practice but rather focus on community assessment, monitoring community health status, and developing policies and program plans are more appropriately considered specialty nurses rather than APNs (Hanson & Hamric, 2003). Community/public health nursing leaders have further differentiated their specialty from this understanding of advanced practice nursing in a recent report on graduate education (Association of Community Health Nursing Educators Task Force on Community/Public Health Master's Level Preparation, 2000). The competencies they list for the community/public health specialty also differ from the core APN competencies. Master's level programs are also being developed for staff development and clinical educators, which are also valuable roles. Some of the students in these programs also take certification examinations in their specialty. However, if the focus of these educator roles is on staff nurses or students, rather than on patients and their families, they would not be considered APN roles according to the definition advanced here. A patient/family-centered focus helps differentiate APNs from other nurses with master's degrees, particularly those in education, administration, and community/public health.

Why limit the definition of advanced practice nursing to roles focused on clinical practice to patients and families? There are many reasons. Nursing is a practice profession. The nurse-patient interface is at the core of nursing practice; in the final analysis, the reason the profession exists is to render nursing services to individuals in need of them. Clinical practice expertise in a given specialty develops from these nurse-patient encounters and lies at the heart of advanced practice nursing. In addition, ongoing direct clinical practice is necessary to maintain and develop an APN's expertise. Without regular immersion in practice, the cutting-edge clinical acumen and expertise found in APN practices cannot be sustained.

The focus of all the APN roles discussed in this book is the patient and family. Emerging roles must be similarly focused on direct clinical practice to be considered advanced practice roles. If every specialized role in nursing were considered advanced practice nursing, the term would become so broad as to lack meaning and explanatory value (see also Cronenwett, 1995). For example, a nurse administrator functions very differently than a CNM does. Distinguishing between APN roles and other specialized roles in nursing can help clarify the concept of advanced practice nursing to consumers, to other health-care providers, and even to other nurses. In addition, the monitoring and regulation of advanced practice nursing are increasingly important issues as APNs work toward more authority for their practices (see Chapter 22). If the definition of advanced practice nursing included nonclinical roles, development of sound regulatory mechanisms would be impossible.

Some nurses with specialized skills in administration, research, and community health have viewed this direct practice requirement as a devaluing of their contributions to the nursing profession. Some faculty who teach clinical nursing but do not themselves maintain an advanced clinical practice have also felt disenfranchised because they are not considered APNs by virtue of this primary criterion. Perhaps this problem has been exacerbated with the term *advanced* used to describe this practice because this term can inadvertently imply that other nurses who do not fit into the APN definition are not "advanced" (i.e., are not as well prepared or highly skilled as APNs). The newest ANA social policy statement draft (2003) deals with this issue by differentiating advanced practice RNs from nurses in other advanced roles. The contention advanced in this book is that there is no value difference between a specialized nurse and an APN: both are equally important to the overall growth and strengthening of the profession. The profession must be able to differentiate its various roles without such differentiation being viewed as a disparagement of any one group. Thus it is critical to understand that this definition of advanced practice nursing is not a value statement, but a differentiation of one group of nurses from other groups for the sake of clarity within and outside of the profession. As the ANA (1995) notes, *all* nurses—whether their focus is clinical practice, educating students, conducting research, planning community programs, or leading nursing service organizations—are valuable and necessary to the integrity and growth of the larger profession. However, all nurses—particularly those with advanced degrees—are *not the same*, nor are they necessarily APNs. Historically, the profession has had difficulty differentiating itself and has struggled with the prevailing lay notion that "a nurse is a nurse is a nurse." This view does not match the reality of the health-care arena, nor does it celebrate the diverse contributions of all the various nursing roles and specialties.

Direct Clinical Practice: The Central Competency

As noted earlier, the primary criteria are necessary but insufficient elements of the definition of advanced practice nursing. Advanced practice is further defined by a set of core competencies that are enacted in each APN role. The first core competency of direct clinical practice is central to and informs all of the others (Figure 3-2). In one sense, it is "first among equals" of the seven core competencies that define advanced practice nursing. Advanced practice nursing is first and foremost characterized by excellence in direct clinical practice. Although APNs do many things in addition to direct clinical practice, direct care expertise provides the foundation necessary for APNs to demonstrate other competencies, such as consultation, patient and staff teaching, and leadership within organizations.

However, clinical expertise alone should not be equated with advanced practice nursing. The work of Patricia Benner and her colleagues (Benner, 1984; Benner, Hooper-Kyriakidis, & Stannard, 1999; Benner, Tanner, & Chesla, 1996) is a major contribution to an understanding of clinically expert nursing practice. The reader will see this important work reflected in various ways throughout the chapters of this book. These researchers extensively studied expert nurses in acute care clinical settings and described the engaged clinical reasoning and domains of practice they observed in clinically expert nurses. Although some of the participants in this research were APNs (in the most recent report [Benner et al., 1999], 16% of the nurse participants were APNs), the majority were nurses with extensive clinical experience who did not have APN preparation. Calkin (1984) characterizes these latter nurses as "experts by experience." (See Chapter 2 for a discussion of Calkin's conceptual differentiation between these levels of nursing practice.) Benner and colleagues have not discussed differences in the practices of APNs as compared with other nurses they have studied. In fact, they state, " 'Expert' is not used to refer to a specific role such as an advanced practice nurse. Expertise is found in the practice of experienced clinicians and advanced practice nurses" (Benner et al., 1999, p. 9).

Although clinical expertise is certainly a central ingredient of the direct practice competency, expertise alone does not provide a complete understanding of the clinical practice of APNs. As noted in Chapter 5, advanced direct care practice includes five

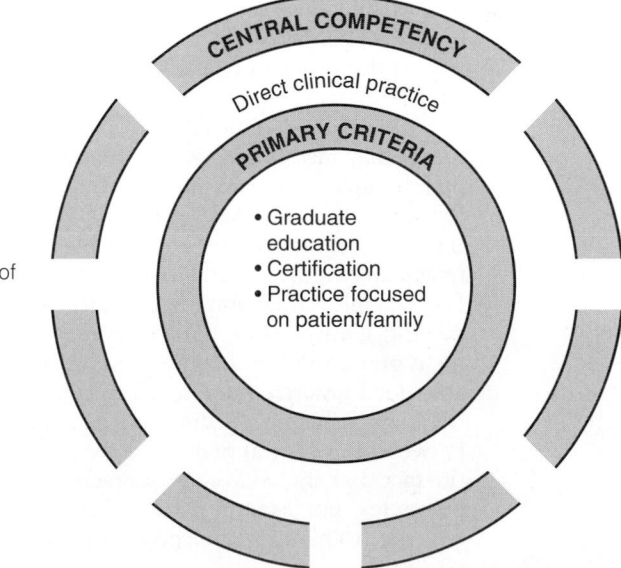

FIGURE 3-2 • Central competency of advanced nursing practice.

characteristics: (1) use of a holistic perspective, (2) formation of partnerships with patients, (3) use of expert clinical thinking and skillful performance, (4) reliance on research evidence as a guide to practice, and (5) use of diverse health and illness management approaches. These characteristics help to distinguish the practice of the expert by experience from that of the APN. As previously noted, experiential knowledge and graduate education work synergistically to develop these characteristics in an APN's clinical practice.

The specific content of the direct practice competency differs significantly by specialty. For example, the clinical practice of a CNS dealing with critically ill children differs from the expertise of an NP managing the health maintenance needs of elderly people or a CRNA administering anesthesia in an outpatient surgical clinic.

Some APNs, particularly CNSs and APN case managers, may spend the majority of their time in activities other than direct clinical practice (see Chapters 12 and 18). So it is important to understand this competency as a central defining characteristic and focus of advanced practice nursing rather than an expectation that APNs only engage in direct clinical practice.

Core Competencies

In addition to the central competency of direct care, six additional competencies further define advanced practice nursing, regardless of role function or setting. These competencies have repeatedly been identified as essential features of advanced practice (American Association of Colleges of Nursing, 1995; ANA, 1995, 2003; Davies & Hughes, 1995; NACNS, 1998; NCSBN, 1993; NONPF, 2002; Spross & Baggerly, 1989). As shown in Figure 3-3, these core competencies are as follows:

1. Expert guidance and coaching of patients, families, and other care providers
2. Consultation
3. Research skills, including use and implementation of evidence-based practice, evaluation, and conduct
4. Clinical and professional leadership, which includes competence as a change agent
5. Collaboration
6. Ethical decision-making skills

These competencies are not unique to advanced practice nursing. Experienced staff nurses may master several of these competencies over time, and this is seen as exemplary performance. These are often the nurses who return to graduate school to become APNs. What distinguishes APN practice is the *expectation* that these competencies are visible in the practice; that is, they are basic elements of the practice. Similarly, many competencies taught in graduate programs are important components of other specialized nursing roles. For example, collaboration, consultation, and leadership are important competencies for nursing administrators. The constellation of competencies and their interaction with the focus on patients and families in direct clinical practice comprise the unique features of advanced practice nursing. Core competencies are similarly learned by all APNs, who then apply them to specific patient populations and settings. In Figure 3-3, the openings between the central practice competency and these additional competencies represent the fact that the APN's direct practice skill interacts with and informs all the other competencies. For example, APNs consult with other providers who seek their practice expertise to plan care for specialty patients. They are able to provide expert guidance and

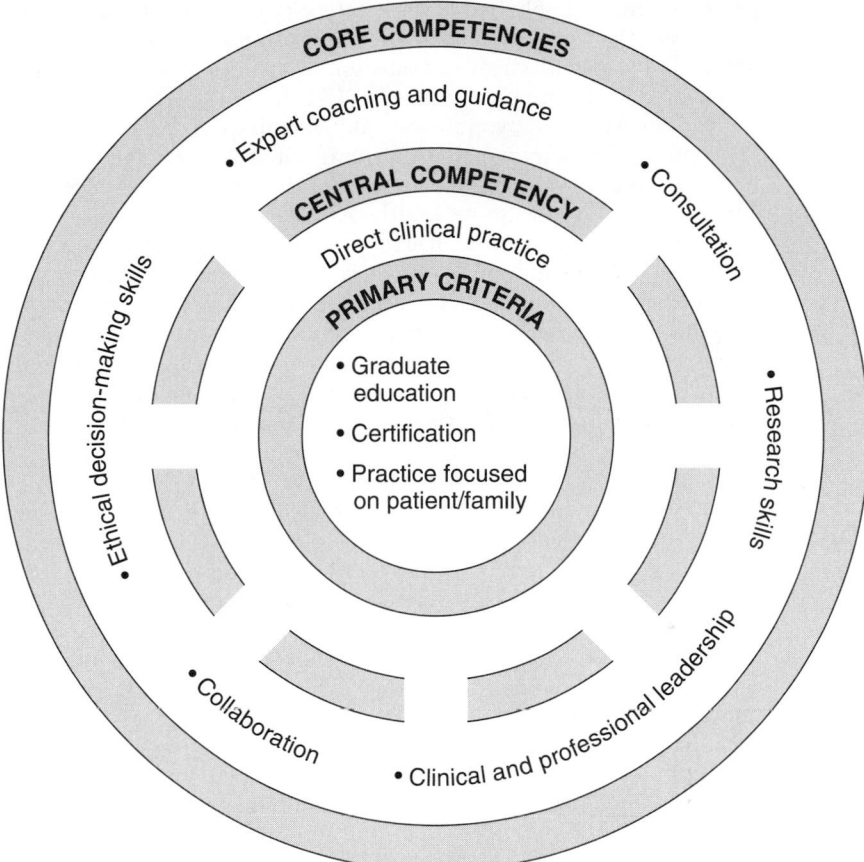

FIGURE 3-3 • Core competencies of advanced practice nursing.

coaching for patients going through health and illness transitions because of their direct practice experience and insight.

It is important to emphasize that these complex competencies develop over time. No APN emerges from a graduate program fully prepared to enact all of them. However, it is critical that graduate programs provide exposure to each competency in the form of didactic content, as well as practical experience so that new graduates can be tested for initial credentialing and be given a base on which to build their practices. These key competencies are described in detail in subsequent chapters and so are not further elaborated here.

Scope of Practice

The term *scope of practice* refers to the legal authority granted to a professional to provide and be reimbursed for health-care services. This authority for practice emanates from many sources, such as state and federal laws and regulations, the profession's code of ethics, and professional practice standards. For all health-care professionals, scope of practice is most closely tied to state statutes; for nursing, these statutes are the nurse practice acts of the various states. As previously discussed, an APN's scope of practice is characterized by specialization; expansion of services provided, including diagnosing and prescribing; and autonomy to practice (ANA, 1996). The scopes of practice differ among the various APN roles; various specialty organizations have provided detailed and specific descriptions for their specialties. Carving out an adequate scope of APN practice authority has been a historic struggle for most of the advanced practice specialties (see Chapter 1), and this continues to be a hotly debated issue among and within the health professions. Significant variability in state practice acts continues such that APNs can perform certain activities, notably prescribing medications and practicing without physician supervision, in some states but may be constrained from performing these same activities if they move to another state (Safriet, 1992, 1994). Safriet (1998) noted that, in the last few years, regulatory challenges have been compounded by changes in the financial restructuring of the health-care delivery system. APNs now face new nongovernmental, market-based barriers to their practices. "These impediments, combined with the remaining restrictions embedded in state licensure laws and state and federal payment schemes, will define nursing's agenda in the next few years" (Safriet, 1998, p. 25).

The Pew Commission's Taskforce on Health Care Workforce Regulation (Finocchio, Dower, Blick, Gragnola, & the Taskforce on Health Care Workforce Regulation, 1998) noted that the tension and turf battles between professions and the increased legislative activities in this area "clog legislative agendas across the country" (p. ii). These battles are costly and time consuming, and lawmakers' decisions related to scope of practice are too often distorted by campaign contributions, lobbying efforts, and political power struggles rather than being based on empirical evidence. The Pew Commission Taskforce Report contains a number of recommendations that directly address scope-of-practice concerns, including the need for a national policy advisory body to research, develop, and publish national scopes of practice and continuing competency standards. The Pew Commission Taskforce noted that this body should develop and press the states to enact model legislative language for uniform scopes of practice authority for the health professions, based on evidence of competence (see Chapter 22 for further discussion).

DIFFERENTIATING ADVANCED PRACTICE ROLES: OPERATIONAL DEFINITIONS OF ADVANCED PRACTICE NURSING

As noted earlier, it is critical to the public's understanding of advanced practice nursing that APN roles and resulting job titles reflect actual practices. Because actual practices differ, job titles should differ. (The following corollary is also true: If the actual practices do not differ, the job titles should not differ.) These differences among roles must be clarified in ways that promote understanding of advanced practice, rather than divide the profession (Davies & Hughes, 1995). This spirit of promoting understanding and clarity informs the ensuing discussion. A key assumption is that *all of these APN roles are valuable* in meeting the needs of patients in current and evolving health-care settings.

Table 3-1 provides National Sample Survey data on RNs prepared to practice as APNs (Spratley Johnson, Sochalski, Fritz, & Spencer, 2001). As of 2000, an estimated 196,279 RNs, or 7.3% of the RN population, were prepared in at least one APN role. Nearly 10% of these individuals were from racial or ethnic minority backgrounds as compared with 13.4% of the overall RN population. The overall number of RNs prepared as APNs represents a 41% increase as compared with 1992 data. CNSs and NPs comprise an estimated

| TABLE 3-1 | NUMBER OF ADVANCED PRACTICE NURSES IN THE UNITED STATES |

	1992*			1996†			2000‡		
APN CATEGORY	TOTAL NO.	% CURRENTLY IN NURSING	% NATIONALLY CERTIFIED	TOTAL NO.	% CURRENTLY IN NURSING	% NATIONALLY CERTIFIED	TOTAL NO.	% CURRENTLY IN NURSING	% NATIONALLY CERTIFIED
CRNAs	25,238	86.3	100	30,386	86.7	84.4	29,844	85.7	84.4
CNMs	7,405	85.9	66	6,534	81.7	87.9	9,232	85.7	88.4
CNSs	58,185	86.5	13.5	53,799	90.5	23.6	54,374	87	36.5
NPs	48,237	88.4	58	63,191	88.2	63.5	88,186	89	74
Blended CNS/ NP Preparation (not included in CNS or NP Nos.)	N/A	N/A	N/A	7,802	100	70.9	14,643	95.7	73.4

CRNAs, Certified registered nurse anesthetists; *CNMs,* certified nurse-midwives; *CNSs,* clinical nurse specialists; *NPs,* nurse practitioners.
*From U.S. Department of Health & Human Services, Division of Nursing. (1992). *National Sample Survey of Registered Nurses, 1992.* Washington, DC: Author.
†From U.S. Department of Health & Human Services, Division of Nursing. (1996). *The registered nurse population March 1996: Findings from the National Sample Survey of Registered Nurses.* Washington, DC: Author.
‡From U.S. Department of Health & Human Services, Division of Nursing. (2002). *The registered nurse population March 2000: Findings from the Seventh National Sample Survey of Registered Nurses.* Washington, DC: Author.

80% of all APNs. When changes in each specialty are compared over time, different patterns are evident in the different APN specialties. CRNA numbers show a small drop from 1996 to 2000, although there has been some growth since 1992. CNMs have also experienced some growth, but the criterion for inclusion in this category did not include a master's degree, so it is not possible to determine how many CNMs are educationally prepared as APNs. CNSs have decreased in overall numbers since 1992, although there has been some stabilization from 1996 to 2000. If the number of CNSs currently in nursing is calculated, a 6.4% decrease can be seen from 1992 to 2000. The APN groups that have shown real growth are NPs and blended CNS/NPs. The number of RNs educated as NPs increased by 44.8% between 1996 and 2000. The number of RNs with dual preparation as a CNS and an NP grew by 88% in those same 4 years.

The NCSBN (1993) notes the differences in scopes of practice in each of the advanced roles. Although the NCSBN recognizes overlapping activities within the four APN roles of CNS, NP, CNM, and CRNA, there are activities unique to each role. In addition to each role's unique competencies, differentiation among APNs occurs in a number of dimensions. The nature of the patient population receiving APN care, organizational expectations, emphasis given to specific competencies, and practice characteristics unique to each role also serve to distinguish the practice of one APN group from others. These differences between APN roles are not rigid demarcations. Nursing's scope of practice is dynamic and continually evolving, and this is especially true at the boundaries of the discipline, where advanced practice occurs (ANA, 1995). "Differences among nurses in their scopes of practice can be characterized as intraprofessional intersections across which collegial, collaborative practice occurs" (ANA, 1995, p. 12). These intersections are not rigid lines, but rather are fluid and involve overlapping areas. The intent of this discussion is not to create stereotypical divisions or to deny the dynamic and evolving nature of advanced practice nursing, but rather to describe key differences that are evident in actual practices at this stage in APN evolution (see Chapter 19 for further discussion of evolving APN roles).

Advanced practice nursing is applied in a variety of roles—some established, some emerging. These roles can be considered to be the operational definitions of the concept of advanced practice nursing. Figure 3-4 shows the differing "shapes" of APN roles. The shapes used in the figure do not have any particular significance; rather, they are meant to illustrate that roles differ along varying dimensions, as noted earlier. Figure 3-4 also shows that although each APN role has the common definition, criteria, and competencies of advanced practice nursing at its center, it has its own distinct form. For example, the American College of Nurse-Midwives (2002), the NONPF (2002), the NACNS (1998), and the American Association of Nurse Anesthetists (1992) have identified additional core competencies for the CNM, NP, CNS, and CRNA roles, respectively. Some of these distinctive features of the various roles are listed here. Differences and similarities among roles are further explored in Part III.

The CNS role has been distinguished by the expectation of practice in four subroles: clinical expert, consultant, educator, and researcher (Hamric & Spross, 1989; see also Chapter 12). CNSs are first and foremost clinical experts who provide direct care to patients with complex health problems. CNSs not only learn consultation processes, as do other APNs, but also function as formal consultants within their organizations. Their multifocal practice in these different subroles means that CNS practice is fluid and changeable. Developing, supporting, and educating nursing staff; managing system change in complex organizations to build teams and improve nursing practices; and "massaging the system" (Fenton, 1985) to advocate for patients are unique role expectations of the CNS. Expectations regarding research activities have been central to this role since its inception. More recently, the NACNS (1998) has distinguished CNS practice by characterizing "spheres of influence" in which the CNS develops competencies. These include the patient/client sphere, the nursing personnel sphere, and the organization/network sphere. NPs, whether in primary care or acute care, possess advanced health assessment, diagnostic, and clinical management skills that include pharmacology management (see Chapters 13 and 14). Their focus is expert direct care, managing the health needs of individuals and their families. Incumbents in the classic NP role provide primary health care

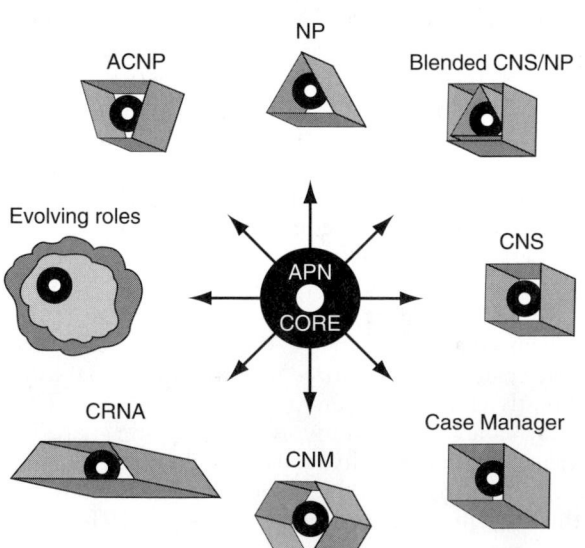

FIGURE 3-4 • Different advanced practice roles. *ACNP,* Acute care nurse practitioner; *NP,* nurse practitioner; *CNS,* clinical nurse specialist; *CNM,* certified nurse-midwife; *CRNA,* certified registered nurse anesthetist.

focused on wellness and prevention; NP practice also includes caring for patients with minor, common, acute conditions and stable chronic conditions. The newer acute care NP (ACNP) brings practitioner skills to a specialized patient population within the acute care setting. The ACNP's focus is the diagnosis and clinical management of acutely or critically ill patient populations in a particular specialized setting. Acquisition of additional medical diagnostic and management skills, such as interpreting computerized tomography and magnetic resonance imaging scans, inserting chest tubes, and performing lumbar punctures, also characterizes this role.

The blended CNS/NP role (see Chapter 15) combines the CNS's in-depth specialized knowledge of a particular patient population with the NP's primary health-care expertise. It is important to clarify that CNSs who acquire NP skills are not necessarily functioning in a blended role. Many work as NPs in either primary care NP or ACNP roles as described earlier. The blended CNS/NP provides primary and specialty care, including clinical management, to a complex patient population, such as children with diabetes. A unique feature of this role is the provision of primary and specialized care such that the blended CNS/NP crosses setting boundaries to provide continuity of care. An additional characteristic that distinguishes this role from that of the ACNP is the expectation of CNS competencies in the three spheres of influence noted earlier. For example, this role combines individual patient management with expectations to develop nursing staff and affect change in complex organizational practices. In addition to acquisition of the advanced practice core competencies, education for this role must include functional role preparation for both the CNS and the NP roles. Blended CNS/NPs must also ensure that their roles are carefully structured to allow time and emphasis in the three spheres of influence.

The CNM (see Chapter 16) has advanced health assessment and intervention skills focused on women's health and childbearing. CNM practice involves independent management of women's health care. CNMs focus particularly on pregnancy, childbirth, the postpartum period, and care of the newborn, but their practices also include family planning, gynecological care, and primary health care for women (American College of Nurse-Midwives, 1997). The CNM's focus is on providing direct care to a select patient population.

CRNA practice (see Chapter 17) is distinguished by advanced procedural and pharmacological management of patients undergoing anesthesia. CRNAs practice independently, in collaboration with physicians, or as employees of a health-care institution. Like CNMs, their focus is providing direct care to a select patient population. Both CNM and CRNA practices are also distinguished by well-established national standards, national examinations, and certification for practice at the advanced specialty level.

APN case managers (see Chapter 18) manage complex care for patients with high-risk or resource-intensive conditions. They identify patient needs for interdisciplinary care and develop and coordinate an integrated plan of care. In addition to direct clinical practice, APN case managers develop interdisciplinary clinical guidelines that support quality and cost outcomes for individual patients and patient populations. Patient management across delivery networks is an expectation of some of these roles. APN case managers are responsible for patient outcome identification and evaluation and share the risk of not accomplishing outcomes with other team members and the institution. It is important to note that many APN roles, particularly the CNS and ACNP, may have case management as a part of their expectations in managing complex patient problems. However, their roles are not structured solely around case management practice, as is the role of the APN case manager.

These differing roles and their similarities and distinctions are explored in detail in subsequent chapters. In addition, newly evolving opportunities for advanced practice nursing are discussed in Chapter 19. This brief discussion underscores the rich and varied nature of advanced practice nursing and the necessity for retaining and supporting different APN roles and titles in the health-care marketplace. At the same time, a consistent definition of advanced practice nursing undergirds each of these roles.

CRITICAL ELEMENTS IN MANAGING ADVANCED NURSING PRACTICE ENVIRONMENTS

The health-care arena is increasingly fluid and changeable: some would even say it is chaotic. Advanced practice nursing does not exist in a vacuum or a singular environment. Rather, the practice takes place in an increasing variety of health-care delivery environments. These diverse environments are complex admixtures of interdependent elements that affect one another. The term *environment* refers to any milieu in which an APN practices, ranging from a community in a rural health-care practice for a primary care NP to a complex tertiary health-care organization for an ACNP. Certain core features of these environments dramatically shape advanced practice and must be managed by APNs for their practices to survive and thrive (see Figure 3-5). Although not technically part of the core definition of advanced practice nursing, these environmental features are included here to frame the growing understanding that APNs must be aware of these key elements in any practice setting. Furthermore, APNs must be prepared to contend with and shape these aspects of their practice environment to be able to fully enact advanced practice nursing.

The environmental elements that affect APN practice include managing reimbursement and business aspects of the practice, dealing with marketing and contracting considerations, understanding regulatory and credentialing requirements, understanding and shaping health policy considerations, strengthening organizational structures and cultures to support advanced practice nursing, and enabling outcome evaluation and performance improvement. Part IV of this book explores these elements in depth. Common to all of these environmental elements are the increasing use of technology and the need for APNs to master a variety of new technologies in implementing procedures. Electronic technology is likewise changing health-care practice in documentation formats, coding schemas, communications, Internet use, and provision of care across state lines through telehealth practices. Learning to use new technologies comfortably is a big challenge for APNs, as it is for all health-care providers in the 21st century.

Managing the business and legal aspects of practice is increasingly critical to survival as a primary care provider in the competitive health-care marketplace. However, APNs who practice primarily in tertiary care settings must also understand the reimbursement issues and legal constraints within their organizations. Given the increasing competition among physicians, APNs, and nonphysician providers, APNs must be prepared to assertively and knowledgeably market their services. Marketing oneself as a new NP in a small community may look different from marketing oneself as a CNS in a large health system, but the principles are the same. Marketing considerations often include the need to advocate for and actively create positions that do not currently exist. Contract considerations are much more complex at the APN level, and all APNs, whether newly graduated or experienced, must be prepared to enter into contract negotiations. Health policy at state and federal levels is an increasingly potent force shaping advanced practice; regulations and policies that flow from legislative actions can enable or constrain APN practices. Variations in the strength and number of APNs in various states attest to the power of this environmental factor. Organizational structures and cultures, whether those of a

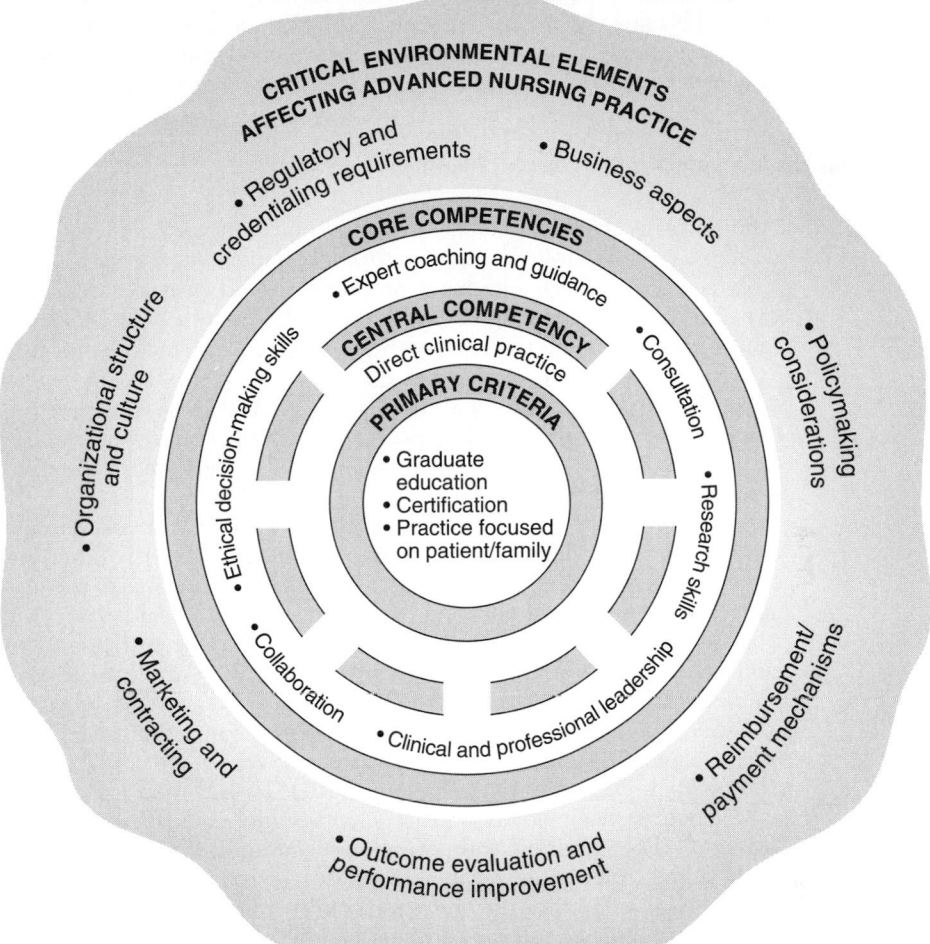

FIGURE 3-5 • Critical elements in advanced nursing practice environments.

community-based practice or a hospital unit, are also important facilitators of or barriers to advanced practice; APN students must learn to assess and intervene to build organizations and cultures that strengthen APN practice. Finally, APNs are accountable for the use of evidence-based practice to ensure positive patient and system outcomes. Measuring the favorable impact of advanced practice nursing on these outcomes and effecting performance improvements are essential activities that all APNs must be prepared to undertake.

IMPLICATIONS OF THE DEFINITION OF ADVANCED PRACTICE NURSING

Many of the implications of the definition of advanced practice nursing presented here have been noted throughout the chapter, such as the necessity for graduate preparation for APN roles and the need for an individual nurse to meet the core definition, criteria, and competencies to be considered an APN. Because of the centrality of direct clinical practice, APNs must hold onto and make explicit their direct patient care activities. In addition, other implications for education, practice, and research flow from this understanding of advanced practice nursing.

Implications for Advanced Practice Nursing Education

APN roles involve many components and competencies. As a result, APNs require a considerable period of role development to fully implement the varied aspects of their practice (see Chapter 4). Graduate programs should provide anticipatory socialization experiences to prepare students for their chosen role. Graduate experiences should include practice in all the competencies of advanced practice, not just clinical practice expertise. For example, students who have no theoretical base or guided practice experiences in consultative skills or clinical leadership will be ill-equipped to demonstrate these competencies on assuming a new APN role. However, even with the best graduate education, no APN new to practice can be expected to perform all the role components and competencies with equal skill.

Other implications concern the education of APNs. Universities must develop articulation programs to help certificate-prepared nurses currently functioning in APN roles obtain master's degrees, and to transition certificate programs to the master's level (this is particularly an issue for nurse-midwifery and women's health NPs). Graduate educators need to support these articulation programs and develop curricula to provide this education. The profession has embraced a wide variety of graduate educational models for preparing APNs, including direct-entry programs for nonnurse college graduates and RN-to-MSN programs. In addition, doctoral preparation for advanced practice nursing has received recent attention (Mundinger et al., 2000; Pearson, Borbasi, & Gott, 1997; Marion et al., 2003; Hanson & Hamric, 2003). These various educational models differ in experience, program length, and academic requirements. Ensuring quality and standardization of APN education in the various specialties is a professional imperative. As previously noted, the variability in some master's programs in terms of both content and clinical hours constrains the profession's ability to regulate advanced practice and guarantee a highly skilled, uniformly educated APN to the public. Likewise, research is needed on the outcomes of these different APN educational pathways in terms of APN graduate experiences and patient outcomes. Such data would be invaluable in continuing to refine advanced practice education.

Schools of nursing must not completely homogenize the preparation for advanced practice nursing. Certainly, all students need exposure to the core definition and competencies of advanced practice described here. However, APNs enact these competencies in widely varying ways in different positions. Schools must provide sufficient functional role preparation so that students are prepared to enter specific work roles. This point seems obvious in a discussion of CNMs and CRNAs, but it is important for CNSs and NPs as well. In a study of NPs who had previously practiced as CNSs, Lindeke et al. (1997) found distinct differences in specific NP and CNS practices that demonstrated that different knowledge and skills were needed to adequately perform each role. They state, "Master's-level educational programs in nursing that combine NP and CNS roles into a single advanced practice role face the danger of diluting the strong competencies of each role" (p. 287). The blended CNS/NP role described in Chapter 15 requires preparation for both roles to enable blended APN practice. Educational standards developed by national specialty organizations for particular APN roles are assuming increasing importance in guiding curricular decisions. These standards have significant differences among them, particularly in the skill set expected for each role. Programs that prepare only a generic APN who has no specific preparation for assuming a particular APN role (or two roles, in the case of the blended CNS/NP) are doing their students, prospective employers of APNs, and the nursing profession a disservice. This role preparation is difficult to ensure when the content is not explicitly addressed but rather "integrated" in clinical coursework. In clinical courses, students are understandably focused on gaining the clinical knowledge base needed for their APN role and often do not concentrate on the other core APN competencies and particular competencies unique to their chosen APN role. Role courses are also extremely helpful in enabling students to differentiate themselves from other APNs and other providers (such as physician assistants) and to explore the many issues surrounding advanced practice nursing (see Chapter 4 and Hamric & Hanson, 2003).

A final educational implication relates to the need for advanced practice nursing students to understand the critical elements in health-care environments that must be managed if their practices are to survive and grow. Beginning graduate students are frequently unaware of the issues involved in enabling advanced practice, particularly the larger policy and regulatory issues. They have often come from clinical environments in which their roles were standardized and focused solely on patient care. Graduate education exposes them to a broader field of vision, and exposure to the issues is invaluable. However, graduate programs must not only include discussion of issues and trends but must also provide students with strategies for managing these issues. Many promising APNs have been unprepared to handle the rough-and-tumble practice environments they entered after graduation, and as a result, their practices have not survived. In some cases, influential leaders in a particular environment have interpreted an individual APN's difficulties to mean that advanced practice was not necessary to achieve desirable patient outcomes and to improve system practices. Such experiences devalue advanced practice nursing and are harmful for individual APNs and the profession. Developing clinically active and astute faculty who understand practice realities and can provide tools for dealing with them is one strategy that graduate programs can use to help students. Providing students with clinical practice experiences that include guided reflection on these key elements is another strategy. Projects designed to focus on the critical elements—such as analyzing regulatory requirements for particular roles, developing an outcome management plan for a complex patient problem, and designing a marketing portfolio—can give students a significant advantage as they enter the marketplace in search of APN positions.

Clearly, graduate program length is an issue with many of these recommendations. Programs that endeavor to shorten clinical practice time or course requirements must balance their desires to be "user friendly" and competitive with other programs with their obligation to prepare APN students who are equipped to enter challenging practice roles in complex settings. As the knowledge base grows and the profession's understanding of advanced practice increases, curricula must also grow. The recognition of this growing knowledge base is one dynamic that fuels interest in the clinical doctorate. Finding a balance remains an ongoing challenge. However, adequate graduate preparation is the necessary foundation for advanced practice nursing to survive and reach its full potential in the 21st century.

Implications for Practice Environments

The fact that new APNs need a period of role development before they can master all of the components and competencies of their chosen role has important implications for employers of new APNs. Employers should provide experienced preceptors, some structure for the new APN, and ongoing support for role development (see Chapter 4 for further recommendations).

"Each individual who practices nursing at an advanced level does so with substantial autonomy and independence requiring a high level of accountability" (NCSBN, 1993, p. 3). Advanced practice roles require considerable autonomy and authority to be fully enacted. Practice settings have not always structured APN roles to allow sufficient autonomy or accountability for achievement of the patient and system outcomes that are expected of advanced practitioners. Federal and state regulations have further limited the potential of APN roles by not recognizing advanced practice or by placing APNs in dependent positions with respect to their physician colleagues. Although encouraging progress has been made, APNs and their advocates must continue to work actively for removal of these barriers if advanced practice nursing is to flourish.

It is equally important to emphasize that APNs have direct and expanded responsibilities to patients. Expanded authority for practice requires expanded responsibility for practice. APNs must demonstrate a higher level of responsibility and accountability if they are to be seen as legitimate providers of care and full partners on provider teams responsible for patient populations. This willingness to be accountable for practice will also promote consumers' and policymakers' perceptions of APNs as credible providers in line with physicians.

The APN leadership competency mandates that APNs serve as visible role models and mentors for other nurses (Cronenwett, 1995; also see Chapter 9). Leadership is not optional in APN practice: it is a requirement. APNs must be a visible part of the solution to the health-care system's problems. For this goal to be realized, each APN must practice leadership in his or her daily activities. In practice environments, the roles need to be structured to allow time and opportunities for this leadership, including mentoring activities with new nurses.

Finally, APN roles must be structured and understood as providing advanced nursing skills rather than as simply substituting for physicians. Advanced practice nursing is a value-added complement to medical practice, not a substitution for it. This is particularly an issue for CRNA, NP, and ACNP roles, which involve additional medical therapeutics in practice. As the number of physicians increases, particularly the number of physicians prepared in family practice and the new "hospitalist" practices, this distinction must be clear in the minds of employers and insurers and must be equally clear in the minds of APNs' staff nurse and physician colleagues. As noted earlier, the advanced practice of nursing is not the junior practice of medicine. The value-added service that APNs provide to patients involves all of the differing perspectives and elements discussed in this chapter. In most cases, advanced nursing practice needs to be understood as complementary to, rather than competing with, medical practice. APNs must be able to clearly and forcefully articulate this critical point if their practices are to survive continued cost cutting in the health-care sector.

Implications for Research

As noted in Chapter 8, the APN may be involved in research at different levels. A baseline expectation is the use of evidence-based practice and the ability to assist others to incorporate research evidence into their practices. Being actively involved in research related to patient care (at whatever level the APN is comfortable) is a crucial ingredient of advanced practice nursing. If research is to be relevant to care delivery and to nursing practice at all levels, APNs must be involved. APNs need to recognize the importance of advancing both the profession's and the health-care system's knowledge about effective patient care practices and to realize that they are a vital link in building this knowledge. APNs are in a key position to uncover the knowledge embedded in clinical practice (Benner, 1984).

Related to this research involvement is the necessity for more research differentiating basic and advanced practice nursing and identifying the patient populations that benefit most from APN intervention. Increasing research evidence that APNs affect or improve outcomes of care is presented in each of the chapters of Part III and in Chapter 25. However, linking advanced practice nursing to specific patient outcomes remains a major research imperative for this century.

CONCLUSION

Today's APNs, future APNs, educators, administrators, and other nursing leaders need to be clear and consistent about the definition of advanced practice nursing so that the profession speaks with one voice. For a profession to succeed, it must have internal cohesion and external legitimacy at the same time (Safriet, 1993). Clarity about the core definition of advanced practice nursing and recognition of the primary criteria and competencies necessary for all APNs will enhance nursing's external legitimacy. At the same time, recognizing the differences among APNs and the legitimacy of different advanced practice roles will enhance nursing's internal cohesion.

REFERENCES

Advanced nursing practice. (2003). *Cumulative Index to Nursing and Allied Health Literature*. Retrieved July 1, 2003.

American Association of Colleges of Nursing. (1995). *The essentials of master's education for advanced practice nursing*. Washington, DC: Author.

American Association of Nurse Anesthetists. (1992). *Guidelines and standards for nurse anesthesia practice*. Park Ridge, IL: Author.

American College of Nurse-Midwives. (2002). *Core competencies for basic midwifery practice*. Washington, DC: Author.

American Nurses Association. (1980). *Nursing: A social policy statement*. Kansas City, MO: Author.

American Nurses Association. (1992). *Nursing facts*. Washington, DC: Author.

American Nurses Association. (1995). *Nursing's social policy statement*. Washington, DC: Author.

American Nurses Association. (1996). *Scope and standards of advanced practice registered nursing*. Washington, DC: Author.

American Nurses Association. (2001). *Code of ethics for nurses with interpretive statements*. Washington, DC: Author.

American Nurses Association. (2003). *Nursing's social policy statement 2003 draft*. Washington, DC: Author.

American Nurses Association. (2003, June 9). *ANA hails introduction of bill to expand access to nurse practitioners* [Press release]. Washington, DC: Author.

Association of Community Health Nursing Educators Task Force on Community/Public Health Master's Level Preparation. (2000, November). *Graduate education for advanced community/public health nursing practice*. Louisville, KY: Author.

Benner, P. (1984). *From novice to expert*. Menlo Park, CA: Addison-Wesley.

Benner, P., Hooper-Kyriakidis, P., & Stannard, D. (1999). *Clinical wisdom and interventions in critical care*. Philadelphia: W. B. Saunders.

Benner, P., Tanner, C. A., & Chesla, C. A. (1996). *Expertise in nursing practice: Caring, clinical judgment, and ethics*. New York: Springer.

Brown, S. J. (1998). A framework for advanced practice nursing. *Journal of Professional Nursing, 14*, 157-164.

Calkin, J. D. (1984). A model for advanced nursing practice. *Journal of Nursing Administration, 14*, 24-30.

Creasia, J. L., & Parker, B. (Eds.). (2001). *Conceptual foundations: The bridge to professional nursing practice* (3rd ed.). St. Louis: Mosby.

Cronenwett, L. R. (1995). Molding the future of advanced practice nursing. *Nursing Outlook, 43*, 112-118.

Davies, B., & Hughes, A. M. (1995). Clarification of advanced nursing practice: Characteristics and competencies. *Clinical Nurse Specialist, 9*, 156-160.

Donley, S. R. (1995). Advanced practice nursing after health care reform. *Nursing Economics, 13*, 84-88.

Fenton, M. V. (1985). Identifying competencies of clinical nurse specialists. *Journal of Nursing Administration, 15*, 31-37.

Finocchio, L. J., Dower, C. M., Blick, N. T., Gragnola, C. M., & the Taskforce on Health Care Workforce Regulation. (1998). *Strengthening consumer protection: Priorities for health care workforce regulation.* San Francisco: Pew Health Professions Commission.

Hamric, A. B. (1996). A definition of advanced nursing practice. In A. B. Hamric, J. A. Spross, & C. M. Hanson (Eds.), *Advanced nursing practice: An integrative approach* (pp. 42-56). Philadelphia: W.B. Saunders.

Hamric, A. B. (2000). A definition of advanced nursing practice. In A. B. Hamric, J. A. Spross, & C. M. Hanson (Eds.), *Advanced nursing practice: An integrative approach* (2nd ed., pp. 53-73). Philadelphia: W.B. Saunders.

Hamric, A. B., & Hanson, C. M. (2003). Educating advanced practice nurses for practice reality. *Journal of Professional Nursing, 19*, 262-268.

Hamric, A. B., & Spross, J. A. (Eds.). (1989). *The clinical nurse specialist in theory and practice* (2nd ed.). Philadelphia: W. B. Saunders.

Hanson, C. M. & Hamric, A. B. (2003). Reflections on the continuing evolution of advanced practice nursing. *Nursing Outlook, 51*, 203-211.

Hickey, J. V., Ouimette, R. V., & Venegoni, S. L. (1996). *Advance practice nursing: Changing roles and clinical applications.* Philadelphia: J. B. Lippincott.

Kitzman, H. (1989). The CNS and the nurse practitioner. In A. B. Hamric & J. A. Spross (Eds.), *The clinical nurse specialist in theory and practice* (2nd ed., pp. 379-394). Philadelphia: W. B. Saunders.

Leddy, S. K. (1998). *Conceptual bases of professional nursing* (4th ed.). Philadelphia: J. B. Lippincott.

Lindeke, L. L., Canedy, B. H., & Kay, M. M. (1997). A comparison of practice domains of clinical nurse specialists and nurse practitioners. *Journal of Professional Nursing, 13*, 281-287.

Lyon, B. L. (2002). The regulation of clinical nurse specialist practice: Issues and current developments. *Clinical Nurse Specialist, 16*, 239-241.

Lyon, B. L. & Minarik, P. A. (2001). Statutory and regulatory issues for clinical nurse specialists: Ensuring the public's access to CNS services. *Clinical Nurse Specialist, 15*, 108-114.

Marion, L., Viens, D., O'Sullivan, A., Crabtree, K., Fontana, S., & Price, M. The practice doctorate in nursing: Future or fringe? *Topics in Advanced Practice Nursing eJournal, 3*, 2. Retrieved May 21, 2003, from http://www.medscape.com/viewarticle/453247.

Mundinger, M., Cook, S., Lenz, E., Piacentini, K., Auerhahn, C., & Smith J. (2000). Assuring quality and access in advanced practice nursing: A challenge to nurse educators. *Journal of Professional Nursing, 16*, 322-329.

National Association of Clinical Nurse Specialists. (1998). *Statement on clinical nurse specialist practice and education.* Glenview, IL: Author.

National Association of Clinical Nurse Specialists. (2003). Position paper on regulatory credentialing of clinical nurse specialists. *Clinical Nurse Specialist, 17*, 163-169.

National Council of State Boards of Nursing. (1993). *Position paper on the regulation of advanced nursing practice.* Chicago: Author.

National Council of State Boards of Nursing. (2002). *Position paper on the regulation of advanced practice nursing.* Chicago: Author.

National Organization of Nurse Practitioner Faculties. (2000). *Challenges and opportunities for integrating community health in nurse practitioner programs.* Washington DC: Author.

National Organization of Nurse Practitioner Faculties. (2002). *Nurse practitioner primary care competencies: Adult, family, gerontologic, pediatric and women's health.* Washington, DC: Author.

O'Malley, J., Cummings, S., & King, C. S. (1996). The politics of advanced practice. *Nursing Administration Quarterly, 20*, 62-72.

Pearson, A., Borbasi, S., & Gott, M. (1997). Doctoral education in nursing for practitioner knowledge and for academic knowledge: The University of Adelaide, Australia. *Image—the Journal of Nursing Scholarship, 29*, 365-368.

Rasch, R. F. R., & Frauman, A. C. (1996). Advanced practice in nursing: Conceptual issues. *Journal of Professional Nursing, 12*, 141-146.

Ray, G. L., & Hardin, S. (1995). Advanced practice nursing: Playing a vital role. *Nursing Management, 26*, 45-47.

Safriet, B. J. (1992). Health care dollars and regulatory sense: The role of advanced practice nursing. *Yale Journal of Regulation, 9*, 417-487.

Safriet, B. J. (1993, February). *Keynote address—one strong voice.* Paper presented at the National Nurse Practitioner Leadership Summit, Washington, DC.

Safriet, B. J. (1994). Impediments to progress in health care workforce policy: License and practice laws. *Inquiry, 31*, 310-317.

Safriet, B. J. (1998). Still spending dollars, still searching for sense: Advanced practice nursing in an era of regulatory and economic turmoil. *Advanced Practice Nursing Quarterly, 4*, 24-33.

Smith, M. C. (1995). The core of advanced practice nursing. *Nursing Science Quarterly, 8*, 2-3.

Snyder, M., & Mirr, M. P. (1995). *Advanced practice nursing: A guide to professional development.* New York: Springer.

Spratley, E., Johnson, A., Sochalski, J., Fritz, M., & Spencer, W. (2001, September). *The registered nurse population March 2000: Findings from the National Sample Survey of Registered Nurses.* Washington, DC: U.S. Department of Health and Human Services, Health Resources and Services Administration, Bureau of Health Professions, Division of Nursing.

Spross, J. A., & Baggerly, J. (1989). Models of advanced practice. In A. B. Hamric & J. A. Spross (Eds.), *The clinical nurse specialist in theory and practice* (2nd ed., pp. 19-40). Philadelphia: W. B. Saunders.

Stimpson, M., & Hanley, B. (1991). Nurse policy analyst: Advanced practice role. *Nursing and Health Care, 12*, 10-15.

Thibodeau, J. A., & Hawkins, J. W. (1994). Moving toward a nursing model in advanced practice. *Western Journal of Nursing Research, 16*, 205-218.

Walker, J., Gerard, P. S., Bayley, E. W., Coeling, H., Clark, A. P., Dayhoff, N., et al. (2003). A description of clinical nurse specialist programs in the United States. *Clinical Nurse Specialist, 17*, 50-57.

CHAPTER 4

Role Development of the Advanced Practice Nurse

KAREN A. BRYKCZYNSKI

INTRODUCTION

What is it like to become an advanced practice nurse (APN)? In the current cost-constrained environment, the pressure to be cost-effective and to make an impact on outcomes is greater than ever. Yet literature indicates that the initial year of practice is one of transition (Brown & Olshansky, 1998; Brykczynski, 1996; Kelly & Mathews, 2001), and an APN's maximum potential may not be realized until approximately 5 or more years in practice (Cooper & Sparacino, 1990). This chapter explores the complex processes of APN role development with the objectives of providing (1) anticipatory guidance for APN students; (2) concepts and strategies for faculty teaching APNs; (3) role facilitation strategies for new APNs, APN preceptors, administrators, and interested colleagues; and (4) guidelines for continued role evolution.

This chapter consolidates literature from all of the APN specialties—including clinical nurse specialists (CNSs), nurse practitioners (NPs), certified nurse-midwives (CNMs), and certified registered nurse anesthetists (CRNAs)—to present a generic process relevant to all APN roles. The discussion is separated into the educational component of APN *role acquisition* and the occupational or work component of *role implementation*. This division in the process of role development is intended to clarify and distinguish the changes occurring during role transitions experienced during the educational component of an APN role (role acquisition) and the changes occurring during the actual performance of the role after program completion (role implementation). Strategies for enhancing APN role development are described. The chapter concludes with summary comments and suggestions regarding facilitation of future APN role development and evolution.

PERSPECTIVES ON APN ROLE DEVELOPMENT

Professional role development is a dynamic, ongoing process that, once begun, spans a lifetime. The concept of graduation as commencement, whereby one's career begins on completion of a degree, is central to understanding the evolving nature of professional roles in response to personal, professional, and societal demands (Gunn, 1998). Professional role development literature in nursing is abundant and complex, involving multiple component processes. These include (1) aspects of adult development, (2) development of clinical expertise, (3) modification of self-identity through initial socialization in school, (4) development and integration of professional subrole components, and (5) subsequent resocialization in the work setting. Like socialization for other professional roles, such as those of attorney, physician, teacher, and social worker, the process of becoming an APN involves aspects of adult development, as well as professional socialization.

The professional socialization process in advanced practice nursing involves identification with and acquisition of the behaviors and attitudes of the "aspired to" advanced practice group (Waugaman & Lu, 1999, p. 239). This includes learning the specialized language, skills, and knowledge of the particular APN group; internalizing its values and norms; and incorporating these into one's professional nursing identity and other life roles (Cohen, 1981). Educational institutions in the United States tend to reflect the dominant European-American culture (Waugaman & Lu, 1999). This is especially true of nursing educational institutions that have not achieved major success in diversifying their faculty or student body. In view of the changing demographics of American society, APN faculty need to carefully examine the values and attitudes conveyed during APN programs and develop strategies to be more culturally sensitive not only to students but to patients as well (Leininger, 1994; Waugaman & Lu, 1999). Gender and age are additional factors that are of particular importance in preparing APNs. Waugaman and Lohrer (2000) observed that there are more men entering nursing graduate programs and that the APN specialty group with the highest percentage of men is nurse anesthesia. APN faculty, who are predominantly female and Anglo- or European-American, must recognize these factors and incorporate them into their educational programs.

NOVICE-TO-EXPERT SKILL ACQUISITION MODEL

Acquisition of knowledge and skill occurs in a progressive movement through stages of performance from novice to expert as described by Dreyfus and Dreyfus (1977, 1986, 1996) who studied diverse groups, including pilots, chess players, and adult learners of second languages. This model has broad applicability and can be used to better understand many different skills, which range from playing a musical instrument to writing a research grant. The most widely known application of this model of skill acquisition is Benner's (1984) observational and interview study of clinical nursing practice situations from the perspective of new nurses and their preceptors in hospital nursing services. Although this study included several APNs, it did not specify a particular education level as a criterion for expertise. As noted in Chapter 3, there has been some confusion about this criterion. The Dreyfus model is a situation-based model, not a trait model; therefore the level of expertise is not an individual characteristic of a particular nurse; rather, it is a function of the nurse's familiarity with a particular situation in combination with his or her educational background. This model could be used to study the level of expertise required for other aspects of advanced practice including coaching and guidance, consultation, collaboration, research, ethical decision making, and leadership. In addition to validating and interpreting the Dreyfus skill acquisition model for nurses, Benner (1984) identified and described domains and competencies for nursing practice that Fenton (1985) adapted for CNSs and Brykczynski (1985, 1999) modified for NPs (see Chapter 2).

According to the Dreyfus model, there is a generic process of skill acquisition through which humans proceed in stages from novice to expert as they acquire new psychomotor, perceptual, and judgment skills (Dreyfus & Dreyfus, 1996). The progression from novice to expert is incremental but not necessarily stepwise or linear. Instead, as with growth and development or healing processes, plateaus, setbacks, and even stagnation can occur, as well as occasional leaps forward. The competent level is a critical juncture in the development of expertise. Some individuals do not advance to expertise because they do not become sufficiently engaged in their practice. A change from "acting like," sometimes referred to as *the imposter phenomenon* (Arena & Page, 1992; Brown & Olshansky, 1997, 1998), to individualized embodiment of the new role occurs as the individual moves up to the proficient level. In other words, it takes time and practice for new skills to become fully owned or embodied. Embodiment of a skill occurs after repeated experiences of performing the skill "as if" one actually could do it skillfully. It is a kind of "going through the motions" until, over time, the skill is transformed from the halting stepwise performance of the novice to the holistic fluid performance of the expert.

The proficient level represents a discontinuous, qualitative leap from the competent level whereby intuition, defined as "holistic situation recognition" (Dreyfus & Dreyfus, 1986, p. 28), replaces analytically reasoned responses. Expertise, according to this model, develops over time through direct personal encounters, which alter preconceptions and prior understanding. The deep situational understanding associated with expertise involves holistic pattern recognition, described as "the intuitive ability to use patterns without decomposing them into component features" (Dreyfus & Dreyfus, 1986, p. 28). Decomposition of situations into abstract attributes is associated with earlier skill levels.

Deliberative rationality, a fine-tuning of intuition, takes place at the expert level, replacing the calculative rationality characteristic of other levels (Dreyfus & Dreyfus, 1986). Deliberative rationality is a kind of detached meditative reflection on goals and possible ways to achieve the goals, whereas calculative rationality is the kind of inferential reasoning exhibited by less-than-expert performers when they apply and modify theoretical principles and rules. Deliberative rationality is involved in distinguishing a novel situation or a situation in which the initial grasp may be incorrect from a situation in which experience can be trusted. Such personal expert knowledge is not totally idiosyncratic; it can be shared in ways such as the identification of maxims, common meanings, and exemplars that convey the contextual understanding of clinical situations (Benner, 1984; Benner, Tanner, & Chesla, 1996; Benner, Hooper-Kyriakidis, & Stannard, 1999; Brykczynski, 1991, 1989, 1999; Horvath et al., 1994).

Figure 4-1 shows a typical APN role development pattern in terms of this skill acquisition model. A major implication of the novice-to-expert model for advanced practice

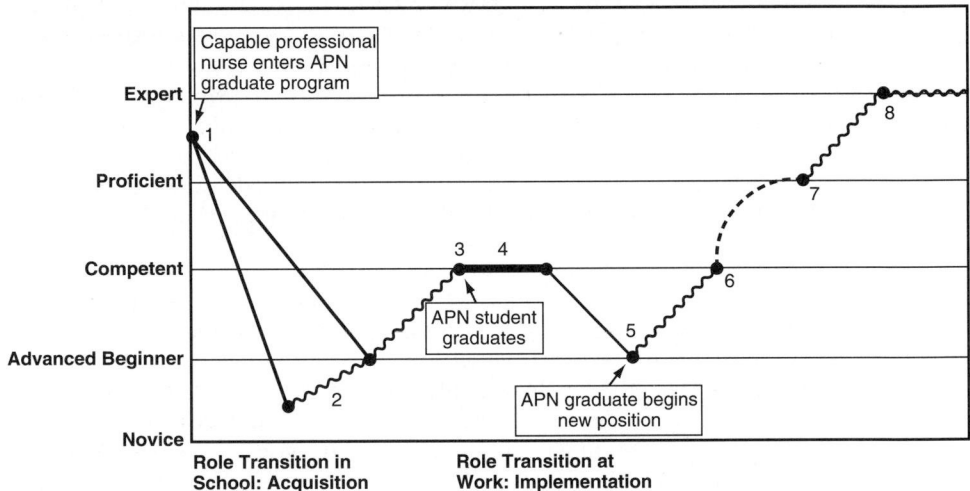

FIGURE 4-1 • Typical advanced practice nurse (APN) role development pattern:
1. APN students typically begin graduate school as proficient or expert nurses.
2. Depending on previous background, the new APN student will revert to novice or advanced-beginner level on assuming the student role.
3. The graduate from an APN program is competent as an APN student but has no experience as a practicing APN.
4. A limbo period is experienced while the APN graduate searches for a position and becomes certified.
5. The newly employed APN reverts to advanced-beginner level in the new APN position as role trajectory begins again.
6. Some individuals remain at the competent level. There is a discontinuous leap from the competent to the proficient level.
7. Proficiency only develops if there is sufficient involvement in practice and embodiment of skills and knowledge.
8. Expertise is intuitive and situation-specific, meaning that not all situations will be managed expertly. Refer to text discussion for details.
NOTE: Refer to Dreyfus skill acquisition model for further details (Benner, Tanner, & Chesla, 1996; Dreyfus & Dreyfus, 1986). For the purpose of illustration this figure is more linear than the individualized role development trajectories that actually occur.

nursing is the claim that even experts can be expected to perform at lower skill levels when they enter new situations or positions. Hamric and Taylor's (1989) report that experienced CNSs starting a new position experience the same role development phases as new graduates, only over a shorter period, supports this claim. Figure 4-1 shows the overall trajectory expected during APN role development; however, each APN experiences a unique pattern of role transitions and life transitions concurrently.

For example, a professional nurse who functions as a mentor for new graduates may decide to pursue an advanced degree as an APN. As an APN graduate student, this nurse will experience the challenges of acquiring a new role, the anxiety associated with learning new skills and practices, and the dependency of being a novice. At the same time, if this nurse continues to work as a registered nurse, his or her functioning in this work role will be at the competent, proficient, or expert level (depending on experience and the situation). On graduation, the new APN may experience a limbo period, during which the nurse is no longer a student and not yet an APN, while searching for a position and meeting certification requirements (see later discussion). Once in a new APN position, this nurse may experience a return to the advanced-beginner stage as he or she proceeds through the phases of role implementation. Even after making the transition to an APN role, progression in role implementation is not a linear process. As Figure 4-1 indicates, there are discontinuities, with movement back and forth as the trajectory begins again. Years later, the APN may decide to pursue yet another APN role. The processes of role acquisition, role implementation, and novice- to-expert skill development will again be experienced (although altered and informed by previous experiences) as the postgraduate student acquires additional skills and knowledge. Role development involves multiple, dynamic, and situational processes, with each new undertaking being characterized by passage through earlier transitional phases with some movement back and forth, horizontally or vertically, as different career options are pursued.

Another significant implication of the Dreyfus model (Dreyfus & Dreyfus, 1977, 1986, 1996) for APNs is the observation that the quality of performance may deteriorate when performers are subjected to intense scrutiny, whether it is their own or that of someone else (Roberts, Tabloski, & Bova, 1997). The increased anxiety experienced by APN students during faculty on-site clinical evaluation visits or during videotaped testing of clinical performance in simulated situations is an example of such intense scrutiny. A third implication of this skill acquisition model for APNs is the need to accrue experience in actual situations over time, so that both practical and theoretical knowledge are refined, clarified, personalized, and embodied, forming an individualized repertoire of experience that guides advanced practice performance.

ROLE CONCEPTS AND ROLE DEVELOPMENT ISSUES

This discussion of professional role issues incorporates role concepts described by Hardy and Hardy (1988) along with the concept that different APN roles represent different subcultural groups within the broader nursing culture (Leininger, 1976). APNs can be described as tricultural and trilingual (Johnson, 1993). They share background knowledge, practices, and skills of three cultures: (1) biomedicine, (2) mainstream nursing, and (3) everyday life. They are fluent in the languages of biomedical science, nursing knowledge and skill, and everyday parlance. Some APNs, CNMs for example, are socialized into a fourth culture as well, that of midwifery. Others are also fluent in more than one everyday language. Just as APN roles can be conceptualized as encompassing skills and knowledge from more than one culture, they can also be seen as encompassing aspects of both male and female occupational sex roles. Because APNs are multicultural, multilingual, and androgynous, they are able to work effectively with many different people in an increasingly diverse world.

The concepts of role stress and strain discussed by Hardy and Hardy (1988) are useful for understanding the dynamics of role transitions (Table 4-1). Hardy and Hardy described role stress as a social structural condition in which role obligations are ambiguous, conflicting, incongruous, excessive, or unpredictable. Role strain is defined as the subjective feeling of frustration, tension, or anxiety experienced in response to role stress. The highly stressful nature of the nursing profession needs to be recognized as the background within which individuals seek advanced education to become APNs (Aiken, Clarke, Sloan, Sochalski, & Saber, 2002; Dionne-Proulz & Pepin, 1993). Role strain can be minimized by the identification of potential role stressors, development of strategies to cope with them, and rehearsal of situations designed for application of those strategies; however, the difficulties experienced by neophytes in new positions cannot be eliminated. As noted previously, expertise is holistic, involving bodily perceptual skills and shared background knowledge, as well as cognitive ability. A school-work, theory-practice, ideal-real gap will remain because of the nature of human skill acquisition.

Spross (personal communication, July 25, 2003) pointed out that Bandura's (1977) social-cognitive theory of self-efficacy may be of interest to APNs in terms of understanding what motivates individuals to acquire skills and what builds confidence as skills are

TABLE 4-1 SELECTED ROLE CONCEPTS		
CONCEPTS	DEFINITION	EXAMPLES
Role stress*	A situation of increased role performance demand	Learning a new role in school
Role strain*	Subjective feeling of frustration, tension, or anxiety in response to role stress	Feeling of decreased self-esteem when performance is below expectations of self or significant others
Role stressors*	Factors that produce role stress	Financial, personal, or academic demands and role expectations that are ambiguous, conflicting, excessive, or unpredictable
Role ambiguity*	Unclear expectations, diffuse responsibilities, uncertainty about subroles	All professional positions have some degree of ambiguity because of the evolving nature of roles and expansion of skills and knowledge.
Role incongruity*	A role with incompatibility between skills and abilities and role obligations or incompatibility between personal values, self-concept, and role obligations	An adult NP in a role requiring pediatric skills and knowledge
Role conflict*	Occurs when role expectations are perceived to be mutually exclusive or contradictory	Intraprofessional role conflict between APNs and other nurses Interprofessional role conflict between APNs and physicians
Role transition*†	A dynamic process of change over time as new roles are acquired	Changing from a staff nurse role to an APN role
Role insufficiency†	Feeling inadequate to meet role demands	New graduate
Role supplementation†	Anticipatory socialization	Role-specific educational components

*Adapted from Hardy, M. E., & Hardy, W. L. (1988). Role stress and role strain. In M. E. Hardy & M. E. Conway (Eds.), *Role theory: Perspectives for health professionals* (2nd ed., pp. 159-239). Norwalk, CT: Appleton & Lange.
†Adapted from Schumacher, K. L., & Meleis, A. I. (1994). Transitions: A central concept in nursing. *Image: The Journal of Nursing Scholarship, 26,* 119-127.

developed. Self-efficacy theory has been used widely to further understanding of skill acquisition with patients, as well as health-care professionals. Application of self-efficacy theory to training health-care professionals in skill acquisition is particularly relevant (Burglehaus, 1997; Clark & Dodge, 1999; Dalton & Blau, 1996; Parle, Maguire, & Heaven, 1997).

Role Ambiguity

Role ambiguity (see Table 4-1) develops when there is a lack of clarity about expectations, a blurring of responsibilities, uncertainty regarding role implementation, and the inherent uncertainty of existent knowledge. According to Hardy and Hardy (1988), role ambiguity characterizes all professional positions. They point out that role ambiguity might be positive in that it offers opportunities for creative possibilities. It can be expected to be more prominent in professions undergoing change, such as those in the health-care field. Role ambiguity has been widely discussed in relation to the CNS role (Chase, Johnson, Laffoon, Jacobs, & Johnson, 1996; Payne & Baumgartner, 1996; Redekopp, 1997; see also Chapter 12), but it is a relevant issue for other APN roles as well, particularly as APN roles evolve (Stahl & Myers, 2002).

Role Incongruity

Role incongruity is intrarole conflict, which Hardy and Hardy (1988) described as developing from two sources. Incompatibility between skills and abilities and role obligations is one source of role incongruity. An example of this is an adult APN hired to work in an emergency department with a large percentage of pediatric patients. Such an APN will find it necessary to enroll in a family NP or pediatric NP program to eliminate this role incongruity. Another source of role incongruity is incompatibility among personal values, self-concept, and expected role behaviors. An APN who hoped for a position with 100% clinical practice may experience this incongruity if the position he or she obtains requires performing administrative functions. An example comes from Banda's (1985) study of psychiatric liaison CNSs in acute care hospitals and community health agencies. She reports that they view consultation and teaching as their major functions, whereas research and administrative activities are associated with role strain.

Role Conflict

Role conflict develops when role expectations are perceived to be contradictory or mutually exclusive. APNs may experience conflict with varying demands of their role, as well as both intraprofessional and interprofessional role conflict.

INTRAPROFESSIONAL ROLE CONFLICT

APNs experience intraprofessional role conflict for a variety of reasons. The historical development of APN roles has been fraught with conflict and controversy in nursing education and nursing organizations, particularly for CNMs (Varney, 1987), NPs (Ford, 1982), and CRNAs (Gunn, 1991; see also Chapter 1). Relationships among these APN groups and nursing as a discipline have improved markedly in recent years, yet difficulties remain.

Communication difficulties among various nursing groups occur in four major areas: (1) at an organizational level, (2) in educational programs, (3) in the literature, and (4) in direct clinical practice. Kimbro (1978) described these communication difficulties in reference to CNMs, but they are relevant for all APN roles. The fact that CNSs, NPs, CNMs, and CRNAs each have specific organizations with different certification requirements, competencies, and curricula creates boundaries and sets up the need for formal lines of communication. Communication gaps occur when courses and textbooks are not shared among APN programs in which more than one specialty is offered in the same school. Specialty-specific journals are another formal communication barrier, because APNs may read only within their own specialty and not keep abreast of larger APN issues. In clinical settings some APNs may be more concerned with providing direct clinical care to individual patients, whereas staff nurses and other APNs may be more concerned with 24-hour coverage and smooth functioning of the unit or the institution. These differences may set the stage for intraprofessional role conflict. Hazle's (1985) descriptive study of interrole conflict between maternity nurses and CNMs indicated that lack of communication is a major source of conflict for nurses in clinical settings. One way to address this issue would be to include APN job descriptions in staff nurse orientation programs.

Hamric and Taylor (1989) point out that staff resistance to change, complacency or apathy, and the fact that nurses have not generally been accustomed to seeking consultation from other nurses as experts can impede CNS role development. Earlier reports of refusals by staff nurses to perform support functions, such as taking vital signs and drawing blood for patients assigned to NPs, and the absence of negative sanctions from nursing supervisors for these behaviors (Brykczynski, 1985; Lurie, 1981) support Hupcey's (1993) observation that NPs continue to feel resistance to their roles from staff nurses. These behaviors are suggestive of horizontal violence (a form of hostility) and may actually be even more common during nursing shortages. Roberts (1983) first described horizontal violence among nurses as oppressed-group behavior wherein nurses who were doubly oppressed as women and as nurses demonstrated hostility toward their own less powerful group instead of toward the more powerful oppressors. Recognizing that intraprofessional conflict among nurses is similar to oppressed-group behavior can be useful in the development of strategies to overcome these difficulties (Brykczynski, 1997; Farrell, 2001; Freshwater, 2000; McKenna, Smith, Poole, & Coverdale, 2003; Rounds, 1997; see also Chapter 9). Such a perspective suggests that, by providing information and support, nurses can learn to value their own worth and significance, become empowered, and consequently practice supportive rather than destructive behaviors toward other nurses. Horizontal violence is less common among APNs (Rounds, 1997).

Curry's (1994) claim that thorough orientation of staff nurses to the APN role (including clear guidelines and policies regarding responsibility issues) is an important component of successful integration of NP practice in an emergency department setting is applicable to other settings as well. Another significant strategy for minimizing intraprofessional role conflict is for the new APN (this holds true for APN students as well) to spend time getting to know the nursing staff to establish rapport and learn as much as possible about the new setting from those who really know what is going on—the nurses. This affirms the value and significance of nurses and nursing and sets up a positive atmosphere for collegiality and intraprofessional role cooperation and collaboration. In Kelly and Mathews' (2001) recent study of new NP graduates, such a strategy was exactly what new NPs regretted not having incorporated into their first positions.

INTERPROFESSIONAL ROLE CONFLICT

Conflicts between physicians and APNs constitute the most common situations of interprofessional conflict. Major sources of conflict for physicians and APNs are the perceived economic threat of competition, limited resources in clinical training sites, lack of experience working together, and the historical hierarchy. The relationship between anesthesiologists and CRNAs is an ongoing exemplar for examination of the issues of interprofessional role conflict between physicians and APNs. The fact that nurse anesthetists predated the first physician anesthesiologists by many years (see Chapter 1) may explain in part why the relationship between anesthesiologists and CRNAs has historically been interpreted by anesthesiologists as one of direct competition, thus creating an adversarial stance. Their relationship over the years might be characterized as a cold war with overt offensives mounted periodically by anesthesiologists. For many years, nurse anesthetists have provided high-quality anesthesia care in a variety of settings, and they are the sole anesthesia providers in more than 65% of rural hospitals (Blumenreich, 2000).

In 1970 CRNAs outnumbered anesthesiologists by 1.5 to 1. Now anesthesiologists outnumber CRNAs (Blumenreich, 2000). This is one of the factors underlying recent conflicts over CRNA autonomy (see the American Association of Nurse Anesthetists' website [www.aana.com] for updates on this issue). Another factor is the decision made, after study of the available evidence in 1997, by the Centers for Medicare and Medicaid Services, to reimburse nurse anesthetists directly under Medicare (Kleinpell, 2001). In response, anesthesiologists and the American Medical Association launched a major campaign against CRNA autonomy in the operating room, claiming that supervision of CRNAs by physicians is essential for public safety (Federwisch, 1999; Kleinpell, 2001; Stein, 2000; see also Chapter 17). This struggle with physicians over limiting the scope of practice of CRNAs is ongoing and reflects the experiences of other APN groups as well.

The complementary nature of advanced practice nursing to medical care is a foreign concept for some physicians who view all health care as an extension of medical care and APNs as physician extenders. This misunderstanding of advanced practice nursing underlies physicians' opposition to independent roles for nurses because they believe APNs want to practice medicine without a license (see Chapter 3). The fact that nursing has its own knowledge and skills is a novel idea for physicians who see nursing as a subset of medicine. When APNs are viewed as direct competitors, as has too often been the case with CRNAs, it is understandable that some physicians would be reluctant to be involved in assisting with APN education (National Commission on Nurse Anesthesia Education, 1990). In a like manner, some nurse educators espouse the belief that physicians should not be involved in teaching or acting as preceptors for APNs. Improved relationships between APNs and physicians will require redefinition of the situation by both groups. Fagin's (1992) assertion that collaboration is imperative holds true today:

Comprehensive health care today requires the broad spectrum of knowledge that no one practitioner can provide. Costs can be reduced by the appropriate utilization of nurses working in teams or in consultative relationships with physicians. Nurses and physicians are not in competition for the patient. As physicians' work roles and autonomy change and more of them are salaried employees, the convergence of issues affecting nurses and doctors will benefit from collaboration. (pp. 357-358)

Nurse-midwives have been in the forefront of developing collaborative relationships with physicians for many years (King, 1990; Long & Sharp, 1982; Rooks, 1983, 1999; Rooks & Haas, 1986). All APN groups would benefit from attention to the progress that CNMs have made in collaboration with physicians. The recent revision of the joint practice statement of the American College of Nurse-Midwives (ACNM) and the American College of Obstetricians and Gynecologists can be used as a model for other APN groups (Roberts, 2001; see also the ACNM's website [www.acnm.org]). Problems with previous joint practice statements were that they included varying interpretations of physician supervision. "The problematic sentence which referred to a maternity care team 'directed by a qualified obstetrician gynecologist' now states that the team 'must include an obstetrician gynecologist with hospital privileges or other physicians with hospital privileges to provide complete obstetric care' " (Roberts, 2001, p. 269). The revised joint practice statement "places responsibility for the outcomes of care with the provider who is directly managing the care" (Roberts, 2001, p. 269).

Collaboration between nurses and physicians is good for both groups, as well as for the public (see also Chapter 10). One way to promote positive interprofessional relationships is to provide education and practice experiences that include APN students, medical students, and both physician and APN faculty to enhance mutual understanding of both professional roles (Kelly & Mathews, 2001). Developing such interdisciplinary experiences is difficult because of different academic calendars and clinical schedules. However, such obstacles can be overcome if these interdisciplinary activities are considered essential for improved health-care delivery and if they have administrative support.

ROLE TRANSITIONS

Role transitions are defined here as dynamic processes of change that occur over time as new roles are acquired (see Table 4-1). Five essential factors found to influence role transitions are noted by Schumacher and Meleis (1994) as follows: (1) the personal meaning of the transition, which relates to the degree of identity crisis experienced; (2) the degree of planning, which involves the time and energy devoted to anticipating the change; (3) environmental barriers and supports, which refer to family, peer, school, and other components; (4) level of knowledge and skill, which relates to prior experience and school experiences; and (5) expectations, which are related to role models, literature, media, and the like. The role strain experienced by individuals in response to role insufficiency (see Table 4-1 for definitions of these terms) that accompanies the transition to APN roles can be minimized, although certainly not completely prevented, by (1) individualized assessment of these five essential factors, (2) development of strategies to cope with them, and (3) rehearsal of situations designed for application of those strategies. Entering graduate school may be associated with a ripple effect of concurrent role transitions in family, work, and other social arenas (Klaich, 1990).

APN Role Acquisition (in School)

The personal meaning of role transitions is a major focus of literature in nursing role development. In a review of APN role development literature from certificate and graduate NP programs, alterations in self-identity and self-concept emerged as a consistent theme, with role acquisition experiences commonly described as identity crises (see Brykczynski, 1996, for a detailed discussion of this earlier work). Most literature on APN role transitions refers to individuals who are already nurses. The process of role transition for people in direct-entry APN master's programs may differ because these individuals were not functioning as nurses before they entered the program. Further investigation is indicated to explore the similarities and differences in the role transition experiences of students in all types of APN programs.

In their study of NP students, Roberts et al. (1997) reported findings very similar to those observed decades earlier by Anderson, Leonard, and Yates (1974). Anderson et al. described the process of role development observed in three NP programs (a graduate program, a postbaccalaureate certificate program, and a continuing education program), whereas Roberts et al. described a current graduate NP program. Anderson and colleagues' (1974) description of NP students' progression from dependence to interdependence being accompanied by regression, anxiety, and conflict, was found to be similar to observations made by Roberts et al. (1997) in graduate NP students over a period of 6 years (Table 4-2). My colleagues and I have consistently observed a similar role transition process in teaching role and clinical courses for graduate NP students for many years. In a recent discussion of role transition experiences for neonatal NPs, Cusson and Viggiano (2002) made the important point that even positive transitions are stressful.

Roberts et al. (1997) observed 100 NP graduate students and reviewed their student clinical journals. They identified three major areas of transition as students progressed from dependence to interdependence: (1) development of professional competence, (2) change in role identity, and (3) evolving relationships with preceptors and faculty. The lowest level of competence coincided with the highest level of role confusion. This occurred at the end of the first semester and the beginning of the second semester in the three-semester program examined (Roberts et al., 1997). My colleagues and I have observed that the most intense transition period comes at the end of the students' first clinical immersion experience. Faculty can help students by identifying such periods of

TABLE 4-2	ROLE ACQUISITION PROCESS IN SCHOOL
STAGE	DESCRIPTIVE CHARACTERISTICS
I: Complete dependence	Immersion in learning medical components of care
	Role transition associated with role confusion and anxiety
	Decreased appreciation for psychosocial components of health and illness concerns
	Loss of confidence in clinical skills; feelings of incompetence
II: Developing competence	Ongoing clinical preceptorship experiences
	Didactic classes that incorporate medical diagnostic and both nursing and medical therapeutic components along with personal experience of illness components
	Renewed sense of appreciation for the value of nursing knowledge and skills
	More realistic self-expectations of clinical performance, although still uncomfortable about accountability
	Increased confidence in ability to succeed in learning and making a valid contribution to care
	Initial formation of own philosophy and standards of practice
III: Independence	Comfortable with ability to conduct holistic assessments (both physical and psychosocial)
	Concentration on intervention and management options
	Conflicts with preceptors occur as student and preceptor challenge one another
	Conflicts with faculty relate to management options, clinical evaluations, exam questions, concern over not being taught all there is to know
IV: Interdependence	Renewed appreciation for the interdependence of nursing and medicine
	Development of individualized version of the advanced practice role

Adapted from Anderson, E. M., Leonard, B. J., & Yates, J. A. (1974). Epigenesis of the nurse practitioner role. *American Journal of Nursing 10,* 12-16; and from Roberts, S. J., Tabloski, P., & Bova, C. (1997). Epigenesis of the nurse practitioner role revisited. *Journal of Nursing Education, 36,* 67-73.

high stress in their particular program so that support can be built in during those periods.

Roberts et al. (1997) have described the first transition as involving an initial feeling of loss of confidence and competence accompanied by anxiety (see Table 4-2, stage I). Initial clinical experiences were associated with the desire to observe rather than to provide care, the inability to recall simple facts, the omission of essential data from history taking, feelings of awkwardness with patients, and difficulty prioritizing data. The students' focus at this time was almost exclusively on acquiring and refining assessment skills and continued development of physical examination techniques. By the end of the first semester, students reported returning feelings of confidence and the regaining of their former competence in interpersonal skills. Although they were still tentative about diagnostic and treatment decisions, students reported feeling more comfortable with patients as some of their basic nursing abilities began to return (see Table 4-2, stage II).

Transitions in nursing role identity occurring during the first two stages were associated with feelings of role confusion. Students were dismayed at how slow and inefficient they were clinically and reported feelings of self-doubt and lack of confidence in their abilities to ever function in the "real world of health care." They sought shortcuts in attempts to increase their efficiency. They reported profound feelings of responsibility regarding diagnostic and treatment decisions and at the same time increasingly realized the limitations of clinical practice when they were confronted with the real-life situations of their patients. They recalled finding it easy to second-guess physicians' decisions in their previous nursing roles, but now they found those decisions more problematic when they were responsible for making them. They joked about feeling like adolescents. This is the point that Cusson and Viggiano (2002) are making when they comment, in reference to neonatal NPs, that the infant really does look different when viewed from the head of the bed rather than the side of the bed. They explain that "rather than taking orders, as they did as staff nurses, NNPs must synthesize incredibly complex information and decide on a plan of action. Experienced neonatal nurses often guide house staff regarding care decisions and in writing orders to match the care that is being given. However, the shift in responsibility to actually writing the orders can be very intimidating" (p. 24).

Roberts et al. (1997) observed that a blending of the new APN and the former nurse developed during stage II as students renewed their appreciation for their previous interpersonal skills as teachers, supporters, and collaborators and again perceived their patients as unique individuals in the context of their life situations. Students developed increased awareness of the uncertainty involved in the process of making definitive diagnostic and treatment decisions. Although these insights served to demystify the clinical diagnostic process, the students' anxiety about providing care increased. In spite of current attempts to reduce diagnostic and treatment uncertainty, evidence-based practice, a certain degree of uncertainty is inherent in clinical practice (see Chapter 5). Learning about strategies to cope with clinical decision making in situations of uncertainty, such as ruling out the worst case scenario, seeking consultation, and monitoring patients closely with phone calls and follow-up visits, can decrease anxiety and promote increased confidence (Brykczynski, 1991).

The transition in the relationships between students and preceptors and students and faculty in the study by Roberts et al. (1997) involved students feeling anxious that they were not learning enough and would never know enough to practice competently. Students felt frustrated and perceived that faculty and preceptors were not providing them with all the information that they needed. Then during the third stage, as they felt more confident and competent, students began to question the clinical judgments of their preceptors and faculty. This process is thought to help students advance from independence to interdependence—the last stage of the transition process. Much of the conflict at this juncture appeared to derive from students' feelings of "ambivalence about giving up dependence on external authorities" (Roberts et al., 1997, p. 71) such as preceptors and faculty and assuming responsibility for making independent judgments based on their own assessments from their clinical and educational experiences and the literature. The relevance of these role acquisition processes for other APN roles has not been reported. This is another area in which research would be helpful.

Strategies to Facilitate Role Acquisition

The anticipatory socialization to APN roles that occurs in graduate education is analogous to immunization (Kramer, 1974). The overall objective is to expose role incumbents to as many real-life experiences as possible during the educational program to minimize reality shock and role insufficiency on graduation and initial role implementation. Role content can be incorporated into APN curricula in a variety of ways such as (1) in the overall framework for designing an APN curriculum, (2) in a specific role course, (3) as part of specific assignments, or (4) in role seminars that span an entire curriculum. Hamric and Hanson (2003) asserted that it is an ethical mandate for all APN educators, regardless of specialty, to provide graduates with up-to-date knowledge of professional role and regulatory issues, in addition to concentration on clinical competence. If there is not a separate role course, careful attention must be paid to this curriculum component so that it does not become integrated out of existence.

Specific strategies for facilitating role acquisition are presented here and categorized according to three major purposes: (1) role rehearsal; (2) development of clinical knowledge and skills, including strategies for dealing with uncertainty; and (3) creation of a supportive network (Table 4-3). For adequate role rehearsal, APN students should experience all aspects of the core competencies (see Chapter 3) directly, while faculty and fellow students are available to help them process or debrief these experiences (Hamric & Taylor, 1989; Hupcey, 1990). APN students should be cautioned that other nurses, physicians, other providers, and administrators in the work setting may only value clinical expertise and not the other core competencies. Strategies for enhancing understanding of how the core competencies are embedded in each APN role include preparation of short-term and long-term goals to use as guides in development of professional portfolios, analysis of existing position descriptions, and development of the ideal position description. These are also helpful for guiding students in their search for an initial APN position.

Portfolio materials (Hawkins & Thibodeau, 1993; see Chapter 21) can be used for learning assignments and seminar discussions by having APN students share drafts of their portfolio components with peers, faculty, and preceptors and then revise them according to the feedback received. These strategies contribute to refinement and modification of definitions and expectations for future APN roles and promote development of students as colleagues and peer evaluators. Learning experiences, such as role negotiation and identification with a role model, that offer students realistic opportunities to apply assessment, management, and role negotiation skills will enhance APN role acquisition (Hunter, Bormann, & Lops, 1996; Kelly & Mathews, 2001). Judith Spross (personal communication, April 11, 1995; September 1, 2003) recommended that beginning APN students conduct "burning question" interviews with experienced APNs to develop a realistic vision and to focus their role acquisition experiences.

A variety of panels can be convened during role seminars to stimulate exploration of issues and to promote greater role clarity. For example, interaction with a panel that

TABLE 4-3 STRATEGIES TO PROMOTE APN ROLE ACQUISITION IN SCHOOL

PURPOSE	STRATEGIES	IMPLEMENTATION
Role rehearsal	Directly experience all core skills	Faculty and students monitor experience in all core competencies
	Create professional marketing portfolio	Prepare a folder containing philosophy of care, résumé, ideal position description, salary data, certification details, APN brochures, etc
	Lifelike role negotiation seminar	Invite interdisciplinary guests to participate
	Identify with a role model	Develop a mentee relationship with an APN and maintain contact throughout APN program
	Burning question interviews	Develop a list of questions of great importance to future role satisfaction to ask APNs
	Panel discussions	Faculty and students can plan discussion with a variety of panels to increase understanding of positions available, practice settings, other health team members, etc.
	Critical incident presentations	Prepare an in-depth self-evaluation of a situation of role conflict experienced in learning the APN role and share this with peers and faculty
Develop clinical knowledge and skills	Realistic clinical immersion experiences	Clinical experiences need to reflect the real world of practice as much as possible
	Clinical conferences	Discussion of clinical experiences with faculty and peers promotes clinical understanding
	Clinical situation narrative seminars	Share full contextual details of situations to promote understanding of aspects of embedded clinical practice knowledge
	Case study analysis	Clinical examples make classroom learning more concrete and memorable
	Clinical logs	Maintain a listing of all patients seen, including pertinent details such as age, diagnosis, etc.
	Final clinical preceptorships	A final semester of clinical practice helps put it all together
	Faculty practice	Maintenance of faculty clinical competence enhances credibility of APN faculty
Create a support network	Establish peer support system	Join local, state, and national APN group
	Share self- and peer evaluations	Learn to be comfortable with giving and receiving feedback for improvement
	Faculty-student-preceptor social functions	Foster an APN supportive environment among faculty, clinicians, students, staff, and administrators
	Establish a pattern for continuing education	Subscribe to selected APN journals, participate in APN conferences, and keep a record of continuing education hours
	Create a virtual community	Establish e-mail and Internet connections
	Establish a self-monitoring system	Select a framework for self-evaluating role performance to keep track of progress in role transition over time

APN, Advanced practice nurse.
Adapted from Brykczynski, K. A. (2000). Chart 1–6: Strategies to promote NP role acquisition in school. In P. Meredith & N. M. Horan (Eds.), *Adult primary care* (p. 16). Philadelphia: W. B. Saunders.

includes APNs in various specialties can help students gain an appreciation of similarities and differences in available roles. Another useful panel is one composed of program graduates and potential employers who can help APN students target their resumes and position descriptions to the existing APN market. An interdisciplinary panel comprising a nurse in an APN role and a physician in a complementary role can be beneficial for clarifying perceptions and discussing strategies for minimizing interprofessional role conflict. The impact and significance of students meeting successful APN graduates cannot be overstated. Establishing collaborative learning experiences between medical students and NP students has been recommended as a strategy to facilitate APN role transition (Kelly & Mathews, 2001).

Two popular role acquisition activities are described here in detail. One activity is a small group discussion wherein APN students present critical incidents encountered while beginning to develop their roles. Critical incident presentations require students to identify an actual role conflict situation from their clinical preceptorship experience. Students analyze these situations using the critical incident format adapted from Gordon and Benner (1980) and present them for discussion in small seminar groups led by APN clinical faculty. Another activity is designed as a social event that specifically focuses on describing the APN role in a social setting. In this second activity, faculty, graduates, APN students, preceptors, and administrators are invited to a reception where Diers' (1992) brief article, in which reader responses to the questions, "You're so smart, why are you just a nurse?" and "Why aren't you a doctor?" are reported, serves as a conversation starter. The purpose of this activity is to provide rehearsal for articulating responses to such questions in future social encounters.

The development of clinical knowledge and skills for APN role acquisition can be promoted by planning for realistic clinical experiences with the support of faculty and preceptors nearby. Clinical conferences can be conducted to share full details of clinical situations so that assessment and management decisions can be presented and refuted or defended in a supportive learning environment. Case studies can be incorporated into didactic classes, assignments, and examinations to enhance their clinical relevance. Clinical logs have been recommended by Hamric and Taylor (1989) to document experiences during the educational program for CNSs. Most current APN programs require that their students maintain clinical logs. Clinical logs provide a record of the variety and types of experiences students have had, which can be useful for documenting their clinical hours to substantiate their qualification to take certification examinations. Clinical logs can also be useful for students in planning future clinical experiences and for graduates in describing their clinical experiences to potential employers. Final clinical preceptorships, sometimes called *capstone experiences*, are important for solidifying the acquisition of role components in actual practice. Exploring ways to manage, synthesize, and retrieve the voluminous clinical literature available is an ongoing challenge for students, educators, clinicians, and researchers (Kelly & Mathews, 2001). Computer literacy is critical for networking and access to the high-quality materials available on websites (Table 4-4), in literature searches, and on personal digital assistants.

Emphasis on realism and a holistic situational perspective are important in clinical experiences for helping students understand that the complex clinical judgments involved in APN assessment and management of patient situations over time are not simply technical medical knowledge, but a hybrid of nursing and medical knowledge and experience. Studies of APN practice demonstrate that advanced practice roles incorporate a holistic approach that blends elements of nursing and medicine (Brown, 1992; Brykczynski, 1989, 1999; Johnson, 1993; see also Chapter 5). Teaching and learning experiences for all of the APN role components should integrate elements of research and theory and be

TABLE 4-4 USEFUL INTERNET SITES FOR CREATING A SUPPORT NETWORK		
WEB ADDRESS	ORGANIZATION	SELECTED HIGHLIGHTS
www.pftweb.org	Partnerships in Training, Association of Academic Health Centers	Standards for Online Instruction, click on "Reach" for links to related websites
www.nonpf.com	National Organization of Nurse Practitioner Faculties	NP competencies, publications, resource centers
www.aanp.org	American Academy of Nurse Practitioners	Certification, legislative news, links to international sites
www.nacns.org	National Association of Clinical Nurse Specialists	Position statement on CNS practice spheres
www.nurse.org/acnp	American College of Nurse Practitioners	End-of-life Project, National NP marketing campaign
www.nursingworld.org	American Nurses Association	Credentialing Center, Nursing news
www.napnap.org	American Association of Pediatric Nurse Practitioners	Scope of practice for PNPs, Immunization updates
www.aana.com	American Association of Nurse Anesthetists	CRNA Standards, Supervision Rule updates, Pain Management forum
www.acnm.org	American College of Nurse Midwives	Legislative alerts, click on "Professionals" for position statements
www.ncsbn.org	National Council of State Boards of Nursing	Institute of Regulatory Excellence, Press releases

CNS, Clinical nurse specialist; *CRNA,* certified registered nurse anesthetist; *NP,* nurse practitioner; *PNPs,* pediatric nurse practitioners.

incorporated into specialty APN courses to build on the knowledge gained in the traditional graduate core and clinical support courses in the curriculum. New APN graduates can benefit from familiarity with role transition processes by not expecting to be able to fully and expertly demonstrate all APN role components immediately on graduation. A useful exercise might be for students to develop projected role implementation trajectories for themselves (see Figure 4-1), which they can use as individualized guides to assess their progress in role transition.

Clinical mentoring by preceptors is an important component of ensuring realistic clinical learning experiences (Kelly & Mathews, 2001; Kleinpell-Nowell, 2001). A survey of 258 graduating NP students at 10 institutions indicated that students who selected their own preceptor scored higher on mentoring and self-efficacy than those whose preceptors were assigned by faculty (Hayes, 1998). Additionally, students with nonnurse preceptors scored lower than those with nurse preceptors. These findings have significant implications for preceptor arrangements. A mix of APN and nonnurse preceptors during the program can be quite valuable. However, requiring students to locate their own preceptors can be associated with problems such as validating the quality of the clinical practice at the new site and possibly producing undue anxiety for some students (Hayes, 2001). The ideal situation is when students become involved in rewarding mentor-mentee relationships and are hired to work in their preceptorship site after graduation.

Careful planning for the first APN position after program completion is important. Reports of the transition experiences of new NP graduates during their first year after graduation suggested that the first position can be critical in terms of solidifying the NP's career (Brown & Olshansky, 1997; Kelly & Mathews, 2001). Preparation of students for fulfillment of APN roles on graduation should be a collaborative effort of students and faculty. The need for position descriptions that clearly outline roles and responsibilities has been emphasized as essential for smooth role transition (Cooper & Sparacino, 1990; Hamric & Taylor, 1989; McMyler & Miller, 1997). The transition to the first position is a process—not an event that needs to be the focus of role content for faculty and students in APN programs (Hamric & Hanson, 2003; Hunter et al., 1996). My colleague Charlene Hanson and I believe that role disillusionment of new APNs may be hidden in multiple job changes and staying in the same registered nurse job after graduation from an APN program (C. Hanson, personal communication, August 30, 2003). Substantial role courses are critical to smooth the path to full APN role implementation (Hamric & Hanson, 2003; Hunter et al., 1996).

Finally and perhaps most importantly, an overall strategy for enhancing APN clinical knowledge and skill is for faculty to maintain competency in clinical practice. Clinical competency enhances the faculty's ability to evaluate students clinically, to discuss clinically relevant examples in classes, to serve as preceptors for students, and to evaluate the care provided in preceptorship sites. The clinical competence of faculty is important to prevent a wide gap between education and practice, to enhance faculty credibility, and to foster realistic expectations for new APN graduates. Faculty practice is also invaluable for establishing and maintaining ongoing interdisciplinary relationships with other healthcare professionals.

Establishing a peer support system, planning social functions with faculty and preceptors, and creating a virtual community can facilitate the development of a support network (see Table 4-3). The importance of forming a network of support people was emphasized by recent study findings (Kelly & Mathews, 2001; Kleinpell-Nowell, 2001). The establishment of a system for self-directed learning activities during the first few years after program completion forms the basis for maintaining competence throughout one's career (Gunn, 1998). The development of a system for lifelong learning should be initiated during the APN educational program as students create a self-monitoring system that includes clinical and role transition experiences over time to serve as a reality check or timetable. On graduation, continuing education program attendance could be incorporated into this monitoring system to facilitate compilation of necessary documentation for certification along with ongoing self-evaluation and role development.

APN Role Implementation (at Work)

After successfully emerging from the APN educational process, new APN graduates face yet another transition from the student role to the professional APN role (see Figure 4-1). APN graduates can be expected to experience attitudinal, behavioral, and value conflicts as they move from the academic world, where holistic care is highly valued, to the work world, where organizational efficiency is paramount. Anticipatory guidance is needed for role transition yet again. The process of APN role implementation is an example of a situational transition (Schumacher & Meleis, 1994), which has been described in the literature as a progressive movement through phases (Baker, 1979; Hamric & Taylor, 1989; Oda, 1977; Page & Arena, 1991). There is general agreement that significant overlap and fluidity exist among the phases. However, for purposes of discussion, the phases are considered sequentially.

Hamric and Taylor's (1989) study of CNS role development and Brown and Olshansky's (1997) study of NP role transition are two major investigations in which APN role implementation processes are described. Other significant studies that contribute to understanding of the transitional processes as APNs implement their roles include the longitudinal survey of acute care NP practice (Kleinpell-Nowell, 1999; 2001), in which the first six cohorts to take the adult acute care national certification examination are being followed up annually for 5 years, and Kelly and Mathews' (2001) qualitative focus group study of 21 recent NP graduates. Findings from these studies will be incorporated into this discussion of APN role implementation.

Hamric and Taylor (1989) described seven phases of CNS role development along with associated characteristics and developmental tasks derived from analysis of questionnaires returned by 100 CNSs (Table 4-5). All but 5% of the 42 CNSs in their first positions for 3 years or less experienced progression through the first three phases (identical to those phases identified by Baker [1979]). Most of the CNS respondents went through these three phases within 2 years. Phase 1, Orientation (Table 4-5, p. 126), is characterized by enthusiasm, optimism, and attention to mastery of clinical skills. The second phase, Frustration, is associated with feelings of conflict, inadequacy, frustration, and anxiety. The next phase, Implementation, is described as one of role modification in response to interactions with others. This phase is associated with a renewed or returning perspective.

CNSs with more than 3 years of experience described their role development experiences in terms very different from Baker's (1979) phases. Content analysis of these data led to a description of four additional phases (see Table 4-5). Experienced CNSs identified the Integration phase, which was characterized by "self-confidence and assurance in the role, high job satisfaction, an advanced level of practice, and signs of recognition and respect for expertise within and outside the work setting" (Hamric & Taylor, 1989, p. 56). Only 10% of the CNSs with less than 5 years of experience in the role met the criteria for this phase, whereas 50% of those with more than 6 years of experience could be categorized as being in this phase. The Integration phase was typically reached after 3 to 5 years in the CNS role. This fourth phase, Integration (thought to be reached only after successful transition through the earlier phases), is characterized by refinement of clinical expertise and integration of role components appropriate for the particular situation.

Hamric and Taylor (1989) also described three negative phases not evident in previous literature. The Frozen phase is described as being associated with frustration, anger, and lack of career satisfaction. The restructuring of role responsibilities and changing organizational expectations characterize the Reorganization phase. The Complacent phase is characterized by comfort, stability, and maintenance of the status quo. Unlike the Integration phase, these additional phases share a negative, nonproductive character. One might speculate that APNs experiencing these negative phases would be more vulnerable to position changes in today's cost-constrained health-care system.

The complexity of APN role development processes is further demonstrated by findings from Brown and Olshansky's (1997) grounded theory study of the role transition experiences of 35 novice NPs during their first year of practice. They described a four-stage process occurring during the first year of practice, which is outlined in Table 4-6 (p. 128) along with developmental tasks and strategies developed for this chapter. The first stage, an "In-between or Limbo" stage was not described in previous literature. During this stage, new graduates take certification examinations, obtain necessary recognition or licensure from state boards of nursing, and look for positions. This stage has been shortened because of the availability of certification examinations by computer.

The second stage, Launching, was defined as beginning with the first NP position and lasting at least 3 months. During this stage the new graduate NP experiences the anxiety associated with the crisis of confidence and competence that accompanies taking on a new position and the return to the advanced-beginner skill level (Benner et al., 1996; Dreyfus & Dreyfus, 1986, 1996). As the advanced beginner becomes increasingly aware of the number of elements relevant to actual performance in the role, he or she may become overwhelmed with the complexity of the skills required for the role and exhausted by the effort required for mastery. This is the at-work version of the crisis of confidence and competence experienced during stage I of the in-school role acquisition process (see Table 4-2). New NPs in Kelly and Mathews' (2001) study described similar experiences of exhaustion and frustration with lack of control over time.

Although Brown and Olshansky (1997, 1998) did not relate their findings about NP role transition to Hamric and Taylor's findings about CNS role development, there appear to be many similarities in the results of the two studies. The characteristics of the Launching stage are very similar to those described by Hamric and Taylor (1989) for the Orientation and Frustration phases. Brown and Olshansky's third stage, "Meeting the Challenge," is associated with feelings of regaining confidence and increasing competence. This stage has much in common with Hamric and Taylor's Implementation phase, which is noted for returning optimism and enthusiasm as expectations are realigned. The last stage, "Broadening the Perspective," is characterized by feelings of legitimacy and competency as NPs. This last stage is quite similar to Hamric and Taylor's (1989) fourth stage of Integration, during which the role is expanded and refined.

Strategies to Facilitate Role Implementation

The four major developmental phases (Orientation, Frustration, Implementation, and Integration) identified by Hamric and Taylor (1989) to describe CNS role development are combined with strategies for facilitating CNS role implementation (see Table 4-5).

I have listed the four stages of NP role implementation and their characteristics as identified by Brown and Olshansky (1997) and added developmental tasks and strategies for facilitating NP role development in an attempt to link this study with those findings from the Hamric and Taylor (1989) study (Table 4-6). The reader is encouraged to compare and contrast Tables 4-5 and 4-6 to glean relevant content for a particular APN role.

The four major phases described by Hamric and Taylor (1989) are used here to structure discussion of strategies to facilitate role implementation. The importance of being patient and recognizing that it takes time to fully develop in a new APN role was stressed by NPs in Kleinpell-Nowell's surveys (1999; 2001). A strategy to facilitate role implementation for all APNs during the Orientation phase is development of a structured orientation plan. Brown and Olshansky (1997, 1998) noted the importance of clarification of values, needs, and expectations and of recognition that transitional experiences are time limited. They also point out the importance of anticipatory guidance and realizing that these transition experiences follow a common pattern in new graduates. An APN in a new position (whether experienced in the role or not) needs to be aware of the importance of being informed about the organizational structure, philosophy, goals, policies, and procedures of the agency.

Networking was emphasized by NPs in Kleinpell-Nowell's surveys (1999; 2001). Peer support both within and outside the work setting is important, as noted by Hamric and Taylor (1989). New NPs stressed the importance of getting to know other nurses in the work setting, gaining their respect, and forming key alliances with them to enhance optimal functioning in their new positions (Kelly & Mathews, 2001). Designating a more experienced APN in the work setting as a mentor would be helpful and provide support for all APNs new to a position. The importance of careful selection of a mentor was reported by NPs in the study by Kelly and Mathews (2001). Additional strategies suggested for networking within the system include developing peer support groups, being accessible to colleagues by beeper, and getting involved in interdisciplinary committees (Page & Arena, 1991). APNs should be encouraged to join local APN groups for both peer support and networking opportunities. Numerous Internet sites are also available for networking as noted earlier.

Page and Arena (1991) recommended that CNSs schedule and devote the major portion of their time during the Orientation phase to direct patient care to substantiate the

TABLE 4-5 PHASES OF ROLE DEVELOPMENT

PHASE	CHARACTERISTICS	DEVELOPMENTAL TASKS	FACILITATION STRATEGIES
Orientation	Enthusiasm, optimism, eager to prove self to setting Anxious about ability to meet self- and institutional expectations Expects to make change	Learn formal and informal organizations Learn key players; begin establishing relationship and power base Explore expectations to see whether compatible with own Identify and clarify role to self and others	Structure an orientation plan Establish mutually agreed upon role expectations Circulate literature on APN role Meetings with key individuals Peer networking Identify with a role model Goal-oriented evaluation Concentrate on clinical mastery Postpone recommendations for major changes Join key committees
Frustration	Discouragement and questioning as a result of unrealistic expectations (either self- or employer); difficult and slow-paced change; resistance encountered Feelings of inadequacy in response to the overwhelming problems encountered, pressure to prove worth	Develop more realistic expectations Work on time management and setting priorities Develop short-term goals or projects to obtain tangible results/feedback Develop support system within and/or outside work setting	Schedule debriefing sessions Practice time management Maintain professional portfolio Continue seeking peer support Maintain communication with administrators Consult with experts Organize resources for easy accessibility
Implementation	Returning optimism and enthusiasm as positive feedback received and expectations realigned Organization and reorganization of role tasks, modified in response to feedback Implementing and balancing new subroles Regaining sense of perspective *May focus on specific project(s)*	Enhance visibility and power base within informal and formal organizations; build coalitions and networks Identify tangible accomplishments Complete transition to advanced practice level, if necessary Continue to reassess and refocus direction	Reassess demands, priorities, goals Plan for performance and impact evaluation Sustain communication with peers, administrators, and others
Integration	Self-confident and assured in role Rates self at advanced level of practice Activities reflect wide recognition, influence in area of specialty Continuously feels challenged; takes on new projects; expands practice Either moderately or very satisfied with present position	Continued role evolution and skill development to strengthen subroles and competencies Share expertise and experience with others through publications, research, professional activities Maintain flexible approach Be alert for signs of complacency or boredom	Continue debriefing sessions Plan for role expansion and refinement Schedule performance and impact evaluations Develop broader professional interests Formulate short-term goals for further development

Congruence between personal and organizational goals and expectations

Stage	Characteristics	Strategies	
Frozen	Self-confident, assured in role; rates self at intermediate or advanced practice level; Experiencing anger/frustration reflecting experience; Conflict between self-goals and those of organization/supervisor; Reports sense of being unable to move forward because of forces outside of self	Obtain feedback from supervisor and peers; Reevaluate self-goals in relation to CNS role and organization; Objective assessment of organization: Is there potential for compatibility?; Attempt to redesign or renegotiate the role; Consider career move/change; If unsuccessful, consider change in position/career direction	Self-assessment and early recognition of problems; Conflict resolution and role clarification discussions; Appraisal of APN goals in relation to organizational goals; Renegotiate role expectations
Reorganization	Reports earlier experiences that represent integration; Organization experiencing major changes; Pressure to change role in ways that are incongruent with own concept of CNS role and/or self-goals	Open discussion with change agents; Attempt compromise to preserve integrity of role and still meet needs of organization; If unsuccessful, change position/title or negotiate job change	
Complacent	Experiences self in role as settled and comfortable; Variable job satisfaction; Questionable impact on organization	Need to reenergize; Reconfigure role to allow growth by identifying new need of patient population or institution	

APN, Advanced practice nurse; *CNS,* clinical nurse specialist.
Adapted from Hamric, A. B., & Taylor, J. W. (1989). Role development of the CNS. In A. B. Hamric & J. A. Spross (Eds.), *The clinical nurse specialist in theory and practice* (2nd ed., p. 48). Philadelphia: W. B. Saunders.

TABLE 4-6　TRANSITION STAGES IN FIRST YEAR OF PRIMARY CARE PRACTICE

STAGE*	CHARACTERISTICS*	DEVELOPMENTAL TASKS	FACILITATION STRATEGIES
Laying the foundation	Period of role identity confusion immediately after graduation Not yet an NP, but no longer a student Feelings of worry, confusion, and insecurity about ability to practice successfully as an NP	Recuperate from school Initiate a job search and secure a position Obtain certification	Take time out to recuperate from the pressures of school Plan rewards for self Maintain peer support network Refine professional portfolio and use it to analyze available positions in terms of future goals
Launching	Discomfort of advanced-beginner level of knowledge and skills Feelings of unreality, insecurity—"the imposter phenomenon" Pervasive performance anxiety Daily stress Time pressure	Develop realistic expectations Incorporate feeling of legitimacy into NP role identity Cope with anxiety Mobilize problem-solving skills Work on time management and setting priorities† Develop support system†	Plan for longer appointments initially Anticipate need for time to feel comfortable in new role Realize that the transition process is time limited Schedule debriefing sessions with experienced MD or APN Seek peer and mentor support regularly Learn time-saving tips Clarify appropriate patient problems to work with initially Monitor internal self-talk—be positive
Meeting the challenge	Decreased anxiety Increased feeling of legitimacy Increased confidence develops along with increased competence Increased acceptance and comfort with the uncertainty inherent in primary care	Expand recognition of practice concerns to include the work environment Gain situational knowledge and skill in managing clinical problems Identify tangible accomplishments† Develop individualized style of approaching patients and organizing care Gain ability to handle uncertainty	Schedule a 6-month evaluation Maintain communication with peers, administrators, and others† Modify expectations to be more realistic Learn from repetitive practice Structure work situation so that resources are readily available Practice strategies to manage uncertainty
Broadening the perspective	Feeling of enhanced self-esteem Solid feeling of legitimacy and competence Realistic and positive feelings about future practice	Acknowledge strengths and identify ways to incorporate additional challenges Identify larger system problems and seek solutions (All the developmental tasks from the Integration phase of Table 4-5 would be appropriate here also.†)	Schedule a 12-month evaluation to reflect on progress and accomplishments Continue to seek verification and feedback from colleagues Make changes in work situation to increase support and effectiveness Inform staff and colleagues about NP role Affirm self-worth (Facilitation strategies from the Integration phase of Table 4-5 would be useful here also.†)

APN, Advanced practice nurse; NP, nurse practitioner.

*Data from Brown, M. A., & Olshansky, E. (1997). From limbo to legitimacy: A theoretical model of the transition to the primary care nurse practitioner role. *Nursing Research 46*, 46-51; and Brown, M. A., & Olshansky, E. (1998). Becoming a primary nurse practitioner: Challenges of the initial year of practice. *The Nurse Practitioner, 23*, 46, 52, 58, 61-66.

†Adapted from Hamric, A. B., & Taylor, J. W. (1989). Role development of the CNS. In A. B. Hamric & J. A. Sross (Eds.), *The clinical nurse specialist in theory and practice* (2nd ed., p. 48). Philadelphia: W. B. Saunders.

clinical expert role. They also suggested making appointments with nursing leaders, physicians, and other health-care professionals during this phase to garner administrative support. They recommended distributing business cards and making the job description available for discussion. They also counseled new CNSs to withhold suggestions for change until they have had the opportunity to more fully assess the system. When a new APN joins the staff of an organization, the administrator should send a letter describing the APN's background experiences and new position to key people in the organization.

Hamric and Taylor (1989) observed that the Frustration phase might come and go and may overlap other phases. They noted that painful affective responses are typical of this very difficult phase. They suggested that monthly sessions for sharing concerns with a group of peers and an administrator might facilitate movement through this phase. Strategies identified as helpful for energizing movement from the Frustration phase to the Implementation phase include obtaining assistance with time management; participating in support groups to ameliorate feelings of inadequacy; engaging in discussions for conflict resolution and role clarification; reassessing priorities and setting realistic expectations; and focusing on short-term, visible goals.

Page and Arena (1991) recommended keeping a work portfolio to document activities so APN progress is more readily visible. This can be an expansion of the portfolio and self-monitoring system begun during the APN program (see also Chapter 21). Brown and Olshansky (1997) pointed out that organized sources of support such as phone calls, seminars, planned meetings with mentors, and scheduled time for consultation can significantly decrease feelings of anxiety. They note that recognition of the discomfort arising from moving from "expert back to novice" and realization that previous expertise can be valuable in the new role may help reduce feelings of inadequacy. They suggest that new APNs request reasonable time frames for initial patient visits, because novices take longer than experienced practitioners, and this may be key to successful adjustment to a new position.

During the Implementation phase, it is important for the APN to reassess demands to prevent feeling overwhelmed. Priorities may need to be readjusted, and short-term goals may need to be reformulated. Brown and Olshansky (1997, 1998) observed that competence and confidence are fostered through repetition. They also recommend scheduling a formal evaluation after approximately 6 months. Feedback about areas of strength and need for improvement should be sought as part of the evaluation process during this phase. Strategies mentioned as important during this time include seeking administrative support through involvement in meetings, maintaining visibility in clinical areas, and developing in-service programs with input from staff (Page & Arena, 1991). After some time in the Implementation phase, APNs may plan and execute small-scale projects to demonstrate their effectiveness in their new roles.

Hamric and Taylor's (1989) survey data indicated that CNSs maximize their role potential during the Integration phase. Satisfactory completion of the earlier phases appears to be essential for passage into the Integration phase. One strategy for enhancing and maintaining optimal role implementation during this phase is having a trusted colleague who can act as a safe sounding board for "feedback, constructive criticism, and advice" (Hamric & Taylor, 1989, p. 79). During this phase, it is important to have a plan to guide continued role expansion and refinement, such as the portfolio mentioned earlier. Seeking appointment to key committees is important to increase recognition of APNs in the organization. Administrative support and constructive feedback from a trusted mentor continue to be important. Development of a promotional system that offers professional advancement in the APN practice role remains a challenge for practitioners and administrators. Page and Arena (1991) observed that less time is required for establishing relationships and assessing the system during this phase; therefore more time can be devoted to areas of scholarly interest. Brown and Olshansky (1995) pointed out the importance of formulating short-term goals to further development.

Whether the Frozen, Reorganization, and Complacent phases are distinct developmental phases or variations of the Implementation and Integration phases, they are clearly negative resolutions for APNs and their organizations. Table 4-5 includes strategies described by Hamric and Taylor (1989) for enhancing role development in these phases. APNs should engage in periodic self-assessment so that they recognize beginning signs associated with these phases, such as feelings of anger or dissatisfaction, conflict between self-goals and those of the organization or supervisor, feeling pressure to change one's APN role in ways that are incongruous with one's concept of the role, and feelings of complacency. Early recognition of problems and taking proactive steps to deal with organizational changes can help prevent or ameliorate the negative feelings associated with these phases.

Hamric and Taylor (1989) stated that honest and open discussions with supervisors or individuals with whom the APN is experiencing conflict should be initiated to resolve conflicts and clarify role issues before they become serious problems. In situations of organizational turmoil that characterize the Reorganization phase, APNs should evaluate their goals in relation to the organizational changes and renegotiate role expectations if necessary. Temporary role realignment may be negotiated to meet a short-term crisis, with explicit negotiated agreement that the APN would return to the original role after an agreed-upon time. In organizations increasingly concerned with cost and patient outcomes, APNs could negotiate to add a component of nurse case management to their practices for patients with complex needs in their specialty. Wells, Erickson, and Spinella (1996) described their experience in developing a CNS role with a major focus on case management as one of role transition.

APNs, along with their colleagues and administrators, need to be on the alert for indicators that one of these negative phases may be emerging and try to take action to change the situation. If discussion, compromise, and negotiations are unsuccessful, the APN should consider a career move, either to another position within the organization or to another organization. Career counseling may be a helpful strategy for the seriously disaffected APN.

Further analysis of the relationships between the stages described by Brown and Olshansky (1997, 1998) for NPs and the phases described by Hamric and Taylor (1989) for CNSs is needed. The relevance of these frameworks for transition processes experienced by other APNs also needs study. Further refinement of these findings could promote their incorporation into APN teaching, research, and practice. For example, two questions of interest are (1) Is the Limbo stage common to other APN groups? and (2) Do the negative phases Frozen, Reorganization, and Complacent appear after 3 years of practice in APN groups other than CNSs?

Facilitators and Barriers in the Work Setting

Aspects of the work setting exert a major influence on APN role definitions and expectations, thereby affecting role ambiguity, role incongruity, and role conflict. Findings from a survey by McFadden and Miller (1994) of CNSs identify access to support services, such as computers, statistical consultation, and secretarial and library services, as facilitators of role development. Factors found to promote NP role development include being recognized as a primary care provider; having one's own examination room; and being supported by co-workers, administrators, and patients (Andrews, Hanson, Maule, & Snelling, 1999; Hupcey, 1993; Lurie, 1981). Factors found to impede NP role development include pressure to manage care for large numbers of patients, resistance from staff nurses, and lack of understanding of the NP role (Andrews et al., 1999; Hupcey, 1993; Lurie, 1981). New constraints operating in today's health-care settings that affect not only APNs but other providers and office staff as well include new billing and coding guidelines, Health Insurance Privacy and Portability Act (HIPAA) regulations, monitoring for fraud and abuse, and sexual harassment.

The ability to incorporate teaching and counseling into the patient visit may be a function of skill development gained with experience in the APN role. This observation may be used as a rationale for structuring more time for visits and fewer total patients for new APNs, with gradual increases in caseloads as experience is accrued. Research indicates that NPs incorporate counseling and teaching into the flow of patient visits—capturing the teachable moment (Brykczynski, 1985; Johnson, 1993; Lurie, 1981; see Chapter 13 for examples).

Administrative factors that should be considered include whether APNs are placed in line or staff positions; whether they are unit based, population based, or in some other arrangement; who evaluates them; and whether they report to administrative or clinical supervisors. Baird and Prouty (1989) maintained that the organizational design should have enough flexibility to change as the situation changes. The placements of various APN positions may differ even within one setting, depending on size, complexity, and distribution of the patient population (Andrews et al., 1999; Baird & Prouty, 1989; see also Chapter 24).

Issues of professional versus administrative authority underlie the importance of the structural placement of the APN within the organization. Effectiveness of the APN role is enhanced when there is a mutual fit between the goals and expectations of the individual and the organization (Cooper & Sparacino, 1990, see also Chapter 24). Clarification of goals and expectations before employment and periodic reassessments can minimize conflict and enhance role development and effectiveness.

Continued APN Role Evolution

CNMs, CRNAs, NPs, and CNSs have attained positive recognition and support or role confirmation for clinical positions in many settings in the United States (Andrews et al., 1999; Oda, 1977). However, in spite of the increasing familiarity and popularity of these APN roles, some health-care settings have employed few if any APNs, and some staff members have had minimal experience working with APNs. In some areas of the United States, physicians or physician assistants are preferred over APNs. Even experienced APNs can expect to encounter resistance to full implementation of their roles if they seek positions in institutions with no history of employing APNs. Andrews et al. (1999) describe their experiences introducing the NP role into a large academic teaching hospital. They delineate helpful strategies for marketing the new NP role to staff, patients, and the surrounding community, as well as ways to set up the necessary infrastructure to support the new role in the institution. They refer to this process as "evolutionary."

The meaning of evolution of established APN roles varies according to the type of APN role. For example, for CNMs, role evolution currently refers to broadening the scope of practice to include primary health care. The Core Competencies for Basic Midwifery Practice have recently been revised to encompass primary care management (ACNM, 1997; see also the ACNM's website [www.acnm.org]). Integrating these competencies into midwifery practice without increasing program length constitutes a threefold challenge for CNMs to (1) incorporate didactic and clinical content into educational programs, (2) address the educational gap between new graduates and practicing CNMs, and (3) define and clarify the appropriate scope of primary health-care practice for CNMs (Stuart & Oshio, 2002, see also Chapter 16).

The emphasis on cost containment in the health-care delivery system has led to increased numbers of APN case managers and the trend of having acute care NPs staff intensive care units because of the shortage of house staff physicians (Sechrist & Berlin, 1998, see Chapters 14 and 18). In addition, evolution of APN roles is also reflected in expansion of practice to multiple areas or sites. Although responsibility for multiple areas in the same facility has been typical of many CNS roles for years, it is an evolutionary process for most other APN roles. Stahl and Myers (2002) explained that multisite roles might signify practice responsibilities at different sites or multiple areas of responsibility in the same site. Multisite roles may combine both inpatient and outpatient responsibilities. Stahl and Myers' clinical practices are exemplars of APN practice evolving to multiple sites, which constitute a strategy for extending APN resources and trying to use them more efficiently. Stahl is a CNS whose practice has evolved from the full range of CNS practice for four medical cardiac units at a tertiary care center to also include support primarily in education, consultation, and program development at two additional hospitals. Myers is an adult NP who directs a hepatitis C program for a specialty physician group with 11 physicians at nine practice locations, and she also provides direct care for patients at four of the sites.

The complexity of multisite roles can be overwhelming if the APN does not develop a certain degree of comfort with ambiguity. Stahl and Myers relied on Quinn's (1996) wisdom for developing the leader within by expecting to "build the bridge as you walk on it" (p. 83) and learning "how to get lost with confidence" (p. 86). Their commitment to being continuous learners is a useful model for APNs to follow as they experience the situational transitions that are inevitable as clinical practices evolve. Stahl and Myers (2002) used the National Association of Clinical Nurse Specialists' (1998) position statement on three spheres of influence to stimulate creativity and guide their APN practices as they evolve into new and multiple practice settings. The three spheres are (1) the individual patient/family, (2) nursing staff, and (3) the system or network.

As individual APNs mature into their respective roles and become comfortable and confident in the more technical components of their roles, greater concentration on the unique nature of APN practice can be expected. In their study of CNSs, Hamric and Taylor (1989) found that freedom to develop their unique APN role, availability of feedback from a mentor, support to broaden their influence and take on new projects, and recognition of their contributions enabled experienced CNSs to stay energized in their clinical practice roles. As Peplau (1997) advocated, nurse leaders must emphasize what nurses do for patients. The claim that nurses provide patient-centered care and that APN practice incorporates patient education, family assessment, involvement, and support, and community awareness and connections (Neale, 1999) needs to be documented. Additional research that demonstrates positive outcomes of APN care is essential for APN practice to make an impact on health-care policy (Brooten et al., 2002; Murphy-Ende, 2002; Russell, VorderBruegge, & Burns, 2002; Ryden et al., 2000; see also Chapter 25). Greater research activity and increasing involvement in the larger arena of health policy may also represent continuing role evolution.

Evaluation of Role Development

Evaluation is fundamental to enhancing role implementation. Evaluation of APNs should comprise both performance and impact (process and outcome) components (see Chapter

25). Development of a professional portfolio to document APN accomplishments can be useful for both performance and impact evaluation. Performance evaluation for APNs should include self-evaluation, peer review, and administrative evaluation (Cooper & Sparacino, 1990; Hamric & Taylor, 1989). Use of a competency profile can be helpful for organizing evaluation in a dynamic way that allows for changes in role implementation over time as expertise, situations, and priorities change (Callahan & Bruton-Maree, 1994). The competency profile can be used to assess performance in each of the core APN competencies. APN programs need to include content and skill development regarding self-evaluation and peer evaluation of role implementation so that individuals can learn to monitor their practice and identify difficulties early to avoid moving into negative developmental phases (Hamric & Hanson, 2003).

Impact evaluation is important to demonstrate the effectiveness of each APN role. Ongoing development of appropriate impact evaluation measures, such as patient outcomes and patient satisfaction, is important (Ingersoll, McIntosh, & Williams, 2000; see Chapter 25). The existence of a reward system to provide for career advancement through a clinical ladder program and accrual of additional benefits is particularly important for retaining APNs in clinical roles. In less structured situations, APNs can negotiate for periodic reassessments and salary increases through options such as profit sharing.

The evaluation process needs to broaden to incorporate interdisciplinary review when APN practice includes hospital privileges, prescriptive privileges, and third-party reimbursement. This expansion of the evaluation process has both positive and negative aspects. Advantages to the review process associated with securing and maintaining hospital privileges include the multiple aspects that are considered in the evaluation, the variety of perspectives, and the visibility afforded APNs. APNs should seek key positions on hospital review committees to promote APN roles within organizations. A major difficulty in implementing interdisciplinary peer review is lack of interaction between and among the incumbents of the various health professional groups during their formative educational programs (Brykczynski, 1989, 1999). The resurgence of interest in developing and implementing interdisciplinary educational experiences between nursing students and medical students is encouraging (Hamric & Hanson, 2003).

CONCLUSION

Role development experiences for APNs encompass role acquisition processes in school and role implementation processes after graduation. The limits of the educational process in preparing graduates for the realities of the work world need to be acknowledged. Students need to be informed about the human skill acquisition process and its stages, the processes of adult and professional socialization, identity transformation, role acquisition, role implementation, and overall career development. Knowing (theoretical knowledge) and actually experiencing (practical knowledge) are very different phenomena, but at least students and new graduates can be forewarned. Anticipatory guidance can be provided through role rehearsal experiences, such as clinical preceptorships and role seminars. Students need to be encouraged to begin networking with practicing APNs through local, state, and national APN groups. This networking is especially important for APNs who will not be practicing in proximity to other APNs. Experienced APNs and new APN graduates can form mutually beneficial relationships.

Although anticipatory socialization experiences in school can facilitate role acquisition, they cannot prevent the transition that occurs with movement into a new position and actual role implementation. APN programs should have a firm foundation in the real world. However, a certain degree of incongruence or conflict between academic ideals and work-world realities will continue to exist (Ormond & Kish, 2001). APNs must take a leadership role in guiding and directing planned change and guard against mere maintenance of the status quo. Establishing mentor programs for new APNs in the work setting is one way to develop and maintain support for the developmental phases of role implementation described here. Networking in local APN organizations is especially useful for enhancing both role acquisition (in school) and role implementation (at work).

APN role development has been described as dynamic, complex, and situational. It is influenced by many factors, such as experience, level of expertise, personal and professional values, setting, specialty, relationships with co-workers, aspects of role transition, and life transitions. Frameworks for understanding APN role development processes have been discussed along with strategies for facilitating role acquisition and role implementation. Ongoing evolution of APN roles, in response to organizational and health-care system changes and demands, has been explored. Future research studies to assess the applicability of this information for all APN specialty groups are needed to further the understanding of APN role development.

REFERENCES

Aiken, L. H., Clarke, S. P., Sloan, D. M., Sochalski, J., & Silber, J. H. (2002). Hospital nurse staffing and patient mortality, nurse burnout, and job dissatisfaction. *JAMA: The Journal of the American Medical Association, 288,* 1987-1995.

American College of Nurse-Midwives. (1997). *The core competencies for basic midwifery practice.* Washington, DC: Author. Retrieved September 1, 2003, from http://www.acnm.org/prof/corecomp.htm

Anderson, E. M., Leonard, B. J., & Yates, J. A. (1974). Epigenesis of the nurse practitioner role. *American Journal of Nursing, 74,* 1812-1816.

Andrews, J., Hanson, C., Maule, S., & Snelling, M. (1999). Attaining role confirmation in nurse practitioner practice. *Clinical Excellence for Nurse Practitioners, 3,* 302-310.

Arena, D. M., & Page, N. E. (1992). The imposter phenomenon in the clinical nurse specialist role. *Image: The Journal of Nursing Scholarship, 24,* 121-125.

Baird, S. B., & Prouty, M. P. (1989). Administratively enhancing CNS contributions. In A. B. Hamric & J. A. Spross (Eds.), *The clinical nurse specialist in theory and practice* (2nd ed., pp. 261-283). Philadelphia: W. B. Saunders.

Baker, V. (1979). Retrospective explorations in role development. In G. V. Padilla (Ed.), *The clinical nurse specialist and improvement of nursing practice* (pp. 56-63). Wakefield, MA: Nursing Resources.

Banda, E. E. (1985). *Role problems, role strain: Perception and experience of clinical nurse specialist.* Unpublished master's thesis, Boston University School of Nursing.

Bandura, A. (1977). Self-efficacy: Toward a unifying theory of behavioral change. *Psychological Review, 84,* 191-215.

Benner, P. (1984). *From novice to expert. Excellence and power in clinical nursing practice.* Menlo Park, CA: Addison-Wesley.

Benner, P., Hooper-Kyriakidis, P., & Stannard, D. (1999). *Clinical wisdom and interventions in critical care: A thinking-in-action approach.* Philadelphia: W. B. Saunders.

Benner, P., Tanner, C. A., & Chesla, C. A. (1996). *Expertise in nursing practice: Caring, clinical judgment and ethics.* New York: Springer-Verlag.

Blumenreich, G. A. (2000). Legal briefs: Supervision. *AANA Journal, 68,* 404-409.

Brooten, D., Naylor, M. D., York, R., Brown, L.P., Munro, B. H., Hollingsworth, A. O., et al. (2002). Lessons learned from testing the quality cost model of advanced practice nursing (APN) transitional care. *Journal of Nursing Scholarship, 34,* 369-375.

Brown, M. A., & Olshansky, E. (1995, July). *Supporting novice nurse practitioners: The experience of the first year of NP practice.* Paper presented at the annual meeting of the National Organization of Nurse Practitioner Faculties, Keystone, CO.

Brown, M. A., & Olshansky, E. F. (1997). From limbo to legitimacy: A theoretical model of the transition to the primary care nurse practitioner role. *Nursing Research, 46,* 46-51.

Brown, S. J. (1992). Tailoring nursing care to the individual client: Empirical challenge of a theoretical concept. *Research in Nursing and Health, 15,* 39-46.

Brykczynski, K. A. (1985). Exploring the clinical practice of nurse practitioners. *Dissertation Abstracts International, 46,* 3789B. (UMI No. DA8600592)

Brykczynski, K. A. (1999). An interpretive study describing the clinical judgment of nurse practitioners. *Scholarly Inquiry for Nursing Practice: An*

International Journal, 13, 141-166. Brykczynski, K. A. (1991). Judgment strategies for coping with ambiguous clinical situations encountered in family primary care. *Journal of the Academy of Nurse Practitioners, 3*, 79-84.

Brykczynski, K. A. (1996). Role development of the advanced practice nurse. In A. B. Hamric, J. A. Spross, & C. M. Hanson (Eds.), *Advanced nursing practice: An integrative approach* (pp. 89-95). Philadelphia: W. B. Saunders.

Brykczynski, K. A. (1997). Holism: A foundation for healing wounds of divisiveness among nurses. In P. B. Kritek (Ed.), *Reflections on healing. A central nursing construct* (pp. 234-241). New York: National League for Nursing.

Burglehaus, M. (1997). Physicians and breastfeeding: Beliefs, knowledge, self-efficacy and counseling practices. *Canadian Journal of Public Health, 88*, 383-387.

Callahan, L., & Bruton-Maree, N. (1994). Establishing measures of competence. In S. D. Foster & L. M. Jordan (Eds.), *Professional aspects of nurse anesthesia practice* (pp. 275-290). Philadelphia: F. A. Davis.

Chase, L. K., Johnson, S. K., Laffoon, T. A., Jacobs, R. S., & Johnson, M. E. (1996). CNS role: An experience in retitling and role clarification. *Clinical Nurse Specialist, 10*, 41-45.

Clark, N., & Dodge, J. (1999). Exploring self-efficacy as a predictor of disease management. *Health Education & Behavior, 26*, 72-89.

Cohen, H. A. (1981). *The nurse's quest for a professional identity.* Menlo Park, CA: Addison-Wesley.

Cooper, D. M., & Sparacino, P. S. A. (1990). Acquiring, implementing, and evaluating the clinical nurse specialist role. In P. S. A. Sparacino, D. M. Cooper, & P. A. Minarik (Eds.), *The clinical nurse specialist: Implementation and impact* (pp. 41-75). Norwalk, CT: Appleton & Lange.

Curry, J. L. (1994). Nurse practitioners in the emergency department: Current issues. *Journal of Emergency Nursing, 20*, 207-215.

Cusson, R. M., & Viggiano, N. M. (2002). Transition to the neonatal nurse practitioner role: Making the change from the side to the head of the bed. *Neonatal Network—Journal of Neonatal Nursing, 21*, 21-28.

Dalton, J., & Blau, W. (1996). Changing the practice of pain management: An examination of the theoretical basis of change. *Pain Forum, 5*, 266-272.

Diers, D. (1992). One-liners. *Image: The Journal of Nursing Scholarship, 24*, 75-77.

Dionne-Proulx, J., & Pepin, R. (1993). Stress management in the nursing profession. *Journal of Nursing Management, 1*, 75-81.

Dreyfus, H. L., & Dreyfus, S. E. (1977). *Uses and abuses of multi-attribute and multi-aspect model of decision making.* Unpublished manuscript, Department of Industrial Engineering and Operations Research, University of California at Berkeley.

Dreyfus, H. L., & Dreyfus, S. E. (1986). *Mind over machine: The power of human intuition and expertise in the era of the computer.* New York: Free Press.

Dreyfus, H. L., & Dreyfus, S. E. (1996). The relationship of theory and practice in the acquisition of skill. In P. Benner, C. A. Tanner, & C. A. Chesla (1996). *Expertise in nursing practice: Caring, clinical judgment and ethics* (pp. 29-47). New York: Springer-Verlag.

Fagin, C. M. (1992). Collaboration between nurses and physicians no longer a choice. *Nursing & Health Care, 13*, 354-363.

Farrell, G. A. (2001). From tall poppies to squashed weeds: Why don't nurses pull together more? *Journal of Advanced Nursing, 35*, 26-33.

Federwisch, A. (1999). CRNA autonomy. Nurse anesthetists fight latest skirmish. *Nursing & Allied Health Week* (Greater Dallas/Fort Worth edition), *4*, 16.

Fenton, M. V. (1985). Identifying competencies of clinical nurse specialists. *Journal of Nursing Administration, 15*, 31-37.

Ford, L. C. (1982). Nurse practitioners: History of a new idea and predictions for the future. In L. H. Aiken (Ed.), *Nursing in the 1980s: Crises, opportunities, challenges* (pp. 231-247). Philadelphia: Lippincott.

Freshwater, D. (2000). Crosscurrents: Against cultural narration in nursing. *Journal of Advanced Nursing, 32*, 481-484.

Gordon, D., & Benner, P. (1984). Guidelines for recording critical incidents. In Benner, P. (Ed), *From novice to expert. Excellence and power in clinical nursing practice* (pp. 299-302). Menlo Park, CA: Addison-Wesley.

Gunn, I. P. (1991). The history of nurse anesthesia education: Highlights and influences. Report of the National Commission on Nurse Anesthesia Education. *Journal of the American Association of Nurse Anesthetists, 59*, 53-61.

Gunn, I. P. (1998). Setting the record straight on nurse anesthesia and medical anesthesiology education. *CRNA: The Clinical Forum for Nurse Anesthetists, 9*, 163-171.

Hamric, A. B., & Hanson, C. M. (2003). Educating advanced practice nurses for practice reality. *Journal of Professional Nursing, 19*, 262-268.

Hamric, A. B., & Taylor, J. W. (1989). Role development of the CNS. In A. B. Hamric & J. Spross (Eds.), *The clinical nurse specialist in theory and practice* (2nd ed., pp. 41-82). Philadelphia: W. B. Saunders.

Hardy, M. E., & Hardy, W. L. (1988). Role stress and role strain. In M. E. Hardy & M. E. Conway (Eds.), *Role theory: Perspectives for health professionals* (2nd ed., pp. 159-239). Norwalk, CT: Appleton & Lange.

Hawkins, J. W., & Thibodeau, J. A. (1993). Negotiating an employment contract. In J. W. Hawkins & J. A. Thibodeau (Eds.), *The practitioner* (3rd ed., pp. 130-140). New York: Tiresias Press.

Hayes, E. (1998). Mentoring and nurse practitioner student self-efficacy. *Western Journal of Nursing Research, 20*, 521-525.

Hayes, E. F. (2001). Factors that facilitate or hinder mentoring in the nurse practitioner preceptor/student relationship. *Clinical Excellence for Nurse Practitioners, 5*, 111-118.

Hazle, N. R. (1985). Perceptions of role conflict between obstetric nurses and nurse-midwives. *Journal of Nurse-Midwifery, 30,* 166-173.

Horvath, K. J., Secatore, J. A., Alpert, H. B., Costa, M. J., Powers, E. M., Stengrevics, S. S., & Aroian, J. (1994). Uncovering the knowledge embedded in clinical nurse manager practice. *Journal of Nursing Administration, 24,* 39-44.

Hunter, L. P., Bormann, J. E., & Lops, V. R. (1996). Student to nurse-midwife role transition process: Smoothing the way. *Journal of Nurse-Midwifery, 41,* 328-333.

Hupcey, J. E. (1990). The socialization process of master's level nurse practitioner students. *Journal of Nursing Education, 29,* 196-201.

Hupcey, J. E. (1993). Factors and work settings that may influence nurse practitioner practice. *Nursing Outlook, 41,* 181-185.

Ingersoll, G. L., McIntosh, E., & Williams, M. (2000). Nurse-sensitive outcomes of advanced practice. *Journal of Advanced Practice, 32,* 1272-1281.

Johnson, R. (1993). Nurse practitioner-patient discourse: Uncovering the voice of nursing in primary care practice. *Scholarly Inquiry for Nursing Practice: An International Journal, 7,* 143-157.

Kelly, N. R., & Mathews, M. (2001). The transition to first position as nurse practitioner. *Journal of Nursing Education, 40,* 156-162.

Kimbro, C. D. (1978). The relationship between nurses and nurse-midwives. *Journal of Nurse-Midwifery, 22,* 28-31.

King, M. B. (1990). Clinical nurse specialist collaboration with physicians. *Clinical Nurse Specialist, 4,* 172-177.

Klaich, K. (1990). Transitions in professional identity of nurses enrolled in graduate educational programs. *Holistic Nursing Practice, 4,* 17-24.

Kleinpell, R. (2001). Nurse anesthetists hold fast under physicians' blast of supervision ruling. *The Nursing Spectrum, 11,* 26-27.

Kleinpell-Nowell, R. (1999). Longitudinal survey of acute care nurse practitioner practice: Year 1. *AACN Clinical Issues, 10,* 515-520.

Kleinpell-Nowell, R. (2001). Longitudinal survey of acute care nurse practitioner practice: Year 2. *AACN Clinical Issues, 12,* 447-452.

Kramer, M. (1974). *Reality shock.* St. Louis: Mosby.

Leininger, M. M. (1976). Two strange health tribes: The Gnisrun and the Enicidem in the United States. *Human Organization. Journal of the Society for Applied Anthropology, 35,* 253-261.

Leininger, M. M. (1994). The tribes of nursing in the United States. *Journal of Transcultural Nursing, 6,* 18-22.

Long, W. N., & Sharp, E. S. (1982). Relationships between professions: From the viewpoint of the physician and nurse-midwife in a tertiary center. *Journal of Nurse Midwifery, 27,* 14-24.

Lurie, E. E. (1981). Nurse practitioners: Issues in professional socialization. *Journal of Health and Social Behavior, 22,* 31-48.

McFadden, E. A., & Miller, M. A. (1994). Clinical nurse specialist practice: Facilitators and barriers. *Clinical Nurse Specialist, 8,* 27-33.

McKenna, B. G., Smith, N. A., Poole, S. J., & Coverdale, J. H. (2003). Horizontal violence: Experiences of registered nurses in their first year of practice. *Journal of Advanced Nursing, 42,* 90-96.

McMyler, E. T., & Miller, D. J. (1997). Two graduating master's students struggle to find meaning. *Clinical Nurse Specialist, 11,* 169-173.

Murphy-Ende, K. (2002). Advanced practice nursing: Reflections on the past, issues for the future. *Oncology Nursing Forum, 29,* 106-112.

National Association of Clinical Nurse Specialists. (1998). Statement on clinical nurse specialists practice and education. Harrisburg, PA: Author.

National Commission on Nurse Anesthesia Education. (1990). Summary of Commission findings: Issues and review of supporting documents. *Journal of the American Association of Nurse Anesthetists, 58,* 394-398.

Neale, J. (1999). Nurse practitioners and physicians: A collaborative practice. *Clinical Nurse Specialist, 13,* 252-258.

Oda, D. (1977). Specialized role development: A three-phase process. *Nursing Outlook, 25,* 374-377.

Ormond, C., & Kish, C. P. (2001). Role acquisition. In D. Robinson & C. P. Kish (Eds.), *Core concepts in advanced practice nursing* (pp. 269-285). St. Louis: Mosby.

Page, N. E., & Arena, D. M. (1991). Practical strategies for CNS role implementation. *Clinical Nurse Specialist, 5,* 43-48.

Parle, M., Maguire, P., & Heaven, C. (1997). The development of a training model to improve health professionals skills, self-efficacy, and outcome expectancies when communicating with cancer patients. *Social Science & Medicine, 44,* 231-240.

Payne, J. L., & Baumgartner, R. G. (1996). CNS role evolution. *Clinical Nurse Specialist, 10,* 46-48.

Peplau, H. (1997, June). *Keynote address.* Presented at International Congress of Nurses, Vancouver, British Columbia, Canada.

Quinn, R. E. (1996). *Deep change—discovering the leader within.* San Francisco: Jossey-Bass.

Redekopp, M. A. (1997). Clinical nurse specialist role confusion: The need for identity. *Clinical Nurse Specialist, 11,* 87-91.

Roberts, J. (2001). Revised "Joint Statement" clarifies relationships between midwives and physician collaborators. *Journal of Midwifery & Women's Health, 46,* 269-271.

Roberts, S. J. (1983). Oppressed group behavior: Implications for nursing. *Advances in Nursing Science, 5,* 21-30.

Roberts, S. J., Tabloski, P., & Bova, C. (1997). Epigenesis of the nurse practitioner role revisited. *Journal of Nursing Education, 36,* 67-73.

Rooks, J. P. (1983). The context of nurse midwifery in the 1980s: Our relationships with medicine, nursing, lay-midwives, consumers and health care economists. *Journal of Nurse-Midwifery, 26,* 3-8.

Rooks, J. P. (1999). The midwifery model of care. *Journal of Nurse Midwifery, 44,* 370-374.

Rooks, J. P., & Haas, J. E. (Eds.). (1986). *Nurse midwifery in America.* Washington, DC: American College of Nurse-Midwives Foundation.

Rounds, L. R. (1997). The nurse practitioner: A healing role for the nurse. In P. B. Kritek (Ed.), *Reflections on healing. A central nursing construct* (pp. 209-223). New York: National League for Nursing.

Russell, D., VorderBruegge, M., & Burns, S. M. (2002). Effect of an outcomes-managed approach to care of neuroscience patients by acute care nurse practitioners. *American Journal of Critical Care, 11,* 353-364.

Ryden, M. B., Snyder, M., Gross, C. R., Savik, K., Pearson, V., Krichbaum, K., et al. (2000). Value-added outcomes: The use of advanced practice nurses in long-term care facilities. *The Gerontologist, 40,* 654-662.

Schumacher, K. L., & Meleis, A. I. (1994). Transitions: A central concept in nursing. *Image: The Journal of Nursing Scholarship, 26,* 119-127.

Sechrist, K. R., & Berlin, L. E. (1998). Role of the clinical nurse specialist: An integrative review of the literature. *AACN Clinical Issues, 9,* 306-324.

Stahl, M. A., & Myers, J. (2002). The advanced practice nursing role with multisite responsibilities. *Critical Care Nursing Clinics of North America, 14,* 299-305.

Stein, T. (2000). Struggling for autonomy: Dispute between CRNAs and anesthesiologists continues. *Nurseweek* (California Statewide Edition), *13,* 31.

Stuart, D., & Oshio, S. (2002). Primary care in nurse-midwifery practice: A national survey. *Journal of Midwifery & Women's Health, 47,* 104-109.

Varney, H. (1987). *Nurse-midwifery* (2nd ed.). Boston: Blackwell Scientific.

Waugaman, W. R., & Lohrer, D. J. (2000). From nurse to nurse anesthetist: The influence of age and gender on professional socialization and career commitment of advanced practice nurses. *Journal of Professional Nursing, 16,* 47-56.

Waugaman, W. R., & Lu, J. (1999). From nurse to nurse anesthetist: The relationship of culture, race, and ethnicity to professional socialization and career commitment of advanced practice nurses. *Journal of Transcultural Nursing, 10,* 237-247.

Wells, N., Erickson, S., & Spinella, J. (1996). Role transition. From clinical nurse specialist to clinical nurse specialist/case manager. *Journal of Nursing Administration, 26,* 23-28.

PART II

Competencies of Advanced Practice Nursing

CHAPTER 5

Direct Clinical Practice

SARAH JO BROWN

INTRODUCTION

In most countries, health-care delivery is constantly being reconfigured. Changing reimbursement structures, integrated delivery systems, new privacy requirements, and population-based management all impose significant changes on clinical practice. As a result, advanced practice nurses (APNs) must alter the way they approach caregiving in general, as well as the specifics of care provided to individual patients.

The challenge many APNs face is how to maintain the characteristics of care that have helped patients achieve positive health outcomes and afforded APN care a unique niche in the health-care marketplace. Characteristics such as use of a holistic perspective and the formation of partnerships with patients to co-produce individualized health care are threatened by care management approaches and cost containment schemas in which the emphasis is on standardization of the processes of care to achieve population-based outcome targets. Conversely, characteristics of APN care such as health promotion, self-care, and low-tech modalities are valued by these managed care programs because they result in low use of health-care system resources. These reasons are, of course, different from the reasons that APNs have valued, and continue to value, these components of care. Throughout the following discussion of the characteristics of APN care, observations are made regarding how each characteristic fits with cost containment goals. Also, suggestions are offered regarding how to incorporate or defend the characteristics within the context of current delivery structures. To balance the picture, the special opportunities to improve care within evolving health-care structures are also noted.

DIRECT CARE ACTIVITIES

Direct care is the central APN competency (see Chapter 3). For the purposes of this chapter, the terms *direct care* and *direct clinical practice* refer to the activities and functions APNs perform within the patient-nurse interface (Hamric, Spross, & Hanson, 2000). Depending on the focus of an APN's practice, the patient may, and often does, include family members/significant others. The activities that occur in this interface, or as direct follow-up to what occurred there, are unique because they are interpersonally and physically co-enacted with a particular patient for the purpose of promoting that patient's health or well-being. Many important processes transpire at this point of care including the following:

- The patient-provider relationship is established.
- Health problems become mutually understood.
- Health or recovery goals are expressed.
- Management and treatment options are explored.
- Physical acts of diagnosis, monitoring, treatment, and therapy are performed.
- Education, support, coaching, counseling, and comfort are provided.
- Decisions regarding future actions to be taken by each party are made.
- Future contact is planned.

Advanced practice nursing activities occurring before and adjacent to the patient-nurse interface have a great influence on the direct care that occurs in the interface; however, they either are not performed with an individual patient or their main purpose is something other than promoting the well-being of the individual patient. For instance, when an APN consults with another provider regarding the nature of a patient's condition or the care that should be recommended to a patient, the APN is engaging in advanced clinical practice, but not in direct care. Even though there may be direct contact with the patient during the consultation, the primary purpose of that contact is to acquire information and understanding to use in formulating recommendations for the patient's direct care provider. Another example is the APN who develops and tests a new assessment method or intervention for a population of patients. Even though this APN may assess patients using the new method or use the new interventions with several patients, the primary purposes of those contacts are to develop and refine a new method of care for the population of patients, not solely to promote the well-being of the individual patients. Thus according to the definition of direct care used in this chapter, the APN is engaged in clinical practice, but he or she is not providing direct care.

Although this delineation may seem too severely drawn to some people, I believe restricting the use of the term *direct care* to what occurs in the patient-nurse interface and as follow-up to it serves heuristic and practical purposes. This delineation is not intended to denigrate clinical activities that occur outside the patient-nurse interface—quite the contrary. I believe these other clinical activities and functions should be recognized as influencing what happens in the interface and as having a significant impact on patient outcomes. Because other clinical activities so significantly affect patient outcomes, they should be valued by the nursing community and by health-care systems. In the current environment of cost containment and technological development, all activities that enhance patients' health, recovery, and adjustment should be valued regardless of whether they are antecedents of direct care, adjuncts to it, or actual direct care itself.

As a result of research investigators are beginning to understand the specific activities that constitute the direct care component of various advanced practice nursing roles. However, it is difficult to make generalizations about these activities because the APNs studied had different roles and worked in different settings with different populations. In addition, different classification schemas were used to categorize APN actions. For instance, in some studies, investigators used the term *activities* to classify APN actions; in others, the term *interventions* was used. The variability in terminology and definitions make it difficult to compare results across studies. Nevertheless a review of these studies yields some insights into the extent and nature of direct care activities in APN roles.

A sample of 724 clinical nurse specialists (CNSs) in traditional roles in the United States reported spending 29% to 91% of their time in *expert practitioner activities*, including the following:

- Diagnosing, treating, and evaluating patient responses to actual or potential health problems
- Managing complex and difficult situations
- Providing direct care to patients with complex problems and their families
- Functioning as case managers
- Prescribing and adjusting medications
- Introducing new technology into the clinical environment (Scott, 1999)

Advanced practice skills performed by these CNSs included family therapy, grief therapy, and crisis intervention. Their ministrations included wound, ostomy, and incontinence management; physical assessment; line insertions; and pain management. Their medical activities included pacemaker programming, suturing and stapling, wound debridement, placement of central lines and chest tubes, and removal of arterial and venous sheaths.

A somewhat similar list of activities emerged from interviews of 10 Canadian acute care NPs (Sidani et al., 2000). The five categories of activities included in the *clinical component* of their role were (1) medical diagnosis and management of symptoms; (2) coordination of the health-care team; (3) assessment, included physical examination and admission history; (4) planning care, including planning for discharge; and (5) direct patient care, which included keeping patients and families informed, teaching patients, performing procedures such as removal of central venous lines, and assisting staff in caring for patients. Although most of these acute care NPs were also expected to be involved in research, committees, staff education, quality management, and program evaluation, they reported spending more than 80% of their time in clinical practice. In another study of 17 employed in five nursing home settings, these APNs reported spending 35% of their working days in *direct patient care* and 26% of their time communicating with nursing home staff, families, and physicians (Kane, Flood, Keckhafer, & Rockwood, 2001).

An analysis of 333 logs kept by APNs who worked with five different patient groups during randomized clinical trials of transitional care from hospital through home follow-up (Brooten, Youngblut, Deatrick, Naylor, & York, 2003) revealed that the most frequent category of *intervention* for all five groups was surveillance. Surveillance accounted for 48% to 65% of the APN interventions across the five groups, with signs and symptoms of physical problems as the most frequent target of surveillance. Health teaching/ guidance/counseling was the second most frequent category of advanced practice nursing intervention in four of the five groups (12%-36%). Case management, including activities such as locating and coordinating postdischarge services and community resources and coordinating specialty medical follow-up, was the third most frequent intervention in four of the five groups. Surprisingly, in all five groups, treatments and procedures accounted for less than 1% of total APN interventions. The proportion of surveillance to teaching was approximately reversed in a study of APNs providing home care to 148 elderly patients with cancer who were recovering from surgery (Hughes et al., 2002). Teaching was the most frequent intervention, comprising 43% of the interventions documented. Care vigilance, which approximates surveillance, comprised 12% of the interventions. Providing psychological support and reassurance was the second most frequent intervention at 16%. In summary, direct care activities comprise a large part of what most APNs do, although there is considerable variation in what activities are performed and how much time is devoted to the direct care function across roles, settings, and patient populations.

FIVE CHARACTERISTICS OF DIRECT CLINICAL CARE PROVIDED BY APNs

In this chapter I propose that there are characteristics of advanced practice nursing care that should, and to a considerable degree already do, extend across advanced practice roles, health-care settings, and populations of patients. These characteristics are as follows:

1. Use of a holistic perspective
2. Formation of partnerships with patients
3. Expert clinical thinking and skillful performance
4. Use of research evidence as a guide to practice
5. Use of diverse approaches to health and illness management

These characteristics have been present in advanced practice nursing for many years, and they constitute the themes one hears when APNs describe what they do. Moreover, there is accumulating research evidence supporting them as features of APN practice and as having positive influences on patient outcomes. Throughout this chapter, the research evidence cited regarding claims about APN practice is illustrative and not based on a systematic review of research on a particular issue. The research regarding outcomes associated with APN practice is addressed comprehensively in Chapter 25.

The five characteristics of advanced direct care practice have their roots in the traditional values of the nursing profession. Nurses in advanced practice roles often have a deep commitment to the values on which these characteristics rest, and are able to persuasively advocate these values in the discourse of daily practice. The expanded scope of practice of APN roles often enables APNs to fully enact these characteristics in their daily interactions with patients. An overview of strategies for enacting these characteristics is provided in Box 5-1.

To maintain these characteristics in daily practice, as opposed to merely holding them as espoused values, APNs must be reflective practitioners. Reflection involves an intentional examination of situations to try to understand what happened and why it happened and to speculate about how the situation might have been managed differently. The goal is to turn experience into personal knowledge by seeking insights that are not available with superficial recall (Rolfe, 1997; Schön, 1984). Kim (1999) has described a method of reflective inquiry involving systematic analysis of personal instances of nursing practice; individual APNs or groups could use this method to monitor and improve practice.

Use of a Holistic Perspective

HOLISM DESCRIBED

Holism has a variety of meanings, both broad and narrow. A broad view is that holism involves a deep understanding of each patient as a complex and unique person who is embedded in a temporally unfolding life. This deep understanding enables the practitioner to view the patient as a sacred and unique person who is in the process of living life as best as she or he can within a particular context. This comprehensive and integrated view of human life and health is enacted in the health-care encounter as attention to the full range of factors influencing patients' experiences (Box 5-2).

Another view is that holism incorporates several perspectives including the following (Newman, 1997; Waite, Harker, & Messerman, 1994):

- Viewing the patient as an integral part of larger social, physical, and energy environments
- Assuming that the mind, body, and spirit are closely related, so that one dimension should not be considered in isolation from the others
- Focusing on the meanings patients assign to health, illness experiences, and health-care choices
- Viewing patients' current behaviors and responses as consistent with their life span patterns of response and choice

Clearly, high-tech care environments with many health-care providers, each focused on one aspect of a patient's condition and treatment, require designated coordinators who have a comprehensive and integrated appreciation of the patient and her or his experience of care as a whole. APNs' capacity to "keep the pieces together" in a way that focuses care on the unique individual is undoubtedly why many high-tech programs (e.g., transplant programs) have an APN member or coordinator (see Management of Complex Situations later in this chapter). In an ethnographic study of one high-tech environment,

---

BOX 5-1 • CHARACTERISTICS OF ADVANCED DIRECT CARE PRACTICE AND STRATEGIES FOR ENACTING THEM

HOLISTIC FRAMEWORK
- Take into account the complexity of human life.
- Recognize and address how social, organizational, and physical environments affect people.
- Consider the profound effects of illness, aging, hospitalization, and stress.
- Consider how symptoms, illness, and treatment affect quality of life.
- Focus on functional abilities and requirements.

FORMATION OF PARTNERSHIP WITH PATIENTS
- Use a conversational style to conduct health care encounters.
- Encourage the patient to actively participate in decision making.
- Look for potential cultural influences on health care discourse.
- Listen to the indirect voices of patients who are noncommunicative.
- Advocate the patient's perspective and concerns to others.

EXPERT CLINICAL REASONING AND SKILLFUL PERFORMANCE
- Acquire specialized knowledge and know-how.
- Seek out supervision when performing a new skill.
- Invest in deeply understanding the patient situations in which you are involved.
- Generate and test alternative lines of reasoning.
- Trust your hunches—check them out.
- Be aware of when you are time pressured and likely to make thinking errors.
- Consider multiple aspects of the patient's situation when you are deciding how to treat.
- Make sure you know how to use technical equipment safely.
- Make sure you know how to interpret data produced by monitoring devices.
- Pay attention to how you move and touch patients during care.
- Anticipate ethical conflicts.
- Acquire computer-related skills for accessing and managing patient data and practice information.

USE OF RESEARCH EVIDENCE
- Learn how to search health care databases for studies related to specific clinical topics.
- Read research reports related to your field of practice.
- Seek out systematic revision of research and research-based clinical guidelines.
- Acquire skills in appraising the various forms of research evidence.
- Work with colleagues to consider research-based improvements in care.
- Be alert for middle-range theories that are applicable to your practice.

DIVERSE APPROACHES TO HEALTH AND ILLNESS MANAGEMENT
- Use interpersonal interventions to influence patients.
- Acquire proficiency in new ways of treating and helping patients.
- Help patients maintain health and capitalize on their strengths and resources.
- Provide preventive services appropriate to your field of practice.
- Know what is allowed under managed care contracts.
- Negotiate with managed care case managers for unallowed services when necessary.
- Coordinate services among care sites and multiple providers.
- Acquire knowledge about complementary and alternative therapies.

---

neonatal intensive care units, APNs were found to emphasize holism, caring, and health (Beal, 2000).

HOLISM AND HEALTH ASSESSMENT

When working with a relatively healthy person, the APN seeks to understand the person's life goals, functional interests, and health risks to preserve quality of life in the future. In

---

BOX 5-2 • FACTORS TO BE CONSIDERED WHEN HELPING THE PATIENT HOLISTICALLY

- The patient's view of his or her health or illness
- Patterns of physical symptoms and amount of distress they cause
- The effect of physical symptoms on the patient's daily functioning and quality of life
- Symptom management approaches that are acceptable to the patient
- Life changes that could affect the patient's physical or psychological well-being (e.g., relationship breakup, job change, intrafamily conflict, retirement, death of a beloved person)
- The context of the patient's life, including the nuclear family unit, social support, job responsibilities, financial situation, health insurance coverage, responsibilities for the care of others (e.g., children, chronically ill spouse or partner, elderly parents)
- Spiritual and life values (e.g., independence, religion, beliefs about life, acceptance of fate)

---

contrast, when working with an ill patient, the APN is interested in what the person views as problems, how she or he is responding to problems, and what the problems and responses mean to the individual in terms of daily living and life goals. In a study of 199 primary care clinical situations (Burman, Stepans, Jansa, & Steiner, 2002), NPs were found to engage in holistic assessment and to ground their decision making within the context of the patient's life.

The ability to function in daily activities and relationships is an important consideration for patients when they evaluate their health, so it is an appropriate and essential focus for holistic, person-centered assessment. Most functional assessment formats focus on (1) how patients view their health or quality of life; (2) how they accomplish self-care and household or job responsibilities; (3) the social, physical, financial, and environmental factors that augment or tax their functioning; and (4) the strategies they and their families use to cope with the stresses and problems in their lives.

Many functional health assessment formats are population specific such as the following:

- Rehabilitation (Dittmar & Grisham, 1997)
- Outpatients (Eisen, Wilcox, Leff, Schaefer, & Culhane, 1999)
- Adults (Gordon, 1994)
- Persons with chronic pain (Vallerand, 1998)
- Home care (Neal, 1998)

In pediatrics, measures of functional status for children with asthma, otitis media, and juvenile rheumatoid arthritis are being field tested (American Academy of Pediatrics, 2003).

A widely used, general tool is the Short Form-36 Health Status Profile (SF-36), which measures general health, functional health status, and well-being in adults and is available in several languages. A brief, open-ended, functional health screening tool that can be used for adult outpatients or hospital inpatients is presented in Box 5-3. This form includes questions that allow the APN to identify problem areas efficiently. The questions can be asked conversationally in interviews with patients to ensure that all functional areas have been considered. Alternatively, patients can complete the questionnaire while waiting to be seen, or support staff can ask the questions of patients before the interview with the APN. The APN can use the answers to focus the interview on problems or

BOX 5-3 • HEALTH SCREENING QUESTIONS

Your answers will help the advanced practice nurse in talking with you about your health and health problems.

1. How has your health been recently?
   Very good _____ Good _____ Fair _____ Poor _____
2. What "new" health problems do you have?
3. What "old" health problems still bother you?
4. Are you physically able to do the activities you would like to be able to do?
   Yes _____ No _____
5. Do you have pain, aches, or discomfort of any type?
   Yes _____ No _____ Not sure _____
6. Do you believe you eat well? Yes _____ No _____ Not sure _____
   Are you satisfied with your weight? Yes _____ No _____ Not sure _____
7. Do you have any problems with your bowels or bladder?
   Yes _____ No _____ Maybe _____
8. Are you satisfied with the amount of sleep and rest you get?
   Yes _____ No _____ Not sure _____
9. Do you notice any problems with your vision, hearing, or feeling in your hands or feet?
   Yes _____ No _____ Maybe _____
10. Are you satisfied with how you handle the problems of daily life and with the decisions you make?
    Yes _____ No _____ Not sure _____
11. Do you generally feel good about yourself?
    Yes _____ No _____ Not sure _____
12. Are you generally satisfied with your relationships with others?
    Yes _____ No _____ Not sure _____
13. Are you satisfied with your sexuality and sexual relations?
    Yes _____ No _____ Not sure _____
14. Do you have beliefs about life that are very important to you and that you think we need to know to provide health care for you?
    Yes _____ No _____ Not sure _____

potential illness areas that need to be explored. The questions provide a time-efficient way of zeroing in on health issues that are of concern to patients while assessing their overall health status.

NURSING MODEL OR MEDICAL MODEL

As APNs take on responsibilities that formerly were in the purview of physicians, concern has been expressed by some that APNs are being asked to function within a medical model of practice rather than within a holistic nursing model. This is particularly true in roles in which APNs replace medical interns or residents. However, some evidence suggests that a nursing orientation is an enduring component of APN practice, even when medical management is part of the role. In a study of 10 collaborative pairs of physicians and NPs in primary care practices in Missouri, the NPs evidenced a holistic approach to care and conscious awareness of using both the medical and nursing models in their thinking (Flesner & Clawson, 1998). In a national survey of 482 randomly selected NPs, conducted in the early 1990s, the NPs were found to be very confident about their practice skills and knowledge and to have a very strong nursing orientation (Thibodeau & Hawkins, 1994). A Canadian study of the practice patterns of acute care NPs revealed that 63% of them reported giving equal weight to nursing and medical perspectives in their practices (Sidani et al., 2000). With a different slant, 188 NPs from the midwestern United States indicated that in their practice they used a wellness/health promotion model frequently and a nursing-theory model and traditional medical model to a minimal degree (Blasdell, Klunick, & Purseglove, 2002). This was true for NPs with master's degrees and those with baccalaureate degrees. In contrast, in another study the educational preparation of NPs was found to affect practice orientation (Beal, Maguire, & Carr, 1996). Certificate-prepared neonatal nurse practitioners (NNPs) aligned themselves with a medical philosophy, whereas master's-prepared NNPs espoused a philosophy of nursing and a strong nursing identity.

Statements from professional organizations indicate that APNs value their nursing orientation and their medical functions. For instance, the description of APNs in the American Nurses Association's (ANA's) Nursing Social Policy Statement includes strong endorsement of both specialized and expanded knowledge and skills within the context of holistic values (ANA, 2003). On the theoretical front, several models of advanced practice blend nursing and medical orientations. The Shuler Nurse Practitioner Practice Model emphasizes wellness and self-care while incorporating the role responsibilities involved in diagnosing and treating acute, episodic diseases and chronic illnesses (Shuler & Huebscher, 1998; see Chapter 2). Similarly, the Circle of Caring model includes traditional elements from both nursing and medicine (Dunphy & Winland-Brown, 1998; see Chapter 2).

HOLISM AND MANAGED CARE

The view of patients as unique, complex, and unitary persons is discordant with how many managed care organizations (MCOs) view patients, that is, as members of a "population" or "subpopulation" having in common a particular health problem. Although "there are compelling reasons to create systems of care to manage subpopulations of patients" (Britt, Schraeder, & Shelton, 1998), *only some* health care needs are predictable on the basis of biostatistics, epidemiology, cost-benefit analysis, outcomes studies, resource utilization tracking, and variance reports. When the care allowed for a certain subpopulation is prescribed by a health-care system, the individuality of each patient is not factored in, and often there is no provision for unique situations, needs, preferences, and beliefs (Ulrich, Soeken, & Miller, 2003).

APNs increasingly find themselves in the position of having to contact case managers who represent the MCO to defend the need for reimbursement for treatment modalities, services, care products, or specific medications that are not paid for under the contract. This form of advocacy on behalf of patients is and will continue to be common in a financing environment that emphasizes cost containment through population-based management. Moreover, many practitioners find themselves in situations in which they believe that their only option is to lie to the system that unjustly constrains their actions. In a survey of 700 NPs in Maryland, 80% of the respondents perceived that it was sometimes necessary to bend managed care guidelines to assist individual patients, and 69% agreed that practitioners must sometimes exaggerate a patient's illness to provide appropriate care (Ulrich et al., 2003). Such duplicity violates personal and professional standards of moral conduct, but then so does the alternative of not providing necessary care. The dilemma can only be resolved by action at both the individual practitioner level and the national level. The individual APN can carefully screen prospective contracts and employers to ensure alliance with an ethically sound system of care. At the national level, action is needed to help health-care systems achieve a fair balance between evidence-based, quality care and fiscal constraint.

Formation of Partnerships with Patients

APNs' person-centered, holistic perspective serves as the foundation for the kinds of relationships they co-create with patients. Research evidence reveals that APNs form collaborative relationships with patients. They do so by engaging in social story exchanges, expressing regard for patients, asking about patients' home lives, and helping patients plan how they can follow health and illness management recommendations (Brown, 1999b; Courtney & Rice, 1997; Flesner & Clawson, 1998; Grando, 1998). Studies of APNs' interactions with patients indicate that advanced nursing practice does embody the ideal of providing "skilled companionship" on illness "journeys" (Pearson, Borbasi, & Walsh, 1997). The collaborative relationship is the ideal medium for providing education and guidance through illness and life transitions, as discussed in Chapter 6.

SHARED DECISION MAKING

In addition to eliciting information that increases understanding of the patient's illness experience, APNs in the studies cited previously encouraged patients to participate in decisions regarding how their disease and illness will be managed. One example of a specific way to involve patients in management decisions was found in a systematic review of educational interventions to improve cancer pain management (Allard, Maunsell, Labbe, & Dorval, 2001). The authors concluded that the most promising avenue might be an intervention in which the nurse works with patients using a pain diary to record fluctuations in pain levels; importantly, documented uncontrolled pain should be followed rapidly by clinical reassessment and dose adjustment.

Substantial evidence indicates that many patients who have cancer want to participate in decisions about their illness management (Degner et al., 1997; Johnson et al., 1996; Petrisek, Laliberte, Allen, & Mor, 1997; Pyke-Grimm, Degner, Small, & Mueller, 1999). Because participatory decision making has been studied most extensively in relation to treatment for cancer, much less is known about the preference of patients facing other kinds of clinical decisions (e.g., hormone replacement therapy or treatment of coronary heart disease). The cancer treatment studies revealed considerable variation in preference for participation; therefore it is possible, and even likely, that patients' decisions regarding other kinds of decisions and decisions made under less threatening circumstances also vary widely. Also, it should be noted that the benefits of patient participation in treatment and management decisions have not been extensively studied (Guadagnoli & Ward, 1998).

Typically, NPs adapt their communication style to individual patients, which is as it should be. In a study of informational and controlling communication styles of MDs and NPs, both groups tended to use an informational style; however, four of the five NPs used a wide range of communication approaches (Lawson, 2002). This finding suggests that, while NPs may have a preferred or casual communication style (i.e., informational), there may be particular patient characteristics that signal the NP to switch to a more controlling style. Adapting communication style to individual preferences and behaviors may be a characteristic of APN communication; however, the research evidence that supports this claim has not been systematically assembled.

Based on current knowledge, providers should be reluctant to make any assumptions about an individual patient's preference for participation in clinical decisions regarding how to prevent and diagnose disease or manage an illness. Instead, they should individually determine each patient's preference for participation in decision making and be sensitive to the fact that patients' preferences may change over time as they get to know the

provider better and as different kinds of health problems arise. Once the patient's preference has been elicited, the provider should tailor his or her communication and decision-
making style to the patient's preference. The importance of this tailoring of
communication style was supported by results of a study of the decision-making preferences of ambulatory veterans in which mismatched patient preference and provider communication style adversely affected patient satisfaction (Harvey, Kazis, & Lee, 1999). The
veterans with a strong preference for involvement in decision making who were offered
fewer decision-making opportunities were significantly less satisfied with medical care
than were veterans in three other groups with different combinations of preference and
offered opportunities. Many patients have not had prior health-care experiences in which
shared decision making was even a possibility, but, when offered the opportunity, many
choose it—tentatively in some cases, enthusiastically in others. "Trying on" a more active
role may require some help from the provider such as explaining how it would work and
which responsibilities are the patient's and which are the provider's. Patients can be
encouraged to bring up issues with open-ended questions such as "So, how have you
been?" and focused-but-open questions such as "So, how are things going at home?"
Patients can be encouraged to participate in decision making by offering them explicit
opportunities in the form of questions such as, "Does one of those approaches sound better
to you than the other?" Gradually, patients approached in this way will learn that health-
care encounters will be organized around their concerns, not around a series of questions
asked by the provider, and that they should express their concerns and preferences.

CULTURAL INFLUENCES ON PARTNERSHIPS

Another important factor affecting whether and how persons want to participate in health-
care decision making is their cultural background. It is easy to forget that not all cultures
value individual autonomy as much as North Americans of Anglo-Saxon ancestry do.
Increasingly, recognizing and respecting the cultural identification of patients is being
viewed as essential to building meaningful partnerships. Cultural groups form along lines of
racial, national origin, religious, professional, organizational, sexual orientation, or age
group identification. Some cultural groups are easier to identify than others. Physical differences in appearance often tip the provider off to the fact that he or she is dealing with a
person of a different cultural orientation. Other cultural identifications are less obvious—
for example, people with religious beliefs about fate, God as healer, or treatment taboos.

Some of these groups have ways of thinking and communication expectations that are
quite different from those of the health-care provider, and possibly unfamiliar to him or
her (Cooper-Patrick et al., 1999; Waite et al., 1994). These differences can cause confusion, misunderstandings, and even conflicts that disrupt the patient-provider relationship
and discourse. Moreover, they often complicate attempts to resolve misunderstandings
because different cultural groups approach conflict negotiation differently. In every
encounter, the provider should expect that the patient may have values that are different
in some ways from his or her own and must make a special effort to ensure that the care
being given meets the patient's needs and is acceptable to him or her.

PARTNERSHIPS WITH NONCOMMUNICATIVE PATIENTS

Some patients are not able to enter fully into partnership with APNs because they are too
young, have compromised cognitive capacity, or are unconscious. Clinical populations
who may be unable to participate *fully* in shared decision making are listed in Box 5-4.
Although these patients may be limited in their abilities to speak for themselves, they are

---

BOX 5-4 • PATIENT POPULATIONS UNABLE TO PARTICIPATE FULLY IN PARTNERSHIP

Infants and preverbal children
Anesthetized patients
Unconscious/comatose patients
People in severe pain
Patients receiving medications that impair cognition
People with dementia
People with psychiatric conditions that seriously impair rational thought
People with conditions that render them incapable of speech and conversation
People with congenital or acquired cognitive limitations
People whose primary language is different from the provider's

---

not entirely without opinion or voice. Situations in which patients will experience temporary alterations in cognition or verbal ability can often be anticipated (e.g., during general anesthesia and during intubation), and the APN can discuss patients' preferences for handling possible events beforehand and elicit their wishes.

In the absence of this kind of prior dialogue, experts who work with patients who cannot verbalize their concerns and preferences learn to pay close attention to how patients are responding to what happens to them; facial expressions, body movement, and physiological parameters are used to ascertain what causes the patient discomfort and what helps alleviate it (Benner, Tanner, & Chesla, 1996; Halliburton, 1998). In a study of persons who had experienced and recovered from unconsciousness (Lawrence, 1995), 27% of the patients reported being able to hear, understand, and respond emotionally while they were unconscious. These findings suggest that nurses should communicate with unconscious patients by providing them with interventions such as reassurance, bodily care, pain relief, explanations, and comforting touch. A naturalistic, interpretive study of critical care nurses revealed that recognizing subtle forms of communication requires perceptiveness and interpersonal involvement with the patient (Benner, Hooper-Kyriakidis, & Stannard, 1999).

Alternative sources of information about patients who are unable to respond physically or to communicate should also be identified. For example, siblings visiting an adolescent male with a major head injury would be able to tell you what kind of music he likes to listen to and would probably even bring you a tape or CD to play for the patient. His mother would know what has caused him to have skin reactions in the past. Responding to his father's offhand comment that he cannot stand to be without his glasses when he is not wearing his contact lenses would most likely help both father and son. All of these are ways of building partnership with an unconscious teenager in an intensive care unit (ICU). In adults and adolescents, advance directives, heath care proxy documents, and organ donation cards are other sources of information regarding patients' wishes. Thus noncommunicative patients are not without voices, but hearing their voices does require presence, attentiveness, and relationship.

Expert Clinical Thinking and Skillful Performance

KNOWLEDGE

APNs' specialized knowledge accrues from a variety of sources including:

- Graduate education
- Experience working with a population of patients

- Professional reading
- Continuing education
- Exchange of information and ideas with colleagues

The integration of knowledge from these sources provides a foundation for the expert clinical thinking that is associated with advanced direct care practice. Once an APN has been in practice for a while, formalized knowledge and experiential knowledge become so mixed together that they are no longer distinguishable. The expert's clinical knowledge is characterized by the ability to make fine distinctions among common features of a particular condition that were not possible during beginning practice. Benner (1984) has studied the practice of nurses who are expert by experience. Although her subjects were not APNs, her studies of expert clinical judgment inform this discussion of APNs' expert clinical judgment. Illness trajectories and presentations of prior patients make an impression and come to mind when a patient with a similar problem is seen later (Benner, 1984). The expert also remembers what interventions worked and did not work in certain situations. Timetables of progress that most patients attain in certain situations (e.g., the time after surgery when patients' energy levels return) create expectations for patients who fit into that population (Benner et al., 1996). Eventually, the expert's clinical knowledge consists of a complex network of memorable cases, prototypic images, research findings, thinking strategies, moral values, maxims, probabilities, behavioral responses, associations, illness trajectories and timetables, therapeutic information, and domain-relevant concepts. Thus, experts have extensive, varied, and complex knowledge networks that can be activated to help them understand clinical situations and events.

CLINICAL THINKING

Clinical reasoning brings together the clinical knowledge of the provider with specific observations, perceptions, events, and facts from the situation at hand to produce an understanding of what is occurring (O'Neill, 1995). Sometimes the understanding is arrived at by using cognitive processes to logically consider evidence and alternative explanations. Other times the insight or understanding "arrives" intuitively, that is, through direct apprehension without recourse to deliberate reasoning (Benner et al., 1996).

Experts have the ability to rapidly scan a situation (e.g., past records, patient's appearance, and the patient's unexpressed concern or discomfort) and identify salient and relevant information. Relying heavily on their perceptions, observations, and physical assessment skills, experts quickly activate one or several lines of reasoning regarding what might be going on. They then conduct a more focused assessment to determine which one best explains the situation at hand. These lines of reasoning are really informal, personal theories about the specific patient situation; their formulation draws from personal knowledge of the particular patient, from personal knowledge acquired from previous experiences, and from formalized domain-specific knowledge (Corcoran-Perry, Narayan, & Cochrane, 1999; Narayan & Corcoran-Perry, 1997; Rolfe, 1997). Often, these lines of reasoning can be tested by performing a clinical intervention and noting how the patient responds. For example, the ventilator settings could be changed in ways suggested by the line of reasoning to determine whether the patient is better able to proceed with weaning (Narayan & Corcoran-Perry, 1997).

Most patient accounts unfold in a fairly predictable way, and the APN arrives at a diagnosis and/or intervention with considerable confidence in her or his clinical inferences.

Other times, however, there is uncertainty and lack of understanding regarding the situation. The uncertainty may pertain to information the patient provides, to the diagnosis, to the best approach to management, or to how the patient is responding (Brykczynski, 1991). When there is ambiguity, experts often break into conscious problem solving or "detective-like thinking and questioning" (Benner et al., 1996; Benner et al., 1999) to try to figure out what is going on.

Knowing the patient as an individual with certain patterns of responses enables experienced nurses to detect subtle changes in a patient's condition (Tanner, Benner, Chesla, & Gordon, 1993). In one study, experienced acute care nurses reported that they often sensed nonspecific changes in patients and experienced a gut feeling that the patient was in transition before they were able to detect significant objective changes (Smith, 1988). These subjective feelings led to "close searching" for confirmatory evidence, which gradually led to detection and recognition of an objective pattern indicating a change in condition. Premonitory feelings were also reported by an NP who reported attending to her "feelings of lack of closure, of uneasiness, incompleteness, or discomfort" because they often indicated that something important was going to come up in the conversation (Brykczynski, 1989).

Knowing the patient may be critical to perceptive and accurate clinical reasoning (Benner et al., 1996). The extent to which a nurse knows the patient may be associated with that nurse's ability to do the following:

- Recognize that risk factors are present
- Detect early indicators of a problem (i.e., a slight change in pattern)
- Take timely preventive action
- Recognize nonfitting and atypical data

Nonfitting data suggest to experts that they need to generate new, or additional, hypotheses because the current observations and parameters do not fully explain the clinical picture as it has been or as it should be. For example, when faced with a nonfitting sign or symptom, the nurse may generate alternative hypotheses pertaining to the onset of a complication or to the worsening of the disease process (Burman et al., 2002).

THINKING ERRORS

The clinical acumen of APNs and the inferences, hypotheses, and lines of reasoning they generate are highly dependable. However, as practice becomes repetitive, APNs may develop routine responses, and they then run the risk of making certain types of thinking errors (Schön, 1984). Errors of expectancy occur when the correct diagnosis is not generated as a hypothesis because there is a set of circumstances, in either the clinician's experience or the patient's circumstances, that predisposes the clinician to disregard it. For example, the NP who over several years has seen an elderly woman for problems associated with chronic pulmonary disease may fail to consider that the most recent onset of shortness of breath and fatigue could be related to worsening aortic stenosis; the NP has come to expect pulmonary disease, not cardiac disease.

Erroneous conclusions are also more likely when the situation is ambiguous, that is, when the meaning or reliability of the data is unclear, the interpretation of the data is not clear-cut, the best approach to treatment is debatable, or one cannot say for sure whether the patient is responding well to treatment (Brykczynski, 1991). To avoid errors in these kinds of situations, experts often revert to the use of maxims to guide their thinking (Brykczynski, 1989). One of the maxims that NPs use to deal with uncertain diagnoses is "When you hear hoof beats in Kansas, think horses, not zebras." This reminds clinicians who are about to make a diagnosis that occurs infrequently to consider the incidence of the condition in the population (i.e., the base rate information). Thus an elderly person with respiratory problems seen in a suburban office is unlikely to have tuberculosis; pneumonia is a more likely diagnosis. Because tuberculosis is rare in the population of which the elderly person is a member, the clinical data for tuberculosis should be quite convincing if that diagnosis is proposed.

To keep the use of axioms in perspective, clinicians must be aware that overreliance on clinical axioms can be a source of error in clinical thinking (Kassirer & Kopelman, 1991). Poor judgment can also result from tunnel vision; overgeneralization; influence by a recent, dramatic experience; premature closure (Croskerry, 2003); and fixation on certain problems to the exclusion of others (Benner et al., 1999). Faulty thinking is not the only source of error in clinical decision making. Other sources include inaccurate observations, misinterpretation of the meaning of data, a sketchy knowledge of the particular situation, and a faulty model of the disease, condition, or response.

TIME PRESSURES

Regardless of setting, practitioners worry about the effect time pressures have on the accuracy and completeness of their clinical thinking and decision making. The Institute of Medicine's report on errors and patient safety cited studies in which between 3% and 46% of hospitalized patients in the United States are harmed by error or negligence (Kohn, Corrigan, & Donaldson, 1999). The wide variation is due to varying definitions of what constitutes adverse events and various methods of detecting their occurrence. Moreover, it is estimated that two thirds of injuries resulting from error or negligence are preventable (Kohn et al., 1999).

A heavy workload is associated with feelings of pressure, being rushed, cognitive overload, and fatigue; these feelings clearly contribute to unsafe acts and omissions in care (Kohn et al., 1999). Evidence in support of this inference comes from studies of nurse staffing in hospitals in which fewer hours of nursing care per patient per day and less care provided by registered nurses were associated with poorer patient outcomes (Kovner, Jones, Zhan, Gergen, & Basu, 2002; Needleman, Buerhaus, Mattke, Steward, & Zelevinsky, 2002). The patient safety movement has led to a variety of efforts aimed at preventing errors: monitoring of sentinel events, improved work processes, redesign of delivery systems, use of technological aids, communication training, and team building. Also, required staffing levels for in-hospital care have been instituted.

The effects of a heavy workload on patient outcomes in nonhospital settings are less well understood; thus actions to address this issue have received less attention. However, as lengths of visit or contact times are decreased or the number of patients practitioners are expected to see in a day is increased, it is logical to assume that the number of errors in clinical thinking will increase. Each contact requires the practitioner to "reset" his or her clinical reasoning process by closing out one thinking project and starting on a whole new one. This resetting, which is done back-to-back many times during a day, is cognitively and physically demanding. How these performance expectations affect clinical reasoning accuracy is unknown.

Moreover, time pressures often get compounded by hassles and interruptions. Hassles come in the form of interruptions, noise in the environment, missing supplies, and system glitches that make clinical data or even whole charts unavailable to providers. These hassles likely interfere with providers' ability to concentrate on what the patient is saying and disrupt their efforts to make clinical sense of patients' accounts. In many settings, providers are required to multitask. They start a task but must attend to another task before completing the original one. This clearly increases the risks of failure to obtain needed information, broken lines of thought, technological missteps, omissions in care, and failure to respond to patients' requests for service. In a descriptive study of emergency department physicians, the number of times physicians were interrupted or required to change to another task while in the process of performing a task was counted (Chisholm, Collison, Nelson, & Cordell, 2001). On average, in a 3-hour period, the physicians saw 12 patients and performed 68 tasks. In the 3-hour period, they were interrupted an average of 31 times and required to change tasks 21 times. The investigators concluded that emergency physicians are "interrupt-driven." Admittedly, the emergency department may be an extreme example of a multitasking environment, but other settings also impose interruptions at a very high rate. As time pressures for clinicians increase, organizational efforts to monitor for errors and potential errors and seek correction when there are system weaknesses is something APNs owe patients—and themselves as providers functioning in busy environments.

Finally, health-care administrators and providers would be naive to think patients are unaffected by practitioners' heavy workloads or tight appointment schedules. Many patients are sensitive to the pace with which staff and providers greet them, talk with them, and do things, particularly those activities that involve verbal interaction and physical contact. Some patients respond to the fast-paced talk and hurried movements of providers by not bringing up some of the questions they had intended to ask. Others may just get flustered and forget to mention important information; still others may become hostile and withhold information. Thus, error in the form of information omission by the patient enters the clinical reasoning and decision-making process.

In summary, clinical thinking is a complex task. It involves drawing on knowledge in memory and attending to multiple sources of situational input, some of which are difficult to interpret. Often, multiple clinical issues must be addressed during a patient encounter, and there are several ways of thinking about each issue. These complexities make clinical thinking a challenging task, even under the best of circumstances.

INFORMATION MANAGEMENT

Undoubtedly, some errors originate as a result of the extensive amount of information and knowledge that must be processed to provide timely, accurate, state-of-the-science care (Kibbe, 1999). Fortunately, electronic information technology is available to assist providers in the retrieval, application, and management of all this information. The Clinical Information Systems (CIS) of many agencies offer a variety of helpful tools including reminders, medication histories, significant event timelines, diagnostic and therapeutic decision support, links to relevant clinical guidelines, and tracking systems. Also, the generation and partial completion of referral forms, reports, and discharge summaries from data already in the information system are reducing the time clinicians spend on paperwork (Yarcey, Given, White, DeVoss, & Coyle, 1998).

To obtain the information they need to take care of patients in the current environment, APNs need to be able to use personal digital assistants (PDAs) and desktop computers to access essential information. Clinical reference software is a rapidly expanding field and is available in desktop and PDA formats; the following is just a sampling of what is available. Drug information guides provide peer-reviewed information on thousands of drugs including information about drug interactions, contraindications, dosage calculators, drug pricing information, and even formularies for health plans in your area. Clinical calculators assist clinicians in a variety of tasks such as drug dosage calculations and determination of pregnancy due dates. Other reference programs provide useful laboratory, diagnostic, and condition management information, as well as a variety of assessment, risk prediction, and probability tools. Online search engines for locating and accessing clinical guidelines, systematic reviews, and research reports are also available; they are discussed in a subsequent section on use of research evidence.

Another important category of electronic tools is patient management software. Many of these programs allow mobile or point-of-care charting, patient data transfer to and from existing clinical information systems, access to appointment scheduling systems, and communication with other providers. In short, for each area of clinical practice, there are reference tools, calculators, information managers, and search engines that make information available to clinicians, support their decision making, and assist them in doing their work.

ETHICAL REASONING

Clinical reasoning is inextricably linked to ethical reasoning. Clinical reasoning generates possibilities of what *could* be done in a situation, whereas ethical reasoning adds the dimension of what *should* be done in the situation. (For a more extensive discussion of ethical decision making, see Chapter 11.) What is possible and what is appropriate in specific situations are furthest apart when dealing with decisions regarding the stopping or withholding of nutrition, hydration, or a treatment; when dealing with reproductive technology; and when cost must figure into clinical treatment decisions. These situations are at high risk for becoming ethically problematic.

The literature regarding how to resolve ethical issues is extensive, but an approach to incorporating ethical considerations into clinical thinking and decision making that makes a great deal of sense is preventive, or prospective, ethics (Forrow, Arnold, & Parker, 1993). This approach places an emphasis on preventing ethical conflicts from developing rather than waiting until a conflict arises; it does so by shaping the process of clinical care so that potential value conflicts are anticipated and discussed before outright conflict occurs. In addition to emphasizing early communication between the patient and the provider(s) about values, preventive ethics requires explicit, critical reflection on the institutional factors that lead to conflict (Forrow et al., 1993). A third aspect of preventive ethics is an effort to create and preserve trust and understanding among providers, as well as between providers and patients (and their families). Thus, preventive ethics is proactive in that it requires providers to consider how the routine processes of care either foster or prevent conflicts from occurring or, at the very least, identify them at an early stage.

Several studies in ICUs have shown that preventive ethics consultations or ethics rounds result in (1) improved communication and decision making (Dowdy, Robertson, & Bander, 1998), (2) shorter time between identification of poor prognosis and the establishment of a comfort care plan (Mion et al., 2003), and (3) reductions in ICU hospital days and life-sustaining treatments (Dowdy et al., 1998; Schneiderman, Gilmer, & Teetzel, 2000). Clearly, some ICU dilemmas would be easier to resolve if discussion of possible future events and decisions were to take place with patients earlier in the course of illness.

Many questions about preventive ethics remain (Dowdy et al., 1998). When in a patient's illness should the values issues be discussed? How can they be raised without frightening patients and families? What information should be discussed? Is it better to discuss specific but hypothetical future clinical scenarios or to discuss a patient's more general goals and values? Even with these unanswered questions, the preventive approach has the potential to avoid conflicts. Preventive ethics also has the potential to integrate ethical reasoning into clinical reasoning at an earlier point in time than when a traditional conflict-based ethics approach is used.

Another approach to ethical reasoning has been uncovered in the research of Benner and associates; in their work they have found that many nurses have a "disposition toward what is good and right" (Benner et al., 1996). These notions of good arise from society, from the nursing profession, from personal and professional experience, and from the work setting. They include commitments to humanizing and personalizing care, promoting comfort and self-care, preventing needless suffering, maximizing patient participation in decision making, responding to the feelings and problems of families, and preventing the patient from experiencing adverse effects in the course of receiving health care (Benner et al., 1996; Benner et al.1999). These notions of good guide the actions of nurses and influence how they see situations. When health care is in conflict with these values and commitments, practitioners experience moral conflict or anguish and often take action to change these kinds of situations. This view of how nurses experience ethical dilemmas suggests that nurses are faced with ethical decisions and conflicts that are very different from those of physicians or those addressed in traditional biomedical ethics.

Ethical issues related to advances in knowledge about human genetics are numerous. APNs working with patients in their childbearing years are most affected by developments in genetics; however, APNs working in various settings experience situations related to patients' genetic information. A pediatric NP might confront the issue of whether to test for a hereditary cancer (MacDonald & Lessick, 2000). A neuroscience CNS might be asked about genetic screening because so many neurological diseases are hereditary (Tazbir, 2001). The following four guidelines indicate how APNs should deal with these kinds of issues (Cassells, Jenkins, Lea, Calzone, & Johnson, 2003).

1. Maintain current genetic knowledge as it pertains to your specialty so you can talk credibly with patients who seek your counsel.
2. Do not go beyond your knowledge when advising patients.
3. Know what genetic testing and counseling services are available in your vicinity and refer patients to the service that best meets their needs.
4. Even though all health-care information should be treated as private and confidential, remember that genetic information is particularly sensitive and demands a special effort to safeguard it.

SKILLFUL PERFORMANCE

Although the health-care professions place high value on knowledge and expert clinical reasoning, it is important to keep in mind that the public values skillful performance in physical examinations, delivery of treatments, diagnostic procedures, and comfort care. Most graduate schools require students to perform a specific set of procedural skills recommended by a national specialty organization before they complete their program. However, little is known about how APNs acquire competency in new or expanded procedural skills once they are in practice. Presumably, competency of APNs to perform specific procedures and treatment is initially ensured through the processes agencies use to credential and grant privileges to APNs. After that, the responsibility for acquiring new competencies lies with the individual APN and the employing agency. When an APN or an agency recognizes that patients would receive better care if the APN would perform a new procedure, an agreement should be reached regarding exactly what new procedure the APN will perform, the conditions under which the procedure will be done, how the APN will acquire the necessary skill, and how supervision will be provided during the learning period.

Use of Research Evidence

An important form of knowledge that must be brought to bear on clinical decision making, for individuals and for populations, is the ever-increasing volume of research findings. For the nursing profession, the use of research findings as a basis for practice is more than the latest trend. The profession has been exploring and considering the issues of research utilization intensively since the early 1970s. Historically, CNSs led efforts in many agencies to move toward research-based practice (Hanson & Ashley, 1994; Hickey, 1990; Mackay, 1998; Stetler et al., 1995). They have brought research findings to the attention of the nursing staff and interdisciplinary teams and worked to develop the research appraisal skills of nursing staffs. The profession, agencies, and APNs themselves view evidence-based practice skills as central to APNs' research competency and as a more appropriate expectation of APNs than the conduct of research itself (see Chapter 8). Research evidence can be used in a variety of ways. Differentiating between research-sensitive practice and research-based practice provides a useful way of thinking about how APNs can incorporate research into their practices.

RESEARCH-SENSITIVE PRACTICE

Research-sensitive practice is practice in which the individual clinician brings research findings to bear on practice in an unstructured way. To do this an APN would (1) read primary research reports and summaries of research findings on a regular basis, (2) informally evaluate the soundness of the methods, and (3) adjust or fine-tune his or her own practice on the basis of credible findings. This is the form of research utilization in which every professional nurse should engage. It is part of staying abreast of new knowledge in one's area of clinical practice.

Research-sensitive practice could take the form of setting time aside to systematically scan clinical journals for reports relevant to one's clinical specialty. Alternatively, an APN could join or form a multidisciplinary group that meets monthly to discuss several research reports on topics of mutual interest. Some APNs keep a small notebook in which to jot down clinical issues and questions about which they have uncertainty. Then once a month, they use the 2 hours of library time that is built into their schedules to find studies about these issues. The recorded questions help them use the limited library time in the most efficient manner. Thus, the APN can constantly refine how she or he delivers care according to new evidence, without undertaking comprehensive reviews of the research.

RESEARCH-BASED PRACTICE

Research-based practice is a more systematic, rigorous, and precise way of translating research findings into practice. The research-based practice process is used within an organization to design a standard of care for a population of patients. The research-based practice process is more formal because research-based care will be widely used as a guide to care, and therefore the scientific conclusions on which it is based must be as free of bias and error as possible. In general terms, the process involves three steps: (1) locating, evaluating, and summarizing the science; (2) translating the science into clinical recommendations; and (3) strategically implementing the recommendations. The recommendations may take the form of a clinical practice guideline, a care map, a decision algorithm, a clinical protocol, or the components of a clinical program.

Although the term *research-based practice* is used in this discussion, most often when APNs are involved in designing care for a population of patients, all forms of objective evidence should be used; this would include quality improvement data, data from internal databases, data from benchmarking partners, and data from state and national databases (e.g., the Centers for Disease Control and Prevention). Agency-specific information, collected to pinpoint the nature of a problem, is particularly useful evidence that should be combined with the more general knowledge gained from research evidence (Brown, 2001; Nelson, Splaine, Batalden, & Plume, 1998).

The easiest means of incorporating research into practice is adoption of research-based guidelines that have been produced by respected organizations. A good starting point in a search for a research-based clinical guideline is the National Guideline Clearinghouse, which can be accessed online at www.guideline.gov. Clinical guidelines can also be located by searching clinical databases such as CINAHL or MEDLINE using the keyword guideline or protocol as a field delimiter. Many professional and specialty associations produce research-based clinical guidelines relevant to the care provided by their members. Thus, one might look for a guideline on a specialty or professional society's website. For example, one might go to the American Pain Society's website to order a guideline on pain management for patients with arthritis, sickle cell disease, or cancer (www.ampainsoc.org). Another group that develops research-based clinical guidelines for problems that nurses manage is the Registered Nurses Association of Ontario (RNAO) in Canada, which is funded by the province of Ontario (www. rnao.org/bestpractices/). The Registered Nurses Association of Ontario is doing an excellent job of producing research-based guidelines and is generous in sharing them.

After finding a research-based guideline produced outside her or his system, the APN (or clinical group) must then decide whether the guideline was produced in a sound way; tools are available to assist in making this determination (Appraisal of Guidelines Research and Evaluation, 2002, www.agreecollaboration.org/; Brown, 1999a). If the guideline was soundly produced, the APNs (or user group) should then consider whether the recommendations are appropriate for their patients and setting; some recommendations may be scientifically justified but may not be realistic to adopt in every setting. The Registered Nurses Association of Ontario's (2003) website provides a great deal of useful information about implementing clinical guidelines.

Also, when an APN engages in a project to design care based on research evidence, she or he should conduct a search for a systematic review on the topic. Systematic reviews summarize the findings from primary studies and can serve as the basis for a clinical guideline. They are being published in clinical journals with increased frequency, and several evidence-based centers around the world specialize in producing them, including:

1. The Cochrane Library (www.update-software.com/cochrane/)
2. The Joanna Briggs Institute (www.joannabriggs.edu.au/about/home.php)
3. The Agency for Healthcare Research and Quality (www.ahrq.gov/)
4. York University Dissemination and Research Centre (www.agatha.york.ac.uk/darehp.htm).

Increasingly, clinicians will be able to locate science summaries or research-based clinical practice guidelines; however, at times, neither will exist. Then the long path to producing a research-based clinical guideline will have to be traversed; this involves the following steps:

1. Identifying research reports on the topic of interest
2. Retrieving the reports
3. Evaluating the credibility of the findings
4. Summarizing the findings
5. Translating the findings into clinical practice guidelines

When production of such a guideline is the goal, it should be undertaken by a group or panel, because the process is arduous, requires a variety of skills, and would be time consuming if it were done by an individual.

Identifying and locating research findings is much easier than it was just 5 years ago. However, clinicians often do not have sufficient experience in use of the various search engines available to retrieve information from databases. APNs in all settings engaging in an evidence-based practice project will be well served by developing a relationship with a health-care librarian who can assist with searches (Pond, 1999). This assistance can save time and prevent the omission of a research-based guideline or systematic review that could be used to develop a setting-specific guideline.

THEORY-BASED PRACTICE

The preceding discussion of research-based practice recognizes how research evidence informs practice but ignores the role of theory. APNs are becoming comfortable with the idea of research evidence as a guide to practice, yet the idea of theory-based practice is less familiar. It should not be, because contrary to common perception, theory can be a very practical tool. Theory often brings together research findings in a way that helps practice be more purposeful, systematic, and comprehensive.

In the past, most discussions of theory-based practice addressed the use of conceptual models of nursing to guide care (Bonamy, Schultz, Graham, & Hampton, 1995; Hawkins, Thibodeau, Utley-Smith, Igou, & Johnson, 1993; Laschinger & Duff, 1991; Sappington & Kelley, 1996). However, more recently, emphasis has shifted to middle-range theories, which guide practice more specifically. Middle-range theories typically address a particular patient experience (e.g., living with rheumatoid arthritis) or problem (e.g., managing chronic pain); thus their range of applicability is relatively narrow. However, this narrow range of applicability allows them to be developed to address specific issues encountered in clinical practice. Schwartz-Barcott, Patterson, Lusardi, and Farmer (2002) make a strong case for developing theories by using fieldwork so that the theories will be more closely aligned to the realities practicing nurses encounter. Another approach to developing theories that are more specific to clinical situations is to generate a middle-range theory from one of the broader conceptual models. For instance, Whittemore and Roy (2002) developed a middle-range theory describing adaptation to diabetes mellitus based on the concepts and theoretical statements of the broader Roy Adaptation Model.

A 1999 analysis of the nursing literature identified 22 middle-range theories that met certain criteria (Liehr & Smith, 1999). The list of theories generated by that analysis is provided in Box 5-5. The list provides a sampling of the middle-range theories currently available to practicing nurses. In looking at this list, the reader can see that the topics of the theories are substantively specific, although some are more specific than others. "Balance between analgesia and side effects" is more specific and less abstract than

BOX 5-5 • MIDDLE-RANGE THEORIES

TOPIC	AUTHOR(S)
Uncertainty in illness	Mishel
Nurse-midwifery care	Thompson et al.
Facilitating growth and development	Kinney
Self-transcendence	Reed
Hazardous secrets and reluctantly taking charge	Burke et al.
Women's anger	Thomas
Caring	Swanson
Negotiating partnership	Powell-Cope
Unpleasant symptoms	Lenz et al.
Cultural brokering	Jezewski
Homelessness-hopelessness	Tollett & Thomas
Balance between analgesia and side effects	Good, Moore, & Good
Chronotherapeutic intervention for postsurgical pain	Auvil-Novak
Nurse-expressed empathy and patient distress	Olso & Hanchett
Interpersonal perceptual awareness	Brooks & Thomas
Resilience	Polk
Individualized music intervention for agitation	Gerdner
Affiliated individuation as a mediator for stress	Acton
Chronic sorrow	Eakes, Burke, & Hainswoth
Acute pain management	Huth & Moore
Psychological adaptation	Levesque et al.
Peaceful end of life	Ruland & Moore

From Liehr, P., & Smith, M. J. (1999). Middle range theory: Spinning research and practice to create knowledge for the new millennium. *Advances in Nursing Science, 14,* 81-91.

"Resilience." An APN in a particular field may find that only one or two of these theories are applicable to his or her area of practice. However, as middle-range theories are developed for other topics, APNs will be able to use several of these types of theories to guide different aspects of practice (Smith & Liehr, 2003).

KNOWLEDGE-BASED PRACTICE

Beyond research-based practice and theory-based practice is the more fundamental issue of knowledge-based practice. Development of useful and dependable knowledge requires both research work and theory work. Research findings are often bits of knowledge, whereas theories are explanatory systems describing how some aspect of the world works. To be most useful, research findings must be brought together into an internally consistent explanatory description. The knowledge development process can, of course, work in reverse. A theory can be based on the experiences of practice; then that theory needs to be tested and refined through research. Research can be used to determine the extent to which a theory holds up across different groups of people and helps identify the circumstances in which it is applicable. The findings of theory-testing research may also reveal ways in which the theory should be modified.

Whether knowledge is generated by theory or research, the goal is meaningful and useful knowledge that has been tested by using scientific methods and found to be an accurate and useful portrayal of certain realities. APNs have the educational background to appreciate how these two knowledge production pathways of science work together and separately to produce useful and dependable clinical knowledge.

Diverse Approaches to Health and Illness Management

APNs' holistic approach to care and their commitment to using research evidence as a basis for care contribute to how they help patients. Generally, APNs use a variety of interventions to effect change in the health status or quality of life of an individual or family and tailor their recommendations, approaches, and treatment to individual patients (Hughes et al., 2002). Interpersonal interventions that are psychosocial in nature are frequently referred to as *support*. Support interventions are somewhat distinct from educational interventions, which are informational in nature. Coaching uses a combination of support and education strategies (see Chapter 6). Then, of course, there are discrete physical actions, which are frequently categorized as nonpharmacological and pharmacological interventions. These distinctions are arbitrary because good clinicians probably craft interventions that are a combination of various types as they seek to alleviate, prevent, or manage specific physical symptoms, conditions, or problems.

INTERPERSONAL INTERVENTIONS

Support is not a discrete intervention; it is a composite of interpersonal interventions based on the patient's unique psychological and informational needs. Supportive interpersonal interventions include providing reassurance, giving information, coaching, affirming, providing anticipatory guidance, guiding decision making, listening actively, expressing understanding, and being available. Each of these interventions can be described in terms of the circumstances under which it is indicated; for example, reassurance is indicated when a patient is experiencing uncertainty, distress, or lack of confidence (Boyd & Munhall, 1989); and active listening is indicated when a patient has a strong need to tell her or his story. The actions that constitute these interventions are not mutually exclusive. For instance, giving factual information can be reassuring, instructional, guiding, or all of these things at the same time.

In practice, these interpersonal interventions are blended, and APNs are not consciously aware of when they are doing one and when they are doing another. This is as it should be. APNs have no need to think "Now I'm doing active listening; now I'm going to do anticipatory guidance." Instead, APNs interact with patients in ways that intermingle the conceptually separate interventions. This crafting of support evolves as the APN talks with patients; infers their worries, fears, and concerns; and, without a great deal of conscious thought, acts to alleviate their distress. A patient may experience the interaction as just a good talk with the APN or as a feeling of being understood. However, support is a complex nursing intervention that is strategically crafted and purposefully administered and often makes a difference in how the patient feels and acts.

DISCRETE MANAGEMENT AND TREATMENT INTERVENTIONS

Preventive Services in Primary Care. Health promotion and disease prevention interventions are tools that APNs in primary care regularly use to help people achieve and maintain a high quality of life. The preventive services include the following:

- Counseling regarding personal health practices that can protect a person from disease or screening for the presence of disease
- Immunization to prevent specific diseases
- Chemoprevention (e.g., use of aspirin for prevention of cardiovascular events)

Discernment is needed in the use of these interventions because time and effort can be wasted if their use is not based on current scientific knowledge and tailored to the individual person or community. In addition, the public is confused regarding many of the preventive recommendations because new research evidence has been unseating long-established recommendations, such as the value of breast self-examination. The U.S. Preventive Services Task Force's *Guide to Clinical Preventive Services* (2003) and the *Canadian Guide to Clinical Preventive Health Care* (Canadian Task Force on the Periodic Health Examination, 1994) provide specific preventive guidelines for many health conditions. These guidelines include valuable summaries of the state of the science for each recommendation, and the U.S. guidelines provide cost-effectiveness analyses, which summarize the benefits, harms, and costs of alternative strategies.

An important point made in an earlier version of the *Guide to Clinical Preventive Services* (U.S. Preventive Services Task Force, 1996) is that primary prevention in the form of counseling aimed at changing health-related behavior may be more effective than diagnostic screening and testing. Many healthy people, as well as people who have had a recent health scare, are quite receptive to, even eager for, information and guidance about how to stay healthy and avoid age-related disabilities. However, other people who engage in one or several unhealthy behaviors can be quite defensive and resistant to talking about their risks and how behavior changes could reduce risks. Introducing behavior change issues with unreceptive people requires a high level of interpersonal skill and a good sense of timing. An APN must consider that it is possible that no health-care provider has previously attempted to discuss the problem (e.g., smoking, lack of exercise, alcohol abuse) with the person, even though signs of a problem have existed for quite a while (Stafford & Blumenthal, 1998). If this is the case, some of these people may welcome the opportunity to be helped in facing the issue.

Talking about the risks of the current behavior and the benefits of the behavior change is not enough. To be effective, counseling regarding these issues should also include a discussion of how the person perceives the burden of changing a personal behavior; that is: what would be lost and what would be required to make the change? The provider must elicit how much effort will be required, what would give the individual the confidence to change, and what forms of self-help assistance are acceptable to the individual. Then, and only then, can a specific recommendation about a strategy or program be made. Theoretical models that can be useful in planning a behavior change program or protocol include the Transtheoretical Model (www.uri.edu/research/cprc/transtheoretical.htm) and the Health Belief Model (www.etr.org/recapp/theories/hbm/index.htm#major-concepts). Both models include provider strategies for building the person's self-efficacy (i.e., confidence in one's ability to take action).

For many risk reduction behaviors, community-based interventions may be more effective than those delivered in a clinical setting. School-based education and media blitzes are being used in attempts to educate children and adolescents about risky behaviors. Small-group discussions about sexual behaviors with adolescents in church programs and community health centers have resulted in less intercourse, greater use of condoms, and less risky sexual behavior in some communities (Kirby, 1994; O'Donnell, 1999). Work-site health education is being used with increased frequency, particularly with regard to occupational risks such as back strain and eye injuries (Volinn, 1999), but also with regard to cancer and heart disease prevention.

Clinicians also have at their disposal a wide array of screening tools, some of which are better with certain populations or age groups than others. For example, the U.S. Preventive Services Task Force (2003) recommends against routinely screening women older than age 65 for cervical cancer if they have had adequate recent screening with normal Papanicolaou test results and are not otherwise at risk; they also recommend against performing routine Papanicolaou tests for women who have had a total hysterectomy as treatment for benign disease. Staying current with the latest screening recommendations in one's area of practice ensures that care is provided in a way that is both scientific and cost-effective.

Preventive Services in Hospitals and Home Care. The preventive services provided in inpatient and home care settings are somewhat different from those provided in primary care. Many of the actions and assessments performed on behalf of acutely ill patients are aimed at early detection and prevention of problems related to treatment, disease progression, self-care deficits, or the hospital environment itself. Nurses assist patients by *preventing* adverse events and complications, including adverse medication reactions, unexpected physiological decline, poor communication, pressure ulcers, and death. This function is also referred to as *surveillance* or *rescuing* (as in rescuing from a bad course of events or death) (Aiken, Sochalski, & Lake, 1997). As mentioned earlier, in five studies of APN interventions with diverse patient groups, surveillance was the predominant APN function (Brooten et al., 2003).

One study of nursing-sensitive outcomes in hospitals identified four types of problems nurses frequently prevent: (1) complications related to treatment, (2) injuries and complications unrelated to treatment (e.g., falls), (3) extension of the disease process, and (4) complications related to a limited ability to engage in self-care activities at home (Stetler & DeZell, 1989). These problems typically result from a complex set of factors, some of which reside in inadequate delivery systems. They also occur when health-care professionals do not assess patients for risk of the problems common to their condition and do not proactively perform interventions that would prevent such problems from developing (Harris, 1997).

Therapeutic Interventions. The decision about whether to treat can be difficult, because the practitioner is faced with several probabilities that do not all lead to the same decision. Moreover, there is often pressure from patients to "do something." When deciding whether and how to treat patients, clinicians consider the following five types of information:

- The degree of certainty about the diagnosis or condition
- What is known about the effectiveness of the various treatment alternatives
- What is known about the risks of the treatment alternatives
- The clinician's comfort with a particular treatment or intervention
- The patient's preference for a certain kind of treatment or management

The most clear-cut situation is when the condition is assuredly present, a particular treatment is known to be highly effective, the treatment can be expected to be low in risk for the particular patient, and both the clinician and the patient are comfortable with the treatment. Unfortunately, many (probably most) therapeutic decisions are not so clear-cut. Instead, the weight of factors in support of a particular treatment and the weight of those against treatment or in support of another treatment are close to equivalent.

The treatment and management interventions that APNs perform include a wide variety of self-care modalities and low-tech, nonpharmacological modalities (Avorn, Everitt, & Baker, 1991; Brown & Grimes, 1993; Brykczynski, 1989). However, even when technological and pharmacological modalities are used, they are used in combination with consideration of many factors (Flesner & Clawson, 1998). For instance, in one study 501 physicians and 298 NPs were asked to describe how they would treat simulated cases involving patients with epigastric pain. The NPs were more likely than the physicians to recommend stopping use of aspirin; changing diet; reducing alcohol, caffeine, and tobacco intake; and obtaining counseling for stress (Avorn et al., 1991). They were also far less likely to recommend a prescription drug.

A slightly different result was found in another study of 10 collaborative pairs of physicians and NPs in which a methodology similar to that of Avorn et al. (1991) was used: NPs and physicians were identical in their final recommendations related to medication management, although the processes used to reach decisions were different (Flesner & Clawson, 1998). The NPs elicited more information about the context of the patients' lives and available resources and collaborated with patients more frequently to work out the details of implementing the management plans.

When prescribing medications, APNs consider the patient's financial status, the patient's previous experience with similar medications, the ease of taking the medication, how many other medications the person is taking, how often the medications must be taken, the side effect profiles of the drugs being considered, and potential drug and disease interactions (Brown & Grimes, 1993). A descriptive study of the safety and effectiveness of APN prescriptive authority revealed that the 33 NPs in the project prescribed medications for 90% of 1,708 patients; 42% had one drug prescribed per visit, and 31% had two drugs prescribed per visit (Hamric, Worley, Lindebak, & Jaubert, 1998). This would seem to be a low number of prescribed medications, but further study of the extent to which APNs recommend prescription drugs as compared with the extent to which other providers who care for similar patients do is needed before it can be established that a lower use of prescription drugs is characteristic of APNs.

Considerable evidence indicates that APNs use a broad range of interventions, with substantial reliance on self-care and low-tech interventions. In Brooten et al.'s (2003) study of advanced practice nursing interventions among five patient groups, surveillance was the most frequently used intervention; however, its range of use varied from 48% in patients with high-risk pregnancies to a high of 65% in patients who had undergone hysterectomies and elderly patients with heart disease. Teaching/guidance/counseling constituted 13% of the interventions in a group of patients who had very low birth weight infants and 36% in a high-risk pregnancy group. Case management activities of coordinating and planning care and care transitions made up 13% of the interventions in a cesarean delivery group and 25% of the interventions in the group of patients with very low birth weight infants. Thus, the frequency with which the various categories of interventions were used varied moderately with patient populations.

APNs in oncology settings report using nonpharmacological interventions such as cognitive activity; imagery; music; relaxation, breathing, and movement techniques; and cutaneous interventions (heat, cold, vibration, and transcutaneous electrical nerve stimulation) for symptom management (McMillan, Heusinkveld, & Spray, 1995; Spross & Wolff-Burke, 1996). Similarly, certified nurse-midwives (CNMs) report teaching perineal massage during late pregnancy (Labrecque et al., 1999) and recommending alternative birthing positions and styles of pushing to avoid having to perform episiotomies (Lydon-Rochelle, Albers, & Teaf, 1995; Sampselle & Hines, 1999). CNMs also use significantly less analgesia and anesthesia; perform less fetal monitoring and fewer episiotomies, forceps deliveries, and amniotomies; use fewer intravenous fluids; and induce labor less frequently than do physicians (Brown & Grimes, 1993; Davis, Riedmann, Sapiro, Minogue, & Kazer, 1994). Another perspective on the use of nonpharmacological management strategies by CNMs is provided by a study in which nurse-midwives' and obstetricians' processes of care were compared; the CNMs emphasized educational and psychosocial care and restrained use of technology, whereas the obstetricians more routinely used state-of-the-art technology (Oakley et al., 1995). In a study of APNs' use of *Current Procedural Terminology* (CPT) codes, family NPs and nurse-midwives used, on average, one third of the codes, a relatively varied usage (Griffith & Robinson, 1993). In summary, APNs clearly use a wide variety of interventions in management of their patients' conditions and problems.

The Nursing Interventions Classification Project (Bulechek & McCloskey, 1999), the Omaha Classification System, and the Home Health Care Classification are well along the road to capturing the full range of treatments and interventions nurses use and are superior to the *CPT* system for categorizing nursing activities (Henry, Holzemer, Randell, Hsieh, & Miller, 1997). These discipline-specific classification systems have the potential to recognize nursing interventions that currently are not recognized by the *CPT* system as contributing to patients' outcomes. Although APNs are not yet able to bill for the full range of services they provide, in February of 2003, the U.S. Department of Health and Human Services authorized the test of a proposed modification to the billing codes used for Medicare and Medicaid. The new codes are called *the Advanced Billing Concept (ABC) codes* and include intervention codes from the intervention classification systems developed and used by nurses. Although this is only a testing phase, it does hold promise for a billing system that will enable APNs to bill for services they provide that are not billable under the current *CPT* system.

The repertoire of interventions used by individual APNs clearly depends on the problems experienced by the population of patients with whom they work. Acute care nurse practitioners (ACNPs), CNMs, certified registered nurse anesthetists (CRNAs), and CNSs use different repertoires of therapeutic interventions than do APNs who provide primary care. The methods of practice an individual APN uses also depend on the methods of practice used by colleagues in their settings and on what is allowed by their reimbursement systems. Nevertheless, APNs must make an effort to constantly extend and refine their repertoire beyond the interventions learned during graduate education.

ALTERNATIVE AND COMPLEMENTARY THERAPIES

Approximately one third of U.S. adults used complementary or alternative therapies in 1999 according to a survey conducted by the Centers for Disease Control and Prevention (Ni, Simile, & Hardy, 2002). The use among certain ethnic groups is undoubtedly considerably higher than the national average. Many patients use alternative therapies in conjunction with conventional medical services; hence, these therapies are also referred to as *integrative therapies*. In a study of visits to complementary and alternative therapy practitioners (Cherkin et al., 2002), the three most commonly used complementary therapies were found to be spiritual healing or prayer (14%), herbal medicine (10%), and chiropractic (8%). Most alternative therapy visits are made by women (two thirds of all visits), and two thirds of the visits are by self-referral.

The effectiveness and safety of alternative and complementary therapies vary widely. Some have been scientifically studied (e.g., relaxation, guided imagery, glucosamine and chondroitin for osteoarthritis), whereas others have not been studied at all. Of concern is that some may interact with other medications the patient is receiving (Scott & Elmer, 2002). A multisite study of patients undergoing surgery revealed that 27% consumed herbs, 39% used dietary supplements, and 54% took vitamins (Norred, 2002). Of concern is that 34% of the patients used alternative therapies that can interact with anesthetics and inhibit coagulation. Another issue particular to dietary supplements and herb therapy is the lack of control over ingredients (Barnes, 2003; Tesch, 2002). Providers are caught between the desire of patients to use alternative therapies and reservations about their safety, often in the face of insufficient scientific evidence.

Nevertheless, APNs are incorporating complementary and alternative treatments into their practices in a variety of ways, albeit with some caution. In one study of 202 NPs in Connecticut, approximately half reported that they usually or sometimes ask patients about their use of these types of therapies (Hayes & Alexander, 2000); 65% of this sample indicated they had referred or recommended alternative therapies to patients. In a study of 151 NPs from Missouri and Oregon (Sohn & Loveland Cook, 2002), 83% said they had recommended complementary or alternative treatments to their patients, with the most frequently recommended being massage therapy, chiropractic care, acupuncture, nutritional therapy, and herbal treatment.

A national survey of CNMs indicated that a little more than half of the respondents used herbal preparations to stimulate labor (McFarlin, Gibson, O'Rear, & Harman, 1999); of those who use herbal preparations, 75% used them first or instead of pitocin. In a sample of 82 CNMs in North Carolina, 94% reported recommending complementary and alternative therapies to their pregnant patients during the last year (Allaire, Moos, & Wells, 2000). The most common forms were herbal therapy (73%), massage therapy (67%), and chiropractic (49%). Herbal therapy was most frequently recommended for relief of nausea and vomiting, labor stimulation, and reduction of perineal discomfort. Although CNSs are less likely to recommend dietary supplements and herbal therapy, they do use complementary therapies to treat patients during hospitalization. For instance, one reviewer found that hypnosis and relaxation, education and information sharing, music therapy, and supportive touch are used by APNs to reduce stress in patients receiving mechanical ventilation (Thomas, 2003). In summary, because patients are using complementary and alternative therapies, APNs seem to believe that it is better that they do so with provider guidance and awareness.

INDIVIDUALIZED INTERVENTIONS

One goal of treatment decision making is to choose from among several possible interventions the one that will have the highest probability of achieving the outcomes the patient most desires. Most often that probability is increased by "particularizing" the treatment or action to the individual patient (Benner et al., 1996, p. 24). Particularizing requires that the recommendation or action take the following into account:

- The acceptability of the treatment to the patient
- What has worked for the patient in the past
- The patient's motivation and ability to use or follow the treatment
- The likelihood that the patient will continue to use the treatment even if side effects are experienced
- The financial burden of the treatment

Nursing has always believed that individualizing nursing care, that is, tailoring care to the unique characteristics of the person and his or her situation, produces the best patient outcomes. In contrast, standardization of care and control of wide variation are important to quality control and cost containment. Clearly, a blending of the two perspectives is required to produce care that is effective for an individual and congruent with available resources. This can be accomplished by adopting evidence-based standards and guidelines to provide a framework for care, while acknowledging that at the point of care (i.e., in the patient-provider interface), interventions and management may need to be tailored to reflect the patient's unique situation and needs (Brown, 2001).

Some research indicates that APNs do individualize care (Brown, 1992; Brykczynski, 1989; Hawkins et al., 1993; Hughes et al., 2002), and many APN-based programs promote individualization of care (Brooten et al., 1994). Unfortunately, research support for the effectiveness of individualized interventions in general is not as strong as most APNs would like. The extent to which the equivocal nature of the evidence is a function of methodological difficulties in studying individualized interventions is unknown. Part of the difficulty stems from the various ways in which health messages may be customized: personalized, targeted, tailored, and individualized (Ryan & Lauver, 2002). An integrative research review of 20 studies in which interventions with varying degrees of customization to the individual were delivered revealed that in only half of the studies were better patient outcomes achieved with tailored interventions as compared with standard interventions (Ryan & Lauver, 2002). The authors of the review proposed that another reason for the modest support for the efficacy of customized interventions is that patients with certain characteristics are more affected by these interventions than others; such uneven effects across subgroups would offset each other and proposed an appearance of little or no benefit. For example, Ryan and Lauver (2002) found that tailored interventions were effective with women who had high barriers to having a mammogram (e.g., affordability or accessibility obstacles), but not with women with low barriers. Even when a tailored intervention does not result in changed behavior or produce better patient outcomes, it may have other benefits. An example of this collateral gain was found in a study of 43 women with gynecological cancer (Ward, Donovan, Owen, Grosen, & Serlin, 2000). The individualized sensory and coping message for pain management intervention did not have a demonstrable effect on analgesic use, pain intensity scores, or pain interference with life, but the women who received the individualized intervention reported that it contained useful information that helped them to feel more comfortable taking pain medication and to discuss pain more openly with a doctor or nurse.

Computer-based health messages hold considerable promise for individualizing patient education because they can be designed in ways that allow patients to choose from several informational pathways and access only information of interest to them (Deyo et al., 2000; Eakin, Brady, & Lusk, 2001). This is important, because patients vary widely in terms of how much information they want and how they want information presented. Allowing them to make choices about how and what they learn should help prevent content overload and enhance relevancy of information given, thus producing better retention and application. Along similar lines, computer-based programs have been developed to counsel patients who are faced with major treatment decisions (Cherkin et al., 2002; Frosch, Kaplan, & Felitti, 2001; Morgan et al., 2000). The program can be designed to allow the patients to acquire information that is most important to them and to help them sort out their values, priorities, and preference in the specific situations they face. Undoubtedly, computer-based learning and decision-making tools will be more acceptable to some groups of patients than others.

MANAGEMENT OF COMPLEX SITUATIONS

APNs' direct care often involves management and coordination of complex situations; many illustrations of this advanced practice nursing characteristic may be found in the chapters on specific advanced practice nursing roles (see Chapters 12 through 18). In some settings, APNs have been designated as the providers responsible for coordination of complex follow-up care (Dellasega & Zerbe, 2002) or for education of patients at high risk for complications (Damato, Dill, Brown, York, & Brooten, 1993; Naylor et al., 1999). APNs manage diverse patient conditions and care requirements, which include the following:

- Confusion in elderly hospitalized patients
- Risk for complications in elders admitted to the emergency department (Mion et al., 2003)
- Pain in patients who are chronically or terminally ill
- Acute pain (Musclow, Sawhney, & Watt-Watson, 2002)
- Transitional care needs of frail rural elders (Dellasega & Zerbe, 2002)
- Long-term mechanical ventilation (Burns & Earven, 2002)
- Skin breakdown or delayed healing
- Organ failure and care needs of patients awaiting transplantation (McNatt & Easom, 2000)
- Trauma injuries (Daleiden, 1993)

Many CNSs have been called in on a consultation and found a need for skilled communication, advocacy, or coordination of the various providers' plans—or some combination thereof. The patient's condition may not be improving because wound care, pain management, and physical therapy have not been well thought out and coordinated. Family members may be angry because plans keep changing and they are receiving conflicting information from various providers. Typically, the CNS talks with the patient and family to become familiar with their concerns and objectives and then brokers a new plan of care that reflects the patient's and family's needs and preferences, as well as the clinical objectives of the involved providers. The agreed-upon plan must also be consistent with the care authorized by the third-party payors for the patient, or a special agreement must be negotiated. This brokering requires broad clinical knowledge regarding the objectives of various providers, interpersonal skill in dealing with the results of misunderstandings, diplomacy to encourage stakeholders to see each other's points of view, and a commitment to keeping the patient's needs at the center of what is being done.

Helping Patients Manage Chronic Illnesses. Another type of complex situation that APNs manage effectively is chronic illness. Chronic diseases such as multiple sclerosis, cognitive degeneration, psoriasis, congestive heart failure, chronic lung disease, cancer, acquired immunodeficiency syndrome, and organ failure with subsequent transplantation affect individuals and families in profound ways. Most chronic illnesses are characterized by a great deal of uncertainty—uncertainty about the future life course, the effectiveness of treatment, the chances of leading a happy life, bodily functions, medical bills, and intimate relationships (Mast, 1995). In addition, spouses and significant others of people with chronic illness often bear considerable emotional and caregiving burdens (Gaynor, 1990; Laizner, Yost, Barg, & McCorkle, 1993; Northouse & Peters-Golden, 1993). For a variety of reasons related to the characteristics of advanced practice nursing, APNs are successful in providing care to persons with chronic conditions and their families.

Among the reasons that APNs are successful in providing care to persons with chronic illness is their advocacy of patient self-care. One example of the value placed on self-care by APNs is found in the core competencies for nurse-midwifery. The American College of Nurse-Midwives (1997) specifies that one of the core competencies is "Providing information and support to enable women to make informed decisions and to assume primary responsibility for their own care" (p. 8). This focus on patients' self-management is also illustrated in a descriptive study of the meaning of advanced practice nursing for APNs (Grando, 1998). One participant, a family NP, believed that her emphasis on patient self-care was one of the biggest differences between her practice and that of a physician. Another participant, a CNM, communicated her support of patient autonomy when she described birthing by saying "the woman gives birth to the baby" rather than referring to the provider "delivering the baby" (Grando, 1998, p. 507).

The benefits of emphasizing self-care are supported by research showing that when patients are given information about illnesses and helped to manage their illnesses, their courses of illness and quality of life are improved (Gifford, Laurent, Gonzales, Chesney, & Lorig, 1998; Lorig, Gonzales, Laurent, Morgan, & Laris, 1998; Von Korff et al., 1998). Moreover, the evidence suggests that health education for self-management works in part by building patients' self-confidence about controlling their lives in spite of the presence of disease (Sobel, 1995). Hence, many self-management, educational interventions for persons with chronic conditions are being designed to bolster patients' sense of self-efficacy related to coping with the associated disabilities and gaining control over the impact of the disease on their lives.

APNs who see chronically ill patients, either in a primary care setting or in a specialty setting, improve care by coordinating the services patients receive from multiple providers. Chronic illnesses often affect several body systems or have numerous sequelae. Thus persons who are chronically ill often receive care from a primary care provider and several other clinicians including physicians and APN specialists, social workers, physical therapists, and dietitians. Without coordination, families coping with chronic illness can find themselves in an "agency maze" (Burton, 1995, p. 457). This vivid phrase captures the confusing experiences that ensue when the agencies and providers rendering care to a family do not communicate with one another. Families do not know where to go for help, and as a result, many resort to a trial-and-error approach to getting what they need. They often suffer the negative effects of misinformation, repetitive intake interviews, denial of service, conflicting approaches, and unsolved problems. A resource-savvy APN can often assess such situations and intervene to reduce stress, improve communications, and benefit patients and families. By contacting other providers to develop a coordinated management plan and by linking patients with suitable agencies, the APN can do much to relieve the burdens of chronic illness on a family.

End-of-life Care. End-of-life care is another realm in which the expanded skills, attentive planning, and coordinating efforts of APNs are required (Weggel, 1997). When a person is nearing death, many decisions need to be coordinated to ensure continuity of care and a peaceful death; these decisions involve issues such as pain control, plans for withholding or initiation of life support measures, where the patient will be cared for, the need for supportive services such as hospice care, and burden on the family. An APN's ability to smooth the patient's and family's experience often depends on knowing the resources of a particular community and how "to work" the patient's health-care insurance system.

The Report of the National Task Force on End-of-Life Care in Managed Care (1999) describes current end-of-life care in the United States as fragmented and inadequate, and points out that special tools and strategies are available within managed care to intervene at the system level to improve it. Examples of these tools include creative case management programs, financing of palliative care programs and referrals, clinical guidelines and education of staff regarding the management of pain at the end of life, collection of population-based data regarding the process of dying, and providing for bereavement counseling (National Task Force on End-of-Life Care in Managed Care, 1999). Thus APNs working within managed care need to consider whether the resources necessary to support patients at the end of life are available within their organization or from the payors with whom they contract. If they are not, an organized lobbying effort to secure palliative care benefits for subscribers should be initiated; the recommendations of national task forces, such as the National Task Force on End-of-Life Care in Managed Care, could be invoked as a standard for end-of-life care.

CONDITIONS CONDUCIVE TO PROVISION OF HIGH-QUALITY DIRECT CARE BY APNs

Supportive Environment

Many forms of system analysis, organizational redesign, planning, and coordination are needed to develop and sustain the processes of direct care that help patients attain good health outcomes at reasonable cost. APNs have long recognized the need for development of organizational systems that support patient care processes and have actively participated in and often led such efforts. In many settings, APN roles are in need of advocacy; this issue is fully addressed in Chapter 24. The following sections briefly describe conditions conducive to sane, high-quality APN care, and several of them are discussed in more detail in subsequent chapters.

Consultation, Collaboration, and Referral

Consultation, collaboration, and referral are crucial to high-quality direct care (Kleinpell et al., 2002). No single clinician can be knowledgeable about all the problems and issues that arise in daily practice, even in a specialized practice. Wise clinicians are aware of the limits of their knowledge and experience. Consulting with other providers who have special expertise, managing complex care as part of a team, and referring patients who have conditions or problems outside their scope of practice—or even outside their comfort zone—are actions that clinicians owe patients. These matters are addressed extensively in Chapters 7 and 10.

Clinical Guidelines

Research-based clinical practice guidelines can be useful decision-making and planning aids for clinicians. Many guidelines have been developed in close association with providers, are based on systematic and thorough reviews of research evidence, and have attained a balance between optimal care and economic reality. However, contractors also use clinical guidelines to ensure quality, limit variation, and control resource use. Guidelines should be based on research evidence summarized by a credible panel, either inside or outside the system, to ensure that the guidelines serve to both incorporate science into practice and contain costs. Providers involved in care of patients with the condition the guideline addresses should have the opportunity to adapt guidelines produced by others. Ideally, contractors and clinicians should review proposed guidelines and negotiate problematic recommendations in advance to avoid situations in which the care of the individual becomes the focus of negotiation. In addition, contractors and clinicians should acknowledge that although the guidelines may serve most patients well, some patients will require treatment and interventions not recommended in the guidelines. An explicit method for advocating for individual needs should be available to clinicians.

A Population Focus

It is no longer possible to serve patients well by providing only good, individual clinical care (Britt et al., 1998). The reality is that, to serve patients well, clinical recommendations must be made within the financial structure of the patient's health-care plan. Thus, APNs may need to familiarize themselves with how several financing systems work, as well as the specifics of several contractual agreements. Most health-care plans use a combination of aggregated individual outcomes, population outcomes, or both to demonstrate value for dollars spent on specified populations of patients (Britt et al., 1998; Grimes & Garcia, 1997). Evaluation of the degree to which desirable outcomes are attained enables health-care systems to compare their effectiveness with that of a comparable system or to evaluate the relative effectiveness of a new program or process of care. These kinds of evaluations and comparisons can lead to the identification of best practice methods at the health-care system level. Use of services, readmission rates, complication rates, and average total cost per case are examples of population outcomes used in these kinds of evaluations and comparisons.

Aggregated, individual clinical outcomes are useful in evaluation of program effectiveness. By requiring that care administered and individual outcomes be documented in standardized ways, the health-care system can conduct programmatic evaluations of clinical outcomes. Population-based evaluations can also be used by APNs to evaluate and improve the care they provide. Such evaluations can help answer questions such as, "Is the specific care I/we provide patients the best way of managing their health or illness?" and "Are my/our patients doing as well as similar patients who are cared for by other providers?" Conducting such an evaluation involves (1) identifying groups of patients (i.e., populations) who have high costs of care, less than optimal outcomes, or both; (2) monitoring and analyzing variances in outcomes and costs; (3) examining processes of care to determine how management of the condition could be improved; and (4) incorporating management methods found to be effective in research or best practice networks.

Contracts

The contractual arrangements APNs' practice groups enter into with various health-care systems have become more complex in recent years. Although the specific nature of these contracts is beyond the scope of this chapter (see Chapter 21 for a more detailed discussion), APNs' direct care delivery is most definitely affected by the terms of these contracts. MCOs, by their very nature, must have some ability to influence how resources are used; it is inevitable that they will acquire this leverage by constraining how providers manage clinical care. This is typically done by monitoring service use, limiting diagnostic and treatment options, and assessing the efficiency and quality of individual provider groups (Britt et al., 1998). Providers are encouraged to practice preventive health care and constrain their use of costly services such as specialty referrals, hospitalization, and expensive technology. A stronger characterization of this constraint is "Every time the physician uses a resource, for example, consultation, diagnostic testing, or surgical procedures, he or she pays an economic penalty" (Chervenak et al., 1996, p. 525). Financial incentives to avoid use of resources create a conflict of interest for providers, which may result in withholding of tests, treatments, and services from patients who really should have them. Thus, the contractual arrangements that integrated health-care delivery systems make between care provider groups along the continuum from acute to long-term care influence what, where, and how illness is managed.

An APN should know who negotiates and manages contracts for advanced practice nursing services in his or her organization. An ongoing relationship and dialogue with this person (often called *a contracting manager*) is essential to ensuring that advanced practice nursing services are fairly and fully represented in negotiations with MCOs (Adams, 1997). From the contracting manager the APN can learn who the top payors for advanced practice nursing services are, what managed care agreements have the most effect on the APN's service line, and how the rate of reimbursement relates to the cost of providing the service (e.g., which services/programs are operating within their reimbursement rate and which are not). The APN should ask to be informed when new contracts are being negotiated and when changes in existing contracts are under discussion so that solutions to problems can be sought and new opportunities can be explored.

EDUCATIONAL STRATEGIES TO DEVELOP THE DIRECT CARE COMPETENCY

The education of APNs should take into account the health-care problems and needs of the population the graduates of the program will serve, the expressed preferences of the public, the health-care policy of the state and the nation, and the competencies set forth by professional nursing organizations and national commissions. In this brief discussion, selected educational issues that pertain directly to the five characteristics of APN practice discussed in this chapter are addressed.

Fostering a Holistic Perspective

When student APNs begin to have learning experiences in the expanded domain of advanced practice (e.g., assessment and management of medical problems), they often experience a deterioration in their comfort level, motor skills, interviewing competency, and clinical problem-solving ability. As they become more competent in the new domain, they eventually realize that they want to retain the holistic perspective from their basic nursing education and career experiences. They do not want to simply diagnose and treat disease; rather, they want to continue to attend to how patients are responding to disease and to the effects patients' social and physical environments have on their illness, and they want to continue to be responsive to the health problems patients experience in their daily lives. Part of the solution may be to address the continued importance of a holistic perspective up front and to encourage students to evaluate the different perspectives they observe in their clinical placements.

Although APNs in practice use both the medical and nursing perspectives, the theoretical, empirical, and educational literatures are rather silent on *how* this is done. Integration of the two perspectives on health and health care may not be possible, or even desirable, because the two perspectives have very different philosophical assumptions, traditions, and assessment interests that inform the design of medical and nursing curricula and affect role socialization. Each perspective has something unique to contribute to health care. Perhaps what should be pursued is facility with both perspectives and awareness of when to use one rather than the other. Although one cannot, and should not, take the nursing perspective out of the APN role, some issues patients raise during health-care encounters may be better addressed by emphasizing the diagnostic processes and therapeutic approaches characteristic of the medical perspective. Other issues are likely to be better addressed by the holistic, functional perspective characterized by the nursing view of the patient. Until the blending of the two perspectives is better understood, the most effective strategy is to approach and think about patient care within a holistic framework but recognize that when disease-related issues surface, it is necessary to think in a more causal way.

Forming Partnerships with Patients

Graduate programs provide an opportunity for students to improve their communication insights, skills, and styles. Some students may not have developed effective communication skills or styles during undergraduate education; whereas others, who once had them, may have acquired bad habits over their time in practice. Graduate students are often willing to reevaluate their communication skills and styles and will reexamine the degree to which they are practicing their person-centered values.

Creating partnerships with patients, refraining from dominating patients, and helping patients be self-determining are some of the values that student APNs need to revisit. After a discussion of person-centered communication and conversational interviewing in my course on assessment and diagnostic reasoning, students reflected on audiotapes of interviews they had held with patients, and several realized how unnecessarily controlling they had been. The assignment moved them to alter drastically their approaches to assessment interviewing.

Developing Expert Clinical Thinking and Skillful Performance

Graduate education for APNs should produce practitioners who think more creatively, more flexibly, more analytically, and more logically than they did before they completed their education. Some combination of the learning experiences listed in Box 5-6 is required to produce broad-based, discriminating, and proficient clinical thinkers.

One approach to developing expert clinical thinking is problem-based learning (PBL), a bottom-up type of case analysis, in which the student is guided through standardized cases by the tutor or teacher (Barrows & Pickell, 1991). The tutor or teacher is responsible

---

BOX 5-6 • LEARNING EXPERIENCES TO DEVELOP CLINICAL REASONING

Exposure to substantive clinical content
Practice using concepts and theories as thinking tools
Reflection on personal episodes of clinical practice (Kim, 1999; Rolfe, 1997a)
Problem-based learning
Experiential learning assignments
Self-directed study
Assignments in appraising research evidence and deciding how to use it in practice
Mentored clinical practice
Computer-based case management simulations

for the process of learning, not for content. In PBL, the tutor guides students through analysis and synthesis by pushing them to identify what they know, what they do not know, and what resources they must use to acquire the information they need to manage a case. During the ensuing week, the students are expected to acquire the needed information so that they can continue analysis and synthesis at a more informed level. Evaluations of PBL indicate that it produces more self-motivated learners than traditional learning methods and that students prefer it to traditional methods (Baker, 2000; Rideout et al., 2002; White, Amos, & Kouzekanani, 1999). The evidence regarding its effect on clinical performance suggests that PBL does result in a higher level of clinical functioning, although this is not a consistent finding across all applications of PBL (Doucer, Prudy, Kaufman, & Langille, 1998; Moore, Block, Style, & Mitchell, 1994).

Competency in performing physical examinations and other advanced practice skills common to particular APN roles should be acquired in graduate school through simulation, practice with peers or standardized patients, and ultimately through supervised performance with patients. Baseline competency in the performance of certain skills can be established before the skill is performed with patients through objective structured competency examinations (OSCEs). Then a documentation system by which authorized persons in the clinical settings verify that the student has performed the skill satisfactorily can be used. This kind of system can be used to document the required skills and additional ones the student has learned and performed under supervision. These kinds of systems assure the public and employing agencies that persons with APN education are competent to perform the basic procedures, treatments, and skills in a specified area of practice.

Using Research Evidence

A research course to prepare APNs to become consumers of research should be taught early in their graduate programs. The focus of the course should be on research-based practice or the research utilization process, not on the conduct of research. They should learn how to (1) locate research evidence, preferably in a synthesized form; (2) appraise the scientific credibility of that evidence; (3) evaluate its clinical significance; and (4) consider its readiness for use in everyday practice. While reading and appraising clinical guidelines, systematic research reviews, and reports of individual studies, students will have an opportunity to revisit and expand their knowledge of basic research methodology.

From the beginning, the expectation should be that APN students will be discerning regarding the amount of research evidence on which an intervention or approach to care is based. The question "Is there any research to guide practice in this area?" should be asked over and over again throughout the program. No clinical course should be taught without appraising the research that has been conducted on the important and recurring issues in that realm of practice. Appraisal of research findings should include the clinical significance of findings and their applicability for practice, as well as the scientific soundness of the study from which the findings came. Textbooks should be chosen based on the degree to which they make explicit the research basis for what is recommended. Research-based practice is a professional value that requires development of search and appraisal skills. Continuing practice of the skills throughout the program increases the likelihood that graduates of the program will have the desire and the competencies to continue updating the scientific basis of their practices after graduation.

An integrated approach to teaching research-based practice is to teach nursing theory and research utilization together in one course. Currently, theory and research are viewed as separate kinds of knowledge rather than as two approaches to nursing knowledge that must influence one another and be used together if meaningful and reliable knowledge for clinical practice is to be produced. With the current emphasis on evidence-based practice, there is a tendency to view empirical findings as the end product of science. This view does not recognize that the ultimate goal of science is to integrate empirical findings in ways that create explanations of how the world works (i.e., create theories). Another form of this integration is to test or explore how empirical findings support or refute existing theories. Creative educational strategies are required to help students see how these various methods of knowledge production work together to provide knowledge that is useful to practitioners.

Implementing Diverse Approaches to Health and Illness Management

Graduate school should be a time when APN students expand their repertoire of therapeutic interventions. They should learn new skills and therapies and refine and expand existing ones. One way to do this is by requiring students to be active learners. There are several approaches for doing this—all aimed at performance-based learning, in contrast to cognitive learning. For instance, students could be required to use an approach to care or an intervention that they have not previously used and then reflect on whether the approach has advantages over the method they are currently using. Other approaches are aimed at building students' self-confidence in performing a particular skill or managing a particular type of clinical situation through practice. The practice can be accomplished by simulation (Cleave-Hogg & Morgan, 2002), by immersion such as working with a prehospital ambulance service (Melby, 2000), or by clinical attachment to a patient or provider (Boakes, Gardner, Yuen, & Doyle, 1999). Experiential learning has the potential to produce (1) insights that cannot be acquired through cognitive learning; (2) knowledge that is linked to real-world situations; and (3) self-efficacy, that is, confidence in one's ability to actually perform a particular action. Thus, experiential learning has a high likelihood of producing lasting change in behavior.

Although the public is using alternative and complementary therapies and many practicing APNs are using and recommending them, a study of NPs showed that only 24% of them learned about these therapies during their graduate education (Sohn & Loveland Cook, 2002). The proportion was even lower in a study of 90 CNMs who use herbal preparations to stimulate labor (McFarlin et al., 1999); 69% learned about them from other CNMs, 4% from formal research publications, and none from their formal education. Attention needs to be given to providing opportunities during graduate education to learn about alternative and complementary therapies, particularly about how to evaluate their effectiveness and safety in a context of insufficient research. Obviously, this is difficult, given the multiple required competencies that compete for time and emphasis in advanced practice nursing curricula.

In summary, if graduate APN students are to begin to demonstrate the five characteristics of direct care described in this chapter, they will require opportunities to think about how to incorporate the characteristics, as well as opportunities to practice using them. Then these characteristics should be included as course and program competencies and evaluated through multiple-station examinations with standardized patients, through video assessment, or in reflective analysis of actual patient-APN encounters (Kim, 1999; Ram, van der Vleuten, Rethans, Grol, & Aretz, 1999).

Interdisciplinary Education

Interdisciplinary educational experiences would seem to be ways of promoting comprehensive patient care and productive professional relationships in health-care workplaces. Educational offerings could bring together students who would subsequently be working together (e.g., APNs, physicians, health-care administrators, physical therapists, dietitians, occupational therapists, social workers, health policy specialists, and others) in ways that promote understanding of each other's views and contributions. Three models of interdisciplinary education have been explicated by Lindeke and Block (1998): (1) elective courses for health science students that are co-taught by teachers from several disciplines, (2) interdisciplinary clinical experiences, and (3) interdisciplinary project-based experiences. The authors of the article caution that, for interdisciplinary education to truly succeed, all the involved faculty must be genuinely open to cross-disciplinary teaching, and each discipline must deliberatively consider how such offerings fit into its curriculum. Issues such as deciding what discipline-specific learning experiences should precede involvement need to be carefully planned. Thoughtful inclusion of interdisciplinary learning into curricula should produce practitioners who bring to interdisciplinary teams strong disciplinary values, skills, and identity combined with a deep commitment to achieving high-quality health care through joint planning, cooperation, and coordination.

CONCLUSION

APNs are currently providing direct health-care services that positively affect patients' health-care outcomes and that are qualitatively different from those provided by other health-care professionals. Importantly, these services are valued by the public and are cost-effective. Research evidence supports each of these claims, and hence, substantiates the nursing profession's and the public's confidence in the care provided by APNs. However, the impact of the full range of APN activities on individual and population outcomes will require ongoing documentation and examination. APNs should continue to build their practices around the holistic perspective, partnerships with patients, expert clinical reasoning and skillful performance, the use of research evidence, and the use of diverse management approaches. Together, these form a solid foundation for providing scientifically based, person-centered, and outcome-validated health care.

REFERENCES

Adams, L. (1997). Perioperative managed care reimbursements. *Nursing Management, 28*(4), 32F, 32H.

Aiken, L., Sochalski, J., & Lake, E. (1997). Studying outcomes of organizational change in health services. *Medical Care, 35*(Suppl.), NS6-NS18.

Allaire, A. D., Moos, M. K., & Wells, S. R. (2000). Complementary and alternative medicine in pregnancy: A survey of North Carolina certified nurse-midwives. *Obstetrics and Gynecology, 95,* 19-23.

Allard, P., Maunsell, E., Labbe, J., & Dorval, M. (2001). Educational interventions to improve cancer pain control: A systematic review. *Journal of Palliative Medicine, 4,* 191-203.

American Academy of Pediatrics. (2003). *Functional Outcomes Project.* Elk Grove Village, IL: Author. Retrieved May 26, 2003, from http://www.aap.org/research/outcome.htm

American College of Nurse Midwives (1997). *The core competencies for basic midwifery practice.* Washington, DC: Author. Retrieved April 12, 2004, from http://www.midwife.org/prof/corecomp.htm

American Nurses Association. (2003). *Nursing's social policy statement* (2nd ed.). Washington, DC: Author.

Appraisal of Guidelines Research and Evaluation. (2002). *AGREE instrument to assess the quality of clinical guidelines.* Retrieved June 23, 2003, from http://www.agreecollaboration.org/

Avorn, J., Everitt, D. E., & Baker, M. W. (1991). The neglected medical history and therapeutic choices for abdominal pain. *Archives of Internal Medicine, 151,* 694-698.

Baker, C. M. (2000). Problem-based learning for nursing: Integrating lessons from other disciplines with nursing experiences. *Journal of Professional Nursing, 16,* 258-266.

Barnes, J. (2003). Quality, efficacy, and safety of complementary medicines: Fashions, facts and the future. Part I. Regulation and quality. *British Journal of Clinical Pharmacology, 55,* 226-233.

Barrows, H. S., & Pickell, G. C. (1991). *Developing clinical problem-solving skills.* New York: Norton.

Beal, J. A. (2000). A nurse practitioner model of practice in the neonatal intensive care unit. *Maternal Child Nursing, 25,* 18-24.

Beal, J. A., Maguire, D., & Carr, R. (1996). Neonatal nurse practitioners: Identity as advanced practice. *Journal of Obstetrical, Gynecological, and Neonatal Nursing, 25,* 401-406.

Benner, P. A. (1984). *From novice to expert: Excellence and power in clinical practice.* Menlo Park, CA: Addison-Wesley.

Benner, P. A., Hooper-Kyriakidis, P., & Stannard, D. (1999). *Clinical wisdom and interventions in critical care: A thinking-in-action approach.* Philadelphia: W. B. Saunders.

Benner, P. A., Tanner, C. A., & Chesla, C. A. (1996). *Expertise in nursing practice: Caring, clinical judgment, and ethics.* New York: Springer-Verlag.

Blasdell, A. L., Klunick, V., & Purseglove, T. (2002). The use of nursing and medical models in advanced practice: Does education affect the nurse practitioner's practice model? *Journal of Nursing Education, 41,* 231-233.

Boakes, J., Gardner, D., Yuen, K., & Doyle, S. (2000). General practitioner training in palliative care: An experiential approach. *Journal of Palliative Care, 16,* 11-19.

Bonamy, C., Schultz, P., Graham, K., & Hampton, M. (1995). The use of theory-based practice in the Department of Veterans' Affairs Medical Centers. *Journal of Nursing Staff Development, 11,* 27-30.

Boyd, C. O., & Munhall, P. L. (1989). A qualitative investigation of reassurance. *Holistic Nursing Practice, 4,* 61-69.

Britt, T., Schraeder, C., & Shelton, P. (1998). *Managed care and capitation: Issues in nursing.* Washington, DC: American Nurses Publishing.

Brooten, D., Roncoli, M., Finkler, S., Arnold, L., Cohen, A., & Mennuti, M. (1994). A randomized trial of early hospital discharge and home follow-up of women having cesarean birth. *Obstetrics and Gynecology, 84,* 832-838.

Brooten, D., Youngblut, J. M., Deatrick, J., Naylor, M., & York, R. (2003). Patient problems, advanced practice nurse (APN) interventions,

time and contacts among five patient groups. *Journal of Nursing Scholarship, 35,* 73-79.

Brown, S. A., & Grimes, D. E. (1993). *Nurse practitioners and certified nurse-midwives: A meta-analysis of studies on nurses in primary care roles.* Washington, DC: American Nurses Publishing.

Brown, S. J. (1992). Tailoring nursing care to the individual client: Empirical challenge of a theoretical concept. *Research in Nursing and Health, 15,* 39-46.

Brown, S. J. (1999a). *Knowledge for health care practice: A guide to using research evidence.* Philadelphia: W. B. Saunders.

Brown, S. J. (1999b). Patient-centered communication. *Annual Review of Nursing Research, 17,* 85-104.

Brown, S. J. (2001). Managing the complexity of best practice health care. *Journal of Nursing Care Quality, 15,* 1-8.

Brykczynski, K. A. (1989). An interpretive study describing the clinical judgment of nurse practitioners. *Scholarly Inquiry for Nursing Practice: An International Journal, 3,* 75-104.

Brykczynski, K. A. (1991). Judgment strategies for coping with ambiguous clinical situations encountered in primary family care. *Journal of the American Academy of Nurse Practitioners, 3,* 79-84.

Bulechek, G. M., & McCloskey, J. C. (Eds.). (1999). *Nursing interventions classification: Effective nursing treatments* (3rd ed.). Philadelphia: W. B. Saunders.

Burman, M. E., Stepans, M. B., Jansa, N., & Steiner, S. (2002). How do NPs make clinical decisions? *The Nurse Practitioner, 27,* 57-64.

Burns, S. M., & Earven, S. (2002). Improving outcomes for mechanically ventilated medical intensive care unit patient using advanced practice nurses: A 6-year experience. *Critical Care Nursing Clinics of North America, 14,* 231-243.

Burton, D. (1995). Agency maze. In I. M. Lubkin (Ed.), *Chronic illness: Impact and interventions* (3rd ed., pp. 457-480). Boston: Jones & Bartlett.

Canadian Task Force on the Periodic Health Examination. (1994). *The Canadian guide to clinical preventive health care.* Ottawa, Ontario, Canada: Health Canada.

Cassells, J. M., Jenkins, J., Lea, D. H., Calzone, K., & Johnson, E. E. (2003). An ethical assessment framework for addressing global genetic issues in clinical practice. *Oncology Nursing Forum, 30,* 383-390.

Cherkin, D. C., Deyo, R. A., Sherman, K. J., Hart, L. G., Street, J. H., Hrbek, A., Davis, R. B., et al. (2002). Characteristics of visits to licensed acupuncturists, chiropractors, massage therapists, and naturopathic physicians. *Journal of the American Board of Family Practice, 16,* 463-472.

Chervenak, F. A., McCullough, L. B., & Chez, R. A. (1996). Responding to the ethical challenges posed by the business tools of managed care in the practice of obstetrics and gynecology. *American Journal of Obstetrics and Gynecology, 175,* 523-527.

Chisholm, C. D., Collison, E. K., Nelson, D. R., & Cordell, W. H. (2001). Emergency department workplace interruptions: Are emergency physicians "interrupt-driven" and "multitasking"? *Academic Emergency Medicine, 7,* 1239-1243.

Cleave-Hogg, D., & Morgan, P. J. (2002). Experiential learning in an anaesthesia simulation centre: Analysis of students comment. *Medical Teaching, 24,* 23-26.

Cooper-Patrick, L., Gallo, J. J., Gonzales, J. J., Vu, H. T., Powe, N. R., & Ford, D. E. (1999). Race, gender, and partnership in the patient-physician relationship. *JAMA: The Journal of the American Medical Association, 282,* 583-589.

Corcoran-Perry, S. A., Narayan, S. M., & Cochrane, S. (1999). Coronary care nurses' clinical decision making. *Nursing and Health Science, 1,* 46-61.

Courtney, R., & Rice, C. (1997). Investigation of nurse practitioner-patient interactions: Using the Nurse Practitioner Rating Form. *Nurse Practitioner, 22,* 46-48, 54-57, 60 passim.

Croskerry, P. (2003). Cognitive forcing strategies in clinical decision-making. *Annals of Emergency Medicine, 41,* 110-121.

Daleiden, E. G. (1993). The CNS as trauma manager: A new frontier. *Clinical Nurse Specialist, 7,* 295-298.

Damato, L. G., Dill, P. Z., Brown, L. P., York, R., & Brooten, D. (1993). The association between CNS direct care time and total time and very low birth weight infant outcomes. *Clinical Nurse Specialist, 7,* 75-79.

Davis, L. G., Riedmann, G. L., Sapiro, M., Minogue, J. P., & Kazer, R. R. (1994). Cesarean section rates in low-risk private patients managed by certified nurse-midwives and obstetricians. *Journal of Nurse Midwifery, 39,* 91-97.

Degner, L. F., Kristjanson, L. J., Bowman, D., Sloan, J. A., Carriere, K. C., O'Neil, J., et al. (1997). Information need and decisional preferences in women with breast cancer. *JAMA: The Journal of the American Medical Association, 277,* 1485-1492.

Dellasega, C., & Zerbe, T. M. (2002). Caregivers of frail rural older adults. Effects of an advanced practice nursing intervention. *Journal of Gerontological Nursing, 28,* 40-49.

Deyo, R. A., Cherkin, D. C., Weinstein, J., Howe, J., Ciol, M., & Mulley, A. G. (2000). Involving patients in clinical decisions: Impact of an interactive video program on use of back surgery. *Medical Care, 38,* 959-969.

Dittmar, S. S., & Grisham, G. E. (Eds.). (1997). *Functional assessment and outcome measures for the rehabilitation health professional.* Rockville, MD: Aspen.

Doucer, M. D., Prudy, R. A., Kaufman, D. M., & Langille, D. B. (1998). Comparison of problem-based learning and lecture format in continuing medical education on headache diagnosis and management. *Medical Education, 32,* 590-596.

Dowdy, M. D., Robertson, C., & Bander, J. A. (1998). A study of proactive ethics consultation for critically and terminally ill patients with extended lengths of stay. *Critical Care Medicine, 26,* 252-259.

Dunphy, L. M., & Winland-Brown, J. E. (1998). The circle of caring: A transformative model of advanced practice. *Clinical Excellence in Nurse Practice, 2,* 241-247.

Eakin, B. L., Brady, J. S., & Lusk, S. L. (2001). Creating a tailored, multimedia, computer-based intervention. *Computers and Nursing, 19,* 152-160.

Eisen, S. V., Wilcox, M., Leff, H. S., Schaefer, E., & Culhane, M. A. (1999). Assessing behavioral health outcomes in outpatient programs: Reliability and validity of the BASIS-32. *Journal of Behavioral Health Services and Research, 26,* 5-17.

Flesner, M., & Clawson, J. (1998). Clinical management by family nurse practitioners and physicians in collaborative practice: A comparative analysis. In T. J. Sullivan (Ed.), *Collaboration: A health care imperative.* New York: McGraw-Hill.

Forrow, L., Arnold, R. M., & Parker, L. A. (1993). Preventive ethics: Expanding the horizons of clinical ethics. *The Journal of Clinical Ethics, 4,* 287-294.

Frosch, D. L., Kaplan, R. M., & Felitti, V. (2001). The evaluation of two methods to facilitate shared decision making for men considering the prostate-specific antigen test. *Journal of General Internal Medicine, 16,* 391-398.

Gaynor, S. E. (1990). The long haul: The effect of home care on the caregiver. *Image: The Journal of Nursing Scholarship, 22,* 208-212.

Gifford, A. L., Laurent, D. D., Gonzales, V. M., Chesney, M. A., & Lorig, K. R. (1998). Pilot randomized trial of education to improve self-management skills of men with symptomatic HIV/AIDS. *Journal of Acquired Immune Deficiency Syndromes and Human Retrovirology, 18,* 136-144.

Gordon, M. (1994). *Nursing diagnosis: Process and application* (3rd ed.). St. Louis, MO: Mosby.

Grando, V. T. (1998). Articulating nursing for advanced practice nursing. In T. J. Sullivan (Ed.), *Collaboration: A health care imperative.* New York: McGraw-Hill.

Griffith, H. M., & Robinson, K. R. (1993). Current procedural terminology (CPT) coded services provided by nurse specialists. *Image: The Journal of Nursing Scholarship, 25,* 178-186.

Grimes, D. E., & Garcia, M. K. (1997). Advanced practice nursing and work site primary care: Challenges for outcomes evaluation. *Advanced Practice Nursing Quarterly, 3,* 19-28.

Guadagnoli, E., & Ward, P. (1998). Patient participation in decision-making. *Social Science and Medicine, 47,* 329-339.

Halliburton, J. R. (1998). Awareness during general anesthesia: New technology for an old problem. *Certified Registered Nurse Anesthetist, 9,* 39-43.

Hamric, A. B., Spross, J. A., & Hanson, C. M. (Eds.). (2000). *Advanced practice nursing: An integrative approach* (2nd ed.). Philadelphia: Elsevier.

Hamric, A. B., Worley, D., Lindebak, S., & Jaubert, S. (1998). Outcomes associated with advanced nursing practice prescriptive authority. *Journal of the American Academy of Nurse Practitioners, 10,* 113-118.

Hanson, J. L., & Ashley, B. (1994). Advanced practice nurses' application of the Stetler Model for Research Utilization: Improving bereavement care. *Oncology Nursing Forum, 21,* 720-724.

Harris, M. R. (1997). Reduced risk of complex response: An invisible outcome. *Nursing Administration Quarterly, 21,* 25-31.

Harvey, R. M., Kazis, L., & Lee, A. F. (1999). Decision-making preference and opportunity in VA ambulatory care patients: Association with patient satisfaction. *Research in Nursing and Health, 22,* 39-48.

Hawkins, J. W., Thibodeau, J. A., Utley-Smith, Q. E., Igou, J. F., & Johnson, E. E. (1993). Using a conceptual model for practice in nursing wellness centre for seniors. *Perspectives, 17,* 11-16.

Hayes, K. M., & Alexander, I. M. (2000). Alternative therapies and nurse practitioners: Knowledge, professional experience, and personal use. *Holistic Nursing Practice, 14,* 49-58.

Henry, S. B., Holzemer, W. L., Randell, C., Hsieh, S. F., & Miller, T. J. (1997). Comparison of nursing interventions classification and current procedural terminology codes for categorizing nursing activities. *Image: The Journal of Nursing Scholarship, 29,* 133-138.

Hickey, M. (1990). The role of the clinical nurse specialist in the research utilization process. *Clinical Nurse Specialist, 4,* 93-96.

Hughes, L. C., Robinson, L., Cooley, M. E., Nuamah, I., Grobe, S. J., & McCorkle, R. (2002). Describing an episode of home nursing care for elderly postsurgical cancer patients. *Nursing Research, 51,* 110-118.

Johnson, J. D., Roberts, C. S., Cox, C. E., Reintgen, D. S., Levine, J. S., & Parsons, M. (1996). Breast cancer patients' personality style, age, and treatment decision-making. *Journal of Surgical Oncology, 63,* 183-186.

Kane, R. L., Flood, S., Keckhafer, G., & Rockwood, T. (2001). How EverCare nurse practitioners spend their time. *Journal of the American Geriatric Society, 49,* 1530-1534.

Kassirer, J. P., & Kopelman, R. I. (1991). *Learning clinical reasoning.* Baltimore: Williams & Wilkins.

Kim, H. S. (1999). Critical reflective inquiry for knowledge development in nursing practice. *Journal of Advanced Nursing, 29,* 1205-1212.

Kinney, C. K., & Erickson, H. C. (1990). Modeling the client's world: A way to holistic care. *Issues in Mental Health Nursing, 11,* 93-108.

Kleinpell, R. M., Faut-Callahan, M., Lauer, K., Kremer, M. J., Murphy, M., & Sperhac, A. (2002). Collaborative practice in advanced practice nursing in acute care. *Critical Care Nursing Clinics of North America, 14,* 307-313.

Kohn, L. T., Corrigan, J. M., & Donaldson, M. S. (1999). *To err is human: Building a safer health system.* Washington, DC: Institute Of Medicine, Committee on Quality of Health Care in America.

Kovner, C., Jones, C., Zhan, C., Gergen, P. J., & Basu, J. (2002). Nurse staffing and postsurgical adverse events: An analysis of administrative data from a sample of U.S. hospitals, 1990-1996. *Health Services Research, 37,* 611-629.

Labrecque, M., Eason, E., Marcoux, S., Lemieux, F., Pinault, J. J., Feldman, P., et al. (1999). Randomized controlled trial of prevention of perineal trauma by perineal massage during pregnancy. *American Journal of Obstetrics and Gynecology, 180,* 593-600.

Laizner, A. M., Yost, L. M., Barg, F. K., & McCorkle, R. (1993). Needs of family caregivers of persons with cancer: A review. *Seminars in Oncology Nursing, 9,* 114-120.

Laschinger, H. K., & Duff, V. (1991). Attitudes of practicing nurses towards theory-based nursing practice. *Canadian Journal of Nursing Administration, 4,* 6-10.

Lawrence, M. (1995). The unconscious experience. *American Journal of Critical Care, 4,* 227-232.

Lawson, M. T. (2002). Nurse practitioner and physician communications styles. *Applied Nursing Research, 15,* 60-66.

Liehr, P., & Smith, M. J. (1999). Middle range theory: Spinning research and practice to create knowledge for the new millennium. *Advances in Nursing Science, 14,* 81-91.

Lorig, K., Gonzales, V. M., Laurent, D. D., Morgan, L., & Laris, B. A. (1998). Arthritis self-management program variations: Three studies. *Arthritis Care Research, 11,* 448-454.

Lydon-Rochelle, M. T., Albers, L., & Teaf, D. (1995). Perineal outcomes and nurse-midwifery management. *Journal of Nurse Midwifery, 40,* 13-18.

MacDonald, D. J., & Lessick, M. (2000). Hereditary cancers in children and ethical and psychosocial implications. *Journal of Pediatric Nursing, 15,* 217-225.

Mackay, M. H. (1998). Research utilization and the CNS: Confronting the issues. *Clinical Nurse Specialist, 12,* 232-237.

Mast, M. E. (1995). Adult uncertainty in illness: A critical review of research. *Scholarly Inquiry for Nursing Practice: An International Journal, 9,* 3-24.

McFarlin, B. L., Gibson, M. H., O'Rear, J., & Harman, P. (1999). A national survey of herbal preparation use by nurse-midwives for labor stimulation. Review of the literature and recommendations for practice. *44, 6,* 205-216.

McMillan, S. C., Heusinkveld, K. B., & Spray, J. (1995). Advanced practice in oncology nursing: A role delineation study. *Oncology Nursing Forum, 22,* 41-50.

McNatt, G. E., & Easom, A. (2000). The role of the advanced practice nurse in the care of organ transplant recipients. *Advances in Renal Replacement Therapy, 7*, 172-176.

Melby, V. (2000). Experiential learning in pre-hospital emergency care: A qualitative study. *Nurse Education Today, 20*, 638-645.

Mion, L. C., Palmer, R. M., Meldon, S. W., Bass, D. M., Singer, M. E., Payne, S. M., et al. (2003). Case finding and referral model for emergency department elders: A randomized clinical trial. *Annals of Emergency Medicine, 41*, 69-71.

Moore, G. T., Block, S. D., Style, C. B., & Mitchell, R. (1994). The influence of the new pathway curriculum on Harvard medical students. *Academic Medicine, 69*, 983-989.

Morgan, M. W., Deber, R. B., Llewellyn-Thomas, H. A., Gladstone, P., Cusimano, R. J., O'Rourke, K., et al. (2000). Randomized, controlled trial of an interactive videodisc decision aid for patients with ischemic heart disease. *Journal of General Internal Medicine, 15*, 685-693.

Musclow, S. L., Sawhney, M., & Watt-Watson, J. (2002). The merging role of advanced nursing practice in acute pain management throughout Canada. *Clinical Nurse Specialist, 16*, 63-66.

Narayan, S. M., & Corcoran-Perry, S. (1997). Line of reasoning as a representation of nurses' clinical decision making. *Research in Nursing and Health, 20*, 353-364.

National Task Force on End-of-Life Care in Managed Care. (1999). *Meeting the challenge: Twelve recommendations for improving end-of-life care in managed care*. Newton, MA: Educational Development Center.

Naylor, M. D., Brooten, D., Campbell, R., Jacobsen, B. S., Mezey, M. D., Pauly, M. V., et al. (1999). Comprehensive discharge planning and home follow-up of hospitalized elders: A randomized clinical trial. *JAMA: The Journal of the American Medical Association, 281*, 613-620.

Neal, L. J. (1998). Current functional assessment tools. *Home Healthcare Nurse, 16*, 766-772.

Needleman, J., Buerhaus, P., Mattke, S., Steward, M., & Zelevinsky, K. (2002). Nurse-staffing levels and the quality of care in hospitals. *New England Journal of Medicine, 346*, 1715-1722.

Nelson, E. C., Splaine, M. E., Batalden, P. B., & Plume, S. K. (1998). Building measurement and data collection into medical practice. *Annals of Internal Medicine, 128*, 460-466.

Newman, M. (1997). Experiencing the whole. *Advances in Nursing Science, 20*, 34-39.

Ni, H., Simile, C., & Hardy, A. M. (2002). Utilization of complementary and alternative medicine by United States adults: Results from the 1999 National Health Interview Survey. *Medical Care, 40*, 353-358.

Norred, C. L. (2002). Complementary and alternative medicine use by surgical patients. *Journal of American Operating Room Nurses, 76*, 1013-1021.

Northouse, L. L., & Peters-Golden, H. (1993). Cancer and the family: Strategies to assist spouses. *Seminars in Oncology Nursing, 9*, 74-82.

Oakley, D., Martland, T., Mayes, F., Hayashi, R., Petersen, B. A., Rorie, C., et al. (1995). Process of care. Comparisons of certified nurse-midwives and obstetricians. *Journal of Nurse Midwifery, 40*, 399-409.

O'Neill, E. S. (1995). Heuristics reasoning in diagnostic judgment. *Journal of Professional Nursing, 11*, 239-245.

Pearson, A., Borbasi, S., & Walsh, K. (1997). Practicing nursing therapeutically through acting as a skilled companion on the illness journey. *Advanced Practice Nursing Quarterly, 3*, 46-52.

Petrisek, A. C., Laliberte, L. L., Allen, S. M., & Mor, V. (1997). The treatment decision-making process: Age differences in a sample of women recently diagnosed with nonrecurrent, early-stage breast cancer. *Gerontologist, 37*, 598-608.

Pond, F. (1999). Searching for studies. In S. J. Brown (Ed.), *Knowledge for health care practice: A guide to using research evidence* (pp. 41-58). Philadelphia: W. B. Saunders.

Pyke-Grimm, K. A., Degner, L., Small, A., & Mueller, B. (1999). Preferences for participation in treatment decision making and information needs of parents of children with cancer: A pilot study. *Journal of Pediatric Oncology Nursing, 16*, 13-24.

Ram, P., van der Vleuten, C., Rethans, J. J., Grol, R., & Aretz, K. (1999). Assessment of practicing family physicians: Comparison of observation in a multiple-station examination using standardized patients with observation of consultations in daily practice. *Academic Medicine, 74*, 62-69.

Registered Nurses Association of Ontario (2003). *Toolkit: Implementation of clinical practice guidelines*. Retrieved April 15, 2004, from http://www.rnao.org/bestpractices/completed_guidelines/BPG-Guide_C1_Toolkit.asp

Rideout, E., England-Oxford, V., Brown, B., Fothergill-Bourbonnais, F., Ingram, C., Benson, G., Ross, M., & Coates, A. (2002). A comparison of problem-based and conventional curricula in nursing education. *Advances in Health Sciences Education 7*, 3-17.

Rolfe, G. (1997). Beyond expertise: Theory, practice, and the reflexive practitioner. *Journal of Clinical Nursing, 6*, 93-97.

Ryan, P., & Lauver, D. R. (2002). The efficacy of tailored interventions. *Journal of Nursing Scholarship, 34*, 331-337.

Sampselle, C. M., & Hines, S. (1999). Spontaneous pushing during birth: Relationship to perineal outcomes. *Journal of Nurse Midwifery, 44*, 36-39.

Sappington, J., & Kelley, J. H. (1996). Modeling and role-modeling theory: A case of holistic care. *Journal of Holistic Nursing, 14*, 130-141.

Schneiderman, L. J., Gilmer, T., & Teetzel, H. D. (2000). Impact of ethics consultations in the intensive care setting: A randomized, controlled trial. *Critical Care Medicine, 28,* 3920-3924.

Schön, D. A. (1984). *The reflective practitioner: How professionals think in action* (2nd ed.). San Francisco: Jossey-Bass.

Scott, G. N., & Elmer, G. W. (2002). Update on natural product-drug interactions. *American Journal of Health-System Pharmacy, 59,* 339-347.

Scott, R. A. (1999). A description of the roles, activities, and skills of clinical nurse specialists in the United States. *Clinical Nurse Specialist, 13,* 183-190.

Shuler, P. A., & Huebscher, R. (1998). Clarifying nurse practitioners' unique contributions: Application of the Shuler Nurse Practitioner Practice Model. *Journal of the American Academy of Nurse Practitioners, 10,* 491-499.

Sidani, S., Irvine, D., Porter, H., O'Brien-Pallas, L., Simpson, B., McGillis Hall, L., et al. (2000). Practice patterns of acute care nurse practitioners. *Canadian Journal of Nursing Leadership, 13,* 296-304.

Smith, M. J., & Liehr, P. R. (2003). *Middle range theory for nursing.* New York: Springer.

Smith, S. (1988). An analysis of the phenomenon of deterioration in the critically ill. *Image: The Journal of Nursing Scholarship, 20,* 12-15.

Sobel, D. S. (1995). Rethinking medicine: Improving health outcomes with cost-effective psychosocial interventions. *Psychosomatic Medicine, 57,* 234-244.

Sohn, P. M., & Loveland Cook, C. A. (2002). Nurse practitioner knowledge of complementary alternative health care: Foundation for practice. *Journal of Advanced Nursing, 39,* 9-16.

Spross, J. A., & Wolff-Burke, M. (1996). Nonpharmacological management of cancer pain. In D. B. McGuire, C. H. Yarbro, & B. R. Ferrell (Eds.), *Cancer pain management* (2nd ed., pp. 159-205). Boston: Jones & Bartlett.

Stafford, R. S., & Blumenthal, D. (1998). Specialty differences in cardiovascular disease prevention practices. *Journal of the American College of Cardiology, 32,* 1238-1243.

Stetler, C. B., Bautista, C., Vernale-Hannon, C., & Foster, J. (1995). Enhancing research utilization by clinical nurse specialists. *Nursing Clinics of North America, 30,* 457-473.

Stetler, C. B., & DeZell, A. (1989). Implementing nursing case management. In M. L. Etheredge (Ed.), *Collaborative care: Nursing case management* (pp. 67-77). Chicago: American Hospital.

Tanner, C. A., Benner, P., Chesla, C., & Gordon, D. R. (1993). The phenomenology of knowing a patient. *Image: The Journal of Nursing Scholarship, 25,* 273-280.

Tazbir, J. (2001). The Human Genome Project: Ethical and legal considerations for neuroscience. *Journal of Neuroscience Nursing, 33,* 180-183.

Tesch, B. J. (2002). Herbs commonly used by women: An evidence-based review. *Disease-A-Month, 48,* 671-696.

Thibodeau, J. A., & Hawkins, J. W. (1994). Moving toward a nursing model in advanced practice. *Western Journal of Nursing Research, 16,* 205-218.

Thomas, L. A. (2003). Clinical management of stressors perceived by patients on mechanical ventilation. *AACN Clinical Issues, 14,* 73-81.

Ulrich, C. M., Soeken, K. L., & Miller, N. (2003). Ethical conflict associated with managed care: Views of nurse practitioners. *Nursing Research, 52,* 168-175.

U.S. Preventive Services Task Force. (1996). *Guide to clinical preventive services: Report of the U.S. Preventive Services Task Force* (2nd ed.). Baltimore: Williams & Wilkins.

U.S. Preventive Services Task Force. (2003). *Guide to clinical preventive services: Report of the U.S. Preventive Services Task Force* (3rd ed.). Baltimore: Williams & Wilkins.

Vallerand, A. H. (1998). Development and testing of the inventory of functional status-chronic pain. *Journal of Pain Symptom Management, 15,* 125-133.

Vernon, D. T., & Blake, R. L. (1993). Does problem-based learning work? A meta-analysis of evaluative research. *Academic Medicine, 68,* 550-563.

Volinn, E. (1999). Do workplace interventions prevent low-back disorders? If so why?: A methodological commentary. *Ergonomics, 42,* 258-272.

Von Korff, M., Moore, J. E., Lorig, K., Cherkin, D. C., Saunders, K., Gonzalez, V. M., et al. (1998). A randomized trial of a lay person-led self-management group intervention for back pain patients in primary care. *Spine, 23,* 2608-2615.

Waite, M. S., Harker, J. O., & Messerman, L. I. (1994). Interdisciplinary team training and diversity: Problems, concepts and strategies. In D. Wieland, D. Benton, B. J. Kramer, & G. D. Dawson (Eds.), *Cultural diversity and geriatric health care: Challenges to the health care professions* (pp. 68-82). New York: Haworth Press.

Ward, S., Donovan, H. S., Owen, B., Grosen, E., & Serlin, R. (2000). An individualized intervention to overcome patient-related barriers to pain management in women with gynecologic cancers. *Research in Nursing and Health, 23,* 393-405.

Weggel, J. M. (1997). Palliative care: New challenges for advanced practice nursing. *Hospice Journal, 12,* 43-56.

White, M. J., Amos, E., & Kouzekanani, K. (1999). Problem-based learning. *Nurse Educator, 24,* 33-36.

Yancey, R., Given, B. A., White, N. J., DeVoss, D., & Coyle, B. (1998). Computerized documentation for a rural nursing intervention project. *Computers and Nursing, 16,* 275-284.

CHAPTER 6

Expert Coaching and Guidance

JUDITH A. SPROSS

INTRODUCTION

Patient education is a central and well-documented function of all nurses in any setting. Patient education provided by advanced practice nurses (APNs) is best conceptualized as interpersonal processes of coaching through life transitions such as illness, childbearing, and bereavement. Teaching and coaching are recognized as core competencies of APNs (e.g., National Association of Clinical Nurse Specialists, 1998, 2004; National Organization of Nurse Practitioner Faculties, 2002; National Panel for Psychiatric Mental Health NP Competencies, 2003). My colleagues and I synthesized our own practice and teaching experiences with theoretical, research, and clinical literature to develop a model of coaching through transitions as the complex, interpersonal process APNs use to enlist patients' active and effective participation in their care (Clarke & Spross, 1996; Spross, Clarke, & Beauregard, 2000). An interdisciplinary perspective informs the discussion of coaching. In this chapter the use of the terms *coach* and *coaching*, rather than *education*, is deliberate because these terms imply the existence of a relationship that is fundamental to effective teaching. Coaching people through transitions is a relatively invisible, intangible, but complex process that must be made more explicit if APNs are to be seen by consumers and policymakers as a solution to health policy concerns such as access to and continuity of care and if they are to secure reimbursement for the care they provide.

Numerous resources exist to help APNs develop and implement educational programs for individuals and groups and therefore are not included here. This chapter focuses on the advanced practice nursing APN competency of coaching, guidance, and teaching. Strategies for acquiring and using the skills needed to coach effectively are presented. Although the primary focus of the chapter is on coaching of patients and families, selected applications of the coaching model to student and staff education are also discussed.

PATIENT EDUCATION AND COACHING BY APNs

Many studies document the nature, focus, content, and amount of time APNs spend in teaching and counseling, as well as the outcomes of these interventions (see Chapter 25 for more detail on studies of APN interventions and outcomes). Teaching and counseling are significant clinical activities in nurse-midwifery (Scupholme, Paine, Lang, Kumar, & DeJoseph, 1994; Scupholme & Walsh, 1994) and clinical nurse specialist (CNS) (Scott, 1999) practices. Studies of nurse practitioners (NPs) indicate that they spend a significant proportion of their direct care time in teaching and counseling (Brown, 1995; Brown & Waybrant, 1988; Draye & Pesznecker, 1980; Mezey, Dougherty, Wade, & Mersmann, 1994). Health promotion topics covered by NPs include diet, exercise, smoking cessation, family planning, and stress management (Brown & Waybrant, 1988). A more recent study of NP students revealed that many of their interventions were also directed toward education. O'Connor, Hameister, and Kershaw (2000) found that for 3,733 patient visits, knowledge deficit was one of the top four nursing diagnoses. Using the Nursing Intervention Classification (NIC) system, O'Connor et al. (2000) also found that patient education was one of the top four intervention classifications used by NP students. An innovative approach to patient education has been developed by The American College of Nurse Practitioners (personal communication, C. M. Hanson, November, 3, 2003). The American College of Nurse Practitioners makes a service available to members whereby NPs can set up their own personal Web pages. They can place personalized directives and patient education materials for their patients on the Web page; they can also choose to have interactive capability with an individual patient or use e-mail to conduct chat room discussions with groups of patients.

Quantitative studies, qualitative studies, and anecdotal reports suggest that coaching patients and staff through transitions is embedded in the practices of nurses, including APNs (Barnsteiner, Gillis-Donovan, Knox-Fischer, & McKlindon, 1994; Benner, Hooper-Kyriakidis, & Stannard, 1999) and that APN-led patient education and monitoring programs for specific clinical populations indicate that patient education and coaching are central to their effectiveness (Crowther, 2003; George et al., 1999; Larson, Neverett, & Larsen, 2001).

The reader should become familiar with studies of the Quality-Cost Model of Early Discharge and Nurse Specialist/APN Transitional Care conducted by Brooten et al. (e.g., 1986, 1988, 1994). These studies provide substantive evidence of the range and focus of teaching activities undertaken by CNSs and NPs who provided interventions to patients across several studies. Controlled trials of APN care that involved teaching and coaching activities have demonstrated statistically significant differences in patient outcomes and resource use for low birth weight infants (Brooten et al., 1986); women undergoing unplanned cesarean deliveries (Brooten et al., 1994); and older patients who were hospitalized (Naylor et al., 1999). Interventions in these studies occurred in hospitals and during the postdischarge period. The interventions used by APNs in these studies indicate that APNs use a holistic focus that requires technical and interpersonal competence. Early work in this program of research documented that APNs provided teaching and counseling during face-to-face contacts in the home and through regular telephone contact, services that were regarded by researchers as critical (Brooten et al., 1986). Analysis of CNSs' interventions revealed that 68% could be categorized as teaching (Brooten et al., 1988, 1991). Other types of interventions were liaison, consultation, and referral; encouragement of self-care and infant care; and reassurance and reinforcement of the patient's actions (Brooten et al., 1988, 1991). Secondary analyses of data collected in studies of The Quality-Cost Model of APN Transitional Care have been conducted in five clinical populations: the elderly, women with high-risk pregnancies or those who have had cesarean deliveries, women who have had hysterectomies, and very low birth weight infants (Brooten et al., 2003; Naylor, Bowles, & Brooten, 2000). Using the Omaha Classification System, the investigators analyzed 9,488 APN interventions. They identified four categories of problems: the environment, psychosocial, physiological, and human-related behavior. They also identified four categories of interventions: health teaching, guidance, and/or counseling; treatments and procedures; case management; and surveillance (Brooten et al., 2003). Physiological problems were most common among the three groups of women; human-related behaviors were most common among the elderly; and psychosocial problems were most common among very low birth weight infants. Across groups, the most frequent intervention was surveillance; health teaching was the second or third most frequent intervention, depending on the patient population. The focus of teaching was usually related to the issues for which the APN was providing surveillance.

Numerous factors in contemporary health care have increased the focus on patient education as a means of improving effectiveness and efficiency and achieving cost and quality outcomes. These include cost containment and reimbursement mechanisms (Barger, 1997; Bauer, 1994; Cook, 1997; Spross & Heaney, 2000; Taylor, Resick, D'Antonio, & Carroll, 1997; The Milbank Memorial Fund and the Center for the Advancement of Health,[1] 1999; The Robert Wood Johnson Foundation [RWJ],[2] 2000;

---

[1]Hereafter called the Milbank report.
[2]Hereafter called the RWJ report.

Weiss, 1998), the evidence-based practice movement (Bero et al., 1998; Porter et al., 1997; Spross & Heaney, 2000; University of York NHS Centre for Reviews and Dissemination, 1999), the educational needs of informal caregivers (Kirk & Glendinning, 1998), efforts to develop interdisciplinary models of health care that are patient-centered (Pew-Fetzer Task Force on Advancing Psychosocial Health Education, 1994), and the widespread use of the Internet for teaching and learning.

Given the research-based evidence of the effectiveness of patient education provided by nurses and APNs, some investigators have questioned why the nature, process, and character-istics of nurse-patient interactions have rarely been the focus of research on patient teaching and patient adherence to therapies (Kasch, 1983; Schwartz-Barcott, Fortin, & Kim 1994; Squier, 1990). More research on the process of patient teaching used by APNs and how it pro-motes adherence to therapies and self-care is needed. The observations that patient education generally improves outcomes and that telephone follow-up has been one of the important APN activities in studies of APN care and patient outcomes (George et al., 1999; Naylor et al., 1999; Brooten et al., 2003) suggest several directions for research. Studies that identify the process and the "dose" of APN-delivered interventions—as well as the differential effects and costs of APN coaching, registered nurse coaching, and the coaching of other clinicians—are needed. The effects of Internet-based information and education and the role of health-care professionals in helping patients use this information effectively should be studied. Finally, effective strategies for teaching patients who are functionally illiterate must be identified.

Although more research is needed, the foregoing review supports the premise that expert guidance and coaching are key foci of the APN's direct care role. In describing APNs' coaching of patients, I assume that APNs understand basic principles of education and are aware of the research on which patient education is based. APNs are responsible for knowing the theoretical and scientific bases for patient teaching in their specialties and practice settings. Examples of APNs' integration of specialty knowledge with princi-ples of patient education to operationalize the coaching competency are incorporated in the chapters on the different APN roles in Part III.

COACHING THROUGH TRANSITIONS: A SYNTHESIS OF THEORETICAL PERSPECTIVES

Coaching: An Interdisciplinary Perspective

The word *coach* is derived from the Middle English word *coche*, meaning "wagon or car-riage, a means of conveyance from one destination to another." Modern use of *coach* to mean a teacher is apt: a coach facilitates the safe passage of a person in transition from one situation to another. Coaching is complex interpersonal work that helps people who are facing personal transitions or journeys. These meanings of coaching can be applied to nurse-patient, faculty-student, preceptor-student, and mentor-protégé relationships.

Coaching has been used by several disciplines to describe interactions between experts and learners that focus on developing the learners' knowledge and skill in an area that is within the coach's expertise (Spross, 1994). A review of the literature supports the use of *coach* and *coaching* as terms that describe the teaching functions of APNs. The fact that *coach* and *coaching* are common terms may also make it easier for APNs to communicate with consumers and policymakers about what they do.

In cognitive psychology, social skills tutoring (Frisch, Elliott, Atsaides, Salva, & Denney, 1982) and interpersonal cognitive problem solving (Hops, 1983) are coaching techniques that have been used to improve individuals' social skills, language skills, and problem-solving abilities. Both techniques include direct verbal instructions in problem-solving principles. Interpersonal cognitive problem solving also emphasizes thinking processes such as identifying problems, generating alternative solutions, and anticipating the consequences of solutions (Pelligrini & Urbain, 1985). A recent review written by two APNs and a psychologist described the process of cognitive therapy and the ways in which nurses can use the therapy to mediate the harmful effects of stress, promote health, and prevent and manage disease (Wells-Federman, Stuart-Shor, & Webster, 2001).

In sports, coaches create and present complex challenges that develop athletes' physical and psychological capacities while providing support and motivation (Lombardo, 1987; Sullivan & Wilson, 1991). Coaches are expected to have technical competence and interpersonal and leadership skills. Lombardo (1987) described humanistic coaches as those who can focus on strengthening athletes' performance and self-concept because the coaches themselves are competent, secure in their self-concepts, and self-accepting. Such coaches help athletes believe in themselves; through coaching, athletes learn that they are trustworthy, responsible, capable of self-direction, and able to identify relevant goals.

Heifetz's (1994) work on leadership illuminated Lombardo's (1987) description of humanistic coaching. According to Heifetz, leadership is "mobilizing people to tackle tough problems" (p. 15). Situations that require leadership or expert coaching are those in which the problems are complex: a technical solution is unavailable and would be inadequate anyway, and the problem demands adaptive work (Heifetz, 1994). Leaders identify the adaptive task. Leadership, as a type of coaching, can be viewed as helping people uncover opportunities for personal growth by helping them clarify their goals, decide what matters most to them, acknowledge trade-offs and losses, and develop coping strategies (see Chapter 9). Becoming a parent, losing a job, adjusting to and living with a chronic illness, coping with national disasters and traumatic losses, and facing impending death are examples of transitions requiring complex, adaptive work that can be facilitated by APNs.

In a qualitative study of nurses' clinical experiences, Benner (1984) identified the teaching-coaching role as one of seven domains of nursing practice. Subsequent studies, based on Benner's work, have confirmed that APNs demonstrate this role as part of their practice (Benner et al., 1999; Fenton, 1984; Fenton & Brykczynski, 1993; Steele & Fenton, 1988). Benner (1985) elaborates on the teaching-coaching role of APNs who work with patients with chronic illness: "Coaches learn what the illness means to the individual, what the adaptive demands, tasks, and resources are for the patient at different stages in the illness" (p. 43). APNs use their knowledge of a patient and knowledge from previous experiences with similar patients to craft patient-specific coaching interventions.

Other nurses have used the term *coaching* to characterize the nature of nurses' relational, therapeutic interventions with patients. In describing coaching as the interpersonal process nurses use to help those who suffer, Spross (1996) summarized the elements of the nurse-patient relationship connoted by the term *coaching*:

Coaching captures the essence of the relationships nurses create with patients on which their effectiveness depends. . . . It is a term that permits the experience of intense emotions on both sides; it captures the temporal nature of the relationship (which may be brief or extended); it suggests both the one-sided aspect (the coach has information and expertise needed by the patient) and the mutuality (opportunities for personal growth) in the relationship; and it conveys the contractual or voluntary nature of the relationship (if the relationship is not working despite the best efforts of both, another coach may need to be found). (pp. 197-198)

Table 6-1 summarizes conceptualizations of coaching just described and those by other nurse clinicians and investigators (Braden, 1990, 1993; Connelly, 1993; Lamm, Dungan,

TABLE 6-1   NURSING CONCEPTUALIZATIONS OF COACHING

	BENNER (1985)	SPROSS (1994)	WILKIE ET AL. (1995)	CARRIERI-KOHLMAN ET AL. (1996)	LEWIS & ZAHLIS (1997)	BENNER ET AL. (1999)
Purpose/focus of coaching	To teach and coach patients	To ameliorate suffering	To teach patients with lung cancer to report pain perception and changes in pain perceptions to clinicians	To increase patients' self-efficacy in performing exercises and decrease anxiety to decrease dyspnea	To help clients (patients and significant others) process thoughts and feelings related to breast cancer experience; to enhance cognitive-behavioral management and self-care skills	An embodied clinical leadership skill in which relational skills are used to help others in their understanding, their judgment, their skilled know-how, and their openness to seeing new possibilities
Characteristics or elements of the coaching interaction or protocol	Capturing readiness to learn Assisting patients to integrate implications of illness and recovery Eliciting patients' understanding of situation Providing interpretation of each patient's condition and giving a rationale for procedures Making culturally avoided aspects of an illness approachable and understandable	Permits the experience of intense emotions on both sides Temporal aspects of the relation-ship (brief or extended) Relationship is both one-sided (nurse has knowledge and skills needed by patient) and mutual (relationship is an opportunity for personal growth for nurse *and* patient) Relationship is, at least theoretically, voluntary and contractual	Encourages patients to mark a self-assessment tool to record pain intensity Encourages patients to report pain characteristics to clinicians Emphasizes and reinforces that pain characteristics reported by patients are important for clinicians' pain treatment decisions	Nurse coach teaches coping skills Nurse coach collaborates with patient to set goals for exercise session based on prior performance and clinical factors Nurse coach teaches relaxation and breathing exercises Nurse coach reinforces information given and encourages patients	Attending to the story Encircling the experience Invites the work Exploring solutions Anchoring the skill through feedback, self-monitoring, and homework Setting up success	Envisions realistic possibilities Makes excellent judgment Is able to balance patient's need for safety with team members' need to learn Is able to help others learn to interpret, forecast, and respond to patient transitions
Type of article/book	Qualitative research	Theoretical synthesis	Quantitative research (pilot study)	Quantitative research (experimental design)	Qualitative research	Qualitative research

& Hiromoto, 1991; Peplau, 1952). These descriptions of coaching by nurses are consistent with the concepts of coaching from other disciplines discussed previously. Thus coaching can be viewed as a relational, multidimensional process that involves all aspects of being human—cognitive, affective, behavioral, physical, social, and spiritual.

Transitions

The word *transition* comes from the Latin *transitus*, meaning, "to go across, to pass over or go through." Transitions—physiological, developmental, situational, and organizational—make up the natural course of human lives. Transitions are paradigms for life and living—"dangerous opportunities" in Chinese culture. Like life, they may be predictable or unpredictable, joyous or painful, obvious or barely perceptible, chosen and welcomed or unexpected and feared. Bridges (1980) described three phases of transition: an ending or leaving; a period of chaos, confusion, and distress; and a new beginning. Bridges indicated that, for some people, "transitionality" might be a semipermanent state. Schumacher and Meleis (1994) asserted that transition is a central concept in nursing, and Chick and Meleis (1986) offered a clinically useful definition of it:

Transition is a passage from one life phase, condition, or status to another. . . . Transition refers to both the process and outcome of complex person-environment interactions. It may involve more than one person and is embedded in the context and the situation. (pp. 239-240)

Chick and Meleis (1986) also characterized the process of transition as having phases during which individuals experience (1) a disconnectedness from their usual social supports, (2) a loss of familiar reference points, (3) old needs that remain unmet, (4) new needs, and (5) old expectations that are no longer congruent with the changing situation. Becoming a parent, giving up cigarettes, learning how to cope with chronic illness, and dying in comfort and dignity are just a few examples of transitions. Transitions can also be characterized according to type, conditions, and universal properties. Schumacher and Meleis (1994) have identified nursing therapeutics that support or facilitate transitions, and education is one of them.

Other models and concepts inform the conceptualization of APN coaching through transition (Table 6-2). Themes that are common across models and studies of particular concepts (Braden, 1990, 1993; Lamm et al., 1991; Peplau, 1952; Travelbee, 1971) include assessment, collaborating with patients, teaching, and mobilizing social support to accomplish health- and illness-related outcomes.

A TYPOLOGY OF TRANSITIONS

Schumacher and Meleis (1994) proposed that there are four categories of transitions in which nurses are involved: *developmental, health/illness, situational,* and *organizational. Developmental transitions* are those that reflect life cycle transitions, such as adolescence, parenthood, and aging. For the purposes of discussing coaching by APNs, developmental transitions are considered to include any transition with an intrapersonal focus, including changes in life cycle, self-perception, motivation, expectations, or meanings.

Health/illness transitions were described by Schumacher and Meleis (1994) primarily as illness related and range from adapting to a chronic illness to returning home after a stay in the hospital. Such transitions can include modifying risk factors, adapting to the physiological and psychological demands of pregnancy, and numerous other clinical

TABLE 6-2	MODELS AND CONCEPTS THAT INFORMED CONCEPTUALIZATION OF COACHING THROUGH TRANSITION	
MODEL OR CONCEPT	**AUTHOR(S)**	**COMMENTS**
Chronic illness trajectory framework	Corbin & Strauss (1992)	• Describes principles of framework • Chronic illness has a course that varies over time • Nurses collaborate with patients to shape the trajectory
Cumulative adversity and posttraumatic stress disorders	Alonzo (2000)	• Describes potential adverse impact of multiple health-care experiences in patients who have had myocardial infarctions • Proposes model for understanding cumulative adversity
Adverse childhood experiences	Felliti (1998, 2002)	• Provides evidence of impact of childhood trauma on adult health
Self-help model	Braden (1990, 1993)	• Describes 5 stages of response to chronic illness • Notes that nursing interventions can facilitate the acquisition of self-help behaviors
Transtheoretical Model of Change	Prochaska et al. (1994)	• Describes phases of behavioral change
Self-care in Chronic Illness Model	Connelly (1993)	• Is an extension of Health Belief Model
Transitional care	Lamm et al. (1991), Brooten et al. (1988), Brooten et al. (2003), Naylor et al. (1999)	• Describes discharge from hospital to home as a transition that can be shaped by nursing interventions
Self-efficacy	Bandura (1977), Carrieri-Kohlman et al. (1996), Clark & Dodge (1999), Lev (1997), McDougall (1999)	• Addresses interaction among factors that influence behavior change • Accounts for changes in motivation, self-confidence, and behavior that result from interventions
Patient-centered communication (PCC)	Squier (1990), Brown (1999)	• Describes empirical support for components of PCC (see Box 6-1)
Comforting-Interaction Relationship Model	Morse et al. (1997)	• Addresses patient and nurse factors • Notes that comforting relationship is negotiated by means of nurse-patient interactions
Therapeutic relationships	Peplau (1952), Travelbee (1971)	• Addresses existential and spiritual aspects of relationship
Transition experiences	Schumacher & Meleis (1994), Chick & Meleis (1986), Benner et al. (1999)	• Delineates types and process of transitions

phenomena. Some health/illness changes are self-limiting (e.g., the physiological changes of pregnancy), whereas others are long term and may be reversible or irreversible. Although Schumacher and Meleis excluded acute self-limiting illnesses (e.g., a cold) from the notion of transition, other variables are likely to influence whether a transition occurs as a result of a self-limiting illness (e.g., if a cold prevents a person from attending an important event). Because health/illness transitions are often the primary incentive for seeking health care, these are discussed in more detail.

In this chapter, *health/illness transitions* are defined as transitions that are driven by an individual's experience of the body in a holistic sense. Recent literature suggests that prior "embodied" experiences may play a role in the expression or the course of health problems. For example, Alonzo (2000), on the basis of results of studies of patients with acute myocardial infarctions, has proposed a model of the impact of cumulative adversity (both personal and illness-related) on the course of chronic illness and individuals' abilities to cope. For example, the memory of the stress of repeated, invasive procedures experienced during one hospitalization for treatment of an acute myocardial infarction (AMI) may prevent a patient from seeking timely health care for a subsequent AMI. Some health-care experiences may elicit or reactivate posttraumatic stress disorder or other significant emotional responses in vulnerable individuals (Alonzo, 2000; Capasso, 1998). In addition, in the Adverse Childhood Experiences (ACE) Study (Felitti et al., 1998; Felitti, 2002), the impact of adverse experiences in childhood, such as abuse and trauma, on adults' health was examined. Health concerns such as smoking and obesity appear to have strong relationships with adverse childhood experiences. In a clinical case study analyzed in light of the ACE Study findings, Felitti (2002) proposed a reordering of the patient's health problems. Although diabetes and hypertension were the "presenting concerns" in a 70-year-old woman, her problem list was as follows:

Childhood sexual abuse
   Chronic depression
   Morbid obesity
   Diabetes mellitus
   Hypertension
   Hyperlipidemia
Macular degeneration
Psoriasis

These studies suggest that APNs' assessment of health/illness transition experiences may be even more complicated than our existing understanding of chronic illness and trauma. Felitti (2002) acknowledged that this understanding of illness, especially chronic conditions, is daunting for providers, especially those in primary care. Nevertheless, theories regarding adverse experiences in childhood and in health care and the potential for cumulative trauma and complex emotional and physical responses may help us better understand the nature and outcomes of coaching.

As just noted, the other types of transitions described by Schumacher and Meleis (1994) are situational transitions and organizational transitions. *Situational transitions* include changes in educational, professional, and family roles and transitions that occur as a result of changes in intangible or tangible structures or resources (e.g., role changes and financial reversals) that are specific to individuals and their relationships. *Organizational transitions* are those that occur in the environment—within agencies, between agencies, or in society—and reflect changes in structures and resources at a system level.

The first three categories of transitions are the ones most likely to lead to clinical encounters between APNs and patients in which expert coaching is required. However, APNs must also be skilled in dealing with organizational transitions, which tend to affect structural and contextual aspects of providing care. Barnsteiner et al. (1994) described an interesting project in which a standard for establishing therapeutic relationships in a pediatric setting was developed. The process was an organizational transition implemented by staff members who were coached by APNs. Wise APNs pay attention to all four types of transitions in their personal and professional lives, because transitions can affect the development and effectiveness of APNs' expert coaching.

In practice, the APN is also aware of the possibility of multiple transitions occurring as a result of one salient transition. While eliciting information on the primary transition that led the patient to seek care, the APN is attending to verbal, nonverbal, and intuitive cues to identify other transitions and meanings associated with the primary one. Attending to the possibility of multiple transitions enables the APN to tailor coaching to the individual's particular needs and concerns. Table 6-3 lists some situations, based on this typology, that require APN coaching.

CHARACTERISTICS, CONDITIONS, AND OUTCOMES OF TRANSITIONS

Transitions can be characterized along the dimensions of time, the nature of the process that occurs, and the type of change that occurs (Schumacher & Meleis, 1994). All transitions seem to unfold over time, as opposed to being one-time events. A single event may precipitate the transition, but the transition is experienced over some period of time. The process that occurs is directional, entailing movement from one state to another, and is often described as occurring in stages. The type of change tends to be substantive and internal, rather than incidental or superficial; transitions affect personal identities, roles, relationships, functional status, and behaviors (Schumacher & Meleis, 1994). The experience of transition can vary considerably for both individuals and groups and from one day to the next as a result of conditions that affect the transition (Corbin & Strauss, 1992; Schumacher & Meleis, 1994).

Outcomes of transitions proposed by Schumacher and Meleis (1994) include subjective well-being, role mastery, and well-being of relationships. Quality-of-care outcomes can also be used as indicators of successful transitions. When one considers the direct, individual effects of coaching by APNs, the most relevant outcomes are those that are patient related. Examples include morbidity; mortality; medical complications; comfort;

TABLE 6-3	TRANSITION SITUATIONS THAT REQUIRE COACHING		
HEALTH/ILLNESS	DEVELOPMENTAL	SITUATIONAL	ORGANIZATIONAL
Pregnancy/labor	Parenting	Job loss or change	Mergers
Hospitalization	Adverse childhood experiences	Divorce	Policy changes
Risk reduction	Puberty	Natural disasters/national	Change in leadership
Lifestyle changes	Suffering	disasters	Change in
Chronic condition	Loss of significant others	Quality of life	organizational
Disability	Caregiving for elderly relatives	Change in social supports	structure
Weight loss or gain	Changes in sexual function or activity	Social isolation	
Symptoms		Financial reversals or windfalls	
Violence		Change in living situations	
		Community trauma	

Note: The situations are categorized according to the initiating change. Many of these transitions have reciprocal impacts across categories.

functional, physiological, or mental status; stress level; coping strategies; quality of life; patient satisfaction; and caregiver burden (Kolcaba, 1992; Lang & Marek, 1992; Naylor, Munro, & Brooten, 1991; Peplau, 1994). Although some researchers have studied intrapersonal phenomena that might be considered outcomes of coaching, such as finding meaning and self-transcendence, more research on how to assess such outcomes is needed. Organizational or cost outcomes that might be affected by coaching processes include lengths of stay, cost of care, proportion of services that receive reimbursement, and use of health-care services (Lang & Marek, 1992; Naylor et al., 1991). This description of transitions as a focus for APN coaching underscores the need for, and the importance of, a holistic orientation when APNs help individuals address their health and illness concerns.

THE FOUNDATIONS OF COACHING THROUGH TRANSITIONS

A Model of APNs' Expert Coaching and Guidance

Coaching by APNs is *a complex, dynamic, collaborative, and holistic interpersonal process that is mediated by the APN-patient relationship and the APN's self-reflective skills.* APNs integrate self-reflection and the technical, clinical, and interpersonal competencies they have acquired through graduate education and experience with patients' understandings, experiences, and goals in order to shape transitional experiences and accomplish therapeutic and educational goals. Graduate education is assumed. Expert coaching by APNs depends on the interaction of four factors: clinical competence, technical competence, interpersonal competence, and self-reflection (Figure 6-1). The interaction of self-reflection with these three areas of competence drives the ongoing expansion and refinement of expertise in advanced practice nursing.

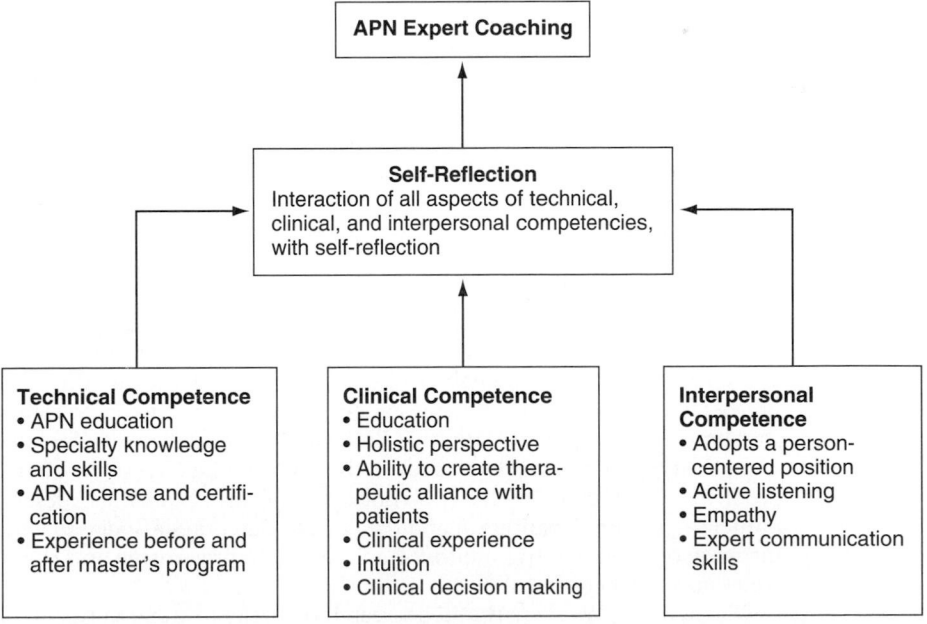

FIGURE 6-1 • Coaching competency of an advanced practice nurse (APN).

Several assumptions that underlie this model of the APN's coaching and guiding must be made explicit. First, in the entire discussion of coaching it is assumed that APNs involve the patient's significant other or the patient's proxy as appropriate. Second, although technical competence and clinical competence may be sufficient for teaching a task, they are insufficient for coaching patients through transitions. For example, patients with diabetes may be taught how to monitor their blood sugar levels and administer insulin with technical accuracy, but if the impact of the transition from health to chronic illness that requires major lifestyle changes is not evaluated, then coaching and guidance cannot occur. Failure to assess the need for coaching when teaching patients about health and illness may influence the outcomes of individual and group teaching approaches. Third, the APN's skill as an expert coach and guide depends on a combination of clinical experience with a particular population and graduate education (see Chapter 3). The clinical and didactic content of graduate education extends the APN's repertoire of assessment skills, technical skills, interpersonal behaviors, and self-reflection abilities, enabling the APN to coach in situations that are broader in scope or more complex in nature. The APN is also able to be more explicit about the processes and outcomes of coaching.

As noted, the basis for expert APN coaching is the interaction of interpersonal, technical, and clinical competence with self-reflection. Expert coaching requires that APNs be self-aware and self-reflective as an interpersonal transaction is unfolding, so that they can shape communications and behaviors to maximize the therapeutic and educational goals of the clinical encounter. The ability to self-reflect and focus on the process of coaching as it is occurring implies that APNs are capable of the simultaneous execution of other skills. While interacting with a patient, APNs integrate physical, cognitive, and intuitive skills such as physical examination, interviewing, attending to their own noncognitive reactions and those of the patient, and interpreting these multiple sources of information. One might compare the process to simultaneous translation of a speech into several languages as it is being given. The difference is that the simultaneous translations are being carried out by one APN, not several translators. De la Cuesta (1994) characterized this as the "'product' [or outcome] taking shape or being 'manufactured' in the very process of the interaction" (p. 457).

The reader might be interested in comparing the model of APN expert coaching proposed here with two other models (Morse, Havens, & Wilson, 1997; Squier, 1990). Given that the goals of health care are preventing future illness, decreasing chronicity, limiting relapses or exacerbations of illnesses, alleviating suffering, and responding to crises, Squier (1990) wondered why the quality of provider-patient relationships is not given more priority—at least as much as is given to technological treatments. To address this question, Squier analyzed existing literature, including studies of physicians and APNs, and has proposed a model linking a clinician's empathic understanding with a patient's adherence to therapeutic regimens. He hypothesized that empathic understanding has two components: cognitive and affective. Clinicians' cognitive ability to accurately take the perspective of the patient enables them to communicate effectively and reflect this understanding back to the patient. Patients are then more likely to elaborate the concerns that brought them to the clinician. Clinicians' emotional sensitivity to patients' emotions and underlying concerns helps reduce the anxiety and stress that often affect the health problems for which patients are consulting clinicians. Squier also described phases of the clinician-patient consultation and the patient outcomes associated with each phase, the ultimate outcomes being improved adherence to preventive and therapeutic strategies (self-care) and better health.

Morse et al. (1997) synthesized research on patient interactions and nurse-patient relationships and proposed a model integrating these findings—the Comforting Interaction-

Relationship Model. The components of the model include nursing actions that represent three interrelated levels: comforting strategies, styles of care, and patterns of relating. Nurses initiate these actions in response to patient actions: signals of distress, indices of discomfort, and patterns of relating. Nurse-patient interactions are the means by which the therapeutic relationship is negotiated and evolves.

Technical Competence and Clinical Competence

Technical and clinical competence are well-defined aspects of established advanced practice nursing roles, and their importance to coaching cannot be overestimated. However, these two factors are not addressed in detail in this chapter. The evolution of specialties in advanced practice nursing has focused on defining and describing the technical and clinical skills required for advanced practice with particular populations. Chapters 1 and 19 document the evolution of these aspects of various advanced practice nursing roles. In addition, the chapters in Part III illustrate the specific technical and clinical skills needed for particular advanced practice nursing roles.

An important part of clinical competence is clinical experience with the populations that are the APN's focus. Pregraduate school experiences, experiences within the clinical practica of graduate programs, and post-master's clinical experiences provide the grist for analyzing, developing, and making visible the coaching competency of APNs. Ongoing development of APNs' coaching competency depends on applying self-reflection to clinical experiences to acquire new coaching knowledge and skills that cannot be found in any textbook. Over the course of caring for patients, nurses learn the many ways people experience and manage health, birth, illness, pain, suffering, and death (Benner, 1985, 1991; Benner et al., 1999). These clinical experiences enable APNs to identify coaching alternatives that help other patients understand, learn, change, modulate, and control experiences of transition.

Interpersonal Competence

Interpersonal competence encompasses the ability to communicate effectively and to establish therapeutic, caring relationships. These two components are briefly described, and theoretical and research support for interpersonal competence as an integral part of coaching is provided. Interpersonal interactions can be characterized as position-centered or person-centered (Bernstein, 1974; Brown, 1999; Kasch & Dine, 1988; Kasch & Knutson, 1985). Position-centered interpersonal interactions are characterized by dependence on roles and rules and the use of power and authority. A person-centered encounter is characterized by an appreciation for the uniqueness of the individuals involved (the nurse and the patient) and attention to the patient's concerns. APNs do not assume they understand the patient's perspective (Kasch, 1983; Kasch & Dine, 1988; Squier, 1990); person-centered communication enables APNs to accurately take the patient's perspective and respond empathically (Squier, 1990). During patient encounters, APNs adopt an open, flexible, nonhierarchical stance and communicate this in words and actions (Brown, 1995); they convey an attitude of openness, elicit and respond to feelings, express concern, confirm the patient's experience, and provide positive reinforcement (Quirk & Casey, 1995). APNs summarize, recap, and interpret as they coach. Verbal and nonverbal skills that characterize a person-centered approach to interviewing are listed in Box 6-1.

Establishing a caring, therapeutic relationship with a patient demands that the APN be emotionally responsive, not distant. The nurse and patient enter the relationship as

BOX 6-1 • SKILLS ASSOCIATED WITH A PERSON-CENTERED STYLE OF COMMUNICATION

- Allowing patients to tell their stories using their own language and chronology
- Using a conversational style of interviewing
- Eliciting patients' thoughts, perspectives, expectations, values, and goals
- Asking about the contexts of patients' lives
- Encouraging self-disclosure
- Responding to patients' indirect and nonverbal clues regarding emotions and problems
- Providing patients with self-care information and enabling patients' participation in health-care decision making
- Creating shared understandings with patients
- Developing health care plans collaboratively with patients
- Expressing concern for patients' well-being
- Responding empathically
- Creating social connectedness with patients by means of humor, touch, and modest personal sharing
- Using open-ended questions and paraphrasing to elicit information and validate patients' communications
- Using a tone of voice and pace of speech appropriate to the topic being discussed
- Making eye contact and using a forward-leaning posture

Data from Brown (1999), Quirk and Casey (1995), and Montgomery (1993).

whole persons, complete with talents, goals, needs, and wishes; but the focus of the interpersonal process is on addressing the patient's potentials and goals (Martocchio, 1987; Montgomery, 1993). Nurses reveal themselves through their eyes, tone of voice, affect, body language, and silences. The APN "who withholds parts of herself [or himself] is unlikely to allow the patient to emerge as a whole, or to comprehend that wholeness if it does emerge" (Gadow, 1980, p. 87). Montgomery (1993) has found that clinicians had predispositional qualities consistent with caring: a person orientation rather than role orientation, concern for the human element in care, person-centered intention, transcendence of judgment, hopeful orientation, lack of ego involvement, and expanded personal boundaries. She also described the properties of caring behaviors (Box 6-2). These properties are consistent with a person-centered style of communication. APNs who rely only on scientific and technical competencies in their relationships with patients are unlikely to appreciate patients' holistic responses or enable patients to express themselves holistically (Gadow, 1980).

Studies of education provided by nurses in basic and advanced practice suggest that a caring, person-centered relationship underlies successful educational interventions (Benner, 1984; Brown, 1999; Fenton, 1984; Lamb & Stempel, 1994; Morgan, 1994; Steele & Fenton, 1988). Selected findings that support the importance of interpersonal competence to APN coaching are summarized here.

In one study of nurses, nurse-patient interaction and the development of rapport were foundational in accomplishing patient education (Morgan, 1994). De la Cuesta (1994) affirmed that therapeutic alliances established by public health nurses with patients have an important enabling function: the relationship is seen as "a medium or vehicle for achieving goals" (p. 452) and as having a mediating function that allows the nurse to adopt conflicting roles (e.g., being able to point out the patient's self-neglect behaviors while supporting the patient as a person or intervening to help the patient accomplish self-care goals).

Patients' experiences with nurse case management offer additional insight. Nurse case management seems to help patients become "their own insider-experts" (Lamb &

BOX 6-2 • PROPERTIES OF CARING EXPRESSED AS BEHAVIORS

- Empowerment through mobilization of resources
- Advocacy
- Authenticity
- Responsiveness
- Commitment
- Being present with
- Creating positive meaning and hope
- Competence

Data from Montgomery (1993).

Stempel, 1994, p. 9). This process consisted of three phases: bonding, working, and changing. Lamb and Stempel noted that bonding or "the demonstration of concern [by nurses] appears to be a key factor in triggering cognitive change" (p. 10). Once the nurse was seen as both expert and insider, the working phase could begin. Patients were willing to examine relationships among their attitudes, behaviors, illness exacerbations, and use of health-care resources. Patients began to see themselves differently and reported changes in self-image, changes in meaning, and mastery of self-care. Many patients became their own insider-experts, skilled at identifying changes in illness patterns, selecting effective self-care interventions, and using the health-care system in a timely and appropriate way.

A caring, person-centered approach demands an involved, current, individualized, contextual understanding of the patient (Tanner, Benner, Chesla, & Gordon, 1993). This understanding serves to bridge the differences between APNs and their patients and enables patients to share power and collaborate with APNs to develop a realistic plan of care. If a patient is to be coached effectively in making transitions that are genuinely his or her own, both the nurse and the patient must enter the relationship as whole persons. Some people will regard this caring, person-centered approach as an unreachable ideal, given the complexity of care and time pressures experienced by clinicians. In most situations, the skilled APN can establish rapport immediately and determine the priorities for assessment and intervention while sustaining this person-centered approach. For example, critical care CNSs are skilled in coaching families facing the loss of a loved one to a traumatic brain injury: they facilitate "bad news" conversations, interpret the intricacies of brain death, and provide comfort to the grief-stricken survivors in rapidly evolving situations. They perform such coaching with skill and compassion, while attending to competing needs, demands, and schedules of other patients and colleagues. APNs must develop strategies for staying personally centered and patient-centered in a variety of circumstances, including those with time constraints.

Self-Reflection

The fourth component of the APN expert coaching model is self-reflection—the deliberate, internal examination of experience in order to learn from it. The APN uses self-reflection during interactions with patients, as well as retrospectively. Schön (1983) described these as "reflection-in-action" and "reflection-on-action." Reflection-in-action is the ability to pay attention to phenomena as they are occurring, giving free rein to one's intuitive understanding of the situation as it is unfolding. The APN is not restricted to using only familiar patterns of thought. APN coaching is analogous to the flexible and inventive playing of a jazz musician; APNs can attend to what is happening in the moment and respond with a varied repertoire of exploratory and transforming actions. The heart of reflective practice is action and paradox, not generalized scripts and certainty (Grimmett, 1988). In the APN-patient relationship, reflective practice is simultaneously doing and learning and coming to know. Reflection-in-action can be compared with the Zen concept of mindfulness (Tremmel, 1993). Mindfulness means paying attention to "right here, right now" and investing the present moment with full concentration. Reflection-in-action, or mindfulness, involves awareness of the world and awareness of multiple aspects of consciousness—thoughts, feelings, behaviors.

Looking within involves listening to one's own thinking processes; it is part of preparing for and demonstrating reflective practice (Bartels, 1998; Pugach & Johnson, 1990). As an extension of the work done by Jackson (1986) on expert teaching, APN coaches might be characterized as those who "see more" than nonexperts do. "Seeing more" refers to the practice of "paying attention" (Jackson, 1986). APNs are sensitive to possibilities— within patients, within the processes of the clinical encounter, and within themselves. They anticipate what might happen during the encounter or after the patient leaves. They are sensitive to incipient difficulty: APNs' sensibilities, processes (including reflection), and skills interact to shape their encounters with patients, to support patients, and to enable patients to navigate transitions to achieve mutually determined goals. Action without reflection becomes automatic; there can be no transformation in the absence of action with reflection (Freire, 1970).

The capacity to reflect mindfully in action and on action is not readily mastered and requires continual practice (Tremmel, 1993). However, certain qualities and characteristics can be developed to facilitate self-reflection. These include motivation, commitment, open-mindedness, self-awareness, the ability to describe phenomena or situations, critical analysis, and the ability to synthesize and evaluate (Atkins & Murphy, 1994). APNs should pay attention to both positive and negative experiences. What made this effective? Why didn't this work? APNs may be more likely to reflect on negative experiences because the feeling of failure is more uncomfortable than the feeling of satisfaction or success. However, reflecting on satisfying, successful experiences can provide clues to interventions that will be effective in future interactions. One of the key aspects of self-reflection is paying attention to feelings. Experienced nurses and APNs are more likely than inexperienced ones to pay attention to feelings or intuition. However, novice APNs need to be taught to recognize that their affective responses to situations are clues to their developing expertise as clinicians and coaches.

COACHING ASSESSMENT, PROCESSES, AND OUTCOMES

Assessment

Patient assessment is the basis for determining which coaching interventions will be used. APNs use whatever physical and psychological assessment procedures, skills, or tools they need to evaluate the patient's concerns. They understand that assessments have multiple purposes: (1) to gain an understanding of the patient and establish a therapeutic relationship, (2) to identify patients' health-related concerns and goals, and (3) to collect data. They make conscious efforts to build a partnership that will work by conveying caring and concern, being honest and dependable, and displaying professional knowledge and self-confidence. The person-centered approach adopted by nurses has been described by several researchers as "knowing the patient" (Jenny & Logan, 1992; Tanner et al., 1993; Radwin, 1996). This entails getting to know the patient as a person and learning the patient's pattern of responses, including experiences, habits, practices, preferences, usual demeanor, and self-presentation (Jenny & Logan, 1992). In addition to getting to know the patient and using strategic communication, APNs use their observations of themselves, the patients, and the interactive process to decode patients' behaviors and the content of their communications for significance (Kasch & Dine, 1988). They need to grasp each patient's perspective, including salient aspects of the patient's self-definition (Olesen, Schatzman, Droes, Hatton, & Chico, 1990). This understanding is critical to the selection of coaching interventions to help people who need to make lifestyle changes, reduce risk, or manage chronic illness.

Assessment must extend beyond the individual to include consideration of the patient's relationships, communities, and social milieu because social and contextual variables often influence the APN's ability to provide effective care. Thus a vital aspect of knowing the patient is what White (1995) calls "sociopolitical knowing." Sociopolitical knowing includes an understanding of the social and political context of the patient, as well as the broader context in which nursing and health care take place. Both the APN's and the patient's cultural and political location powerfully influence their understanding of health, illness, language, identity, social roles, and historical issues. For example, domestic violence, child abuse, malnutrition, substance abuse, and stress-induced illnesses are responses to political, social, and personal problems. Both Steven (1989) and Chopoorian (1986) emphasized the need for nurses to provide a vocal critique of how domination, alienation, poverty, homelessness, and unemployment affect the health of persons and communities. APNs may find that coaching their patients requires that they expose and problematize social and political inequities that affect people's health (Hagedorn, 1995; Kendall, 1992). Otherwise, the core issues in many patients' transitions will be invisible and unidentified, and the coaching strategies used will be superficial, unfocused, and ineffective.

Several conditions influence the experience of transition and its unfolding (Corbin & Strauss, 1992; Schumacher & Meleis, 1994) and should be assessed. Meaning and expectations are subjective phenomena that affect the anticipation and experience of transition (Schumacher & Meleis, 1994; Neimeyer, 2001). Although many transition conditions can be affected by prior experience, meanings and expectations may be the ones most colored by memories and previous experiences. Meanings may be positive, negative, or neutral. Transitions may require the reconstruction of meaning. Regardless of whether the meaning is positive or negative, patients may experience uncertainty, grief, guilt, stress, or other emotional responses. Expectations may be accurate and realistic, or they may be unrealistic and even fantastic. Cognitive variables such as knowledge, self-care skills, motivation, coping style, habitual stressors, and personal preferences for control affect people's experience of and ability to accept, adjust to, or adapt to transitional experiences (Alonzo, 2000; Brooten et al., 1991; Corbin & Strauss, 1992; Jenny & Logan, 1992; Kasch & Dine, 1988; Neimeyer, 2001; Schumacher & Meleis, 1994). The environment—including resources, relationships, social support, setting of care, and contextual variables—can mediate transitions (Brooten et al., 1991; Corbin & Strauss, 1992; Schumacher & Meleis, 1994). Role demands and responsibilities that may interfere with therapeutic self-care must be identified (Connelly, 1993). Level of planning—including problem and need identification, organization of phase-related interventions, and communication—influences the success of the transition. Physical and emotional well-being also determine how the transition process is experienced (Schumacher & Meleis, 1994). The nature of the health concern; the severity of symptoms, perceived vulnerability, and seriousness; and the degree of predictability or certainty about one's experience of the body can make for smooth or chaotic transitions.

APNs identify missing information that they might need for coaching and variables that might enhance or hinder coaching. Throughout the interaction, they try to regulate distress (Heifetz, 1994), respond to patients' needs for information, and create a physically and interpersonally comforting environment (Kasch & Lisnek, 1984). For example, an APN might observe that a patient is becoming fatigued during an examination. In addition to providing for rest and changing the pace of the examination, the APN will explore the causes, duration, and significance of the fatigue.

Several points can be made about the assessment aspects of coaching through transitions. First, not every encounter will involve a transition; many encounters will be self-limiting. Even in these more routine situations, the APN's coaching competence can result in efficient care delivery, improved patient satisfaction, and return business—all valued outcomes in managed care environments. Second, not every individual immersed in a transitional situation is interested in moving or adjusting; a person can become stuck or immobilized by the demands of the transition, the underlying nature of the illness (such as borderline personality disorder), or personal factors such as limited social support or cognitive ability. Even so, APNs can often help patients who are immobilized. These are often the patients for whom physicians, staff nurses, or novice APNs seek the help of an experienced APN. By working effectively with difficult cases, APNs expand their repertoire of coaching interventions (see Exemplar 6-1). Some patients who are stuck simply need a new coach—someone with a different approach or personality. A smaller population may be help rejecters; in this case, coaching is unlikely to be effective, and such patients can only be "maintained." Third, although some conscious patients may reject help, noncommunicative patients can often be coached effectively. For example, the APN who is providing palliative care may talk to the dying person about letting go, review aspects of the patient's life, and provide comforting touch interventions. The APN observes responses that indicate relaxation and peace (e.g., less restlessness and moaning).

EXEMPLAR 6-1

Ms. A. was a 35-year-old African American woman who came to the anesthesia pain unit for an outpatient procedure—a stellate ganglion block for treatment of chronic pain. Assessment revealed that she understood the procedure, including the purposes and the risks. She knew that an intravenous (IV) line would be placed. As the anesthesiology fellow was inserting the IV line, Ms. A began to cry, shake, and sweat and said she felt afraid. The clinical nurse specialist (CNS) asked the fellow to stop the procedure and give the CNS an opportunity to further assess the patient. The patient indicated that she had not expected such a reaction and had had IV lines placed before. However, after further questioning by the CNS, the patient indicated that the last time she had had an IV line placed was while she was in the emergency department, 10 years before, after she had been raped and beaten. The experience of having the IV started reproduced the distress and fear she felt then. Ms. A. was offered the option of rescheduling the procedure, but she did not want to do that because she was counting on having the procedure to ameliorate her pain. Ms. A chose to receive additional antianxiety medication, and she was also coached in the standard relaxation exercise that was part of the stellate ganglion block protocol and was reassured that the CNS would remain with her throughout the procedure. Postprocedure discharge planning included referral to a counselor she had seen in the past who had been helpful. In addition, a debriefing session was held with Ms. A. She was advised that future invasive procedures could reproduce the reaction of the prior trauma and that she should include both the original traumatic event and the reaction to the block procedure when relaying her health history.

Processes and Outcomes

Coaching processes used by APNs focus on fostering involvement, choice, and independence. The results of one study of patient education suggest that a continuum of nurse-patient interactions exists, from simple interactions, such as preoperative teaching, to decrease anxiety to complex ones such as counseling to enhance problem-solving skills (Morgan, 1994). Intervention mapping, a strategy for tailoring educational interventions to the needs of the population, has been proposed as a strategy for planning health education initiatives (Bartholomew, Parcel, & Kok, 1998). The concept of intervention mapping may also be used to plan care for individuals; an individualized assessment often leads APNs to tailor the usual treatment to improve adherence and the likelihood of reaching a desired outcome.

Benner (1985) elaborated on APNs' coaching behaviors. In coaching a patient, APNs have four main tasks: interpreting unfamiliar diagnostic and treatment demands, coaching the patient through alienated stances (e.g., anger and hopelessness), identifying changing relevance as demands or symptoms of the illness change, and ensuring that cure is enhanced by care. These tasks can be accomplished through coaching processes. Both processes and outcomes can be categorized by focus: bodily or physical, affective/interpersonal/spiritual, cognitive/behavioral, and social. Coaching processes and outcomes derived from the literature review presented earlier and in a review by Spross (1996) are listed in Table 6-4.

APNs attend to issues of timing and sequencing in teaching and counseling patients. Thus they may need to coach a patient to become motivated before beginning to teach him or her a particular task. APNs integrate coaching into processes of consultation, collaboration, and referral. They use their knowledge of the patient to mobilize resources and interpret the patient's needs to team members, consultants, and family caregivers. Knowing the patient enables APNs to take risks, adopt stances that are unusual or unpopular, and make the system work to shape patients' transitional experiences, a quality of the APN direct care competency that has been described as "fearlessness" (Koetters, 1989). Therefore coaching is a holistic process, and although there is a primary focus or target, coaching behaviors often have effects across all dimensions of the patient's experience.

The case in Exemplar 6-2 (p. 206) illustrates the following aspects of coaching: recognizing the need for coaching early in a patient encounter and the risks of not coaching (poor pain management, poor rehabilitation outcome, alienation between staff and patient), identifying the multiple levels of coaching needed (patient, staff, postdischarge caregivers), and using relationships with patients and colleagues to shape a positive outcome in a complex situation.

DEVELOPMENT OF APNs' COACHING COMPETENCE

Becoming an expert coach requires a combination of education, experience, interpersonal competence, and self-reflection on one's practice. It is not a technical skill; technical skill is insufficient "in the swampy lowland [of clinical practice] where situations are confusing 'messes'" (Schön, 1983, p. 42). Although scientific and technical knowledge are essential for effective coaching, it is in the coaching of patients that the art of advanced practice nursing is fully expressed. APNs need a highly nuanced range of interpersonal skills to coach people through multifaceted transitions. The strategies used to develop coaching expertise are designed to prepare APNs for reflective practice and a person-oriented interactive style, which are foundational abilities that APNs must develop to become skilled coaches.

TABLE 6-4	ADVANCED PRACTICE NURSES' COACHING PROCESSES AND POSSIBLE OUTCOMES	
DOMINANT FOCUS	COACHING PROCESSES	POSSIBLE OUTCOMES*
Physical	Demonstrating self-care or self-monitoring skills Describing the likely physical trajectory of the health or illness concern, including physical and psychological demands, tasks, and resources Describing the possibilities inherent in the physical transitions experienced Identifying risk factors Implementing pain and symptom management Interpreting the person's experiences of the body Offering alternative (e.g., more hopeful) interpretations of bodily sensations/functions Offering strategies to modify risk factors Providing assistance with hygiene and toileting and conducting invasive procedures and other physical interventions while preserving dignity Using comforting touch	Effective self-care (e.g., fewer symptoms) Improved functional status Improved mental status (e.g., as a result of decreased pain or normalized blood sugar levels) Increased physical comfort
Affective, interpersonal, spiritual	Accepting the person as he or she is Acknowledging the person's courage, strength, or other personal qualities Acknowledging both expressed and possible fears and concerns Attuning oneself to patient's needs and goals Being available/presencing Being honest Bonding, establishing a therapeutic alliance Comforting through touch, behavior, and interactions Counseling Eliciting expectations, fears, meanings, and values Enabling Encouraging, praising Ensuring safe passage Expressing confidence in patients and their abilities Inspiring/inspiriting Listening Keeping a vigil Making a commitment to help Offering hope Reassuring Supporting Validating	Acceptance of help from others Decreased anxiety, stress, or uncertainty Decreased spiritual distress Finding meaning Hope Improved quality of life Increased ability to initiate self-care Increased comfort, decreased suffering Revised future agendas Self-acceptance Self-report of satisfaction with decision making Self-transcendence

Cognitive, behavioral	Challenging Coaching in communication and technical skills Communicating strategically Confronting and identifying contradictions Dealing with conflict Demonstrating and role-modeling Explaining Guiding, offering a map Identifying adaptive tasks Identifying the goals of interventions Improving problem-solving skills Intervention mapping Mediating Monitoring Motivating Negotiating Offering options Organizing goals Presenting challenges Providing cognitive strategies to alter negative thought patterns Providing feedback Reframing expectations, goals, and meanings Setting tasks Using a variety of teaching strategies Using humor Using cognitive coping strategies	Behavior change Change in beliefs or attitudes Decreased stress Effective self-care and problem solving related to clinical issues Improved functional status Improved quality of life Increased self-efficacy
Social	Advocating Bonding Collaborating with the patient and with other providers Facilitating important relationships Interpreting patients' behaviors, needs, and goals to members of the health care team and patients' families Keeping tradition Mobilizing community, financial, and social resources Strengthening social supports through teaching, consultation, and referral	Affection Alienation and stigmatization averted or minimized Comfort Decreased caregiver burden Decreased costs of care Improved satisfaction with care Improved self-care Satisfaction with social support

Adapted from Spross, J. A. (1996). Coaching and suffering: The role of the nurse in helping people face illness. In B. R. Ferrell (Ed.), *The human dimensions of suffering* (Table 8.3, pp. 198-199). Boston: Jones & Bartlett; reprinted with permission. (The reader is encouraged to refer to this publication for additional references from which the coaching processes were derived.)

†Although most outcomes are patient and family related, some systems outcomes are included to help the reader connect the individual coaching by advanced practice nurses with organization-level outcomes.

EXEMPLAR 6-2

A clinical nurse specialist (CNS), collaborated with a psychologist in the care of a patient with complex care needs named Jack, who had been admitted to a rehabilitation hospital after a left hip arthroplasty and left tibial traction pin. His immediate postoperative course had been complicated by a staphylococcal infection at the surgical site, for which he was still receiving intravenous antibiotics. Jack had a history of substance abuse and had been in a methadone maintenance program. Jack was well known to the staff because he had been in the rehabilitation hospital 1 year earlier after a girdlestone surgical procedure was performed on his right hip. During both admissions, pain management was a significant problem. He became easily frustrated and impatient and expressed his anger verbally. These characteristics were exacerbated when he was in moderate to severe pain. For example, requests for pain medications were made in demanding and insistent tones. Jack currently reports pain in his left hip and left lower leg, as well as some right shoulder and paralumbar pain. According to the nursing assessment, his pain intensity data are as follows: worst pain is 10/10, least is 9/10, and average pain is 9/10. Despite administration of Percocet, 2 tablets every 6 hours, his pain is never below 9/10. Jack did not complete high school and is disabled. His parents are divorced. He has nieces and nephews he adores and has been motivated to stay clean because he is not permitted to see them if he is abusing drugs.

The CNS, performed an initial, thorough assessment of Jack's pain. During this assessment, she initiated coaching by reviewing with him what they had learned during the prior admission about how to manage his pain by using a combination of scheduled opioids and nondrug interventions. Jack expressed frustration that he was not as independent as he had been during the prior admission. The CNS explained that during the prior admission, he had had the use of his "good" leg to compensate for what the treated leg could not do. Although he had made a good recovery, the leg treated last year was not functional enough to support his weight and compensate for the temporary loss of function in the leg being treated during this admission. He acknowledged that this made sense. The CNS knew from having reviewed the admission orders that she would need to talk to the physicians to get the analgesics changed to an around-the-clock schedule so Jack could participate effectively in therapies.

The CNS and the psychologist conferred and agreed to share responsibility for coaching, with the CNS having a primary focus on the patient and the psychologist having a primary focus on the staff. The CNS had been working with the staff for more than a year to improve pain management practices in the unit. However, the staff would need coaching because they were being challenged to apply what they learned about pain management to a patient whose history they believed made use of opioids for pain risky. The psychologist would help the staff understand this patient and the reasons for treating pain with opioids in an addict who had had surgery, and, if needed, help staff see when their attitudes and misconceptions might be interfering with Jack's care. Jack needed coaching regarding appropriate ways to communicate his pain and response to pain management interventions to avoid alienating staff and to maximize participation in therapy. In addition, the CNS would work with the nurses and physicians on titrating analgesia to effect. Given Jack's history, he was likely to need more analgesia, not less.

The psychologist noticed during the course of working with Jack that staff often assumed that Jack was "drug seeking" if he requested medications for pain. Staff had other concerns that needed attention: fear of giving too much pain medication, weaning Jack from analgesics as soon as possible (regardless of pain intensity level or impact of unrelieved pain on progress in rehabilitation), and concern that Jack would relapse with regard to substance abuse. The psychologist listened to and acknowledged the staff's issues. He offered them new information to encourage them to modify their thinking about how pain in addicts should be managed. Both the psychologist and the CNS were able to show staff the effectiveness of their interventions: when Jack's pain was well managed, his participation in therapy was better. If someone had withheld or forgotten Jack's medication, it showed in a decreased level of activity during physical and occupational therapy.

The CNS coached Jack in effective ways to communicate his frustration and explained why angry and blaming communications might make it harder for some staff to help him. Both the psychologist and the CNS used cognitive restructuring strategies to help Jack think differently about his problems and learn ways to increase his threshold for frustration. For example, when Jack reported that nothing was going right or that he could not do anything, events of the day were reviewed for evidence of some progress. The links between his thinking and behavior

EXEMPLAR 6-2—cont'd

were identified. When Jack became an outpatient, the psychologist and the CNS praised his self-care and adherence to treatment plans. Jack had been discharged 4 weeks after admission with an effective analgesic regimen so he could continue to make progress at home. Before his discharge, the psychologist and the CNS collaborated with the social worker to find, and then coach, a primary care physician in the most effective strategies to help Jack because Jack was at high risk of being lost to follow-up. The staff also gained a better understanding of how to manage pain in a patient with a history of substance abuse. The staff's success with managing Jack's pain enabled them to better manage the pain of the occasional future patient who happened to have a co-morbid addiction.

Graduate Nursing Education: The Influence of Faculty and Preceptors

Graduate faculty and clinical preceptors are highly influential models for APN students seeking to develop coaching skills. Faculty can assist APN students to develop as coaches by being reflective themselves. In particular, faculty need to name and evaluate the processes and pedagogies to which they were exposed, distinguishing between effective, respectful experiences of being taught or coached and ineffective, disrespectful ones. Students who have been effectively coached by teachers and preceptors will know experientially what respectful coaching "feels like." They will be more likely to reproduce these behaviors with patients. Schön (1987) called this the "hall of mirrors" effect. The teacher, in the very process of supervising and coaching the student, exemplifies the coaching repertoire that the student is attempting to acquire. If disrespectful, ineffective teaching is recognized for what it is—a position-centered style—then students also learn how *not* to coach.

Clinical preceptors play a particularly salient role with APN students. In effect, there is a "double exposure" to coaching: the student experiences being coached and observes how patients are coached by the preceptor. Similarly, preceptors need to be able to coach students while coaching patients. A person-centered style of interaction on the part of the preceptor is just as important to developing APN students' coaching skills as it is to helping patients accomplish their health goals. It is possible to have preceptors who use a person-centered style of interaction with patients yet, because of their own student experiences, adopt a position-centered style of interacting with students. Very experienced APNs can be novice preceptors (Meng & Morris, 1995), so that preceptors themselves may need coaching by faculty to develop in their preceptor roles. Davis, Sawin, and Dunn (1993) have identified three strategies that preceptors should employ to create the best conditions for learning: (1) using orientation strategies; (2) managing the clinical environment to decrease student anxiety; and (3) optimizing patient, student, and preceptor interactions. Just as APNs tailor their coaching to meet individual patient needs, so APN preceptors need to tailor their coaching of students to the level of the student and the situation (Davis et al., 1993).

Faculty and APN preceptors need to be explicit with students in articulating the range of coaching strategies used in the classroom and the clinical area. In this way, students learn the components of coaching. What was ineffable and undervalued in the process of coaching becomes defined, contextualized, reproducible, and valued (McKinnon & Erickson, 1988). Developing coaching competence requires attention to all ways of knowing, including personal knowing (Diemert Moch, 1990). Therefore faculty and APN preceptors need to encourage students to pay close attention to their experiences. APN students should reflect on their previous educational experiences, identifying and evaluating effective and ineffective coaching. Bringing these educational moments to full consciousness and naming them is a key first step to envisioning coaching processes that students will want to emulate or discard.

Strategies for Developing Coaching Competence

Coaching activities can be conceptualized along two dimensions: the degree of structure and the focus. Activities may be very structured (e.g., a lecture) or unstructured (e.g., storytelling). The focus of the APN's coaching may be individuals or groups. Table 6-5 organizes teaching activities and strategies along these dimensions. These strategies can be used to foster the development of coaching processes and can also be used to evaluate the APN's competence in coaching.

Less traditional teaching strategies must be used if the advanced practice nursing student's interpersonal repertoire and self-reflective abilities are to be enlarged. Expressive writing (Fulwiler, 1987; Sorrell, 1994; Van Manen, 1989) enables the student to recapture important experiences in nursing and reflect on them to arrive at new insights and interpretations. Keeping a journal, storytelling, and writing poetry are other examples.

TABLE 6-5	EDUCATIONAL STRATEGIES TO DEVELOP THE COACHING SKILLS OF THE ADVANCED PRACTICE NURSE

INDIVIDUAL	GROUP
	UNSTRUCTURED
Coaching	Discussion group
Debriefing	Grand rounds
Discovery	Online chat rooms, LISTSERV discussions
Experiential learning	Online communication
Expressive writing (e.g., poetry)	Storytelling
Use of humor	Support groups
Individual clinical supervision	Use of movies/media with a health-care theme
Journal keeping	Walking rounds
Mentoring	
Peer coaching	
Reading about others' health-care experiences	
Support for risk taking	
	STRUCTURED
Chart review	Classroom-as-clinic (videotapes)
Critical incidents/exemplars	Continuing education programs
Demonstrations	Group patient education
Clear, immediate feedback on strengths *and* areas for growth	In-services
Competency-based instruction	Lecture
Computer-assisted learning	Orientation
Individualized media (e.g., patient education booklets and self-study programs)	Staff development
Intervention mapping	Standardized curricula
Objective tests	Standardized patient teaching plans
Practice laboratories	Virtual courses
Precepting	Teaching undergraduate students
Self-learning modules	Interdisciplinary team meetings

I included journal writing as a teaching strategy in courses on role development. The journals were not graded. Through the students' writings and the instructor's responses, salient experiences were debriefed, a process described by Davies (1995). Sometimes debriefing consisted of the instructor's written response to the student's reflections. Other times, with the student's permission, the journal entries became the focus of a seminar discussion. Students' reflections on the experience of being new or uncertain of their skills led to discussions of developmental tasks such as embracing novicehood or learning to trust one's hands, heart, gut, and observations. Storytelling is another expressive strategy in which stories, the products of reflection, are relayed orally (Mattingly, 1998). Storytelling can build community and mutual respect among nurses (Lindesmith & McWeeny, 1994). Sharing stories from practice enables advanced practice nursing students to establish a shared history and provides a means of offering and receiving support. The process promotes critical thinking, strengthens collegiality, and builds self-esteem and rapport (Lindesmith & McWeeny, 1994). Through journals and storytelling, cues and strategies for coaching used by different advanced practice nursing students and preceptors became available to a larger group of learners.

Aesthetic approaches to developing interpersonal competence can also enhance APNs' coaching skills. The intense insights that can come from reading poetry and literature or watching a movie are often unexplored ways of knowing. Some of the most profound aesthetic experiences in which nurses are involved can never be known through scientific and transactional writing because of the limitations of these styles of writing. The acutely personal, reflective nature of poetry especially captures for nurses the person-oriented stance of interpersonal interaction that is required in APN coaching. Poetry and literature have been potent triggers for reflective practice. Spross et al. (2000) related that when Clarke was a graduate student, an instructor invited students to bring a short piece of prose, a poem, or a song that was meaningful to them. When she volunteered to share the piece with the class, the teacher provided coaching in the process of delivering the piece effectively by focusing and calming the student, demonstrating the process, standing close to the student, and offering encouragement. Similarly, movies with plots involving illness or disability, such as *Heartsounds, Passion Fish, Marvin's Room,* and *Regarding Henry,* can help students assess needs for coaching, evaluate clinicians' ineffective and effective interpersonal styles, and articulate the gaps in care that might require advanced practice nursing intervention.

Faculty should examine the curriculum for opportunities to incorporate aesthetic educational approaches into courses that tend to be structured. One instructor integrated aesthetics into a three-credit graduate course on pathophysiology (Clarke & Spross, 1996). The basic sciences and clinical features of various pathologic conditions were presented to teach students "what disease is." Poetry and literature were used to help students understand the lived experience of illness—"what it is like for a person to have this disease." Patients' stories were integrated with scientific principles in the course activities and take-home tests. These strategies enabled students to acquire a holistic understanding of disease and illness as experienced by patients and families.

Another strategy for developing students' coaching competence is to participate in developing and implementing patient education. For example, a student could initiate or co-lead a self-management group for patients with a chronic condition, an activity that would be informed by the recommendations in the Milbank report (1999) and the RWJ report (2000). Other activities could include developing limited literacy tools or evaluating existing patient education materials with regard to the appropriateness of content and health literacy level (Foltz & Sullivan, 1999; Quirk, 2000; Hahn Winslow, 2001); assessing the cost-effectiveness of a patient education initiative (Welch, Fisher, & Dayhoff,

2002); or evaluating the reliability and appropriateness of health information on the Internet (Clark & Gomez, 2001; Health Summit Working Group, 1999). The Internet is a resource used by many health-care consumers. Students should know the health information resources likely to be used by their patient populations and be able to advise patients on those that are reliable and regularly updated. Students and faculty are urged to consult the paper titled, *Criteria for Assessing the Quality of Health Information on the Internet: Policy Paper, Miritek Systems* (Health Summit Working Group, 1999). In addition, the Health Summit Working Group has an information quality tool that can be used by students to assess the quality of health-care information found on the Internet (1999).

Additional strategies and resources that are available to APNs interested in refining their coaching skills include peer coaching (Aviram, Ophir, Raviv, & Shiloah, 1998; Robbins, 1991), thinking aloud (Corcoran & Moreland, 1988), teaching diagnostic reasoning with the classroom-as-clinic approach (Neistadt & Smith, 1996), and mentoring (Daloz, 1986).

PATIENT EDUCATION AND COACHING: SELECTED ISSUES

Contemporary Health Care

Numerous factors in contemporary health care have increased the focus on patient education as a means of improving effectiveness and efficiency and achieving cost and quality outcomes. The Joint Commission on Accreditation of Healthcare Organizations (JCAHO) (1997) mandates that patient education be given so that the patient can understand the information. Other factors include cost containment initiatives (Cook, 1997; Spross & Heaney, 2000; Taylor et al., 1997; Barger, 1997; Bauer, 1994; Smith, 1989; Weiss, 1998); the evidence-based practice movement (Bero et al., 1998; Porter et al., 1997; Spross & Heaney, 2000; University of York NHS Centre for Reviews and Dissemination, 1999); the educational needs of informal caregivers (Kirk & Glendinning, 1998); and the widespread use of the Internet for teaching and learning. The emphasis in health-care networks on risk reduction (Harris, 1997), disease management (Weiss, 1998; see Chapter 18), and implementation of evidence-based practices (Chapters 8 and 25) requires that nurses establish partnerships with patients so that nurses can coach patients in self-care and tailor interventions to the needs of patients and the situational context. However, insurers' willingness to pay for programs that teach self-management of chronic conditions may be limited because turnover among plan members may limit the return on investment (Milbank report, 1999).

Policy Initiatives Aimed at Helping Patients Manage Chronic Illness

As the incidence of chronic conditions such as asthma and diabetes has increased, various government and philanthropic agencies have begun to examine strategies that can assist in preventing illness or medication-related complications and in improving quality of life for consumers while reducing use of health-care resources and costs. National organizations such as the JCAHO (1997), the National Council on Patient Information and Education (NCPIE) (2003), and the Agency for Healthcare Research and Quality (AHRQ) have initiatives aimed at promoting patient safety and reducing medical errors. Consumer involvement in preventing errors is one strategy that is being used. For example, through collaboration between the National Council on Patient Information and Education (2003) and the Agency for Healthcare Research and Quality, a brochure titled, "Your Medicine: Play it Safe" is being distributed (www.ahrq.gov/news/press/pr2003/safemedpr.htm). This brochure advises patients to discuss both prescription and over-the-counter medications with their health-care providers.

APNs involved in helping patients manage chronic illness, particularly APNs involved in programs to promote self-care, are encouraged to become familiar with the three reports briefly described here. Evidence that better self-management of chronic conditions reduces morbidity and mortality rates and health-care resource use and improves health outcomes such as functional ability, quality of life, and productivity is presented in the Milbank report (1999). Despite the evidence that patients can collaborate effectively with providers to manage chronic conditions, insurers and health-care organizations have been slow to adopt programs to improve self-management of chronic disease because of cost disincentives. Only recently have health-care purchasers begun to recognize the benefits of investing in programs that foster self-management of chronic conditions. The authors of the Milbank report recommended that standards to accredit self-management programs be adopted so that purchasers will include self-management programs as a covered benefit. A similar report has been published by the Department of Health of the United Kingdom (2001). Although the report from the United Kingdom is based on the same evidence as the Milbank report (1999), it places more emphasis on patient-centeredness, types of self-management programs, and the need to ensure that health-care providers are trained in the importance of self-management of chronic illness. Finally, the RWJ report was prepared by a panel of expert clinicians, patient advocates, and researchers who were convened to "identify a range of strategies and tactics to help individuals with chronic conditions become more active participants in their health and health care" (2000, p. 1). In addition to recommendations for research to understand and foster what the panel called "consumer activation," other recommendations that are relevant to teaching and coaching individual patients and developing education and support groups for patients with chronic conditions were identified.

Research Utilization and Research

Chapter 5 addresses the role of APNs in applying middle-range theories to practice, highlighting theories APNs are likely to use. Middle-range theories that have informed health education and counseling interventions for many clinical populations include self-efficacy (Bandura, 1977; Clark & Dodge, 1999; Lev, 1997), the Transtheoretical Model of Behavior Change (Prochaska, Norcross, & DiClemente, 1994), and the Health Belief Model (Becker, 1974; see Chapter 18). Given the importance of behavior change to improving health and coping with illness, applying these theories to better understand the expert coaching and guidance competency could yield important insights from both a nursing perspective and an interdisciplinary perspective.

One of the problems in discerning the impact of APN education on patient care is the inconsistency with which the nurse or APN "dose" of the intervention is described (Brooten et al., 2003). In updating the literature review for this chapter, it was difficult to ascertain the characteristics of the nurse delivering the intervention. Of the dozen review articles or studies in which teaching and coaching interventions were examined (Brooten et al., 1994; Carrieri-Kohlman, Gormley, Douglas, Paul, & Stulbarg, 1996; Eller, 1999; Forshee et al.,

1998; George et al., 1999; McDougall, 1999; Naylor et al., 1999; Pettersson, Gardulf, Nordstrom, Svanberg-Johnsson, & Bylin, 1999; Ryan, 1999; Schwartz-Barcott et al., 1994; Taylor et al., 1997; Wilkie, Williams, Grevstad, & Mekwa, 1995), only those by Brooten et al. (1994), George et al. (1999), Naylor et al. (1999), and Taylor et al. (1997) specified that the nurse was an APN. APNs who participate in the design and execution of such studies should ensure that the characteristics of the clinicians delivering the interventions are included in descriptions of intervention protocols and, when appropriate, that analyses account for clinician characteristics when the interventions are evaluated. Such analyses are important for determining the most efficacious and cost-effective approaches to patient education and coaching. If patient education is effective and if efficient patient education is one of the means of reducing the costs of health care, better understanding of the teaching/coaching processes used by APNs and how they promote adherence to therapies and self-care is needed.

Health Literacy

An important consideration in implementing the APN coaching and guidance competency is the extent of health illiteracy in the United States. Literacy is defined as "an individual's ability to read, write, and speak in English, and compute and solve problems at levels of proficiency necessary to function on the job and in society, to achieve one's goals, and develop one's knowledge and potential" (1991 National Literacy Act passed by the U. S. Congress and cited in Ad Hoc Committee on Health Literacy for the Council on Scientific Affairs, American Medical Association, 1999, p. 552). The National Adult Literacy Survey revealed that nearly one quarter of the U.S. population (40 to 44 million people) is functionally illiterate. The large number of individuals with marginal literacy skills (about 50 million) means that almost one half of adults in this country have reading and computational skills that are inadequate to meet the demands of daily life (Kirsch, Jungeblut, Jenkins, & Kolstad, 1993). To further understand health literacy, investigators studied 3,260 Medicare enrollees older than 65 years to assess functional health literacy (Gazmararian et al., 1999). They found that one third of English-speaking subjects (n = 2,956) and more than one half of Spanish-speaking subjects (n = 304) had inadequate or marginal health literacy. Reading ability declined with age, even when results were adjusted for variables such as cognitive impairment and years of school completed.

Assessment of functional health literacy must be done sensitively. Years of education completed may not be an adequate indicator of reading and computational literacy (Davis, Michielutte, Askov, Williams, & Weiss, 1998). In addition, people with higher levels of education who experience a new diagnosis or other stresses may be unable to process complex information and consequently may benefit from use of limited literacy materials (Foltz & Sullivan, 1999). A variety of tools are available to assist clinicians in assessing patient literacy (Davis et al., 1998; Quirk, 2000). APNs involved in developing programmatic approaches to patient education must ascertain that materials are appropriate to the literacy level of participants in educational programs. A variety of Internet resources on health literacy exist including *Harvard School of Public Health, Health Literacy Studies* (www.hsph.harvard.edu/healthliteracy/), *National Networks of Libraries of Medicine* (www.nnlm.gov/scr/conhlth/hlthlit.htm), and *Eastern LINCS Health and Literacy Home* (www.worlded.org/us/health/lincs/links.htm#hl). The Harvard School of Public Health site is particularly useful: it includes slides documenting the problem of health literacy and its effects on health, as well as links to numerous resources. As APNs work to improve the quality of educational materials for patients with limited literacy, they may encounter resistance to simplifying language and educational tools (Root & Stableford, 1999); therefore slides and other resources that document the extent and impact of health illiteracy may be useful.

Selected Literature Review on Patient Education

Redman (1988) described patient education as a complex set of interactions that include a diversity of subtasks and approaches. What and how to teach patients and how to help them cope with or master their health concerns have long been concerns of nurses in basic and advanced practice (Redman, 1997; Sparks, 1995; Walsh & Bernhard, 1998). Studies on patient education were among the earliest types of clinical research performed by nurses. Much of what is considered standard practice in nursing, such as preparing patients for procedures and surgery by providing sensory, procedural, and other information, is based on a program of research initiated by Johnson and colleagues (Johnson, Rice, Fuller, & Endress, 1978; Leventhal & Johnson, 1983) and replicated and extended by subsequent investigators (Hathaway, 1986).

Sufficient research on patient education has been done to indicate that teaching influences outcomes. In an integrative review of research on patient education, Lindemann (1988) found that most teaching strategies are effective. Although this may be an artifact of various research designs, it may also underscore the strength of patient education as an intervention. A meta-analysis of patient teaching strategies revealed that nine strategies had small to moderate effect sizes (Theis & Johnson, 1995). The largest effect sizes were associated with structured approaches, reinforcement, independent study, and multiple strategies. Regardless of a strategy's effect size, all subjects in experimental groups had better outcomes than did those in control groups. In a meta-analysis of 84 experimental studies, Heater, Becker, and Olson (1988) evaluated the effectiveness of patient education for 4,000 subjects, including neonates, preterm infants, preschool children, grade school children, adolescents, new parents, parents and infants, adults, and the elderly. They concluded that the average subject in an experimental group had a better outcome than did 72% of the subjects in comparison groups. Improved outcomes occurred in the cognitive (knowledge), behavioral, physiological, and psychosocial areas. A literature search for this edition with the key words *patient education* and *advanced practice nurses* and specific advanced practice roles did not identify more recent meta-analyses. However, an integrative review of patient and clinician education interventions to improve cancer pain management suggested that of all the types of interventions reviewed, nurse counseling interventions aimed at patients seem more likely to affect pain-related outcomes and are seen as a promising area for further research (Allard, Maunsell, Labbe, & Dorval, 2001).

Studies of telephone nursing interventions are promising, demonstrating beneficial effects on pain management (Ahles et al., 2001) and depression (Hunkeler et al., 2000). An integrative review of 74 randomized, controlled trials of telephone-delivered interventions (TDIs) indicated that TDIs have been used to broaden the reach of health-care interventions, promote health behavior change, and increase the efficacy of health-care services delivery (McBride & Rimer, 1999). In 27 studies, nurses delivered interventions; of these,

TABLE 6-6	TYPES OF TELEPHONE-DELIVERED INTERVENTIONS	
GOAL	PURPOSES	TYPES OF TDIs
Reaching the underserved	• Smoking cessation • Pain management • Treatment adherence	• Hotline • Helpline • Callbacks • Counseling
Sustaining health behavior changes in populations with addictions or chronic diseases or in groups at risk for health problems	• Smoking cessation • Relapse prevention • Complication prevention (e.g., patients with diabetes, patients with asthma) • Cancer screening • Appropriate use of services	• Helpline • Counseling • Booster calls (reminders, encouragement)
Increasing the effectiveness of health-care services	• Decrease system burdens • Decrease patient burdens • Increase/improve outpatient support for those with health problems • Improve treatment/medication adherence (e.g., patients with hypertension, elderly patients)	• Callbacks • Helpline

TDIs, Telephone-delivered interventions.

in only three could interventions be clearly identified as having been delivered by APNs. Table 6-6 lists the areas in which TDIs have been associated with improvements in patient outcomes and better use of health-care services. This review article should be of interest to APNs who wish to understand the ways in which TDIs have been used effectively and who want to incorporate systematic use of TDIs in clinical programs. The review concluded with some of the unanswered questions about TDIs. These questions could be modified to guide research regarding the use of the Internet for patient education.

CONCLUSION

APNs coach patients through transitions. In the APN, graduate education and technical, clinical, and interpersonal competence interact with self-reflection to produce a diverse set of coaching skills and the ability to invent new coaching processes during novel clinical encounters. Coaching is an extremely complex skill that depends on APNs' personal and professional qualities. Although coaching processes occur simultaneously, they are not automatic. APNs can usually describe the intent of coaching interventions and explain their selection of one approach over another. What may seem automatic is actually very deliberate: the APN has learned what has worked in similar encounters and uses it over and over. In using a person-centered style with a patient, the APN remains open to cues that the approach may not work in this particular encounter, thereby remaining flexible and aware of alternatives. An observer seeing the APN in action may think these processes are automatic because of how natural they seem. That such interactions appear to occur naturally arises from the APN's mindfulness of the encounter and the patient's and the APN's own responses.

In many arts and sports, coaches no longer perform the skill they coach and yet are still able to coach effectively. The nature of the health-care environment and the delivery of clinical services are dynamic and complex. A nurse's coaching expertise can still develop when the nurse's primary responsibility shifts from direct care to another area within nursing, such as teaching or administration. However, the coaching processes that are developed will be related to the learners—students or staff. The ability to coach patients depends on direct care experiences in which new human responses, possibilities for growth, and new coaching strategies are revealed through APNs' encounters with patients and families as they experience health and illness and new technologies and therapies. There is evidence that nursing care, whether provided by staff nurses or APNs, has salutary effects on patient outcomes. The challenge for APNs is to determine the most efficient and effective means of adopting these best practices related to patient education and coaching that will enable patients and their families to cope with transitions and improve health and health-related quality of life.

REFERENCES

Ad Hoc Committee on Health Literacy for the Council on Scientific Affairs, American Medical Association. (1999). Health literacy: Report of the Council on Scientific Affairs. *JAMA: The Journal of the American Medical Association, 281,* 552-557.

Ahles, T., Seville, J., Wasson, J., Johnson, D., Callahan, E., & Stukel, T. (2001). Panel-based pain management in primary care: A pilot study. *Journal of Pain and Symptom Management, 22,* 584-590.

Allard, P., Maunsell, E., Labbe, J., & Dorval, M. (2001). Educational interventions to improve cancer pain control: A systematic review. *Journal of Palliative Medicine, 4,* 191-203.

Alonzo, A. (2000). The experience of chronic illness and post-traumatic stress disorder: The consequences of cumulative adversity. *Social Science & Medicine, 50,* 1475-1484.

Atkins, S., & Murphy, K. (1994). Reflective practice. *Nursing Standard, 8,* 49-54.

Aviram, M., Ophir, R., Raviv, D., & Shiloah, M. (1998). Experiential learning of clinical skills by beginning nursing students: "Coaching" project by fourth-year student interns. *Journal of Nursing Education, 37,* 228-231.

Bandura, A. (1977). Self-efficacy: Toward a unifying theory of behavioral change. *Psychological Review, 84,* 191-215.

Barger, S. (1997). Building healthier communities in a managed care environment: Opportunities for advanced practice nurses. *Advanced Practice Nursing Quarterly, 2,* 9-14.

Barnsteiner, J. H., Gillis-Donovan, J., Knox-Fischer, C., & McKlindon, D. D. (1994). Defining and implementing a standard for therapeutic relationships. *Journal of Holistic Nursing, 12,* 35-49.

Bartels, J. E. (1998). Developing reflective learners—student self-assessment as learning. *Journal of Professional Nursing, 14,* 135.

Bartholomew, L. K., Parcel, G. S., & Kok, G. (1998). Intervention mapping: A process for developing theory- and evidence-based health education programs. *Health Education & Behavior: The Official Publication of the Society for Public Health Education, 25,* 545-563.

Bauer, J. (1994). *Not what the doctor ordered: Reinventing medical care in America.* Chicago: Probus.

Becker, M. (1974). *The health belief model and personal health behavior.* Thorofare, NJ: Charles B. Slack.

Benner, P. (1984). *From novice to expert: Excellence and power in clinical nursing practice.* Menlo Park, CA: Addison-Wesley.

Benner, P. (1985). The oncology clinical nurse specialist as expert coach. *Oncology Nursing Forum, 12,* 40-44.

Benner, P. (1991). The role of experience, narrative, and community in skilled ethical comportment. *Advances in Nursing Science, 14,* 1-21.

Benner, P., Hooper-Kyriakidis, P., & Stannard, D. (1999). *Clinical wisdom and interventions in critical care: A thinking-in-action approach.* Philadelphia: W. B. Saunders.

Bernstein, B. (1974). *Class, codes, and control: Theoretical studies towards a sociology of language.* New York: Schocken Books.

Bero, L., Grilli, R., Grimshaw, I. M., Harvey, E., Oxman, A. D., & Thomson, M. A. (1998). Closing the gap between research and practice: An overview of systematic reviews of interventions to promote the implementation of research findings. *BMJ, 317,* 465-468.

Braden, C. (1990). Learned self-help response to chronic illness experience: A test of three alternative learning theories. *Scholarly Inquiry for Nursing Practice, 4,* 23-41.

Braden, C. (1993). Research program on learned response to chronic illness experience: Self-help model. *Holistic Nursing Practice, 8,* 38-44.

Bridges, W. (1980). *Transitions: Making sense of life's changes.* Reading, MA: Addison-Wesley.

Brooten, D., Brown, L., Hazard Munro, B., York, R., Cohen, S., Roncoli, M., et al. (1988). Early discharge and specialist transitional care. *Image: The Journal of Nursing Scholarship, 20,* 64-68.

Brooten, D., Gennaro, S., Knapp, H., Jovene, N., Brown, L., & York, R. (1991). Functions of the CNS in early discharge and home follow-up of very low birthweight infants. *Clinical Nurse Specialist, 5,* 196-201.

Brooten, D., Kumar, S., Brown, L., Butts, P., Finkler, S., Bakewell-Sachs, S., et al. (1986). A randomized clinical trial of early hospital discharge and home follow-up of very low birthweight infants. *New England Journal of Medicine, 315,* 934-939.

Brooten, D., Roncoli, M., Finkler, S., Arnold, L., Cohen, A., & Mennutti, M. (1994). A randomized clinical trial of hospital discharge and nurse specialist home follow-up of women with unplanned cesarean birth. *Obstetrics and Gynecology, 84,* 832-838.

Brooten, D., Youngblut, J., Deatrick, J., Naylor, M., & York, R. (2003). Patient problems, advanced practice nurse (APN) interventions, time and contacts among five patient groups. *Journal of Nursing Scholarship, 35,* 73-79.

Brown, M., & Waybrant, K. (1988). Health promotion, education, counseling, and coordination in primary health care nursing. *Public Health Nursing, 5,* 16-23.

Brown, S. J. (1995). An interviewing style for nursing assessment. *Journal of Advanced Nursing, 21,* 340-343.

Brown, S. J. (1999). Patient-centered communication. *Annual Review of Nursing Research, 17,* 85-104.

Capasso, V. (1998). The theory is the practice: An exemplar. *Clinical Nurse Specialist, 12,* 226-229.

Carrieri-Kohlman, V., Gormley, J. M., Douglas, M. K., Paul, S. M., & Stulbarg, M. S. (1996). Exercise training decreases dyspnea and the distress and anxiety associated with it: Monitoring alone may be as effective as coaching. *Chest, 110,* 1526-1535.

Chick, N., & Meleis, A. (1986). Transitions: A nursing concern. In P. Chinn (Ed.), *Nursing research methodology: Issues and implementation* (pp. 237-258). Rockville, MD: Aspen.

Chopoorian, T. (1986). Reconceptualizing the environment. In P. Moccia (Ed.), *New approaches to theory development.* New York: National League for Nursing.

Clark, N. M., & Dodge, J. A. (1999). Exploring self-efficacy as a predictor of disease management. *Health Education & Behavior: The Official Publication of the Society for Public Health Education, 26,* 72-89.

Clark, P., & Gomez, E. (2001). Details on demand: Consumers, cancer information, and the Internet. *Clinical Journal of Oncology Nursing, 5,* 19-24.

Clarke, E. B., & Spross, J. A. (1996). Expert coaching and guidance. In A. B. Hamric, J. A. Spross, & C. M. Hanson (Eds.), *Advanced practice nursing: An integrative approach* (pp. 139-164). Philadelphia: W. B. Saunders.

Connelly, C. (1993). An empirical model of self-care in chronic illness. *Clinical Nurse Specialist, 7,* 247-253.

Cook, S. S. (1997). Configuring childbirth education to survive in managed care. *Advanced Practice Nursing Quarterly, 2,* 22-26.

Corbin, J., & Strauss, A. (1992). A nursing model for chronic illness management based upon the trajectory framework. In P. Woog (Ed.), *The chronic illness trajectory framework: The Corbin and Strauss model* (pp. 9-28). New York: Springer-Verlag.

Corcoran, S., & Moreland, H. (1988). "Thinking aloud" as a strategy to improve clinical decision making. *Heart & Lung: The Journal of Critical Care, 17,* 463-468.

Crowther, M. (2003). Optimal management of outpatients with heart failure using advanced practice nurses in a hospital-based heart failure center. *Journal of the American Academy of Nurse Practitioners, 15,* 260-265.

Daloz, L. (1986). *Effective teaching and mentoring: Realizing the transformational power of adult learning experiences.* San Francisco: Jossey-Bass.

Davies, E. (1995). Reflective practice: A focus for caring. *Journal of Nursing Education, 34,* 167-174.

Davis, M., Sawin, K., & Dunn, M. (1993). Teaching strategies used by expert nurse practitioner preceptors: A qualitative study. *Journal of the American Academy of Nurse Practitioners, 5,* 27-33.

Davis, T. C., Michielutte, R., Askov, E. N., Williams, M. V., & Weiss, B. D. (1998). Practical assessment of adult literacy in health care. *Health Education & Behavior: The Official Publication of the Society for Public Health Education, 25,* 613-624.

de La Cuesta, C. (1994). Relationships in health visiting: Enabling and mediating. *International Journal of Nursing Studies, 31,* 451-459.

Department of Health, United Kingdom. (2001). *The expert patient: A new approach to chronic disease management for the 21st century.* Retrieved November 1, 2003, from United Kingdom, National Health Service, Department of Health Web site: http://www.doh.gov.uk/healthinequalities/ep_report.pdf

Diemert Moch, S. (1990). Personal knowing: Evolving research and practice. *Scholarly Inquiry for Nursing Practice, 4,* 155-170.

Draye, M., & Pesznecker, B. (1980). Teaching activities of nurse practitioners. *Nurse Practitioner, 5,* 28-33.

Eller, L. S. (1999). Effects of cognitive-behavioral interventions on quality of life in persons with HIV. *International Journal of Nursing Studies, 36,* 223-233.

Felitti, V. (2002). The relationship between adverse childhood experiences and adult health: Turning gold into lead. *The Permanente Journal, 6*, 1-7.

Felitti, V., Anda, R., Nordenberg, D., Williamson, D., Spitz, A., Edwards, V., et al. (1998). Relationship of childhood abuse and household dysfunction to many of the leading causes of death in adults. The Adverse Childhood Experiences (ACE) Study. *American Journal of Preventive Medicine, 14*, 245-258.

Fenton, M. (1984). Identification of the skilled performance of master's prepared nurses as a method of curriculum planning and evaluation. In P. Benner (Ed.), *From novice to expert* (pp. 262-274). Menlo Park, CA: Addison-Wesley.

Fenton, M., & Brykczynski, K. (1993). Qualitative distinctions and similarities in the practice of clinical nurse specialists and nurse practitioners. *Journal of Professional Nursing, 9*, 313-326.

Foltz, A., & Sullivan, J. (1999). Limited literacy revisited. *Cancer Practice, 7*, 145-150.

Forshee, J. D., Whalen, E. B., Hackel, R., Butt, L. T., Smeltzer, P. A., Martin, J., et al. (1998). The effectiveness of one-on-one nurse education on the outcomes of high-risk adult and pediatric patients with asthma. *Managed Care Interface, 11*, 82-92.

Freire, P. (1970). *Pedagogy of the oppressed.* New York: Continuum.

Frisch, M., Elliott, C., Atsaides, J., Salva, D., & Denney, D. (1982). Social skills and stress management training to enhance patients' interpersonal competencies. *Psychotherapy Theory, Research and Practice, 19*, 349-358.

Fulwiler, T. (1987). *Teaching with writing.* Upper Montclair, NJ: Boynton/Cook.

Gadow, S. (1980). Existential advocacy: Philosophical foundations of nursing. In S. Spicker & S. Gadow (Eds.), *Nursing: Images and ideas* (pp. 79-101). New York: Springer-Verlag.

Gazmararian, J. A., Baker, D. W., Williams, M. V., Parker, R. M., Scott, T. L., Green, D. C., et al. (1999). Health literacy among Medicare enrollees in a managed care organization. *JAMA: The Journal of the American Medical Association, 281*, 545-551.

George, M. R., O'Dowd, L. C., Martin, I., Lindell, K. O., Whitney, F., Jones, M., et al. (1999). A comprehensive educational program improves clinical outcome measures in inner-city patients with asthma. *Archives of Internal Medicine, 159*, 1710-1716.

Grimmett, P. (1988). The nature of reflection and Schön's conception in perspective. In P. Grimmett & G. Erickson (Eds.), *Reflection in teacher education* (pp. 5-15). New York: Teacher's College Press.

Hagedorn, S. (1995). The politics of caring: The role of activism in primary care. *Advances in Nursing Science, 17*, 1-11.

Harris, M. (1997). Reduced risk of complex response: An invisible outcome. *Nursing Administration Quarterly, 21*, 25-31.

Hathaway, D. (1986). Effect of preoperative instruction on postoperative outcomes: A meta-analysis. *Nursing Research, 35*, 269-275.

Health Summit Working Group. (1999). Criteria for assessing the quality of health information on the Internet: Policy Paper, Mitretek Systems. Retrieved November 2, 2003, from http://hiti web.mitretek.org/docs/policy.html

Heater, B., Becker, A., & Olson, R. (1988). Nursing interventions and patient outcomes: A meta-analysis of studies. *Nursing Research, 37*, 303-307.

Heifetz, R. (1994). *Leadership without easy answers.* Cambridge, MA: Belknap Press.

Hops, H. (1983). Children's social competence and skill: Current research, practices, and future directions. *Behavioral Therapy, 14*, 3-18.

Hunkeler, E., Meresman, J., Jargreaves, W., Fireman, B., Berman, W., Kirsch, A., et al. (2000). Efficacy of nurse telehealth care and peer support in augmenting treatment of depression in primary care. *Archives of Family Medicine, 9*, 700-708.

Jackson, P. (1986). *The practice of teaching.* New York: Teacher's College Press.

Jenny, J., & Logan, J. (1992). Knowing the patient: One aspect of clinical knowledge. *Image: The Journal of Nursing Scholarship, 24*, 254-258.

Johnson, J., Rice, V., Fuller, S., & Endress, M. (1978). Sensory information, instruction in a coping strategy, and recovery from surgery. *Research in Nursing and Health, 1*, 4-17.

Joint Commission on Accreditation of Healthcare Organizations. (1997). *Accreditation manual for hospitals.* Oakbrook Terrace, IL: Author.

Kasch, C. (1983). Interpersonal competence and communication in the delivery of nursing care. *Advances in Nursing Science, 5*, 71-88.

Kasch, C., & Dine, J. (1988). Person-centered communication and social perspective taking. *Western Journal of Nursing Research, 10*, 317-326.

Kasch, C., & Knutson, K. (1985). Patient compliance and interpersonal style: Implications for practice and research. *Nurse Practitioner, 10*, 52-64.

Kasch, C., & Lisnek, P. (1984). Role of strategic communication in nursing theory and research. *Advances in Nursing Science, 6*, 56-71.

Kendall, J. (1992). Fighting back: Promoting emancipatory nursing actions. *Advances in Nursing Science, 15*, 1-15.

Kirk, S., & Glendinning, C. (1998). Trends in community care and patient participation: Implications for the roles of informal carers and community nurses in the United Kingdom. *Journal of Advanced Nursing, 28*, 370-381.

Kirsch, I., Jungeblut, A., Jenkins, L., & Kolstad, A. (1993). *Adult literacy in America: A first look at the findings of the National Adult Literacy Survey.* Washington, DC: U.S. Department of Education, National Center for Education Statistics.

Koetters, T. L. (1989). Clinical practice and direct patient care. In A. B. Hamric & J. A. Spross (Eds.),

The clinical nurse specialist in theory and practice (2nd ed., pp. 107-124). Philadelphia: W. B. Saunders.

Kolcaba, K. (1992). Holistic comfort: Operationalizing the construct as a nurse-sensitive outcome. *Advances in Nursing Science, 15*, 1-10.

Lamb, G., & Stempel, J. (1994). Nurse case management from the client's view: Growing as insider-expert. *Nursing Outlook, 42*, 7-13.

Lamm, B., Dungan, J., & Hiromoto, B. (1991). Long-term lifestyle management. *Clinical Nurse Specialist, 5*, 182-188.

Lang, N., & Marek, K. (1992). Outcomes that reflect clinical practice. In *Patient outcomes research: Examining the effectiveness of nursing practice* (NIH Publication No. 93-3411, pp. 27-38). Washington, DC: Department of Health and Human Services.

Larson, L., Neverett, S., & Larsen, R. (2001). Clinical nurse specialist as facilitator of interdisciplinary collaborative program for adult sickle cell population. *Clinical Nurse Specialist, 15*, 15-22.

Lev, E. (1997). Bandura's theory of self-efficacy: Applications to oncology. *Scholarly Inquiry for Nursing Practice, 11*, 21-37.

Leventhal, H., & Johnson, J. (1983). Laboratory and field experimentation: Development of a theory of self-regulation. In P. Woolridge, M. Schmitt, J. Skipper, & P. Leonard (Eds.), *Behavioral science and nursing theory* (pp. 189-262). St. Louis, MO: C. V. Mosby.

Lewis, F. M., & Zahlis, E. (1997). The nurse as coach: A conceptual framework for clinical practice. *Oncology Nursing Forum, 24*, 1695-1702.

Lindemann, C. (1988). Nursing research in patient education. *Annual Review of Nursing Research, 6*, 29-60.

Lindesmith, K., & McWeeny, M. (1994). The power of storytelling. *Journal of Continuing Education in Nursing, 25*, 186-187.

Lombardo, B. (1987). *The humanistic coach: From theory to practice*. Springfield, IL: Charles C Thomas.

Martocchio, B. (1987). Authenticity, belonging, emotional closeness, and self representation. *Oncology Nursing Forum, 14*, 23-27.

Mattingly, C. (1998). Healing dramas and clinical plots: The narrative structure of experience. Cambridge, United Kingdom: Cambridge University Press.

McBride, C. M., & Rimer, B. K. (1999). Using the telephone to improve health behavior and health service delivery. *Patient Education and Counseling, 37*, 3-18.

McDougall, G. J., Jr., (1999). Cognitive interventions among older adults. *Annual Review of Nursing Research, 17*, 219-240.

McKinnon, A., & Erickson, G. (1988). Taking Schön's ideas to a science teaching practicum. In P. Grimmett & G. Erickson (Eds.), *Reflection in teacher education* (pp. 113-137). New York: Teacher's College Press.

Meng, A., & Morris, D. (1995). Continuing education for advanced nurse practitioners: Preparing nurse-midwives as clinical preceptors. *Journal of Continuing Education in Nursing, 26*, 180-184.

Mezey, M., Dougherty, M., Wade, P., & Mersmann, C. (1994). Nurse practitioners, certified nurse-midwives, and nurse anesthetists: Changing care in acute care hospitals in New York City. *Journal of the New York State Nurses' Association, 25*, 13-17.

The Milbank Memorial Fund and Center for the Advancement of Health. (1999). *Patients as effective collaborators in managing chronic conditions*. Retrieved November 1, 2003, from The Milbank Memorial Fund Website: http://www.milbank.org/990811chronic.html

Montgomery, C. L. (1993). *Healing through communication*. Newbury Park, CA: Sage.

Morgan, A. (1994). Client education experiences in professional nursing practice—a phenomenological perspective. *Journal of Advanced Nursing, 19*, 792-801.

Morse, J. M., Havens, G. D., & Wilson, S. (1997). The comforting interaction: Developing a model of nurse-patient relationship. *Scholarly Inquiry for Nursing Practice, 11*, 321-343.

National Association of Clinical Nurse Specialists. (1998). *Statement on clinical nurse specialist practice and education*. Harrisburg, PA: Author.

National Association of Clinical Nurse Specialists. (2004). *Statement on clinical nurse specialist practice and education* (2nd ed.) Harrisburg, PA: Author.

National Council on Patient Information and Education. (2003). Your medicine: Play it safe. Retrieved November 2, 2003, from http://www.talkaboutrx.org/playitsafe_bro.pdf

National Organization of Nurse Practitioner Faculties (NONPF), & American Association of Colleges of Nursing (AACN). (2002). *Nurse practitioner primary competencies in specialty areas: Adult, family, gerontological, pediatric, and women's health*. Prepared for the US Department of Health and Human Services, Health Resources and Services Administration, Bureau of Health Professions, Division of Nursing. Retrieved November 2, 2003, from http://www.nonpf.com/finalaug 2002.pdf

National Panel for Psychiatric Mental Health NP Competencies. (2003). *Psychiatric-mental health nurse practitioner competencies*. Retrieved November 2, 2003, from http://www.nonpf.com/finalcomps03.pdf

Naylor, M., Bowles, K., & Brooten, D. (2000). Patient problems and advanced practice nurse interventions during transitional care. *Public Health Nursing, 17*, 94-102.

Naylor, M., Munro, B., & Brooten, D. (1991). Measuring the effectiveness of nursing practice. *Clinical Nurse Specialist, 5*, 210-215.

Naylor, M. D., Brooten, D., Campbell, R., Jacobsen, B. S., Mezey, M. D., Pauly, M. V., et al. (1999). Comprehensive discharge planning and home follow-up of hospitalized elders. *JAMA: The Journal of the American Medical Association, 281*, 613-620.

Neimeyer, R. (2001). Traumatic loss and the reconstruction of meaning. *Innovations in End of Life Care, 3*. Retrieved April 16, 2004, from http://www2.edc.org/lastacts/archives/archives Nov01/editorial.asp

Neistadt, M. E., & Smith, R. E. (1996). Teaching diagnostic reasoning: Using a classroom-as-clinic methodology with videotapes. *American Journal of Occupational Therapy, 51*, 361-368.

O'Connor, N. A., Hameister, A. D., & Kershaw. T. (2000). Developing a database to describe the practice patterns of adult nurse practitioner students. *Journal of Nursing Scholarship, 32*, 57-63.

Olesen, V., Schatzman, L., Droes, N., Hatton, D., & Chico, N. (1990). The mundane ailment and the physical self: Analysis of the social psychology of health and illness. *Social Science and Medicine, 30*, 449-455.

Pelligrini, D., & Urbain, E. (1985). An evaluation of interpersonal cognitive problem solving training with children. *Journal of Psychology and Psychiatry, 26*, 17-41.

Peplau, H. (1952). *Interpersonal relations in nursing: A conceptual frame of reference.* New York: G. P. Putnam.

Peplau, H. (1994). Quality of life: An interpersonal perspective. *Nursing Science Quarterly, 7*, 10-15.

Pettersson, E., Gardulf, A., Nordstrom, G., Svanberg-Johnsson, C., & Bylin, G. (1999). Evaluation of a nurse-run asthma school. *International Journal of Nursing Studies, 36*, 145-151.

Pew-Fetzer Task Force on Advancing Psychosocial Health Education. (1994). *Health professions education and relationship-centered care.* San Francisco: Pew Health Professions Commission.

Porter, C. P., Pender, N. J., Hayman, L. L., Armstrong, M. L., Riesch, S. K., & Lewis, M. A. (1997). Educating APNs for implementing the guidelines for adolescents in Bright Futures: Guidelines of health supervision of infants, children, and adolescents. *Nursing Outlook, 45*, 252-257.

Prochaska, J. O., Norcross, J. C., & DiClemente, C. C. (1994). *Changing for good.* New York: William Morrow.

Pugach, M., & Johnson, L. (1990). Developing reflective practice through structured dialogue. In R. Clift, W. Houston, & M. Pugach (Eds.), *Encouraging reflective practice in teacher education* (pp. 186-207). New York: Teacher's College Press.

Quirk, M., & Casey, L. (1995). Primary care for women: The art of interviewing. *Journal of Nurse-Midwifery, 40*, 97-103.

Quirk, P. (2000). Screening for literacy and readability: Implications for the advanced practice nurse. *Clinical Nurse Specialist, 14*, 26-32.

Radwin, L. E. (1996). "Knowing the patient": A review of research on an emerging concept. *Journal of Advanced Nursing, 23*, 1142-1146.

Redman, B. (1988). *The process of patient education.* St. Louis, MO: Mosby–Year Book.

Redman, B. K. (1997). *The practice of patient education* (8th ed.). St. Louis, MO: Mosby–Year Book, Inc.

Robbins, P. (1991). *How to plan and implement a peer-coaching program.* Alexandria, VA: Association for Supervision and Curriculum Development.

The Robert Wood Johnson Foundation. (2000). *Patient education and consumer activation in chronic disease. Report of the Planning Meeting on Patient Education and Consumer Activation in Chronic Conditions, Princeton, NJ.* Retrieved November 1, 2003, from http://www.rwjf.org/publications/publicationsPdfs/patient_educati

Root, J., & Stableford, S. (1999). Easy-to-read consumer communications: A missing link in Medicaid managed care. *Journal of Health Politics, Policy and Law, 24*, 1-26.

Rudd, R. E. *Literacy and implications for navigating health care.* Retrieved November 2, 2003, from the Harvard School of Public Health, Health Literacy Website. 2002. http://www.hsph.harvard.edu/healthliteracy/slides/2002/2002_01.html

Ryan, A. A. (1999). Medication compliance and older people: A review of the literature. *International Journal of Nursing Studies, 36*, 153-162.

Schön, D. (1983). *The reflective practitioner: How professionals think in action.* New York: Basic Books.

Schön, D. (1987). *Educating the reflective practitioner: Toward a new design for teaching and learning in the professions.* San Francisco: Jossey-Bass.

Schumacher, K., & Meleis, A. (1994). Transitions: A central concept in nursing. *Image: The Journal of Nursing Scholarship, 26*, 119-127.

Schwartz-Barcott, D., Fortin, J., & Kim, H. (1994). Client-nurse interaction: Testing for its impact in preoperative instruction. *International Journal of Nursing Studies, 31*, 23-35.

Scupholme, A., Paine, L., Lang, J., Kumar, S., & DeJoseph, J. (1994). Time associated with components of clinical services rendered by nurse-midwives: Sample data from phase II of nurse-midwifery care to vulnerable populations in the United States. *Journal of Nurse-Midwifery, 39*, 5-12.

Scupholme, A., & Walsh, L. (1994). Home-based services by nurse-midwives: Sample data from phase II of nurse-midwifery care to vulnerable populations in the United States. *Journal of Nurse-Midwifery, 39*, 358-362.

Smith, C. (1989). Overview of patient education: Opportunities and challenges for the twenty-first century. *Nursing Clinics of North America, 24*, 583-587.

Sorrell, J. (1994). Remembrance of things past through writing: Esthetic patterns of knowing in nursing. *Advances in Nursing Science, 17*, 60-70.

Sparks, R. K. (1995). Client education. In M. Snyder & M. P. Mirr (Eds.), *Advanced practice nursing: A guide to professional development* (pp. 117-133). New York: Springer-Verlag.

Spross, J. (1994). *Coaching: An interdisciplinary perspective*. Unpublished manuscript, Doctoral Program in Nursing, Boston College.

Spross, J. (1996). Coaching and suffering: The role of the nurse in helping people face illness. In B. Ferrell (Ed.), *Suffering* (pp. 173-208). Boston: Jones & Bartlett.

Spross, J. A., Clarke, E. B, & Beauregard., J. (2000). Expert coaching and guidance. In A. B. Hamric, J. A. Spross, C. M. Hanson (Eds.), *Advanced nursing practice: An integrative approach* (pp.183-215). Philadelphia: W. B. Saunders.

Spross, J. A., & Heaney, C. A. (2000). Shaping advanced nursing practice roles in the new millennium. *Seminars in Oncology Nursing, 16,* 12-24.

Squier, R. (1990). A model of empathic understanding and adherence to treatment regimens in practitioner-patient relationships. *Social Science and Medicine, 30,* 325-339.

Steele, S., & Fenton, M. (1988). Expert practice of clinical nurse specialists. *Clinical Nurse Specialist, 2,* 45-52.

Steven, P. (1989). A critical social reconstruction of environment in nursing: Implications for methodology. *Advances in Nursing Science, 11,* 55-68.

Sullivan, P., & Wilson, D. (1991). The coach's role. In G. Cohen (Ed.), *Women in sport: Issues and controversies* (pp. 230-237). Newbury Park, CA: Sage.

Tanner, C., Benner, P., Chesla, C., & Gordon, D. (1993). The phenomenology of knowing the patient. *Image: The Journal of Nursing Scholarship, 25,* 273-280.

Taylor, C. A., Resick, L., D'Antonio, J. A., & Carroll, T. L. (1997). The advanced practice nurse role in implementing and evaluating two nurse-managed wellness clinics: Lessons learned about structure, process, and outcomes. *Advanced Practice Nursing Quarterly, 3,* 36-45.

Theis, S., & Johnson, J. (1995). Strategies for teaching patients: A meta-analysis. *Clinical Nurse Specialist, 9,* 100-105, 120.

Travelbee, J. (1971). *Interpersonal aspects of nursing.* Philadelphia: F. A. Davis.

Tremmel, R. (1993). Zen and the art of reflective practice in teacher education. *Harvard Educational Review, 63,* 434-458.

University of York NHS. Centre for Reviews and Dissemination. (1999). Getting evidence into practice. *Effective Health Care, 5,* 1-16. Retrieved September 1, 2003, from http://www.york.ac.uk/inst/crd/ehc51.pdf

Van Manen, M. (1989). By the light of anecdote. *Phenomenological Pedagogy, 7,* 232-253.

Walsh, M., & Bernhard, L. A. (1998). Selected theories and models for advanced practice nursing. In C. M. Sheehy & M. McCarthy (Eds.), *Advanced practice nursing: Emphasizing common roles* (pp. 88-113). Philadelphia: F. A. Davis.

Weiss, M. (1998). Case management as a tool for clinical integration. *Advanced Practice Nursing Quarterly, 4,* 9-15.

Welch, J., Fisher, M., & Dayhoff, N. (2002). A cost-effectiveness worksheet for patient education programs. *Clinical Nurse Specialist, 16,* 187-192.

Wells-Federman, C., Stuart-Shor, E., & Webster, A. (2001). Cognitive therapy: Applications for health promotion, disease prevention, and disease management. *Nursing Clinics of North America, 36,* 93-113.

White, J. (1995). Patterns of knowing: Review, critique, and update. *Advances in Nursing Science, 17,* 73-86.

Wilkie, D. J., Williams, A. R., Grevstad, P., & Mekwa, J. (1995). Coaching persons with lung cancer to report sensory pain: Literature review and pilot study findings. *Cancer Nursing, 18,* 7-15.

Additional Readings

Alexander, J., Younger, R., Cohen, R., & Crawford, L. (1988). Effectiveness of a nurse managed program for children with chronic asthma. *Journal of Pediatric Nursing, 3,* 312-317.

Beheshti, P., & Fonteyn, M. (1988). Role of the advanced practice nurse in continence care in the home. *AACN Clinical Issues, 9,* 389-395.

Brown, S. (1998). A framework for advanced practice nursing. *Journal of Professional Nursing, 14,* 157-164.

Brykczynski, K. (1989). An interpretive study describing the clinical judgment of nurse practitioners. *Scholarly Inquiry for Nursing Practice, 3,* 75-112.

Fenton, M. (1985). Identifying competencies of clinical nurse specialists. *Journal of Nursing Administration, 15,* 31-37.

Hodnett, E. (1999). *Continuity of caregivers for care during pregnancy and childbirth* (Cochrane Review). Retrieved March 7, 2004, from http://www.cochrane.org/cochrane/revabstr/AB000062.htm

Leigh, S. (1998). The long-term cancer survivor: A challenge for nurse practitioners. *Nurse Practitioner Forum, 9,* 192-196.

Lipman, T. (1986). Length of hospitalization of children with diabetes: Effect of a clinical nurse specialist. *Diabetes Educator, 14,* 41-43.

Office of Technology Assessment. (1986). *Nurse practitioners, physician assistants, and certified nurse-midwives: A policy analysis* (Health Technology Case Study 37, No. OTA-HCS-37). Washington, DC: U. S. Congress.

Pozen, M., Stechmiller, J., Harris, W., Smith, S., Fred, D., & Voight, G. (1977). A nurse rehabilitator's impact on patients with myocardial infarction. *Medical Care, 15,* 830-837.

Priest, A. R. (1989). The CNS as educator. In A. B. Hamric & J. A. Spross (Eds.), *The clinical nurse specialist in theory and practice* (2nd ed., pp. 147-168). Philadelphia: W. B. Saunders.

Reiger, P. (1998). Overview of cancer and genetics: Implications for nurse practitioners. *Nurse Practitioner Forum, 9,* 122-133.

Scott, R. A. (1999). A description of the roles, activities, and skills of clinical nurse specialists in the United States. *Clinical Nurse Specialist, 13,* 183-190.

Younger, J. (1995). The alienation of the sufferer. *Advances in Nursing Science, 17,* 53-72.

CHAPTER 7

Consultation

ANNE-MARIE BARRON • PATRICIA A. WHITE

Continued

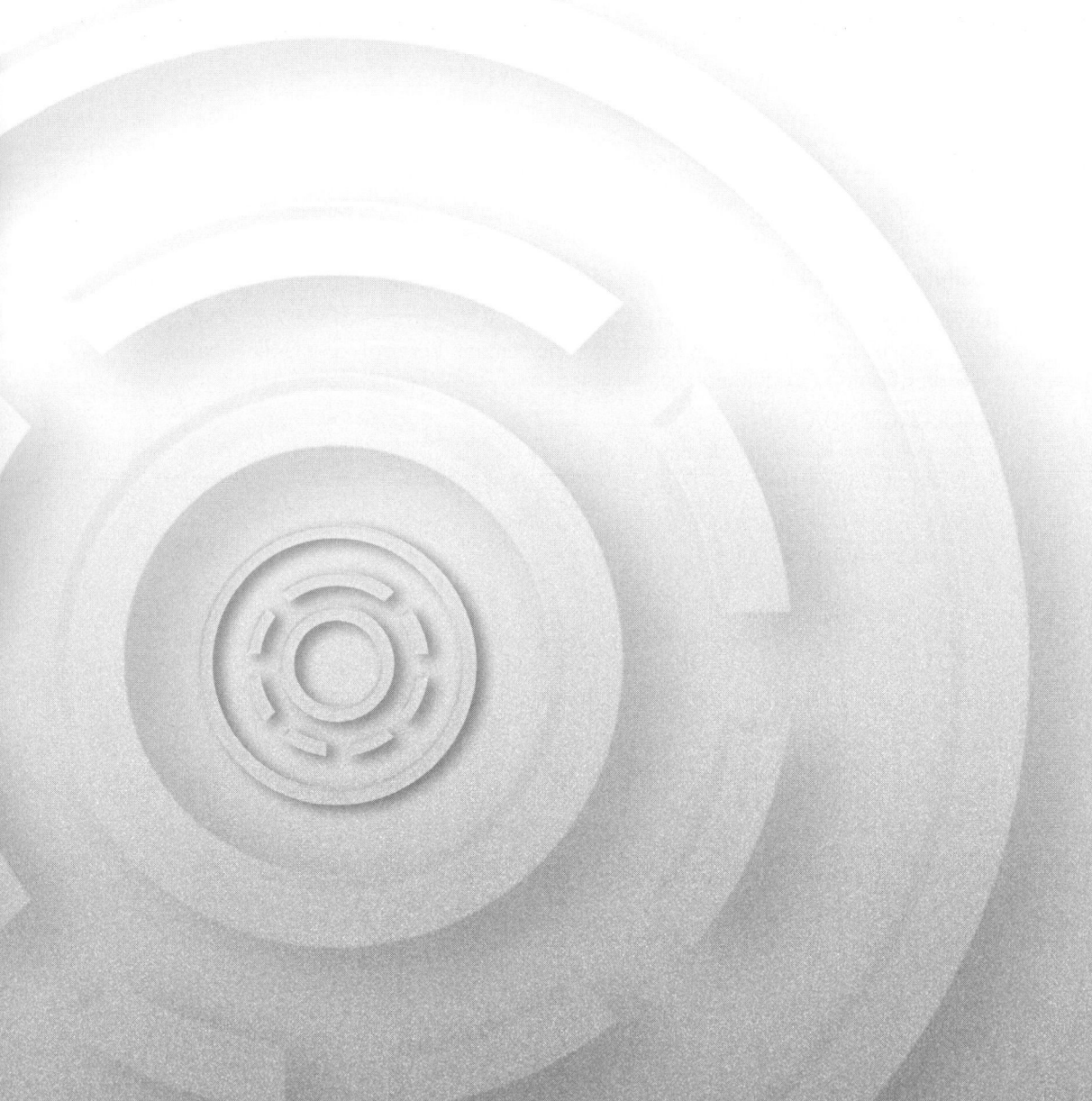

INTRODUCTION

Consultation is an important aspect of advanced practice nursing. Historically, the nursing literature on consultation focused on the clinical nurse specialist (CNS) role. As advanced practice nursing has evolved, the consultation competency has received more attention and is explicitly addressed as a role expectation. Because the profession of nursing considers the educational and practice issues relevant to all advanced practice, consultation should be considered an essential core competency of all advanced practice roles. In practice, all advanced practice nurses (APNs) offer and receive consultation.

We are a psychiatric CNS with a background in psychiatric liaison nursing who is currently working as a part-time CNS in an oncology and bone marrow transplant inpatient unit and a primary care nurse practitioner (NP) with a gerontology and adult health emphasis. Both of us are currently nursing faculty members. The synergy that developed from our collaboration and the sharing of experiences and perspectives were enriching and energizing and perhaps underscores the most fundamental points of this book—that there is much common ground across roles, that APNs have much to offer one another, and that together they can effect important changes.

This chapter has several goals. First, consultation is distinguished from supervision, collaboration, referral, and co-management. We are concerned that these terms continue to be used interchangeably in practice without clear distinctions. Each term suggests very distinct relationships and responsibilities. For example, consultation is a role function used by APNs to offer their own clinical expertise to other colleagues or to seek additional information to enhance their own practice. Because consultation is often confused with co-management, supervision, and referral in practice settings, these terms are defined to distinguish them from consultation. We then describe our model of consultation in advanced practice, and the purposes and processes of consultation are discussed. Current realities of practice are considered and issues are explored. Our goal is to provide more clarity regarding the nature of consultation because it has the potential to increase APNs' expert nursing care. APNs can also develop their own consultative skills and use their expertise to enhance their colleagues' nursing practice.

Although all APNs seek and provide consultation, specific attention has rarely been directed to this competency as it relates to NP practice. Certified nurse-midwives (CNMs), for example, specifically address consultation as an expectation, and consultation has long been a specific expectation for those in CNS positions. We highlight the importance and value of incorporating consultation as a core competency of the NP role. NPs have much to offer one another, as well as other colleagues, in consultation. Many NPs have developed important expertise in specific areas of their practice that can be of enormous benefit to other practitioners. We draw on the more extensive literature on CNS consultation to discuss APN consultation in general and use our experiences as a CNS and an NP, respectively, to illustrate the consultation competency in practice. Provision of care to patients with complex needs requires continual development of practice. The sharing of expertise through a consultative relationship is an important way to enhance understanding and promote development.

The enduring works of Caplan (1970), Caplan and Caplan (1993), and Lipowski (1974, 1981, 1983) continue to inform our thinking, writing, and practice. A number of the sources used to prepare this chapter are considered classics and are currently relevant despite their early publication dates. We reviewed the literature using the following search terms in combination with the term *consultation*: *documentation guidelines*; *Medicare*; *reimbursement*; *professional practice*; *quality standards*; *information control*; *legal issues; benefit-cost analysis; psychiatry; billable services and nursing; telemedicine;* and *technology.* Citations to the literature are included in the relevant sections of the chapter.

CONSULTATION AND ADVANCED PRACTICE NURSING

Much of the recent literature related to consultation continues to be found in the CNS literature (Ingersoll & Jones, 1992; Norwood, 1998; Scott & Beare, 1993), with the notable exceptions of the work of Monicken (1995) and Manley (1998). Barron and White (2000) emphasized the importance of consultation across advanced practice nursing roles. More recently, Sabatier (2002) described a creative partnership between a university nursing school and a medical center. An institute was developed to enhance shared activities between clinicians and academicians. Nursing consultation is a primary means of offering access to expertise within the medical center, the university, and the larger community of nurses. The institute brokers the sharing of nursing expertise and coordinates the consultation activities locally, regionally, and even internationally. Forsyth, Rhudy, and Johnson (2002) described the consultation role of the nurse educator in staff development and outlined how the principles of consultation described by Barron and White (1996) and Caplan (1970) can be adapted for educational consultation. Stichler (2002) described the role of the nurse as independent consultant. She focused on practical issues to be considered by nurses who want to share their expertise and leadership skills through consultation. She did not address APNs directly, although she acknowledged that the consultants to whom she posed her questions emphasized that a graduate level degree in an area related to the consultation need was important.

Although consultation is part of every APN's practice (Barron and White, 1996, 2000), the CNS and CNM role expectations seem to address the competency most specifically (American College of Nurse-Midwives [ACNM], 1992, 1997; Barron, 1983, 1989; Barron & White 1996, 2000; National Association of Clinical Nurse Specialists, 2004; see Chapters 12 and 16). Faut-Callahan and Kremer (2000) (see also Chapter 17) discuss consultation in the certified registered nurse anesthetist (CRNA) role. Skalla and Hamric (2000) and Skalla, Caron, and Hamric (see Chapter 15) discuss the importance of consultation for the blended role of the CNS and NP. Similarly, Mahn and Zazworsky (2000; see Chapter 18) described the consultation competency of the APN case manager role. For other advanced nursing practice roles, consultation seems to have been less formally described. In CNS roles, consultation is often directed toward staff nurses as a way of directly or indirectly influencing patient care. Although CNSs might serve as consultants to physicians and other clinicians, staff nurses and their patients are their primary clients.

APNs should be aware that state laws and regulations may mandate a "consulting" or "collaborating" physician as a requirement for advanced practice and prescriptive privileges. The wording of such mandates often directly states or implies a hierarchical relationship between APN and physician, which is contrary to the description of consultation being put forth here. Minarik and Price (1999) described the critical importance of conceptual clarity for legislative and regulatory reform. At the state and federal levels, medical societies have attempted to limit advanced practice nursing, so the terminology included in the legislation describing the relationship between physicians and APNs is of enormous significance. Minarik and Price (1999) make the compelling argument that the practical effect of legislation related to financing of health care can be devastating to advanced practice nursing, even though state boards of nursing are clear in their regulations about the appropriateness of the expanded scope of practice for APNs. APNs must be sophisticated readers of legislative proposals that include mandated relationships between physicians and APNs. Because legislation is drafted regarding both scope of practice and direct reimbursement for practice, APNs need to be clear and articulate about the implications of such terms as *collaboration*, *supervision*, *direction*, and *consultation*. Medical societies may propose such terminology with a clear intent to mandate hierarchical relationships with physicians in order to limit advanced practice nursing. Because mandated relationships between APNs and physicians may constrain advanced practice nursing consultation, APNs should be aware of the statutes and norms that regulate their practices.

The goals and outcomes of consultation are relevant to ongoing efforts to reform health care. APNs can help to bring about the national goal of high-quality, cost-effective health care for every American. Through consultation, APNs create networks with other APNs, physicians, and other colleagues, offering and receiving advice and information that can improve patient care and their own clinical knowledge and skills. Interacting with colleagues in other disciplines can enhance interdisciplinary collaboration (see Chapter 10). Consultation can also help to shape and develop the practices of consultees and protégés, thereby indirectly but significantly improving the quality, depth, and comprehensiveness of care available to populations of patients and families. Consultation offers APNs the opportunity to positively influence health-care outcomes beyond the direct patient care encounter.

Given the importance of consultation for all APNs, it is surprising that so little emphasis is reflected in other advanced practice nursing literature. With the exception of CNS practice, consultation within advanced practice nursing may be less visible, less common, or just not a major publication emphasis; but consultation activities may be an important variable in explaining the effectiveness of APNs. We urge all APNs to recognize the significance of consultation within their practices and to communicate the issues, concerns, and successes of this aspect of practice. Advanced practice nursing researchers must also study the role that timely consultations play in the high-quality, cost-effective care delivered by APNs. Consultation is a variable that ought to be considered in health-care outcomes research. Looking specifically at advanced practice nursing consultation in relation to outcomes may shed some light on the elusive phenomenon of nurse-sensitive outcomes in care.

DEFINING CONSULTATION

The term *consultation* is used in many ways. It is sometimes used to describe direct care: the practitioner is in consultation with the patient. It is also used interchangeably with the terms *referral* and *collaboration*. For example, a staff nurse might request consultation with the oncology CNS so that the CNS would assume management of the patient's pain, which really is a referral. The term *consultation* is also used when there is a hierarchical or supervisory relationship and the person without decision-making authority presents an issue to the person with such authority for a decision. For example, a psychiatric CNS might consult with the psychiatrist regarding admission of a person to the hospital for inpatient treatment. Some consultants always see the patient being considered, and some consultants never see the patient being considered. Thus how the term is being used in a given situation may be unclear, and it may be difficult to determine exactly what is being requested and what is expected. The more precisely the word *consultation* is defined, the more likely consultation will be utilized for its intended purposes. Because consultation is a core competency of advanced practice nursing, such precision is needed for communication within and outside the profession regarding advanced practice nursing roles and patient care. Consultations can enhance patient care and promote positive professional relationships; however, it is important to understand the differences between consultation and other types of professional interactions. Table 7-1 summarizes these differences, which are further described in the remainder of this section.

Distinguishing Consultation from Co-management, Referral, and Collaboration

Providing direct care involves a variety of interactions with colleagues. The terms *consultation*, *collaboration*, *co-management*, and *referral* are, at times, used interchangeably but should not be. Lack of clarity about the specific process being used for clinical problem solving leads to confusion about roles and clinical accountability. The primary characteristic that distinguishes consultation from co-management, referral, and supervision is the degree to which one assumes responsibility for the direct clinical management of a problem that falls within one's area of expertise. *Consultation* is an interaction between two professionals in which the consultant is recognized as having specialized expertise (Caplan, 1970; Caplan & Caplan, 1993). The consultee requests the assistance of that expert in the handling of a problem that he or she recognizes as falling within the expertise of the consultant. *Co-management* is the process whereby one professional manages some aspects of a patient's care while another professional manages other aspects of

| TABLE 7-1 | CLARIFYING DEFINITIONS OF CLINICAL CONSULTATION, CO-MANAGEMENT, REFERRAL, AND SUPERVISION |

TYPE OF INTERACTION	GOALS	FOCUS	RESPONSIBILITY FOR CLINICAL OUTCOMES
Clinical consultation	To enhance patient care and/or improve skills and confidence of consultee	Consultant may or may not see patient directly Degree of focus on consultee's skill is negotiated with consultee	Remains with consultee, who is free to accept or reject the advice of consultant
Co-management	To enhance patient care through availability of expertise of two (or more) professionals working together to optimize outcomes	Both professionals see patient directly and coordinate their care with one another (e.g., physician may monitor complex medication regimen while APN focuses on adaptation and human responses)	Shared
Referral	To enhance patient care by relinquishing care (or aspects of care) to another professional whose expertise is perceived to be more essential to care than that of the professional making the referral	Establish connection between patient and professional who is accepting referral Negotiate responsibilities for outcomes	Negotiated, but responsibility is often assumed (at least for aspects of care) by professional accepting referral
Supervision	To enhance patient care by overseeing the work of a less senior professional	On developing the skill of the supervisee	Supervisor and supervisee

the same patient's care. Often, co-management takes place between professionals who consider themselves part of the same interdisciplinary team. Effective co-management requires excellent communication, coordination, and collaborative skills.

The ACNM (2003) distinguishes among consultation, collaboration, and referral in the care of the high-risk patient in its position statement on collaborative management. When the CNM requests the advice of a physician or other health-care team member in a consultative relationship, he or she maintains primary responsibility for the patient's care. The ACNM uses the term *collaboration* to describe the process whereby the CNM and physician jointly manage the care of the woman or newborn.[1] *Referral,* another frequently encountered term, describes a situation in which the clinician making the referral relinquishes responsibility for care (or aspects of care), either temporarily or permanently.

Caplan and Caplan (1993), Spross (1989), Hanson and Spross (1996), and Hanson, Spross, and Carr (2000) discuss collaboration in some depth. Collaboration is raised as an issue for consideration in relation to consultation because it has been the authors' experience that APNs are confused about the differences between collaboration and consultation. In Chapter 10, Hanson and Spross offer a thoughtful definition of *collaboration,* which is slightly modified from the one they proposed in 1996:

A dynamic, interpersonal process in which two or more individuals make a commitment to each other to interact authentically and constructively to solve problems and to learn from each other to accomplish identified goals, purposes, or outcomes. The individuals recognize and articulate the shared values that make this commitment possible. (Chapter 10, p. 340)

This definition suggests that collaboration is a process that underlies the professional interactions involved in consultation, co-management, referral, and supervision. Therefore in the discussion of consultation, collaboration is assumed to be essential to the process.

Distinguishing Consultation from Clinical and Administrative Supervision

Caplan and Caplan (1993), Critchley (1985), and Lewis and Levy (1982) described clinical supervision in mental health practice. The term *clinical supervision,* as used in mental health, describes an ongoing supportive and educational process between a more senior and expert clinician and a less senior, more novice clinician. The goals of clinical supervision are to develop the knowledge, skills, self-esteem, and autonomy of the supervisee (Caplan & Caplan, 1993). Unlike the consultant, the supervisor is generally responsible for safeguarding the care of the supervisee's patients and is accountable in that respect for the work of the supervisee (Caplan & Caplan, 1993). Thus the process of supervision can be helpful for enhancing the practice of clinicians, especially novice clinicians, regardless of specialty area. In this sense of the term, APNs can be competent supervisors. Some characteristics of clinical supervision distinguish it from consultation, and it is important that the supervisor and supervisee understand that supervision is different from consultation. Also unlike the consultant, who is often an outsider to the organization or unit

---

In this chapter, we use the term *collaboration* to refer to a specific advanced practice nursing competency (Chapter 10) and the term, *co-management,* to refer to a specific type of collaborative interaction (Table 7-1). Thus we consider co-management one of many collaborative processes used by APNs. In ACNM documents, the terms *co-management, collaboration,* and *collaborative management* are used synonymously (ACNM, 1992, 1997).

where the consultation occurs, the supervisor and supervisee are commonly employed by the same organization and work together in the same clinical area. The clinical supervisor and supervisee are generally in hierarchical positions, with the supervisor being in a higher position (Caplan & Caplan, 1993). Although the ultimate goal of clinical supervision and consultation is the same—namely, assisting another professional to enhance knowledge, skills, and abilities as he or she cares for patients and families—the processes, relationships, and responsibilities are different.

Administrative supervision (e.g., vice president for nursing for APN employees) has much in common with clinical supervision (e.g., hierarchical relationship, responsibility for professional development of APNs). However, in administrative supervision, interactions are likely to focus on operations and the APN's ability to meet job responsibilities rather than the day-to-day clinical management of patients.

BACKGROUND

Consultation in Mental Health Practice

Gerald Caplan, the father of mental health consultation theory (Simmons, 1985), recognized that there were many more needs to be addressed in the Israeli community in which he worked than could possibly be met by available mental health professionals (Caplan & Caplan, 1993). In the late 1940s, Caplan and a small team of psychologists and social workers were expected to meet the mental health needs of 16,000 new immigrant children in Jerusalem. He developed his consultation model in response to these pressing needs. By consulting with other professionals, such as teachers and counselors, he found that the recipients of consultation could effectively meet many of the mental health needs of the children. Both the need that gave rise to this model and the model itself are relevant to APNs, who must consider strategies that enable patients and families, beyond their direct practice reach, to benefit from advanced practice nursing knowledge and skills.

Lipowski (1981) also developed a model of mental health consultation for use in the general hospital setting. He stressed that it is essential for consultants to understand the context of the consultation situation. He recommended that consultation include an evaluation of the patient, the patient's interactions with the staff, and the specific needs of the consultee (the staff member). The family and social supports are considered as well. The consultant carefully communicates with the staff and provides regular follow-up of the patient for the course of the hospitalization. Although the Caplan and Lipowski models were developed for application in mental health, they have informed our evolving model of advanced practice nursing consultation.

Types of Consultation

According to Caplan (1970), there are four different types of consultation. *Client-centered case consultation* is the most common type of consultation. The primary goal of this type of consultation is assisting the consultee to develop an effective plan of care for a patient who has a particularly difficult or complex problem. In client-centered case consultation, the consultant often sees the patient directly to complete an assessment of the patient and to make recommendations to the consultee for the consultee's management of the case. This is often a one-time evaluation. Follow-up by the consultant is sometimes needed.

The primary goal is to assist the consultee in helping the patient. A positive experience with handling that specific case will enhance the consultee's ability so that future patients with similar problems can be treated more effectively.

In *consultee-centered case consultation*, improving patient care is important, but the emphasis is focused directly on the consultee's difficulty in handling the situation. Thus the primary goals are to assess the consultee's needs and address the problem effectively. In consultee-centered case consultation, the task for the consultant is to understand and remedy the problems of the consultee in managing a particular case. Usual problems are lack of knowledge, skill, confidence, or objectivity. Thus the consultant may educate the consultee further on the issues presented by the patient or may suggest alternative strategies for dealing with the problem. This is probably the most common type of consultation sought by APNs. The consultant may seek to bolster the confidence of the consultee in handling the problem, if, in the opinion of the consultant, the consultee has the ability and potential to do so. If the problem presented by the consultee is a lack of professional objectivity, the consultant can help the consultee to identify the factors interfering with the consultee's ability to see the patient realistically. The consultee may hold a stereotyped view of the patient, or perhaps the patient's difficulties in some way mirror or symbolize the consultee's personal difficulties and cloud the consultee's ability to see the reality of the situation. Effective consultation can foster orderly reflection and extend the frames of reference used by the consultee to solve clinical problems (Caplan & Caplan, 1993). Both client-centered and consultee-centered case consultations have been important activities in traditional CNS practice. The extent to which other APNs engage in these types of consultation has rarely been described.

Program-centered administrative consultation focuses on the planning and administration of clinical services. *Consultee-centered administrative consultation* focuses on the consultee's (or group of consultees') difficulties as they interfere with the organization's objectives. APNs may be involved in all four types of consultation at various times. This chapter specifically considers client-centered case consultation and consultee-centered case consultation, because the focus of this chapter is the process of interacting with other professionals regarding the care of individual patients.

A MODEL OF ADVANCED PRACTICE NURSING CONSULTATION

Principles of Consultation

The model of advanced practice nursing consultation that we propose is based on the following principles of consultation derived from the field of mental health (Caplan, 1970; Caplan & Caplan, 1993; Lipowski, 1981):

1. The consultation is usually initiated by the consultee.
2. The relationship between the consultant and consultee is nonhierarchical and collaborative.
3. The consultant always considers contextual factors when responding to the request for consultation.
4. The consultant has no direct authority for managing patient care.
5. The consultant does not prescribe but makes recommendations.
6. The consultee is free to accept or reject the recommendations of the consultant.
7. The consultation should be documented.

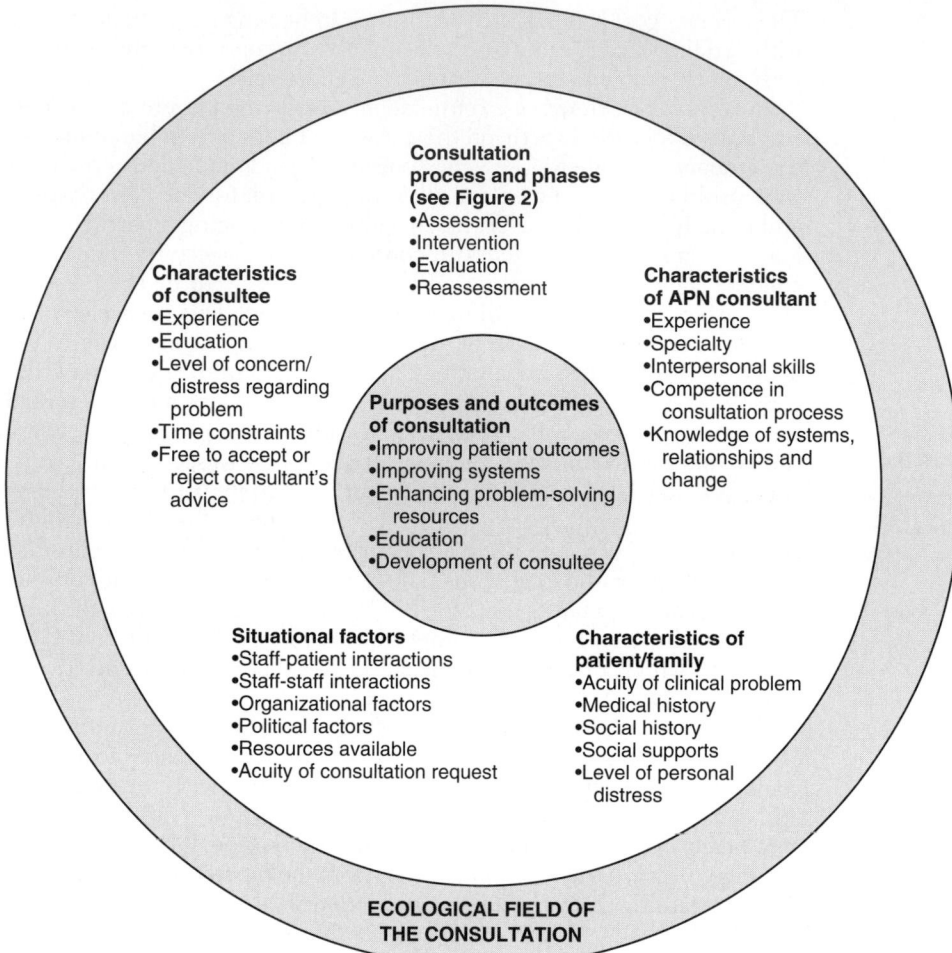

Consultation process and phases (see Figure 2)
•Assessment
•Intervention
•Evaluation
•Reassessment

Characteristics of consultee
•Experience
•Education
•Level of concern/ distress regarding problem
•Time constraints
•Free to accept or reject consultant's advice

Characteristics of APN consultant
•Experience
•Specialty
•Interpersonal skills
•Competence in consultation process
•Knowledge of systems, relationships and change

Purposes and outcomes of consultation
•Improving patient outcomes
•Improving systems
•Enhancing problem-solving resources
•Education
•Development of consultee

Situational factors
•Staff-patient interactions
•Staff-staff interactions
•Organizational factors
•Political factors
•Resources available
•Acuity of consultation request

Characteristics of patient/family
•Acuity of clinical problem
•Medical history
•Social history
•Social supports
•Level of personal distress

ECOLOGICAL FIELD OF THE CONSULTATION

FIGURE 7-1 • A model of APN consultation.

Description of the Model

Barron (1989) proposed a model of consultation for CNSs that was based on the nursing process and incorporated principles from the work of Caplan (1970) and Lipowski (1974, 1981, 1983). This model, expanded by Barron and White (1996), has evolved into the model of advanced practice nursing consultation shown in Figure 7-1. APNs tend to have a holistic orientation and an understanding of systems theory that will enable them to apply this consultation model in practice. At the center of Barron and White's proposed model are the purposes and outcomes of consultation that are essentially the same. Surrounding the center is the ecological field of the consultation. Consultations are embedded in the context of the specific circumstances surrounding the consultation request, so the ecological field in which the consultation takes place must be understood to provide effective consultation (Caplan & Caplan, 1993). This involves an appreciation of the interconnection and interrelatedness of the systems and contexts influencing the consultation problem and

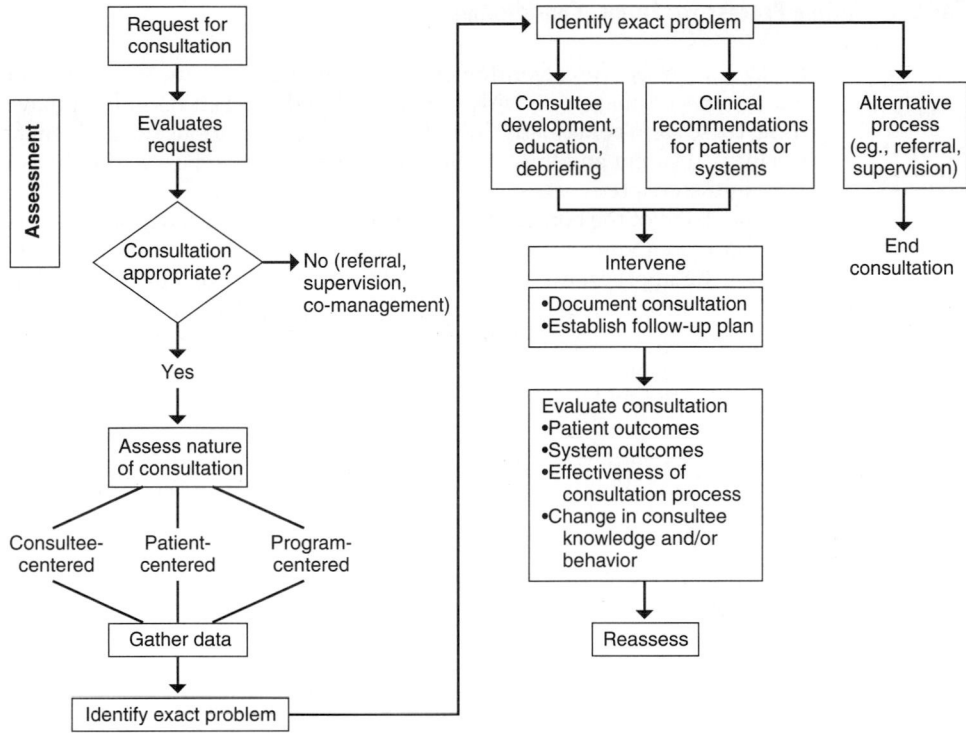

FIGURE 7-2 • Algorithm for consultation process.

process. Thus the consultation process is an integral part of the ecological field. The process—in which the consultant evaluates the request, performs an assessment, determines the skills required to address the problem, intervenes, and evaluates the outcome—is expanded in Figure 7-2. Other elements of the ecological field include the characteristics of the consultant, characteristics of the consultee, characteristics of the patient and family, and situational factors. We assume that there are reciprocal influences among the purposes, process, and contextual factors that can affect consultation processes and outcomes. Each component of the model is elaborated in the following sections.

Purpose and Outcomes

The purpose of a consultation may be to improve patient outcomes, enhance health-care delivery systems, extend the knowledge available to solve clinical problems, foster the ongoing professional development of the consultee, or a combination of these goals. Consultants should be aware that the purposes for which they have been consulted may contract or expand during the process of consulting. Often, APN consultants accomplish several purposes at once. If additional purposes and possible outcomes are uncovered during consultation, these should be made clear to the consultee. The consultee may want the consultant's assistance with a patient but does not have the time or interest to focus on his or her own development. Patients may also reveal information that requires a shift in the consultation's focus, purpose, and outcome. Over the course of the consultation, being explicit about the goal or outcome of the consultation is essential if APNs are to evaluate the impact of consultation on practice.

The Consultation Process for Formal Consultation

Figure 7-2 presents an algorithm of the consultation process. With experience and expertise, the process may occur fairly rapidly so that the expert consultant may not be aware of using these steps consciously. In addition, in some situations the problem for which help is sought is clear-cut and the consultation is brief. These types of consultations are discussed later in the chapter.

Assessment of the consultation problem begins with evaluation of the request itself. An important component of assessment is confirming with the consultee that consultation is, in fact, the appropriate strategy for addressing the problem (rather than a referral, for example). At this stage, the consultant and consultee may decide that an alternative process is needed (e.g., a shift to co-management or referral). The consultant confirms that the problem has been accurately identified and falls within the realm of the consultant's expertise and clarifies the nonhierarchical nature of the relationship between the consultant and consultee. The consultant also confirms that the consultee will remain clinically responsible for the patient who is the focus of the consultation. The consultant must remember that the consultee is ultimately free to accept or reject his or her recommendations. Once the request itself has been considered, the consultant gathers information from the consultee about the specific nature of the problem. The consultant tries to determine whether the patient has unusually difficult and complex problems (patient-centered consultation) and whether the problem results from the consultee's lack of knowledge, skill, confidence, or objectivity (consultee-centered consultation). Once the request, the nature of the relationship, and appropriateness of consultation have been established, the consultant focuses on gathering data related to the consultation problem. This may include direct assessment of the patient. The consultant considers the ecological field of the consultation, which includes the systems and contexts that may influence the patient and family, the consultee and staff, and the setting in which the consultation takes place. Some requests for consultation are quite focused and require that the consultant identify aspects of the ecological field that are priorities for assessment and attention.

The consultant uses available resources such as patient records, direct assessment of the patient, and interviews with staff to *identify the exact problem* or problems that are to be the focus of consultation. This may or may not be the problem for which help has been sought. Some consultation problems are simple and do not require extensive data collection. Others are complex and may require extensive chart review for a longstanding problem or calls to referring clinicians when incomplete data have been provided. The consultant shares the identified problem with the consultee and validates this with the consultee. If part of the problem is the consultee's lack of expertise, the consultant will want to use tact as the problem is identified and discussed. Interpersonal qualities of the consultant are crucial and are discussed later in this chapter.

Once the specific problem or problems have been identified, the consultant and consultee *consider interventions* that will address the problem(s). The consultant may intervene directly with the consultee by using such approaches as education, assistance with reinterpretation of the problem, or identification of appropriate resources if the problem is the consultee's lack of experience. If the problem results from a particularly difficult patient situation, the consultant may assist with the process of clinical decision making by providing alternative perspectives on the problem and recommending specific interventions. More data may be needed to further analyze the situation, and a decision may need to be made about whether the consultee or consultant will gather more data. If the consultee accepts the recommendations of the consultant, together they negotiate how the interventions will be carried out and by whom. If the consultant is to intervene directly with the patient, the consultee must understand his or her ongoing responsibility for the patient and agree to the consultant's interventions. Together they identify additional resources and determine the time frame for the consultation (one time or ongoing).

After the intervention, the consultant and consultee engage in *evaluation*. Evaluation of the success or lack of success of the intervention and the overall consultation is essential to the consultation process. If the problem is resolved, evaluation offers an opportunity for review, confirmation of the enhanced effectiveness of the consultee in managing the problem (underscoring the new skills and abilities or understanding of the situation by the consultee), and closure. If problems remain, reassessment offers the consultant and consultee another opportunity for problem solving.

Formal and Informal Consultation

The process of consultation described previously is comprehensive and formal. The consultant brings clinical expertise, as well as an understanding and appreciation of the process of consultation, to the problem presented. According to the model, the consultant considers all elements of the nursing process in relation to the consultation problem. However, what about the quick questions to the consultant, when what is needed is a piece of information and a quick description of how to apply the information? Are these brief interactions, sometimes called *corridor consultations*, related to a circumscribed problem true consultations? Absolutely, but the consultant needs to make a conscious decision about responding in a brief and simple way to the request and needs to consider with the consultee whether the quick response addresses the problem. There are times when the problem presented oversimplifies a complex concern requiring a more comprehensive approach. If the consultant and consultee consider the problem together, they can determine whether the quick response is adequate or whether consultation is needed. Conversely, there are times when what is truly needed is a short answer to a clinical question or validation that the approach to the problem is appropriate.

Staff nurses, at times, equate this brief type of consultation with consultation in general because they have experienced only this type of consultation with physicians, who quickly impart information and are then off to the next patient. The idea of the roving clinical expert dropping by with tidbits of expert advice is indeed the notion non-APNs can have of a consultant. That is another reason that it is important to make a conscious decision about responding in a brief way to the consultation request. In the informal situation, the consultee may not realize that a more comprehensive and thorough investigation of the problem and solutions with the consultant is possible. Also, some clinical situations require a more formal approach to the consultation problem. We suggest that APNs consider the kinds of problems in practice that require a formal approach and develop a system for integrating nurse-nurse and interdisciplinary consultations that make advanced practice nursing skills more visible and extend their knowledge and skills.

Ecological Field of the Consultation Process

CHARACTERISTICS OF THE APN CONSULTANT

In addition to theoretical understanding, self-awareness and interpersonal skills are essential for the consultant (Barron, 1989; Barron & White, 1996, 2000). For a model of consultative practice to be implemented, it is critical that APNs first value themselves and the specialized expertise they have developed. One must appreciate one's skills and knowledge before the possibilities for consultation can be envisioned (see Chapter 3). APNs have developed specialized expertise in the direct care of underserved populations, such as the homeless; the frail elderly; persons who are chronically mentally ill, home-bound, or institutionalized; and patients with human immunodeficiency virus infection. The knowledge and skills acquired by APNs could serve to inform and expand the practices of staff nurses, other APNs, and health-care professionals of various disciplines involved in the care of these populations of patients. However, APNs must first appreciate that they have valuable understanding and knowledge to share.

Ideally, consultants know themselves well: they are aware of their own personal issues, strengths, weaknesses, and motives. A good consultant must be able to suspend judgment and avoid stereotyping. When consultation is sought, often what is needed is a fresh perspective. Self-understanding allows the consultant to see consultation issues realistically and without prejudice. It is not uncommon for a consultant to step into a highly emotionally charged situation. Self-awareness, understanding, and being able to remain centered and self-possessed are key to remaining objective and clear. It can be meaningful and helpful for the consultant to have a trusted colleague or supervisor with whom to share and review consultation situations. Such discussions can offer support and enhance the consultant's understanding of personal and interpersonal responses to the consultation material.

The consultant should also be able to establish warm, respectful, and accepting relationships with consultees. The initiation of a consultation request is often associated with a sense of vulnerability on the part of the consultee, who recognizes that assistance is required to help manage the situation at hand. The consultant must communicate (and sincerely believe) that the problem and the consultee are important and worthy of consideration. The consultant must also communicate confidence in the consultee's ability to overcome the difficulties resulting in the consultation request. When the consultant creates a climate of trust and acceptance, the consultee can then be willing to risk vulnerability and genuineness with the consultant. When a respectful, trusting connection is made between the consultant and consultee, a deep examination of the problem, implications, and solutions is possible.

An APN is sometimes the consultee, and often, the consultation is requested from a physician. As a consultee, the APN should be able to identify and articulate the nature of the problem for which help is being sought. It may be necessary to clarify the collegial, nonhierarchical nature of the consultation relationship. When consulting with an APN colleague or physician, an APN has often already tried alternative plans or is thinking about possible directions to take based on knowledge of the patient or clinical situation. Consultants find such information useful in planning their approaches to the consultation. Dialogue with APN colleagues and physicians can improve the effectiveness and efficiency of the consultation and can strengthen collaboration among colleagues. In addition to their intrapersonal knowledge and interpersonal skills, APNs must be competent in the consultative process. To be an effective consultant, an APN must be knowledgeable about systems, relationships, and change. Although skill in consultation develops over time, the consultant attributes and consultation process described here can help novice APNs who are open to learning approach consultation with confidence (see the section on developing consultation skills later in this chapter).

CHARACTERISTICS OF THE CONSULTEE

The consultee identifies a problem that exists in a clinical situation because of uncertainty or a lack of knowledge on his or her part and believes that increased knowledge and assistance with clinical decision making would enhance practice. Characteristics of the consultee may need to be considered. Education, experience, level of distress (the consultee's) regarding the clinical problem for which help is sought, organizational skills, and availability to problem solve with the consultant are factors that can influence the consultation.

PATIENT AND FAMILY FACTORS

Among factors to consider are the acuity and complexity of the clinical problem; the patient's medical history, social history, and social supports; and other resources. Depending on the nature of the problem, it may be important to consider concurrent stresses being experienced by the patient and family. An acute problem may demand the consultant's immediate assistance, requiring a shift in the consultant's priorities. A complex or unusual problem may take more time to solve.

SITUATIONAL FACTORS

In this model, situational factors refer to those inherent within the organization and staff caring for the patient. Numerous situational factors can affect the consultation process. The quality of relationships and interactions between staff and patients or among staff members themselves may be important issues. For example, a patient perceived as being nonadherent to some therapy may be responding to conflicts among team members that the patient has inferred from clinicians' behaviors. A clinician may seek validation from a consultant as a way of getting support for an unpopular but potentially productive approach to a clinical problem. Time pressures and lack of adequate resources can affect consultation. Organizational politics, power imbalances, and rapid or frequent system changes are other things to consider. All of these factors can affect the consultee's view of the importance of the request.

For APNs, the status of advanced practice nursing and APNs in a particular agency or state may influence consultation. For example, organizational policies and procedures regarding consultation, statutes regarding APN-physician "consulting" relationships, reimbursement policies, and degree of prescriptive authority may affect the consultation process.

COMMON APN CONSULTATION SITUATIONS

Depending on one's particular advanced practice nursing role, certain consultation situations may be more common than others. APNs are most likely to receive requests for patient- and consultee-centered case consultations. These types of consultations are described in this section. Experienced APNs may extend their consultative skills into other types of consultations, such as program-centered consultations. The exemplars included here vary in the complexity of consultations and the extent to which aspects of the consultation model are made explicit. The reader is encouraged to examine the ways in which the proposed model of advanced practice nursing consultation is applied and consider ways in which it can be applied in his or her own practice.

APN-APN Consultation

Within their specialty or setting, APNs may take for granted the available APN consulting resources. They may not think of their interactions regarding patient care as consultation because they occur in the hallway or over coffee. Consultation among APNs may be more or less formal, depending on the culture of the unit or clinic, the relationships among the APNs, and the specialty populations seen in the facility. Consultations are likely to involve specific patient issues, for example: "Could you look at this rash? I've never seen one quite like this before," or "I've done everything I can think of to try to make sure this pregnant teen comes to her prenatal visits and she still misses them. Here's what I've done . . . can you think of anything else before I get the city department of social services involved?" An example of a formal APN-to-APN consultation follows.

Norwood (1998) discussed the importance of and practicalities related to APNs seeking consultation from other APNs. She noted that APNs readily think of themselves as consultants but may overlook opportunities for seeking consultation. She outlined the following factors as relevant when APNs consider the use of a consultant: cost savings, objectivity, politics, when not to seek consultation, and issues to consider in choosing a consultant.

In many settings, APNs may have some clinical and supervisory responsibilities. For example, a senior NP may supervise other APNs and staff and also have a patient caseload. The supervisory relationship may constrain the consultation process as it is described here. An NP seeking consultation from a supervisor may worry that such a request reflects poorly on his or her clinical competency. The nature of the relationship (i.e., whether it is with a colleague or a supervisor) can affect the consultation process. Given our belief that a nonhierarchical relationship is essential for true consultation, it may be more accurate to refer to interactions with a supervisor as *problem solving*. Regardless of what the interaction is called, these types of interactions are important for professional development and optimal patient care. As APNs integrate consultation more explicitly into their practices and reflect on the process and outcomes of consultation, future discussions might illuminate this consultation dilemma.

Exemplar 7-1 describes a formal CNS-to-CNS consultation that is both client-centered and consultee-centered. Exemplar 7-2 describes an informal consultee-centered

EXEMPLAR 7-1

The medical-surgical clinical nurse specialist (CNS) consulted the psychiatric liaison CNS regarding the care of a young man with severe burn injuries who had been transferred to the surgical service from the intensive care unit (ICU). An initial problem to be addressed was the frequent and painful dressing changes. The patient disliked the lingering effects of narcotic analgesia for the dressing changes but clearly needed assistance with pain relief during the dressing changes. The medical-surgical CNS asked whether the psychiatric liaison nurse could teach the patient relaxation and imagery strategies for use during the dressing changes (and if the strategies proved to be helpful for the patient, could also teach the staff to coach the patient with these tools). The medical-surgical CNS also recognized that there were many complex and difficult psychosocial issues to be confronted by the patient as he recovered. His hands and face were significantly burned. He would likely be permanently disfigured and disabled. She requested that the liaison nurse provide additional supportive care to the patient and be available to the staff as they planned for the psychosocial dimension of his care.

The patient and staff found relaxation and imagery techniques to be quite helpful for the dressing changes. The liaison CNS and staff planned the patient's care together with the clear intention of providing a climate of trust, acceptance, and openness with the hope that the patient would experience himself as whole and respected and worthwhile in his relationships with them. In spite of his severe and disfiguring burns, the nurses could experience the beauty of the patient's humanity as they established intentional relationships with him. They helped him to experience the depths of himself, which transcended the limits established by the burns. They helped him plan his first visit with his young child, preparing the patient for potential reactions and helping the patient to prepare his child for his first visit. Follow-up mental health care was arranged at the time of discharge.

consultation between a primary care NP and a psychiatric/mental health NP. Exemplar 7-3 illustrates a formal consultee-centered consultation that is between a primary care NP and a CNS specializing in HIV/AIDS; this consultation also led to a plan to co-manage the patient. Exemplar 7-4 illustrates an informal consultation that led to a referral.

EXEMPLAR 7-2

A primary care NP caring for an adolescent patient was concerned about the high-risk sexual practices her patient reported. Despite the rapport and long-standing nature of the relationship with her patient, the NP felt the need for additional expertise in order to facilitate caring for this patient. The APN sought the consultation of a psychiatric NP colleague with clinical and research expertise in the area of adolescent health care. The consultant provided some of the latest research on adolescents and high-risk sexual activities and advised the primary care NP to consider other factors that could be influencing the adolescent's behavior. The consultant advised the primary care NP of findings that would warrant further evaluation by a psychiatrist or psychiatric APN to determine the adolescent's need for more specialized care. The NP scheduled a visit with the adolescent and incorporated the consultant's suggestions into her assessment. Specifically, she elicited new information about factors that might be motivating the teenager to engage in high-risk sexual activities, and the NP modified her communications with the teen to focus more on nurturing her and promoting self-care.

The exchange between a primary care NP and psychiatric NP in Exemplar 7-2 depicts consultee-centered consultation. The expert provided important knowledge and suggestions aimed at enhancing the NP's practice, yet was not responsible for how the NP used this information. The consultant provided important perspectives and new information that indirectly affected the patient's care, yet was not responsible for the consultee's

EXEMPLAR 7-3

Ms. L. is a 29-year-old female who has been followed regularly for primary care through her young adulthood in the family practice. She presented 2 years ago with symptoms initially thought consistent with bronchitis. Her symptoms worsened, and she was eventually hospitalized and diagnosed with pneumocystis pneumonia. A diagnosis of acquired immunodeficiency syndrome (AIDS) was then made. Ms. L. was subsequently referred to the infectious disease specialists in a tertiary setting for ongoing management of AIDS; she continued to have her general primary care needs met at the family practice. The primary care NP was pleased that her patient wanted to continue to be cared for in the family practice but was challenged by the increasing complexities in management of her new illness and the patient's struggles in coping with this disease. The primary care NP scheduled a telephone consultation with the APN in the infectious disease clinic where Ms. L. received her care for AIDS. The APN was a blended role CNS/NP who had extensive knowledge and experience in the care of clients with HIV and AIDS. She was able to provide the primary care NP with specific knowledge regarding expected and unusual side effects of the medication regimen and commonly encountered drug-drug interactions. While the CNS/NP would continue to prescribe and oversee the medication regimen, they discussed what they would do to co-manage Ms. L.'s care. The NP agreed that she felt comfortable with managing common side effects and would collaborate to monitor Ms. L. for any problems with adherence to the treatment regimen between visits to the specialty clinic. When discussing how the patient was coping, the CNS/NP reassured the NP that her patient's response was appropriate for her stage of illness and suggested communication strategies that might further assist the patient in dealing with the reactions of family, co-workers, and friends. In addition, they acknowledged that the NP was likely to have more opportunities to help Ms. L. with coping with the disease so the CNS/NP agreed to send the NP some recent, relevant literature on the unique challenges of integrating the experience of living with AIDS into one's life. The CNS/NP provided information on a support group and other resources that the patient might find helpful.

EXEMPLAR 7-4

> Mr. S is a 56-year-old man residing in a group home. He has a diagnosis of mental retardation with an IQ consistent with a mild range of mental retardation. In addition, he has a seizure disorder requiring daily medications and laboratory monitoring of the medication. He attends a sheltered workshop 5 days a week and is able to manage his activities of daily living; however, he requires supervision for cooking, shopping, and managing money. The staff at the group home provides the needed support but has noticed over the past few months that he has become agitated and less cooperative around the house. The patient and his caseworker presented to the family practice where he receives his ongoing care. After a careful workup ruled out a physical cause of the behavior change, it was determined that he would need additional monitoring and support, as well as a behavior modification intervention. The primary care APN sought the consultation of an APN expert in the care of the older mentally retarded population. The consultant shared clinical experiences in caring for this population and cited the lack of research in the area of behavioral change in the mentally retarded population. She also recommended a physician colleague whose subspecialty is assessing and treating these issues in the mentally retarded population.

decision making or outcomes of care. If a psychiatric consultation was necessary and had been initiated by the primary care NP and was accepted by the patient, this would be an example of how this informal, consultee-centered consultation led to a referral for a formal, client-centered case consultation.

Exemplar 7-3 highlights both formal consultation and co-management of a client whose needs are chronic and complex and require the resources of many professionals. The CNS/NP specialist in HIV/AIDS provided consultee-centered consultation enhancing the knowledge base of the primary care APN and providing insight into the expected course of adjustment of patients with AIDS as well as suggestions for community-based support. The primary care NP continued providing ongoing primary care and monitoring the patient's response to treatment and adjustment to the illness, co-managing Ms. L's illness with the HIV/AIDS CNS/NP and her colleagues at the specialty clinic.

Exemplar 7-4 demonstrates that an informal consultation may lead to a change in care. In this case, the APN expert's recommendation of a referral illustrates how a consultation may lead to a referral to a third party for assessment, treatment, and co-management when it may be more beneficial for the patient. Although the consultant's role was an important first step, additional care was determined to be the best course of action, since neither the consultant nor the primary care APN could provide the range of services deemed necessary for the patient.

APN-Physician Consultation

When consulting with other APNs or physicians, an APN is likely to be fairly far along in the problem-solving process. The need for consultation is often related to the consultee's level of diagnostic uncertainty (Colman, 1992). Experienced APNs often have a clear definition of the problem and a preliminary plan to address it that they wish to validate or reformulate, depending on the consultant's advice.

The need for statutory language that clearly describes the autonomous nature of advanced practice nursing has been addressed (Safriet, 1992; Birkholz & Walker, 1994) and continues to inform regulation of practice. The ACNM (1992; 2003) was deliberate in describing the various kinds of interactions CNMs have, primarily with physicians. Unfortunately, as noted earlier, APN-physician consultative relationships have often been structured by laws and regulations that mandate or imply a supervisory relationship, which can reinforce stereotypical nurse-physician relationships. Many organizational cultures reinforce traditional nurse-physician relationships and the behavioral norms associated with them. One of the major challenges facing advanced practice nursing educators is to explicitly address students' prior socialization to nurse-physician relationships that may undermine full expression of autonomous advanced practice nursing. When a hierarchical relationship exists between an APN and a physician, the APN who consults with a physician may defer to the physician's decisions, downplaying or ignoring firsthand knowledge of the patient. However, numerous descriptions of successful collaborative practices between physicians and APNs exist (Barron & White, 1996). Such practices embrace the collaborative relationships we believe are key to effective consultations (see Chapter 10).

In some APN-physician exchanges, true consultation occurs; however, much of the language that defines relationships between APNs and physicians involve the terms *co-management*, *referral*, and *supervision*. Physicians in primary care often consult APNs regarding such issues as assisting patients in making lifestyle changes or in coping with the effects of chronic illness. Many APNs in primary care have special expertise in women's health care and are sought out by physicians for consultation on such issues. Physicians might then choose to co-manage patients with APNs so that patients benefit from the expertise of both professionals. APNs in turn might consult a physician regarding a patient in a medically unstable condition, which evolves into co-management by the physician and APN, with each assuming responsibility for the outcomes of decision making. Consultation between APNs and physicians can highlight the strengths of each, that is, the APN's deep appreciation for the human responses related to health and illness and the physician's deep understanding of disease and treatment. When both areas of expertise are available to patients and their families, truly holistic, comprehensive, and individualized care is offered.

As APN knowledge evolves and deepens, an emerging issue in relation to APN-physician consultation is the crossing of traditional nurse-physician boundaries. As APNs become more and more specialized, the knowledge embedded in practice may be more closely related to what is generally thought of as medical practice. For example, an oncology CNS may have very highly developed skills in the area of pain management. As a physician consults with the CNS regarding an individual patient, the CNS may make recommendations for specific medications. Regardless of whether the APN has prescriptive authority, an appreciation for the inherent shifts in the usual "professional territories" of nurses and physicians and the need for flexibility is helpful. Tact and understanding of the longstanding boundaries that are being crossed can bring the consultation relationship to a new level.

APN-Staff Nurse Consultation

As CNSs implemented their consultative roles, it became apparent that the culture of nursing had not adopted consultation as an important strategy in providing patient care (Barron, 1983). Staff nurses were expected to take care of the patients themselves. A novice might consult a head nurse or more senior nurse, but staff members were expected to know how to solve problems and use the policy and procedures manual. Part of implementing consultation meant teaching staff members how and when to consult. In the early days, CNSs often engaged in active case finding to identify the patients who needed the knowledge and skills they had, because CNSs were not "assigned" to patients and staff nurses. By building this kind of clinical caseload, they demonstrated to staff how consultation might be helpful. Of note, CNSs tended to do direct consultation with patients, as well as to consult with other professionals to assist the staff with problem solving and enhancing patient care. For example, staff nurses might call the medical-surgical CNS regarding a patient with Guillain-Barré syndrome because they had had no previous experience caring for patients with this disorder. The CNS may have had little or no experience as well but would mobilize the resources needed, such as arranging in-services by the neuroscience or rehabilitation CNS, providing articles, being available to staff on all shifts as they implement unfamiliar assessments, and assisting with care plan development. The CNS would initiate processes (including additional consultation) and provide knowledge directly.

Once relationships are established and staff perceive that the APN consultant is approachable, respectful, and helpful, then staff will initiate contact with the consultant when complex clinical issues arise. In Exemplar 7-5, intensive care unit nurses requested a psychiatric liaison nursing consultation. The staff and consultant had a well-established relationship.

EXEMPLAR 7-5

A young man had been admitted to the intensive care unit several hours before consultation was sought, after he had taken an overdose of acetaminophen. Unfortunately, a large quantity of acetaminophen had been ingested the night before, and many hours had passed before he and his family sought medical assistance. His medical condition was grave. The psychiatric service and liaison CNS had been consulted to assess the suicidal risk and make recommendations for the treatment of the patient. The nurses were very concerned about the young man and his family. The patient was expressing regret about the overdose, saying he was no longer suicidal. He was terrified by the potential for slipping into liver failure and dying. His mother was beside herself with guilt. The night before admission, the patient had come home intoxicated, telling his mother that he had taken the acetaminophen. She did not believe him; she thought he was looking for sympathy to avoid getting into trouble in relation to his drinking. She also reasoned that if he had taken the acetaminophen, it was no big deal; after all, it was a relatively mild and safe drug. When he woke up in the morning very ill, she brought him to the local emergency department for care. He was treated initially and sent by ambulance to the medical center.

The gastroenterologist was not at all confident that liver failure could be prevented. The psychiatrists assessed the patient to no longer be at risk of suicide. Everyone involved was deeply moved and distressed by the tragedy they were witnessing. The nurses requested that the liaison CNS be available for additional supportive care for the patient, support and referral for the family, and assistance in planning nursing care for the patient.

After about a day and a half, the patient slipped into a coma. It became clear that he was dying. His mother had accepted referral to her local mental health center, which was arranged by the psychiatric consult service and liaison nurse. For the first 2 days, the mother was in the unit most of the time. She spoke openly with staff and the liaison CNS about her guilt, regret, and pain. After her son became comatose, she did not spend much time in the unit. She said it was just too painful for her to see him deteriorate. Other family members and friends spent a great deal of time in the unit. The liaison CNS stopped by the unit frequently, talking with staff and with family members. Everyone (including the liaison nurse) had a great need to talk through the sorrow and sense of impotence in the situation. Everything that could be done was being done, but that was not enough to change the outcome.

The patient had lived for 5 days, but on Friday evening, when the liaison CNS was leaving for the weekend, it was clear that death was not far away. She invited the staff to call her if they needed her over the weekend. The nurses called her and asked her to come very late on Friday evening. They sensed that the patient would die within a matter of minutes or hours, and they were concerned about how to respond to his mother when he actually died.

The CNS came in and was present with the family and friends to support the patient in the process of dying. His mother did not return to the hospital. Hands were held; songs, chanted; and tears shed as the patient peacefully died. Unit nurses were in and out of the room also, being present as time allowed. After the emotionally tumultuous week with the young patient, there was some sense of satisfaction in knowing that if his death could not be prevented, a

EXEMPLAR 7-5—cont'd

> peaceful death could be facilitated. The family and friends expressed their deep gratitude for that facilitation.
>
> The client-centered consultation focused primarily on the needs of the patient and family. The consultant and staff regularly shared their own feelings of impotence and despair with one another as they discussed the care of the patient. That sharing and planning helped to shape the nursing perspective in the situation and clarify the goal of promoting a peaceful and comfortable death, once cure was no longer a viable goal. The consultation contributed to an active and compassionate nursing presence in the midst of tragedy and pain.

MECHANISMS TO FACILITATE CONSULTATION

Mechanisms to facilitate consultation need to be considered by all APNs, regardless of setting. Traditionally, CNSs have offered consultation to staff in institutions where they are employed. Consultation is an explicit role expectation for CNSs and often a daily activity for these APNs. Consultation services are usually not considered directly reimbursable activities. As health care becomes more community focused and as APNs provide care to increasingly diverse and vulnerable populations, the breadth and depth of skills required for these newer roles will be considerable. APN-APN consultation is an important means of developing consultative skills.

In some situations an APN may refer a patient to another provider, and the APN who is consulted may be reimbursed. For example, if the primary care NP in Exemplar 7-2 referred the teen to a psychiatric CNS, or a geriatric NP referred an elderly female patient to another NP who specializes in urinary incontinence management, these consultants would be likely to be reimbursed. However, current mechanisms do not provide for reimbursement of indirect patient care activities, even though those activities may improve outcomes for patient care (Sebus, 1994), such as the initial, informal consultation with the psychiatric CNS described in Exemplar 7-2. To the extent that APNs and other disciplines can demonstrate the benefits of consultation, this shortcoming of the current payment system for health-care services should be addressed as part of reform efforts. With the current focus on reimbursement for direct care activities and capitation-based reimbursement, it seems unlikely that additional, specific funds will be available in the near future for consultative activities. Creative strategies for funding consultation need to be developed. For example, incorporating APN consultation into critical pathways for selected populations may be one strategy for ensuring the cost-effectiveness of capitation-based reimbursement and of building in bottom-line consideration of consultation services. We were unable to find any current payors that provide reimbursement for any advanced practice nursing consultation activities related to indirect care. Although Medicare provides some reimbursement for case management activities of primary care providers, consultation activities are currently not included.

Boyd et al. (1991) described CNS revenue-generating activities at their hospital in Columbia, South Carolina. They described relevant strategies for APNs as they creatively consider sources of funding for consultation services. They obtained third-party reimbursement for patient education and direct patient care. Other revenue was generated by selling instructional and informational tapes and books written and produced by CNSs. Notably, they also received substantial funding from grants.

Another strategy is bartering of services among APN colleagues. Members of the Sara Beth Harris Clinical Nurse Specialist Group (A. Spang, personal communication, fall 1994) described exchanging consultative services with a network of other providers. They had an informal understanding that consultation could be sought with reciprocal availability of consultees as consultants when the need arose in the future. APNs may also need to look to professional organizations for assistance in developing mechanisms to market and facilitate nursing consultation. Until the issues of financing and reimbursement in the health-care delivery system are resolved and include mechanisms to reimburse consultative activities, creative strategies for this activity will be the responsibility of the profession.

In addition to funding considerations, it is important to consider new settings and potential beneficiaries of advanced practice nursing consultation (see Chapter 21). When the APN is involved in collaborative relationships, clarification of the possibilities for consultation could be discussed and negotiated. The consultant's services could be made available to interdisciplinary teams—even teams of which the APN is a member. Interdisciplinary teams exist in many settings. In addition to working collaboratively on such teams, APNs can offer valuable consultative services. Staff nurses in these settings may be without the benefit of abundant resources to enhance practice and professional development. APNs could offer such opportunities through consultation.

When APNs are the primary providers of care, such as in nursing homes and community health centers, opportunities for consultation may be missed because the most common interactions are collaborative or co-managerial or because of time constraints. Yet in these settings the outcome of consultation is often improved patient care. APNs should consider documenting their consultations in somewhat standard and easily retrievable forms such as computerized databases. If such consultations were easy to access, their potential usefulness for research would be greatly enhanced, and the effectiveness of consultation could be studied.

As APNs move into innovative practices, they should determine which consultative services they will market and what types of APNs and other consultants are available and will be needed. Consultation between APNs offers the additional benefit of collegial networking. Certified registered nurse anesthetists are establishing private independent practices (see Chapter 17). As independent practitioners, they are offering their services in home health (particularly to assist in the respiratory care of patients who require ventilators), in pain clinics, and in obstetrical care settings. Consultation with other APNs in those settings, in addition to the direct care they offer, has the potential to enhance the knowledge and practice of APNs and creates co-management and collaborative possibilities for all of the APNs involved.

ISSUES IN APN CONSULTATION

Developing Consultation Skills in APN Students

For APNs to learn the theoretical and practical issues involved in the development of consultative abilities, relevant content must be included in graduate education curricula. Focusing on the theoretical issues in a seminar and engaging in a project as a clinical consultant were helpful for Barron in her graduate program and has been a strategy that some of her mental health CNS colleagues have described as part of their graduate programs. Development of consultative skill should ideally be considered during the educational process as role identity is beginning to be formed. Although this aspect of skill development may be more commonly part of CNS education, it is relevant for all advanced practice nursing graduate programs if APNs are to integrate the consultation competency into their practices.

Encouraging students to consider how the process of consultation differs from the direct care role and discussing the process and methods can be easily accomplished in a professional seminar. The students complete assigned readings ahead of time and engage in a faculty-led discussion of the process and issues. Course requirements should include a clinical consultation project. Students could approach individuals or organizations that might benefit in some way from the sharing of their area of expertise. They would negotiate a consultation issue to focus on and engage in a consultation. In previous experiences with this model, students were surprised by how well they were received and had a positive experience trying out these skills in a practical way. The entire focus on consultation was limited to two seminar discussions and the project, yet it was influential later in terms of position choice and role preparation. Judith A. Spross (personal communication, May 19, 1995) recommended having graduate advanced practice nursing students from different specialty areas consult one another. She allotted the first 20 minutes of the graduate role seminar she facilitated for APN students to consult with one another.

Students can also be asked to report on their observations of consultation in clinical settings. Students could reflect on the type of consultation offered, the skills demonstrated, the process in which they were engaged, the problem focus, and the outcome. Having students consider actual situations in which consultation evolved into co-management or referral provides faculty with an opportunity to explicate the differences in the terminology and implications of each type of interaction.

Graduate educators and APNs could collaborate on much-needed research to evaluate the effects of consultative activities on patient outcomes. Documentation of the value and cost-effectiveness of consultation could help to inform curricular decisions. It could also be presented by APNs to insurers and policymakers who determine policy and payment for health-care services. Gurka (1991) suggested that some research questions could emerge from analysis of one's own consultations. In an analysis of her own practice, there were three major outcomes of CNS consultation. The first was prevention of complications. The CNS was able to identify high-risk situations and intervene to prevent complications. The second was the maintenance of standards of care and the development of new standards. The CNS's consultation activities ensured that high-quality standards of care were consistently maintained. The third outcome she identified was improvement in staff nurses' clinical judgment skills. Students could be required to reflect on the outcomes of their consultation projects as an aspect of the assignment. Encouraging the process of reflection on practice, with a focus on outcomes of care, can help to build important practice "habits" with benefits to the students beyond acquisition of consultation skills.

Developing comfort with seeking, providing, and evaluating consultation is an important goal of advanced practice nursing graduate education. APNs are expected to influence patients, other providers, and the systems within which they work. Therefore when APNs graduate, they should be equipped with knowledge, skill, and confidence in the consultation process. Effective consultation, whether it is sought or provided, enables APNs to establish credibility and build collaborative relationships with other members of the health-care team.

Using Technology to Provide Consultation

The use of new technologies to enhance care delivery has affected every aspect of the health-care delivery system. APNs should review how consultation activities delivered through these new modalities can potentially enhance the capacity to affect care. Equally important is thoughtful consideration of the potential concerns that might arise in the embracing of these mechanisms to enhance patient care through consultation. In a recent review of literature, Roine, Ohinmaa, and Hailey (2001) critiqued more than 1000 studies and found little evidence to support positive outcomes or cost-effectiveness related to consultation activities using technology. No studies that reported outcomes occurring over time were found; however, examples of successful programs were reported anecdotally. Most of the studies documented the use and application of telemedicine but did not link use to outcome or cost savings. The most well studied telemedicine technologies were the submission of recent diagnostic studies in advance of a patient transfer to another facility, videoconferencing, electronic referrals with subsequent e-mail communication, and telepsychiatry with psychiatrists providing phone consultation.

Use of telemedicine in the treatment of patients with injuries related to trauma in rural areas was reported to be lifesaving in a recent study by Ricci et al. (2003). The authors analyzed 41 tele-trauma consults in a rural emergency department, and results of the study suggest that at least three lives were saved and overall enhancement of clinical care was considered improved. Death rates for patients involved in trauma in rural areas are reported at twice the rate of those in urban areas, justifying the continued study of such consultation activities in emergency settings.

Telenurse practice has been described in the literature, and some initial research has linked phone call follow-up to quality of care and patient outcomes. Larson-Dahn (2001) reported an analysis of quality indicators of telephone contact with patients and identified many of the complexities of providing care through the use of telephone contact. She identified such indicators as critical thinking, use of established protocols, and issues of continuity of care in her pilot study involving analysis of 10 telephone encounters for each of the five nurses recruited for her study. Patient outcomes were not measured but were recommended as a critical measure to be studied in the future. In addition, entrepreneurs in health care are designing business models around telephonic coaching of patients by nurses, although being an APN is not a requirement.

Risks involved in the application of telecommunication in health care have been highlighted by Ohler and Daine (2001). Security involving the use of e-mail was highlighted, with confidentiality being a major issue in the provision of care. The issues of miscommunication in reading or applying information obtained by means of an e-mail message were also addressed as a concern. Providing information through telecommunication across state lines raised concerns about liability and about differences in nurse practice acts regarding scope of practice. Ohler and Daine suggested that documentation guidelines and protocols be established for the application of any telecommunication and recommended further research on confidentiality and security issues in telehealth practice.

The application of technology in delivering health-related information has not been well studied in terms of process and outcomes. APNs should consider the potential opportunities that exist to enhance consultation activities with these modalities, but they should exercise caution regarding their implementation until future research elucidates specific processes, outcomes, and concerns.

Documentation and Legal Considerations

Although it has been stressed that the consultee remains clinically responsible for the patient who is the focus of the consultation, it is also critical to appreciate that APN consultants are also accountable for their practices relative to the consultation problem. Marie Snyder, RN, MS, JD (personal communication, June 14, 1995), described the overall responsibilities of the consultant as gathering accurate data about the consultation problem (or letting the consultee know that the data are incomplete), making reasonable recommendations, and giving good advice. She stressed that APN consultants who are working within the same organization as the consultees have a higher degree of accountability in relation to the patient care situations for which they are consulted than do consultants who come from outside the organization. APNs consulting within their own organizations would be expected to identify and follow through on urgent concerns and particularly problematic situations in ways that outside consultants would not be. APNs who are consulting should therefore know the organizational structure well and be certain that the advanced practice nursing consultation responsibilities are consistent with the overall job description of the APN. That is, if the job description required that APNs be in a line position of authority for a unit or a clinic (thereby being ultimately responsible for clinical care), for example, responsibility would constrain their ability to function as consultants as defined here. The hierarchical/supervisory relationship could interfere with the consultation process.

Kathleen Moore, RN, JD (personal communication, June 16, 1999) stressed that APNs be cognizant of their responsibility to adhere to the standard of practice for their specialty areas in all aspects of practice, including consultation. In terms of liability for consultation, Moore stated that an initial issue to be determined in the event of litigation would be whether a nurse-patient relationship exists in the consultation situation and thus invokes the duty of care. Although there are no clear-cut legal answers to the question of liability for consultation services, Moore emphasized the importance of the question as to whether a relationship exists between the clinician and the patient. In a court of law, whether a relationship exists would be a question of fact. If a relationship exists, then liability attaches. The likelihood of determining that a nurse-patient relationship exists increases when the consultant sees the patient directly, receives payment for the consultation, or becomes aware of gross negligence in clinical care.

When the APN consultant sees the patient directly, documentation of the consultation in the patient's record is appropriate and important. Ingersoll and Jones (1992) comprehensively described the elements of the consultation note. The consultant's assessment of the problem and recommendations for clinical problem solving should be clearly articulated in the documentation. When the patient is not seen directly, the consultant will want to decide whether it is appropriate to document the consultation in the patient's record. If the primary focus of the consultation is on education of the consultee in relation to the consultation problem, documentation in the patient's chart is not necessary. However, consultants should document all consultations in their own records, outlining the issues, the assessment data, and the recommendations (M. Snyder, personal communication, June 14, 1995). Such records provide important data. They enable APNs to make consultation visible and to analyze the nature, volume, and effects of consultation on patient care outcomes.

Snyder recommended documenting informal consultations (see the section on formal and informal consultation earlier in this chapter) only if they seem to raise particularly problematic situations (personal communication, June 14, 1995). The APN should keep in mind that an informal consultation may be inadequate in relation to the problem described. For example, there may not be enough assessment data to clearly identify the problem for the consultant, or the problem may be particularly complex or urgent. When that is the case, it is important to acknowledge the lack of sufficient information with the person seeking the informal consultation and recommend that a formal consultation be sought to consider the problem comprehensively. If the situation seems to be potentially urgent or emergent, the consultant should recommend the immediate initiation of an emergency consultation.

Kim Larkin, RN, JD (personal communication, June 18, 2003) stressed the importance of APN consultants clearly defining the consultation relationship. Consultants need to be clear when they do not see patients directly that they are not actually caring for the patient. When they do see patients directly, consultants need to be clear that they offer knowledge but that the practitioner requesting the consultation has the established duty to the patient and is ultimately responsible for assessments and recommendations. Larkin also emphasized the importance of nurse consultants understanding professional standards of practice, state regulations, nurse practice acts, and institutional policies as they relate to consultation because they would be used in a court of law to determine the elements of a malpractice claim (duty of care, standards, breach of standards, and damages), should the nurse consultant be sued. APNs also need to know when a consultation with a physician, rather than with another APN, would be considered as the standard of care. Lastly, Larkin cautioned that nurse consultants be aware of the Health Insurance Portability and Accountability Act (HIPAA) rules as they apply to consultations, especially informal consultations.

The increased responsibilities inherent in advanced practice nursing expose APNs to increased liability (Poteet, 1989; Scott & Beare, 1993; Survillo & Levine, 1993). Specialists may be held to a higher standard than generalists (Survillo & Levine, 1993). Thus APNs should be cognizant of legal issues in all areas of advanced practice nursing, including consultation.

Stepping Out of the Consultation Process

The APN must recognize that unusual circumstances could necessitate abandoning the consultation process and assuming the stance of clinically responsible expert (Barron, 1983, 1989). If the APN became aware that the patient being considered during the consultation was in a dangerous situation and the consultee was unable or unwilling to intervene on behalf of the patient, the consultant would then assume direct responsibility for ensuring that safety needs were addressed. It is unusual that consultees, once aware of safety concerns, are unable or unwilling to address them, but it does happen. Barron described such a circumstance (1989). She was consulted by the coronary care unit (CCU) nursing staff because of a patient's unwillingness to adhere to the safety guidelines of his care protocol. The patient had had a myocardial infarction 2 days earlier. It became apparent during the consultant's psychosocial assessment of the patient that he was delirious. Recognizing the potentially dangerous implications of the delirium, the consultant went directly to the intern (having discussed her plan with the consultee, who fully supported her direct action) to share her concern and to recommend that the cause of the delirium be evaluated. The intern and then the resident minimized the delirium and attributed the patient's symptoms to psychological distress. The consultant then initiated a psychiatric consultation by discussing her concerns with one of the psychiatrists on the consultation and liaison service and asked that he contact the attending CCU physician and offer psychiatric consultation. The psychiatrist consultant agreed with the liaison nurse consultant, and an investigation into the causes of the delirium revealed that the patient's digitalis level exceeded the therapeutic range. A potentially dangerous and correctable problem was identified.

Developing the Practice of Other Nurses

An outcome of nursing consultation, especially consultation over time, is to enhance the professional development and practice of nurse consultees. Consultation can clearly enhance the clinical knowledge and practice of nurses requesting consultation. One of the most satisfying aspects of the consultative process is to watch consultees master new skills and become more clinically expert.

A goal for consultation is to enable the consultee to manage future similar situations effectively. When the consultant and consultee evaluate the effectiveness of the consultation, they can recognize and reinforce helpful problem-solving strategies, which can then be applied in the future. As APNs engage in self-reflection and include staff in that reflection, they model a critical aspect of practice.

Evaluation of the consultation itself with the consultee is enormously important. It can enhance the learning and skill of both the consultee and the consultant. APNs can contribute to the development of other APNs in a meaningful way through the consultation process. APNs can also enhance their own professional development and practices by receiving nursing consultation.

Consultation Practice over Time

For APNs whose work includes substantial consultation, observations can be made about its evolution. Initially, consultants must market their services to potential consultees. Setting, niche identification, workload, and experience are all issues that contribute to the time and focus an APN may have for consultation efforts. For novice APNs, marketing may consist of demonstrating expertise and offering consultation services. Over time, staff and colleagues will recognize the APN's skill, and the APN may need to develop strategies to deal with large numbers of requests. Setting priorities and identifying alternative resources when the consultant's caseload is full are important activities as the consultation practice becomes more and more recognized and valued. Identifying other APNs who can consult on similar issues may be a useful strategy for balancing requests with availability.

Clarifying availability and the timing of responses to requests is essential if consultees are to continue to consider consultation as a helpful, timely option for assistance with complex clinical situations. Negotiating directly with the consultee at the time of the request (or shortly thereafter) allows the consultant to express to the consultee the importance and worth of the request, even if the consultant cannot meet the need directly. It also provides the opportunity to consider appropriate alternative resources to assist the consultee in addressing the clinical problem. The consultant must have established backup resources who are available to handle emergencies when the consultant is not available. Establishing such resources at the beginning of the consultant's practice is essential. Consultees should always know whom to contact in the event of a clinical emergency.

Over time, the number of consultee-centered requests may increase. After trust has been established with the consultant, the consultee may feel more comfortable and able to focus on specific problems in the clinical situation. The consultee may also feel more comfortable to focus on the needs of the patient. Over time, the consultee may be willing to examine lack of understanding, skill, or objectivity. Wonderful professional development can result from that level of self-examination, but trust usually needs to be firmly developed before such self-examination can take place with the consultant.

The consultant may find that the consultees' requests become more sophisticated over time. The consultee who often requested basic assistance with care may develop skill, understanding, and confidence with basic issues such that future requests for consultation reflect more expert levels of concern and understanding. Such requests may involve more complex or unusual situations and can be catalysts for the consultant's ongoing professional growth. Experiencing the development of the consultee's professional practice is exciting and satisfying.

Conversely, boredom with requests may be an issue for the established consultant. Particularly in settings where there is high turnover of staff, the consultant may focus time and time again on the same clinical concerns. Seeking support from a trusted colleague may help the consultant cope with frustration and avoid communicating frustration to consultees in inappropriate ways. Communicating a lack of interest with concerns presented by consultees is a sure way to derail both the specific consultation and the use of consultation as a means to address clinical problems. The consultant may also consider developing an educational program to address, in a different way, the needs commonly being expressed in consultation requests. If the problem is common, the consultant may also want to develop written guidelines, protocols, or care plans to share with consultees.

As the APN's consultation skills become widely appreciated in the system and in the community, the nature and types of consultation requests may change. Using different types of consultation, such as programmatic or administrative consultation, can be stimulating, and indeed APN consultants have much to contribute in these areas. APNs should be careful to consider the impact of such shifts, however, because such requests move them away from their original purposes. Such requests can lead to job restructuring or new positions, which may or may not be advanced practice roles. Initially, the request to move into new professional areas can be seductive. Furthermore, the shifts can be time and energy consuming, leading the APN away from direct practice and ultimately creating job dissatisfaction.

The message that skills and perspectives are valued and that new avenues are available for exploration is gratifying. Developing new ideas and plans can also be helpful to both the institution and the consultant. Recognizing the significance of new directions for consultees who have grown to rely on the consultant is critical. Planning with the consultees when such shifts occur can assure consultees that their concerns will continue to be considered even if the resource person changes temporarily or the response from the consultant is not going to be immediate.

EVALUATION OF THE CONSULTATION COMPETENCY

APNs evaluate individual consultations as the final step of the consultation process. Overall evaluation of the consultative process and skills is also important. Barron (1989) discussed both aspects of evaluation. APNs should consider strategies that will help them to determine their overall effectiveness (see Chapter 25) and their specific effectiveness in relation to consultation. Data may be obtained from consultees, peers, administrators, review of the APN's documentation of consults, and the APN's self-evaluation.

Practices of individual APNs will vary considerably as to what questions and criteria are considered relevant to evaluation of consultation skills. (See Chapter 25 for a comprehensive discussion of evaluation of advanced practice nursing.) Some questions that may be useful in eliciting data regarding consultation have been suggested by Lewis and Levy (1982) and Barron (1989). Is the consultant re-contacted after the initial consultation? Are consultation requests becoming more sophisticated over time (Lewis & Levy, 1982)? Was the APN able to respond to all requests for consultation? Do glaring issues or needs seem to be going unaddressed? Do there seem to be patterns in terms of the theme, number, or location of consultations (Barron, 1989)?

The subjective experiences of the consultant are also important (Barron, 1989). Sensing openness and enthusiasm on the part of consultees can provide the APN with data. However, sensing resistance or unwillingness to implement consultation recommendations can also provide data. One would not want to rely solely on subjective data, but the feelings of the consultant can yield important information.

Clinical competency, competency in applying the consultation process, interpersonal skills, and professionalism are all areas to be considered in the evaluation process. Identifying the appropriate people to be involved in the evaluation and developing a systematic approach to data collection regarding the consultation aspects of an APN's practice are important. Evaluation can guide the APN's individual professional growth and can ultimately validate the need for the APN's service and skill in the specific work setting and beyond.

SUMMARY

APNs have had a long tradition of being involved in various aspects of direct and indirect patient care activities, including consultation. Consultation has the potential to influence patient care directly and beyond the direct care encounter. The power of consultative activities to inform and advance practice compels all APNs to consider consultation as an integral aspect of role performance. Consultation offers APNs the opportunity to both share and acquire the clinical expertise necessary to meet the increasingly challenging and diverse demands of patient care. This chapter has defined consultation; identified various types of consultation; and distinguished consultation from co-management, referral, and supervision. We have offered an ecological model of the APN consultation competency and have highlighted issues related to implementation of the consultative process. We encourage the reader to apply the model in practice and welcome input from APNs in all roles with regard to its utility. It remains imperative that the term *consultation* be used appropriately and that APNs participate in further defining this competency and understanding its impact on care processes and patient outcomes. We have attempted to clarify the concept of consultation because conceptual clarity will enhance its appropriate use in practice and in the literature.

We believe that APN consultation contributes to positive patient outcomes and may promote more appropriate use of scarce health-care resources. These assumptions must be tested through quality improvement studies, cost-benefit studies, and research that examines the processes and outcomes of care. Outcomes of consultation activities can then be effectively measured. Ongoing discussion regarding this important topic will assist in the much-needed clarification of the other terms used to characterize relationships with other professionals. APNs can contribute to this discussion, as well as to the research, by sharing their experiences as both recipients and providers of consultation. We believe that consultation by and for APNs in all settings can enhance and extend quality nursing care and improve outcomes of care. Consultation can facilitate having comprehensive and specialty-related knowledge available to all patients who might need it and therefore should be an expected and integral aspect of APN role performance.

REFERENCES

American College of Nurse-Midwives. (1992). *Clinical practice statement: Collaborative management in nurse-midwifery practice for medical, gynecological and obstetrical conditions.* Washington, DC: Author.

American College of Nurse-Midwives. (1997). *Position statement: Clinical practice statement: Collaborative management in nurse-midwifery practice for medical, gynecological and obstetrical condi-* tions. Retrieved June 9, 2003, from http://www.midwife.org

Barron, A. M. (1983). The clinical nurse specialist as consultant. In A. B. Hamric & J. A. Spross (Eds.), *The clinical nurse specialist in theory and practice* (pp. 91-113). New York: Grune & Stratton.

Barron A. M. (1989). The clinical nurse specialist as consultant. In A. B. Hamric & J. A. Spross (Eds.),

The clinical nurse specialist in theory and practice (2nd ed., pp. 125-146). Philadelphia: W. B. Saunders.

Barron, A. M., & White, P. (1996). Consultation. In A. B. Hamric, J. A. Spross, & C. M. Hanson (Eds.), *Advanced nursing practice: An integrative approach* (pp. 165-183). Philadelphia: W. B. Saunders.

Barron, A. M., & White, P. (2000). Consultation. In A. B. Hamric, J. A. Spross, & C. M. Hanson (Eds.), *Advanced nursing practice: An integrative approach* (2nd ed., pp. 217-243). Philadelphia: W. B. Saunders.

Birkholz, G., & Walker, D. (1994). Strategies for state statutory language changes granting fully independent nurse practitioner practice. *Nurse Practitioner, 19,* 54-58.

Boyd, J. N., Stasiowski, S. A., Catoe, P. T., Wells, P. R., Stahl, B. M., Judson, E., et al. (1991). The merit and significance of clinical nurse specialists. *Journal of Nursing Administration, 21,* 35-43.

Caplan, G. (1970). *The theory and practice of mental health consultation.* New York: Basic Books.

Caplan, G., & Caplan, R. (1993). *Mental health consultation and collaboration.* San Francisco: Jossey-Bass.

Colman, N. S. (1992). Variability in consultation rates and practitioner level of diagnostic certainty. *Journal of Family Practice, 35,* 31-38.

Critchley, D. L. (1985). Clinical supervision. In D. L. Critchley & J. T. Maurin (Eds.), *The clinical specialist in psychiatric mental health nursing* (pp. 495-510). New York: John Wiley & Sons.

Faut-Callahan, M., & Kremer, M. (2000). The certified registered nurse-anesthetist. In A. B. Hamric, J. A. Spross, & C. M. Hanson (Eds.), *Advanced nursing practice: An integrative approach* (2nd ed., pp. 521-548). Philadelphia: W. B. Saunders.

Forsyth, D., Rhudy, L. & Johnson, L. (2002). The consultation role of a nurse educator. *Journal of Continuing Education in Nursing, 33,* 197-204.

Gurka, A. M. (1991). Process and outcome components of clinical nurse specialist consultation. *Dimensions of Critical Care Nursing, 10,* 169-175.

Hanson, C. M., & Spross, J. A. (1996). Collaboration. In A. B. Hamric, J. A. Spross, & C. M. Hanson (Eds.), *Advanced practice nursing: An integrative approach* (pp. 229-248). Philadelphia: W. B. Saunders.

Hanson, C. M., Spross, J. A., & Carr, D. B. (2000). Collaboration. In A. B. Hamric, J. A. Spross, & C. M. Hanson (Eds.), *Advanced practice nursing: An integrative approach* (2nd ed., pp. 315-347). Philadelphia: W. B. Saunders.

Ingersoll, G., & Jones, L. (1992). The art of the consultation note. *Clinical Nurse Specialist, 6,* 218-220.

Larson-Dahn, M. (2001). Tele-Nurse practice: Quality of care and patient outcomes. *Journal of Nursing Administration, 31,* 145-152. Retrieved May 22, 2003, from http://www.80-gateway2.ovid. com)

Lewis, A., & Levy, J. (1982). *Psychiatric liaison nursing: The theory and clinical practice.* Reston, VA: Reston.

Lipowski, Z. J. (1974). Consultation-liaison psychiatry: An overview. *American Journal of Psychiatry, 131,* 623-630.

Lipowski, Z. J. (1981). Liaison psychiatry, liaison nursing and behavioral medicine. *Comprehensive Psychiatry, 22,* 554-561.

Lipowski, Z. J. (1983). Current trends in consultation-liaison psychiatry. *Canadian Journal of Psychiatry, 28,* 329-338.

Mahn, V. A., & Zazworsky, D. J. (2000). The advanced practice nurse case manager. In A. B. Hamric, J. A. Spross, & C. M. Hanson, *Advanced nursing practice: An integrative approach* (2nd ed.). Philadelphia: W. B. Saunders.

Manley, K. (1998). A conceptual framework for advanced practice: An action research project operationalizing an advanced practitioner/consultant role. In G. Rolfe & P. Fulbrook (Eds.), *Advanced nursing practice* (pp. 118-135). Boston: Butterworth Heinemann.

Minarik, P., & Price, L. (1999). Collaboration? Supervision? Direction? Independence? What is the relationship between the advanced practice nurse and the physician? States legislative and regulatory reform III. *Clinical Nurse Specialist, 13,* 34-37.

Monicken, D. R. (1995). Consultation in advanced practice nursing. In M. Snyder & M. Mirr (Eds.), *Advanced practice nursing* (pp. 183-195). New York: Springer-Verlag.

National Association of Clinical Nurse Specialists. (2004). *Statement on clinical nurse specialist education and practice* (2nd ed.) Harrisburg, PA: Author.

Norwood, S. L. (1998). When the CNS needs a consultant. *Clinical Nurse Specialist, 12,* 53-58.

Ohler, L., & Daine, V. (2001). Potential telecommunication risks: Cautions and suggestions for the team. *Progress in Cardiovascular Nursing, 16,* 172-176. Retrieved May 22, 2003, from http://www.0-prpquest.umi.com

Poteet, G. W. (1989). Consultation. *Clinical Nurse Specialist, 3,* 41.

Ricci, M., Cauto, M., Amour, M., Rogers, F., Sartorelli, K., Callas, P., et al. (2003). Telemedicine reduces discrepancies in rural trauma care. *Telemedicine Journal and e-Health, 9,* 3-11.

Roine, R., Ohinmaa, A., & Hailey, D. (2001). Assessing telemedicine: A systematic review of the literature. *Canadian Medical Association, 165,* 765-773.

Sabatier, K. (2002). The Institute for Johns Hopkins Nursing: A collaborative model for nursing practice. *Nursing Education Perspective, 23,* 178-182.

Safriet, B. J. (1992). Health care dollars and regulatory sense: The role of advanced practice nursing (special issue). *Yale Journal on Regulation, 9,* 417-488.

Scott, L., & Beare, P. (1993). Nurse consultant and professional liability. *Clinical Nurse Specialist, 7*, 331-334.

Sebus, M. (1994). Developing a collaborative practice agreement for the primary care setting. *Nurse Practitioner, 19*, 44-51.

Skalla, K., & Hamric, A. (2000). The blended role of the clinical nurse specialist and the nurse practitioner. In A. B. Hamric, J. A. Spross, & C. M. Hanson (Eds.), *Advanced nursing practice: An integrative approach* (2nd ed., pp. 459-490). Philadelphia: W. B. Saunders.

Simmons, M. K. (1985). Psychiatric consultation and liaison. In D. L. Critchley & J. T. Maurin (Eds.), *The clinical specialist in psychiatric mental health nursing* (pp. 362-381). New York: John Wiley & Sons.

Spross, J. A. (1989). The clinical nurse specialist as collaborator. In A. B. Hamric & J. A. Spross (Eds.), *The clinical nurse specialist in theory and practice* (2nd ed., pp. 205-226). Philadelphia: W. B. Saunders.

Stichler, J. (2002). The nurse as consultant. *Nursing Administration Quarterly, 26*, 52-68.

Survillo, A. I., & Levine, A. T. (1993). Strategies to limit CNS malpractice liability exposure. *Clinical Nurse Specialist, 7*, 215-220.

CHAPTER 8

Research

JUDITH A. DePALMA • DEBORAH B. McGUIRE

INTRODUCTION

CURRENT TRENDS
 Variable Quality of Care and Efforts to Improve It
 Scientific and Technological Advances
 The Increasing Uninsured Population and Increasing Consumer Financial Burden
  for Health Care
 The Nursing Shortage
 Interrelationships among Research Competencies and Trends

COMPETENCY I: INTERPRETATION AND USE OF RESEARCH IN PRACTICE
 Evidence-Based Practice
 Fundamental and Expanded Levels of Research Competency I
 Phases of Competency I

COMPETENCY II: EVALUATION OF PRACTICE
 Identifying Key Goals/Desired Outcomes of Practice
 Ensuring Collection of Appropriate and Accurate Data
 Comparing Data with Internal and External Benchmarks
 Changing Practice Based on Evaluation Results

COMPETENCY III: PARTICIPATION IN COLLABORATIVE RESEARCH

ACQUIRING AND DEVELOPING RESEARCH COMPETENCIES
 Graduate Education
 Postgraduate Research Development

SUMMARY AND CONCLUSION

INTRODUCTION

The role of "researcher" has long been considered integral to the practice of clinical nurse specialists (CNSs) (Hamric & Spross, 1989; Hodgman, 1983; McGuire & Harwood, 1989) and reflects the critical contribution they have made to nursing knowledge and to scientifically based practice. With the emergence of professional consensus on the definition, preparation, and practice of the advanced practice nurse (APN) (Cronenwett, 1995; Hamric, 1996, 2000; American Association of Colleges of Nursing [AACN], 1996, 1999; National Association of Clinical Nurse Specialists, 2004), the "research role" is now considered a "core competency" for APNs (McGuire & Harwood, 1996, 2000; see Chapter 3). More important, the requirement for evidence-based outcomes as a basis for competent and reimbursable advanced practice nursing makes this competency a critical component of advanced practice nursing education and practice.

The purpose of this chapter is to describe an updated set of three individual competencies that comprise the core advanced practice nursing research competence (described in Chapter 3). These competencies are (1) interpretation and use of research in practice, (2) evaluation of practice, and (3) participation in collaborative research (Table 8-1). These research competencies are presented on two levels. The *fundamental level* includes activities that are reasonable to expect at graduation from a master's program in nursing (e.g., appraising scientific literature as a step to incorporating research findings in the nurse's own practice), and the expanded level consists of activities that are acquired through experience and individual initiative in the advanced practice nursing role (e.g., developing institutional mechanisms for implementing evidence-based practice [EBP]).

Documents published by professional and federal organizations provide definitive support for research competence within the advanced practice nursing role (see role chapters in section III). A position statement by the AACN (2002) indicates that master's degree

TABLE 8-1	OVERVIEW OF RESEARCH COMPETENCIES AND LEVELS	
COMPETENCY	FUNDAMENTAL LEVEL	EXPANDED LEVEL
I. Interpretation and use of research in practice	Use an EBP process to incorporate research into one's individual practice and assist others to incorporate research into their individual practices.	Develop EBP process at the unit, program, department, or organization level to incorporate research into practice.
II. Evaluation of practice	Design and implement a process to evaluate relevant outcomes of the individual's advanced practice nursing.	Design and implement a process to evaluate relevant outcomes of basic or advanced practice nursing at a group (e.g., group of APNs, clinic, or unit) or system (e.g., program, department) level. *(Please note: This is not the same thing as traditional "outcomes research.")*
III. Participation in collaborative research	Function as a clinical expert/ consultant in a collaborative knowledge-generating research project.	Function as an investigator or co-investigator in a collaborative knowledge-generating research project.

APNs, Advanced practice nurses; *EBP,* evidence-based practice.

programs should " . . . prepare nurses to critique research and to implement changes in practice based on research data. Their (nurses) leadership skills enable them to form teams of professionals, and to initiate and evaluate new practice policies and programs within their agencies and professional groups" (p. 2). And further, the AACN notes that master's prepared nurses ". . . identify practice and systems problems that need to be studied and collaborate with other scientists to generate new studies based on their expertise" (2002, p. 2). A document describing nurse practitioner (NP) competencies, developed by the National Organization of Nurse Practitioner Faculties (NONPF) and AACN, notes that NPs manage a patient's illness using "an action plan based on scientific rationale, evidence-based standards of care and practice guidelines" (NONPF & AACN, 2002, p. 42). Other NP practice competencies that are consistent with research competence are those that call for monitoring and ensuring quality health care by using an "evidence-based approach to patient management that critically evaluates and applies research findings pertinent to patient care management and outcomes" and monitoring "quality of own practice" and practicing "continuous quality improvement based on professional practice standards and relevant statutes and regulation" (NONPF & AACN, 2002, p. 47).

These research competencies need to become a major focus in academic programs, individual advanced practice nursing, and administrative planning and implementation of advanced practice nursing positions across clinical settings. The activities described in the AACN position statement—critiquing and using research in practice, evaluating practices and programs, and identifying researchable problems and collaborating in research to address them—require specific knowledge and skills related to the conduct and utilization of research. Thus these research competencies must be clearly defined and feasible to teach within the context of typical advanced practice nursing curricula. Moreover, they must be flexible enough to meet the needs of all types of APNs in a wide variety of settings.

As the review in the preceding section suggests, research competencies are integral to advanced practice nursing and quality care. In addition, APNs are commonly viewed as key links between research and the patient when they function as direct care providers and between research and other providers of care when they function in programmatic or leadership positions.

Although the three research competencies that are proposed for APNs are outlined as individual entities, in reality there is overlap across all three competencies. Focusing on EBP (Competency I) and evaluating an individual's practice (Competency II) are based on best available evidence, and therefore experience and proficiency in Competency III strengthen APNs' ability to assess evidence and interpret data.

Some other examples of such overlap include the following:

1. In the final step of Competency I, when the outcomes of the EBP change are being evaluated, the conclusion may be that further change is required, possibly with a subset of the patient population or the management of a particular symptom, but evidence may not be sufficient to guide the additional change. Therefore an actual research study would be needed (Competency III).
2. The same decision may be made when outcomes of practice are evaluated (Competency II). If a significant difference in outcomes is obvious when compared with the benchmarks, further study may be needed to determine the reason for the difference or to determine why certain patient groups are experiencing different outcomes from the same treatment.
3. Evaluating the value of advanced practice naturally leads to further questioning about what particular aspects of care make a difference, but accomplishment of this

next step requires a good knowledge of the formal research process (Competency III). An example is assessment of the relationship between a particular intervention or the timing of an intervention and desirable outcome variables such as prevention of readmission, decreased complications, or improved functional status.

4. When evidence is sought to answer clinical questions (Competency I), a dearth of published research studies may lead to a decision to replicate one of the few studies available or to design a new study to determine the effectiveness of a proposed intervention (Competency III).

In this chapter, current health-care trends that support the importance of and critical need for advanced practice nursing research competencies are briefly discussed, and the three competencies are presented in tables that outline the phases or steps in the specific competency, the knowledge required, and the key activities inherent in each phase. The corresponding narrative for each phase within the competency provides a concrete description of the competency with examples.

The tables can be used in a variety of ways, depending on the perspective of the user. APNs can use the tables as an outline of steps in an appropriate project or as professional development checklists to determine whether they have acquired the needed knowledge from their formal education programs and experience. Nurses considering graduate programs can use them as a basis for comparing programs or as discussion points during entrance interviews. Educators can use the knowledge and activities in the tables when they design courses to support research competence in graduate programs. Managers can use the knowledge and skills for a given competency as the basis for a checklist in a performance evaluation or, during the interview process, to determine the readiness of an applicant for an advanced practice nursing role. The latter portion of the chapter provides recommendations for academic curricula and teaching strategies to assist faculty in the development of the fundamental competencies during graduate education and mechanisms for enabling APNs to develop expanded levels of the research competencies after graduate school. Examples of using and teaching the competencies are presented so that both students and faculty may see how they can be operationalized.

CURRENT TRENDS

Current trends in health-care delivery dramatically affect how and where APNs practice, as well as the demands placed on them. Moreover, such trends support the need for research competence within the advanced practice nursing role. Trends addressed in the report, *Crossing the Quality Chasm,* by the Institute of Medicine (IOM) (2001) include variable quality of care and efforts to improve it; scientific and technological advances; the increasing uninsured population and rising consumer financial burden for health care; and the current nursing shortage. These trends are briefly described in the following sections, followed by a discussion of interrelationships among the trends and advanced practice nursing research competencies.

Variable Quality of Care and Efforts to Improve It

The health-care delivery system needs to be redesigned to improve patient safety and quality of care. Health-care leaders must focus attention on identifying the types of changes that will ensure well-designed care processes and contribute to safe, effective care

(Richardson & Corrigan, 2003). Health care has not always tracked or rewarded quality, but recently, numerous health-care report cards have been published that facilitate the comparison of the quality of care across providers (Mehrotra, Bodenheimer, & Dudley, 2003).

The IOM (2001) has recommended a partnership with the U.S. Department of Health and Human Services and professional and health-care associations interested in quality to develop a program that supports clinicians' evidence-based decision making. According to the IOM's report (2001), six aims on which to base quality improvement goals are safety, effectiveness (services based on scientific knowledge), timeliness, efficiency, equitable access and treatment, and a patient-centered emphasis. In partial response to these recommendations, various accrediting and regulating agencies have integrated quality measurement into their expectations. Examples include the ORYX initiative of the Joint Commission on Accreditation for Healthcare Organizations (JCAHO) (2003b), the National Committee for Quality Assurance's Health Plan Report Card (2000), and Medicare's Quality Initiatives with quality indicators by type of provider (Jencks, Huff, & Cuerdon, 2003).

Scientific and Technological Advances

New roles and opportunities exist for telehealth practitioners who consult electronically (Masys, 2002). Such innovative video-interactive patient-provider encounters offer effective and satisfying health care to underserved populations (Connors, 2002). Electronically entered, stored, transported, and accessed information has the potential to improve the quality of care, increase the efficiency of clinical practice, and reduce human error (Masys, 2002). Electronic data allow for trending of quality improvement processes and clinical outcomes, and therefore, the evaluation of practice by both the individual practitioner and the total organization.

Another important advance is the quantity of online resources that exist to support evidence-based care and evaluation of practice. Practice guidelines, benchmark data, quality indicators, bibliographical databases, online journals, and online reports from accrediting and regulatory agencies are all available to APNs through the Internet.

The Increasing Uninsured Population and Increasing Consumer Financial Burden for Health Care

The number of people with no health insurance coverage in 2002 rose to 43.6 million, reflecting an increase of 2.4 million (0.6%) (Mills & Bhandari, 2003). Some of this increase can be explained by the continued economic downturn and rising unemployment. People who left jobs involuntarily had a 25% higher rate of being uninsured (Kapur & Marquis, 2003). The Health and Retirement Study indicated that average annual out-of-pocket spending for the elderly or near elderly was $2022 in 1998, with those having employer supplements or Medicare managed care plans spending less than those with only traditional Medicare (Goldman & Zissimopoulos, 2003). Since 2000, the trend has been to decrease benefits and increase the copayments for pharmaceuticals and physician visits (Goldman & Zissimopoulos, 2003).

It is projected that personal health-care spending will decrease from 7.9% in 2001 to 6.1% in 2012. However, the health-care share of the nation's gross domestic product is projected to increase from 14.1% in 2001 to 17.7% in 2012, indicating where the cost shift will occur (Heffler et al., 2003).

The Nursing Shortage

Estimates from the Bureau of Health Professions of the U.S. Department of Health and Human Services documented a national shortage of 110,700 full-time registered nurses (RNs) in 2000. Retirement of baby-boomer nurses is projected to create 331,000 RN vacancies between 1998 and 2008 (Sochalski, 2002). According to a Health Resources and Services Administration report (2002), in 2000, 30 states were estimated to have shortages of RNs. The shortage is projected to intensify over the next 2 decades, and 44 states plus the District of Columbia are expected to have RN shortages by the year 2020. Nursing schools turned away 5283 qualified applicants across the United States in 2002 because of budget constraints and insufficient faculty, clinical sites, classroom space, and clinical preceptors. Almost two thirds (62%) of the nursing schools that responded to the 2002 survey pointed to faculty shortages as a reason for not accepting all qualified applicants into entry-level baccalaureate programs (AACN, 2003).

Evidence that the shortage of nurses contributes to decreased patient safety and negative clinical outcomes has been documented (Aiken, Clarke, Sloane, Sochalski, & Silber, 2002; Blendon et al., 2002; JCAHO, 2002, 2003a; Needleman, Buerhaus, Mattke, Stewart, & Zelevinsky, 2002).

Interrelationships among Research Competencies and Trends

The trends described previously demonstrate the need for the research competencies and how they might affect the competencies implemented by APNs. Each competency is presented as it interrelates to one or more of the trends: quality of care, scientific and technological advances, uninsured population, and the nursing shortage.

- Competency I: The interpretation and use of the best current evidence should be used to justify and develop any proposed new approaches to care, whether those approaches are based on new technologies initiated to meet the six improvement aims identified by the IOM, or designed to meet the needs of the medically uninsured. Implementing evidence-based care should make the IOM's six improvement aims feasible to accomplish. Because unnecessary services and treatments can do harm and offer no benefits, ethical principles dictate that clinicians avoid recommending or prescribing treatment that is of uncertain benefit (IOM, 2001). Evidence-based care is known to make a difference in patient outcomes; APNs' research competencies, especially those that foster the adoption of EBP, are even more important in the face of clinician workforce shortages.
- Competency II: The evaluation of practice will be a critical competency for the new advanced practice nursing roles that result from the nursing shortage or new technologies. Expectations of accrediting and regulatory agencies can be met by means of appropriate data collection and evaluation of practice—specifically in terms of cost-effectiveness, quality indicators, and nursing sensitive outcomes. Data included in health-care report cards dictate the types of quality data organizations must collect and should be included in any evaluation of advanced practice nursing. Online access to benchmarks, quality indicators, practice guidelines, and clinical databases facilitates this evaluation of practice.
- Competency III: Formal research projects are often needed when sufficient evidence does not exist to guide practice, to determine the effect of new technological approaches to care, to evaluate new advanced practice nursing roles, or to address

the nursing shortage in specific settings. Other areas in which formal research projects are needed include determination of the most effective care delivery models for the growing number of uninsured and examination of decision-making approaches used by the elderly related to out-of-pocket expenses, especially the cost of medications, and the impact of these decisions on outcomes.

COMPETENCY I: INTERPRETATION AND USE OF RESEARCH IN PRACTICE

Before Competency I is discussed in detail, it is necessary to address the process that is integral to this competency: EBP.

Evidence-Based Practice

The research role for master's-prepared nurses initially focused on the conduct of research, exemplified by numerous graduate programs that taught the research process and required formal, original research theses for graduation. As doctoral education developed and the American Nurses Association (1981, 1996) recommended specific research roles for graduate nurses prepared in various academic programs, the research role of the master's-prepared nurse became focused on use of research findings in practice (McGuire & Harwood, 1989), commonly referred to at that time as *research utilization* (RU) (Stetler, 1985). RU has been defined broadly as "basing the practice, education, and management of nursing on research findings" (Stetler, 1985, p. 40). Most definitions of this process only mention nursing practice (Stevens & Cassidy, 1999). The RU models and projects that were initiated in the 1970s (Stetler & Marram, 1976; Dracup & Breu, 1977; Conway, 1978; Horsley, Crane, & Bingle, 1978; Krueger, 1978) paved the way for EBP and are often cited by other health-care disciplines.

The term *evidence-based* was coined at McMaster University Medical School in Canada to describe a teaching-learning strategy designed to shape clinical decision making (Evidence-Based Medicine Working Group, 1992; Guyatt & Rennie, 2002; Sackett, Straus, Richardson, Rosenberg, & Haynes, 2000). The definition of Sackett and his colleagues (1997) is often considered a classic for medicine and consists of three primary factors: (1) best research evidence, (2) applied with clinical expertise, and (3) applied with an appreciation of the patient's values and expectations. Despite Sackett's definition, the primary emphasis of evidence-based medicine (EBM) has continued to be on use of medical research with little discussion of clinical expertise or adaptation for individual patient values and expectations.

The term *evidence-based practice* (EBP) has evolved from EBM and acknowledges the interdisciplinary nature of health care, of which medical care is a part. EBP has been defined in a variety of ways, including the following.

- White (1997) defined it as a method of problem solving that involves identifying a clinical problem, searching the literature, evaluating the research evidence, and deciding on the intervention.
- Brown (1999) defined research-based practice as "health care practitioners' considered use of research findings and collective research evidence to shape general approaches to care, specific courses of action and recommendations made to individual patients" (p. 4).

- On the Academic Center of Evidence-Based Nursing website (www.acestar.uth-scsa.edu/Goals/terminolgy1325.html), it is defined as "A process of finding, apprais-ing and applying scientific evidence to the treatment and management of health care. EBP is the discovery of underlying trends and principles developed from the accumulation and refinement of a large body of studies. The processes of EBP create new, state of the science knowledge, summarized and clarified for translation into best practice for clinical policy" (Ledbetter & Stevens, 2000).

Two points of discussion that surface in the literature are (1) the differences between RU and EBP (Brown, 1999; Jennings & Loan, 2001; McGuire & Harwood, 2000) and (2) the definitions of EBM, evidence-based nursing, and EBP (Jennings & Loan, 2001). Both RU and EBP are forms of knowledge utilization (Hunt, 2002), but EBP is more than RU (Jennings & Loan, 2001). EBP is considered a total process, beginning with knowing what clinical question to ask, knowing how to find the best current evidence—which may or may not be research—and knowing how to critically appraise the evidence for validity and applicability to the particular care situation. The best evidence is then applied by the clinician and influenced by the clinician's knowledge drawn from experience and the inter-pretation of the needs and perspectives of the patient. The final aspect of the process is an evaluation of the effectiveness of care after implementation of the practice change and the continual improvement of the process from both the caregiver's and patient's perspectives (Pearson & Craig, 2002; DePalma, 2000; Goode & Piedalue, 1999; White, 1997).

Key differences in the definitions of EBM, evidence-based nursing, and EBP are (1) the range or levels of evidence that are inherent in each, that is, whether evidence other than results of research or randomized controlled trials (RCTs) is included and (2) whether any mention is made of patients and clinical expertise of the health-care provider in the defi-nition or the discussion of the scope of the term. To define evidence is really to indicate the levels of evidence that are deemed acceptable by an individual or group involved in the process of EBP. Levels or hierarchies of evidence identify types of evidence and rank-order them according to credibility or strength. Levels or hierarchies of evidence differ in the scope of evidence included, with some primarily limited to research methodologies (Ball et al., 2001; Guyatt et al, 2000; Hadorn, Baker, Hodges, & Hicks, 1995; Harris et al., 2001). Some evidence hierarchies rank-order the evidence on the basis of research design alone. Other hierarchies include nonresearch evidence such as quality or risk data, clini-cal experience, and expert opinion (Goode, 2000; Rutledge & Grant, 2002; Stetler et al., 1998). The RCT methodology is considered the "gold standard" of research and is usually high in any hierarchy. Unfortunately, not all research areas have RCTs, and in fact, some areas of study are not appropriate for RCTs. Rutledge and Grant's (2002) hierarchy of evi-dence differs from some other levels of evidence because it includes all types of research designs, systematic reviews, and nonresearch or practice-based evidence such as bench-mark, quality, risk, and infection control data.

Nursing's broader view of evidence may be due to its tradition of using a variety of research methods, necessitated by "the concepts and situations that constitute the phe-nomena of interest to the nursing profession" (Pravikoff & Donaldson, 2001, p. 589). Because nursing involves a wide range of interventions and a perspective of care that focuses on the individual patient's experience with a disease or symptom, nurses draw on a diverse evidence base. This diverse evidence base spans the medical sciences, including the behavioral and social sciences, but also extends to public health, wellness, communi-cations, and organizational change and management evidence (Pearson & Craig, 2002).

EBP is a natural process for the inquiring nurse who wants to provide the highest qual-ity, cost-effective care; however, adopting an evidence-based approach to practice is a time-consuming and resource-intensive process. Practice settings that value the use of new knowledge are most likely to provide resources for access and application of that new knowledge (Rosswurm & Larrabee, 1999). Advantages of adopting an evidence-based approach to practice exist from administrative, regulatory, and legal perspectives. The importance of EBP is evident in the new requirements from regulatory and accrediting agencies, such as the JCAHO Core Measures phase of the ORYX initiative requirement, which fosters use of evidence-based performance measures in health-care settings (JCAHO, 2003b). The National Quality Forum—a private, not-for-profit membership organization created to develop and implement a national strategy for health-care quality measurement and reporting (www.qualityforum.org/)—endorses most of the JCAHO's core measures.

EBP has a rationale that can be stated and a credibility that is needed in the present health-care environment when there is no time to administer care that does not make a difference. APNs are the ideal facilitators of EBP in any clinical setting because they possess the necessary clinical expertise; have an awareness of patient, family, and health-care provider needs; and know the system well enough to be able to negotiate for both the basic process and the resultant practice changes.

Fundamental and Expanded Levels of Research Competency I

Adopting an evidence-based foundation for practice can be actualized on several levels within any clinical setting. First, APNs should internalize the use of evidence as a value and make an individual commitment to practice in this manner through learning about it during graduate school. APNs can demonstrate the fundamental level of this competency by fostering EBP when they function as preceptors or begin a journal club with colleagues. APNs can demonstrate the expanded level of competency I when they develop and promote system changes based on evidence and advocate for the proper environment and resources to support EBP in a particular clinical setting or organization. This level of promoting EBP may occur in a clinical inpatient unit or outpatient clinic to which the APN is assigned; it may be done by a group of APNs employed in a particular setting; or it may be an initiative that involves the entire department of nursing or a total clinical organization. For example, a certified nurse-midwife (CNM) might distribute the Maternity Center Association's guidelines on pain management during childbirth (www.maternitywise.org/pdfs/laborpainexecsum.pdf) within a birthing center to nursing and medical colleagues as a means of evaluating current practices and determining whether changes are needed to improve the standard of care. If a group of colleagues agrees that change is needed, they might decide to begin by developing an interdisciplinary critical pathway to ensure timely and effective use of pharmacological and nonpharmacological measures throughout the delivery.

Phases of Competency I

EBP at any level of commitment requires a particular knowledge base and a set of core skills. There are numerous models of EBP (Brown 1999; Guyatt et al, 2000; Rosswurm & Larrabee, 1999; Rutledge et al., 2001; Stetler et al., 1998; Titler, Mentes, Rakel, Abbott, & Baumler, 1998), but they all contain similar phases or steps. The phases of the EBP process begin with understanding the clinical issues and being able to state a researchable problem or clinical question succinctly; followed by finding, evaluating, and synthesizing evidence; and finally implementing appropriate practice changes and evaluating those changes.

The clinical expertise of the APN is critical in the phases of the competency that require an understanding of clinical care issues and processes within a particular clinical system. Table 8-2 lists the phases of Competency I and the knowledge and activities appropriate to each. Each phase of the competency is discussed.

TABLE 8-2	COMPETENCY I: INTERPRETATION AND USE OF RESEARCH IN PRACTICE	
PHASE	**KNOWLEDGE/SKILLS**	**ACTIVITIES**
1. Stating the problem/ clinical question	• Critical thinking skills • Team-building skills • Ability to prioritize clinical issues • Ability to guide a discussion toward the development of a problem statement/clinical question with key words that can focus the evidence search • Ability to locate and interpret internal data to validly describe current practice	• Facilitate collaborative brainstorming with all stakeholders to list and prioritize clinical issues • Determine the status of current practice • Write a detailed problem statement with key words that can be searched
2. Searching for and retrieving evidence	• Understanding the continuum of evidence, especially research sources and evidence-based guidelines • Ability to do or direct a computerized search for evidence • Ability to rephrase or focus the problem statement or clinical question when problems with the search occur	• Do a computerized search of bibliographical databases • Do a computerized search of guideline resources • Focus and refocus search to obtain the most relevant evidence • Create an electronic library of citations by using bibliographical software
3. Evaluating evidence	• Ability to critique individual research study for scientific merit and applicability • Ability to critique systematic reviews, practice guidelines, and quality improvement reports • Understanding of the concept of a hierarchy of evidence • Ability to apply hierarchy of evidence in evaluating evidence • Awareness of tools to facilitate evaluation of evidence • Ability to calculate and differentiate between clinical and statistical significance	• Select a hierarchy of evidence to use • Select tools to help sort and compile evidence • Rate the level of evidence by using the chosen hierarchy • Critique evidence from a variety of sources (individual studies, meta-analyses, integrated reviews, guidelines) for credibility, applicability, and feasibility to clinical practice • Display summary of evidence in format that facilitates synthesis

TABLE 8-2	COMPETENCY I: INTERPRETATION AND USE OF RESEARCH IN PRACTICE—cont'd	
PHASE	KNOWLEDGE/SKILLS	ACTIVITIES
	• Ability to teach, guide others in evidence evaluation • Ability to facilitate group discussion to reach consensus	
4. Synthesizing evidence and recommending appropriate practice changes	• Concept and process of synthesis • Components of a synthesis report • Ability to determine clinical relevance of evidence • Ability to assess clinical environment for barriers and facilitators for specific practice change • Evaluation of applicability and feasibility of evidence to particular practice setting • Ability to write an effective report that presents evidence synthesis, practice change recommended, and implementation strategy	• Facilitate a collaborative multidisciplinary group to develop synthesis • Determine the status of current practice • Sort evidence by using tables of tools used in evaluating • Identify key areas/themes addressed across all evidence • Compare key areas/themes with current practice • Determine whether there is sufficient evidence to recommend practice change • Develop specific practice recommendations • Determine feasibility of change and risks and benefits • Determine strategy for proposing practice change recommendation to stakeholders • Write a synthesis report, including practice recommendations, risks/benefits, and implementation strategy • Develop a visual presentation of the report to influence acceptance of practice change recommendation
5. Implementing the recommended evidence-based practice change plan	• Theoretical and practical approaches to institutional and clinical behavior change • Systems/processes within setting • Organizational assessment of potential barriers and facilitators • Team-building skills • Principles of education readiness • Communication skills • Motivational skills	• Update baseline data on current practice • Develop plan that includes implementation, maintenance, and evaluation of practice • Include additional stakeholders to ensure further engagement and to have their unique clinical expertise • Identify expected outcomes of the change • Reflect patient values and expectations • Determine costs and resources needed • Identify potential barriers and facilitators • Seek approval for practice change

Continued

TABLE 8-2	COMPETENCY I: INTERPRETATION AND USE OF RESEARCH IN PRACTICE—cont'd	
PHASE	KNOWLEDGE/SKILLS	ACTIVITIES
		• Educate staff and other stakeholders • Set data collection methods to allow for evaluation of outcomes
6. Evaluating practice change	• Principles of evaluation • CQI process • Communication skills • Ability to conceptualize valid data collection methods • Work with appropriate departments (e.g., Information Services, Infection Control, Risk) to create data collection methods that prevent duplication • Ability to interpret data • Ability to determine relevant clinical, caregiver, and organizational outcomes	• Implement evaluation plan simultaneously with implementation plan • Identify tools with which to collect data to monitor outcomes/quality indicators • Monitor process and outcomes (include points that address ability to use clinical expertise and individualize for patient) • Compare data with internal and external benchmarks • Facilitate ongoing review of data with commitment to continual improvement • Coordinate a process for dissemination of evaluation data to stakeholders at regular intervals • Coordinate ongoing education and periodic review of practice change

CQI, Continuous quality improvement.

STATING THE PROBLEM OR CLINICAL QUESTION

The first step is to define the problem or question because a clearly stated clinical problem or question is critical to focusing one's efforts on selecting, appraising, and synthesizing evidence and making a practice recommendation. When information about a particular treatment or intervention is being sought, the clinical problem or question is often easier to develop than in cases in which problems are more complex and involve both physical and psychosocial aspects of care (Glanville, Schirm, & Wineman, 2000). An ideal statement is succinct and includes the patient population, the setting, the intervention or treatment, and a desired outcome (Brown, 1999; Craig, 2002; Gibbs 2003). The PICO (population, intervention, comparison, and outcome) framework can be helpful in formulating the statement and serve as a reminder of the key aspects to include (Craig, 2002).

When an APN looks for evidence about a current clinical situation, the process of forming a clinical question is informal, and the question may change as the APN searches the literature. At the very start of the search, consultation with a librarian is often helpful (Pond, 1999). If the APN is working with a librarian to conduct a literature search and retrieve the most relevant articles, a clear problem statement ensures that the most appropriate key words are used to direct the search. The search itself—looking at titles and abstracts—may lead to refinement of the question.

When a group of clinicians is seeking evidence, the process of developing and reaching consensus on the statement of the problem is more formalized. The group often works to refine the question before starting the literature search. Ideally, an interdisciplinary group of stakeholders should ultimately develop the statement or clinical question and follow through with the remaining steps in the process. APNs are the ideal leaders or co-leaders with a physician for such a planning group because of their clinical expertise, their knowledge of the systems within the workplace, and their ability to facilitate group discussion and practice changes (Barnsteiner & Prevost, 2002) (see Box 8-1 for examples of problem statements or clinical questions).

SEARCHING FOR AND RETRIEVING EVIDENCE

Before searching for evidence, the APN must have an understanding that "evidence exists on a continuum of rigor" (Stevens & Ledbetter, 2000, p. 93) and a familiarity with levels or hierarchies of evidence. Ideally, the choice of a particular level of evidence is determined before searching begins to help focus the search and dictate the searching strategy. Starting with broader evidence levels will ensure that research reviews, guidelines, and consensus statements—as well as individual published studies—are accessed (Rutledge & Grant, 2002). Therefore in addition to bibliographical databases such as MEDLINE and CINAHL, sites that offer systematic reviews, clinical guidelines, or specialty-specific standards are valuable resources and should be included in the search strategy (Hunt & McKibbon, 1997; McSweeney, Spies, & Cann, 2001). (See Box 8-2 on p. 270 for a list of online sources.) Some of the resources require that the user be a subscriber or pay a fee to either search or obtain a document.

Review articles should be the initial focus of the literature search. There are two types of reviews—systematic reviews and meta-analyses. An integrated or systematic review of the literature provides a narrative or qualitative synthesis of quantitative research findings about a clinical problem (Ropka & Spencer-Cisek, 2001). A meta-analysis can be thought of as a quantitative analysis and synthesis of quantitative research findings—a "study of studies." In a meta-analysis, statistical analyses are performed with the data from already published studies (LoBiondo-Wood & Haber, 2002) to calculate measures such as effect sizes. A meta-analysis may confirm existing findings from individual studies or clarify

---

BOX 8-1 • **EXAMPLES OF PROBLEM STATEMENTS OR CLINICAL QUESTIONS FOR COMPETENCY I**

- What is the best treatment for urinary dysfunction in patients with multiple sclerosis?
- What are the key factors to include in education of patients with cancer and their families regarding pain management?
- What is the best way to monitor complications of diabetes?
- What is the best method for collecting a urine culture from an infant during a clinic visit?
- What is the best tool to use to assess dehydration in elderly nursing home patients?
- Can length of stay in the trauma unit be reduced by performing tracheotomies on ventilator-dependent patients in the first 24 hours after admission?
- What are the most valid indicators of child abuse for emergency department nurses to be aware of?
- Which smoking cessation program works best with pregnant women?
- Do family caregivers of patients with Alzheimer's disease benefit from support groups?
- Is povidone-iodine best to use on vascular catheter sites to prevent infections?

BOX 8-2 • EVIDENCED-BASED PRACTICE RESOURCE AREAS

SITE/URL

DESCRIPTION

SYSTEMATIC REVIEWS

Cochrane Library
   www.cochranelibrary.com/cochrane/

Systematic reviews and guidelines; generally medically oriented but considered the gold standard of such reviews (can browse titles and get abstracts for free but need subscription or must pay fee for documents)

Database of Abstracts of Reviews of Effects (DARE)
   www.nhscrd.york.ac.uk/welcome.htm

Systematic reviews produced and maintained by the National Health System's Centre for Reviews and Dissemination

ONS EBP Online Resource Center
   www.ons.org

Integrated review area provides a list of integrated reviews pertinent to cancer care

CLINICAL PRACTICE GUIDELINES

Agency for Healthcare Research and Quality (AHRQ)
   www.ahcpr.gov/
National Guideline Clearinghouse (NGC)
   www.guideline.gov/
National Quality Measures Clearinghouse
   www.qualitymeasures.ahrq.gov/

Evidence report topics, evidence technical reviews, and clinical guidelines
A public resource for evidence-based clinical practice guidelines and measurement tools. NGC is sponsored by the Agency for Healthcare Research and Quality (AHRQ)

SPECIALTY-SPECIFIC GUIDELINES

National Comprehensive Cancer Network (NCCN)
   www.nccn.org/index.html
Primary Care Clinical Practice Guidelines
   www.medicine.ucsf.edu/resources/guidelines/
Internet Stroke Center, Washington University
   www.strokecenter.org/ebtcd-03/
   index.html
American Academy of Pediatrics
   www.aap.org/ policy/ paramtoc.html
AGREE Collaboration
   www.agreecollaboration.org/

Cancer care guidelines

Guidelines and resources

Evidence-based guides to specific aspects of stroke care

Guidelines for pediatric specialty

Guideline appraisal instrument and list of guidelines that have been appraised

GENERAL SITES WITH EXCELLENT LINKS TO OTHER EBP SITES

Academic Center for Evidence-based Nursing (ACE), University of Texas Health Center, San Antonio
   www.acestar.uthscsa.edu/
Centre for Health Evidence, Canadian Office of Health
   www.cche.net/che/home.asp
Centre for Evidence-Based Nursing, University of York
   www.york.ac.uk/healthsciences/centres/
   evidence/cebn.htm
Centre for Evidence-Based Medicine (CEBM)
   www.cebm.net/
Joanna Briggs Institute
   www.joannabriggs.edu.au/about/home.php

Comprehensive list of EBP resources

Users' guides for EBP series from JAMA; how to critique and use different types of evidence articles
Lists of pertinent systematic reviews and research reports
How-to's for every step in EBP process
Australia-based, privately owned EBP site—some free pages and some pages only by subscription; nursing and allied health topics

---

BOX 8-2 • EVIDENCED-BASED PRACTICE RESOURCE AREAS—cont'd

SITE/URL	DESCRIPTION
GENERAL SITES WITH EXCELLENT LINKS TO OTHER EBP SITES—cont'd	
Advanced Practice Nursing www.enursescribe.com/ advanced_practice_nursing.htm	Privately owned site with many pertinent sources
ONLINE JOURNALS	
Bandolier Evidence-Based Health Care www.jr2.ox.ac.uk/bandolier/	Independent journal about evidence-based health care, written by Oxford scientists
Evidence-Based Nursing (EBN) Online www.ebn.bmjjournals.com/	Online version of the journal (requires subscription)
Online Journal of Clinical Innovations (OJCI), CINAHL www.cinahl.com	Online journal of research reviews and clinical innovations (requires subscription)
WorldViews on Evidence Based Practice, Sigma Theta Tau International www.nursingsociety.org/	New online journal as of 2004 (requires subscription)

EBP, Evidence-based practice; *JAMA,* Journal of the American Medical Association; *ONS,* Oncology Nursing Society.

---

conflicting findings. More recently, the term meta-synthesis has been used to describe narrative, qualitative syntheses of findings from qualitative studies (Brown, 1999). Finding a review in current literature can "jump-start" an evidence-based project because the published synthesis may be all that is needed if it is current and comprehensive enough; someone else has done the work. Or the review can be used as a blueprint, and the planning group can add the most current evidence in a similar pattern. (See Box 8-3 for advantages of using published evidence summaries.)

APNs should become proficient and efficient in searching for evidence. With each search, APNs will become more skilled at focusing and refocusing the topic so that the

---

BOX 8-3 • ADVANTAGES OF PUBLISHED EVIDENCE SUMMARIES

- Reduce large quantities of information into a manageable form
- Establish generalizability across participants, settings, treatment variations, and study designs
- Assess consistency and explain inconsistencies of findings across studies
- Increase power in suggesting the cause-and-effect relationship
- Reduce bias from random and systematic error, improving true reflection of reality
- Integrate existing information for decisions about clinical care, economic decisions, future research design, and policy formation
- Increase efficiency in time between research and clinical implementation
- Provide a basis for continual updates with new evidence (Mulrow & Oxman, 1997)

most pertinent evidence is identified and retrieved. Basic searching strategies that should have been taught in undergraduate programs are reinforced and expanded for use in comprehensive searches through assignments in the graduate program. Strategies for comprehensive searching can be found in the literature and can help APNs remain current in this skill (Beaven, 2002; Burns & Grove, 2003; Conn et al., 2003; Helmer, Savoie, Green, & Kazanjian, 2001; Morrisey & DeBourgh, 2001; Pond, 1999; Shojania & Bero, 2001; Schulmeister & Vrabel, 2002).

If an interdisciplinary planning group is involved, the APN is frequently the most appropriate person to rework the search strategies because he or she has an expert view of the clinical topic and a clear focus on what is being sought. Ideally, this process is a collaboration between the APN and a reference librarian (Burns & Grove, 2003; Pond, 1999). This collaborative searching incorporates the expertise of each and can strengthen the process, but access to a librarian may not always be possible.

The final decision regarding the body of literature or evidence to be reviewed and the criteria for evaluation need to be a consensus of the stakeholder planning group so that all perspectives on the clinical issue are adequately represented. For example, a group of APNs did a synthesis project on sleep disturbances in patients with cancer for the Oncology Nursing Society, and the following is a list of criteria that were used for selection of articles (Clark, Cunningham, McMillan, Vena, & Parker, 2004).

- **Time frame:** articles from past 5 years preferred but in some instances there are classic citations that need to be considered
- **Sample:** adult patients; patients undergoing treatment for cancer preferred but sleep disturbances during treatment of other chronic illnesses were considered because of the small number of studies
- **Setting:** any setting
- **Measurement:** must have assessed sleep disturbances or sleep patterns as a primary variable, not ancillary analyses or results
- **Types of evidence:** opinion articles omitted; had to be research or review

EVALUATING EVIDENCE

Once research studies, reviews, guidelines, and other information have been selected by the planning group, the evidence needs to be reviewed, rated, and compiled in a format that will facilitate creation of a narrative synthesis and practice recommendations. These activities depend on the ability of the planning group members to critique evidence, establish a hierarchy of evidence, select available tools with which to critique the evidence, and compile or summarize the results. First, the planning group needs to determine which members will read the literature collected. Some groups choose several people to read all of the literature; other groups divide the literature evenly among all members of the group. At least two people should read each item to allow for discussion and consensus (Papadopoulos & Rheeder, 2000). Three factors must be considered when all evidence is evaluated: scientific merit, applicability to clinical practice, and feasibility for the setting. Critiquing and recording tools are especially important when the reading is shared by the group to provide some basis for consistency.

Literature reviews, meta-analyses, and guidelines require different evaluation processes. The critique of a review is unique because not only does the credibility of the research need to be evaluated but also the feasibility and applicability of the findings to a particular clinical practice or health-care setting. Guides have been developed to facilitate such evaluations for application to practice (Brown, 1999; Cullum, 1999;

Smyth, 2002; Stetler et al., 1998; Titler et al., 1999). These guides usually deal with methodological attributes of the review and evaluation of the applicability of the findings to the particular clinical setting (e.g., Are the sample, setting, and technology comparable to those found in the planning group's agency?) and the feasibility of applying the findings to the particular clinical setting (e.g., issues of risk/benefit, needed resources, cost, and readiness to adopt the practice change need to be considered) (Stetler et al., 1998).

Clinical practice guidelines are systematically developed statements to assist practitioner and patient with decisions about what is the most appropriate heath care for specific clinical circumstances (IOM, 1990). The most valid guidelines are the result of gathering, appraising, and synthesizing evidence; considering risks and benefits; and reflecting on "value judgments about the relative importance of various health and economic outcomes in specific clinical situations" (Hayward, Wilson, Tunis, Bass, & Guyatt, 1995, p. 571). Guidelines make explicit recommendations for the clinical situation, which may include screening or treatment interventions, symptom management, and education. Evaluating clinical practice guidelines is also unique and involves determining the credibility of the author or authoring organization, timeliness (Shekelle, Eccles, Grimshaw, & Woolf, 2001), validity of the evidence base and methods of development, cost-effectiveness in implementation (Thomas & Hotchkiss, 2002), and applicability to the particular practice setting. Questions to ask in evaluation of clinical practice guidelines are available in both the medical and nursing literature (AGREE Collaboration, 2001; Brown, 1999; Hayward et al., 1995; McSweeney et al., 2001; Shaneyfelt, Mayo-Smith, & Rothwangl, 1999; Thomas & Hotchkiss, 2002).

The evaluation of individual research studies for scientific merit is the same as the research critique process taught in undergraduate program research courses and reinforced in graduate programs. Guides for critiquing individual research articles can be found in most research books (Brown, 1999; Burns & Grove, 2003; Fain, 2003; Norwood, 2000; Polit, Beck, & Hungler, 2001). Some resources provide guides for critiquing specific types of studies (Gibbs, 2003; Guyatt & Rennie, 2002), and Rosswurm and Larrabee (1999) have designed a worksheet that can be used to evaluate individual studies. Evidence tables are helpful tools and can be completed by the planning group to visually display the findings of multiple studies. An evidence table clearly highlights relevant features of individual research studies, including those that affect use of findings. Columns in the table may vary according to topic of interest and purpose of the table (e.g., methodological factors or utilization factors) but usually include citation information, study purpose, measurement tools, sample, design, procedures, outcome variables, results/findings, limitations, and implications of the project (Brown, 1999; Norwood, 2000). A good example of a table of evidence can be found in an article by Wakefield, Johnson, Kron-Chalupa, & Paulsen (1998, pp. 1507-1508). This table includes columns for study (citation information), purpose, sample, outcome variables (including the measurement tools used), and results. Other examples of evidence tables can be found in well-developed systematic reviews. After members of the planning group have read and critiqued the evidence, they will have impressions about applicability and feasibility. The final step in the evaluation phase is completion of an evidence table for the proposed practice change.

SYNTHESIZING EVIDENCE AND RECOMMENDING PRACTICE CHANGES

A collective evidence table will help the planning group compare and synthesize evidence. Members of the planning group who have evaluated research and other evidence contribute to completion of the evidence table. For the purposes of the planning group, an evidence table may include the citation, sample and setting descriptions, methods, interventions, findings, level of evidence, and a comment column. In addition to an evidence table that summarizes published findings, the planning group may also prepare another table that summarizes internal data derived from quality improvement, benchmarking, and accreditation activities. Time will be needed to present and discuss the evidence reviewed by individuals, and then the group will need to consider the evidence in total. Having stakeholders in the group is especially important to this aspect of evaluation because each stakeholder can see the clinical situation from his or her perspective and should be able to offer unique views and comments regarding the applicability of the evidence and the feasibility of making any practice changes.

The actual synthesis product may resemble an outline for a systematic review article. Some items that may be included are as follows:

- Statement of the clinical problem or question
- Overview of the search strategy and results
- Narrative summary of commonalities and differences across evidence
- Proposed practice recommendations when the strength of evidence is sufficient
- Practices that can and should remain the same because the evidence affirms existing practice or is insufficient for recommendation of changes
- Comparison of new practice recommendations with current practice in the clinical setting (e.g., patient outcomes, costs, risks)
- Feasibility of practice changes in the clinical setting
- Proposed implementation strategies for practice change recommendations (e.g., algorithm, protocol, clinical guideline, standing orders, staff education)
- Resources needed to implement recommendations (e.g., budget, personnel, equipment, software)

The planning group needs to consider all of these items before formal recommendations are made.

For each practice recommendation that is different from existing practice, the planning group should document the following in its report:

- That there is sufficient evidence to justify a practice change
- Any contradictory evidence that supports existing practice and possible ways to resolve the contradiction(s)
- Whether practice changes recommended by the evidence are likely to make a significant difference in patient outcomes

Examples of articles that describe the process of synthesizing evidence and making practice recommendations include a protocol for preventing opioid-induced constipation (Robinson et al., 2000), appropriate use of transdermal fentanyl for chronic pain management (Wakefield et al., 1998), and development of an evidence-based procedure for the maintenance of central venous catheters, including use of dressings and flushing (Newell-Stokes, Broughton, Guiliano, & Stetler, 2001).

IMPLEMENTING THE RECOMMENDED EVIDENCE-BASED PRACTICE CHANGE

The implementation plan actually begins to emerge during the process of synthesis and becomes part of the synthesis report. All that may need to be done to ensure adoption of the recommendations is to add detail to the synthesis plan outlined previously. The members of the planning group should reach consensus as to the practice changes that they will recommend for adoption. It may be necessary to invite a few more individuals who will be key change facilitators to the planning group at this time. These may be administrators or clinicians from the areas where the change will begin or areas where it is anticipated that there will be the most resistance.

Planning groups should ideally base the rollout of the implementation plan on some theoretical model of institutional (e.g., Shortell, Bennett, & Byck, 1998) or clinician behavior change (e.g., Rogers, 2003). A theoretical approach to change combined with an objective assessment of the organization will help the planning group anticipate and address barriers to adoption of the new practice and enlist the support of informal and formal leaders in the process (Carson, 2002; Rutledge et al., 2001).

An implementation plan should expand on the last two sections of the synthesis report: strategies for practice change recommendations and resources needed to implement recommendations. A possible outline for such a plan is as follows:

- Current practice (based on internal data)
- Proposed change with evidence-based rationale and risks/benefits that can be anticipated
- Potential barriers and facilitators identified through an organizational assessment
- Necessary resources and costs to implement and monitor outcomes
- Step-by-step protocol for applying the practice change (reflect patient values and expectations and flexibility related to caregiver expertise)
- Evaluation plan—outcome measures (based on internal data and external benchmarks)
- Education—content and timing
- Timeline (including implementation, education, and evaluation)

When possible, a trial implementation or pilot in one or two units should be done. A trial or pilot provides concrete information on the feasibility of the practice change in the target setting and allows practitioners to influence adaptation of the change, providing a sense of ownership of the change process and contributing to a smoother integration of the change (Rosswurm & Larrabee, 1999, Titler et al., 1994). An area, service, or unit should be chosen to initiate the implementation to offer the best opportunity for successful adoption. On the basis of an evaluation of the pilot, the practice change, implementation plan, or both can be modified and rolled out across the institution. Evaluation of the impact of the practice change completes the process of interpretation and use of research and other evidence. Evaluation provides essential data for decision making and assists staff in determining whether the practice change is making a difference and should be continued (Goode, 1995).

EVALUATING THE RECOMMENDED EVIDENCE-BASED PRACTICE CHANGE PLAN

A practice change evaluation plan has many similarities to the evaluation of practice that is addressed in Competency II. Therefore understanding evaluation as it relates to Competency I will facilitate the APN's implementation of Competency II. Key steps in the development of any evaluation plan are as follows:

- Develop the evaluation plan simultaneously with the implementation plan once the outcomes have been determined.
- Determine short-term and long-term timetables: identify what should be measured, how it should be measured, and when.

- Determine baseline outcomes by using internal and external benchmark data, as well as goals of the program for patients and staff; include patient, caregiver, and organizational outcomes (Jennings, Staggers, & Brosch, 1999).
- Compare the measured outcomes with the baseline benchmark data collected before the practice change implementation.
- Monitor the process, including utilization of the practice change (Wakefield et al., 1998), as well as outcomes; ensure that the plan allows for flexibility to accommodate variations in providers' clinical expertise and judgments and patients' characteristics, values, and expectations.
- Evaluate the implementation process, including identification of any unforeseen barriers; determine adequacy of education and availability of support (Wakefield et al., 1998).
- Monitor effects of practice changes on patient outcomes and staff for at least two consecutive quarters after implementation (Wakefield et al., 1998).
- Monitor cost/benefit ratio (Polit et al., 2001).
- Evaluate staff's level of knowledge about the new practice, determine ongoing educational needs, and plan educational updates periodically (Robinson et al., 2000).
- Ensure a process (ideally one is already in place within the clinical setting) for continual review.
- Review evaluation data regularly to identify trends, to determine that goals are being met, or to determine a subsequent need for revision of the practice change.
- Share the results both internally and externally.

Progress in the practice change plan should be reviewed within the first quarter of implementation to ensure that no major problem exists and to deal with any major issues that may have arisen. Significant differences in patients' clinical outcomes may not be apparent by that time. However, the process, including the extent to which the practice change is being accepted and used, can be evaluated, and the opinions of the clinicians concerning the practice change can be determined. If the practice change has not been adopted readily, additional measures may be needed to promote the change.

An evaluation report should be written when sufficient time for assessment of clinical outcomes has elapsed. In the interim, quarterly reports that document evaluation activities may be required by the appropriate administrative or clinical committees. Writers of the formal evaluation report should do the following:

- Be succinct and present major points clearly.
- Incorporate graphic representation of outcomes.
- Include outcomes for patient population, clinicians, and organization.
- Be tailored to the audience receiving the report.
- Provide data for continuation or revision of the practice change (Sudduth, 1999).
- Specify what resources are needed for continuation or revision.

On the basis of the evaluation report, outcomes may continue to be monitored, or a new plan may be developed and implemented as a result of disappointing outcomes. Alternatively, a new plan may be generated or a decision may be made to adopt the plan more widely if outcomes have exceeded expectations. Finally, if the report identifies significant variations in outcome attainment, research projects may be developed to determine why some patients are achieving better outcomes than others or why certain areas in the setting are achieving better outcomes (Competency III). Exemplar 8-1 provides examples of fundamental and expanded levels of Competency I.

EXEMPLAR 8-1

COMPETENCY I

These are examples of the improvement of practice by the application of research evidence to the development of evidence-based procedures, protocols, or programs. Some of these may exemplify one or more of the levels of Competency I—the *fundamental* level if applied to individual practice and the expanded level if the practice change was adopted by a group, unit, or entire clinical setting.

- Development of an evidence-based procedure for the maintenance of central venous catheters, including dressings and flushing (Newell-Stokes et al., 2001); *this exemplifies the fundamental competency level if it is applied to individual practice and the expanded level if it is adopted by the entire clinical setting.*
- Development of an evidence-based oncology oral care clinical practice guideline, by using the 1989 National Institutes of Health consensus statement, comprehensive search of biomedical literature, and expert panel input (Stricker & Sullivan, 2003); *exemplifies the expanded competency because the effort was led by an APN and was done in the context of several inpatient oncology units.*
- A research-based practice protocol to prevent constipation in hospitalized older adults undergoing surgery (Titler, Mentes, Rackel, Abbott, & Baumler, 1999); *exemplifies expanded level because it is a protocol adopted by entire setting.*
- Implementing a pain management program based on national standards (Bookbinder et al., 1995, 1996); *exemplifies expanded level because it is a program for an entire clinical setting.*
- Model of evidence-based practice at an academic, tertiary health-care organization and three examples of projects to improve oncology practice (Payne, 2002); *exemplifies expanded level because a practice setting is implementing the projects.*

COMPETENCY II: EVALUATION OF PRACTICE

Advanced practice nursing should be evidence-based and should be evaluated; this is especially important in the current health-care environment. With the current nursing shortage and the managed care environment, only roles that have a positive influence on patient outcomes and health-care costs can afford to be continued in any clinical setting. Clinicians must demonstrate that they make a difference and document their value to the population being served and to those who pay for health care. This can be accomplished in a variety of ways (see Chapters 18 and 25). For the purposes of this research competency, the emphasis is on how APNs can incorporate evaluation into their individual practice, rather than on sophisticated outcomes research using large datasets (see Table 8-3, Competency II).

Documenting the value and effectiveness of advanced practice not only assists clinicians in improving their own practices but also provides valuable information for stakeholders including consumers, administrators, insurers, managed care companies, health-care systems, and regulatory and accrediting agencies such as the JCAHO (Byers & Brunell, 1998, Humphris, 1999). If employment of an individual APN or a group of APNs is cost-effective and results in improved clinical care, the APN role can be more easily justified when cost-cutting or quality improvement decisions are made by administrators (see Chapter 24).

The implementation and maintenance of an evaluation process, whether it be for an individual APN's practice (fundamental level of the competency), for a total department of APNs (expanded level of the competency), or for a nursing or interdisciplinary team is complex, requiring extensive planning, knowledge, and skills. This competency is outlined in Table 8-3.

Assessment of the impact of advanced practice on clinical outcomes and quality indicators is appearing more commonly in the professional literature. For instance, the Advanced Practice Work Group of the American Association of Critical Care Nurses is developing a database of information on ways that APNs influence patient care and health-care costs (Ahrens, 2000). This process is feasible at any level of advanced practice

TABLE 8-3 COMPETENCY II: EVALUATION OF PRACTICE		
PHASE	**KNOWLEDGE/SKILLS**	**ACTIVITIES**
1. Identifying key goals/ desired outcomes of practice	• Key goals of practice or desired clinical outcomes of patients and the organization • Ability to articulate goals in measurable terms	• List major desired goals or impacts of practice on patients' clinical outcomes, both short-term and long-term • List major desired goals or impacts of practice on the organization, both short-term and long-term • Ensure that the impacts are stated in a manner so that they are feasible and measurable
2. Ensuring collection of appropriate and accurate data	• Methodological approaches to evaluation • Data collection and storage techniques • Basic research principles of data collection to avoid bias • Principles of data management including quality assurance of data	• Indicate what actual data will indicate proof of the achievement of desired practice goals • Review external benchmarks from established standards of care, clinical guidelines, quality indicators, or published research to validate what data points are appropriate and feasible • Review documentation for inclusion of all data points, with emphasis on point-of-service data collection and no duplication • Identify and secure established data collection tools as needed • Design or revise current documentation tools to include all data points
3. Comparing data with internal and external benchmarks	• Concept and principle of benchmark data • Basic statistical analysis techniques	• Establish a process to compare data from individual or collaborative practice, ideally electronically, on a short-term and long-term basis • Establish a process that provides a periodic, user-friendly report of the benchmark comparisons
4. Changing practice based on evaluation results	• Theoretical and practical approaches to implementing institutional and clinician behavior change • Systems and processes within the setting • Process and outcome evaluation strategies • Verbal and written communication skills	• Establish a process that facilitates all appropriate stakeholders reviewing the data and making recommendations for practice changes based on the data • Disseminate process and results within clinical setting

and in any setting because data collection can be done as an integral part of point-of-service documentation or by incorporating quality indicators that are already collected and reported to regulatory and accrediting agencies (DePalma, 2000).

In the next section, each component of Competency II is discussed relative to the knowledge and activities required to accomplish each step in the process of evaluating advanced practice. Examples are also included to demonstrate application to practice.

Identifying Key Goals/Desired Outcomes of Practice

APNs must be aware of and able to articulate the primary goals of their practices. Primary goals for any specific role can be broadly guided by standards and competencies that have been developed and distributed by professional organizations or accrediting and licensing agencies. For example, NONPF, in partnership with AACN, developed consensus-based primary care competencies for adult, family, gerontological, pediatric, and women's health NPs (NONPF & AACN, 2002). Job descriptions or key program objectives or services that involve APNs are also starting points for determining primary goals. These primary goals will most likely focus on improved clinical outcomes for patient populations, but the impact of the APN's role on the particular clinical environment and co-workers must also be included (Jennings et al., 1999). Four dimensions to consider in evaluation of an APN role are quality, access, education, and economy (Humphris, 1999). Although these four dimensions overlap, they are discussed individually, and reference is made to the impact on patients, clinical environment, and co-workers for each dimension.

The *quality* dimension of evaluation can include data on improved clinical outcomes for patients and families, as well as patient satisfaction. One example of a quality evaluation is a comparison of national data on women with high-risk pregnancies cared for by CNMs or obstetricians. Those women who received care from CNMs had significantly higher rates of spontaneous delivery (Davidson, 2002). In addition, patients of CNMs were less likely to have instrument-assisted deliveries and had fewer cesarean deliveries than the comparison group. Finally, a significantly higher percentage of women who had had prior cesarean deliveries had vaginal deliveries when they were under the care of CNMs. Based on this national database and the findings of the comparison study, an individual CNM could select the quality indicators that should be monitored in his or her own practice—specifically, numbers of spontaneous deliveries, cesarean deliveries, instrument-assisted deliveries, and vaginal deliveries after prior cesarean deliveries.

The *access* dimension refers to direct care provided by APNs; this may include services made available, facilitated, or coordinated by APNs or information to facilitate decision making by patients that is provided by APNs. APNs may be providing a level of care that would not be otherwise accessible or may be improving health-care access by improving coordination of care. Data documenting such improvements are necessary for evaluation of advanced practice nursing. For example, an APN-led, community-based program of breast and cervical cancer screening for medically underserved, low-income women (Schulz, Ludwick, Cukr, & Kelly, 2002) improved access by removing barriers to health care. The accessible, acceptable, and appropriate services that were provided resulted in an increased attendance rate with each screening program. Investigators attributed the high minority participation (20% of the screening programs' attendees were women of color from a predominantly white [96.1%] geographical area) to their emphasis on minority recruitment and the supportive informal network that emerged during the project (Schulz et al., 2002).

The *education* dimension refers to both patients and the health-care workforce and may include formal and informal teaching. APNs may assist staff educators in the development of patient teaching materials, obtain materials that already exist externally, and provide important information to patients and their families while administering care. Because APNs are often involved with patients for whom care is complex or complicated, those staff who have the primary responsibility for such patients can learn from the APN as a role model, as well as from a discussion with the APN about priority aspects of care. A specialized home care intervention provided by APNs for older patients with cancer who had undergone surgery and their families included comprehensive clinical assessments, monitoring, and teaching over a 4-week period (McCorkle et al., 2000). The information needs for this patient population after discharge were assessed and found to be extensive and varied. Forty percent of the teaching for home care patients was provided during telephone contacts in response to urgent problems or to requests for clarification of information originally provided during home visits (Hughes, Hodgson, Muller, Robinson, & McCorkle, 2000). The patients with late-stage cancer in the specialized home care intervention group had improved survival rates when compared with those in the usual care group who had routine follow-up in outpatient clinics.

The *economy* dimension can include evaluation of costs; cost-effectiveness; the impact of underuse, overuse, or misuse of evidence-based interventions (IOM, 2001); and assessment of underuse of APNs. Cost-effectiveness may be demonstrated by reductions in lengths of stay, complications, or readmissions. Other cost savings may be dependent on specific patient populations. For example, CNMs' positive impact on costs of care might be measured by using data that demonstrate a decreasing number of cesarean deliveries and premature births. An annual cost analysis is another strategy for evaluating the economic dimension of advanced practice nursing (Vincent, 2002). Vincent (2002) recognized the improved patient satisfaction and effectiveness of care associated with nurse-managed clinics but made the point that survival of such clinics would depend on the combination of financial stability and a reputation for clinical excellence. A cost analysis of the academic-based nursing center was conducted and resulted in the identification of services that were profitable and those that were not (Vincent, 2002). On the basis of the analysis, recommendations were made to decrease administrative costs, increase the number of primary care visits, and decrease the variable costs of the Women, Infants and Children (WIC) program to break even financially.

Ensuring Collection of Appropriate and Accurate Data

A key aspect of the data collection component of Competency II is determining whether relevant data already exist. If existing data or databases cannot be used, then the APN should ensure that the most relevant data are being collected and that the data collection is being done in the most expeditious manner according to sound research principles. Priorities for data collection must be established. Only data that are essential and can be used to change practice or compared with established standards should be collected. The question that should be asked in determining whether more information should be collected is "How will I use this information?" If the answer is not clear, then the additional information should not be collected. Ideally, the goals of practice are stated in a manner that indicates clearly what type of information is needed. The reader is referred to Chapter 18, p. 659, for an illustration of a data collection plan established to monitor outcomes of congestive heart failure.

Exactly what data should be collected can be determined by answering the question, "What information is needed to demonstrate that a particular goal has been met or an outcome achieved?" Review of external benchmarks from established standards of care, clinical guidelines, quality indicators, or published research can assist in validating what data points are appropriate and feasible.

Information collection should be done as an integral part of the APN's practice and point-of service documentation to ensure appropriateness, currency, and accuracy and to avoid redundancy. Special data collection sheets are not needed in the ideal process. Flow sheets and progress notes should provide all necessary information whenever possible. This may require the revision of documentation tools to include the priority information or a shift to electronic documentation. If information is truly pertinent, it should be included as a part of the usual documentation in some form. Data that need to be collected in addition to usual documentation are often incomplete or inaccurate because of clinicians' time constraints. Therefore data that are necessary for evaluation should be collected as part of care delivery. Collection of additional, project-specific data should be kept to a minimum.

If formal measures are deemed necessary, well-established instruments should be considered for use. When valid and reliable instruments are used, the data collected can be compared with findings from other settings or practices in which the instruments were used. Health surveys such as the Short Form-36 Health Status Profile (SF-36) can be used to determine how programs of care are improving the overall health of patients (Eisen, Leff, & Schaefer, 1999; Wyrwich, Tierney, & Wolinsky, 1999). Total scores or subscale scores of the SF-36 may be relevant to an APN's individual, group, or interdisciplinary practice. However, disease-specific outcome instruments are more likely to be able to detect changes in the disease that are a result of advanced practice nursing interventions. For example, a symptom index for benign prostate disease was developed after researchers determined that men with identical symptoms from benign prostate disease had very different opinions about how much the disease bothered them. Furthermore, urine flow rate, the measure most commonly used to evaluate the need for treatment, had almost no relationship to patients' perceptions of their symptoms or need for treatment (Jacobsen et al., 1995).

Knowledge and skills related to the handling of data are similar regardless of whether data are collected for evaluation or for generation of knowledge through research. Such techniques are included among the knowledge and skills necessary for the third research competency, participating in collaborative research (see next section). Because these techniques may be complex and require computer hardware and software with which many APNs may not be familiar, APNs should seek appropriate resources or consultants. For example, the institution may have quality improvement or data management personnel who can assist with the design of a data system for the evaluation project (see Chapter 25 for further discussion of data management).

Cost and feasibility of collecting the data must also be considered. When APNs are selecting measures to collect data, they must be aware of data available through existing resources and databases to avoid unnecessary effort and duplication. Therefore APNs need an understanding of the types of data that are stored and retrievable within the particular clinical setting and must also know how to plan for the development of additional databases (Wu, Crosby, Ventura, & Finnick, 1994). A wide variety of institutional databases, such as administrative databases for billing and medical records, can provide APNs with clinical data (Bozzo, 1999; Minarik, 1999). Many clinical settings maintain databases that include data related to patient satisfaction after hospitalizations and clinic visits, patients' perceptions of the adequacy of education provided, and assessments of level of pain and functional status. Such databases can be invaluable in the evaluation of practice. Existing databases and computerized documentation make it easier to generate summaries and allow APNs to request routine reports regarding processes and outcomes of care.

Comparing Data with Internal and External Benchmarks

Once a data collection process has been established, APNs need an adequate understanding of research methodology to interpret data appropriately and to recognize the potential for confounding variables. For example, when analyzing the impact of advanced practice nursing interactions on patients, it is also important to consider the influence of disease status over time. Decreasing functional status in a patient with stable disease has different implications than it would in a patient with progressive cancer.

The internal and external benchmark data that served as guides for establishing what data should be collected will also serve as comparison data. Internal reports can be requested on a regular basis (e.g., monthly or quarterly). External data, such as those received from Medicare and Medicaid, can also be used. Reports should be reviewed for what they reveal about current practice and what comparisons can be made with previous reports for trending.

Changing Practice Based on Evaluation Results

As with Competency I, the next step is to determine whether practice needs to change. Collected and reported data may reaffirm that current practice is effective or indicate that a change in practice is needed to improve the quality of care. Data trended over a specific period will be most useful to indicate whether practice changes are needed. For example, if complication or readmission rates are increasing, an EBP change can be implemented and then tracked for several months to look for improvement. Accomplishment of this step therefore requires the knowledge and skills of Competency

Also included in this phase of the competency is the effective dissemination of results, including cost and resource implications, to administrators and other key decision makers. Effective dissemination requires that the APN be able to clearly and comprehensively describe the process, explain the results, articulate how or why the results are related to advanced practice nursing, and link the findings with current practice or proposals for revised practice.

A variety of research skills are essential for evaluation of practice. Some of these skills are acquired during development of the other two research competencies, whereas others must be acquired separately to identify key aspects of care, select appropriate measures, implement evaluation within one's practice, and interpret and apply the results appropriately. Exemplar 8-2 provides examples of practice evaluation.

EXEMPLAR 8-2

COMPETENCY II

Published accounts of evaluation of practice are often within the activities described for Competency III, because they tend to be formal studies evaluating a program or comparing advanced practice nursing outcomes with physician outcomes. Findings from such articles can be used by APNs, however, in designing their own practice evaluation projects related to standards, quality indicators, or outcomes of their care, which are the focus of Competency II activities.

EXEMPLAR 8-2

COMPETENCY II—cont'd

- Midwives tracked maternal and infant outcomes based on the American College of Nurse-Midwives Standards (www.midwives.com), including patient satisfaction, clinical outcomes, population-specific care, appropriate use of technology and resources, and access to care.
- An NP position was added to a multidisciplinary stroke team in a small community hospital as a facilitator. The NP is notified of admission by MD; NP calls stroke team, orders basic scans and laboratory testing, and begins implementation of protocols. Outcomes improved: decreased mortality and complication rates, especially urinary tract infections and pneumonia, and decreased lengths of stay. Protocols were based on American Stroke Association's Scientific Statement, "Guidelines for the Early Management of Patients with Ischemic Stroke" (Adams et al., 2003).
- Evaluation of an APN-led worksite disease management program (Carioti, Lavigne, Stone, Tortoretti, & Chiverton, 2001)
- NP community-based breast and cervical screening program for medically underserved, low-income women (Schulz et al., 2002)
- APN-directed heart failure program—tracking of readmission rates, treatment, and mortality rate (Dahl & Penque, 2000)
- Evaluation of weekend on-call nurse anesthetist coverage—costs and risks/benefits (Dexter, Epstein, & Marsh, 2002)
- CNS-led smoking cessation program—designed and evaluated according to the National Advisory Committee on Health and Disability's guidelines (2002) and a Cochrane systematic review (Bigotti, Munafo, Murphy, & Stead, 2003).

APN, Advanced practice nurse; *CNS,* clinical nurse specialist; *NP,* nurse practitioner.

COMPETENCY III: PARTICIPATION IN COLLABORATIVE RESEARCH

This third research competency involves participation in collaborative nursing or interdisciplinary research studies undertaken to generate knowledge that enhances understanding of clinical phenomena, to define optimal nursing or other interventions for particular populations and specific clinical problems (Brooten & Naylor, 1995), or to examine outcomes of care (Whitman, 2002b). This competency is consistent with the AACN's (2002) position that master's prepared nurses "... identify practice and systems problems that need to be studied and collaborate with other scientists to generate new studies based on their expertise" (p. 2). In addition to being consumers of research (Competency I) and users of the research process to examine their own practice (Competency II), APNs need to recognize the value of conducting research, understand the research process and their unique and essential contributions to this process, and make collaborative participation in knowledge-generating or outcomes research a priority (Martin, 1995).

The importance of this research competency for APNs cannot be emphasized enough, for it is through their direct participation in research studies that APNs can help to (1) ensure the clinical relevance of the research questions (Polit & Beck, 2004), (2) participate in selection of nursing-sensitive outcomes or outcomes that are critical components of quality patient care (Whitman, 2002a), (3) ensure feasibility of the methods in a given clinical setting (McGuire et al., 2000; Nail, 1990), and (4) ultimately influence the clinical applicability of the results (McGuire et al., 2000; Polit & Beck, 2004). Two areas of research are critically important for advanced practice nursing research collaboration. First, knowledge-generating research elucidates useful descriptive information for clinical practice or subsequent research, produces the evidence that is used in evidence-based clinical practice guidelines, and ultimately "... helps push the limits of current practice so that patients receive evidence-based care" (Curley, 1998, p. 68). Second, outcomes research examines the quality of patient care or validates the role of selected personnel such as APNs (Clochesy, 2002; Jastremski, 2002; see Chapter 25).

Regardless of an APN's work setting or position description, we view this competency as essential rather than optional. However, it must be individualized, as are the other two competencies, to a particular APN's setting; position description; sociopolitical climate; and personal desires, goals, and values. Perhaps most importantly, this competency is a logical extension of research-related activity for APNs when Research Competency I reveals insufficient evidence in a given area or when Research Competency II does not yield the anticipated outcomes of one's practice, especially when the practice is based on existing research. In other words, when there is no evidence or when outcomes are less than optimal, it is likely that additional knowledge-generating research is necessary, and the APN is an ideal individual to participate in such research by virtue of educational preparation.

Competency III has both fundamental and expanded levels of activity (see Table 8-1). At the fundamental level, defined as occurring on completion of a graduate program, the APN is capable of assuming a role as a consultant or clinical expert in a research study. The expanded level, developed after graduation, positions the APN who has acquired additional education and/or experience in conducting research as a principal investigator or co-investigator in knowledge-generating research. The APN's work setting and position description may greatly influence his or her involvement in Competency III activities because research may or may not be a major component of the position description and clinical environment.

The ways in which APNs can participate in collaborative research are many, but two foundational elements are necessary. First, an APN must possess general knowledge about research paradigms and the phases of the research process, which should initially be acquired in a graduate program and continually developed over time (see next section). This basic research knowledge is thoroughly detailed in the typical nursing research textbooks used in most graduate nursing programs (Burns & Grove, 2003; Polit & Beck, 2004). Therefore it is important that APNs avail themselves not only of such textbooks but also of other resources such as a network of professional colleagues knowledgeable about research (e.g., a professor from the APN's graduate program or other school of nursing, an APN colleague who is active in research, or a practice partner who is engaged in research) and internal and external sources of information and materials on research (e.g., libraries, websites, professional organizations).

The second foundational element the APN needs is knowledge of how to identify, meet, and develop collaborations with active researchers who are studying areas of interest to the APN. This can be easy or challenging, depending on the APN's work setting, geographical area, and other factors such as motivation, interest, and support of superiors. A detailed description of strategies is beyond the scope of this text, but several general suggestions may be helpful to the reader. If the APN works in an academic health center or academically affiliated setting, research may already be an integral component of the position description, and collaborative participation may be a given. If APNs are not involved in research, there are likely to be clinical researchers in affiliated schools of nursing and medicine, some of whom may already be collaborating with others in the APN's setting. The APN can learn more about such individuals and their research from personal contacts; networking; examining Web pages (e.g., research activities of faculty); or attending research presentations, journal clubs, and other research-related offerings. If the APN is not in an academic setting, it is possible to explore potential collaborative opportunities with faculty and researchers in nearby academic settings (as described previously) or to talk with local representatives of pharmaceutical or medical device companies, which are increasingly seeking research partners in the community, about participating in one or more of their studies. Other willing and useful collaborators might include rural health, migrant, and other federal, state, and local agencies that provide care to vulnerable populations. Another tactic for identifying collaborative opportunities might be exploration of professional society research initiatives, such as the American Association of Critical-Care Nurses' Thunder and Thunder 2 projects (Thompson et al., 2001; White, 1996) or the Association of Women's Health (Church-Balin & Damus, 2003; Sampselle et al., 2000). Technological advances in communication, computer support, and networking allow research partners to collaborate virtually; they do not all need to reside and work in the same geographical location. The bottom line is that it is important for the APN to "put out the word" about his or her interest in collaboration, because many researchers are interested in finding good clinical partners for their research projects and in having access to new clinical settings and will appreciate hearing of interested APNs.

The scope of specific research activities in which APNs can become engaged within this research competency is wide-ranging. These activities are not only important to collaborative research but are also commensurate with existing advanced nursing practice standards (American Association of Critical-Care Nurses & ANA, 1995; ANA 1996; Jacobs, 2003) and accrediting organizations' recommendations regarding research (AACN, 2002). In most settings, the APN is the individual most likely to understand the clinical issues and questions in a given patient population and to be familiar with the routines and culture of the clinical setting. Thus, the APN is ideally positioned to make meaningful contributions to all phases of the research process, regardless of whether the research is focused on generating descriptive knowledge, testing interventions, or examining outcomes of care.

Tables 8-4 and 8-5 outline the major phases of the quantitative and qualitative research processes and list, for each phase, specific activities in which APNs can become engaged, along with any special knowledge or skills that might enhance their performance of the activities. These activities are assumed to complement the solid foundation of general research knowledge mentioned previously, and further, they are not exhaustive because APNs engage in numerous additional activities, depending on the context of their work environment. The activities shown in Tables 8-4 and 8-5 are focused primarily at the fundamental level of activity for this research competency (see Table 8-1). After graduation, expanded levels of activity will depend on the individual APN's interests and opportunities and cannot be thoroughly detailed here. An excellent resource for APNs who are moving into the expanded level of activity for this research competency is the text by Mateo and Kirchhoff (1999), which deals with designing and conducting research in the clinical setting and is targeted to the practicing nurse.

In conclusion, participation in collaborative research is an essential competency for APNs, although clearly less critical to the quality and effectiveness of their own personal professional practices than are Competencies I and II. Participation by APNs in knowledge-generating or outcomes research builds on research Competencies I and II and contributes to the broader goal of evidence-based, high-quality care. Exemplar 8-3 (p. 287) provides examples of Competency III.

ACQUIRING AND DEVELOPING RESEARCH COMPETENCIES

This final section discusses the important roles that graduate education and postgraduate research development play in APNs' achievement of meaningful and realistic research competencies that can coexist with the demands placed on them as practitioners. Faculty in APN graduate programs should introduce research competencies to their students by

TABLE 8-4 — COMPETENCY III: SELECTED ADVANCED PRACTICE NURSING ACTIVITIES IN COLLABORATIVE QUANTITATIVE RESEARCH

PHASE OF THE RESEARCH*	KNOWLEDGE/SKILLS	ACTIVITIES
1. Conceptual—formulating the problem, selecting a conceptual framework, developing study purposes, questions, and hypotheses	• Expert clinical knowledge of the topic, setting, and population • Good grasp of what constitutes appropriate and feasible nursing-sensitive outcomes in the setting	• Identify nursing practice problems • Consult with researchers to translate problems into researchable questions • Assist in identifying relevant clinical variables and nursing-sensitive outcomes
2. Design and Planning—deciding on the design and methods and developing procedures	• Understanding of quantitative research process and the importance of study rigor, expert clinical knowledge of population, setting, and benchmark data • Understanding and ensuring ethical conduct of research including protection of human subjects and implications for patients, staff, and agency • Understanding of setting's personnel needs and policies, and mechanisms that facilitate good communication with administrators and relevant others in the setting	• Help determine appropriate study sample and selection criteria • Help ensure clinical feasibility of design and methods, assist in selecting appropriate instruments for the population, minimize study burden to patients and staff • Facilitate presentation of study to the agency's IRB • Help develop processes to ensure rigor, participate in developing protocols or procedure manuals for study implementation • Help refine protocols for delivering interventions (if relevant) and collecting data; assist with access to the site and study subjects • Help determine roles of staff and other relevant personnel, including self
3. Empirical—collecting the data and preparing it for analysis	• Knowledge of existing databases and data resources within the institution where research will be conducted	• Collaborate in designing a data collection plan that is practical, most likely to be accurate, and minimizes burdens on clinical staff • Help ensure accurate and consistent collection of data; participate in actual collection of data (if relevant) • Assist researchers in cleaning and coding data (if needed)
4. Analytic—analyzing the data and interpreting it	• Expert knowledge of topic, patients, and setting • Understanding of the research process and research questions being asked in the study • Knowledge of external benchmark data for comparison	• Work with investigators in reviewing the analyses and ensuring that they make sense clinically • Help to provide clinical explanations for findings if needed • Put the findings into the real clinical context of the setting, comparing results with appropriate external benchmark data • Determine the implications for practice or the need for further research
5. Dissemination—communicating research findings	• Expert knowledge of the clinical setting, administration, and other relevant groups to whom research should be disseminated	• Assist in identifying how and where results should be disseminated (both internal and external) • Work with researchers to develop possible clinical, research, and methodological dissemination topics • Help develop abstracts, posters, slide shows, and manuscripts; take responsibility for arranging internal dissemination meetings

*Adapted from Polit, D. F., & Beck, C. T. (2004). *Nursing research: Principles and methods* (7th ed). Philadelphia: Lippincott, Williams, & Wilkins. *IRB*, Institutional review board.

TABLE 8-5	COMPETENCY III: SELECTED ADVANCED PRACTICE NURSING ACTIVITIES IN COLLABORATIVE QUALITATIVE RESEARCH

PHASE OF THE RESEARCH*	KNOWLEDGE/SKILLS	ACTIVITIES
1. Conceptualizing and planning the study—deciding on the focus, approach, site, and participant recruitment	• Understanding of the differences between quantitative and qualitative studies • Expert knowledge of the setting and population • Good communication with administrative and other relevant groups • Understanding of ethical issues including protection of human subjects (as in Table 8-4)	• Identify nursing practice problems • Consult with researchers to translate problems into researchable questions • Facilitate presentation to the agency's IRB • Assist with access to the site and study participants • Help develop procedures that are compatible with the site
2. Conducting the study *(Please note: In qualitative research, the conduct of the study and analysis of the data are often simultaneous or interrelated activities; thus this phase of "conducting the study" refers to both.)*	• Understanding of the emergent process-oriented nature of qualitative research designs and analyses • Expert knowledge of the population under study	• Assist researchers in identifying and contacting potential participants • Facilitate interviews or other data collection processes • Provide information to researchers in the ongoing process of data reduction and analysis • Provide expert clinical insight and knowledge to the interpretative phases of the study • Assist in identifying clinical implications
3. Disseminating the findings	• Expert knowledge of the clinical setting, administration, and other relevant groups to whom research should be disseminated	• Assist in identifying how and where results should be disseminated (both internal and external) • Work with researchers to develop possible clinical, research, and methodological dissemination topics • Help develop abstracts, posters, slide shows, and manuscripts; take responsibility for arranging internal dissemination meetings

*Adapted from Polit, D. F., & Beck, C. T. (2004). *Nursing research: Principles and methods* (7th ed). Philadelphia: Lippincott, Williams, & Wilkins. *IRB*, Institutional review board.

EXEMPLAR 8-3

COMPETENCY III

The following are examples of formal research studies in which APNs played key roles as clinical experts or co-investigators. The examples were chosen to illustrate the variety of ways APNs can participate in research as well as the influence of nursing on complications and quality indicators.

• National survey to determine whether nurse anesthetists demonstrate gender bias in treating pain (Criste, 2003)
• Evaluation of a risk reduction program for cancer-surviving adolescents (Hollen, Hobbie, & Finley, 1999)
• Determination of the time spent by home care APNs in providing prenatal care to women with high-risk pregnancies (Brooten, Brooks, Madigan, & Youngblut, 1998)
• Assessing whether advanced practice nursing intervention would promote positive physical and emotional outcomes in caregivers of frail older adults who reside in rural areas and were recently discharged from urban-based hospitals (Dellasega & Zerbe, 2002)
• Quality improvement initiative, led by CNS, evaluating the impact of clopidogrel on cardiac surgical bleeding (evidence-based protocol [Ley, 2001])

Continued

EXEMPLAR 8-3

COMPETENCY III — cont'd

- Study to describe patient problems and advanced practice nursing interventions in five clinical trials (very low birth weight infants; women with unplanned cesarean deliveries or high-risk pregnancies; women who had undergone hysterectomy; and elders with cardiac medical and surgical diagnoses) and establish links among patient problems (Brooten, Youngblut, Deatrick, Naylor, & York, 2003)
- Descriptive study of incidence of specific high-risk factors of the population cared for by a group of certified nurse-midwives (CNMs) in an inner-city clinic (Davidson, 2002)
- Evaluation of the effectiveness of a hospital-based disease management program for diabetes mellitus (Maljanian et al., 2002)

APNs, Advanced practice nurses; *CNMs,* certified nurse-midwives; *CNS,* clinical nurse specialist.

designing curricula and learning experiences that foster the development of knowledge and skills necessary for participation in fundamental activities. They should also provide learning activities that help APNs understand how to strive for expanded activities after graduation. Thus prepared, APNs can more easily take on the personal and professional responsibility of continuing to develop their research competency knowledge and skills after graduation.

It is unrealistic to expect that any graduate program can, with its temporal and structural constraints, prepare APNs for the full spectrum of possible research competency activities (i.e., both fundamental and expanded levels) (see Table 8-1). APNs will initially begin to acquire their research competencies in graduate school but will continue to develop them throughout their careers, as described previously. Thus on graduation, APNs should be able to perform at the fundamental levels of activity shown in Table 8-1 for all three competencies. Achievement of the expanded levels of activity for the three competencies will depend on the APN's own commitment and on additional experience, continuing education, mentoring, motivation, professional goals, and factors within the clinical setting.

Graduate Education

Graduate programs and their faculty bear the primary responsibility for teaching the knowledge and skills necessary for the fundamental levels of activity in the three research competencies. Thus in addition to teaching new clinical skills and knowledge, faculty in graduate programs should foster, in their advanced practice nursing students, an appreciation of both levels of activity and motivate them to seek the expanded levels of activity for these three research competencies, once they assume advanced practice nursing roles in the workplace. Furthermore, graduate faculty should be role models for all three competencies in their respective areas of didactic and clinical expertise. A discussion of this issue is beyond the scope of this chapter, but such role modeling is critical to the successful teaching of research competencies. Graduate faculty should be adept in interpreting and using research, designing ways to evaluate individual advanced nursing practice, and participating in collaborative research. They should not only have the expertise needed for the three research competencies but should also be able to communicate this to students in their teaching (through both content and assignments) and in clinical activities in a manner that clearly emphasizes the implications of research competencies for advanced practice nursing.

Nursing educators have noted the importance of using EBP as a foundation for advanced practice nursing programs and have addressed some of the curricular issues (Glanville et al., 2000; Sebastian et al., 2000). However, it is not clear whether the notion of advanced practice nursing research competencies has been used as a foundational concept in curricular design and teaching. Adoption of this set of research competencies for APNs will require, for many schools, a rethinking of how "research" is conceptualized and taught at the master's level. If research is indeed a core competency for APNs, as presented in Chapter 3, then it must be taught in a manner that enables students to internalize the research competencies so that they become second nature or part of the APN's repertoire of knowledge, skills, and behaviors. Internalization of any body of knowledge or set of skills does not occur as a result of brief exposure or admonitions to engage in self-study, but rather when important material is introduced early, repeated regularly, and integrated into other components of the curriculum at every possible opportunity.

Teaching research competencies effectively may require a careful examination of and possible overhaul of the APN curriculum in a given program, because these competencies need to be integrated throughout the curriculum, not just isolated in the "research" course(s). That said, the first order of business is still a well-designed foundational research course that focuses on research competencies and the knowledge and skills necessary to carry them out. Because the major emphasis of these research competencies is centered on EBP and evaluation of one's individual practice, the research course should clearly address these areas, and faculty should use teaching techniques that are interesting, relevant, and ultimately helpful to students in developing, practicing, and refining specific skills that they can take away from graduate school and into the workplace. Table 8-6 shows how the advanced practice nursing research competencies are used as a framework for teaching the required research course in a graduate nursing program. Major emphasis is placed on research Competencies I and II, with specific course objectives and assignments and evaluation methods that flow from these competencies. A current research textbook provides a basic reference, with the addition of a packet of carefully selected articles to enhance understanding of content and skills and to enable students to carry out assignments.

In addition to a solid beginning in research competencies through the required research course, which should be placed as early in a graduate program as possible, opportunities to practice and refine these competencies should be available as students progress through the program. A hypothetical curriculum is shown in Table 8-7 to demonstrate how research competencies can be integrated throughout an advanced practice nursing curriculum. In some courses, such as research, the specific knowledge and skills related to research competencies (Tables 8-2, 8-3, 8-4, 8-5) can be used to develop and organize course content, as well as assignments, as shown in Table 8-6 (the research course). In other courses, it may be more appropriate to design student assignments and classroom experiences that use and reinforce the knowledge and specific skills shown in the tables. A specific example may help to clarify how research competencies can be integrated into the curriculum and taught to student APNs (McGuire & Harwood, 2000). As a member of the graduate faculty at the Emory University Nell Hodgson Woodruff School of Nursing (1993–1999), Deborah McGuire worked with a number of other faculty members to introduce research competencies into the required core research course and integrate them into subsequent clinical courses. In the required research course, the following three major assignments tapped into the fundamental level of activities for research Competencies I and II:

1. Students wrote individual quantitative and qualitative research critiques that focused on scientific merit and application of findings to practice (Competency I).

TABLE 8-6	USING RESEARCH COMPETENCIES AS A FRAMEWORK FOR TEACHING RESEARCH AT THE MASTER'S LEVEL		
RESEARCH COMPETENCY	RELEVANT COURSE OBJECTIVES	ASSIGNMENTS/ EVALUATION METHODS	COMMENTS
Interpretation and use of research	1. Identify criteria for evaluating the scientific merit and clinical relevance of research reports 2. Identify sources available for obtaining a synthesis of research concerning a particular nursing procedure or problem 3. Develop skills to critically evaluate nursing and other research for use in practice by using evaluation schemas derived from research utilization and evidence-based practice	1. Each student finds a set of evidence-based clinical practice guidelines on the Web and evaluates them using criteria related to quality, type, and feasibility of clinical application and potential impact on setting, patients, practice, and practitioners. 2. Small groups of students critique a research article with an emphasis on quality of the research and applicability of the results.	These two assignments enable students to begin learning the process of how to evaluate research for use in practice; one focuses on finding and then analyzing available guidelines that are evidence based, and the other focuses on scientific and applicability appraisals of individual research articles.
Evaluation of individual practice	1. Develop beginning skills in using the components of the research process to identify a clinical problem of interest to APNs, to formulate an intervention to address the problem, and to design a project to evaluate a relevant outcome that results from the intervention	1. Small groups of students develop a proposal for a project that addresses a clinical problem relevant to advanced nursing practice and amenable to an improved outcome through advanced practice nursing intervention; they select a problem and an outcome, then design an advanced practice nursing intervention and devise sound methods to assess the outcome.	This assignment provides practice, on a small scale, in selecting relevant clinical outcomes and designing approaches to evaluate those outcomes; it is intended to help APNs learn how to evaluate outcomes of their own individual practice; it is not an outcomes or clinical research project.
Participation in collaborative research	1. Analyze the relationships between research, theory, research design, research questions, data collection, results, and implications for clinical practice	1. All students complete a take-home mid-term exam that covers the phases of the research process, with an emphasis on the design and implementation of rigorous research studies.	This exam helps solidify learning that occurs in assigned reading, didactic content, and classroom discussion; the intent is to develop a solid foundation of knowledge about research.

From McGuire, D. B. (Fall 2003). *Nursing 637: Introduction to research methods and design:* Philadelphia: University of Pennsylvania School of Nursing.

TABLE 8-7	INTEGRATING RESEARCH COMPETENCIES INTO AN ADVANCED PRACTICE NURSING GRADUATE CURRICULUM	
COURSES	**COMPETENCY**	**ASSIGNMENTS**
CORE COURSES		
Theory/knowledge generation	I. Interpretation and use of research in practice	• Integrative review of literature supporting or testing a given theory or identifying a gap in knowledge where theory would be helpful • Analyzing a midrange theory for its relevance to advanced practice
Research/statistics	I. Interpretation and use of research in practice	• Research-based policy, procedure, or protocol • Use computer lab to orient to evidence-based websites, use Web-based calculators to assess clinical significance
	II. Evaluation of practice	• Critique the methodology of a published article on evaluation of advanced practice nursing • Short-term individual or group project evaluating a specific intervention and its effects on selected outcomes
	III. Participation in Collaborative Research	• Design a data collection protocol; develop research questions • Determine clinical problems or issues that can be addressed by a qualitative study (e.g., factors associated with why a particular vulnerable population may or may not participate in available cancer screening programs)
Health policy/professional issues	I. Interpretation and use of research in practice	• Write research-based clinical guidelines for a selected problem and make recommendations for implementation at a policy level
	II. Evaluation of practice	• Develop an evaluation plan for a set of clinical guidelines or a health policy program
Ethics	I. Interpretation and use of research in practice	• Write a research-based paper exploring dimensions of a selected ethical issue (e.g., advance directives, genetics testing, studying vulnerable populations) • Complete the institution's requirements for protection of human subjects
Pharmacology	I. Interpretation and use of research in practice	• Case reports describing selection and use of pharmacological agents based on existing research
	II. Evaluation of practice	• Written evaluation plan for use of specific pharmacological agents or protocol in treating selected clinical problems (e.g., nonopioid and opioid analgesics for cancer pain)
Role theory	I. Interpretation and use of research in practice	• Conduct a literature review and critique selected research on the role of APNs (e.g., studies that compare nurse practitioners with physician assistants)
	II. Evaluation of practice	• Design a project to evaluate the outcomes of a given APN's role in a given setting • Have students do a content analysis of their clinical journals for themes

Continued

TABLE 8-7	INTEGRATING RESEARCH COMPETENCIES INTO AN ADVANCED PRACTICE NURSING GRADUATE CURRICULUM—cont'd

COURSES	COMPETENCY	ASSIGNMENTS
CLINICAL COURSES Advanced practice nursing/ nurse practitioner I, II, III, etc. (includes didactic sessions and clinical practice)	I. Interpretation and use of research in practice	• Retrieve an existing evidence-based guideline in the specialty area and write a paper comparing existing practice with guideline recommendations • Description of comprehensive assessment and intervention plan for individual cases or groups derived from current research; can include critical pathways, care maps, algorithms, protocols, etc.
	II. Evaluation of practice	• Design and implement an evaluation "study" of a specific intervention; include APN-relevant outcomes; make recommendations for practice based on findings • Critique benchmarks/outcomes used in published practice evaluation projects
	III. Participation in collaborative research	• Problem identification, selection of research sample, development of data collection procedures

APN, Advanced practice nurse.

2. Working in small groups, students read about and then selected either an RU model (e.g., Stetler, 1994) or a research application approach such as EBM and used it to evaluate a small body of research and make decisions about applicability to practice (Competency I).
3. Again working in small groups (usually aggregated by programmatic specialty, such as family NPs, oncology APNs, or CNMs), students conceptualized and designed an advanced practice nursing outcomes project in which they identified key outcomes attributable to advanced practice nursing and then selected methods for measuring the outcomes (Competency II).

Integration of research competencies also occurred in one of the clinical courses required of advanced practice nursing students. The course focused on long-term care and included two assignments based on research competencies. The assignments were as follows:

1. Students wrote a paper describing the formulation and management of a set of data they could use in examining their practice (Competency II).
2. Students worked with an APN in a clinical setting to conduct a collaborative project that resulted in a discrete product, such as a component of a critical pathway or selection of a pain assessment tool for a specific patient population. The assignment required students to identify, retrieve, interpret, and make recommendations for use of the research literature relevant to the problem at hand (Competency I).

This example of a graduate faculty's effort to introduce core research competency content early and then reinforce it later in the curriculum was challenging and required strong collaboration and shared ownership and responsibility. However, it is a viable model for how other graduate faculty might attempt to integrate research competencies throughout the curriculum.

Postgraduate Research Competency Development

Much of graduate education is geared toward providing general knowledge and skills that support future learning and development, with faculty providing guidance and oversight. Postgraduate development of research competencies, on the other hand, falls more directly into the purview of the APN. This development is highly individualized to the APN's practice setting, specialty, position expectations, and professional goals and serves to move the APN toward the expanded levels of activity in all three research competencies (see Table 8-1).

Areas in which the APN can develop include augmenting his or her knowledge of appropriate clinical research literature, appropriate outcome measurement techniques, and EBP and research methodologies. Further, the APN can develop and maintain proficiency in computer applications related to information access (e.g., websites) and database management (e.g., to evaluate practice outcomes) and hone personal skills as a change agent in complex, fluid environments (see also Chapter 9). There are numerous ways in which an APN can seek further development in these areas, including collaboration with experienced colleagues, formal academic study, mentorship, membership in professional societies that emphasize EBP and specialty-related research, and independent self-study.

Membership in professional nursing specialty organizations is a good way to expose oneself to current thought and activities related to research competencies. For instance, many nursing specialty organizations such as the Association of Women's Health, Obstetrics and Neonatal Nurses; the Oncology Nursing Society; and the American Association of Critical-Care Nurses have very active resources and programs for members that focus specifically on development and use of clinical practice guidelines, implementation and evaluation of EBP, and collaborative research aimed at improving practice. Often, the annual conferences of these organizations offer continuing education credit for participation in workshops related to expanded levels of research competencies. In these workshops, presentations often provide examples of APNs who are functioning at the expanded level.

Formal coursework in an academic environment offers another avenue for development in selected research-related areas. Relevant courses may be found within graduate programs in nursing, public health, epidemiology, basic sciences (e.g., physiology), social sciences (e.g., psychology), computer sciences, business management, and others. Appropriate courses or workshops may also be offered for professional development within one's work environment or by private companies specializing in professional development. In fact, institutions that employ APNs should demonstrate that these research competencies are valued by incorporating them into position descriptions and performance evaluations. Further, administrators should provide resources to help APNs maintain, refine, and develop these competencies. For example, they can develop and support a formalized program of EBP, by creating an organizational structure that provides personnel and resources to develop, implement, and evaluate EBP (Stricker & Sullivan, 2003).

APNs can also gain needed skills by pursuing an additional academic degree. Obtaining a doctoral degree in nursing or a related field is one means by which an APN can acquire additional research knowledge and skills that will enhance performance of research competencies. After completion of doctoral work, APNs may assume a variety of research-related roles in the workplace. For instance, some APNs will obtain a doctorate in order to have a more advanced set of skills that they can apply directly to their practice, providing more evidence-based care, evaluating their own individual practices, and engaging in collaborative research or even conducting independent research within their specialty areas. Others will choose to obtain a doctorate with its attendant advanced research skills so that they can become clinical researchers, collaborating with active clinicians such as other APNs to address important clinical problems and research questions (Haller, 1990; Kirchhoff, 1993; McGuire et al., 2000).

The mentor-protégé relationship (Vance & Olson, 1998) offers another opportunity for development of expanded-level research competencies. Mentoring is defined as the professional and personal nurturing of a less experienced person (Kinsey, 1990; Vance & Olson, 1998). Mentor-protégé relationships occur on a continuum, ranging from passive role modeling or active precepting of the APN who is new in a role or new in an institution to the classic mentoring relationship. APNs can identify role models and potential mentors both within their organizations and within their practice specialties. For instance, it is possible to develop mentoring relationships that enhance research competencies within the context of institution-wide EBP programs. In one example, an APN who was a novice with EBP was mentored by the director of research and other experts to lead an oral care task force that developed, implemented, and evaluated an evidence-based oral care protocol for inpatients with cancer (Stricker & Sullivan, 2003).

Within the mentoring continuum, the classic mentor-protégé relationship offers the maximum opportunity for developing expanded-level research competencies. These relationships are typically initiated by the nurse identifying an individual to be emulated and then approaching the individual with a request for mentorship. If the mentor agrees, he or she then provides teaching, guidance, and feedback in broad areas relative to the protégé's development. The protégé sustains the relationship by providing feedback on how the guidance has been used and by giving status or outcome reports on activities undertaken in this mentoring process. These relationships often provide an opportunity for collaborative research in which the APN's clinical expertise and the mentor's research expertise are used. APNs may find appropriate mentors among nursing colleagues within their agencies, specialties, professional nursing organizations, or academic faculties. Colleagues from other disciplines may also become research mentors for APNs. Watching and reading about how others have incorporated research findings into their practice, evaluated their practice, or participated in research can be both instructive and motivating. An APN may thus be able to identify a preceptor to assist in the development of a specific skill or group of skills related to any of the research competencies. For example, an APN may request guidance and feedback from an experienced individual when seeking resources to develop evidence-based care protocols, selecting or incorporating a new outcome measurement technique, or designing a database for the collection of outcome data.

Regardless of the methods chosen to advance one's research competencies, self-study is essential to the continued development of research competencies. This self-study is carefully focused on the individual's specialty area and practice. For instance, one APN who was interested in determining appropriate treatment of chemotherapy extravasation (McGuire & Harwood, 2000) engaged in extensive self-study to supplement her graduate education and mentorship support. In addition to graduate work in pharmacology, chemistry, and physiology, she did focused readings in areas such as doxorubicin pharmacology, free radicals and free radical scavenging techniques, and wound healing. She then used this knowledge to identify potential antidotes for evaluation in a research project (Harwood, Straumann, & Gonin, 1994). Determining appropriate animal models for antidote testing required focused self-study in comparative anatomy and physiology. Although this self-study was related to a specific issue, the multifaceted and increasingly interdisciplinary nature of clinical practice, research, and EBP will always require APNs to pursue in-depth knowledge and skills beyond their graduate education to meet research competency needs and other practice requirements

SUMMARY AND CONCLUSION

Research competence for APNs comprises three specific research competencies that are required for APNs to meet the various research-related demands of the advanced practice role in today's health-care delivery system: Competency I, interpretation and use of research; Competency II, evaluation of practice; and Competency III, participation in collaborative research. These competencies are operationalized at two levels—fundamental activities learned through graduate education and expanded activities acquired through postgraduate research development. These competencies are essential to APNs as they define, implement, refine, validate, and evaluate their practices and as they take visible leadership positions in the health-care system of the future.

REFERENCES

Adams, H. P., Adams, R. J., Brott, T., del Zoppo, G. J., Furlan, A., Goldstein, L. B., et al. (2003). Guidelines for the early management of patients with ischemic stroke. *Stroke, 34,* 1056-1083.

AGREE Collaboration. (2001). *Appraisal of Guidelines Research, and Evaluation (AGREE) Instrument.* Retrieved November 4, 2003, from http://www.agreecollaboration.org

Ahrens, T. (2000). Share outcome data and tools demonstrating the value of APNs. *AACN News, 17,* 6.

Aiken, L. H., Clarke, S. P., Sloane, D. M., Sochalski, J., & Silber, J. H. (2002). Hospital nurse staffing and patient mortality, nurse burnout, and job dissatisfaction. *JAMA: The Journal of the American Medical Association, 288,* 1987-1993.

American Association of Colleges of Nursing. (1996). *The essentials of master's education for advanced practice nursing.* Washington, DC: Author.

American Association of Colleges of Nursing. (1999). Certification and regulation of advanced practice nurses. *Journal of Professional Nursing, 15,* 130-132.

American Association of Colleges of Nursing. (2002) *Position statement on nursing research.* Retrieved November 3, 2003, from http://www.aacn.org

American Association of Critical-Care Nurses & American Nurses Association. (1995). *Standards of*
clinical practice and scope of practice for the acute care nurse practitioner. Washington, DC: American Nurses Association.

American Nurses Association. (1981). *Guidelines for the investigative function of nurses.* Kansas City, MO: Author.

American Nurses Association. (1996). *Scope and standards of advanced practice registered nurses.* Washington, DC: Author.

Ball, C., Sackett, D., Phillips, B., Haynes, B., Straus, S., & Dawes, M. (2001). *Levels of evidence and grades of recommendations.* Retrieved March 21, 2004, from http://www.cebm.net/levels_of_evidence.asp

Barnsteiner, J., & Prevost, S. (2002). How to implement evidence-based practice. *Reflections on Nursing Leadership, 28*(2), 18-21.

Beaven, O. (2002). Searching the literature. In J. V. Craig & R. L. Smyth (Eds.), *Evidence-based practice manual for nurses* (pp. 45-85). Edinburgh: Churchill-Livingstone.

Blendon, R. J., DesRoches, C. M., Brodie, M., Benson, J. M. Rosen, A. B., Schneider, E., et al. (2002). Views of practicing physicians and the public on medical errors. *New England Journal of Medicine, 347,* 1933-1940.

Bookbinder, M., Coyle, N., Kiss, M., Goldstein, M. L., Holritz, K., Thaler, H., et al. (1996). Implementing national standards for cancer pain management: Program model and evaluation. *Journal of Pain and Symptom Management, 12,* 334-337.

Bookbinder, M., Kiss, M., Coyle, N., Brown, M., Gianella, A., & Thaler, H. (1995). Improving pain management practices. In D. B. McGuire, C. H. Yarbro, & B. R. Ferrell (Eds.), *Cancer pain management* (2nd ed., pp. 321-361). Boston: Jones & Bartlett.

Bozzo, J. (1999). Databases and nursing outcomes. *American Journal of Nursing, 99*(4), 22.

Brooton, D. Books, L., Madigan, E. A., & Youngblut, J. M. (1998). Home care of high risk pregnant women by advanced practice nurses: Nurse time consumed. *Home Healthcare Nurse, 16*(12), 823-830.

Brooten, D., & Naylor, M. D. (1995). Nurses' effect on changing patient outcomes. *Image: The Journal of Nursing Scholarship, 27,* 95-99.

Brooton, D., Youngblut, J. M., Deatrick, J. Naylor, M. & York, R. (2003). Patient problems, Advanced Practice Nurse (APN) interventions, time and contacts among five patient groups. *Journal of Nursing Scholarship, 35*(1), 73-79.

Brown, S. J. (1999). *Knowledge for health care practice: A guide to using research evidence.* Philadelphia: W. B. Saunders.

Burns, N., & Grove, S. K. (2003). *The practice of nursing research: Conduct, critique, & utilization* (4th ed.). Philadelphia: W. B. Saunders.

Byers, J. F, & Brunell, M. L. (1998). Demonstrating the value of the advanced practice nurse: An evaluation model. *AACN Clinical Issues, 9,* 296-305.

Carioti, C. A., Lavigne, J. E., Stone, P., Tortoretti, D. M., & Chiverton, P. (2001). Work site disease management outcomes: Expanding the role of the APN. *Outcomes Management for Nursing Practice, 5,* 179-184.

Carson, S. (2002). Organizational change. In J. V. Craig & R. L. Smyth, (Eds.), *Evidence-based practice manual for nurses* (pp. 175-196). Edinburgh: Churchill-Livingstone.

Church-Balin, C., & Damus, K. (2003). Preventing prematurity: AWHONN, March of Dimes partner for national campaign. *AWHONN Lifelines, 7,* 97-101.

Clark, J., Cunningham, M., McMillan, S., Vena, C., & Parker, K. (In press). Sleep-wake disturbances in people with cancer (Part II): Evaluating the evidence for clinical decision making. *Oncology Nursing Forum, 31.*

Clochesy, J. M. (2002). Research designs for advanced practice nursing outcomes research. *Critical Care Nursing Clinics of North America, 14,* 293-298.

Conn, V. S., Isaramalai, S., Rath, S., Jantarakupt, P., Wadhawan, R., & Dash, Y. (2003). Beyond MEDLINE for literature searches. *Journal of Nursing Scholarship, 35,* 177-182.

Connors, H. R. (2002). Telehealth technologies enhance children's health care. *Journal of Professional Nursing, 18,* 311-312.

Conway, M. E. (1978). Clinical research: Instrument for change. *Journal of Nursing Administration, 8,* 27-32.

Craig, J. V. (2002). How to ask the right question. In J. V. Craig & R. L. Smyth, (Eds.), *Evidence-based practice manual for nurses* (pp. 21-44). Edinburgh: Churchill-Livingstone.

Criste, A. (2003). Do nurse anesthetists demonstrate gender bias in treating pain? A national survey using a standardized pain model. *AANA Journal, 71,* 206-209.

Cronenwett, L. R. (1995). Molding the future of advanced practice nursing. *Nursing Outlook, 43,* 112-118.

Cullum, N. (1999). How to decide if review articles are trustworthy and relevant for practice. *NT Learning Curve, 3,* 4-6.

Curley, M. A. Q. (1998). Patient-nurse synergy: Optimizing patients' outcomes. *American Journal of Critical Care Nursing, 7,* 64-72.

Dahl, J., & Penque, S. (2000). The effects of an advanced practice nurse–directed heart failure program. *The Nurse Practitioner, 25,* 61-77.

Davidson, M. R. (2002). Clinical practice exchange. Outcomes of high-risk women cared for by certified nurse-midwives. *Journal of Midwifery & Women's Health, 47,* 46-49.

Dellasega, C., & Zerbe, T. M. (2002). Caregivers of frail rural older adults: Effects of an advanced practice nursing intervention. *Journal of Gerontological Nursing, 28*(10), 40-49.

DePalma, J. A. (2000). Evidence-based clinical practice guidelines. *Seminars in Perioperative Nursing, 9,* 115-120.

Dexter, F., Epstein, R. H., Marsh, H. M. (2002). Costs and risks of weekend anesthesia staffing at 6 independently managed surgical suites. *AANA Journal, 70,* 377-381.

Dracup, K. A., & Breu, C. S. (1977). Strengthening practice through research utilization. In M. Batey (Ed.), *Community Nursing Research.* Boulder, CO: Western Interstate Commission for Higher Education.

Eisen, S. V., Leff, H. S., & Schaefer, E. (1999). Implementing outcome systems: Lessons from a test of the BASIS-2 and the SF-36. *Journal of Behavioral Health Services & Research, 26,* 18-27.

Evidence-Based Medicine Working Group. (1992). Evidence based medicine: A new approach to teaching the practice of medicine. *JAMA: The Journal of the American Medical Association, 268,* 2420-2425.

Fain, J. A. (2003). *Reading, understanding, and applying nursing research: A text and workbook* (2nd ed.). Philadelphia: F. A. Davis.

Gibbs, L. E. (2003). *Evidence-based practice for the helping professions.* Toronto, Ontario, Canada: Thomson Brooks/Cole.

Glanville, I., Schirm, V., & Wineman, N. M. (2000). Using evidence-based practice for managing clinical outcomes in advanced practice nursing. *Journal of Nursing Care Quality, 15,* 1-11.

Goldman, D. P., & Zissimopoulos, J. M. (2003). High out-of-pocket health care spending by the elderly. *Health Affairs, 22,* 194-202.

Goode, C. J. (1995). Evaluation of research-based nursing practice. *Nursing Clinics of North America, 30,* 421-428.

Goode, C. J. (2000). What constitutes the "evidence" in evidence-based practice? *Applied Nursing Research, 13,* 222-225.

Goode, C. J., & Piedalue, F. (1999). Evidence-based clinical practice. Journal of Nursing Administration, 29, 15-21.

Guyatt, G. H., Haynes, R. B., Jaeschke, R. Z., Cook, D. J., Green, L., Naylor, C. D., et al. (2000) Users' guides to the medical literature: XXV Evidence-based medicine: Principles for applying the users' guides to patient care. JAMA: *The Journal of the American Medical Association, 284,* 1290-1296.

Guyatt, G., & Rennie, D. (Eds.). (2002). *Users' guides to the medical literature.* Chicago: AMA Press.

Hadorn, D. C., Baker, D., Hodges, J. S., & Hicks, N. (1995). Rating the quality of evidence for clinical practice guidelines. *Journal of Clinical Epidemiology, 49,* 749-754.

Haller, K. B. (1990). The clinical nurse researcher role in a practice setting. In N. L. Chaska (Ed.), *The nursing profession: Turning points* (pp. 194-201). St. Louis, MO: C. V. Mosby.

Hamric, A. B. (1996). A definition of advanced nursing practice. In A. B. Hamric, J. A. Spross, & C. M. Hanson (Eds.), *Advanced nursing practice: An integrative approach* (pp. 42-56). Philadelphia: W.B. Saunders.

Hamric, A. B. (2000). A definition of advanced nursing practice. In A. B. Hamric, J. A. Spross, & C. M. Hanson (Eds.), *Advanced nursing practice: An integrative approach* (pp. 53-73). Philadelphia: W.B. Saunders.

Hamric, A. B. & Spross, J. A. (Eds.). (1989). *The clinical nurse specialist in theory and practice* (2nd ed.). Philadelphia: W. B. Saunders.

Harris, R. P., Helfand, M., Woolf, S. H., Lohr, K. N., Mulrow, C. D., Teutsch, S. M., et al. (2001). Current methods of the U.S. Preventative Services Task Force: A review of the process. *American Journal of Preventative Medicine, 20,* 21-35.

Harwood, K., Strauman, J., & Gonin, R. (1994). Short-term vs. long-term local cooling after doxorubicin (DOX) extravasation: An Eastern Cooperative Oncology Group (ECOG) study [Abstract]. *Proceedings of the American Society of Clinical Oncology, 13,* 447.

Hayward, R. S. A., Wilson, M. C., Tunis, S. R., Bass, E. B., & Guyatt, G. (1995). How to use a clinical practice guideline. JAMA: *The Journal of the American Medical Association, 274,* 570-574.

Health Resources & Service Administration (HRSA). (2002). *Nurse practitioner primary care competencies in specialty areas: Adult, family geronto-logical, pediatric, and women's health.* Retrieved November 3, 2003, from http://www.aacn.org

Heffler, S., Smith, S., Keehan, S., Clemens, M. K., Won, G., & Zessa, M. (2003). Health spending projections for 2002-2012. *Health Affairs, 22,* 12.

Helmer, D., Savoie, I., Green, C., & Kazanjian, A. (2001). Evidence-based practice: Extending the search to find material for the systematic review. *Bulletin of Medical Library Association, 89,* 346-352.

Hodgman, E. C. (1983). The CNS as researcher. In A. B. Hamric & J. A. Spross (Eds.), *The clinical nurse specialist in theory and practice* (pp. 73-2). New York: Grune & Stratton.

Hollen, P. J., Hobbie, W. L., & Finley, S. M. (1999). Testing the effects of a decision-making and risk-reduction program for cancer-surviving adolescents. *Oncology Nursing Forum, 26,* 1475-1486.

Horsley, J., Crane, J., & Bingle, J. (1978). Research utilization as an organizational process. *Journal of Nursing Administration, 8,* 4-6.

Hughes, L. C., Hodgson, N. A., Muller, P., Robinson, L. A., & McCorkle, R. (2000). Information needs of elderly postsurgical cancer patients during the transition from hospital to home. *Journal of Nursing Scholarship, 32,* 25-30.

Humphris, D. (1999). A framework to evaluate the role of nurse specialists. *Professional Nurse, 14,* 37-39.

Hunt, D. L., & McKibbon, K. A. (1997). Locating and appraising systematic reviews. *Annals of Internal Medicine, 126,* 532-538.

Hunt, J. M. (2002). Future perspectives of evidence-based practice. *Seminars in Oncology Nursing, 18,* 79-81.

Institute of Medicine. (1990). *Clinical practice guidelines: Directions for a new program.* Washington, DC: National Academy Press.

Institute of Medicine. (2001). *Crossing the quality chasm: A new health system for the 21st century.* Washington, DC: National Academy Press.

Jacobs, L. A. (Ed.). (2003). *Statement on the scope and standards of advanced practice nursing in oncology* (3rd ed.). Pittsburgh: Oncology Nursing Society Publishing Division.

Jacobsen, S. J., Girman, C. J., Guess, H. A., Panser, L. A., Chute, C. G., Oesterling, J. E., et al. (1995). Do prostate size and urinary flow rates predict health care seeking behavior for urinary symptoms in men? *Urology, 45,* 64-69.

Jastremski, C. A. (2002). Using outcomes research to validate the advanced practice nursing role administratively. *Critical Care Nursing Clinics of North America, 14,* 275-280.

Jencks, S. F., Huff, E. D., & Cuerdon, T. (2003). Change in the quality of care delivered to Medicare beneficiaries, 1998-1999 to 2000-2001. JAMA: *The Journal of the American Medical Association, 289,* 305-312.

Jennings, B. M. & Loan, L. A. (2001). Misconceptions among nurses about evidence-based practice. *Journal of Nursing Scholarship, 33,* 121-127.

Jennings, B. M., Staggers, N., & Brosch, L. R. (1999). A classification scheme for outcome indicators. *Image: The Journal of Nursing Scholarship, 31*, 381-388.

Joint Commission on Accreditation of Healthcare Organizations (JCAHO). (2002). *Nursing shortage poses serious health care risk: Joint Commission expert panel offers solutions to national health care crisis.* Retrieved November 3, 2003, from http://www.jcaho.org/news+room/ news+release+archives/ nursing+shortage.htm

Joint Commission on Accreditation of Healthcare Organizations (JCAHO). (2003a). *Health care at the crossroads: Strategies for addressing the evolving nursing crisis.* Oakbrook Terrace, IL: Author.

Joint Commission on Accreditation of Healthcare Organizations (JCAHO). (2003b). *Specification manual for national implementation of hospital core measures version 2.0.* Oakbrook Terrace, IL: Author.

Kapur, K., & Marquis, M. S. (2003). Health insurance for workers who lose jobs: Implications for various subsidy schemes. *Health Affairs, 22*, 203-213.

Kinsey, D. C. (1990). Mentorship and influence in nursing. *Nursing Management, 45*, 45-46.

Kirchhoff, K. T. (1993). The role of nurse researchers employed in clinical settings. *Annual Review of Nursing Research, 11*, 169-181.

Krueger, J. (1978). Utilization of nursing research: The planning process. *Journal of Nursing Administration, 8*, 6-9.

Ledbetter, C. A., & Stevens, K. R. (2000). Basics of evidence-based practice part 2: Unscrambling the terms and processes. *Seminars in Perioperative Nursing, 9*, 98-104.

Ley, S. J. (2001). Quality care outcomes in cardiac surgery: The role of evidence-based practice. *AACN Clinical Issues, 12*(4), 606-617.

LoBiondo-Wood, G., & Haber, J. (2002). *Nursing research: Methods, critical appraisal & utilization,* 5th ed. St. Louis: Mosby.

Maljanian, R. Grey, N. Staff, I., Cruzmarino de Aponte, M. (2002). Improved diabetes control through a provider-based disease management program. *Disease Management & Health Outcomes, 10*(1), 1-8.

Martin, P. A. (1995). Finding time for research. *Applied Nursing Research, 8*, 151-153.

Masys, D. R. (2002). Effects of current and future information technologies on the health care workforce. *Health Affairs, 21*, 33-41.

Mateo, M. A., & Kirchhoff, K. T. (Eds.). (1999). *Using and conducting nursing research in the clinical setting* (2nd ed.). Philadelphia: W.B. Saunders.

McCorkle, R., Strumpf, N. E., Nuramah, I. F., Adler, D. C., Cooley, M. E., Jepson, C., et al. (2000). A specialized home care intervention improves survival among older post-surgical cancer patients. *Journal of the American Geriatrics Society, 48*, 1707-1713.

McGuire, D. B., DeLoney, V. G., Yeager, K. A., Owen, D. C., Peterson, D. E., Lin, L. S., et al. (2000).

Maintaining study validity in a changing clinical environment. *Nursing Research, 49*, 231-235.

McGuire, D. B., & Harwood, K. V. (1989). The CNS as researcher. In A. B. Hamric & J. A. Spross (Eds.), *The clinical nurse specialist in theory and practice* (2nd ed., pp. 169-203). Philadelphia: W.B. Saunders.

McGuire, D. B., & Harwood, K. (1996). Research interpretation, utilization, and conduct. In A. B. Hamric, J. A. Spross, & C. M. Hanson, (Eds.), *Advanced nursing practice: An integrative approach* (pp. 184-211). Philadelphia: W.B. Saunders.

McGuire, D. B., & Harwood, K. V. (2000). Research. In A. B. Hamric, J. A. Spross, & C. M. Hanson (Eds.), *Advanced nursing practice: An integrative approach* (2nd ed.) (pp. 245-278). Philadelphia: W.B. Saunders.

McSweeney, M., Spies, M., & Cann, C. J. (2001). Finding and evaluating clinical practice guidelines. *The Nurse Practitioner, 26*, 30, 33-34, 39, 43-47.

Mehrotra, A., Bodenheimer, T., & Dudley, R.A. (2003). Employers' efforts to measure and improve hospital quality: Determinants of success. *Health Affairs, 22*, 60-71.

Mills, R. J., & Bhandari, S. (2003). *Health insurance coverage in the United States: 2002.* Washington, DC: U.S. Department of Commerce, U.S. Census Bureau.

Minarik, P. (1999). Using hospital databases. *American Journal of Nursing, 99*, 54.

Morrisey, L. J., & DeBourgh, G. A. (2001). Finding evidence: Refining literature searching skills for the advanced practice nurse. *AACN Clinical Issues, 12*, 560-577.

Mulrow, C. D., & Oxman, A. D. (1997). Cochrane collaboration handbook. *The Cochrane collaboration,* Issue 4, Chichester, UK: John Wiley & Sons, Ltd.

Nail, L. M. (1990). Involving clinicians in nursing research. *Oncology Nursing Forum, 17*, 621-623.

National Association of Clinical Nurse Specialists. (2004). *Statement on clinical nurse specialist practice and education* (2nd ed). Harrisburg, PA: Author.

National Committee for Quality Assurance's Health Plan (NCQA). (2000). *NCQA unveils free on-line consumer resource to rate health plans on clinical care, member satisfaction, overall quality.* Retrieved November 3, 2003, from http://www.ncqa.org/ communications/news/hprcrel.htm

National Organization of Nurse Practitioners Faculties (NONPF) & American Association of Colleges of Nursing (AACN). (2002). *Nurse practitioner primary care competencies in specialty areas: Adult, family gerontological, pediatric, and women's health.* Washington, DC: U.S. Department of Health and Human Services.

Needleman, J., Buerhaus, P., Mattke, S., Stewart, M., & Zelevinsky, K. (2002). Nurse-staffing levels and the quality of care in hospitals. *New England Journal of Medicine, 347*, 1118-1119.

Newell-Stokes, V., Broughton, S., Guiliano, K. K., & Stetler, C. B. (2001). Developing an evidence-based procedure: Maintenance of central venous catheters. Clinical Nurse Specialist, 15, 199-206.

Norwood, S. L. (2000). *Research strategies for advanced practice nurses.* Upper Saddle River, NJ: Prentice Hall Health.

Papadopoulos, M., & Rheeder, P. (2000). How to do a systematic literature review. *Journal of Physiotherapy, 56,* 3-6.

Payne, J. K. (2002). An integrated model of nursing using evidence-based practice. *Oncology Nursing Forum, 29,* 463-465.

Pearson, M., & Craig, J. V. (2002). In J. V. Craig & R. L. Smyth, (Eds.), *Evidence-based practice manual for nurses* (pp. 3-20). Edinburgh: Churchill-Livingstone.

Polit, D. F., & Beck, C. T. (2004). *Nursing research: Principles and methods* (7th ed.). Philadelphia: Lippincott Williams & Wilkins.

Polit, D. F., Beck, C. T., & Hungler, B. P. (2001). *Essentials of nursing research* (5th ed.). Philadelphia: Lippincott Williams & Wilkins.

Pond, F. (1999). Searching for studies. In S. J. Brown (Ed.), *Knowledge for health care practice: A guide to using research evidence* (pp. 41-58). Philadelphia: W.B. Saunders.

Pravikoff, D. S., & Donaldson, N. E. (2001). Online journals: Access and support for evidence-based practice. *AACN Clinical Issues, 12,* 588-596.

Richardson, W. C., & Corrigan, J. M. (2003). Provider responsibility and system redesign: Two sides of the same coin. *Health Affairs, 22,* 116-118.

Rigotti, N. A., Munafo, M. R., Murphy, M. F., & Stead, L. F. (2003). Interventions for smoking cessation in hospitalized patients. In *The Cochrane Library,* Issue 1. Chichester, UK: John Wiley & Sons, Ltd.

Robinson, C. B., Fritch, M., Hullett, L., Petersen, M. A., Sikkema, S., Theuninck, L., et al. (2000). Development of a protocol to prevent opioid-induced constipation in patients with cancer: A research utilization project. *Clinical Journal of Oncology Nursing, 4,* 79-84.

Rogers, E. M. (2003). Diffusion of innovations (5th ed.). New York: The Free Press.

Ropka, M. E., & Spencer-Cisek, P. (2001). PRISM: Priority Symptom Management Project. Phase I—Assessment. *Oncology Nursing Forum, 28,* 1585-1594.

Rosswurm, M. A., & Larrabee, J. H. (1999). A model for change to evidence-based practice. *Image: The Journal of Nursing Scholarship, 31,* 317-322.

Rutledge, D., Cope, D., Haas, M., Hinds, P., Moore, K., & Van Gerpen, R. (2001). *EBP Process Model.* Retrieved October 4, 2003, from http://www.onsopcontent.ons.org/toolkits/ebp/index.htm

Rutledge, D. N., & Grant, M. (2002). Evidence-based practice in cancer nursing, Introduction. *Seminars in Oncology Nursing, 18,* 1-2.

Sackett, D. L., Straus, S. E., Richardson, W. S., Rosenberg, W., & Haynes, R. B. (1997). *Evidence-based medicine: How to practice and teach EBM.* Edinburgh: Churchill Livingstone.

Sackett, D. L., Straus, S. E., Richardon, W. S., Rosenberg, W., & Haynes, R. B. (2000). *Evidence-based medicine: How to practice and teach EBM* (2nd ed.). Edinburgh: Churchill Livingstone.

Sampselle, C. M., Wyman, J. F., Thomas, K. K., Newman, D. K., Gray, M., Dougherty, M., et al. (2000). Continence for women: Evaluation of AWHONN's third research utilization project. *JOGNN: Journal of Obstetric, Gynecologic, & Neonatal Nursing, 29,* 9-17.

Schulmeister, L., & Vrabel, M. (2002). Searching for information for presentations and publications. *Clinical Nurse Specialist, 16,* 79-84.

Schulz, M. A., Ludwick, R., Cukr, P. L., & Kelly, D. (2002). Outcomes of a community-based three-year breast and cervical screening program for medically underserved, low income women. *Journal of the American Academy of Nurse Practitioners, 14,* 219-224.

Sebastian, J. G., Christman, N. J., Howard, P. B., Lock, S. E., Free, T. A., Chlebowy, D. O., et al. (2000). Evidence-based practice and the advanced practice nurse: A curriculum for the future. *Seminars in Perioperative Nursing, 9,* 143-148.

Shaneyfelt, T. M., Mayo-Smith, M. F., & Rothwangl, J. (1999). Are guidelines following guidelines? The methodological quality of clinical practice guidelines in the peer-reviewed medical literature. *JAMA: The Journal of the American Medical Association, 281,* 1900-1905.

Shekelle, P. G., Eccles, M. P., Grimshaw, J. M., Woolf, S. H. (2001). When should clinical guidelines be updated? *British Medical Journal, 323,* 155-157.

Shojania, K. G., & Bero, L. A. (2001). Taking advantage of the explosion of systematic reviews: An efficient MEDLINE search strategy. *Effective Clinical Practice, 4,* 157-162.

Shortell, S. M., Bennett, C. L., & Byck, G. R. (1998). Assessing the impact of continuous quality improvement on clinical practice: What it will take to accelerate progress. Milbank Quarterly, 76, 755-757.

Smyth, R. L. (2002). Systematic reviews: What are they and how can they be used? In J. V. Craig & R. L. Smyth (Eds.), *Evidence-based practice manual for nurses* (pp.164-187). Edinburgh: Churchill-Livingstone.

Sochalski, J. (2002). Nursing shortage redux: Turning the corner on an enduring problem. *Health Affairs, 21,* 157-164.

Stetler, C. B. (1985). Research utilization: Defining the concept. *Image: The Journal of Nursing Scholarship, 17,* 40-44.

Stetler, C. B. (1994). Refinement of the Stetler/Marram Model for application of research findings to practice. *Nursing Outlook, 42*(1), 15-25.

Stetler, C. B. & Marram, G. (1976). Evaluating research findings for applicability in practice. *Nursing Outlook, 24,* 559-563.

Stetler, C. B., Morsi, D., Rucki, S., Broughton, S., Corrigan, B., Fitzgerald, J., et al. (1998). Utilization-focused integrative reviews in nursing service. *Applied Nursing Research, 1*, 195-206.

Stevens, K. R., & Cassidy, V.R. (1999). *Evidence-based teaching: Current research in nursing education.* Boston: Jones & Bartlett.

Stevens, K. R., & Ledbetter, C. A. (2000). Basics of evidence-based practice. Part 1: The nature of the evidence. *Seminars in Perioperative Nursing, 9*, 91-97.

Stricker, C. T., & Sullivan, J. (2003). Evidence-based oncology care clinical practice guidelines: Development, implementation, and evaluation. *Clinical Journal of Oncology Nursing, 7*, 222-227.

Thomas, L., & Hotchkiss, K. (2002). Evidence-based guidelines. In J. V. Craig & R. L. Smyth (Eds.), *Evidence-based practice manual for nurses* (pp. 187-210). Edinburgh: Churchill-Livingstone.

Thompson, C. L., White, C., Wild, L. R., Morris, A. B., Perdue, S. T., Stanik-Hutt, J., et al. (2001). Translating research into practice: Implications of the Thunder Project II. *Critical Care Nursing Clinics of North America, 13*, 541-546.

Titler, M. G. (1998). Use of research in practice. In G. Lobiondo-Wood & J. Haber (Eds.), *Nursing research* (4th ed., pp. 467-498). St. Louis, MO: Mosby.

Titler, M. G., Kleiber, C., Steelman, V., Goode, C., Rakel, B., Barry-Walker, J., et al. (1994). Infusing research into practice to promote quality care. *Nursing Research, 43*, 307-313.

Titler, M. G., Mentes, J.C., Rakel, B.A., Abbott, L., & Baumler, S. (1999). From book to bedside: Putting evidence to use in the care of the elderly. *Journal of Quality Improvement, 25*, 545-556.

Vance, C., & Olson, R. K. (Eds.). (1998). *The mentor connection in nursing.* New York: Springer-Verlag.

Vincent, D. (2002). Using cost-analysis techniques to measure the value of nurse practitioner care. *International Nursing Review, 49*, 243-249.

Wakefield, B., Johnson, J., Kron-Chalupa, J., & Paulsen, L. (1998). A research-based guideline for appropriate use of transdermal fentanyl to treat chronic pain. *Oncology Nursing Forum, 25*, 1505-1512.

Welch, L. B. (1979). Planned change in nursing: The theory. *Nursing Clinics of North America, 14*, 307-321.

White, C. A. (1996). A study of pain: Site enrollment for Thunder Project II concluding. *ASPMN Pathways, 5*, 9.

White, S. J. (1997). Evidence-based practice and nursing. The new panacea? *British Journal of Nursing, 6*, 175-178.

Whitman, G. R. (2002a). Outcomes research in advanced practice nursing: Selecting an outcome. *Critical Care Nursing Clinics of North America, 14*, 253-260.

Whitman, G. R. (2002b). Outcomes research: Getting started, defining outcomes, a framework, and data sources. *Critical Care Nursing Clinics of North America, 14*, 261-268.

Wu, Y. W. B., Crosby, F., Ventura, M., & Finnick, M. (1994). In a changing world: Database to keep the pace. *Clinical Nurse Specialist, 8*, 104-108.

Wyrwich, K. W., Tierney, W. M., & Wolinsky, F. D. (1999). Further evidence supporting an SEM-based criterion for identifying meaningful intra-individual changes in health-related quality of life. *Journal of Clinical Epidemiology, 52*, 861-873.

CHAPTER 9

Clinical and Professional Leadership

CHARLENE M. HANSON • JUDITH A. SPROSS

Continued

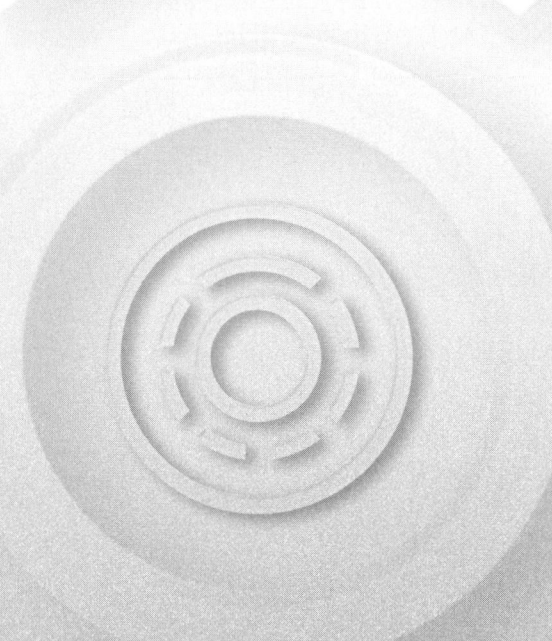

INTRODUCTION

Leadership is a core competency of the advanced practice nurse (APN). In this chapter, the definition of advanced practice nursing leadership is expanded beyond the traditional understanding of clinical leadership. The age of communication and high-tech information systems has markedly changed the milieu in which APNs practice and interact with others. Change is the only constant in the current environment. The abilities to effectively manage change, to empower others, and to influence political processes are three reciprocal elements of the advanced practice nursing competency of leadership. In short, effective change agents must be leaders, and effective leaders require the skills of a change agent. In this chapter, this broader concept of leadership is explored. The essential elements and skills needed for successful leadership are defined, and strategies for applying them in both clinical and professional arenas are presented. Obstacles frequently encountered by APNs are examined, along with strategies to manage these barriers and thus move the leader toward successful outcomes. An Additional Readings section is included, which directs readers to the extensive literature that defines traditional leadership and change concepts and strategies.

APNs may exercise leadership at local, regional, and national levels and in clinical environments, within nursing and across disciplines. Leadership activities of APNs may range from taking a stand on behalf of a patient to advocating for a change in health-care policy at the national level. The leadership competency depends on APNs' other competencies (e.g., direct care and collaboration). Specific leadership skills should be discussed, nurtured, and developed during graduate education through refinement of communication skills; supported risk-taking; reflective learning; and interactions with nurse leaders, mentors, and role models. The purposes of this chapter are to describe leadership domains and activities of APNs, provide useful literature and resources on leadership and change, describe characteristics of effective leaders, identify obstacles to effective leadership, and discuss strategies for developing leadership skills.

LEADERSHIP DOMAINS OF ADVANCED PRACTICE NURSES

Though the need for leadership in health-care settings is well-recognized (National Organization of Nurse Practitioner Faculties [NONPF] & American Association of Colleges of Nursing [AACN], 2002; National Association of Clinical Nurse Specialists [NACNS], 2004; Spencer & Jordan, 2001), the topic has not been well studied, and research on effective leadership is needed (Thomson et al., 1999; Vance & Larson, 2002). Not all APNs are comfortable with the idea of being leaders, but leadership is *not* an optional activity. Advanced practice nursing leadership can be conceptualized as occurring in three primary domains: in clinical practice with patients and staff, within health-care institutions and professional organizations, and in health-care policymaking arenas. The extent to which individual APNs choose to lead in each of these areas depends on patients' needs; APNs' personal characteristics, interests, and commitments; institutional or organizational priorities; and priority health-care policy issues in nursing as a whole and within one's specialty. This chapter will help APNs define their need for leadership skills and embark on a plan for acquiring the necessary skills appropriate to their particular positions and professional goals. Some aspects of empowerment, change agency, and political activism are discussed separately to help readers grasp the different domains of leadership. However, there is considerable overlap in the knowledge and skills needed to lead in each domain.

Leadership in Clinical Practice with Patients and Staff

Leadership experiences are most likely to arise in clinical practice with patients and colleagues. The most common leadership roles APNs can expect to play are those of advocate, group leader, and change agent. APNs may advocate for a particular patient or family, as when an acute care nurse practitioner (NP) consults with a psychiatric clinical nurse specialist (CNS) to assist in explaining a grave prognosis to family members. Group leadership may be informal, as when an APN agrees to coordinate multiple referrals for a patient with complex care needs or when an APN has expertise in a particular clinical problem such as pain management. APNs may also have more formal leadership responsibilities: for example, an APN may agree to convene a group and lead the development of a new practice protocol to bring care into line with new standards.

A change agent is one who motivates colleagues and facilitates their use of new knowledge and/or the adoption of new practices. Historically, explicit responsibilities for change agency were an integral component of only the CNS role. As conceptualizations of advanced nursing practice have evolved, it is apparent that all APNs have responsibilities and opportunities to improve clinical practice.

Leadership in Health Care and Professional Organizations

Within health-care organizations, APNs may lead clinical teams, chair committees, and direct other initiatives aimed at improving the clinical practice of nurses and other professionals and patient care. In Chapter 15, for example, Skalla, Hamric, and Caron describe the evolution of leadership within a group of APNs (NPs and blended-role CNS/NPs). APNs may identify an increase in the rate of patient falls and create a task force to evaluate the problem and intervene to correct it. A critical care CNS may initiate interdisciplinary rounds to monitor patients on mechanical ventilation and gather data on clinical variables such as complication rate and time to weaning. APNs may be asked to participate in or lead standing or ad hoc interdisciplinary committees such as Medical Credentialing, Ethics, Institutional Review Boards, or Pharmacy and Therapeutics to ensure that a nursing perspective will be articulated. APNs may be asked by administrators to participate in organizational reengineering or other activities aimed at improving the environment in which nurses practice (see Chapters 11 and 24).

Most APNs are members of one or more nursing and interdisciplinary organizations. These memberships provide myriad leadership opportunities that include organizing a continuing education offering, presenting at national conferences, chairing a committee, and running for the board of directors. In these situations APNs exercise more choice as to whether and when they will participate in leadership activities than in their employee roles.

Empowering Others to Provide Leadership

Closely aligned to, but somewhat different from, the mentoring process APNs use to lead others is the process of empowerment. As the word implies, *empowerment* is defined as giving power to another, enabling, or giving authority. APNs operationalize empowerment by sharing power with other nurses, colleagues, and patients or by enabling them to access or assert their own power. Empowerment as a leadership strategy is guided by the shared vision of the leader and follower and a willingness of the leader to delegate authority to others. Visionary leaders who empower their followers greatly increase the influence of APNs both within nursing and beyond nursing's boundaries. Empowerment of other nurses fosters change, provides new opportunities for practice, and enhances the ability to influence health-care policy decisions.

Leadership in Health-Care Policy Arenas

Although some APNs may not see themselves as being particularly interested in or talented at political advocacy, all APNs have a vested interest in policymaking that affects nursing generally and advanced practice nursing more specifically. APNs should be aware of, and must often respond to, local, state, and national policymaking efforts likely to affect laws and regulations that affect their scopes of practice.

By outlining these various leadership activities early in the chapter, we want to encourage readers to reflect on leadership opportunities they encounter, consider those that align with their clinical interests and personal characteristics, and begin to develop a leadership portfolio. We hope the chapter will challenge readers to rethink their ideas about leadership and help students begin to integrate a personally meaningful concept of leadership into their identities as APNs.

To be a leader in the current health-care arena requires an ability to analyze health-care systems, an understanding of the personal qualities that are associated with effective leadership, and the skill to use this understanding to act strategically.

LEADERSHIP, EMPOWERMENT, CHANGE, AND ACTIVISM: SELECTED LITERATURE

The nursing, sociology, and business literatures are rich sources of leadership definitions, concepts, and models that help APNs develop as effective and dynamic leaders and role models. Concepts such as vision, sharing power, and action-oriented strategies are well defined in nursing's leadership vocabulary. Multiple conceptual models exist for understanding the interactions that occur in the leadership process. Leadership models that empower followers, include others outside of nursing, and allow for change to occur seem to "fit" the best in these unsettled times. Some of these frameworks and related concepts are briefly explained here and are meant as a guide for skill development; however, it is beyond the scope of this chapter to provide an in-depth discussion of the breadth and depth of nursing leadership. Readers can use the Additional Readings section to broaden their understanding of the evolution of nursing leadership throughout the 20th century.

Definitions of Leadership

Definitions of leadership generally fit into one of two categories—transactional or transformational (Vance & Larson, 2002). More traditional notions of leadership tend to be transactional. For example, Burns (1978) defined *transactional leadership* as occurring when one person takes the initiative to foster the exchange of something of economic, psychological, or political value with another person. The leader and follower may have related purposes, but they are not necessarily connected by common goals. With this definition, Burns implied that change is a component of leadership.

Barker (1994) defined *transformational leadership* as a process whereby "the purposes of the leader and follower become fused, creating unity, wholeness and a collective purpose" (p. 83). Collins (2001) suggested that businesses that adhere to team approaches move their companies from "good" to "great" status. Transformational leadership can lead to changes in values, attitudes, perceptions, and/or behaviors on the part of the leader, as well as the follower, and lays the groundwork for further positive change and improvement in outcomes. Thus transformational leadership occurs when people interact in ways that raise each other to higher levels of motivation and morality. Leaders motivate, stimulate, share with, conciliate, and satisfy their followers in an interdependent, interactional exchange. DePree (1989) described leadership as an art form that frees (empowers) people "to do what is required of them in the most effective and humane way possible" (p. 1) and contended that contemporary leadership may be simply viewed as a process of moving the self and others toward a shared vision that becomes a shared reality. Successful transformational leadership is relational, driven by a common goal or purpose, and satisfies the needs of both leader and follower. It is the leadership style often associated with effective change agents. Other authors who describe a transformational approach to leadership include Heifetz (1994), Senge, (1990, 1999), and Covey (1989).

In addition to these two broad definitions, other commentators have explored additional dimensions of leadership. The role of follower is important and relevant to any discussion about leadership. Grohar-Murray and DiCroce (1992) included the role of follower in research in which they explored the *situational* approach to leadership, which was first defined by Stogdill in 1948 and expanded by Fiedler, Chermers, and Mahar in 1976. Their approach suggested that leadership is situationally dependent, with identified leaders and followers in interchangeable roles according to environmental demands. DePree (1989) enlarged on this idea and used the term *roving leadership* to describe a participatory process that legitimizes the situational leadership of empowered followers through the support and approval of the hierarchical leader. This concept has great relevance for the APN, who continually works in collaborative health-care teams that require that the roles of leader and follower be interchangeable to meet the complex needs of the patient. APNs will assume both leader and follower roles and need to develop skills to know when these different roles are indicated and when a situation warrants their moving from the role of follower to that of leader.

Inherent in the discussion of transformational and situational leadership is the importance of vision. The APN as a leader who has a vision of collaboration among health-care team members may facilitate an atmosphere that supports individuals (followers) in assuming the leadership role in various situations. The APN does not cease being the leader by empowering colleagues to appropriately assume a leadership role. In fact, this important approach may be an effective way of both sharing a vision and sharing power, issues discussed later in the chapter.

Types of Leadership

Certain situations require distinct types of leadership that allow leadership styles to emerge in several unique forms and settings. Leadership begins at the micro level, with patients. *Clinical leadership* occurs when APNs learn with and from others about how to build appropriate working relationships with health-care team members, how to instill confidence in patients and colleagues, and how to problem solve as part of a team (Engebretson & Wardell, 1997). Clinical leaders are role models and mentors who empower patients and colleagues. They serve as change agents who implement change strategies that improve patient care and enhance others' perceptions of the value of advanced practice nursing. Some of the direct clinical leadership skills are part of the competencies of consultation (Chapter 7) and collaboration (Chapter 11) and are portrayed in the exemplars in the role chapters (Part III) as well. Clinical leadership often moves beyond nursing's discipline into the realm of *interdisciplinary leadership,* which occurs across the boundaries of other disciplines. Covey (1989) suggested that interdisciplinary leadership occurs at a very high level because it requires the ability to understand issues in another profession's domain. An example is an APN who serves as chairperson for a national task force of health-care professionals that is developing practice guidelines for the treatment of asthma. The ability to provide interdisciplinary leadership requires a firm grasp of the issues and differences within the nursing profession while responding to the challenges of other disciplines and the larger society. As clinical leaders gain skill, they develop the attributes needed to interact at this level with other members of the health-care team.

Organizational leadership refers to situations in which leaders are formally elected or appointed to positions of power within defined organizations and groups. As with clinical leadership, organizational leadership begins at the grass-roots level and proceeds upward to state, national, and international levels. To acquire leadership skills and experience, novice APNs need to become involved in the leadership and committee work of local advanced practice nursing coalitions and organizations and move into state and regional leadership roles as they develop their style and strengths as advanced practice nursing leaders. Situations in which leaders are formally elected or appointed to positions of power within defined organizations and groups are very important to the growth and vitality of advanced practice nursing. The ability to place nurse leaders in key positions is critical to the visibility and credibility of APNs and to the establishment of roles for APNs within nursing and within the larger health-care community. *Entrepreneurial leadership* refers to those leaders who go outside of traditional employment systems to create new opportunities to exercise their special abilities (Ballein, 1998). Chapter 1 clearly depicts the role that entrepreneurial nurse leaders have played in creating advanced practice roles in nursing. Creative, entrepreneurial leadership is necessary for APNs to navigate in today's complex health-care systems. Ballein (1998) studied entrepreneurial leadership skills as defined by corporate executive officers and senior nurse executives. High-level leadership and communication skills were ranked as most important in the study, followed by the ability to build coalitions and to interact with political savvy. Other leadership characteristics of successful entrepreneur nurses were ranked as follows: confident, team player, persistent, innovative, risk taker, adjusts to change, decisive, strategic thinker, high integrity, and possesses vision. A conclusion of the study was that nurse leaders must have strong entrepreneurial skills to succeed in today's marketplace. The need to reach out to the community was also perceived as a core requirement. Entrepreneurial leadership is best explained in Exemplar 9-1, which also illustrates the evolving nature of the advanced practice nursing leadership competency and how it expands in breadth over time.

Models of Leadership and Change

Models that deal with leadership and change processes are well substantiated in the literature across all disciplines. The models of leadership and change described here are derived from differing perspectives and provide useful frameworks for APNs who want to understand basic leadership concepts and how to acquire leadership and change agent skills.

EXEMPLAR 9-1

> Ellie's dream and goal upon entering a graduate family nurse practitioner (NP) program was to open a practice in the rural community where she and her family lived. She used her health policy course requirements to conduct a needs assessment and to set up interviews with the regional hospital to propose an outreach clinic that would be sponsored by the hospital. She planned to see patients independently and would contract with her physician preceptor to visit once a week for collaboration and to see patients who were beyond her scope of practice. Ellie's entrepreneurial leadership skills allowed her to negotiate with the managed care owner of the hospital and with the medical staff. Her community-based practice was viewed as a model of excellence for other NPs, and she served as a mentor and role model for many. As her clinic gained prominence, Ellie was nominated by the governor to represent APNs and rural interests on the state board of nursing. She also wrote a column for the local weekly newspaper about prevention and wellness.
>
> After 3 years in practice, Ellie wanted to use extra space in her clinic to broaden the services she offered, so she set up a meeting with the members of the midwifery group in an adjoining town to invite them to use her office as a satellite clinic once a week. She also invited two clinical nurses specialists (CNSs) who were seeing mental health and oncology patients in the area to do the same. Her vision and excellent communication skills offered new alliances with other APNs and brought new services for rural patients. The visibility of her successful clinic led to her nomination to membership on the National Rural Health Advisory Committee, which advises the Secretary of Health and Human Services on matters of rural health care. This nationally based committee work allowed Ellie to use her well-developed leadership skills to influence the health-care system.

THE FIFTH DISCIPLINE (SENGE)

Peter Senge has written about leadership from a business perspective (1990). *The Fifth Discipline* (Senge, 1990), identified in 1997 by the *Harvard Business Review* as one of the most influential business books of the last two decades, contains concepts that are very useful to APNs as they engage in the important work of mastering the competencies of advanced practice nursing leadership. Senge described a discipline as "a developmental path for acquiring certain skills or competencies" (p. 10). He contended that, although certain people may have innate gifts for playing a musical instrument or running with a football, others can develop these proficiencies through practice and commitment to the task. This definition implies that to practice a discipline is to be a lifelong learner. In this case, leadership is a good example because good leaders are constantly striving to become better, to empower others, and to facilitate change.

The five disciplines outlined by Senge provide a framework that effectively integrates the descriptions of leadership provided in the previous paragraphs with the components of learning as they relate to leadership. Because empowerment is key to leadership models, Senge's concepts serve as a useful base upon which understanding leadership and change within complex structures and environments can be understood. The following five disciplines (Senge, 1990) are easily adapted to provide the structure for the leadership competency identified for advanced practice nursing.

Personal mastery is the important work of continually redefining and clarifying one's personal vision, refocusing energies, maintaining objectivity, and committing to personal goals and objectives. The importance of personal growth and development is vital to attaining the competency of leadership. *Mental models* are the images that influence how one views the world and attains new insights; one must be willing to examine one's internal views and hold them up for inquiry and scrutiny by others. This discipline speaks to the need for clear vision about advanced practice nursing and the ability to defend this viewpoint. *Building shared vision* refers to the leader's ability to help a team develop and sustain a common image of what one seeks to create in the future: it is the ability to share a vision with others rather than to dictate that vision. The ability to empower others to share the dream and implement change is critical to this discipline. *Team learning* is the ability to suspend one's own assumptions, listen to other viewpoints, and genuinely "think together." *Systems thinking* is the "fifth discipline"—a conceptual framework for leadership based on the ability to see the whole picture rather than the isolated parts. This last discipline is an important concept for APNs, who must be able to view advanced practice within the context of health care collectively as one member of a team of professionals and patients. More recently, in *The Dance of Change*, Senge et al. (1999) noted that there are challenges inherent in the change process: by nature, change is dynamic, nonlinear, and interdependent. These characteristics can make it difficult to predict the trajectory a change initiative will take and highlight the importance of a flexible, responsive leadership style. Such a style fosters cohesion, collaboration, and communication among team members, enabling them to approach problem identification and solving with candor, commitment, and creativity.

THE TIPPING POINT (GLADWELL)

Another perspective on change is offered by Gladwell (2000). In *The Tipping Point: How Little Things Make a Difference*, Gladwell posited social change as the "biography of an idea" (p. 7) using questions like How does something catch on and become popular? What tips a phenomenon from being uncommon to common, unpopular to popular? Using the public health notion of epidemics, he helps readers understand how phenomena as diverse as health problems (teenage smoking, acquired immunodeficiency syndrome [AIDS]) and successful products (Hush Puppies shoes) and programs (Sesame Street) arise. He outlined three elements that seem to push an event or phenomenon to the tipping point: the "Law of the Few," the "Stickiness Factor," and the "Power of Context." The Law of the Few refers to the fact that it doesn't take many people to move things forward, but one needs exceptional people who are persuasive—people he describes as *mavens*. Mavens can be described as experts or self-appointed leaders who have charisma. Thus within nursing, one might think of Florence Nightingale as a maven. The Stickiness Factor refers to the fact that one can package a message, a program, or a product to make it "irresistible" (p. 132); the challenge is to find what makes it stick. Writers of television commercials do this all the time by coining new phrases and adopting new technology to appeal to a wide variety of viewers. In health care, although pain continues to be undertreated, one might consider patient-controlled analgesia (PCA) and other high-tech pain interventions that are widely and effectively used as an illustration of the Stickiness Factor. The Power of Context is also important to consider. Our social and physical environments shape our thoughts and behavior to a significant degree so that what we see and hear around us defines what decisions we make. It may take many small movements to create "one contagious movement" (Gladwell, 2000, p. 192). The three elements defined by Gladwell are important to developing the leadership potential of APNs. It takes only a few APN mavens with the right message at the right time to make changes in health care.

THE SEVEN HABITS OF HIGHLY EFFECTIVE PEOPLE (COVEY)

Stephen Covey's 1989 best seller presented both personal and interdependent characteristics that foster leadership acquisition. In creating a personal view of leadership, Covey suggested that the most effective way to "keep the end in mind" is by creating a personal mission statement that becomes a personal standard to live by as one progresses to new levels of independence and subsequent interdependence. In Covey's model, interdependence is achieved only after one has defined and integrated this personal mission/standard into one's practice. He described attributes of those who lead from a philosophy of interdependence: listening twice as much as you speak, remaining trustworthy by never compromising honesty, maintaining a positive attitude, and keeping a sense of humor. Interdependence allows one to hear and understand the other person's viewpoint, leading to a synergistic or win-win level of communication.

These are three of many leadership models that readers may find helpful; other models are listed in the Additional Readings section at end of the chapter. As readers may notice, throughout this discussion are the themes of movement, wholeness, and goals. Yet one can also trace, from the work of Burns (1978) to more recent definitions, the inclusion of integrity, empowerment, and caring, which are more directly related to leadership provided by APNs. Delivering care to patients in an effective and humane way requires a host of learning organizations with multidisciplinary providers. Nursing is not a solo endeavor, and leadership can be viewed as a way to professionalize nursing within a larger context. Bernhard and Walsh (1995) provided a useful way to understand leadership as a competency within the professional role of APNs. They included eight criteria identified by Pavalko (1971) that are essential to the leadership process irrespective of profession: a theoretical base, social values, knowledge, motivation, autonomy, commitment, community, and a code of ethics (Bernhard & Walsh, 1995; Pavalko, 1971). These generic leadership criteria are integral to advanced practice nursing education and subsumed within the essentials of leadership that follow.

The Change Process

As noted, the competency of being a change agent is embedded in leadership. Change is constant in professional and personal lives and in today's health-care system. Change does not have a discrete beginning and ending, but instead appears to be a series of continuous transitions that overlap one another. This phenomenon requires leadership that is continuous and flexible and demands ongoing attention to and redefinition of appropriate strategies. At this point in time, change is a never-ending process that must be woven into the fabric of everyday life and work. Being a successful change agent requires many of the skills and attributes that are needed to be a successful advanced practice nursing leader. However, it is important to understand the complex concepts and forces that drive the health-care system and how APNs take on the important activity of change agency every time they enact leadership (Klein, Gabelnick, & Herr, 1998).

With the emphasis on evidence-based practice and the knowledge that evidence-based guidelines and therapies are underused (Institute of Medicine, 2001; McGlynn et al., 2003), overused, or misused (Institute of Medicine, 2001), APNs have an important leadership/change agent role in improving care by leading and collaborating with nurses and interdisciplinary colleagues to ensure adoption of best practices (Duffy, 2002; Spencer & Jordan, 2001; Spross & Heaney, 2000). Implementing change depends on identifying stakeholders—those who have vested interests in the change and/or the power to promote or thwart change—and developing change strategies that take into account a variety of driving and restraining factors that can influence change.

A specific change-agent strategy associated with leading a change initiative is "opinion leadership" (Soumerai et al., 1998; Thomson et al., 1999; Oxman, Thomson, Davis, & Haynes, 1995; Locock, Dopson, Chambers, & Gabbay, 2001). Opinion leaders are clinicians who are identified by their colleagues as educationally influential (Oxman et al., 1995): a clinician would listen to the opinion leader and might make a change in practice based on what he or she learned from the opinion leader. The role of an opinion leader parallels that of the maven described by Gladwell (2000). One study of opinion leaders in several different clinical settings indicated that contextual factors influenced the ability of an opinion leader to promote guideline adoption by colleagues (Locock et al., 2001), suggesting the importance of attending to environmental cues when change is planned. Although studies of opinion leaders have been done, findings from studies of their effectiveness are mixed, in part, because the activities of opinion leaders are not well described (Oxman et al., 1995).

Steven Covey's work with interdisciplinary groups is also very instructive as one studies change and change strategies. Change occurs at both the system and the personal level, and Covey (1989) proposed that one must deal with core values to successfully change or serve as an agent for change:

People can't live with change if there is not a changeless core inside them. The key to the ability to change is a changeless sense of who you are, what you are about, and what you value. Real change comes from the inside out. (p. 108)

There is an affective dimension to change. Although many people are excited by the prospect of change, some changes are difficult and painful. At best, change can be described as challenging and invigorating (Norton & Grady, 1996). To understand change within today's health-care environment, the dynamics of change and the culture within which it occurs must be explored. Seminal research by Senge (1990) and Senge et al. (1999) suggests that systems thinking, which takes into account the notion that change is a given, is what integrates personal mastery, mental modeling, shared vision, and team learning. Taken together this discussion of change models and processes suggests that APNs must consider several factors when they are experiencing or trying to introduce change: the relevance of power and influence, stakeholders' concerns and interests, contextual factors, and the affective dimensions of change. These are all important constructs in dealing with change and demonstrate that change is an integral part of the leadership process.

FORCE FIELD ANALYSIS: DRIVING AND RESTRAINING FORCES OF CHANGE

Traditional models of the change process are insufficient for addressing change today because these models conceived of change as a linear process that occurred over time. Although they are less useful, certain concepts from these traditional models are still relevant. Lewin (1976) described a state of equilibrium between driving and restraining forces that encourage or discourage movement. Driving forces are usually perceived as positive, reasonable, and conscious forces; whereas restraining forces are perceived as negative, illogical, and often subconscious. It is the effect of these opposing forces that makes change, especially rapid change, so difficult (Lewin, 1976). These external and internal forces or tensions may also account for the cognitive dissonance (the conflict between actions and values) that may be evident during change and that causes the uncomfortable feelings that people undergoing change often experience. Driving and restraining forces are useful concepts for APNs as they plan for change and evaluate both planned and unplanned changes as they unfold. For example, as APNs extend their practices across state lines, the movement toward multistate licensure is gaining momentum (see Chapter 22).

Depending on existing policies and procedures for reimbursement and presciptive authority within states, these forces can serve as driving or restraining influences for APNs. As multistate licensure for APNs evolves, telehealth may be considered a driving force, and states' rights may be a restraining force. Driving and restraining forces are also useful for analyzing the organizational settings in whcih APNs work. For example, an organizational assessment of these forces is useful in determining the institution's level of commitment to diversity.

THE DEMISE OF PLANNED CHANGE: CHANGE AS A CONSTANT, CHANGE AS EVOLUTION

A major concern for health-care stakeholders at all levels is the rapidity with which change is occurring in health care. Change is no longer episodic; indeed, planned change may be somewhat of a misnomer. Even when one plans a change, for example rolling out a new advanced practice nursing program or service, events may occur that reshape the program: the program that was conceptualized and the one that gets implemented may not be exactly the same. For example, funding available for the program may fall short of what had been anticipated because of a change in reimbursement structures, and thus services or personnel may be eliminated. Thus although planning for change is not useless, such planning requires change agents and leaders to adopt a flexible and responsive approach to planning change, seeing it as an evolutionary process.

As the time frame to accomplish change strategies shortens, changes become more and more difficult for individuals and organizations to manage and therefore require enhanced strategies to support both leaders and followers. Many of the traditional theory-based models for implementing change do not work because of the speed with which change is occurring. The issues of planned versus unplanned change are based predominately on issues of *time:* time to plan for and think through the desired change, time to orient and allow stakeholders to become comfortable with change, and time to educate and allow the change process to occur. Senge (1999) identified time as one of ten challenges to initiating change and suggested looking at the issue of insufficient time as an opportunity to reexamine the ways workplaces are organized in order to consider a redesign that allows for flexibility, reflection, and innovation.

Unplanned and constant change is the reality of today's health-care environment, and this factor is the basis of the leadership discussion that follows. O'Connell (1999) questioned whether health-care organizations can sustain fast-paced change unless there is a "culture of change" in place that assists and supports adaptation to new systems and ways of knowing and doing. O'Connell proposed the following strategies for developing a culture of change within an organization:

- Maintain momentum
- Emphasize managerial support in the process of changing work flow and practice patterns
- Encourage the question "why" and exercise tolerance for the results
- Emphasize the importance of concerns on the personal level
- Find new and different ways to demonstrate administrative support

It is also helpful to consider the techniques used for implementing change outlined by Norton and Grady (1996) and in Chapter 6 of this text as they relate to providing a positive culture for change. Senge's (1990) analogies, in which leading is compared with athletic coaching or playing in a jazz ensemble, speak to the importance of individuality, sensitivity, and faith in leading change efforts and creating an environment that supports change. Leaders need to understand the personal implications of change if a culture of change is to be realized. APNs with highly developed interpersonal and psychosocial skills are poised to lead institutional change initiatives.

Political Activism and Advocacy

Political activism and advocacy are other critical components of advanced practice nursing leadership. Many of the skills needed to successfully navigate in political waters are closely associated with good leadership. The core elements that define contemporary leadership—such as shared vision, systems thinking, and the ability to engage in high-level communication within the context of a changing environment—are all basic to political effectiveness. Again, change is the common denominator that drives APNs to advocate for advanced practice and patient issues. In fact, there is little room for discussion about whether APNs need to take on the mantles of policymaker and patient advocate as part of their leadership role (see Chapter 22). For many, this falls within the context of a moral imperative: to meet the needs of patients and society, APNs must position themselves strategically at the policy table to advocate for access to care and appropriate interventions for everyone. There is also little question about whether APNs are up to the task. There have been great strides in nurses' skill and acuity as policymakers. Strong mentors have helped along the way, and trial by fire has always been an effective learning tool. The Developing Skills as Advanced Practice Nursing Leaders and Change Agents section of this chapter offers strategies for developing policy advocacy skills.

ATTRIBUTES OF EFFECTIVE ADVANCED PRACTICE NURSING LEADERS AND CHANGE AGENTS

Several personal attributes are deemed necessary for successful leadership (Box 9-1). These qualities are very broad and support the concept that all leadership today is required to be interdisciplinary. No longer do nurse leaders have the luxury of leading only in nursing circles. The history of advanced practice nursing (Chapter 1) demonstrates the roles that nurse leaders have played outside the realm of organized nursing education and practice. The role that certified registered nurse anesthetist (CRNA) leaders played in improving care for anesthetized patients early in the century and the multifaceted roles that APNs have played during times of war are good examples of the opportunities APNs have to exercise leadership in interdisciplinary settings.

Vision

Vision is often perceived as the most important component of leadership and the talent that is most coveted. The ability to anticipate the future and communicate that image to others is a valuable aptitude. Vision encompasses a long-range view of both personal and collective goals that can be shared and that empower others to move forward. Innovation is associated with and closely linked to vision. It is the ability to "think big" or to "think

BOX 9-1 • ATTRIBUTES OF NURSE LEADERS

EXPERT COMMUNICATION SKILLS
- Articulate in speech and in writing
- Ability to get one's point across
- Excellent listening skills
- Desire to hear and understand another's point of view
- Staying connected to other people

COMMITMENT
- Giving of self personally and professionally
- Listening to one's inner voice
- Balancing professional and private life
- Planning ahead, making change happen
- Self-reflection

DEVELOPING ONE'S OWN STYLE
- Getting involved
- Staying involved
- Setting priorities
- Managing boundaries

- Using technology
- Lifelong learning
- Creating a learning environment for self and others
- A good sense of humor

RISK TAKING
- Getting involved at any level
- Self-confidence and assertiveness
- Thinking "big"
- Willingness to fail and begin again
- A sense of timing
- Coping with change

WILLINGNESS TO COLLABORATE
- Respect for cultural diversity
- Desire to team build
- Sharing power
- Willingness to mentor

Adapted from Hanson, C., Boyle, J., Hatmaker, D., & Murray, J. (1999). *Finding your voice as a leader*. Washington, DC: American Academy of Nursing; reprinted with permission.

outside the box," the capacity to see alternatives to the current thinking on a given issue. Vision is also grounded in a deep knowledge of the subject and brings with it the responsibility to stay abreast of trends and issues in the field. However, having vision is not enough. A leader must be able to articulate and develop a shared vision, one that others can embrace as their own. Christopher, Miller, Beck, and Toughill (2002) described the visionary leader as one who remains tenacious and decisive while being caring and flexible in the process. To do this well, a visionary leader must not get too far out in front of his or her followers because teamwork is critical to shared vision. Tornabeni (1996), a nurse leader, noted that she would not have been able to "hold onto the vision" (p. 65) had she not broadened her scope of influence to include others outside of the discipline of nursing. An important element of vision is the ability to set priorities so that there is a clear path to the ultimate goal.

Timing

A good sense of timing may be an inherent gift, but for most people, it requires painstaking development and practice. Timing is the ability to know when to act and when to hold back. It acknowledges a sense of urgency at times as, for example, during an unexpected legislative vote in Congress, or the need, during a change in scope of practice, to take the time to develop a carefully thought-out plan with careful strategy. The notion of timing is implied in the change agent's axiom to use mandated change as opportunities to introduce other changes. For example, institutions applying for accreditation by the Joint Commission on Accreditation of Healthcare Organizations (JCAHO) were expected to demonstrate compliance with the JCAHO's evidence-based standards for pain management in 2000 (JCAHO, 2000). Many institutions used this mandated change to launch a variety of initiatives aimed at improving pain and symptom management.

Self-Confidence and Risk Taking

Taking risks is inherent in the leadership process and is tied inextricably to self-confidence and vision. The willingness to take a chance, to try, and to fail occasionally is the mark of a true leader. The mantra "take a risk, make a decision, pay the price," coined by Helen Mannock in 1959, is worth keeping in mind (Norton & Grady, 1996). Risk-taking behaviors differentiate APNs who will be recognized as leaders and agents for change from other capable APNs. By learning to take risks, APNs enhance their leadership repertoire, allowing for more spontaneity and flexibility in response to conflict, resistance, anger, and other reactions to change and high-risk situations (Norton & Grady, 1996). Motivation, which can be described as the desire to move forward, can also be viewed as a component of risk. Staying put is rarely as risky as taking the chance to move ahead.

Expert Communication and Relationship Building

The relevance of good communication and collegial relationships to quality health care has received significant attention in the last few years (Houghton, 2003; King, 2002; McAvoy & Murtagh, 2002; Rider, 2002). APNs must be able to communicate effectively to collaborate with other professionals (see Chapter 10) and participate in the identification and resolution of clinical and ethical conflicts among team members (see Chapter 11). The successful leader must have superb communication skills to build the trust and cooperation necessary to negotiate difficult intra- and interprofessional issues. The ability to understand another's viewpoint and respect opposing views is key to effective communication and ultimately reaching a mutually satisfactory outcome. Covey (1989) suggested that one should "seek first to understand and then to be understood" (p. 235). Good leaders listen and really try to hear the other person's viewpoint before they speak. The charisma that is associated with many natural-born leaders is often simply outstanding listening and communication skills. The ability to influence, a key power strategy used to gain the cooperation of others, is an outcome of excellent communication.

A second part of expert communication is relationship building. The art of building strong alliances and coalitions with others and staying connected with colleagues and groups is basic to the sense of community needed within the leadership process. This is true at all levels of leadership, whether it occurs at the highest levels of international policymaking or at the local level in building coalitions of APNs to solve patient problems. Building relationships is central to the effectiveness of the team that cares for patients. Not only must APNs establish effective relationships with their co-workers, they are often in a position to strengthen relationships among other members of the team through role modeling and mediation.

Building relationships is central to another advanced practice nursing communication skill, conflict negotiation. Advanced practice nursing students may come to their graduate programs having been socialized to be silent or suppress their opinions in situations of conflict. Specific approaches to identifying conflicts and resolving them successfully have been identified and used successfully in business (Fisher, Ury, & Patton, 2002) and in health care (Marcus, Dorn, Kritek, Miller, & Wyatt, 1999). Readers are referred to the following URLs for resources and information on conflict negotiation: The Conflict

Resolution Network (www.crnhq.org/) and The Program on Negotiation at Harvard Law School (www.pon.org/).

Boundary Management

Managing boundaries refers to the ways in which APNs limit or extend various aspects of advanced nursing practice such as scope of practice, workload, and interpersonal boundaries. Sometimes APNs are in the position of "guarding" the boundary such as when they are approached to undertake a task that is not within their scope of practice. Boundaries also need to be managed when there is a risk of *scope creep*, a term used to characterize the "one more good idea or task" that should be done to perfect some initiative—an idea or task that is likely to delay or compromise the intended goal. Often, managing boundaries means extending them—building a bridge that enables the APN to partner with other groups or expanding a boundary as other patient or health-care needs are identified. Extending the boundary may mean leveraging human or other resources so that partners can move forward toward a goal. Extending a boundary may also mean expanding one's scope of practice at an agency or regulatory level so that patient needs can be better met. Knowing where the current boundaries of nursing practice are and making strategic decisions about going beyond them is another way to define risk taking.

As boundary managers, APNs recognize communications and behaviors that breach or enhance interpersonal relationships. APNs may be the ones with the influence to identify and address unacceptable or unprofessional behavior in the workplace. For example, a licensed practical nurse relayed to the clinical nurse specialist (CNS) that an alert and oriented patient had touched her inappropriately while she was giving care. The licensed practical nurse wanted to avoid trouble and was inclined to let it go but agreed to have the CNS intervene. The CNS worked with the nurse manager and physician to communicate with the patient, establish that the behavior was inappropriate, and specify the consequences if it were to occur again. The employee was referred to human resources to obtain counseling for the incident and learn strategies for addressing such behavior, should it occur again. As boundary managers, APN leaders also teach others how to collaborate (see Chapter 10) with other disciplines and colleagues, build coalitions, and set limits while maintaining their own boundaries—a fine distinction, but strategically important. For example, a certified nurse-midwife (CNM) may delicately negotiate the boundaries among the neonatologist, the obstetrician, and the nurse-midwifery staff. Both clinical leadership and professional leadership require the negotiation of boundaries, regardless of whether the borders are drawn around professional roles, patient populations, or organizations.

Self-Reflection

Self-reflection is an important activity for APNs who aspire to be leaders. Self-reflection enables APNs to make sense of and learn from experience. One must recognize that there often is a chasm between the rhetoric and the reality of nursing. Self-reflection as a strategy for refining direct care and coaching competencies is addressed in Chapters 5 and 6. For one to lead successfully it is especially instructive to reflect on one's experiences of socialization and acculturation as a member of a particular family, peer group, and discipline. For example, the need to group together along some continuum of sameness is the basis of family structure, as well as the basis for stereotyping. For the APN, self-assessment of his or her valuing of diversity needs to be a continuous, evolving activity.

Respect for Cultural Diversity

Cultural competence and valuing diversity are significant attributes for advanced practice nursing leaders. These attributes require sensitivity to one's own biases and the awareness of damaging attitudes and behaviors that surface at all levels of interaction and in all settings. An advanced practice nursing leader needs to be responsive to and serve as role model by demonstrating respect for the cultural, racial, and ethnic differences of followers and constituencies in any given situation. When a systems framework is used for understanding a complex concept such as culturally competent leadership, four levels can be identified: societal, professional, organizational, and individual. For the APN, the responsibility for culturally competent care includes all four levels of the diversity system. Culturally competent care is care delivered with knowledge, sensitivity, and respect for the patient's and family's cultural, racial, and ethnic background and practices. This definition is built on the assumption that care providers are fully aware of, sensitized to, and able to integrate their own cultural, racial, and ethnic backgrounds into their professional delivery of care services. The interactive nature of caregiving requires the engagement and synchrony of the provider's own background with the backgrounds of those receiving care.

Differences are an issue for every member of the human race, and they become even more important when one becomes a leader and role model. Working with colleagues who are different gives APNs opportunities for soliciting information about others' experiences. Box 9-2 provides strategies for enhancing cultural awareness.

Balance in Personal and Professional Life

Most people know when they have overextended themselves: their bodies give clues such as fatigue, stress signals, and feelings of frustration. One of the negative aspects of being a good leader is the provocative realization that one is being asked to play many important cutting-edge roles at the same time. It is very easy to overextend one's abilities well beyond manageable, realistic boundaries. The skills of being able to delegate tasks; mentor others to take on some of the load; and enlarge the circle of leaders, strategists, and followers are integral to effective leadership. Unfortunately, the inability to set realistic personal boundaries paves the way to stress, frustration, and burnout. It is not easy to be both a leader and a competent advanced practice nursing care provider, but it can be done.

BOX 9-2 • STRATEGIES TO ACHIEVE CULTURAL COMPETENCE

1. Explore and learn about your own racial/ethnic culture and background.
2. Explore and learn about the different racial/ethnic cultures most frequently encountered in your practice.
3. Read ethnic newspapers, magazines, and books.
4. Listen to the music from a different culture.
5. Learn the language of the culture. Become bilingual with the verbal and the nonverbal behavior of the different culture.
6. Take advantage of training opportunities for increasing your cultural awareness and sensitivity.
7. Be able to identify personal biases and develop strategies to manage, eliminate, or sublimate those potentially damaging attitudes and behaviors.
8. When faced with a difficult patient, consider whether unconscious biases may be operating for you or your colleagues.

Adapted from Hanson, C. M., & Malone, B. (2000). Leadership: Empowerment, change agency, and activism. In A. B. Hamric, J. A. Spross, & C. M. Hanson (Eds.), *Advanced nursing practice: An integrative approach* (2nd ed., pp. 279-313). Philadelphia: W. B. Saunders.

APNs need to engage in a process of self-reflection to see what personal and work characteristics seem to set off imbalances. We offer three strategies, which are simple in concept but can be complicated in execution. First, expecting perfection is often a setup for imbalance. "If I just do this one more thing, everything will be fine, " one thinks. Keeping in mind the axiom, "Perfect is the enemy of good," may help APNs establish realistic expectations. Another strategy is for APNs to examine what makes them say "yes" or "no." One CNS kept a Post-it note on her phone that read "The answer is no." This reminded her to either decline something that would tip the scales to overcommitment or to buy time by asking "Can I think about it and call you tomorrow?" One colleague avoids commitments that are perceived as distant elephants; they are not threatening a year in advance when one's usual commitments, such as class and writing, are not looming. As the time to fulfill a commitment approaches, the distant elephants become as threatening as an impending stampede. The third strategy is to make appointments with oneself for important personal and professional activities. By putting such appointments on a calendar, APNs can lessen the risk of giving away time that they need to maintain balance.

It is not accidental that several of the key attributes in Box 9-1 incorporate the word *willingness*. The abilities to be open and willing, to take what comes, and to work through differences are key to all levels of leadership. Leadership is about negotiation and interactions with others to reach common goals. To do this may mean failing and trying again and again to reach the desired outcome. This quality of personal hardiness—the ability to "pick oneself up and start again"—is seen repeatedly in biographies of successful leaders who have made change happen in difficult times.

Leaders are involved with change at many points in the change process. Visionary change makers intervene early in the change process, before change occurs, and set the stage for the events that follow. They provide the guiding principles and assumptions for the proposed change and begin to introduce themes that position the organization and its members in a positive direction toward the new events. Change implementers—as defined by Kantor, Stein, and Jick (1992)—have the difficult task of "making it happen." Two critical attributes that define change makers are that they are culturally competent and that they have the ability to mentor and empower their colleagues and others with whom they come in contact.

Mentoring and Empowerment

Two major proficiencies, mentoring and empowerment, stand out as important skills in the processes of leadership, change, and advocacy. The responsibility to mentor and empower is central to all of the definitions of leadership and change outlined earlier. The ability to help others to grow and to encourage them toward self-actualization requires competent, caring leaders who are interested in the success and well-being of their followers. Coaching and guiding with an awareness and attentiveness to the needs and concerns of followers are basic characteristics of successful leaders. The ideas behind the colloquial statements "taking someone under your wing" or "giving a colleague a leg up" are grounded in the mentoring process. Leading by example, role modeling, enabling followers, and encouraging them to move upward are all leadership aptitudes that must be disseminated.

Mentors have been defined by many as having those qualities that epitomize success in their own careers and the ability and desire to help others achieve success. Most important, mentors are role models who help those with less experience gain expertise through example (Fawcett, 2002). Mentors are seen as self-confident and competent, with a willingness to share their expertise. Mentees, or protégés, are viewed as those people who exhibit a desire to learn, are committed to the long course of events, and are open to the process of trial and error. It is important to note that there are two parts to the advanced practice nursing mentorship equation: APNs who are seeking to be mentored by those they aspire to emulate and APNs who can serve as mentors. "The learning curve [to leadership] is vastly facilitated by exposure to those who display mastery, those who have wisdom" (Koerner, 1997, p. 78). The reward for the mentor is to step back and enjoy the success and achievements of the protégé. Unfortunately, some APNs are reluctant to mentor, perhaps thinking that the protégé will compete with the APN, overshadow his or her expertise, or will not work as hard as they did to be successful. Vance and Olson (1998) suggested the following requirements for APNs who want to attract mentors: be dedicated to your cause, market yourself, seek opportunities for networking and meeting other APNs, reach out to possible mentors who are both leaders and peers, and cultivate an attitude of openness. The best way for novice APNs to move into the leadership arena is to be guided by an experienced nurse advocate. However, the mentoring process is often deterred by the environment within which APNs and other nurses practice. In a more recent publication, Vance (2003) asserted that the current chaotic health-care environment makes mentoring support more important than ever. She suggested that mentors and protégés adopt a mentoring philosophy that encourages collaboration, in contrast to competition, with others. Only in this way can new leaders emerge.

DEVELOPING SKILLS AS ADVANCED PRACTICE NURSING LEADERS AND CHANGE AGENTS

Factors Influencing Leadership Development

A common myth is that leaders are born not made, that there is an inborn leadership trait that some people have and others do not. Trent (2003) asserted that this is not true and that individuals can learn to lead by understanding and using "power resources" as described by Rost (1993). Power resources include many of the attributes described in this chapter such as education, experience, expert communication, networking, assertiveness, and collaboration and are clearly demonstrated in the studies of leadership discussed in the following sections.

Allen (1998) explored perceptions of 12 nurse leaders regarding the primary factors and individual characteristics that influenced their leadership development. *Self-confidence*, traced to childhood and subsequent risk-taking behaviors, was perceived as a critical factor. Feedback from significant others led to enhanced self-confidence over time. The nurse leaders also spoke about having *innate qualities and tendencies of leaders*, such as being extroverted or bossy and wanting to take charge, and about having roles as team captains and officers in organizations. They were seen as people who "rise to the occasion." A third important factor was a *progression of experiences and successes* that were pivotal in moving them forward. Being at "the right place at the right time" and taking advantage of opportunities that were presented in those situations allowed them to grow as leaders. Closely aligned with this factor was the *influence of significant people* such as mentors, role models, faculty, and parents who had the ability to encourage and provide opportunities for advancement. A final set of factors identified in this study was *personal life factors*, defined as situations in which time, family, health, and work schedules influenced their development to a greater or lesser degree. For example, study participants who had supportive spouses and relatives who assisted with family and home responsibilities and employers who were flexible found these factors to be important to the leadership development process. Allen's findings clearly support the definitions and elements of leadership described in the first part of this chapter.

Educational Strategies for Preparing Advanced Practice Nursing Leaders

Formal educational opportunities such as those experienced during graduate school fit well into the process of leadership development. Opportunities to work with role models and mentors help students to acquire leadership skills and further reinforce their self-confidence. Community-based projects such as coordinating health fairs or the Special Olympics offer rich resources for building interpersonal skills and create new opportunities for influence and visibility. Running for graduate student office or local leadership positions in professional organizations and serving on local boards and coalitions are other good strategies. Also, leadership conferences that foster effective communication and interaction are beneficial. Exemplar 9-2 shows how students can practice their leadership development during graduate education.

EXEMPLAR 9-2

Joan was beginning her second year as a student APN. She had completed her core courses, which gave her a good foundation in the theoretical concepts related to role development, health policy, and research. Now, she was ready to move on to the clinical component of her program and to complete her scholarly project. Joan had thought carefully about this and wanted to focus her project on developing her leadership skills in the policy arena. She knew that one of her faculty, Dr. Wesson, who had taught her health policy course, was a respected state and national leader who was actively engaged in the process of gaining primary care provider (PCP) status for advanced practice nurses (APNs). Joan made an appointment to talk with Dr. Wesson about how she could help with the PCP issue and at the same time complete her scholarly project. Dr. Wesson suggested three things. Joan should use the Internet to become familiar with and articulate about the proposed legislation; she could accompany Dr. Wesson to the next statewide meeting of APNs and offer to carry out the phone survey of APNs that was needed by this group; and she could develop the research proposal, implement the survey methodology, and present the findings as part of testimony at the hearing at the state capitol in the spring. These activities would allow Joan to interact with leader role models, try out her new leadership skills, and complete her research assignment. Dr. Wesson also suggested that Joan apply for the student scholarship offered by a national advanced practice nursing organization to attend the Washington, DC–based APN Summit.

Throughout the fall and winter, Joan implemented the phone survey with the advanced practice nursing community. She interacted with many practicing APNs and learned a great deal about advanced nursing practice. The advanced practice nursing leaders at the state meeting were excellent role models, and Dr. Wesson served as an excellent mentor throughout the year. Joan was extremely proud of her contribution to advanced practice nursing when she presented her findings at the hearing. Throughout the process, she had used many of the skills that she had read about in her leadership class, such as communication, networking, vision, and timing. Because Joan has a husband and a 4-year-old child, she also learned about balance and boundary management. Her most lasting recollection was how important it was to have a mentor to guide her through the process.

In 1999, the American Academy of Nursing funded a distance learning educational project that brought together four nursing leaders from Georgia to share their ideas about the skills needed to develop successful nurse leaders. These leaders "attended" class over interactive television and offered their experience and expertise to novice APNs. Many of the skills they shared are part of the essentials of leadership as described earlier in this chapter. Box 9-1 (p. 314) contains a list of their joint suggestions for students and others who desire to become leaders (Hanson, Boyle, Hatmaker, & Murray, 1999).

Leadership skills are developed and perfected over time and in myriad ways. Communication is one of the strengths often attributed to nurses, and it is a skill that can be augmented through practice. Many of the other skills and attributes shared by Hanson et al. (1999) in Box 9-1 (p. 314) are familiar to APNs and just need to be framed within the context of leadership. For example, the notion of staying connected is important for busy APNs and was operationalized by these leaders in a variety of ways, from electronic mailing lists and shared projects to planning to attend conferences that allowed for time to interact and problem solve with colleagues about similar professional issues. A sense of timing was described by one leader as negotiating ahead of time with her spouse for time to lobby for prescriptive authority, with the understanding that she would lessen her load at the end of the legislative session. The need for faculty and students in graduate programs to become involved in raising the visibility of advanced practice nursing roles in their institutions and communities is extremely important to building a community of advanced practice nursing leaders. Faculty need to serve as resource persons to keep students informed about key legislative issues and introduce them, through role modeling, to the role of political advocacy. Inviting APNs to accompany faculty who are giving testimony at a legislative hearing is an appropriate way to model the advocacy role. Gaining local visibility is accomplished when APN students and faculty participate in local health-care activities for special populations such as Special Olympics, AIDS awareness, and after-school programs for high-risk youth.

DEVELOPING LEADERSHIP IN THE POLITICAL ARENA

Health-care policy issues affecting APNs and their patients are explored in Chapter 23. The following section describes how APNs can develop skills to influence health-care policy through creative leadership and political advocacy, whether by means of local grass-roots endeavors or directly through congressional involvement. Advocacy can be defined as the act of pleading another person's cause; it is multifaceted with diverse activities (Halpern, 2002). APNs are being called on, collectively and individually, to make their voices heard as the nation and individual states struggle with budget constraints and difficult decisions about health-care programming. Major changes are driving the nursing and health-care agenda and demand APNs' attention. These changes include the increasing numbers of older adults with chronic diseases, the increasing cultural diversity of the U.S. population, and the increased use of costly new technologies (Wakefield, 2003a).

Becoming an Astute Political Activist: The Growth Process

In the political arena, developing power and influence is an imperative that tests one's leadership skills. Leadership strategies used by APNs in the political arena include developing power, influencing contacts, motivating colleagues to stay abreast of current issues, and providing bridges to other leaders who have access to important resources. Mentoring APNs to understand their power and influence in the health-care policy arena is a serious role for the advanced practice nursing leader. Taking on the mantle of policy advocate requires a commitment to advanced nursing practice and education issues.

The developmental process for becoming a political activist begins during primary school when children are first introduced to government and the political system. Field trips to Washington, DC, and the state capitol are the first sparks toward political activism. Throughout secondary education and by way of the nightly news, young adults continue to be bombarded with policy decisions in many venues. Then, in basic nursing education, fledgling nurses are further exposed to specific policies related to health-care, and they are introduced to professional nursing and specialty nursing organizations. However, serious involvement often begins in graduate school, when health-care policy is offered as one of the "core" courses leading to the role of APN. During master's education, advanced practice nursing students are coached to better understand the power inherent in policymaking, the power of policies to influence practice, and ways that they can influence the system, both individually and collectively, to better their own practice and to be high-level patient advocates. This is accomplished both though classroom teaching and experientially through interaction with policymakers and nursing leaders and mentors. Exemplar 9-2, presented earlier in the chapter, exemplifies this educational strategy.

DEPTH OF INVOLVEMENT

There is no question that influencing policy is costly in terms of time and energy. Timing is an important consideration for APNs who want and need to be health-care policy advocates. Therefore it is important for APNs to ask themselves several personal and professional questions to determine the degree of involvement and level of sophistication at which advocacy is to be undertaken. These questions are as follows:

- What are my responsibilities related to wage earning, small children, dependent parents, single parenthood, health issues, school, and gaining initial competence as an APN?
- How can I best serve the advanced practice nursing community at this time?
- What are the learning opportunities that will help me to be most effective?
- How can I develop a long-term plan and a short-term plan for becoming a more politically astute advocate for myself and for my patients?
- What am I able to commit to based on the response to these questions?

Once APNs have made a decision about the depth of involvement to which they can commit, they need to find an appropriate mentor. Advanced practice nursing has a wealth of strong nursing leaders and advocates who are willing and able to move new advocates into positions to make positive changes in health-care policy. Opportunities for input and influence exist at various levels of the legislative process from the time a bill is first introduced, through committee and subcommittee meetings and the conference stage, until it is presented on the floor of the Senate or House of Representatives (Winterfeldt, 2001).

USING PROFESSIONAL ORGANIZATIONS TO BEST ADVANTAGE

For APNs, close contact with their professional organization is an important link for staying abreast of national and state policy agendas, for finding a support network of like-minded colleagues, and for accessing information about changes in credentialing and practice issues. Unfortunately, in today's complex world, this means being an active member of more than one affiliate organization in order to stay on the cutting edge of pertinent issues. Most APNs are aligned with one or more professional nursing organizations, and those APNs who aspire to an active role in influencing policy often have membership in several. Basic membership brings with it the newsletters, journals, and Internet access needed to stay current; and active membership requires committee assignments and more involvement. As new graduates move from the educational milieu into diverse practice settings, they must align with the advanced practice nursing organizations that best meet their needs and offer the strongest support, choosing to actively engage in some and remain on the periphery in others.

Membership can be maintained at different levels, from simple financial support through dues to high-level leadership and committee work. Choosing the "right" organizations to belong to is a very personal decision based on particular needs, comfort level, specialty, and experience. Many APNs belong to one organization that meets their particular clinical needs (e.g., the Oncology Nursing Society or the American Association of Nurse Anesthetists) and to another that offers cutting-edge access to pressing professional issues such as the NONPF or Sigma Theta Tau International. Others use their professional organization as a support group that offers nurturing and professional sustenance, a group that "understands" local advanced practice nursing concerns. Regional and state affiliates of national organizations often serve this purpose.

The critical factor in interfacing with organizations is getting and staying involved in a very definitive way. Being part of an electronic mailing list or chat room, attending meetings and conferences, reading newsletters and journals, participating on committees, and working up the ladder to leadership positions represent different levels of involvement. Professional organizations offer the source of leadership and collective wisdom necessary to stay the course in today's political and policy arena. The notions of strength in numbers and speaking with one strong voice are not new concepts but are essential to the success of advanced practice nursing. The state and national organizations that are tied to advanced practice nursing education and practice are too varied and numerous to describe here, but it is safe to say that there is something for everyone.

POLITICAL ACTION COMMITTEES

A political action committee (PAC) is the arm of an organization, structured as a separate entity that finances political campaigns. PAC contributions do not buy votes, but they do buy access to candidates (Malone, Chafee, & Wachter, 2002), which is critical to the advocacy process. Federal guidelines dictate how donations and funds are raised and administered (deVries & Vanderbuilt, 1992). Decisions about endorsements are complex and are made at the national professional organization level based on careful research and candidates' past support for nursing and health-care interests that align with nursing's professional priorities and values. Fund-raising to support candidates is a major function of PACs and requires nursing support at every level. PACs are important to APNs because the decisions about Medicare and Medicaid that undergird advanced practice nursing reimbursement are at stake when support is provided to political nominees running for national office. Advanced practice nursing leaders are in key positions to influence the endorsement of political candidates who are aligned with advanced nursing practice and education issues.

INTERNSHIPS AND FELLOWSHIPS

One excellent way to develop the necessary skills to move into the role of advanced practice nursing policy advocate is to apply for a national or state policy internship or fellowship. These appointments, which last from several days to 1 or 2 years, offer a wide range of health-care policy and political experiences that are targeted to both novice and expert APNs. For example, the Nurse in Washington Internship is a 4-day internship that introduces nurses to policymaking in Washington, DC. The Nurse in Washington Internship is sponsored by the Nursing Organizations Alliance (see www.nursing-alliance.org). This internship serves as an excellent beginning step in fulfilling the advanced practice nursing policy role. Federal fellowships and internships that link nurses to legislators or to the various branches of federal and state government are invaluable in assisting APNs to understand how leaders are developed and how the system for setting health-care policy is operationalized.

Raising Awareness through Communication

The ability of APNs to influence public policy rests with the individual nurse, as well as with collective groups of APNs. The ability to communicate with others accurately and efficiently and in a timely manner is a driving force in the world of policy and politics. Never before have people had such an opportunity to share information in its original form and to engage with others at a distance (Wakefield, 2003b). Face-to-face, one-on-one interaction and on-site networking are always the best ways to ensure successful communication that satisfies all parties. However, time and distance make these modes of communication a luxury rather than a reality. Few APNs have the time or inclination to serve as full-time policymakers. The reality is that APNs rely on other modalities such as the Internet to stay connected to the larger professional world.

THE INTERNET, E-MAIL, FAX, AND TELEPHONE COMMUNICATION

Today's communication networks are wonderful resources for gaining awareness and keeping current on policy initiatives and concerns from a wide variety of perspectives. Probably the most useful tool available to APNs is the World Wide Web, which makes it possible for APNs to influence policy change from their own homes. It is possible to follow committee sessions in Congress via television or computer as they happen or later the same day via CNN. Box 9-3 contains a partial list of Internet sites that offer excellent resources for staying abreast of advanced practice nursing policy and practice issues.

E-mail, fax, and cell phone modalities have revolutionized the ability to communicate rapidly and effectively throughout the world. Board and committee meetings can be conducted at any time, day or night. Augmenting skills that are required to intercept attached documents and faxes via computer greatly expands the ability to do business. TeleWeb conferencing offers yet another mode of communication. Conference calls save countless hours on the road or in the air. Often, APNs at the grass-roots level must push for this type of interaction with major policy activists and organizations. It is important for APNs in busy practices to press for distance access in order to directly engage in policy activities while caring for patients.

THE MEDIA

The Woodhull Study of Nurses and the Media, a work commissioned by Sigma Theta Tau titled "Healthcare's Invisible Partner," (Woodhull, 1998) makes the point that nurses do not use the media to their best advantage. Mundt (1997) conducted a research study exploring how nurses were represented in 35 books about health policy and health-care reform from 13 disciplines. The findings were significant because more than half of the

BOX 9-3 • COMMON URLS FOR INTERNET ACCESS	
Agency for Healthcare Research and Quality (formerly Agency for Health Care Policy and Research [AHCPR])	www.ahcpr.gov
American Academy of Nurse Practitioners	www.aanp.org
American Association of Colleges of Nursing	www.aacn.nche.edu
American Association of Nurse Anesthetists	www.aana.org
American College of Nurse-Midwives	www.acnm.org
American College of Nurse Practitioners	www.nurse.org/acnp
American Medical Association	www.ama-assn.org
American Nurses Association	www.ana.org
American Nurses Credentialing Center	www.nursingworld.org/ancc
Thomas: Legislative Information on the Internet	www.thomas.loc.gov
National Association of County and City Health Officials	www.naccho.org
National Association of Neonatal Nurses	www.nann.org
National Association of Pediatric Nurse Practitioners	www.napnap.org
National Certification Board of Pediatric Nurse Practitioners/Nurses	www.pnpcert.org
National Council of State Boards of Nursing	www.ncsbn.org
National Institute of Nursing Research	www.nih.gov/ninr
National Institutes of Health	www.nih.gov
National League for Nursing	www.nln.org
National Organization/Nurse Practitioner Faculties	www.nonpf.com
National Rural Health Association	www.nrharural.org
Oncology Nurses Society (ONS)	www.ons.org
Reuters Health Information Services	www.reutershealth.com
State Government	www.state.[insert abbreviation].us
U. S. Government Printing Office	www.access.gpo.gov
U. S. Government White House Publications, Executive Orders Search Site	www.pub.whitehouse/gov/search/executive-orders.html
U. S. House of Representatives	www.house.gov
U. S. Senate	www.senate.gov
World Health Organization	www.who.int

Adapted from Hebda, T., Czar, P., & Mascara, C. (1998). *Handbook of informatics for nurses and health care professionals*. New York: Addison-Wesley; reprinted with permission.

books reviewed had no reference to nurses at all, and only four books contained more than 10 references to nurses throughout the text. More recently, journalists have reported that information about nurses rarely comes forward, that nurses are reluctant to make their voices heard and that they have expressed fear about being misquoted (Buresh & Gorden, 2000). The outcomes of these studies are clear. APNs must write, speak, and publish broadly, integrating nursing's influence into policy decisions (Mundt, 1997). The media in all forms—whether newsprint, television, the Internet, books, or journals—serve as important links to information and opinions. Furthermore, the media serve as a springboard for policy initiatives and as a means to communicate with policymakers, stakeholders, and constituents. The critical issue is how can APNs use the media as an instrument to enhance policy and professional influence?

Multiple resources that provide strategies and pointers for using the media appropriately are available. Several very basic communication concepts emerge, as shown in Box 9-4. APNs should use the media strategy that works best for them. Most APNs know how to present themselves most effectively and most comfortably. Is it easier to conceive of doing a speech or a radio or television spot or writing an article for the newspaper? In which mode are you best able to communicate your point using the strategies in Box 9-4?

BOX 9-4 • BASIC COMMUNICATION STRATEGIES

Understand how the system works.
Make your point.
Get the facts straight.
Use data to back up your statements.
KISS it (Keep it short and simple).

Do your homework.
Ask for what you want.
Tell the truth.
Personalize the message.

What venue will get the most visibility at the best time? How controversial is the issue? Is it important to pave the way with other stakeholders, in and outside of nursing, before you go public? Is it important to reach many people (the public), or do you need to focus on educating a particular legislator or committee? If you are speaking publicly, are you ready to see your remarks in print the next day? Can you back up what you say? (deVries & Vanderbuilt, 1992; Hassmiller, 1995; Mason, Leavitt, & Chaffee, 2002).

EDUCATING POLICYMAKERS AND LEGISLATORS

Educating influential leaders and policymakers requires special consideration. They are usually dealing with a multitude of issues at once and use staffers and aides to stay abreast of the issues. Their work is structured around committees, and so they are much closer to and more informed about some issues than others. They have personal goals, as well as responsibilities to their constituents. They are bombarded on every side by multiple special interest groups who want their attention and their vote. The *sine qua non* of educating and influencing busy policymakers can be summed up in the following four basic strategies:

1. Use their staff to the fullest degree possible. The staffers are following the legislation and have the best insight on the strengths and weaknesses of getting what you want.
2. Be clear; understand the issue fully; know what you hope to gain and what you are willing to give up.
3. Use multiple strategies, such as face-to-face communication, letter writing, e-mail campaigns, and fact sheets.
4. Garner support from others who have a like mission.

EDUCATING THE PUBLIC

A common misconception among APNs is that the public in general is aware of the roles and issues surrounding health care and advanced practice nursing. APNs are often amazed to discover that physicians, legislators, and their patients really have very little understanding of what APNs are about, what they can do, and how they fit into the overall scheme of health care. Each APN has a primary responsibility for educating people he or she encounters and for conducting this education in a clear and articulate manner. This may seem to be an easy task, but in fact it is fraught with political complexities and varying levels of sophistication. Again, using the strengths of professional associations is key to getting out a message that is clear and appropriate. Most advanced practice nursing organizations have packaged materials and references that APNs at the grass-roots level can access from Internet pages or can order hard copies.

The ways in which APNs gain visibility are based on personal style. One APN may write a weekly column in the local newspaper, another may be very visible on local planning and advisory boards, and a third may host a radio talk show. Volunteering for community service or as a member of the local or state speakers' bureau also works well. Written materials or videotapes in office waiting rooms provide patients and families with an important introduction to advanced practice nursing health care. In addition, personal visits to legislators, policymakers, and health-care leaders are critical components for gaining needed visibility. The epitome of gaining visibility is to run for professional or public office.

PLAYING BOTH SIDES OF THE STREET

Judy Buckalew, who was the first nurse to be a special assistant to the President of the United States, reminded us that nurses have long been criticized for being very self-serving and not "playing both sides of the street" (Pearson, 1987). This phrase refers to the need for the APN to be able to see beyond the issues at hand and to look at the larger picture and the differing perspectives on health-care legislation of the other stakeholders. It requires careful monitoring of legislation and regulation both in and beyond nursing and knowing the policymakers' philosophy and interests. Buckalew stated further, "playing both sides of the street is just smart politics. No matter who is currently in power, you should divide your energy and your power evenly" (Pearson, 1987, p. 54).

Becoming an insider who has a place at the policy and political table happens over time and is predicated on a collegial approach based on mutual respect and valuing of others' points of view.

SPECIAL INTEREST GROUPS

One way to offer advocacy and become more visible with the public is to align with and keep abreast of issues that have high priority with special interest groups. Special interest groups or key stakeholders are often the deciding factor in policy decisions. For example, using the American Association of Retired Persons' (AARP's) website is a good way to track the policy and legislative agenda of senior citizens and to share the expertise of APNs with senior citizens. A feature story on the role of the NP in retirement communities or offering information about polypharmacy problems in *Modern Maturity*, the journal for the AARP, can provide needed visibility. Likewise, exploring the linkages for the American College of Nurse-Midwives online can lead you to the issues surrounding home births or birthing center care provided by APNs. Special interest groups have important connections to legislators and high-ranking policymakers, and these groups serve as stepping stones to ensure that APNs are positioned to influence policy.

General Political Strategies

APNs have come a long way in developing their political acumen at both state and national levels and have considerable power to achieve positive change if they capitalize on their newfound status. An important cohesiveness within nursing has emerged in response to health-care system changes. The nursing profession as a whole is beginning to recognize its strength at the policy table. As far back as 1984, Nancy Milio cautioned that nurses must be prepared to forge alliances, do their homework, and bring their case before the public; and she predicted that it would be APNs who carry the message forward (Milio, 1984). More than 10 years later, Towers (1995) cautioned the same thing: "It is clear that the contribution that nursing makes in the health-care arena must be brought forward. Nurses need to be heard, their data must be shared, their leadership enhanced. Nurses must take responsibility for educating and communicating with legislators" (p. 44). Politics and ethics are inherent in relationships at all systems levels and most obviously in policy development. Therefore nursing's ethical stance on social mandates that support poor and underserved populations needs to be clearly articulated (Aroskar, 1987; Sarikonda-Woitas, 2002). Advanced practice nursing leaders have a responsibility to bring their views and perspectives to decision-making and policy forums. They need to turn competitors into partners to make changes that will result in a more interdisciplinary system.

Professional turf issues have plagued APNs since the early days of their clinical practice. A lack of legal empowerment to practice to the fullest extent of knowledge and skills has been a dominant barrier to the optimal practice of NPs (Dempster, 1994). CNMs and CRNAs have the longest track record in dealing with these issues and have many successes to their credit. Health-care reform and managed care dialogue have caused physicians and other important health-care stakeholders to retrench, which has heightened the perception of APNs as a threat. This has made the current political arena extremely sensitive.

The political agenda that is carried out at the professional level (American Nurses Association/American Medical Association) and between advanced practice nursing specialty organizations is much different from the agenda played out at the grass-roots level. There is evidence that locally practicing physicians and nurses have strong collaborative relationships and that they are frustrated by the lack of cohesion at the professional level at which policy is made. APNs must closely monitor policy issues through phone trees, newsletters, and regional meetings. There is no question that an important strategy for the removal of barriers is through enlistment of support from physician and APN teams who are practicing successfully in a collegial manner.

Another strategy to assist in the improvement of practice environments for advanced practice is to create local networks of APNs within state structures that will help to remove barriers and develop workable practice guidelines. Close interaction with local collaborating physicians and leaders of local health-care entities is crucial. States that have made the greatest strides in removing practice barriers need to help states that have more serious constraints to advanced nursing practice. There are a myriad of recent textbooks on the market, as well as a plethora of journal articles, that deal with the issue of grooming APNs with political savvy and know-how to circumvent the landmines of political and legislative action. Most of these resources are well targeted toward helping the nurse gain confidence and expertise as a policymaker. The Additional Readings section at the end of this chapter includes some of these resources. It is recommended that all APNs, as part of their basic graduate program and through continued seminars and workshops, take advantage of these tools of the trade. Nurses have a formidable voting power base of more than 2.2 million. This is an incredible strength for nurses but requires cohesiveness within the ranks in order to make positive change for advanced nursing practice. The notion that someone else will carry the flag is not realistic. Developing political acumen and competence is a required skill for all practicing APNs, and most certainly for advanced practice nursing leaders, that is nurtured through time and experience. Lescavage (1995) offered several important points of entry for APN leaders: Develop political allies in Congress and inform them of APNs' changing goals, ambitions, and needs; champion causes for special interest groups that are cared for by APNs; serve on national boards and commissions; work on campaigns or better still, run for office. Peters (2002) asserted that nursing is facing an important "policy window" triggered by the nursing shortage, decreased access to care, and skyrocketing health-care costs that provides an opportunity for nurses to gain leverage in the policy arena. It will be important for APNs to take advantage of this window of opportunity.

OBSTACLES TO LEADERSHIP DEVELOPMENT AND EFFECTIVE LEADERSHIP

Professional and System Obstacles

There are several obstacles to achieving competence as an advanced practice nursing leader. Most of the obstacles result from conflict or competition between individuals, groups, or organizations. Competition can be both intraprofessional, as between advanced practice nursing groups, and interprofessional, as between physicians and nurses. Grensing-Pophal (1997) identified several barriers to good leadership and offered some advice. She suggested that being respected rather than being "liked" is one desired criterion for leadership. For most people, this is a difficult reality because being accepted and popular with others is important. Trying to "do it all" rather than delegating to others is a common trap that plagues busy leaders. A good leader is able to encourage a shared workload that recognizes the talents and abilities of followers. Two other pitfalls include avoiding the direct confrontation of difficult issues and a lack of communication with the resulting failure to keep others informed.

Oppressed Group Behavior and Dysfunctional Leadership Styles

Although there are many barriers to leading effectively and creating community, three constellations of behavior that are particularly destructive have been identified. Nurses may be vulnerable to these destructive behaviors because of the profession's historic marginalization as a female and relatively powerless group within health care. Three manifestations of oppressed group behavior limit the ability of APNs to lead: the star complex, the Queen Bee Syndrome, and failure to mentor ("eating one's young"). These behaviors are of particular concern during a nursing shortage when the profession needs to recruit and mentor younger nurses to help them create satisfying careers and pass this legacy on to future generations of nurses. Faculty and advanced practice nursing preceptors need to be alert to the appearance of such behaviors in students and coach the students to understand the impact of such behaviors on patients and colleagues. Readers are referred to the articles by King (2002) and Rider (2002) for specific suggestions on strategies for communicating with students and colleagues who demonstrate these interpersonal styles.

ABANDONING ONE'S NURSING IDENTITY: THE STAR COMPLEX

An effective advanced practice nursing leader is proud of his or her identity as a nurse. Those with the star complex deny their nursing identity or minimize their affiliation with nursing when being identified as a nurse might diminish their influence (e.g., some nurse authors use only their academic credential in publications within and outside of nursing). The star complex is a condition that may be associated with the experienced APN. Although the psychology of this phenomenon is beyond the scope of this chapter, individuals with the star complex are those whose sense of self and identity depend a great deal on the opinions of powerful others. Acknowledging or promoting their identity as a nurse might diminish their power or the opinions powerful others hold about them. As an example, consider the case of Janice, an APN who over the years has become identified with superior patient-focused care. Physician colleagues considered her to be a partner in the delivery of care, but staff and other APNs gave up consulting with her because her self-promotion often interfered with getting the job of the consultation done. In a recent conversation, a well-respected physician colleague told her how impressed he was with her practice. "In fact," he stated, "you're really not a nurse. You're different from all the other nurses I know." Janice graciously accepted this compliment, knowing that stardom, although overdue, had finally arrived. She had ascended to the heights of provider status and crashed through the nursing ceiling into a zone beyond nursing. Clearly, Janice's understanding of herself as an APN was dormant.

APNs are particularly vulnerable to being seduced into believing they are something other (more) than a nurse. Advanced practice nursing specialties that have expanded roles may seek the "status" of medicine. This vulnerability stems from the historical lack of recognition of nursing by physicians, other disciplines, and nurses; the need for approval; and a lack of personal mastery. The star complex can also represent inadequate socialization to nursing as a profession and/or to advanced practice nursing.

A primary strategy for the management of this obstacle is effective mentoring by a powerful APN with an intact nursing identity. An APN with the star complex has often been mentored exclusively by individuals outside of nursing, such as physicians. Mentors tend to select protégés who remind them of themselves (Bowen, 1985) and then mold their protégés in their own images. The affirmation of the APN's expert clinical skills and even personal mastery are thus validated by a reference group outside of nursing. An additional essential strategy is to use clear and concise communication skills to provide an appropriate response to a colleague who believes that it is a compliment to be identified as other than a nurse. Grohar-Murray and DiCroce's (1992) guidelines for effective communication, discussed earlier in this chapter, are applicable. An appropriate response for Janice to have made would have been, "Thank you, but I'm proud to be an advanced practice nurse." The existence of the star complex may represent a more fundamental problem for the APN than good communication skills can address. The issue is whether the APN truly desires to be identified as a *nurse*, performing at the boundaries of nursing practice and accepted by other nurses as a valued member of the nursing profession. The resolution of this issue may require counseling and/or group experiential exploration and training. Self-exploration within the context of organizations is provided by various agencies. For example, the Public Health Policy Fellowship at the Health Resources and Services Administration gives individuals opportunities to focus disciplined attention on their role, particularly in terms of authority, power, and leadership, in both small and large interdisciplinary groups. This type of experiential training may prove invaluable to APNs attempting to identify with their professional reference group.

HOARDING OR MISUSING POWER: THE QUEEN BEE SYNDROME

An effective leader is generous, looking for opportunities to lift colleagues up by sharing opportunities, knowledge, and expertise and acknowledging the contributions of others. Queen bees are leaders who hoard all of the visible leadership tasks for themselves. Like those with the star complex, the effort to garner power is a theme. In this case, power derives not from powerful others, but from their own knowledge and expertise. These APNs are threatened by strong individuals and tend to denigrate them instead of sharing power. This type of leader prefers to be surrounded by servile individuals who will not challenge his or her authority. For example, although Jackie, a wound and ostomy APN has been at her agency for many years, very few staff nurses are as competent as they want or need to be at managing wounds and ostomies. Jackie makes sure she sees every patient and that the patients know she is the authority on wounds and ostomies. Staff nurses who are competent in these skills report that Jackie undermines them with patients by saying the care should have been done a certain way. Jackie was not happy when the staff on a surgical unit, who had tried to involve her in the project unsuccessfully, conducted a quality improvement project during which both physicians and patients identified some service delivery issues relative to ostomy care. These staff members had the support of an assertive (new) CNS and a nurse manager and over time slowly changed the way wound and ostomy services were managed.

The antidote to the queen bee syndrome is to use knowledge and expertise to move away from hoarded leadership toward collaborative, empowered leadership. Queen bee behavior is the antithesis of good leadership, and unfortunately, is not uncommon among women and nurses. As noted, it is an illustration of oppressed group behavior. As advanced practice nursing leaders become more confident in their leadership abilities and as more APNs join the circle of leaders, Queen Bees will have more difficulty remaining as leaders and keeping positions of stature. All effective leaders empower others.

FAILURE TO MENTOR: LEAVING OTHER NURSES BEHIND

Nurses who advance in their profession may forget their roots and leave young nurses behind or, worse, actively undermine the advancement of young nurses. This latter behavior is sometimes referred to by the horrific phrase *eating one's young*. For example, nurses are often criticized by other nurses for continuing their education and moving into advanced practice nursing roles. This horizontal violence from colleagues hampers others from moving forward, in their careers. During orientation to a new position, the process too often becomes a survival test to see whether the new APN can survive without mentoring or a supportive network. This phenomenon is another illustration of oppressed group behavior. Because perceived powerlessness is at the root of this behavior, an important antidote is empowerment. Leaders who are aware of this phenomenon can foster mentoring opportunities that can enhance the transition of colleagues in new positions in both practice and leadership roles. APNs need to lead their organizations in a thoughtful evaluation of the nursing environment. Are nurses being supported and mentored to develop their capabilities and professional investment? Are unsupportive comments confronted and addressed? Nurses need to be responsible and held accountable for statements and actions that denigrate their colleagues. It is not an overstatement to claim that the future health of the profession depends on overcoming this barrier and relegating it to history.

STRATEGIES FOR IMPLEMENTING PROFESSIONAL AND CLINICAL LEADERSHIP

Developing a Leadership Portfolio

Throughout the chapter, definitions, attributes, and components of leadership and key strategies for becoming a political advocate have been presented. These approaches will help new APNs assimilate the leadership competency. Developing a leadership component as part of a marketing portfolio is helpful to novice APNs who desire to individualize the components of the leadership competency within their personal vision, goals, timeline, and advanced practice nursing role in the practice setting. Falter (2003) suggested the use of a strategy map that includes vision, goals, and objectives that outline steps to achieve a particular strategy. Portfolios are designed to meet the needs of individual APNs and should be consistent with clinical and personal interests and professional goals, and provide and a timeline that allows for personal and professional balance and boundary setting. Chapter 21 provides the elements of a marketing portfolio.

Promoting Collaboration: Unity Versus Fragmentation

At different times, each subgroup of APNs has emerged as a leader for the nursing profession. Psychiatric CNSs were among the first entrepreneurial APNs to hang out their shingles, despite the litigious climate in which they could be threatened with lawsuits for "practicing medicine." CNMs and CRNAs have led the way in powerfully using data to justify their existence. Early in their history, both groups began to record the results of their practices, showing the quality and suitability of their care (Diers, 1992; Chapter 1). In the 1990s, NPs, with their flexible, community-based primary care practices, stood at the forefront of the changing health-care delivery system. Although these subgroups of APNs have made impressive strides for advanced practice nursing, an obstacle to effective leadership is the tendency for APNs to separate and establish rigid boundaries that distinguish them from one another, thereby fragmenting APN groups and blocking opportunities for the increased power that unity would bring.

With the tension and fragmentation created by rigid boundaries, there is a need for leadership that transcends APN role boundaries. APNs must both manage and bridge boundaries among other nursing groups and within the ranks of the various APN constituencies. Although the uniqueness of each type of APN must be protected, a professional structure that provides a forum for discussing issues pertinent to all types of APNs also needs to be created. This structure may be simply an annual meeting for APNs, or it may be a permanent entity residing within an existing or new professional organization. Progress was made in this area during the 1990s. Consensus groups at the national level are meeting to discuss policy issues. At the policy level, the power of collective numbers of all advanced practice nursing groups speaking with one voice cannot be overemphasized. APN specialty groups have joined to speak out collaboratively about state regulations regarding reimbursement, prescriptive authority, and managed care regulation.

The opportunity to unify practice and collaborate is calling to every APN. It is critical that each APN, regardless of specialty, take on the burden of moving toward unification. One of the most important things that APNs do as leaders is to create community. Creating community in the current health-care environment is particularly challenging because of the realignment of clinical decision making, scopes of practice for APNs and physicians, and new roles that blur boundaries between nursing and medicine. Although it was developed for community health partnerships, readers are encouraged to become familiar with the Community Tool Box, a URL sponsored by the University of Kansas (http://www.ctb.ku.edu/). APNs will find many useful resources on leadership, promoting change, and cultural competence in the forms of narrative descriptions, checklists, and other tools for building community. In addition, the following guidelines, adapted from Heifetz (1994), may help APNs at both individual and group levels to move from fragmentation to unity:

- Because leadership is a core competency for the APN, the goal of unification must be translated into a shared vision. This is the case whether leadership occurs at high-level policy meetings or in the grass-roots clinical setting.

- APNs and their various professional associations need a forum in which to explore, identify, and regulate the stress related to crossing and perhaps merging boundaries previously viewed as impenetrable. A specific example of this is the blended CNS/NP role discussed in Chapter 16. This redefinition of reality will require taking risks with and without the benefit of a safety net.
- With a legitimate forum established, APNs can direct disciplined attention to the issue of unity. Examples are the national coalitions that have been formed to implement program standards and to explore the issues surrounding interstate compacts.
- Each NP, CNS, CNM, and CRNA will return to his or her referent professional association for continuing dialogue and support of the outcomes from forum discussions. This involves giving the work and dialogue back to colleagues at the grassroots level.
- Each APN will listen with respect to leaders in the advanced practice nursing and nursing professional communities and in the communities of care recipients, providers, payors, legislators, and citizens.
- Each APN will emerge from this systematic, inclusive exploration of unity with a clear trajectory for building a learning organization to support the continued development of a unified vision of advanced practice nursing.

These strategies lead to the structures on which unity is built—an understanding of change, effective communication, coalition building, and collaborative practice. These four building blocks form the foundation of interdisciplinary leadership and practice.

Motivating and Empowering Others

Earlier in the chapter, empowerment was defined as the ability of the leader to give followers the freedom and authority to act. However, truly empowering others requires more than just giving them permission to act on their own. Empowerment is a developmental process that a good leader fosters over time that encourages constituents to feel competent, responsible, independent, and authorized to act. Rajotte (1996) offered a useful six-step method for advanced practice nursing leaders to use to empower other nurses. The first step involves *education*, which in itself provides power through increasing the individual's knowledge base. The process of *leading* by inspiring, motivating, and encouraging is the second step. Providing *structure* is a third step of empowering. Structure provides a framework that offers protection and security as one moves into new territory. The fourth step for enhancing empowerment in followers involves *providing resources* with which one can grow and develop. *Mentoring*, a key skill for leaders, provides the support and direction necessary for change toward empowerment to happen. The final step is *actualization*, in which others—whether nurses, patients, or colleagues—are empowered to evoke change. For example, CNMs empower pregnant women by putting them in control of the birthing process through education, mentoring, and providing resources for parenting that nurture self-esteem and enhance family structure.

Networking

Networking is an integral technique used by leaders to stay informed and connected regarding advanced practice nursing issues. Networking, both formal and informal, is not a new strategy for advanced practice nursing leaders. Formal networks take the form of committees, coalitions, and consortia of people who come together to share information and plan strategy regarding mutual issues. Formal networks open doors to new opportunities and provide shared resources. Informal networking is a behind-the-scenes format that allows for contact with APNs and others who "speak the same language," have the same viewpoints, and can offer support and feedback at critical times. The ability of APNs to stay connected to important practice and education issues through networking is a key component of leadership. Networking has long been credited as a powerful tool for successful leaders and strategists. The Internet has markedly augmented the busy APN's ability to informally network with professional colleagues and organizations around the world. The most highly effective strategy for becoming an insider is networking with colleagues within the circle of APN peers and with other health-care providers who have a stake in the outcomes.

Planning and Implementing Change

Jick (1993) suggested an inventory of "10 commandments" that provide a strong base for the APN who is preparing to become an effective change agent (Box 9-5). Many of the skills that were outlined in the earlier section on personal attributes of successful leaders, such as shared vision, expert communication, and risk-taking behaviors, are the same tenets offered by Jick. However, there are other strategies that assist in the process as follows. First, it is important to analyze the situation and explore the need for change. Second, one must craft an implementation plan that involves everyone. Third, there must be support for capable leadership. Desired change does not happen without strong leadership, from both individuals and teams (Jick, 1993). In these 10 commandments, one can clearly see the organic link between leadership and change agency.

Box 9-6 provides a list of leadership strategies that are useful for moving through these transitions. These strategies are key leadership activities in times of ongoing change. Bonalumi and Fisher (1999) suggested that an important component of leadership in an atmosphere of change is the ability to foster and encourage resilience in change recipients. O'Connell (1999) defined the characteristics of resilient people as follows: being positive and self-assured in the face of life's complexities; having a focused, clear vision of what

---

BOX 9-5 • 10 COMMANDMENTS OF IMPLEMENTING CHANGE

1. *Analyze the organization and its need for change.*
2. *Create a shared vision and common direction.*
3. *Separate from the past.*
4. *Create a sense of urgency.*
5. *Support a strong leader role.*
6. *Line up political sponsorship.*
7. *Craft an implementation plan.*
8. *Develop enabling structures.*
9. *Communicate, involve people, and be honest.*
10. *Reinforce and institutionalize the change.*

BOX 9-6 • LEADERSHIP STRATEGIES FOR MOVING THROUGH THE TRANSITION OF CHANGE

Developing interim procedures and policies . . . *to create structure*
Fostering group cohesion . . . *so people can draw strength from each other*
Anticipating that old issues/rumors will surface . . . *allow them to be acknowledged*
Reminding folks over and over why change is necessary . . . *to gain support for change*
Creating new communication channels . . . *being honest about uncertainty*
Minimizing unnecessary changes . . . *which can lead to frustration and resistance*
Reminding and showing people what they can count on . . . *to build confidence*

Adapted from Mason, D. J., & Leavitt, J. K. (1998). *Policy and politics in nursing and health care* (pp. 280-293). Philadelphia: W. B. Saunders; reprinted with permission.

they want to achieve; and having the abilities to be organized but flexible and proactive rather than reactive. Helping colleagues and followers to develop resilience is a major achievement for advanced practice nursing leaders who seek to facilitate the growth of their followers.

SUMMARY

The health-care system is constantly changing, but despite the challenges of change, the future is bright for APNs as clinical and professional leaders. APNs can define the scope of their leadership influence. They can focus on improving clinical care by adopting best practices, building teams committed to evidence-based practice, and modeling effective interpersonal and communication skills at the clinic, unit, department or agency level—leadership with a lower case *l* (Norton & Grady, 1996). They can extend their leadership into communities, professional organizations, and national and international health policy arenas—leadership with a capital *L* (Norton, & Grady, 1996).

The evolution of APNs, particularly CNMs, CNSs, CRNAs, and all NPs, has had far-reaching influence on this country's health-care system, as well as on nursing itself—at every level. Strengthening interdisciplinary collaboration and communication within caregiving teams may eventually translate to better cooperation among national organizations. APNs exercise leadership when they present ideas or dilemmas to colleagues, whether on an electronic mailing list or at a national meeting. As Gladwell (2000) noted, many small changes contribute to a big change, so APNs should not underestimate the potentially far-reaching impact of leadership exercised at the bedside or in the clinic and with patients, colleagues, and administrators. It is important to consider the ways in which you can lead—make a difference—and commit to doing so, knowing that you can redefine the scope of your leadership influence in response to opportunities or changing life circumstances.

Nursing care is based on an interactive style that empowers patients and colleagues. This foundation holds advanced practice nursing leaders in good stead as they move into the interdisciplinary paradigm of the future. It is very important for new graduates to begin the trajectory for growth and development as leaders and for existing APN leaders to mentor their protégés into leadership positions.

As APNs contemplate the demands and opportunities for leadership that the future holds, they must work toward identifying, clarifying, and demystifying the health-care system of today, for within today's reality lies the basis of tomorrow's change. APNs are change specialists who operate at the boundary between today's health-care system and tomorrow's. Effective leadership positions APNs and their colleagues to meet the health-care needs of individuals, families, and communities (Malone, 1996).

REFERENCES

Allen, D. W. (1998). How nurses become leaders: Perceptions and beliefs about leadership development. *Journal of Nursing Administration, 28,* 15-20.

Aroskar, M. A. (1987). The interface of ethics and politics in nursing. *Nursing Outlook, 35,* 268-272.

Ballein, K. M. (1998). Entrepreneurial leadership characteristics of SNEs emerge as their role develops. *Nursing Administration Quarterly, 22,* 60-69.

Barker, A. (1994). An energy leadership paradigm: Transformational leadership. In E. I. Hein & M. J. Nicholson (Eds.), *Contemporary leadership* (4th ed., pp. 81-86). Philadelphia: J. B. Lippincott.

Bernhard, L. A., & Walsh, M. (1995). *Leadership: The key to the professionalization of nursing* (3rd ed.). St. Louis, MO: Mosby.

Bonalumi, N., & Fisher, K. (1999). Health care change: Challenge for nurse administrators. *Nursing Administration Quarterly, 23,* 69-73.

Bowen, D. (1985). Were men meant to mentor women? *Training and Development Journal, 39,* 30-34.

Bridges, W. (1991). *Managing transitions: Making the most of change.* Reading, MA: Addison-Wesley.

Buresh, B., & Gordon, S. (2000). From silence to voice: What nurses know and must communicate to the public. Ottawa, Ontario, Canada: Canadian Nurses Association.

Burns, J. M. (1978). *Leadership.* New York: Harper & Row.

Christopher, M. A., Miller, J., Beck, T., & Toughill, E. (2002). Working with the community for change. In D. Mason, J. Leavitt, & M. Chaffee (Eds.), *Policy and politics in nursing and health care* (4th ed.). Philadelphia: W. B. Saunders.

Collins, J. (2001). *Good to great: Why some companies make the leap…and others don't.* New York: Harper Business.

Covey, S. (1989). *The seven habits of highly effective people: Powerful lessons in personal change.* New York: Simon & Schuster.

Dempster, J. S. (1994). Autonomy: A professional issue of concern for nurse practitioners. *Nurse Practitioner Forum, 5,* 227-232.

DePree, M. (1989). *Leadership is an art.* New York: Doubleday/Currency.

DeVries, C. M., & Vanderbuilt, M. W. (1992). *The grassroots lobbying handbook: Empowering nurses through legislative and political action.* Washington, DC: American Nurses Association.

Diers, D. (1992). Nurse midwives and nurse anesthetists: The cutting edge in specialist practice. In L. Aiken & C. Fagin (Eds.), *Charting nursing's future* (pp. 159-180). Philadelphia: J. B. Lippincott.

Engebretson, J., & Wardell, D. W. (1997). The essence of partnership in research. *Journal of Professional Nursing, 13*(1), 38-47.

Falter, E. (2003). Successful leaders map and measure. *Nurse Leader: From Management to Leadership, 1*(4), 40-42, 45.

Fawcett, D. (2002). Mentoring—what it is and how to make it work. *AORN Journal, 75,* 950-954.

Fiedler, F. E., Chermers, M. M., & Mahar, L. C. (1976). *Improving leadership effectiveness: The leader match concept.* New York: John Wiley & Sons.

Fisher, R., Ury, W., & Patton, B. (2002). *Getting to yes: How to negotiate an agreement without giving in* (2nd ed.). New York: Penguin Putnam.

Gladwell, M. (2000). *The tipping point: How little things can make a big difference.* New York: Little Brown & Co.

Grensing-Pophal, L. (1997). Improving your leadership skills: Seven common pitfalls to avoid. *Nursing 97, 27,* 41-42.

Grohar-Murray, M. E., & DiCroce, H. R. (1992). *Leadership and management in nursing.* Norwalk, CT: Appleton & Lange.

Halpern, I. M. (2002). Reflections of a health policy advocate: The natural extension of nursing activities. *Oncology Nursing Forum, 29,* 1261-1263.

Hanson, C. M., Boyle, J., Hatmaker, D., & Murray, J. (1999). *Finding your voice as a leader.* Washington, DC: American Academy of Nursing.

Hassmiller, S. (1995). *Legislative logistics for leaders.* Washington, DC: Health Resources and Services Administration.

Hebda, T., Czar, P., & Mascara, C. (1998). *Handbook of informatics for nurses and health care professionals.* New York: Addison-Wesley.

Heifetz, R. (1994). *Leadership without easy answers.* Cambridge, MA: Belknap Press.

Houghton, A. (2003). Bullying in medicine. *British Medical Journal, 326,* S125.

Institute of Medicine. (2001). *Crossing the quality chasm: A new health system for the 21st century.* Washington, DC: National Academy Press.

Joint Commission on Accreditation of Healthcare Organizations. (2000). *Joint commission focuses on pain management.* Retrieved April 7, 2004, from http://www.jcaho.org

Jick, T. D. (1993). *Managing change: Cases and concepts.* Burr Ridge, IL: Irwin.

Kantor, R. M., Stein, B. A., & Jick, T. D. (1992). *The challenge of organizational change: How companies experience it and leaders guide it.* New York: The Free Press.

King, J. (2002). Dealing with difficult doctors. *British Medical Journal, 325,* S43.

Klein, E., Gabelnick, F., & Herr, P. (1998). *The psychodynamics of leadership.* Madison, CT: Psychosocial Press.

Koerner, J. E. (1997). Profiles of leadership: A dialogue with two nursing revolutionaries. *Nursing Administration Quarterly, 22,* 1-7.

Lescavage, N. J. (1995). Nurses, make your presence felt: Taking off the rose colored glasses. *Nursing Policy Forum, 1,* 18-21.

Lewin, K. (1976). *Field theory in social science.* Chicago: University of Chicago Press.

Locock, L., Dopson, S., Chambers, D., & Gabbay, J. (2001). Understanding the role of opinion leaders in improving clinical effectiveness. *Social Science and Medicine, 53,* 745-757.

Malone, B. L. (1996). Clinical and professional leadership. In A. B. Hamric, J. A. Spross, & C. M. Hanson (Eds.), *Advanced nursing practice: An integrative approach* (pp. 213-228). Philadelphia: W. B. Saunders.

Malone, P., Chafee, M., & Wachter, M. (2002). The power and influence of special interest groups in health care. In D. J. Mason, J. K. Leavitt, & M. Chaffee (Eds.), *Policy and politics in nursing and health care* (4th ed., pp. 627-638.) Philadelphia: W. B. Saunders.

Marcus, L., Dorn, B. C., Kritek, P., Miller, V. & Wyatt, J. (1999). *Renegotiating health care: Resolving conflict to build collaboration* (2nd ed.). San Francisco: Jossey Bass.

Mason, D. J., Leavitt, J. K., & Chaffee, M. (2002). *Policy and politics in nursing and health care.* Philadelphia: W. B. Saunders.

McAvoy, B., & Murtagh, J. (2003). Workplace bullying: The silent epidemic [Letter]. *British Medical Journal, 326,* 776-777.

McGlynn, E. A., Asch, S. M., Adams, J., Keesey, J., Hicks, J., DeCristofaro, A., et al. (2003). The quality of health care delivered to adults in the United States. *New England Journal of Medicine, 348*(26), 2635-2645.

Milio, N. (1984). The realities of policymaking: Can nurses have an impact? *The Journal of Nursing Administration, 14,* 18-23.

Mundt, M. H. (1997). Books on health policy and health reform: How is nursing represented? *Journal of Professional Nursing, 13,* 19-27.

National Association of Clinical Nurse Specialists. (2004). *Statement on clinical nurse specialist practice and education.* Harrisburg, PA: Author.

National Organization of Nurse Practitioner Faculties & The American Association of Colleges of Nursing. (2002). *Nurse practitioner primary care competencies in specialty areas: Adult, family, gerontological, pediatric, and women's health.*

Washington DC: U.S. Department of Health and Human Services. [HRSA Contract 00-0532(P)].

Norton, S. F., & Grady, E. M. (1996). Change agent skills. In A. B. Hamric, J. A. Spross, & C. M. Hanson (Eds.), *Advanced nursing practice: An integrative approach* (pp. 249-271). Philadelphia: W. B. Saunders.

O'Connell, C. (1999). A culture of change or a change of culture. *Nursing Administration Quarterly, 23,* 65-68.

Oxman, A. D., Thomson, M. A., Davis, D. A., & Haynes, R. B. (1995). No magic bullets: A systematic review of 102 trials of interventions to improve professional practice. *Canadian Medical Association Journal, 153,* 1423-1431.

Pavalko, R. M. (1971). *Sociology of occupations and professions.* Itasca, IL: Peacock.

Pearson, L. (1987). Judi Buckalew: Learning to play political hardball. *The Nurse Practitioner: The American Journal of Primary Health Care, 12,* 49-50, 52, 54.

Peters, R. M. (2002). Nurse administrators' role in health care policy: Teaching the elephant to dance. *Nursing Administration Quarterly, 26,* 1-8.

Rajotte, C. A. (1996). Empowerment as a leadership theory. *Kansas Nurse, 71,* 1.

Rider, E. (2002). Twelve strategies for effective communication and collaboration in medical teams. *British Medical Journal. 325,* S45.

Rost, J. C. (1993). *Leadership for the 21st century.* Westport, CT: Praeger.

Sarikonda-Woitas, C. (2002). Ethical health care policy: Nursing's voice in allocation. *Nursing Administration Quarterly, 26,* 72-80.

Senge, P. (1990). *The fifth discipline: The art and practice of the learning organization.* New York: Doubleday.

Senge, P., Kleiner, A., Roberts, C., Ross, R., Roth, G., & Smith, B. (1999) *The dance of change: The challenges of sustaining momentum in learning organizations.* New York: Doubleday/Currency.

Soumerai, S. B., McLaughlin, T. J., Gurwitz, J. H., Guadagnoli, E., Hauptman, P. J., Borbas, C., et al. (1998). Effect of local medical opinion leaders on quality of care for acute myocardial infarction: A randomized controlled trial. *JAMA: The Journal of the American Medical Association, 279,* 1358-1363.

Spencer, J., & Jordan, R. (2001). Educational outcomes and leadership to meet the needs of modern health care. *Quality and Safety in Health Care, 10*(Suppl)2, 38-45.

Spross, J. A., & Heaney, C. A. (2000). Shaping advanced nursing practice in the new millennium. *Seminars in Oncology Nursing, 16*(1), 12-24.

Stogdill, R. M. (1948). Personal factors associated with leadership in a survey of the literature. *Journal of Psychology, 25,* 35-71.

Thomson, M. A., Oxman, A. D., Haynes, R. B., Davis, D. A., Freemantle, N., & Harvey, E. L. (1999). *Local opinion leaders to improve health professional practice and health care outcomes.* The Cochrane Library. Oxford: Update Software.

Tornabeni, J. (1996). Changes in the advanced practice of administration: A personal perspective of the changes affecting the role. *Advanced Practice Nursing Quarterly, 2,* 62-66.

Towers, J. (1995). A call to action: The GNE-GME-NEA debate. *Nursing Policy Forum, 1,* 40-45.

Trent, B. A. (2003). Leadership myths. *Reflections on Nursing Leadership, 29,* 8.

Vance, C. (2003, January/February). Mentoring at the edge of chaos. *Nurse Leader,* 42-43.

Vance, C., & Larson, E. (2002). Leadership research in business and health care. *Journal of Nursing Scholarship, 34,*165-171.

Vance, C., & Olson, R. K. (1998). *The mentor connection in nursing.* New York: Springer-Verlag.

Wakefield, M. K. (2003a). Change drivers for nursing and health care. *Nursing Economics, 21,* 150-151.

Wakefield, M. K. (2003b). The more things change. *Nursing Economics, 20,* 44-45.

Winterfeldt, E. (2001). Influencing public policy. *Topics in Clinical Nutrition, 16,* 8-16.

Woodhull, N. (1998). *Healthcare's invisible partner. The Woodhall Study on nursing and the media.* Indianapolis, IN: Sigma Theta Tau International.

Additional Readings

Abreu, B. C. (1997). Interdisciplinary leadership: The future is now. *OT Practice, 2,* 20-23.

Anderson, R. (1997). Future organizational leadership. *Journal of Professional Nursing, 13*(6), 334.

Antrobus, S., & Brown, S. (1997). The impact of the commissioning agenda upon nursing practice: A pro-active approach to influencing health policy. *Journal of Advanced Nursing, 25,* 309-315.

Barczak, N. L. (1996). How to lead effective teams. *Critical Care Nursing Quarterly, 19,* 73-82.

Bessent, H. (Ed.). (1997). *Strategies for recruitment, retention, and graduation of minority nurses in colleges of nursing.* Washington, DC: American Nurses Association.

Bowen, W., & Bok, D. (1998). *The shape of the river: Long term consequences of considering race in college and university admissions.* Princeton, NJ: Princeton University Press.

Boykin, A. (1995). *Power, politics and public policy.* New York: National League for Nursing Press.

Buppert, C. (1999). *Nurse practitioner's business practice and legal guide.* Gaithersburg, MD: Aspen.

Carpenito, L. J. (1998). Redefining the gold standard of health care aka medical care. *Nursing Forum, 33,* 3-4.

DePree, M. (1992). *Leadership is an art* (2nd ed.). New York: Doubleday/Currency.

Duffy, J. R. (2002). The clinical leadership role of the CNS in the identification of nursing-sensitive and multidisciplinary quality indicator sets. *Clinical Nurse Specialist 16*(2), 70-76

Ellis-Stoll, C. C., & Popkess-Vawter, S. (1998). A concept analysis on the process of empowerment. *Advances in Nursing Science, 21,* 62-68.

Hamric, A. B., & Spross, J. A. (Eds.). (1989). *The clinical nurse specialist in theory and practice* (2nd ed.). Philadelphia: W. B. Saunders.

Hamric, A. B., Spross, J. A., & Hanson, C. M. (Eds.). (1996). *Advanced nursing practice: An integrative approach.* Philadelphia: W. B. Saunders.

Hanson, C. M. (1998). Regulatory issues will lead advanced practice nursing challenges into the new millennium. *Advanced Practice Nursing Quarterly, 4,* v-vi.

Ketefian, S. (1999). Knowing good and doing good—is there a difference? *Journal of Professional Nursing, 15,* 4.

Kissinger, J. A. (1998). Overconfidence: A concept analysis. *Nursing Forum, 33,* 18-26.

Kleinpell, R. M., & Piano, M. R. (1998). *Practice issues for the acute care nurse practitioner.* New York: Springer-Verlag.

Mahaffey, T. L. (1998). A nursing fellowship: Building leadership skills. *Nursing Management, 29,* 30-32.

Malby, B. (1998). Clinical leadership. *Advanced Practice Nursing Quarterly, 3,* 40-43.

Manfredi, C. M. (1996). A descriptive study of nurse managers and leadership. *Western Journal of Nursing Research, 18,* 314-329.

Mason, D. J., & Leavitt, J. K. (1998). *Policy and politics in nursing and health care* (3rd ed.). Philadelphia: W. B. Saunders.

McGuire, C. A., Stanhope, M., & Weisenbeck, S. M. (1998). Nursing competence—an evolving regulatory issue in Kentucky. *Nursing Administration Quarterly, 23,* 24-28.

Mellon, S., & Nelson, P. (1998). Leadership experiences in the community for nursing students: Redesigning education for the 21st century. *Nursing and Health Care Perspectives, 19,* 120-123.

Michaels, C. (1997). Leading beyond traditional boundaries: A community nursing perspective. *Nursing Administration Quarterly, 22,* 30-37.

Milstead, J. A. (1997). A social mandate: APN leadership for the whole policy process. *Advanced Practice Nursing Quarterly, 3,* 1-8.

Milstead, J. A. (1998). *Health policy and politics: A nurse's guide.* Gaithersburg, MD: Aspen.

Newell, M., & Pinardo, M. (1998). *Reinventing your nursing career: A handbook for success with the age of managed care.* Gaithersburg, MD: Aspen.

Penney, N. E., Campbell-Heider, N., Miller, B. K., Carter, E., & Bidwell-Cerone, S. (1996). Influencing health care policy: Nursing research and the ANA social policy statement. *Journal of the New York State Nurses Association, 27,* 15-19.

Pew Health Professions Commission. (1995). *Critical challenges: Revitalizing the health professions for the twenty-first century, third report.* San Francisco: University of California–San Francisco Center for the Health Professions.

Safriet, B. (1998). Still spending dollars, still searching for sense: Advanced practice nursing in an era of regulatory and economic turmoil. *Advanced Practice Nursing Quarterly, 4,* 24-33.

Simpson, R. L. (1999). Changing world, changing systems: Why managed health care demands information technology. *Nursing Administration Quarterly, 23*, 86-88.

Starfield, B. (1997). Primary care and health policy: The future of primary care in a managed care era. *International Journal of Health Services, 27*, 687-696.

Sullivan, T. J. (1998). *Collaboration: A health care imperative. Part III, intraorganizational collaboration.* New York: McGraw-Hill.

Triolo, P. K., Pozehl, B. J., & Mahaffey, T. L. (1997). Development of leadership within the university and beyond: Challenges to faculty and their development. *Journal of Professional Nursing, 13*, 149-153.

Whitman, M. (1998). Nurses can influence public health policy. *Advanced Practice Nursing Quarterly, 3*, 67-71.

Williams, R. P. (1998). Nurse leaders' perceptions of quality nursing: An analysis from academe. *Nursing Outlook, 46*, 262-267.

Williamson, S. H., & Hutcherson, C. (1998). Mutual recognition: Response to the regulatory implications of a changing health care environment. *Advanced Practice Nursing Quarterly, 4*, 86-93.

CHAPTER 10

Collaboration

CHARLENE M. HANSON • JUDITH A. SPROSS

Continued

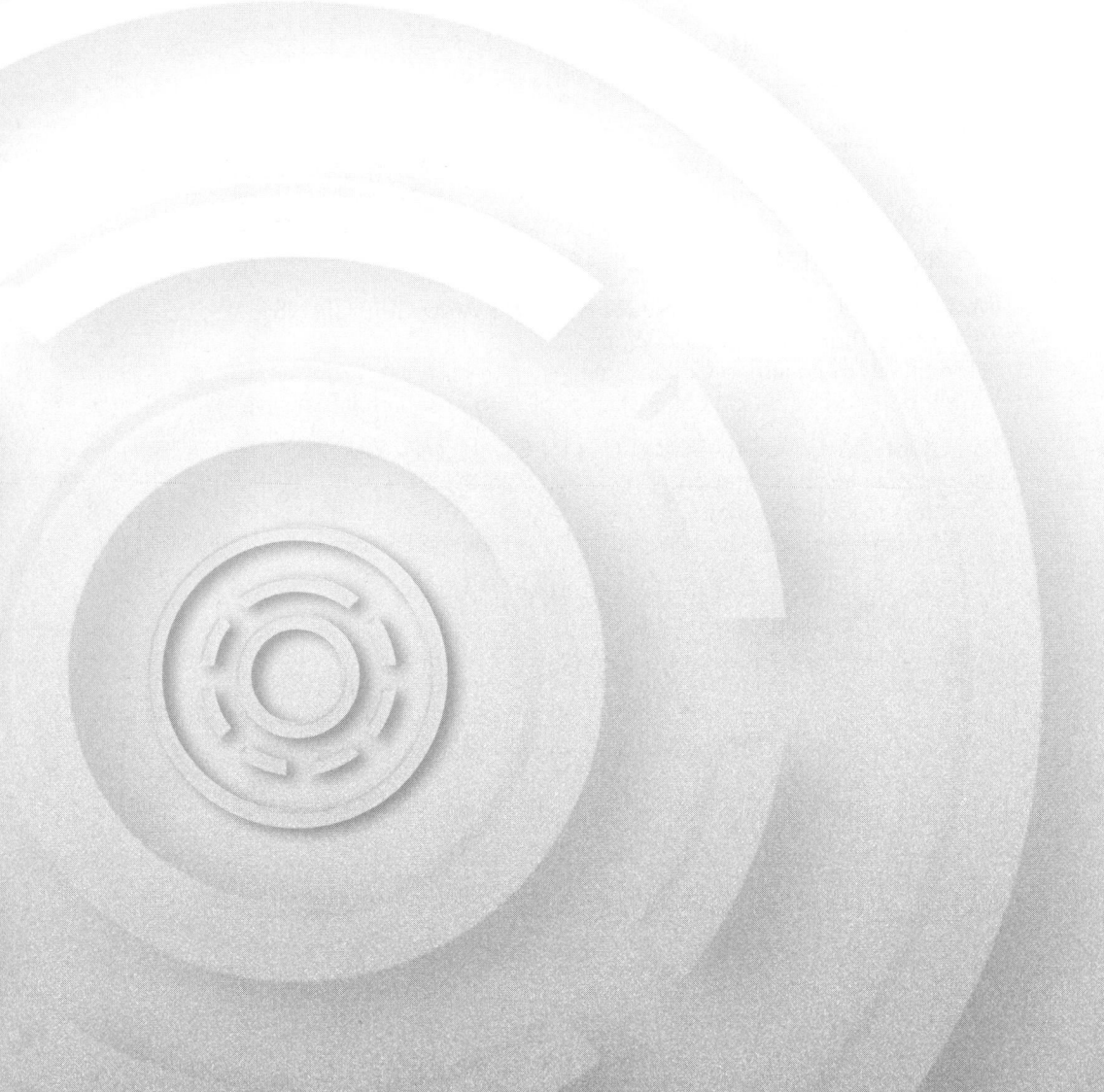

INTRODUCTION

Collaboration works. This simple statement belies the complexity of the phenomenon and the significant interpersonal commitment involved in building collaborative relationships. Collaboration can be conceptualized as occurring between or among individuals, work groups, and organizations. Research supports the premise that collaboration results in better patient outcomes, including patient satisfaction, and provides personal and professional satisfaction for clinicians. Advanced practice nurses (APNs) must have or acquire interpersonal communication skills and behaviors that make collaboration possible among a broad range of professionals and patients. Today, more than ever before, collaboration between health-care providers is an essential component of effective patient care. Historically, discussions about collaboration in the health field have focused on the relationship between physicians and nurses because that is where the most serious tensions have occurred. Although this chapter's discussion is often framed within the context of collaboration between APNs and physicians, it is important that any discussion of collaborative relationships address intradisciplinary collaboration among nurses, interdisciplinary collaboration between nurses and members of other disciplines, and collaboration among work groups and agencies.

The presence or absence of collaborative relationships affects patient care. Patients assume that their health-care providers communicate and collaborate effectively. Patient dissatisfaction with care, unsatisfactory clinical outcomes, and clinician frustration can often be traced to a failure to collaborate. The ability to collaborate is a core competency of advanced practice nursing (Brown, 1998; see Chapter 3). Collaboration depends on clinical and interpersonal expertise and an understanding of factors that can promote or impede efforts to establish collegial relationships. The primary focus of this chapter is on collaboration between and among individuals and work groups.

A paradox of the contemporary health-care system is that both incentives and disincentives exist for members of different disciplines, work groups, and organizations to collaborate. Incentives and disincentives may be equally powerful, so that motivation to collaborate can be diminished or eliminated by a compelling counterforce. An understanding of this paradox can help APNs and their colleagues approach opportunities for collaboration strategically and build and sustain clinical environments that support collaboration. As pressures to change mount in response to ongoing health-care inequities and as the proportion of nonphysician health care professionals increases, interdisciplinary collaboration at educational, clinical, and institutional levels is essential (Lindeke & Block, 1998; American Council of Graduate Medical Education, 2002; Cramer, 2002).

In this chapter, a conceptualization of collaboration is presented, followed by evidence that collaboration works. Incentives and disincentives for collaborating are identified. A definition and characteristics of collaboration that more fully address values, interpersonal aspects, and goals are offered; and strategies for developing and evaluating this competency are suggested. Key collaborative relationships for the APN are those with nurses, physicians, physician assistants, social workers, and other members of interdisciplinary teams. These relationships are used to illustrate important aspects of this core competency. In addition, selected aspects of organizational collaboration within and outside of nursing are explored.

A CONCEPTUALIZATION OF COLLABORATION

In 1997, the American College of Nurse-Midwives revised an earlier document and established definitions of collaboration, consultation, and referral to clarify their practice relationships with obstetricians (American College of Nurse-Midwives, 1997). These definitions inform the discussion of collaboration in this chapter. Collaboration can be thought of as one of several modes of interaction that occur between and among clinicians during the delivery of care. It is useful to describe the variety of interactions that can occur so that the complexity of collaboration can be appreciated. These include parallel communication and functioning, information exchange, coordination, consultation, co-management, referral, and collaboration. We assume that these interactions represent a hierarchy that proceeds from simple to complex *and* from less effective to more effective. Thus parallel communication may be the simplest form of communication but is likely to be the least effective for facilitating optimal outcomes, and collaboration is the most complex and most effective.

Parallel communication: Providers interact with a patient separately; they do not talk together before seeing a patient, nor do they see the patient together. There is no expectation of joint interactions. For example, the staff registered nurse, the medical student, and the attending physician all ask the patient about the medications the patient is taking.

Parallel functioning: Providers care for patients, addressing the same clinical problem, but do not engage in any joint or collaborative planning. For example, nurses, physical therapists, and physicians document their interventions for pain in separate parts of the patient record.

Information exchange: Informing may be one- or two-sided and may or may not require action or decision making. If action is needed, the decision is unilateral, not a result of joint planning.

Coordination: The establishment of structures to minimize duplication of effort and to maximize efficient use of patients' and providers' resources.

Consultation: The process whereby the clinician who is caring for a patient seeks advice regarding a patient concern but retains primary responsibility for care delivery (see Chapter 7).

Co-management: This refers to the process in which two or more clinicians provide care and each professional retains accountability and responsibility for defined aspects of care. This process usually arises from consultation in which a problem requires management that is outside the scope of practice of the referring clinician. One clinician usually retains responsibility for the majority of care (as in primary care settings) while the second provider is accountable for managing the problem that is outside the primary provider's expertise. Providers must be explicit with each other about their responsibilities. Co-management may also characterize well-functioning interdisciplinary teams.

Referral: The process by which the APN directs the patient to a physician or another practitioner for management of a particular problem or aspect of the patient's care when the problem is beyond the APN's expertise (see Chapter 7).

With the exceptions of parallel communication and parallel functioning, the above processes require some level of interaction and communication among providers but may not involve collaboration.

Collaboration is a dynamic, interpersonal process in which two or more individuals make a commitment to each other to interact authentically and constructively to solve problems and to learn from each other to accomplish identified goals, purposes, or outcomes. The individuals recognize and articulate the shared values that make this commitment possible (Hanson & Spross, 1996; Hanson, Spross, & Carr, 2000).

Some background on our definition of collaboration is warranted. According to the dictionary, *collaboration* means "to work together, especially in a joint intellectual effort";

it also means to cooperate with the enemy (McKechnie, 1983). The term *collaborative* has often been used with other words, such as *teamwork* and *partnership*. The description of collaboration in the American Nurses Association's (ANA's) Social Policy Statement (ANA, 1995, ANA, 2003) informed the definition and discussion of collaboration in this chapter. The ANA recognized that the boundaries of each health-care professional's practice change and that high-quality care depends on a common focus, a recognition of each other's expertise, an appreciation for the skills and knowledge shared across disciplines, and the collegial exchange of ideas and knowledge. Yet none of these meanings adequately represented the concept of collaboration as it exists, or should exist, in the provision of health and illness care.

On the basis of a review of the literature and our experiences, we developed this definition of collaboration as a dynamic, interpersonal process. This definition implies shared values, commitment, and goals and yet allows for differences in opinions and approaches. It also acknowledges that collaboration requires individuals to interact holistically (strengths, weaknesses, and emotions), to share power, and to remain open to the possibilities for personal and professional transformation that exist within a collaborative relationship. This definition captures the complexity and challenge of collaboration. Including the notions of shared values and commitment makes it clear that collaboration is a process that evolves over time. Tjosvold (1986) and Hughes and Mackenzie (1990) emphasized the importance of goal interdependence to collaboration. By definition, collaboration describes relationships that are positive and work well for professionals and patients. There is room for disagreement in collaborative relationships; partners develop strategies for dealing with disagreement that are mutually satisfactory and enhance collaboration. Information exchange, coordination, consultation, co-management, and referral do not require collaboration as it is described here, although collaboration is likely to enhance these interactions. It is important to note that collaboration is an interpersonal and developmental process; it cannot be mandated.

IMPACT OF COLLABORATION ON PATIENTS AND CLINICIANS

Experience and evidence suggest that collaboration works, yet effective collaboration eludes many clinicians. Why? Some authors link barriers to the history of the health-care professions, traditional gender roles, and hierarchical relationships (Christman, 1998; DeAngelis, 1994; Larson, 1999; Wells, Johnson, & Salyer, 1997). Over the years, there have been many reports of successful collaborative relationships involving APNs (Ryan, Edwards, & Rickles; 1980; Steele, 1986; Littell, 1981; Crowley & Wollner, 1987; Hilderley, 1991; Kavesh, 1993; Dressler, 1994; Kedziera & Levy, 1994; Siegler & Whitney, 1994a; Brita-Rossi et al., 1996; Hales, Karshmer, Montes-Sandoval, & Fiszbein, 1998; Grimaldi & Cousins, 1998). The importance of collaboration in various aspects of advanced practice nursing to APNs continues to be recognized (Kleinpell et al., 2002; Ingersoll, McIntosh, & Williams, 2000; Jackson et al., 2003).

In a review of the literature on collaboration, Sullivan (1998) noted that collaboration is widely perceived as useful and desirable. Although there are few studies of collaboration that have measured patient outcomes systematically (Sullivan, 1998; Torres & Dominguez, 1998), both patient and provider benefits have been documented. Sullivan (1998) found no reports indicating that collaboration failed when the models or practices had been jointly developed and implemented. Table 10-1 illustrates the types of patient and provider benefits that have been ascribed to clinical collaboration. Of all the publications on collaboration, few are found in the medical literature. Larson (1999) noted that

TABLE 10-1	BENEFITS OF COLLABORATION
FOR PATIENTS	**FOR PROVIDERS**
• Improved quality of care • Increased patient satisfaction • Lower mortality rate • Improved patient outcomes • Patients feel more secure, cared for, closer to nurses.	• Increased sharing of responsibility • Increased sharing of expertise • More mutually satisfying problem solving • Improved communications • Increased personal satisfaction • Increased quality of professional life • Enhanced mutual trust and respect • Bridges care-cure dichotomy • Expands horizons of providers • Avoids redundant care and ensures coverage • Empowers providers to influence health policy

Adapted from Sullivan, T. J. (1998). *Collaboration: A health care imperative* (pp. 26-27). New York: McGraw-Hill Health Professionals Division; reprinted with permission.

of 61 citations on nurse-physician collaboration published between 1990 and 1995, only 29.5% were published in medical journals. It is noteworthy that new competencies required by the American College of Graduate Medical Education for participants in medical residency programs have included behaviors related to interdisciplinary teamwork, group problem solving, and communication across boundaries. Over time, these behaviors may lead to positive changes in health-care clinical guidelines and in the literature on collaboration.

Evidence That Collaboration Works

THE NATIONAL JOINT PRACTICE COMMISSION

In the 1970s, the ANA and the American Medical Association collaborated to form the National Joint Practice Committee (NJPC) (1979). The committee was created to respond to tension and conflict between physicians and nurses that was perceived to be due to increased patient loads and cost constraints, which were placing excessive demands on both groups. The NJPC funded several demonstration projects to implement joint practice arrangements within four different hospital settings that were attempting to improve nurse-physician relationships. The NJPC identified five critical elements of collaborative practice in hospital settings: primary nursing, integrated patient records, encouragement of nurse decision making, a joint practice committee, and a joint record review (Devereux, 1981; NJPC, 1979). The NJPC demonstration project was one of the earliest studies to document that collaboration benefited clinicians and patients. Although the data from these NJPC projects indicated improved communication and improved patient care outcomes, the work was never completed. Unfortunately, there has not been widespread implementation of the NJPC's recommendations (Crowley & Wollner, 1987; Fagin, 1992).

OUTCOMES OF INTENSIVE CARE UNIT STAYS

One of the first studies to identify the impact of nurse-physician communication on patient outcomes indicated that the most significant factor associated with excess mortality rates in intensive care units (ICUs) was nurse-physician communication patterns (Knaus, Draper, Wagner, & Zimmerman, 1986). The investigators reported that another factor associated with lower mortality rates was the presence of a comprehensive nursing education support system in which clinical nurse specialists (CNSs) had responsibility for staff development. Hospitals with lower mortality rates had systems that ensured excellent nurse-physician communication.

In an extension of this research, a study of 17,440 patients in 42 ICUs provided additional evidence that interactions among caregivers affect patient care (Shortell et al., 1994). Effective caregiver interactions were associated with lower risk-adjusted length of stay, lower nurse turnover, better quality of care, and greater ability to meet family member needs. In the analytical model the investigators used, caregiver interaction included the culture, leadership, coordination, communication, and conflict management abilities of the unit's staff. Greater technological availability, a measure of state-of-the-art treatments, was also associated with lower risk-adjusted mortality rates. Hospitals that were more profitable, that were involved in teaching activities, and in which the unit leaders were more involved in quality improvement activities had greater technological availability.

In another study of ICU outcomes, a threefold increase in in-hospital mortality rates was associated with not having daily rounds made by an ICU physician (Pronovost et al., 1999). Lack of daily rounds was also associated with an increased risk of complications such as cardiac arrest, acute renal failure, and septicemia. Increased resource utilization was associated with several factors, including lack of daily rounds, having an ICU nurse/patient ratio of less than 1:2, not having monthly review of morbidity and mortality data, and the extubation of patients in the operating room. The authors did not cite nurse-physician communication and collaboration in their interpretation of findings. However, absence of daily rounds—an opportunity for nurses and physicians to communicate and plan care—indirectly supports the findings that nurse-physician communication and collaboration affect patient care.

MORTALITY RATES AMONG MEDICARE PATIENTS

Before undertaking an analysis of mortality rates in magnet and nonmagnet hospitals, Aiken, Smith, and Lake (1994) reviewed the literature on two independent streams of research, magnet hospitals and Medicare mortality rates. Aiken et al. (1994) examined institutional characteristics in conjunction with characteristics of nurses and physicians working in the same institution. *Magnet hospital* is a term used to describe a hospital that has a reputation for being a good place in which to practice nursing. In the analysis of organizational characteristics of magnet and nonmagnet hospitals, Aiken et al. (1994) concluded that the designation of *magnet hospital* was an indication that three characteristics of nursing practice were present in a hospital: nurse autonomy, nurse control over practice, and positive relations between nurses and physicians. When mortality data in both types of hospitals were analyzed, these authors found that magnet hospitals had a 5% reduction in excess mortality rates. They concluded that the difference in mortality rates between the two groups of hospitals was attributable to the organization of nursing care within magnet hospitals. Although this study did not look at advanced practice nursing specifically, the results suggest that organizational characteristics may influence the quality of collaboration between nurses and physicians.

OTHER EVIDENCE

In studies of clinical expertise in nurses, Benner, Hooper-Kyriakidis, and Stannard (1999) identified the myriad ways in which expert nurses, including APNs, contribute to collaboration and teambuilding. Box 10-1 lists the behaviors of expert nurses that

---

BOX 10-1 • COLLABORATIVE ACTIVITIES USED BY EXPERT CRITICAL CARE NURSES

Diagnosing and managing life-sustaining physiological functions in unstable patients
- Coordinating and managing multiple, instantaneous therapies

The skilled know-how of managing a crisis
- Organizing the team and orchestrating their actions during a crisis
- Exhibiting experiential leadership when a physician is present
- Taking necessary medical action to manage a crisis when a physician is absent
- Recognizing clinical talent and skilled clinicians and marshaling these for the particular situation
- Modulating one's emotional responses and facilitating the social climate

Communicating multiple clinical, ethical, and practical perspectives
- Teambuilding: developing a community of attentiveness, skill, and collaboration

Monitoring quality and managing a breakdown
- Front-line quality improvement, monitoring, and risk management
- Teambuilding in the context of breakdown
- Minimizing health-care system failures in destabilized work environments

The skilled know-how of clinical leadership and the coaching and mentoring of others
- Facilitating the clinical development of others
- Building and preserving collaborative relationships
- Transforming care delivery systems

Data from Benner, P., Hooper-Kyriakidis, P., & Stannard, D. (1999). *Clinical wisdom and interventions in critical care* (p. 3). Philadelphia: W. B. Saunders; reprinted with permission.

represent collaborative activities within specific domains of nursing practice. Wells et al. (1997) examined interdisciplinary collaboration in seven inpatient units over time. They hypothesized that (1) staff in units using different interdisciplinary strategies would report different levels of collaboration and (2) staff who perceived high physician involvement in collaborative practice would report greater collaboration than staff who perceived low physician involvement. This study was done at a time when critical pathways were being developed by CNSs. Over time, CNSs became APN case managers, and the process of critical path development became a collaborative one between APNs and physicians. Degree of use of critical paths was used to categorize collaborative practice strategies. Although there were differences in perceived collaboration based on critical pathway use, the findings suggested that physician involvement was more strongly associated with degree of collaboration than with the type of strategy used.

Collaboration has also been associated with decreased costs of care. Lassen, Fosbinder, Minton, and Robins (1997) reported that the complex diagnosis and treatment of neonates with sepsis was enhanced by collaborative nurse-physician relationships and that cost of care was reduced while quality was improved. Additional anecdotal benefits of this study included decreased parental anxiety and confusion, enhanced continuity and consistency of care, and a reduction of the need for further consultation. Brita-Rossi et al. (1996) demonstrated better patient outcomes and reduced costs when nurses and physicians collaborated to improve orthopedic care. Urgent care visits to a geriatric primary care clinic were enhanced through collaborative care provided by nurse practitioners (NPs) and physicians (Sears, Maxwell, & Townsend, 2003). Jackson et al. (2003) reported that fewer fiscal resources were required when obstetricians and certified nurse-midwives worked within a collaborative care birth center model.

The importance of collaboration to effective, accessible health care has been recognized by several philanthropies that support health-care initiatives. The report of the Pew Health Professions Commission identified the following core competencies for health professionals of the future: community health focus; delivery of contemporary, evidence-based clinical care; expanded accountability; appropriate and cost-effective use of technology; preventive care and promotion of healthy lifestyles; patient and family involvement in decision making; and information management, including lifelong learning (Pew Health Professions Commission, 1995; Gelman, O'Neil, Kimmey, & the Task Force on Accreditation of Health Professions Education, 1999). In an earlier initiative, the Pew-Fetzer Task Force on Advancing Psychosocial Health Education Health Professions and Relationship-Centered Care (hereafter cited as Pew-Fetzer Task Force) (1994) advocated a relationship-centered approach to health care. A relationship-centered approach is thought to foster health care that integrates biomedical and psychosocial approaches. The Pew-Fetzer Task Force (1994) described three dimensions of such care: the patient-practitioner relationship, the community-practitioner relationship, and the practitioner-practitioner relationship. The importance of clinician collaboration is illustrated in the following description of the practitioner-practitioner relationship:

Effective, empathic care requires a community of practitioners who commit themselves to working together to serve the complex matrix of individuals' needs in health and illness. . . . Such relationships serve the needs of practitioners as well as patients: building communities enables health care providers to care for one another and give and receive the support and encouragement that produces personal and professional maturation and more effective patient care. (p. 27)

A guiding principle of this group's work has been that the quality of relationships formed with patients, communities, students, and fellow practitioners across disciplines "is of primary importance to ensuring effective, comprehensive education and health care" (Pew-Fetzer Task Force, 1994, p. 48).

The Robert Wood Johnson Foundation (RWJF) has supported projects that encourage interdisciplinary collaboration. RWJF's Partnerships for Quality Education (PQE) Project, conducted from 1998 to 2003, included a program that helped NPs and medical residents learn how to work together. In addition, projects aimed at helping interdisciplinary clinical teams collaborate to improve patient care were undertaken (RWJF, PQE, 2004; see the following URL for more information: http://www.pqe.org/about.html).

RWJF's Partnerships for Training (PFT) was established in 1994 to train APNs and physicians to work in underserved areas (Johnson-Pawlson, Posey, Dalal, & Page, 2003). Many aspects of this project illustrate how collaboration works. Readers are encouraged to visit the PFT website to learn how eight interdisciplinary grantee groups worked to improve collaboration (www.pftweb.org). Readers can click on each individual state's site to see examples of collaboration (RWJF, Partnerships for Training, 2003).

The Effects of Failure to Collaborate

FOR ORGANIZATIONS

Failure to collaborate has implications for organizations and individuals. The aftermath of September 11, 2001, including the anthrax scare, provided health-care professionals with compelling examples of the failure of organizations and agencies to collaborate. The Centers for Disease Control and Prevention and other parts of the U.S. Public Health Service failed to share data and resources with other agencies that would have ensured timely, broad-based solutions to the anthrax problem. Conversely, in February 2003, effective collaboration and coordination between the World Health Organization and several nations in dealing with the SARS (severe acute respiratory syndrome) outbreak received worldwide acclaim (Hotez, 2003).

FOR INDIVIDUALS

The failure to communicate and collaborate affects individual patients and clinicians. The absence of collaboration has been identified as a source of distress to nurses (Larson, 1999). Lack of collaboration and the diminished autonomy that often accompanies it may contribute to job dissatisfaction and staff turnover. Job dissatisfaction and turnover among staff nurses are serious concerns, especially during a nursing shortage, and are particularly relevant to CNSs and blended-role APNs. While APNs may experience these effects of failure to collaborate, they usually have more autonomy and can work to improve collaboration.

In addition, failure to collaborate may contribute to inefficiencies in the delivery of patient care (Cooper, Henderson, & Dietrich, 1998; Grumbach & Coffman, 1998). Alpert, Goldman, Kilroy, and Pike (1992) found that job satisfaction and attitude were negatively affected when collaboration failed and that territoriality and competitiveness increased. However, the most important result of failure to collaborate is its negative effect on patient care. The studies of intensive care cited previously and the Study to Understand Prognosis and Preferences for Outcomes and Risks of Treatments (SUPPORT, 1995), described next, are among the few that document the effects of failure to collaborate on patients.

THE SUPPORT STUDY

The primary purpose of this randomized, controlled trial was to improve end-of-life decision making by improving physician-patient communication and clinical care. This study is relevant because it attempted to manipulate nurse-physician interactions to improve end-of-life care by structuring an intervention using CNSs. The study was conducted at five teaching hospitals across the United States. The intervention consisted of providing physicians with information on the likelihood of specific outcomes for seriously ill patients and the involvement of a specially trained nurse who, although clearly identified as a member of the research team, "had the role and appearance of a typical clinical specialist" (SUPPORT Principal Investigators, 1995, p. 1593). The nurse was free to implement the role to achieve the best possible care and outcomes. While the CNSs' involvement required the approval of physicians, which in all cases was provided, physicians were free to limit the intervention in any way that they believed would be best for the patient, and they sometimes did. In general, SUPPORT nurses made relevant information from their interactions with patients and clinicians available to physicians and other caregivers

This expensive clinical trial had no impact on any of the designated outcomes. Data for 4,742 patients were abstracted from medical records and interviews with patients and families. The authors concluded that providing additional resources, such as the time and expertise of nurses, did not improve collaborative decision making in end-of-life care. Collaboration, or the lack of it, between nurses (APNs) and physicians was not identified as a possible barrier to implementation, nor was it mentioned as an explanation of the findings (Oddi & Cassidy, 1998). The study appears to have been conceptualized from a physician perspective: all of the principal investigators were physicians. The lists of the study team members indicated that nurses delivering the intervention had various education credentials, suggesting that not all SUPPORT nurses were, in fact, CNSs. No data were reported regarding how nursing was organized within the hospital. The failure to analyze and report data on the relationships between organizational characteristics and patient outcomes may contribute to the interpretation that the intervention had no effect and thus weakens the conclusions drawn by the authors.

Collaboration as an Ethical, Institutional, and Research Imperative

THE ETHICAL IMPERATIVE TO COLLABORATE

Some writers have suggested that the failure to collaborate is an ethical issue. Compassionate, ethical patient care that provides a healing environment requires collaborative working relationships between physicians and nurses (Aroskar, 1998; Larson, 1999; Smith, Hiatt, & Berwick, 1999). As noted in Chapter 11, communication and collaboration problems are often a component of ethical dilemmas. Thus environments that foster collaboration may also create a more supportive context for addressing ethical issues.

Larson (1999) identified key beliefs about collaboration on which nurses and physicians differ: the importance of relationships, what constitutes effective and desirable communication, the degree to which communication and shared decision making occur, the authority nurses have to make decisions, and what strategies would improve communication. The failure of physicians and nurses to understand each other's perspectives, a prerequisite for collaboration, results in a difficult work environment and contributes to uncoordinated, unsafe care (Larson, 1999).

Gianakos (1997) identified three reasons for nurses and physicians to collaborate and asserted that the ethical imperative to collaborate is the most important. The reasons are as follows:

- Collaboration is a moral imperative—good patient care requires it.
- Collaboration reinforces commitment to a common goal and reaffirms the message that patient welfare is the goal.
- Collaboration enhances shared knowledge as physicians and nurses educate each other repeatedly about the patient.

Smith et al. (1999) suggested that collaboration is essential to improving quality of care and included interdisciplinary cooperation as one of several shared ethical principles they proposed for adoption by health-care teams.

THE INSTITUTIONAL IMPERATIVE TO COLLABORATE

The evidence that collaboration works suggests that there are structural as well as interpersonal dimensions to collaboration. That is, although institutional policies or standards do not guarantee collaboration, they can establish expectations for communication and collaboration. As suggested in a study by Knaus et al. (1986), such institutional expectations can provide a structure that facilitates interpersonal communication and relationship building. Pellegrino (1996), a physician and medical ethicist, concluded that human organization and relationships are more important than mutual concerns over resources and technologies. The mutual goal of good patient care and the ethical imperative to collaborate should be at the center of any interdisciplinary effort to plan care or resolve conflicts in approaches to care. Institutions that apply for magnet status are expected to have a structure in place for effective communication among nurses, physicians, and administrators, as one of five key characteristics (North Shore Long Island Jewish Health System, 2001).

THE RESEARCH IMPERATIVE TO STUDY COLLABORATION

Schmitt (2001) suggested that collaboration be examined as an intermediate outcome when health care is evaluated. In a review of the literature, Schmitt cited a number of challenges health services researchers face in trying to understand collaboration and its impact on outcomes. Methodological challenges include the need for more robust, well-designed studies, including clinical trials to provide more conclusive evidence about the impact of collaboration on patient outcomes. In addition, sample selection, measurement of collaboration, and outcome measurement pose dilemmas for those interested in studying the phenomenon. A major limitation of existing knowledge is that much of it comes from hospital-based practice, and according to Schmitt, studies of collaboration and its outcomes are underdeveloped (2001). Schmitt noted: "If there is an important place for interprofessional collaboration in health care delivery then it is a high priority task to get on with the research, difficult as it is, that demonstrates what mix of collaborators, for what purposes, for whom, with what outcomes and at what costs matters" (2001, p. 63).

Taken together, the studies and reports on the topic of collaboration suggest that the degree of collaboration is determined in part by one's own personal and professional characteristics, by institutional structures and processes, and by the culture of the systems in which one practices. Collaboration among providers with different perspectives results in a creative and multidimensional intelligence that is emotionally rewarding because patients do better and clinicians derive personal and professional gratification from this work. This conclusion has implications for APNs, administrators, physicians, researchers, and others. APNs and their administrative and clinical colleagues need to assess the collaborative climate, determine facilitators and barriers, and work together to strengthen relationships and build an organizational culture that values collaboration. Researchers must help APNs and administrators understand the structures and processes that are associated with collaboration and the extent to which collaboration affects patient and utilization outcomes. This work is essential and should be a priority for institutions and individuals.

THE CONTEXT OF COLLABORATION IN CONTEMPORARY HEALTH CARE

The pressures on APNs, physicians, and others to improve quality, work more efficiently, and allow others (e.g., insurers) to be involved in decisions about patient care could be expected to foster collaboration among clinicians. Paradoxically, these same factors may undermine collaboration. In mathematics, there is a phenomenon in which the closer that organisms, atoms, or attractors move to critical transition, the greater is the risk of a catastrophe. In this sense, *catastrophe* means a sudden transition to a qualitatively different type of organization or state. Catastrophe theory offers a metaphor for understanding the complexity of collaborating effectively in a constantly changing system.

As APNs have acquired more education and have become better prepared to practice autonomously and collaboratively, physicians have experienced multiple pressures, including the increasing supply of APN providers (Cooper, Henderson, & Dietrich, 1998; Cooper, Laud, & Dietrich, 1998), which apparently or actually encroach on the physicians' autonomy and willingness to collaborate. The mounting pressures on physicians may lead them to fear "undifferentiation"—that no one will be able to tell them from physician assistants, APNs, or other providers—which could be perceived as a sudden transition to a qualitatively different state. These same pressures generate concern about relinquishing authority and power, fears that may cause individuals to withdraw from or sabotage efforts to collaborate. Thus the transition to a (presumably) more effective, accessible, and efficient health-care system may actually undermine collaboration, a process many leaders believe is central to achieving the goal of a health-care system that is accessible, effective, and affordable.

Confusion about scope of practice can be damaging to collaboration for all involved. Physicians' assistants may be asked to distinguish their role from that of the NP (see Chapter 13). Physicians may ask themselves: What's in it for me to collaborate? What areas of my work do I get to expand because other providers can do things I have traditionally done? What do I get to keep that's different from other providers? What do I keep that "looks similar" to what other providers are offering? One physician acknowledged, "Certain individuals in our group would have a problem with it ...saying a nurse can do our job. It bruises egos ...but I would love [to work with a nurse practitioner]" (Cairo, 1996, p. 415). APNs may be uncertain about their scope of practice when a physician or institution asks them to assume responsibility for a new skill, such as performing an invasive procedure. The reality is that managed care and regulatory initiatives are rearranging practice boundaries almost daily. These changes are often at the heart of the tension associated with collaboration between players as roles and boundaries of disciplines blur and expand.

Opportunities for Collaboration

There are numerous incentives for providers to collaborate. APNs, physicians, and other providers share a common purpose—the desire to provide good patient care. This mutual goal should be enough to ensure that collaboration occurs consistently. Each group of clinicians has unique, complementary, and overlapping skills that benefit patients, and APNs are eager to make their skills and knowledge available. Although the changes in health care have resulted in numerous pressures that can constrain collaboration, certain opportunities for promoting collaboration exist.

Although it may not be immediately apparent, efforts to reduce costs of health care actually provide APNs and physicians with a common goal toward which to work and with opportunities for learning from each other. Medicare guidelines that are used to document care for coding and billing purposes encourage physicians and nurses to work together to provide the appropriate level of care necessary to meet the standards for reimbursement. National, interdisciplinary guidelines and standards of care are intended to reduce unwarranted, often expensive, variation in health care. Many guidelines specify interdisciplinary collaboration as a critical component of effective care (Acute Pain Management Guideline Panel, 1992; Management of Cancer Pain Guideline Panel, 1992). Standards and guidelines developed and agreed upon by interdisciplinary groups, whether at the local (office or institution) or national level, offer a sound starting point for jointly determining patient care goals, processes, and outcomes. Reports of interdisciplinary teams charged with developing or adopting clinical practice guidelines indicate that these initiatives have had beneficial effects on interdisciplinary relationships and collaboration (Brita-Rossi et al., 1996; Weinstein, McCormack, Brown, & Rosenthal, 1998; Weisman, Griffie, Gordon, & Dahl, 1997).

Accreditation activities offer another opportunity to build collaborative relationships. The Joint Commission on Accreditation of Healthcare Organizations' *Agenda for Change* (1992) requires documentation that demonstrates collaborative, interdisciplinary practice. The premise of this initiative was that quality patient care is driven by collegial relationships between members of the health-care disciplines (Lumpkins & Veal, 1995). The requirement to document these activities can help providers to develop stronger interdisciplinary approaches to care. Other opportunities for improving interdisciplinary relationships and fostering collaboration include case management (Mahn & Spross, 1996; see Chapter 18), development and implementation of clinical pathways, and interdisciplinary rounds (Felton, Cady, Metzler, & Burton, 1997; Weissman, 1988).

The move toward a more community-based, health promotion/disease prevention model of care is also creating new opportunities for collaborative practice in primary care (Simpson, 1998). New alliances, both among advanced practice nursing groups and between advanced practice nursing groups and physician groups, need to be developed and nurtured.

Barriers to Collaboration

Although it is easy to discuss professional liaisons and to draw up collaborative arrangements on paper, there are many obstacles to actually implementing effective collaborative professional relationships in the workplace. Research by Sands, Stafford, and McClelland (1990) suggested that team members see themselves primarily as representatives of their own discipline, rather than as members of a collaborative team. Several barriers to collaboration exist and can be characterized as professional, sociocultural, organizational, and regulatory.

PROFESSIONAL BARRIERS

Disciplinary Differences. Silos in medical and nursing education have long been barriers to successful collaboration. Each profession is a culture with its own values, knowledge, rules, and norms (Benoliel, 1995; Bray & Rogers, 1997). Often, clinicians differ in their basic philosophy of care based on how they have been socialized into the system. For example, medicine is oriented toward biomedical research, technical solutions, hierarchical relationships, and a strong sense of personal responsibility for patient outcomes (Bray & Rogers, 1997). This sense of responsibility is apparent even among physicians who support APNs but imply or explicitly indicate that physician oversight of APNs' practice is necessary (Cairo, 1996; DeAngelis, 1994). Fagin (1992) asserted that the stance preferred by physicians is not to collaborate with anyone. This is a strong statement and might seem inflammatory. Yet the Pew-Fetzer Task Force (1994) (the majority of whose members were physicians) also acknowledged that collaboration was a particular challenge for physicians. In a study of 80 NPs, physician acceptance and support was the most frequent factor facilitating NP performance (Hupcey, 1993). Knaus et al. (1986) cited prior efforts by organized medicine to discredit APNs. Current efforts to place certified registered nurse anesthetists under physician supervision (see Chapter 17) and the review of the literature by Larson (1999) also suggest that collaboration is difficult for physicians.

As medical practice and nursing practice evolve, scopes of medical and nursing practice may seem to overlap, largely a result of shifting skills and responsibilities. In the early days of advanced practice nursing, this overlap was often addressed by requiring "physician supervision" of aspects of an APN's practice (an issue discussed in the section on regulatory barriers and in Chapter 22). An outcome of this historical "accident" is that supervision of APNs by physicians is often mentioned explicitly or implicitly in some of the literature on collaboration and advanced practice nursing. The view advanced here is that supervision precludes the development of a collaborative relationship and that physicians cannot truly supervise advanced practice nursing. A study of physicians' supervision of pediatric NPs (Cruikshank & Chow, 1984) suggested that what is called *supervision* is actually consultation or referral as these terms are defined in this chapter. Rather than supervision, in this dynamic environment, we believe these terms are preferable to define the scope of autonomous nursing management and identify high-risk populations within a particular population or practice that would require consultation, collaboration/co-management, or referral.

Collaboration and the Nursing Shortage. The current severe nursing shortage, especially in hospital-based nursing, has been linked to lack of collaboration in the workplace. The conflicts and stresses engendered by lack of collaboration and the accompanying diminished autonomy have a negative impact on nursing as a career choice for college students and are significant reasons that nurses choose to leave the profession for new careers. Tensions between physicians and nurses and between nurses and other nurses rank high in reasons that nurses are dissatisfied with their work environment (Hanson & Beverly, 2001). The current nursing shortage and the negative effects of failure to collaborate suggest that the need for productive models of collaboration that benefit patients, nurses, and physicians is urgent.

Professional Education and Role Socialization. We believe that barriers to collaboration can be attributed, in part, to the few opportunities there are for interdisciplinary education as health-care providers learn their professions. The RWJF Partnerships in Training initiative (1996) identified many of the stresses inherent in building and sustaining interdisciplinary, academic-community partnerships. Stresses encountered by participants as they developed partnerships centered on money, differing agendas, systems that were not integrated, varying philosophies, and long-held beliefs about "how things should be done." This report suggested that building relationships between disciplines would be difficult unless there is a high level of commitment among all participants for collaboration to succeed (RWJF, 1996).

Despite efforts to foster interdisciplinary collaboration among individuals and organizations, challenges remain. Still, there is evidence of progress. New work with outcomes at the national level shows great promise as medicine and nursing begin to come together to craft management guidelines in areas of family practice and prevention. The U.S. Preventive Services Task Force, which is part of the federal Agency for Healthcare Research and Quality, is made up of an interdisciplinary group of providers and researchers who develop and disperse evidenced-based recommendations on screening and prevention for a variety of health-care concerns (U.S. Preventive Services Task Force, 2003). Also, in the past 15 years there has been a slow but steady movement away from language requiring physician supervision and reference to protocols and toward emphasizing consultation, collaboration, peer review, and use of referral (Grimaldi & Cousins, 1998). However, the American Medical Association (1995) reaffirmed a policy that *supports* supervision of APNs by physicians and claims that physicians have the responsibility for managing health-care needs of patients, a policy that continues to inform its organizational activities. Despite rhetoric to the contrary, such a policy does not promote a philosophy of collaboration and reinforces stereotyped views of nurse-physician relationships. Because of such initiatives by organized medicine, the need for nursing to standardize advanced practice nursing educational programs, national certification, and state credentialing is particularly urgent. In Chapter 22 these issues are explored in greater depth.

SOCIOCULTURAL ISSUES

Tradition, role, and gender stereotypes and ineffective communication styles are obstacles to collaboration (Rafferty, Ball, & Aiken, 2001). Safriet (1992, 1998) suggested that the field of medicine staked out broad turf early on and considered any movement into this turf by nurses at any level to be unacceptable. Thus turf issues have been a major stumbling block to successful interactions between nurses and physicians. Although nurses are highly valued for the physical care, nurturing, and psychosocial support they provide for patients, it is clear that the physician is perceived and valued as the decision maker about treatment. One writer suggested that physicians are at risk of losing their roles as "quarterbacks" of the health-care team (Kuraitis, 1999). Many people think of APNs as second best providers or as caregivers for the unfortunate or indigent. Such attitudes perpetuate the view that the physician is the supervisor and the nurse is the subordinate. Nursing remains a predominantly female profession and, despite the influx of women into medicine and efforts to recruit men into nursing, these role stereotypes still exist. Unfortunately, because of barriers to practice that are difficult to break, APNs may buy into this view, which further hampers collaborative, collegial relationships (Lenz, 1994).

SEXISM, STEREOTYPES, AND INEFFECTIVE COMMUNICATION

Sexism affects collaboration (Coeling & Wilcox, 1994; Siegler & Whitney, 1994b). Gender stereotypes dominate images of staff nurses in the media, and APNs are rarely portrayed on television. With few exceptions, APNs' contributions are not profiled in healthcare reports in the lay press. Media bias and the nursing profession's inability to market itself adequately make nursing and advanced practice nursing invisible (Fagin, 1992). The "doctor-nurse game," a phenomenon that is influenced by roles and gender and was first described in the 1970s, continues to operate in many institutions; however, it is apparent that the rules are changing and nurses do not want to play anymore (Stein, Watts, & Howell, 1990; Rafferty et al., 2001).

Stereotypical images and the invisibility of APNs influence how nursing is viewed by both health-care professionals and consumers: at best nurses are viewed as kind and nice; at worst, as unintelligent and incompetent. Thus APNs often find that they must actively counter low expectations with interactions and practices that convey their intelligence, competence, confidence, and trustworthiness.

Communication styles may also be a barrier to collaboration. Recent literature has begun to recognize styles of interactions among health-care professionals that particularly undermine collaboration, which have been described as "being difficult," "bullying," or abusive (Anonymous, 2001; Houghton, 2003; King, 2002; McAvoy & Murtagh, 2003; Rider, 2002; Rosenstein, 2002). Difficult colleagues are those who display attitudinal and behavioral problems such as arrogance, rudeness, and poor communication and those who are unable to work as part of a team (King, 2002). While such individuals may be clinically competent, if their behavior is harassing, coercive, or abusive, they put patients at risk, in part, because other clinicians may be unwilling to deal with these individuals around nonclinical behaviors or actions (King, 2002). We encourage APN readers to recognize this risk to collaboration and patient care and develop a repertoire of interpersonal and system strategies with which to address such behaviors directly and promptly.

ORGANIZATIONAL BARRIERS

Competitive situations arise that can interfere with collaboration among APNs and between APNs and other disciplines at the level of systems and organizations. In her extensive work in the field of health policy, Hanson has observed one group of APNs who aligned around a common viewpoint early in a debate, while members of other advanced practice nursing groups used precious time debating fine points, delaying or eliminating the possibility of unity on a policy issue that would affect all advanced practice nursing groups (Hanson, Unpublished data, 1986, 1989). Competitive stances and polarizing statements, whether they occur within or between disciplines, are barriers to collaboration. Managed care has been perceived to have a negative effect on both physician-patient and physician-APN relationships. The inability of APNs to be part of managed care panels has, in many settings, made collaboration difficult at best and may contribute to unproductive competition. Medicare billing requirements also discourage collaborative relations between health-care providers and may actually serve as disincentives. "Incident-to" billing (see Chapter 20) requires that patient care services provided by APNs be directly supervised by physicians, severely hampering a collaborative environment. (Wolf, 2003).

Patients, as the consumers of health care, are important players in the quest for successful collaboration. Patients are sensitive to the relationships between caregivers and are quick to pick up on the lack of respect or trust between their providers. Some research suggests that collaborative relationships among interdisciplinary health-care providers can ameliorate some of these negative effects (Afflitto, 1997; Stichler, 1995; Weinstein et al., 1998). Successful collaborative practices are those in which patients easily move back and forth between providers as their care and situations dictate. Collaboration requires an ability to transform competitive situations into opportunities for working together that are mutually beneficial, where all parties can imagine the possibility of creating a win-win situation.

REGULATORY BARRIERS

As noted previously, societies of medical professionals continue to try to limit advanced practice nursing (e.g., eligibility for reimbursement, prescriptive authority) through legislative and regulatory reform (Minarik & Price, 1999). Legislation and regulations have been barriers to the implementation of collaborative roles (Fagin, 1992; Inglis & Kjervik, 1993). Although major strides have been made in some states, statutes and regulations often support a hierarchical structure that impedes collaboration between nurses and physicians (Hodnick, Dietz, McNeil, & Miles, 2004; see Chapter 22). Language that mandates the nature of APN-physician relationships can undermine collaborative practice. Use of such language to regulate interprofessional relationships presents risks to professional autonomy and effective collaboration for APNs and physicians. Collaboration cannot be mandated; it is a process that develops over time. The discussion in a recent monograph by Barbara Safriet of the scope of practice for APNs is an excellent example of innovations based on joint purposes and public interest principles fostering collaboration between the professions (Safriet, 2002). A good illustration of this collaboration is provided by psychiatric APNs, Grimaldi and Cousins (1998), with regard to their collaboration with a psychiatrist on psychopharmacological interventions.

Opportunities to create collaborative relationships are lost in the morass of money, political power, and control issues that arise when too-rapid changes in health-care delivery systems occur (Dziabis & Lant, 1998). Furthermore, nurses and other stakeholders who are confronting their own professional concerns may not fully appreciate the stresses physicians experience in today's volatile market. This factor is a serious deterrent to collaborative relationships.

Organized Medicine and Nursing Versus Practice Environment

In an analysis of the evolution of the APN and physician assistant roles, Christman (1998) suggested that the responses of organized nursing (e.g., the ANA and the National League for Nursing) to physician efforts to extend advanced practice roles to other specialties in the 1970s were not constructive and contributed to the development of the physician assistant role in medicine. This conclusion is likely to be debated by others who witnessed the same events. However, like the history of the NJPC described earlier, these events suggest that decisions made by leaders of nursing and medical organizations can shape the context and process of interdisciplinary collaboration.

It is fairly well accepted by both medicine and nursing that collaboration at the community "grass-roots" level is easier to implement and maintain than at the professional organizational level. Lack of commitment on the part of organizational leaders and continued power inequities create a negative milieu and discourage productive interactions between representatives of organized medicine and nursing (Stichler, 1995). Although collaboration happens daily among practicing clinicians, at national levels, where it is really needed, collaboration may be nonexistent, impeding efforts to move toward a coordinated health-care system. The positions espoused by "old guard" policymakers from all disciplines may be based on stereotyped beliefs about disciplinary roles and responsibilities, not reflective consideration of the issues or what is best for consumers. This factor makes it increasingly important for APNs and physicians practicing at local levels, who have learned the art of collaboration, to take an active role in bringing their perspectives and experiences to policymaking at institutional, community, state, and national levels that foster collaboration. According to Gianakos (1997), "[f]or physicians and nurses to become more collegial, major medical and nursing organizations must make interdisciplinary collegiality a priority" (p. 58). A broader statutory definition of professional autonomy for APNs than currently exists in many states is necessary if the more complex autonomy of interdependent collaborators is to be exercised effectively (Forbes & Fitzsimmons, 1993; Inglis & Kjervik, 1993).

CHARACTERISTICS OF EFFECTIVE COLLABORATION

Effective collaboration between and among APNs, physicians, and other nurses in an ever-changing health-care environment depends on many factors. The definition of collaboration proposed in this chapter demands a radical rethinking of how APNs, physicians, and others are prepared for their roles and how clinicians interact to ensure positive patient outcomes. The definition also invites exploration of the characteristics that make up a successful collaborative relationship and the personal and setting-specific attributes that are pivotal to successful professional collaborations.

Some characteristics of collaboration have long been recognized and promulgated, but, as the work of the NJPC has indicated, clinicians and organizations have resisted adopting the philosophy and behaviors that promote collaboration. The five components of collaborative practice, cited earlier in this chapter, that the NJPC (1979) identified as critical, nurse autonomy and authority for nursing practice, are still important today. Steele's (1986) analysis of collaboration among NPs and physicians revealed several characteristics: mutual trust and respect, an understanding and acceptance of each other's disciplines, positive self-image, equivalent professional maturity arising from education and experience, recognition that the partners are not substitutes for each other, and a willingness to negotiate. Hughes and Mackenzie (1990) outlined four characteristics of NP-physician collaboration: collegiality, communication, goal sharing, and task interdependence. Spross (1989), based on a review of CNS and interdisciplinary literature, described three essential elements of collaboration: a common purpose, diverse and complementary professional knowledge and skills, and effective communication processes. In their program of research, Baggs (1989), Baggs and Schmitt (1997), and Baggs et al. (1999) noted the following characteristics of collaboration between registered nurses and physicians: assertiveness, shared decision making, communication, planning together, and coordination. Although this is not an exhaustive summary of the literature on collaboration, it is clear that shared values, effective interpersonal communication, and organizational structures can promote productive alliances among clinicians and create environments in which collaboration is valued and practiced.

The discussion of characteristics of collaboration that follows elaborates on the definition of collaboration proposed in this chapter. The ability to "make a commitment to interact authentically and constructively" suggests that there are characteristics that are prerequisites—qualities that prospective partners must bring to initial and ongoing encounters. To interact authentically means that partners do not leave some part of themselves behind. For example, partners share the emotional satisfactions and frustrations of clinical work and develop ways of supporting each other. Although it is not discussed in the literature, we have observed that successful collaboration can lead to an intimacy that arises from working closely together over time. In her sixth year in a collaborative practice, one NP compared the relationship to a marriage in terms of the interpersonal ups and downs that occurred and the challenge of dealing with the same person daily over matters of great or negligible, albeit clinical, import. Thus mature collaboration can be both rewarding and challenging.

Other essential characteristics are a common purpose, clinical competence, interpersonal skills (or a willingness to learn them), and a sense of humor. Trust, respect, and valuing each other's knowledge and skills reflect the nature of collaboration as an "interpersonal process." They are equally important but only develop fully over time. However, in order for these characteristics to develop, prospective partners must approach encounters with a commitment to respect each other, a willingness to trust, and an assumption that the other's knowledge and skills are valuable. In this sense, these characteristics are also prerequisites, but they are fully realized only after many constructive and productive interactions have occurred. Evans (1994) discussed collaboration as a force for achieving desired outcomes. She confirmed that clinicians who collaborate engage in a communal, intellectual effort on behalf of patients and share problem solving, goal setting, and decision making. Thus collaboration occurs when prospective partners recognize that a problem can be solved *only* when each party's input, expertise, and participation are solicited (Stichler, 1995).

Common Purpose

The notion that a common purpose must be the basis for collaboration is well supported in the literature (Alpert et al., 1992; Arslanian-Engoren, 1995; Spross, 1989; King, 2002; Rider, 2002). Even if partners have not discussed the purposes and goals of their interactions, the organizations in which they work usually have an explicit mission and goals. These can be the starting point for identifying the goals and purposes of clinical collaboration. Collaboration involves a bond, a union, a commitment to caring for patients that goes beyond a single approach to care and represents a synergistic alliance that maximizes the contributions of each participant (Evans, 1994). In implementing a model of nurse-physician collaboration at a tertiary care institution, Alpert et al. (1992) affirmed that a special synergy arising from collaborative work improves patient outcomes. A collaborative management birth center care model in which physicians and nurse-midwives collaborated on treatment options resulted in safe outcomes for mothers and babies with fewer operative deliveries (Jackson et al., 2003).

Collaboration, by definition, implies that the participants are interdependent. Recognizing their interdependence, team members can combine their individual perceptions and skills to synthesize more complex and comprehensive care plans (Forbes & Fitzsimmons, 1993). Each member brings a particular set of skills and unique expertise to the table for a combined strength that cannot be matched by individuals working alone. Like other characteristics, the common purpose(s) that initially brought partners together may change over time. For example, the organizational goal or situation that brought two clinicians together becomes subordinate to the deep, personal commitment to work together in ways that improve patient care and are interpersonally satisfying.

Clinical Competence

Clinical competence is perhaps the most important characteristic underlying a successful collaborative experience among clinicians, for without it, the trust and desire needed to work together are not possible. Trust and respect are built on the assurance that each member is able to carry out her or his role and function in a competent manner. That clinical competence is a prerequisite for collaboration has been validated in research (Cairo, 1996; Hanson, Hodnicki, & Boyle, 1994; Prescott & Bowen, 1985). Yet stereotyped views of nursing and medical practice may interfere with collaborative efforts. Physicians are perceived as all-knowing and having ultimate responsibility for patient care; whereas nurses may be viewed as nonintellectual, second-best substitutes for excellent health care (Cairo, 1996; Fagin, 1992; Petronis-Jones, 1994; Sands, Stafford, & McClelland, 1990) and as having little authority or responsibility for patient care outcomes (Larson, 1999). The status of advanced practice nursing is still such that nurses must prove their competence to the profession and to society (Fagin, 1992; Prescott & Bowen, 1985, Hodnicki et al., 2004). When collaborating clinicians can rely on each other to be clinically competent, mutual trust and respect develop. Partners recognize that leadership is problem based, not team or role based, and are open to sharing power. Instead of one person always being the team leader, in a departure from the traditional "captain of the team" approach, leadership can shift among partners. Thus the person with the most expertise, interest, or talent can respond to the particular demands of the situation or problem. The trust and respect among collaborators are such that they can count on satisfactory resolution of the problem even when they know as individuals that they might have approached the issue differently. In fact, this openness to shared leadership and alternative solutions allows partners to learn from each other. For example, APNs usually have expertise in educating patients about their illnesses and lifestyle choices. Physicians are often expert diagnosticians. Thus collaboration offers APNs and physicians opportunities to model their varied assessment and intervention strategies for each other, fostering mutual learning and appreciation for the contributions of each to the care of patients and families. Because consumers and physicians underestimate nurses' expertise, competence, and authority, APNs need to showcase their competent and exemplary practice to build nursing's reputation for competence (Fagin, 1992; Lenz, 1994; see Chapter 25).

Interpersonal Competence and Communication Skills

Interpersonal competence is the ability to communicate effectively with colleagues in a variety of situations, including uncomplicated, routine interactions; disagreements; value conflicts; and stressful situations. It requires a level of self-esteem and assertiveness that nurses have begun to acquire only recently (Norton & Grady, 1996). It is imperative that nurses understand and articulate what they bring to clinical practice as members of the health-care team. Communication must be open and dynamic (Wolf, 2003). The key to demonstrating interpersonal competence is the APN's ability to communicate clearly and convincingly, both orally and in writing. This attribute was identified by Hanson et al. (1994) in their analysis of the attributes that physicians most valued in their NP colleagues. The ability to communicate well with physicians, other staff members, the patient, and the patient's family was highly regarded by the physicians in this study. After clinical competence, interpersonal competence may be the most important individual characteristic needed for APNs to establish collaborative relationships.

Trust

Implicit in discussions of collaboration is the presence of mutual trust, mutual respect, and personal integrity—qualities evinced in the nature of interactions between partners. In fact, distrust is often cited as a major barrier to successful collaborative relationships (Alpert et al., 1992; Cairo, 1996; Evans, 1994). The development of trust and respect depends on clinical competence; it is very difficult to trust and respect a colleague whose clinical competence is questionable. This does not mean that novice APNs cannot establish collaborative relationships. However, the environments in which advanced practice nursing students and new graduates work must support their "novicehood" so that they can learn and mature clinically. Partners must recognize and appreciate their overlapping and diverse skills and knowledge (Nugent & Lambert, 1996; Spross, 1989; Stichler, 1995) so that mutual trust and respect can develop and deepen over time. Partners observe that each other's clinical competence is consistent; that their interactions—even those that involve significant conflict over goals of care and interventions—are respectful, productive, and satisfying; and that patients benefit from their combined talents and efforts. They come to depend on each other to use good clinical judgment and to take appropriate actions.

A lack of knowledge about another's discipline is thought to be a barrier to developing effective teamwork (Gilbert et al. 2000). Thus a central theme of the development of trust is *sharing*. Partners are guided by a shared vision of the possibilities inherent in collaboration; they believe in the value of collaboration, and they are committed to achieving the relationship's potential (Krumm, 1992; Nugent & Lambert, 1996). Collaboration also means sharing in planning, decision making, problem solving, goal setting, and assuming responsibility (Baggs & Schmitt, 1988). Conger and Craig (1998) suggested that shared vision and collaboration between NPs and CNSs could be used to implement a cost-effective model of community-based health care. Thus even though partners' ideas, opinions, and actions might be different, their belief in each other and their shared vision permit—even value—such differences.

The issue of developing trust presents a particular challenge to APNs because it has been observed that the competence of physicians is assumed and medical incompetence must be proven, whereas nurses must prove themselves and their competence in each new encounter (Fagin, 1992; Prescott & Bowen, 1985). APNs encounter numerous physicians in the course of practice; a lack of positive expectations and the potential assumption of incompetence of APNs until they demonstrate otherwise are major barriers to collaboration (Fagin, 1992). This means that APNs require courage and fortitude to challenge such assumptions assertively when they become apparent in disconfirming or aggressive encounters with colleagues (Coeling & Wilcox, 1994).

Valuing and Respecting of Diverse, Complementary Knowledge

In a conversation with a group of psychiatric APNs, an APN reported that the medical director of psychiatry "loved APNs," and, apologizing in advance for how it might sound, he said he thought of them as "discount physicians." Although such a perspective may be intended as a compliment, it diminishes advanced practice nursing contributions and impedes the development of the mutual respect that we view as essential. Respect for others' practice and knowledge is key to successful collaboration, because it enhances shared decision making. A great deal of successful collaborative work is self-driven. There must be a desire, at a very personal level, to collaborate and to value and respect others' ideas and actions, as well as a personal belief that complementary knowledge will enhance one's own personal plan for patient care. Initially, collaborators have limited knowledge of each other as individuals and as professionals; collaboration is a "conscious, learned behavior" that improves as team members learn to value and respect one another's practice and expertise (Alpert et al., 1992). Medicine and nursing, although overlapping disciplines, are culturally distinct and have diverse goals for patient care. In many cases, they complement each other in their quest to restore patients to health. This complementarity extends beyond the disciplines of medicine and nursing. The Linkages Project, an interdisciplinary educational initiative to promote collaboration between physicians and psychologists, was instrumental in shaping collaborative approaches to clinical care (Bray & Rogers, 1997). Collaboration is built on the respect and valuing of the contributions of each profession to the common goal of optimal health-care delivery (Stichler, 1995).

Humor

Another important aspect of the collaborative process is humor. Humor, in which the intent is positive and nonthreatening, is a creative way to set the stage for effective communication and problem solving between members of different disciplines (Balzer, 1993). In collaborative practice, humor serves to decrease defensiveness, invite openness, relieve tension, and deflect anger. It helps individuals keep perspective and acknowledge the lack of perfection, and it sets the tone for trust and acceptance among colleagues so that difficult situations can be reframed (Balzer, 1993). The use of humor helps to diffuse the need for persons to argue their own point of view and allows them to refocus on how they can work together to meet common goals (Hill & Hewlett, 2002). Graduate students can be encouraged to observe the ways in which humor is used by preceptors and colleagues and identify those uses that seem effective in improving communication and defusing conflict situations.

Processes Associated with Effective Collaboration

RECURRING INTERACTIONS

In addition to the attributes discussed previously, there are several processes that enable effective collaboration. A theme implicit in the reports of those who have written about their experiences with collaboration is that establishing a trusting and collaborative relationship is a developmental process (Alpert et al., 1992; Bray & Rogers, 1997; Krumm, 1992; Nugent & Lambert, 1996; Wells et al., 1997). Although this notion of development over time is relevant to all aspects of collaboration, it is particularly important to establishing trust. The fact that effective collaboration is developmental and time dependent explains why collaborative relationships are difficult to develop in organizations where there is a high staff turnover or frequent rotation of clinicians, such as house physicians. A physician wrote that the process seemed to be related to how well the nurse and physician know each other (Alpert et al., 1992).

It seems likely that a series of less complicated interactions, such as information exchange and coordination, that has been satisfactory clinically or personally contributes to the development of collaborative relationships. Team members need recurring interactions to acquire an understanding of each other's backgrounds, roles, and functions and to develop patterns of interaction that are constructive, productive, and supportive. Several reports illustrate the developmental aspects of interactions that lead to collaborative relationships (Alpert et al., 1992; Bray & Rogers, 1997; Dickinson, Mateo, Jackson, & Swartz, 1995; Hilderley, 1991). Redmond, Riggleman, Sorrell, and Zerull (1999) suggested that projects focused on quality and outcomes of care that involve joint collection and analysis of data build collegiality and foster collaboration. In our experiences, membership on such interdisciplinary committees as pharmacy and therapeutics, performance improvement, institutional review boards, ethics committees, and others with a patient-care focus also fosters communication and collegiality. Recurring interactions help clinicians learn the similarities and differences in each discipline's practice. Understanding each other's scope of practice and responsibility enables APNs, physicians, and other colleagues to use their knowledge and skills to benefit patients.

BRIDGING

Krumm (1992) noted that bridging is a component of collaboration. She did not define bridging but implied that it is the ability to develop connections that support positive outcomes for individuals and populations of patients. She described one bridging skill as the "ability to recognize and rearrange boundaries within the practice setting" (Krumm, p. 24). Exemplars 10-1 and 10-2 illustrate the concept of bridging.

 EXEMPLAR 10-1

> Nurse practitioners (NPs) in a gynecological practice noted the length of time it took for patients to get an appointment for colposcopy and the disadvantages to the practice of having only one physician who could do the procedure. They proposed that two of the NPs become trained to do the procedure. They outlined the precedents for such a change in practice and the benefits in terms of clinical outcomes, patient satisfaction, productivity, and cost-effectiveness. The proposal was adopted, two NPs acquired the training, and many of the advantages they anticipated for both patients and the practice have been realized.

 EXEMPLAR 10-2

> While a clinical nurse specialist (CNS) at a tertiary hospital, Spross noted that patients who were admitted directly from the oncology clinic for a short admission were receiving their chemotherapy late at night because members of the house staff were not taking the patients' histories and performing physical examinations until last. Lengths of stay were longer, treatments that could have been prepared and given during the better staffed day shift were burdening the evening and night staff, and patients were dissatisfied. House staff left these

Continued

EXEMPLAR 10-2—cont'd

admissions until last because the patients tended to be clinically stable, and to the interns, this was an appropriate way of triaging their workload. The CNS and nurse manager met with the physician director of hematology/oncology to propose that short-stay chemotherapy admissions be handled differently from other admissions—an idea for which there was no precedent. All admissions had been done by the interns and residents. Under the new arrangement, patients would come to the unit directly from the clinic with their admission orders written by the attending physician. Intravenous lines could be initiated immediately, prescriptions could be filled by the pharmacy as the orders came down, and nurses could initiate teaching and other interventions in a timely fashion.

An important aspect of these exemplars is that the APNs understood both medical and nursing aspects of care. Brown (1989) referred to this as *shuttle diplomacy*. She described the CNS as the person capable of speaking the languages of both medical and nursing subcultures, understanding the problems of each, and assisting in clinical and organizational problem solving. In both cases, boundaries were rearranged in ways that improved patient care and staff job satisfaction, suggesting that bridging creates conditions conducive to collaboration.

CONSULTATION

Consultation is another process that can promote collaboration among clinicians (see Chapter 7). The process of consultation can promote collaboration in several ways. First, it gives the consultant an opportunity to make visible her or his knowledge, competence, and expertise; and the interaction can be used to counter stereotypical views of what APNs and physicians do and how they interact. It is also a situation, when approached with collegiality and an open mind, in which one can teach and be taught. CNSs have developed this form of communication to an art form and use it very successfully to interact with nurse colleagues within the hospital setting (Barron, 1989). As APNs mature in their roles, they can observe the ways in which consultation has contributed to a collaborative environment and share these observations with graduate students and staff.

IMPLEMENTING COLLABORATION

Socialization to Collaboration during Graduate Education

Although one might be able to identify a core set of clinical skills that all health professions should possess, it is unusual for graduate health professional students to learn these skills together (Larson, 1995; Stumpf & Clark, 1999; Gilbert et al., 2000). The absence of a common socialization process for health professionals is thought to impede collaboration and teamwork (Larson, 1995; Pew-Fetzer Task Force, 1994; Gilbert et al., 2000). Predictions about changes in the health-care workforce suggest that undertaking initiatives to evaluate and improve interdisciplinary collaboration is critical. Cooper, Henderson, and Dietrich (1998) suggested that medicine and nursing are all in the same "leaky boat" and would do well to pull together. Health-care professionals who have been socialized early to value cooperation and collaboration are much better able to understand the strengths and concerns of other groups. The need to focus on collaboration was highlighted in a series of articles on predictions about the interdisciplinary workforce in the new millennium (Cooper, Henderson, & Dietrich, 1998; Grumbach &

Coffman, 1998). Reflecting on how patients, policymakers, and educators will deal with the future composition of the interdisciplinary workforce, Cooper, Henderson, and Dietrich (1998) concluded that "it is time for interdisciplinary regulation and clinical integration so that a health care workforce that includes a diversity of disciplines can be assured of providing a uniform level of care in the future" (p. 802).

As part of the socialization process toward building collaboration, it is important that APNs add to the communication skills they learned in their undergraduate nursing programs. Advanced practice nursing curricula need to offer a foundation for collaborative interactions throughout the entire graduate program. Course objectives and specific content should be based on the characteristics of effective intradisciplinary and interdisciplinary collaboration and the development of skills to achieve this goal. Professional roles and issues courses need to include content that profiles not only the role sought by the students but also the roles of the health-care providers with whom the students will interact, such as physicians, other nurses, pharmacists, physical therapists, social workers, and other providers (Hamric & Hanson, 2003). It is important that APNs be able to articulate the roles of nurse, NP, CNS, certified nurse-midwife, and CRNA and to explain the nursing profession to consumers and nonnurse health-care providers. Content that leads the novice APN through team interaction, networking, conflict negotiation (The Conflict Resolution Network, 2003), and other concepts that build personal self-esteem and confidence is crucial. The theme of collaboration can be woven throughout the major coursework, as well as the graduate core curriculum, by including objectives that build collaborative skills within other class requirements. For example, an objective for a role development core course that requires the student to create a collage depicting collaborative relationships within nursing would help the student grasp the concept of collaboration.

The curriculum should include content on group dynamics, role theory, organizational theory, change theory, and negotiation strategies to prepare learners for collaborative roles. Students should discuss examples of collaboration and noncollaboration from their own clinical experiences and should be able to identify what factors accounted for success or failure. Furthermore, students need to be aware of the forces, both positive and negative, that influence collaborative efforts. Innovative classroom strategies that allow for interactions, such as role playing and storytelling, are extremely worthwhile. Students need opportunities to debrief with peers and faculty their positive and negative experiences of collaboration. This is vital if students are to be able to analyze the personal, social, and organizational variables that affect collaboration.

Most importantly, curricula should include interdisciplinary seminars in which students can learn from colleagues in other disciplines. Although it is necessary and valuable for each discipline to structure and clarify role development issues and to socialize its members into the profession, it is extremely useful for students in role and policy core courses to be able to discuss and interact with individuals who see policy and practice issues from another perspective. In this way they learn to value each other's contributions and are more able to view differences at a higher level. Furthermore, it is very important for students to observe faculty in collaborative relationships with their interdisciplinary peers. New funding initiatives that allow for interdisciplinary education in both the classroom and the clinical setting offer great promise for improved collaborative relationships among health-care providers from different disciplines.

Peer learning can foster socialization to collaboration. New technologies such as distance interactive television and online Web-based instruction enable students from various disciplines to interact through problem-based case learning. Such strategies help students learn about and value the styles and models used by other health-care providers to manage patients. The team approach to problem solving and the approach to patient care are enhanced as students learn in interdisciplinary venues. Behaviors that undermine collaboration are often dispelled before they take root if interdisciplinary learning is started early in the education process. Gilbert et al. (2000) described an effective approach to fostering these interactions based on teambuilding theory. This intervention included teamwork simulation, activities designed to foster better understanding of each other's professions, communication facilitation, development of team agreements, clarification of responsibilities, case analyses, debriefing, and interprofessional discussions.

Peer learning also helps to correct myths and misunderstandings physicians and nurses may harbor about the perceived deficits in advanced practice nursing and medical education. Interdisciplinary courses in pharmacotherapeutics, pathophysiology, and the like provide useful tools to dispel myths and provide accurate information. The ways in which health-care professionals are socialized in medical school and nursing school are also important. The underlying principle taught in medical school that physicians must present themselves as confident and "take charge" flies in the face of collaboration. A "captain of the ship," authoritarian leadership style and the interactive, caring, and collaborative style that nurses are expected to model make for strange bedfellows in practice. Furthermore, the hierarchies present in hospital and academic environments provide difficult hurdles to overcome.

One of the factors that is critical to socialization is time. Collaborative relationships based on competence, trust, and respect are built as players learn and practice together in various settings and situations, both as students and as peers in practice settings. Collaboration cannot be forced and must be allowed to develop over time. Activities such as group rounds, team conferences, and joint decision making in which advanced practice nursing preceptors and students actively participate can assist in this process.

Clinical placements for advanced practice nursing students have the potential to set the stage for long-term successful collaboration between APNs and physicians. The key is careful assessment of sites during the preplacement phase in order to match advanced practice nursing students and students from other disciplines with preceptors who support collaboration. Good interdisciplinary clinical educational experiences should be characterized not by parallel processes but by true team approaches to the diagnosis, management, and education of patients and families. Faculty who practice collaboratively with colleagues play a key role in setting up these experiences and can serve as important role models and mentors. Supportive debriefing through journals, patient rounds, and postclinical seminars is an excellent way to instill the concepts of collaboration into long-term student learning, especially when efforts to collaborate are unsuccessful or unsatisfactory.

Final preceptorships and practica offer additional opportunities for advanced practice nursing students to try out collaborative relationships with physicians and to practice newfound collaborative skills. Currently, there is broad support for interdisciplinary models of clinician education. There is a need to restructure curricula in order to better understand training and education strategies in nonnursing education models (Bray & Rogers, 1997; Cooper, Henderson, & Dietrich, 1998; Evans, 1994; Fagin, 1992; Larson, 1995; Pew-Fetzer Task Force, 1994; RWJF, 1999). The resurgence of interdisciplinary training for physicians and nurses for primary care practices should have a positive effect on collaboration. A recent article in the *New York Times* (April 18, 2004) by a Yale primary care MD, Lisa Sanders, called "The End of Primary Care" makes the case for interdisciplinary models of care using APN collaborators.

Assessment of Personal Factors

Professionals bring many personal attributes to a professional partnership. Personal characteristics such as clinical and interpersonal competence and well-developed communication skills are vital to the collaborative relationship. Good clinical judgment and a well-developed sense of ethics promote trust. Most important for a good collaborative experience is a shared vision of the desired outcome.

In *The Fifth Discipline: The Art and Practice of the Learning Organization*, Senge (1990) used the metaphors of a superlative basketball team and a fantastic jazz ensemble to illustrate the power of people working in collaboration. It is clear that it takes more than professionals with expert skills, who may have different strengths, working side by side. Senge discussed the energy and power that are produced when teams become aligned to purpose, when they are able to combine energies and harmonize to produce a synergistic effect. Although individuals may come to the team with great skills and expertise, it is the shared vision and the commonality of purpose that lead to success and improved outcome (Senge, 1990). These ideas can inform the work of teams who want to improve collaboration and achieve targeted patient outcomes.

Successful professional collaboration requires work and practice in the same way that personal relationships require time and effort. According to Senge (1990); Senge, Kleiner, Roberts, Ross, and Smith (1994); and Senge et al. (1999), practice is the hallmark of teamwork. Successful professional relationships—regardless of whether they are formed within a basketball team, a team of primary care physicians and nurses, a birthing center group, or a team of anesthesiologists and CRNAs—need continued work and practice to grow and succeed. Self-assessment is one important component to consider when one is embarking on a new professional relationship or evaluating the success or failure of current or potential collaborative relationships. The self-directed questions in Box 10-2 may help team members identify their personal strengths and weaknesses vis-à-vis collegiality. For a synopsis of Senge's work on teambuilding and leadership, readers are referred to the following URL: www.infed.org/thinkers/senge.htm.

Covey (1989) offered another perspective on moving toward a higher level of interdependence with colleagues. He portrayed interdependence as a higher level of performance than independence. Only individuals who have gained competence and confidence in their own expertise are able to move beyond autonomy and independence toward the higher synergistic level of collaboration. Collaboration appears to have the same meaning as interdependence in Covey's work. This view is provocative when one considers the hierarchical context that often frames clinical collaboration.

Assessment and Monitoring of Environmental Factors

Administrative leadership plays a key role in the development of collaborative relationships between organizational members. Administrators who support team and interdisciplinary

---

BOX 10-2 • PERSONAL STRENGTHS AND WEAKNESSES QUESTIONNAIRE

Am I clear about my role in the partnership?
What values do I bring to the relationship?
What do I expect to gain or lose by collaborating?
What do others expect of me?
Do I feel good about my contribution to the team?
Do I feel self-confident and competent in the collaborative relationship?
Are there anxieties causing repeated friction that have not been addressed?
Has serious thought been given to the boundaries of the collaborative relationship?

administrative models and who are good communicators themselves can do a great deal to increase the momentum of new collaborations. Differing philosophies and standards of care within organizational settings can cause conflict between team members and need to be resolved early (Spross, 1989). The common vision of quality patient care and staff satisfaction that makes collaboration possible should bring APNs and nursing administrators together to create administrative structures that support collaboration (Krumm, 1992; see Chapter 24).

Increased acuity of illness in both inpatient and outpatient settings is an obstacle to collaboration. As professionals move from one crisis to another, there is little time to sit down, communicate, analyze data, and make joint decisions (Spross, 1989). The lack of time to communicate remains a significant barrier to collaboration (Coeling & Wilcox, 1994).

Power inequities between medicine and nursing are often apparent. However, power issues also exist among nurses. Elitist stances by APNs set up roadblocks to collaboration with staff nurses. Balancing power differences between groups equalizes the hierarchical differences between members and makes collaboration possible if there is sufficient expertise among players (Stichler, 1995).

STRATEGIES FOR SUCCESSFUL COLLABORATION

Many of the barriers to successful collaboration occur because of values, beliefs, and behaviors that have, until recently, gone unchallenged in society and in the organizations in which nurses practice. There is a need for radical change if the conditions conducive to collaboration are to become the norm. APNs may feel as if they are the only ones with an active commitment to collaboration (Spross, 1989). Of all the competencies required for advanced practice, collaboration may be the most difficult to accomplish because it is mediated by social processes (Siegler & Whitney, 1994b) that are ingrained in the larger culture. Efforts to change the environment to one that is more collaborative involve proving oneself over and over and challenging colleagues' behaviors that restrain attempts to work together. These intrapersonal demands, along with the clinical demands of one's job, can be exhausting. Therefore APNs need to evaluate the potential for collaboration when seeking employment opportunities. Questions about how clinicians work together—the interpersonal climate as well as organizational structures that support collaboration—should be a high priority. A realistic appraisal of the existence of or potential for collaboration is needed to determine whether APNs can provide the standard and quality of care that are characteristic of advanced practice nursing and whether they can expect a reasonable level of job satisfaction.

Individual Strategies

The abilities to listen to and encourage others and to experience someone else's success or failure and the capability to *know* a colleague well foster the ability to successfully work as an interactive team (Dziabis & Lant, 1998). The strategies offered by Norton and Grady (1996) for developing and implementing the change agent competency are useful in developing collaborative skills.

Box 10-3 provides a list of strategies (Rider, 2002) that are thought to promote collaboration. Students and practicing APNs can examine their interactions for opportunities to implement these ideas and strengthen their interpersonal competence.

One strategy is for APNs to promote their exemplary nursing practices to help other health professionals and consumers better understand the strengths of APNs as

---

BOX 10-3 • STRATEGIES TO PROMOTE EFFECTIVE COMMUNICATION AND COLLABORATION

1. Be respectful and professional
2. Listen intently
3. Try to understand the other person's viewpoint
4. Acknowledge the other person's thoughts and feelings
5. Be cooperative
6. Look for shared goals and concerns
7. State your feelings using I statements
8. Don't take things personally
9. Learn to say "I was wrong" or "You could be right"
10. Don't feel pressure to agree instantly
11. Think about possible solutions before meeting
12. Think of conflict negotiation and resolution as a helical process, not a linear one; recognize that negotiation may occur over several interactions.

Adapted from Rider, E. (2002). Twelve strategies for effective communication and collaboration in medical teams. *British Medical Journal, 325*, S45.

health-care providers (Fagin, 1992; see Chapter 25). In today's health-care environment, participating in critical pathway development is one way to do this. Within advanced nursing practice, it is useful for nurses to role model their practice strategies for other nurses to facilitate intranursing collaboration and consultation. One way to share excellence in practice is to include in grand rounds or team conferences the opportunity for each care team member to describe her or his own decision making about patients and suggest new strategies for care to the team. Furthermore, Garcia, Bruce, Niemeyer, and Robbins (1993) suggested that integrated patient records provide a means to communicate formally about patient care. Joint review of patient care is an important component of collaboration in practice.

Working together on joint projects is another way to facilitate good collaboration. Collaborative research and scholarly writing projects, as well as community service projects that tap into the strengths of various members, open people's eyes to the benefits of collaboration. Federal and private agencies are currently supporting interdisciplinary collaborative studies. Reporting the results in the literature will illustrate the considerable advantages of collaborative interactions. In addition, social opportunities at conferences and receptions allow camaraderie to grow and help reinforce the bond between members of the partnership (Fitzpatrick, Wykle, & Morris, 1990; Hanson, 1993). These strategies move across lines from personal life to organizational settings and from education to practice arenas. New models that foster joint medical and nursing care are needed in primary care, as well as within specialty practice in all settings. More importantly, collaboratively developed practice guidelines improve communication and clarify clinicians' roles in patient treatment (Weinstein et al., 1998).

Organizational Strategies

Fagin (1992) and Hanson (1993) identified several strategies that foster successful collaboration at all levels. As noted previously, there needs to be a move toward interdisciplinary educational programs that allow for face-to-face interaction between medical and nursing students. Definitive changes in the structure of clinical hours and sequencing of content will be required. Given the entrenched bureaucracies involved, this will be a difficult task requiring stronger interactions between schools of medicine and schools of nursing. Health-care providers need to be learning about health policy issues from a perspective that offers broad-stroke solutions to health care issues. Faculty in both nursing and medicine need to be evaluating and treating patients and supervising students together. It is important to introduce joint appointments of nursing faculty to medical school clinics (and medical faculty to nursing schools) to give faculty opportunities to role model advanced practice nursing care and build rapport (Fitzpatrick et al., 1990).

National and state medical and nursing organizations must endorse the shift toward a more collaborative model (Fagin, 1992; Hanson, 1993). Strategies that facilitate this shift—such as retreats, social interactions, communication workshops, joint practice committees, and sensitivity training sessions—are imperative. Again, sharing exemplary nursing innovations is a major factor. Until strategies for this type of change are instituted, barriers to successful interprofessional collaboration will remain.

EXEMPLARS OF SUCCESSFUL COLLABORATIVE PRACTICE

Exemplars 10-3 and 10-4 illustrate successful collaboration.

EXEMPLAR 10-3

THE CLINICAL NURSE SPECIALIST IN PAIN MANAGEMENT

One of the authors (JS) was hired to start a cancer rehabilitation program. The director of nursing made it clear that she also wanted to improve pain management for all patients in the rehabilitation hospital, not just oncology patients. The clinical nurse specialist (CNS) began by developing collaborative relationships with the staff on the unit for which she had primary responsibility. As the staff on the unit got to know the CNS's skills, they began to consult her for pain management problems. As the CNS worked with patients, she learned that one of the pharmacists, who was full-time, was very interested in pain management and the two began to work together regularly—jointly evaluating patients and proposing pharmacological interventions to physicians. This collaboration was particularly beneficial for patients and staff because the CNS only worked half-time. Over time, the head nurse, the unit physician, and the consulting neurologist and physiatrist with whom the CNS and pharmacist had worked on some difficult pain issues began to ask the two clinicians to see patients in other units. The neurologist, in particular, seemed interested in learning more about pain management. The neurologist was also the chairperson of quality improvement. At the CNS's suggestion, the neurologist attended an all-day seminar on pain management that was being offered locally by a nationally known nurse leader in pain management. When the neurologist came back from the conference, where she learned about the clinical problems associated with using meperidine, she immediately sent a memo to clinical staff about its dangers. She then worked with the CNS, the quality improvement committee, and the pharmacy and therapeutics committee to limit the use of the drug for pain management by creating a policy and making the prescription of meperidine a sentinel event, to be evaluated by the CNS, the pharmacist, or the neurologist.

Over time, the CNS—with the support of the director of nursing, the neurologist, and the pharmacist—created an interdisciplinary team for pain management that included—in addition to the initial three disciplines of nursing, medicine, and pharmacy—two nurse educators, a head nurse, a psychologist, a physical therapist, a physical therapy assistant, an occupational therapist, a social worker, and a nurse case manager. Staff from all disciplines learned techniques to assess and treat pain. The team learned more about each other's skills and developed a "transdisciplinary" consultation model so that, regardless of discipline, each member knew the critical elements of patient and chart assessment. An interdisciplinary assessment

EXEMPLAR 10-3

THE CLINICAL NURSE SPECIALIST IN PAIN MANAGEMENT — cont'd

tool and core interventions that could be initiated by any member of the team were developed. This meant that any member of the team could do an initial evaluation of the patient to determine what steps needed to be taken. For example, although the CNS and psychologist could not make a pain diagnosis, they recognized when one was needed to guide treatment planning. In these situations, they would recommend to the internal medicine (IM) physician or nurse practitioner (NP) that a neurology consult be made if the primary physician or NP could not make such a diagnosis. All team members learned how to look at a medication Kardex to evaluate how well prescribed analgesics were being used. If undertreatment was evident from the Kardex review, the psychologist or physical or occupational therapist would involve the CNS or pharmacist. All team members knew some simple nondrug pain management techniques and the criteria for using them.

In an analysis of why this collaborative effort worked, several organizational and professional factors were found to be facilitators. Organizationally, the support provided by the director of nursing and the neurologist, who also had administrative responsibilities, was central. The neurologist's "buy-in" occurred about 6 months after the CNS was hired, resulting from a combination of her personal commitment to improve patient care and the knowledge she acquired at the pain management conference she attended. The fact that she chaired the quality improvement committee was also useful. The interdisciplinary team came together as a team about 18 months after the CNS had begun to work at the hospital. A structural factor that facilitated the development of the pain management program was the existence of weekly team meetings held to discuss each patient. The team meetings provided an opportunity for the CNS to identify pain management issues and report progress on decreasing pain for particular patients. This structure enabled the team, as a team, to see that managing pain well actually improved patients' participation in therapy, contrary to the widely held belief that patients in rehabilitation should not be receiving analgesics. This shift in attitude occurred over several months. In addition, the CNS could identify those staff members who had a particular interest in pain management and were open to being coached regarding pain management, thus building a community commitment to relieving pain.

Another structural factor was the presence of an NP in each of the patient care units. Units were organized such that an internal medicine (IM) physician and an NP were responsible for the medical management of the patients. In fact, some of the IM physicians were among the last to buy in to the institutional efforts to improve pain management. The close collaboration that occurred among NPs and IM physicians facilitated the collaboration of the CNS when she worked with the IM physicians to address patients' pain management issues.

From a process standpoint, the hospital philosophy and staff behavior reflected a commitment to patients. The fact that team meetings were "institutionalized" enabled clinicians to maintain a patient-centered focus even when there were disagreements about how to manage pain. In the beginning of the CNS's tenure, there was great reluctance to use opioids for relief of noncancer pain. Both experiences with patients and discussion of results of pain management efforts in team meetings reinforced the emphasis on patient comfort and progress in therapy as outcomes. Repeated experience with the CNS, in which her competence and the positive results for patients were observed, served to modify the attitudes of many of the staff members. One IM physician's buy-in occurred after the CNS effectively used relaxation, guided imagery, and therapeutic touch to treat the physician's own chronic back pain. (He was against use of medication for his own pain, although he had come to prescribe analgesics more frequently for patients because of the advocacy of the staff nurses for their patients.)

This was a situation that evolved to an unusually high level of collaboration. Had the team never evolved, the pharmacist and CNS would have still made a contribution to improving pain management. However, the level of interdisciplinary collaboration that ultimately resulted would not have occurred without the administrative, professional, and personal factors that contributed to the success of the initiative.

EXEMPLAR 10-4

THE NURSE PRACTITIONER IN PRIMARY CARE: PHYSICIANS' OBSERVATIONS ABOUT COLLABORATION

For several years, Syntex Corporation sponsored a Nurse Practitioner of the Year Award to honor nurse practitioners (NPs) who had achieved high levels of success in their practice. The letters of the physicians and nurses who nominated successful NPs for the award all appeared to say the same thing: "The individual exhibits a high level of collaboration." The following is a composite of the nomination letters received by Syntex from physician nominators.

I would like to tell you about Mary Q., a nurse practitioner who is a member of our group primary care practice. Mary is an extremely competent nurse practitioner and an able diagnostician. I would trust her to care for my own wife and children. She is totally committed to her patients, strives to give them the best possible care, and has many of the same values and ideas about good patient care that my physician partner and I do. Although Mary carries her own panel of patients very successfully, she seems to want and need to consult with me and our other physicians if she is concerned about a complex patient. We all function as a team and we have all learned from Mary's nursing expertise, as she has from ours. All of us work together to give high-quality care. Most importantly, Mary is a team player; all the members of our group practice enjoy her quick wit and willingness to share her expertise. At first, one of the partners did not want a nurse practitioner to join the group, but Mary won him over with her professional and interpersonal competence. I guess that the most important quality that I would share is that Mary is a people person; she works hard to communicate at a high level and it pays off. We trust her as a professional colleague and a friend.

Although Exemplar 10-4 is a composite of typical physician nominations, the content affirms what the literature on collaboration suggests: the burden of proof that collaboration works often depends on the APNs' skills and initiatives. APNs and their employers need to recognize that an important component of clinical practice is investing time and energy to build a collaborative climate: immediate results will not be apparent (a disadvantage, given the economics shaping health care), but collaboration should pay off over time in the form of improved patient outcomes.

CONCLUSION

Collaborative relationships are not only professionally satisfying (Alpert et al., 1992; Fagin, 1992; Weinstein et al., 1998), they improve access to care (Siegler & Whitney, 1994a; Waugaman & Foster, 1995) and patient outcomes (Knaus et al., 1986; Lassen et al., 1997; Rubinstein et al., 1984, Sears et al., 2003). Although APNs collaborate with many individuals within and outside of nursing and do so successfully, APNs may find that one of their most important collaborative relationships—that with physicians—may also be the most challenging. Despite the fact that there are many successful individual APN-physician collaborative practices, many with data that demonstrate their beneficial effects on health care, tradition and stereotypes are often powerful negative influences on policy-making and in health-care and professional organizations.

To meet the demands for cost-effectiveness and quality, clinicians from all disciplines are meeting together to discuss the care they provide and to define ways to deliver it so as to maximize quality and minimize duplication of effort. It is these interactions that foster the trust and respect required for mature collaboration. They enable collaborators to recognize their interdependence and value the input of others, thus creating a synergy that improves the quality of clinical decision making (Lassen et al., 1997; Stichler, 1995; Weinstein et al., 1998). APNs will find that their success as clinicians and leaders often depends on their proficiency as collaborators.

In the current health-care environment, collaboration may flourish regardless of the barriers identified. However, there is an urgent need to better understand the organizational structures, communications, and interactive styles that enable clinicians to collaborate in ways that benefit patients and health-care agencies. APNs can contribute to this understanding in several ways: (1) by documenting and analyzing their experiences with collaboration in published case studies, (2) by precepting students and helping them develop the skills essential for collaboration, and (3) by working with researchers who are studying the characteristics and clinical implications of collaboration. Effective collaboration must be at the heart of any redesign of the health-care delivery system, whether that redesign occurs in a unit, in a clinic, or within and between organizations.

REFERENCES

Acute Pain Management Guideline Panel. (1992). *Acute pain management: Operative or medical procedures and trauma* (Clinical Practice Guideline 92-0032). Rockville, MD: Agency for Health Care Policy and Research.

Afflitto, L. (1997). Managed care and its influence on physician-patient relationship: Implications for collaborative practice. *Plastic Surgical Nursing, 17,* 217-218.

Aiken, L. H., Smith, H. L., & Lake, E. T. (1994). Lower Medicare mortality among a set of hospitals known for good nursing care. *Medical Care, 32,* 771-787.

Alpert, H., Goldman, L., Kilroy, C., & Pike, A. (1992). 7 Gryzmish: Toward an understanding of collaboration. *Nursing Clinics of North America, 27,* 47-59.

American College of Graduate Medical Education. (2002). *ACGME outcome competencies.* Retrieved September 20, 2003, from http://www.ACGME.org

American College of Nurse-Midwives. (1997). *Collaborative management in nurse-midwifery practice for medical, gynecological, and obstetrical conditions.* Retrieved September 20, 2003, from http://www.midwife.org/prof/display.cfm?id=117

American Medical Association. (1995). *Board of Trustees report 6-A-95.* Chicago: Author.

American Nurses Association. (1995). *Nursing's social policy statement.* Washington, DC: Author.

American Nurses Association. (2003). *Nursing's social policy statement (new draft language)* (2nd ed.). Washington, DC: Author.

Anonymous. (2001). Bullying in medicine. *British Medical Journal, 323,* 1314.

Aroskar, M. (1998). Ethical working relationships in patient care. *Nursing Clinics of North America, 33,* 313-324.

Arslanian-Engoren, C. M. (1995). Lived experiences of CNSs who collaborate with physicians: A phenomenological study. *Clinical Nurse Specialist, 9,* 68-73.

Baggs, J. G. (1989). Intensive care unit use and collaboration between nurses and physicians. *Heart & Lung: The Journal of Acute and Critical Care, 18,* 332-338.

Baggs, J. G., & Schmitt, M. H. (1988). Collaboration between nurses and physicians. *Image: The Journal of Nursing Scholarship, 20,* 145-149.

Baggs, J. G., & Schmitt, M. H. (1997). Nurses' and resident physicians' perceptions of the process of collaboration in an MICU. *Research in Nursing and in Health, 20,* 71-80.

Baggs, J. G., Schmitt, M. H., Mushlin, A. L., Mitchell, P. H., Eldredge, D. H., Oakes, D., et al. (1999). Association between nurse-physician collaboration and patient outcomes in three intensive care units. *Critical Care Medicine, 27,* 1991-1998.

Balzer, J. (1993). Humor—a missing ingredient in collaborative practice. *Holistic Nursing Practice, 7,* 28-35.

Barron, A. M. (1989). The clinical nurse specialist as consultant. In A. B. Hamric & J. A. Spross (Eds.), *The clinical nurse specialist in theory and practice* (2nd ed., pp. 125-146). Philadelphia: W. B. Saunders.

Benner, P., Hooper-Kyriakidis, P., & Stannard, D. (1999). *Clinical wisdom and interventions in critical care: A thinking-in-action approach.* Philadelphia: W. B. Saunders.

Benoliel, J. Q. (1995). Multiple meanings of pain and complexities of pain management. *Nursing Clinics of North America, 30,* 583-596.

Bray, J. H., & Rogers, J. C. (1997). The Linkages Project: Training health professionals for collaborative practice with primary care physicians. *Families, Systems & Health, 15,* 55-62.

Brita-Rossi, P., Adduci, D., Kaufman, J., Lipson, S. J., Totte, C., & Wasserman, K. (1996). Improving the process of care: The cost-quality value of interdisciplinary collaboration. *Journal of Nursing Care Quality, 10,* 10-16.

Brown, S. J. (1989). Supportive supervision of the CNS. In A. B. Hamric & J. A. Spross (Eds.), *The clinical nurse specialist in theory and practice* (2nd ed., pp. 285-286). Philadelphia: W. B. Saunders.

Brown, S. J. (1998). A framework for advanced practice nursing. *Journal of Professional Nursing, 14,* 157-164.

Cairo, J. M. (1996). Emergency physicians' attitudes toward the emergency nurse practitioner role: Validation versus rejection. *Journal of the American Academy of Nurse Practitioners, 8,* 411-417.

Christman, L. (1998). Advanced practice nursing: Is the physician's assistant an accident of history or a failure to act? *Nursing Outlook, 46,* 56-59.

Coeling, H., & Wilcox, J. (1994). Steps to collaboration. *Nursing Administration Quarterly, 18,* 44-55.

The Conflict Resolution Network. (2003). *12 Skills summary: Conflict resolution skills.* Retrieved October 5, 2003, from http://www.crnhq.org/twelveskills.html

Conger, M., & Craig, C. (1998). Advanced nurse practice: A model for collaboration. *Nursing Case Management, 3,* 120-127.

Cooper, R. A., Henderson, T., & Dietrich, C. L. (1998). Roles of nonphysician clinicians as autonomous providers in patient care. *JAMA: The Journal of the American Medical Association, 280,* 795-800.

Cooper, R. A., Laud, P., & Dietrich, C. L. (1998). Current and projected workforce of nonphysician clinicians. *JAMA: The Journal of the American Medical Association, 280,* 788-794.

Covey, S. R. (1989). *The seven habits of highly effective people.* New York: Simon & Schuster.

Cramer, M. E. (2002). Factor influencing organized political participation in nursing. *Policy, Politics, and Nursing Practice, 3*(2), 97-107.

Crowley, S. A., & Wollner, I. S. (1987). Collaborative practice: A tool for change. *Oncology Nursing Forum, 14,* 59-63.

Cruikshank, B., & Chow, T. (1984). Physician supervision/collaboration as reported by PNPs in practice settings. *Pediatric Nursing, 10,* 13-18.

DeAngelis, C. (1994). Nurse practitioner redux. *JAMA: The Journal of the American Medical Association, 271,* 868-871.

Devereux, P. (1981). Nurse/physician collaboration: Nursing practice considerations. *Journal of Nursing Administration, 9,* 37-39.

Dickinson, C. P., Mateo, M., Jackson, D., & Swartz, W. (1995). OB-GYN Consultants and Sharp The BirthPlace: An exemplar of nurse-midwife and obstetrician independence and integration. *Advanced Practice Nursing Quarterly, 1,* 40-48.

Dressler, D. (1994). The critical care clinical nurse specialist in joint practice with physicians. In A. Gawlinski & L. Kern (Eds.), *The clinical nurse specialist in critical care* (pp. 51-61). Philadelphia: W. B. Saunders.

Dziabis, S. P., & Lant, T. W. (1998). Building partnerships with physicians: Moving outside the walls of the hospital. *Nursing Administration Quarterly, 22,* 1-5.

Evans, J. A. (1994). The role of the nurse manager in creating an environment for collaborative practice. *Holistic Nursing Practice, 8,* 23-31.

Fagin, C. (1992). Collaboration between nurses and physicians: No longer a choice. *Nursing and Health Care, 13,* 354-363.

Felton S., Cady, N., Metzler, M. H., & Burton, S. (1997). Implementation of collaborative practice through interdisciplinary rounds on a general surgery service. *Nursing Case Management, 2,* 122-126.

Fitzpatrick, J., Wykle, M., & Morris, D. (1990). Collaboration in care and research. *Archives of Psychiatric Nursing, 4,* 53-61.

Forbes, E., & Fitzsimmons, V. (1993). Education: The key for holistic interdisciplinary collaboration. *Holistic Nursing Practice, 7,* 1-10.

Garcia, M. A., Bruce, D., Niemeyer, J., & Robbins, J. (1993). Collaborative practice: A shared success. *Nursing Management, 24,* 72-79.

Gelman, S., O'Neil, E., Kimmey, J., & the Task Force on Accreditation of Health Professions Education. (1999). *Strategies for change and improvement: The report of the Task Force on Accreditation of Health Professions Education.* San Francisco: Center for the Health Professions, University of California at San Francisco.

Gianakos, D. (1997). Physicians, nurses and collegiality. *Nursing Outlook, 45,* 57-58.

Gilbert, J. H. V., Camp, R. D., Cole, C. D., Bruce, C., Fielding, D. W., & Stanton, S. J. (2000). Preparing students for interprofessional teamwork in health care. *Journal of Interprofessional Care, 14:* 223-235.

Grimaldi, D., & Cousins, A. (1998). Establishing a collaborative psychopharmacology practice: Practical considerations. *Journal of Psychosocial Nursing and Mental Health Services, 36,* 32-35.

Grumbach, K., & Coffman, J. (1998). Physicians and nonphysician clinicians. *JAMA : The Journal of the American Medical Association, 280*, 825-826.

Hales, A., Karshmer, J., Montes-Sandoval, L., & Fiszbein, A. (1998). Preparing for prescriptive privileges: A CNS-physician collaborative model. Expanding the scope of the psychiatric-mental health clinical nurse specialist. *Clinical Nurse Specialist, 12,* 73-80.

Hamric, A. B., & Hanson, C. M. (2003). Educating advanced practice nurses for practice reality. *Journal of Professional Nursing, 19*(5), 262-268.

Hanson, C. M. (1993). Our role in health care reform: Collegiality counts. *American Journal of Nursing, 93,* 16A-16E.

Hanson, C. M., & Beverly, K. B. (2001, May). *Code blue: Workforce in crisis.* Atlanta: Georgia Department of Community Health: State of Georgia Health Strategies Council.

Hanson, C. M., Hodnicki, D. R., & Boyle, J. S. (1994). Nominations for excellence: Collegial advocacy for nurse practitioners. *Journal of the American Academy of Nurse Practitioners, 6,* 471-476.

Hanson, C. M., & Malone, B. L. (2000). Leadership: Empowerment, change agency, and activism. In A. B. Hamric, J. A. Spross, & C. M. Hanson, (Eds.), *Advanced nursing practice: An integrative approach* (2nd ed., pp. 279-313). Philadelphia: W. B. Saunders.

Hanson, C. M., & Spross, J. A. (1996). Collaboration. In A. B. Hamric, J. A. Spross, & C. M. Hanson (Eds.), *Advanced nursing practice: An integrative approach* (pp. 229-248). Philadelphia: W. B. Saunders.

Hanson, C. M, Spross, J. A., & Carr, D. B. (2000). Collaboration. In A. B. Hamric, J. A. Spross, & C. J. Hanson, (Eds.), *Advanced nursing practice: An integrative approach* (2nd ed., pp. 315-347). Philadelphia: W. B. Saunders.

Hilderley, L. (1991). Nurse-physician collaborative practice: The clinical nurse specialist in a radiation oncology private practice. *Oncology Nursing Forum, 18,* 585-591.

Hill, M. N., & Hewlett, P. O. (2002). Getting to the top: Martha Hill, President American Heart Association. In D. J. Mason, J. K. Leavitt, & M. W. Chaffee. (Eds.), *Policy and politics in nursing and health care* (pp. 621-625). Philadelphia: W. B. Saunders.

Hodnicki, D. R., Dietz, A., McNeil, F., & Miles, K. (2004). Prescriptive authority: Medication-ordering patterns of advanced practice registered nurses in Georgia. *American Journal for Nurse Practitioners, 8*(1), 9-24.

Hotez, P. (2003, April 13). For the latest disease, a faster response. *The Washington Post,* pp. B1, B4.

Houghton, A. (2003). Bullying in medicine. *British Medical Journal, 326,* S125.

Hughes, A., & Mackenzie, C. (1990). Components necessary in a successful nurse practitioner-physi-cian collaborative practice. *Journal of the American Academy of Nurse Practitioners, 2,* 54-57.

Hupcey, J. (1993). Factors and work settings that may influence nurse practitioner practice. *Nursing Outlook, 41,* 181-185.

Ingersoll, G. L., McIntosh, E., & Williams, M. (2000). Nurse-sensitive outcomes of advanced practice. *Journal of Advanced Nursing Practice, 32,* 1272-1281

Inglis, A., & Kjervik, D. (1993). Empowerment of advanced practice nurses: Regulation reform needed to increase access to care. *Journal of Law, Medicine & Ethics, 21,* 193-205.

Jackson, D. J., Lang, J. M., Swartz, W. H., Ganiats, T. G., Fullerton, J., Ecker, J., et al. (2003). Outcomes, safety, and resource utilization in a collaborative care birth center program compared with traditional physician-based perinatal care. *American Journal of Public Health, 93,* 999-1006.

Johnson-Pawlson, J., Posey, L., Dalal, A., & Page, J. (2003). *Educating primary care practitioners in their home communities: Partnerships for training.* Washington, DC: Partnerships for Training, Association for Academic Health Centers.

Kavesh, W. (1993). Physician and nurse practitioner relationships. In M. Mezey & D. McGivern (Eds.), *Nurses, nurse practitioners: Evolution to advanced practice* (pp. 171-184). New York: Springer-Verlag.

Kedziera, P., & Levy, M. (1994). Collaborative practice in oncology. *Seminars in Oncology, 21,* 705-711.

King, J. (2002). Dealing with difficult doctors. *British Medical Journal, 325,* S43.

Kleinpell, R. M., Faut-Callahan, M., Lauer, K., Kremer, M., Murphy, M., & Sperhac, A. (2002). Collaborative practice in advanced nursing in acute care. *Critical Care Nursing Clinics of North America, 14,* 307-313.

Knaus, W. A., Draper, E. A., Wagner, D. P., & Zimmerman, J. E. (1986). An evaluation of outcome from intensive care in major medical centers. *Annals of Internal Medicine, 104,* 410-418.

Krumm, S. (1992). Collaboration between oncology clinical nurse specialists and nursing administrators. *Oncology Nursing Forum, 19*(Suppl. 1), 21-24.

Kuraitis, V. (1999). Physicians and care management: MBAs practicing medicine, or doctors controlling their own destiny? *Better Health Technologies* (May 6, 1999). Retrieved May 3, 2004, from http://www.bhtinfo.com/5_6_99.htm

Larson, E. (1999). The impact of physician-nurse interaction on patient care. *Holistic Nursing Practice, 13,* 38-46.

Larson, E. L. (1995). New rules for the game: Interdisciplinary education for health professionals. *Nursing Outlook, 43,* 180-185.

Lassen, A. A., Fosbinder, D., Minton, S., & Robins, M. (1997). Nurse/physician collaborative practice: Improving health care quality while decreasing cost. *Nursing Economics, 15,* 87-91.

Lenz, C. (1994). Multidisciplinary community-based education and practice. In J. C. McCloskey &

H. K. Grace (Eds.), *Current issues in nursing* (pp. 586-602). St. Louis, MO: Mosby.

Lindeke, L. L., & Block, D. E. (1998). Maintaining professional integrity in the midst of interdisciplinary collaboration. *Nursing Outlook, 46,* 213-218.

Littell, S. (1981). The clinical nurse specialist in private medical practice. *Nursing Administration Quarterly, 6,* 77-85.

Lumpkins, R., & Veal, J. (1995). Interdisciplinary collaboration: Strengthening documentation. *Nursing Management, 26,* 48L, 48N, 48P.

Management of Cancer Pain Guideline Panel. (1994). *Management of cancer pain* (Clinical Practice Guideline No. 9, AHCPR Publication No. 95-0592). Rockville, MD: Agency for Health Care Policy and Research.

McAvoy, B., & Murtagh, J. (2003). Workplace bullying: The silent epidemic [Letter]. *British Medical Journal, 326,* 776-777.

McKechnie, J. L. (Ed.). (1983). *Webster's new universal unabridged dictionary.* New York: Simon & Schuster.

Minarik, P. A., & Price, L. C. (1999). Collaboration? Supervision? Direction? Independence? What is the relationship between the advanced practice nurse and the physician? States' legislative and regulatory forum III. *Clinical Nurse Specialist, 13,* 34-37.

National Joint Practice Commission. (1979). *Brief description of a demonstration project to establish collaborative or joint practice in hospitals* (pp. 2-6). Chicago: Author.

North Shore Long Island Jewish Health System. (2001). *Magnet award.* Retrieved May 3, 2004, from http://www.northshorelij.edu/body.cfm?id=1081

Norton, S. F., & Grady, E. M. (1996). Change agent skills. In A. B. Hamric, J. A. Spross, & C. M. Hanson (Eds.), *Advanced nursing practice: An integrative approach* (pp. 249-271). Philadelphia: W. B. Saunders.

Nugent, K. E., & Lambert, V. A. (1996). The advanced practice nurse in collaborative practice. *Nursing Connections, 9* 5-14.

Oddi, L. F., & Cassidy, V. R. (1998). The message of SUPPORT: Change is long overdue. *Journal of Professional Nursing, 14,* 165-174.

Pellegrino, E. D. (1996). What's wrong with the nurse-physician relationship in today's hospitals? A physician's view. *Hospitals, 40,* 70-80.

Petronis-Jones, R. A. (1994). Nurse-physician collaboration: A descriptive study. *Holistic Nursing Practice, 8,* 38-53.

Pew Health Professions Commission. (1995). *Critical challenges: Revitalizing the health professions for the twenty-first century, third report.* San Francisco: University of California–San Francisco Center for the Health Professions.

Pew-Fetzer Task Force on Advancing Psychosocial Health Education. (1994). *Health professions education and relationship-centered care.* San Francisco: Pew Health Professions Commission.

Prescott, P., & Bowen, S. (1985). Physician-nurse relationships. *Annals of Internal Medicine, 103,* 127-133.

Pronovost, P. J., Jenckes, M. W., Dorman, T., Garrett, E., Breslow, M. J., Rosenfeld, B. A., et al. (1999). Organizational characteristics of intensive care units related to outcomes of abdominal aortic surgery. *JAMA: The Journal of the American Medical Association, 281,* 1310-1317.

Rafferty, A. M., Ball, J., & Aiken, L. H. (2001). Are teamwork and professional autonomy compatible and do they result in improved hospital care? *Quality in Health Care, 10* (Suppl. II), ii32-ii37.

Redmond, G., Riggleman, J., Sorrell, J. M., & Zerull, L. (1999). Creative winds of change: Nurses collaborating for quality outcomes. *Nursing Administration Quarterly, 23,* 55-64.

Rider, E. (2002). Twelve strategies for effective communication and collaboration in medical teams. *British Medical Journal, 325,* S45.

Robert Wood Johnson Foundation. (2003). *Partnerships for training: Educating primary care practitioners in their home communities.* Retrieved May 3, 2004, from http://www.pftweb.org/pft_brochure_web.pdf

Robert Wood Johnson Foundation. (2004). *Partnerships for quality education (PQE): About PQE.* Retrieved May 3, 2004, from http//www.pqe.org/about.html

Ryan, L., Edwards, R., & Rickles, F. (1980). A joint practice approach to the care of persons with cancer. *Oncology Nursing Forum, 8,* 8-11.

Safriet, B. J. (1992). Health care dollars and regulatory sense: The role of advanced practice nursing. *Yale Journal on Regulation, 9,* 417-487.

Safriet, B. J. (2002). Closing the gap between "can" and "may" in health care providers' scopes of practice: A primer for policymakers. *Yale Journal on Regulation, 19,* 301.

Sanders, L. The end of primary care. (2004, April 18). *The New York Times.*

Sands, R., Stafford, J., & McClelland, M. (1990). "I beg to differ": Conflict in the interdisciplinary team. *Social Work in Health Care, 14,* 55-72.

Schmitt, M. H. (2001). Collaboration improves the quality of care: Methodological challenges and evidence from US health care research. *Journal of Interprofessional Care, 15*(1), 47-66.

Sears, L., Maxwell, W., & Townsend, C. (2003). Urgent-care visits to a geriatric primary care clinic. *American Journal for Nurse Practitioners, 7,* 15-18.

Senge, P. M. (1990). *The fifth discipline: The art and practice of the learning organization.* New York: Doubleday.

Senge, P., Kleiner, A. Robert, C., Ross, R., & Smith, B. J. (1994) *The fifth discipline fieldbook: Strategies and tools for building a learning organization.* New York: Doubleday.

Senge, P., Kleiner, A., Roberts, C., Ross, R., Roth, G., & Smith, B. (1999) *The dance of change: The challenges of sustaining momentum in learning organizations.* New York: Doubleday/Currency.

Shortell, S. M., Zimmerman, J. E., Rousseau, D. M., Gillies, R. R., Wagner, D. P., Draper, E. A., et al.

(1994). The performance of intensive care units: Does good management make a difference? *Medical Care, 32,* 508-525.

Siegler, E. L., & Whitney, F. W. (Eds.). (1994a). *Nurse physician collaboration: Care of adults and the elderly.* New York: Springer-Verlag.

Siegler, E. L., & Whitney, F. W. (1994b). Social and economic barriers to collaborative practice. In E. L. Siegler & F. W. Whitney (Eds.), *Nurse-physician collaboration: Care of adults and the elderly* (pp. 21-32). New York: Springer-Verlag.

Simpson, R. L. (1998). Bridging the nursing-physician gap: Technology's role in interdisciplinary practice. *Nursing Administration Quarterly, 22,* 87-90.

Smith, R., Hiatt, H., & Berwick, D. (1999). Shared ethical principles for everybody in health care: a working from the Tavistock group. *British Medical Journal, 318,* 248-51.

Spross, J. A. (1989). The CNS as collaborator. In A. B. Hamric & J. A. Spross (Eds.), *The clinical nurse specialist in theory and practice* (2nd ed., pp. 205-226). Philadelphia: W. B. Saunders.

Steele J. E. (Ed.). (1986). *Issues in collaborative practice.* Orlando, FL: Grune & Stratton.

Stein, L. I., Watts, D. T., & Howell, T. (1990). The doctor-nurse game revisited. *New England Journal of Medicine, 322,* 546-549.

Stichler, J. F. (1995). Professional interdependence: The art of collaboration. *Advanced Practice Nursing Quarterly, 1,* 53-61.

Stumpf, S. H., & Clark, J. Z. (1999). The promise and pragmatism of interdisciplinary education. *Journal of Allied Health, 28,* 30-32.

Sullivan, T. J. (1998). *Collaboration: A health care imperative.* New York: McGraw-Hill Health Professions Division.

SUPPORT Principal Investigators. (1995). A controlled trial to improve care for seriously ill hospitalized patients: The Study to Understand Prognosis and Preferences for Outcomes and Risks of Treatment (SUPPORT). *JAMA: The Journal of the American Medical Association, 274,* 1591-1598.

Tjosvold, D. (1986). The dynamics of interdependence in organizations. *Human Relations, 39,* 517-540.

Torres, S., & Dominguez, L. M. (1998). Collaborative practice: How we get from coordination to the integration of skills and knowledge. In C. M. Sheehy & M. C. McCarthy (Eds.), *Advanced practice nursing: Emphasizing common roles* (pp. 217-240). Philadelphia: F. A. Davis.

U.S. Preventive Services Task Force. (2003). *About USPSTF* (AHRQ Publication No. 00-P046). Retrieved May 3, 2004, from http://www.ahrq.gov/clinic/uspstfab.htm

Waugaman, W. R., & Foster, S. D. (1995). CRNAs: An enviable legacy of patient service. *Advanced Practice Nursing Quarterly, 1,* 21-28.

Weinstein, M. E., McCormack, B., Brown, M. E., & Rosenthal, D. S. (1998). Build consensus and develop collaborative practice guidelines. *Nursing Management, 29,* 48-52.

Weisman, D., Griffie, J., Gordon, D. B., & Dahl, J. (1997). A role model program to promote institutional change for management of acute and cancer pain. *Journal of Pain and Symptom Management, 14,* 274-279.

Weissman, D. (1988). Cancer pain education: A call for role models. *Journal of Clinical Oncology, 6,* 1793-1794.

Wells, N., Johnson, R., & Salyer, S. (1997). Interdisciplinary collaboration. *Clinical Nurse Specialist, 12,* 161-168.

Wolf, A. (2003). Collaborative APN practice. In Fitzpatrick, J. J., Glascow, A., & Young, J. N. (Eds.), *Managing your practice: A guide for advanced practice nurses.* New York: Springer

Additional Readings

American Association of Colleges of Nursing. (1999). Certification and regulation of advanced practice nurses. *Journal of Professional Nursing, 15,* 130-132.

Bauer, J. C. (1994). *Not what the doctor ordered: Reinventing medical care in America.* Chicago: Probus.

Cooper, R. A., Laud, P., & Dietrich, C. L. (1998). Current and projected workforce of nonphysician clinicians. *JAMA: The Journal of the American Medical Association, 280,* 788-794.

Joel, L. A. (1998). Advanced practice nursing in the current sociopolitical environment. In C. Sheehy & M. McCarthy (Eds.), *Advanced practice nursing: Emphasizing common roles* (pp. 47-68). Philadelphia: F. A. Davis.

Joint Commission on Accreditation of Healthcare Organizations. (1992). *Agenda for change.* Oakbrook Terrace, IL: Author.

Jones, P. E., & Cawley, J. F. (1994). Physicians assistants and health system reform. *JAMA: The Journal of the American Medical Association, 271,* 1266-1272.

McCloskey, J. C., & Maas, M. (1998). Interdisciplinary team: The nursing perspective is essential. *Nursing Outlook, 46,* 157-163.

McCoy, S. T., Cope, K. A., Joy, S. J., Baker, R. T., & Brugler, C. I. (1997). Interdisciplinary documentation of patient education: How collaboration can effect change. *Rehabilitation Nursing, 22,* 235-238.

Miller, S., King, T., Lurie, P., & Choitz, P. (1997). Certified nurse-midwife and physician collaborative practice. *Journal of Nurse-Midwifery, 42,* 308-315.

Mitchell, P. H., & Shortell, S. M. (1997). Adverse outcomes and variations in organization of care delivery. *Medical Care, 35,* NS19-NS32.

Mundinger, M. (1994). Sounding board: Advanced-practice nursing—good medicine for physicians? *New England Journal of Medicine, 330,* 211-214.

Mundinger, M. (1999). Can advanced practice nurses succeed in the primary care market? *Nursing Economics, 17,* 7-14.

Mundt, M. H. (1997). Books on health policy and health reform: How is nursing represented? *Journal of Professional Nursing, 13,* 19-27.

Reynolds, P. P., Giardino, A., Onady, G. M., & Siegler, E. L. (1994). Collaboration in the preparation of the generalist physician. *Journal of General Internal Medicine, 9*(Suppl. 1), S55-S63.

Safriet, B. J. (1997). Still spending dollars, still searching for sense: Advanced practice nursing in an era of regulatory and economic turmoil. *Advanced Practice Nursing Quarterly, 4,* 24-33.

University of York NHS Centre for Reviews and Dissemination. (1999). Getting evidence into practice. *Effective Health Care, 5,* 1-16.

Verschuren, P. J. M., & Masselink, H. (1997). Role concepts and expectations of physicians and nurses in hospitals. *Social Science and Medicine, 45,* 1135-1138.

Walker, P. H., Baldwin, D., Fitzpatrick, J. J., Ryan, S., Bulger, R., DeBasio, N., et al. (1998). Commentary: Building community: Developing skills for inter-professional health. *Nursing Outlook, 46,* 88-89.

Wocial, L. D. (1996). Collaborative practice: Achieving collaboration in ethical decision making: Strategies for nurses in clinical practice. *DCCN: Dimensions of Critical Care Nursing, 15,* 150-159.

Wood, M., Ferlie, E., & Fitzgerald, L. (1998). Achieving clinical behaviour change: A case of becoming indeterminate. *Social Science and Medicine, 47,* 1729-1738.

Woods, L. P. (1998). Implementing advanced practice: Identifying factors that facilitate and inhibit the process. *Journal of Clinical Nursing, 7,* 265-273.

CHAPTER 11

Ethical Decision Making

ANN B. HAMRIC • JUANITA REIGLE

INTRODUCTION

Various factors, including changes in interprofessional roles, advances in medical technology, availability of information online, revisions in patient care delivery systems, and heightened economic constraints, have increased the complexity of ethical issues in the health-care setting. Nurses in all areas of health care routinely encounter disturbing moral issues, yet the success with which these dilemmas are resolved varies significantly. Because nurses have a unique relationship to the patient and family, the moral position of nursing in the health-care arena is distinct. As the complexity of issues intensifies, the role of the advanced practice nurse (APN) becomes particularly important in the identification, deliberation, and resolution of complicated and difficult moral problems. While all nurses are moral agents, APNs are expected to be leaders in both resolving moral problems and working to create ethical practice environments. It is a basic tenet of the central definition of advanced practice nursing (see Chapter 3) that skill in ethical decision making is one of the core competencies of all APNs. This chapter explores the distinctive ethical decision-making competency of advanced practice nursing, the process of developing and evaluating this competency, and barriers to ethical practice that APNs can expect to confront.

CHARACTERISTICS OF ETHICAL DILEMMAS IN NURSING

In this chapter, the terms *ethics* and *morality* or *morals* are used interchangeably. A problem becomes an ethical or moral problem when issues of core values or fundamental obligations are present. An *ethical or moral dilemma* occurs when obligations require or appear to require that a person adopt two (or more) alternative actions, yet the person cannot carry out all the required alternatives. The agent experiences tension because the moral obligations resulting from the dilemma create differing and opposing demands (Beauchamp & Childress, 2001; Purtilo, 1999). In some moral dilemmas, the agent must choose between equally unacceptable alternatives; that is, both may have elements that are morally unsatisfactory. For example, a family nurse practitioner (NP) may oppose mandatory screening of pregnant women for human immunodeficiency virus (HIV) because it violates the central concept of patient autonomy. However, vertical transmission of HIV is often preventable with new therapies, and to exclude screening the mother for HIV may result in transmission of the virus to the fetus. This choice violates the NP's central tenet to promote good, and thus to choose either alternative results in an unsatisfactory effect on one of the involved parties.

Jameton (1984, 1993) distinguished two additional types of moral problems in nursing from the classic moral dilemma, which he called *moral uncertainty* and *moral distress*. In situations of *moral uncertainty*, the nurse experiences unease and questions the right course of action. In *moral distress*, nurses believe they know the ethically appropriate action but feel constrained from carrying out that action because of institutional obstacles such as lack of time or supervisory support, physician power, institutional policies, or legal constraints. The phenomenon of moral distress has received increasing attention in the last few years (Brown, 2003; Corley, 1995, 2002; Hamric, 2000; Tiedje, 1999; Meaney, 2002) as a potentially negative influence on nurses' decisions to remain in clinical practice. APNs play an important role in decreasing the incidence of both moral uncertainty and moral distress in nursing staff through education, empowerment, and problem solving.

Although the scope and nature of moral problems experienced by nurses reflect the varied clinical settings in which they practice, three general themes emerge when ethical issues in nursing practice are examined. These themes are problems with communication, the presence of interdisciplinary involvement, and nurses' difficulties with managing multiple commitments and obligations.

Communication Problems

The first theme encountered in many ethical dilemmas is the erosion of open and honest communication. Clear communication is an essential prerequisite for informed and responsible decision making. In fact, some ethical disputes reflect inadequate communication rather than a difference in values (LaMear-Tucker & Friedson, 1997). Clear and definitive communication with patients and families will increase understanding and lead to more knowledgeable decision making and may improve compliance with current therapies. The APN's communication skills are applied in several arenas. Within the multidisciplinary health-care team, discussions are most effective when members are accountable for presenting information in a precise and succinct manner. The skill of listening is just as crucial in effective communication as having proficient verbal skills. Listening involves recognizing and appreciating various perspectives. To listen well is to allow others the necessary time to form and present their thoughts and ideas. In this way, good communication may be an effective tool in preventing ethical dilemmas.

It is also the case that understanding the language used in ethical deliberations helps the APN frame the concern. This framing can help parties see the components of the ethical problem rather than be mired in their emotional responses. This ability to communicate the problem can lead to productive decision making. When ethical dilemmas arise, effective communication is the first key to negotiating and facilitating a resolution.

Interdisciplinary Involvement

Second, most ethical dilemmas that occur in the health-care setting are interdisciplinary in nature. Issues such as refusal of treatment, end-of-life decision making, cost containment, and confidentiality all have multidisciplinary elements interwoven in the dilemmas; and therefore an interdisciplinary approach is necessary for successful resolution of the issue. Health-care professionals bring varied viewpoints and perspectives into discussions of ethical issues (Shannon, 1997). These differing positions can lead to creative and collaborative decision making or to a breakdown in communication and lack of problem solving. Thus an interdisciplinary theme is prevalent in both the presentation and resolution of ethical problems.

The moral dilemmas that often surround end-of-life decision making provide an excellent example of interdisciplinary issues that call for a collaborative approach. In the Study to Understand Prognosis and Preferences for Outcomes and Risks of Treatments (SUPPORT) investigation, study nurses provided patients and families opportunities to discuss preferences for medical treatments at end-of-life hospitalization (SUPPORT Principal Investigators, 1995). Although the SUPPORT study nurses communicated the patients' and/or families' wishes about resuscitation to the multidisciplinary team, the physicians often neglected to discuss these treatment preferences further with the patient or family. Moreover, when the patient's preferences were known, the multidisciplinary team (which did not include the SUPPORT nurses) often did not act in accordance with these wishes. In the 2,534 intervention patients, the prevalence of do-not-resuscitate (DNR) orders and the timing of the orders did not vary significantly from those in the 2,208 control patients. Even terminally ill patients who specifically requested to be designated DNR did not have DNR orders written early in their hospitalization (SUP-PORT Principal Investigators, 1995). In such situations, nurses experience a moral dilemma with several dimensions. If the patient arrested, the nurses would be obligated to initiate resuscitative interventions and thereby violate the patient's moral and physical boundaries. Additionally, because the physicians failed to acknowledge the nurses' understanding of the patient's wishes, the nurses were excluded from the decision-making process and became marginalized health-care providers. In their critique of the SUP-PORT study, Oddi and Cassidy (1998) noted that the lack of interdisciplinary professional collaboration and the lack of physician understanding of nursing's professional roles, particularly advanced practice roles, were key problems underlying the findings that were not addressed by the researchers.

Multiple Commitments

The third theme that frequently arises when ethical issues in nursing practice are examined is the issue of balancing commitments to multiple agents. Nurses have numerous and, at times, competing fidelity obligations to various stakeholders within the health-care and legal systems (Saulo & Wagener, 1996; Hamric, 2001). Fidelity is an ethical concept that requires persons to be faithful to their commitments and promises (see Box 11-1). For the APN, these obligations start with the patient and family but also include physicians and other colleagues, the institution or employer, the larger profession, and oneself. Ethical deliberation involves analyzing and dealing with the differing and opposing demands that occur. For example, an acute care nurse practitioner (ACNP) is writing discharge orders for an elderly woman who is terminally ill with heart failure. The plan of care, agreed upon by the interdisciplinary team, the patient, and her family, is to continue oral medications but discontinue intravenous inotropic support and all other aggressive measures. Just prior to discharge, the social worker informs the ACNP that medical coverage for the patient's care in the long-term care facility will only be covered by the insurer if the patient has an IV in place. Now the ACNP is faced with an ethical dilemma created by multiple commitments and the need to balance obligations. The responsibilities to the patient are to ensure that care is provided in a manner that is consistent with the patient's wishes and to minimize the cost burden to the patient. However, the ACNP also has a responsibility to society to practice as a responsible steward of limited resources and to prevent fraud and abuse in the health-care system.

The general themes of communication, interdisciplinary involvement, and balancing multiple commitments are prevalent in most ethical dilemmas. Although these characteristics emerge as common elements, specific ethical issues may be unique to the specialty area and clinical setting in which the APN practices.

ETHICAL ISSUES AFFECTING APNs

Primary Care Issues

Issues in which personal values contradict professional responsibilities often confront NPs in a primary care setting. Issues such as abortion, teen pregnancy, patient nonadherence to treatment, childhood immunizations, regulations and law, and financial constraints that interfere with care are cited as ethical issues frequently encountered (Turner, Marquis, & Burman, 1996). In one study, primary care NPs interpreted their moral responsibilities as balancing obligations to the patient, family, colleagues, employer, and society (Viens,

1994). Often APNs in a rural setting have fewer resources than their acute care colleagues do to assist with resolution of ethical dilemmas. Studies of primary care NPs suggest that the quality of the patient-practitioner relationship is the central feature in facilitating or hindering ethical decision making (Turner et al., 1996; Viens, 1994, 1995).

Issues of quality of life and symptom management traverse primary care and acute health-care settings (Calkins, 1993; Omery, Henneman, Billet, Luna-Raines, & Brown-Saltzman, 1995; Solomon et al., 1993; Winters, Glass, & Sakurai, 1993). It is not surprising that these issues are central moral concerns for nurses. Typically, the nurse monitors the patient, interprets symptoms, and administers medication to provide optimal relief of undesirable and intolerable symptoms. Pain relief and symptom management become problematic for nurses when physicians are reluctant to acknowledge the patient's problem and/or to prescribe adequate amounts of medication to alleviate the patient's pain and suffering (Turner et al., 1996; Omery et al., 1995; Solomon et al., 1993). APNs must confront the various and sometimes conflicting goals of the patient, family, and other health-care providers regarding the plans for treatment, symptom management, and quality of life. The APN is often the individual who coordinates the plan of care and thus is faced with clinical and ethical concerns when the goals among the participants of care are not consistent or appropriate.

Acute and Chronic Care

In the acute care setting, APNs struggle with moral dilemmas involving pain management, end-of-life decision making, advance directives, assisted suicide and dealing with medical errors (Hall, 1996; O'Connor, 1996; Schlenk, 1997; Hebert, Levin, & Robertson, 2001). The prevalence of these issues was described in a 1994 survey of practicing nurses conducted by the American Nurses Association's (ANA's) Center for Ethics and Human Rights. Nurse participants from a variety of practice domains and roles identified 10 areas in which moral issues surfaced: issues of cost containment that jeopardized patient welfare; end-of-life decisions; breaches of patient confidentiality; incompetent, illegal, or unethical practices of colleagues; pain management; use of advance directives; informed consent for procedures; access to health care; issues in the care of persons with HIV infection or acquired immunodeficiency syndrome (AIDS); and providing "futile" care (Scanlon, 1994). Many of the same ethical issues are embodied in three themes that emerged from discussions with oncology nurses (O'Connor, 1996). The theme of suffering was most frequently cited and involved the issues of pain management and symptom relief. Keeping secrets, the second theme, was a common experience for the study participants. In many situations, the physician communicated information to the patient or family about the patient's condition in a dishonest manner via incomplete disclosure of information or outright dishonesty. Finally, the theme of struggle arose from the oncology nurses' descriptions of situations involving disagreements. Conflict occurred between the nurse and family, nurse and physician, and nurse and other professional colleagues.

APNs bring a distinct perspective to collaborative decision making and often find themselves bridging communication between the medical team and patient or family. For example, the neonatal nurse practitioner (NNP) is responsible for the day-to-day medical management of the critically ill neonate and may be the first provider to respond in emergency situations (Juretschke, 2001). While at the bedside, the NNP is able to observe the family's interactions with the infant. The NNP establishes a trusting relationship with the family and becomes aware of the values, beliefs, and attitudes that shape the family's decisions. Thus the NNP has insight into the perspectives of both the health-care team and family. This position, however, can be accompanied by moral distress, particularly when the treatment decision carried out by the NNP is not congruent with the NNP's professional judgment or values. Waltman and Schenk (1999) conducted an informal survey of NNPs and found that they felt inadequately prepared to deal with ethical issues that arise in the neonatal intensive care unit. Knowing the best interests of the infant and balancing those obligations to the infant with the emotional, cognitive, financial, and moral concerns that face the family struggling with a critically ill neonate is a complex undertaking. Care must be guided by an NNP and health-care team who understand the ethical principles and decision making related to issues confronted in neonatal intensive care unit practice.

Societal Issues

The arrival of managed care has significantly changed the traditional practice of delivering health care. Managed care goals of reduced expenditures and services and increased efficiency may compete with enhanced quality of life for patients and improved treatment and care, creating conflict and tension among nurses, physicians, and employers with diverse goals (Rowdin, 1995). A study of 254 NPs with some affiliation with managed care systems revealed that 80% of the sample perceived that it was sometimes necessary to bend managed care guidelines to help patients; many respondents were moderately to extremely ethically concerned with managed care (Ulrich, Soeken, & Miller, 2003). An example of how managed care goals can create conflict is a situation in which a certified nurse midwife (CNM) practices in a managed care organization where routine obstetrical ultrasound examination is not approved. This decision by the organization was based on a large randomized study that showed no improvement in perinatal outcome when ultrasound examination was performed before 24 weeks' gestation (Ewigman et al., 1993). Although this decision meets the objective of reducing costs and expenditures, by limiting options for the woman, it may conflict with the goal of enhancing care (Chervenak & McCullough, 1995). In some cases, a woman's decision to continue a pregnancy is based on the presence or absence of serious fetal anomalies detected on routine ultrasound examination. In a managed care environment, the CNM may be faced with several alternatives. The CNM could simply not offer a woman routine ultrasound and thus exclude the option for early detection of fetal anomalies by this test. Another option would be to offer ultrasound examination to the woman but state at the outset that this diagnostic test would not be covered by the managed care plan. A third option involves dishonesty on the part of the CNM and would require devising some reason for the woman to be considered at high risk for carrying a fetus with congenital anomalies, thereby sanctioning the use of and reimbursement for ultrasound examination. Each option places the CNM in conflict with some other party, either the patient or the managed care organization.

Technological advances, such as the rapidly expanding field of genetics, will further challenge APNs in the near future. The completion of the Human Genome Project promises to usher in a new era in biomedical research and clinical medicine (Collins & Mansoura, 2001). As Hopkinson and Mackay (2002) noted, while the potential impact of this information is immense, the challenge of how to rapidly translate genetic data into improvements in prevention, diagnosis, and treatment of disease remains. APNs may be faced with discussing the need for, and perhaps results of, predictive testing for genetic disorders. Issues such as inadvertent detection of nonpaternity, expanded reproductive choices, denial of reimbursement for genetic testing, loss of eligibility for insurance, and the potential for discrimination may surface as the use of genetic technology increases (Williams & Lea, 1995; Dwyer, 1998). Because genetic information is crucially linked to the concepts of privacy and confidentiality and the availability of this information is increasing, it is inevitable that APNs will encounter legal issues and ethical dilemmas related to the use of genetic data.

APNs engage in research as principal investigators, co-investigators, or data collectors for clinical studies and trials. Ethical issues abound in clinical research, including recruiting and retaining patients in studies, ensuring informed consent, protecting vulnerable populations from undue risk, ensuring fair access to research, and ensuring study subjects' privacy (Grady, 1991; Sadler, Lantz, Fullerton, & Dault, 1999). Regardless of the level of involvement, the APN must support the best interests of the patient and uphold the ethical concepts of informed consent and truthfulness. In addition to the risks and benefits of their participation, patients must understand that they are in a research study, which may not be therapeutic for them, and that they may withdraw from any study at any time without penalty. The use of incentives, such as money or a reduced cost of care, must be balanced with the interests of the subject so as not to exert an undue coercive influence on patients (Eisenberg, 1999).

Access to Resources and Issues of Justice

As cost containment continues unabated in health-care systems, issues of access to resources and equitable distribution of resources create powerful dilemmas for APNs, many of whom care for underserved populations. Issues of social justice and equitable access to resources continue to present formidable challenges in clinical practice. Whether in community or acute care settings, APNs must, on a daily basis, balance the profession's obligation to provide holistic and individualized care with pressures to contain costs and the reality that some patients do not have access to needed health care. For example, in her study of primary care NPs' moral dilemmas, Viens (1994) noted that issues of justice were ever present in some primary care NP practices. One of her study participants commented, "How do I make an income, generate an income for the clinic, and at the same time be able to provide a service to patients who were poor and still offer quality coverage[?] That straddle within our society of those who can afford insurance, those who can't afford insurance to me is not fair, so what can I do about it?" (p. 210).

One of the value-added components that APNs bring to any practice setting is creativity and a wide range of patient management strategies, but this is exhausting business in a society with large numbers of uninsured and underinsured persons. In addition, situations that arise when APNs deal with the uninsured and underinsured are often morally unsettling. Many underinsured patients with chronic conditions are faced with mounting medical costs and dwindling resources. It is not uncommon for an APN to encounter a patient who has been forced to omit medications for financial reasons. Although many practitioners prescribe generic forms of medications if they are available, some patients still face exorbitant prices for their medications. For example, an ACNP managing an underinsured patient with chronic lung disease and heart failure discovers that the patient is unable to pay for all the medications prescribed and has elected to forego the diuretic and angiotensin-converting enzyme inhibitor (ACE-I). Because the ACNP knows the reduced morbidity and mortality rates associated with benefits of the ACE-I and the importance of the diuretic in symptom management and preventing rehospitalization, these choices are discouraged. Instead, the ACNP helps the patient make more suitable choices when altering his medications, such as dosing some medications on an every-other-day basis. Thus a less optimal plan of care is proposed to help the patient make better decisions about medications when confronted with unmanageable costs. The ACNP has helped the patient cope with the situation but is troubled by promoting an inferior plan of care.

Legal Issues

Over the last 30 years, the complexity of ethical issues in the health-care environment and the inability to reach agreement among parties has resulted in participants turning to the legal system for resolution. A body of legal precedent has emerged, reflecting changes in society's moral consensus. Ideally, moral rights are upheld or protected by the law, and in some cases it is necessary to have these rights affirmed. For example, the Patient Self-Determination Act (part of the Omnibus Budget Reconciliation Act of 1990) upholds the rights of patients to enact an advance directive to guide future medical treatments. More recently, the Health Insurance Portability and Accountability Act's (HIPAA's) 2003 compliance deadline has mandated a new set of privacy regulations related to use or disclosure of protected health information (see Chapter 22). The APN must understand the relevance of current laws and regulations to clinical practice.

In some cases, public policies and legal guidelines may infringe on the process of ethical decision making. It is important to recognize that the law is open to interpretation, and current laws surrounding an issue in conflict may be overemphasized or misunderstood. Misinterpretation of legal decisions in precedent-setting cases may diminish the chances of successful negotiation. For example, an APN in Virginia may be involved with a case of withdrawing nutrition and hydration. Parties involved in the case may misunderstand the U.S. Supreme Court ruling in the case of Nancy Cruzan (*Cruzan v. Missouri Department of Health et al.*, 1990) and incorrectly assume that nutrition and hydration cannot be withdrawn. If the APN is familiar with the Cruzan case, general misconceptions can be explained and clarified. APNs who are knowledgeable about relevant case law and pertinent state and federal policies are better able to take moral action when dilemmas arise.

Unfortunately, in the current health-care climate, there is an increasing tendency to look to the law for the final word. The tendency to resort to the courts for guidance in ethical decision making is troubling because clinical understanding may be absent from the judicial perspective. It is important that APNs not conflate legal perspectives with ethical decision making. In many cases, there is no relevant law, and thoughtful deliberation of the ethical issues offers the best hope of resolution.

NNPs practice in a setting that illustrates how ethical knowledge and legal regulations are interwoven in clinical practice. An NNP must understand the current laws and regulations regarding parental rights and resuscitation of preterm newborns. Paradigm cases, such as the cases of "Baby Doe" and "Baby Jane Doe" (United States Child Abuse Protection and Treatment Amendments of 1984) serve as important tools to help the NNP frame ethical dilemmas in neonatal care (Kopelman, Irons, & Kopelman, 1988; Waltman & Schenk, 1999). Other guidelines regarding the care of this patient population, such as the American Academy of Pediatrics' guidelines for the care of critically ill newborns (American Academy of Pediatrics, Committee on Bioethics, 1996), expand the NNP's understanding and anticipation of ethical issues that arise in these situations.

THE ETHICAL DECISION-MAKING COMPETENCY OF APNs

As described previously, the current challenges facing APNs in all practice settings give rise to numerous ethical concerns. At the APN level, ethical involvement follows and evolves from clinical expertise. Ethical involvement requires APNs to extend beyond the technical demands of clinical practice and enter the patient's world (Dreyfus, Dreyfus, & Benner, 1996). As experienced clinicians, APNs are capable of relinquishing this exclusive focus on clinical skills and blending clinical knowledge with humanistic and spiritual knowledge (Dreyfus et al., 1996; Leavitt, 1996).

Another reason that advanced practice nursing includes involvement in clinical ethics is the expanded collaborative skills that APNs develop (see Chapter 10). APNs practice in a variety of settings and positions, but in most cases the APN is part of an interdisciplinary team of caregivers for the patient. The team may be loosely defined and structured, as in a rural setting, or more definitive, as in the acute care setting. Regardless of the structure, the APN has knowledge and skills to avoid power struggles, broker interdisciplinary communication, and facilitate consensus among interdisciplinary team members.

Phases of Core Competency Development

The core competency of ethical decision making for APNs can be organized into three phases. Each phase depends on the acquisition of the knowledge and skills embedded in the previous level. Thus the competency of ethical decision making is understood as an evolutionary process in an APN's development. Phase 1 and beginning exposure to Phase 2 should be explicitly taught in the APN's graduate education. Phase 3 evolves as APNs mature in their roles and become comfortable in the practice setting; this phase represents a leadership behavior and the full enactment of the ethical decision-making competency. The essential elements of each phase are described in Table 11-1.

TABLE 11-1 PHASES OF DEVELOPMENT OF CORE COMPETENCY FOR ETHICAL DECISION MAKING		
	KNOWLEDGE	SKILL/BEHAVIOR

Phase 1: Knowledge Development—Moral Sensitivity	Ethical theories
	Ethical issues in specialty
	Professional code
	Professional standards
	Legal precedent
		Sensitivity to ethical dimensions of clinical practice
		  -values clarification
		  -sensitivity to fidelity conflicts
		Gather relevant literature related to problems identified
		Evaluate practice setting for congruence with literature
		Identify ethical issues in the practice setting and bring to the attention of other team members

Phase 2: Knowledge Application—Moral Action	Ethical decision-making models Mediation/facilitation strategies	Apply ethical decision-making models to clinical problems Use of skilled communication regarding ethical issues Facilitate decision making by using select strategies
Phase 3: Creating an Ethical Environment	Preventive ethics Awareness of environmental barriers to ethical practice	Role-model collaborative problem solving Mentor others to develop ethical practice Address barriers to ethical practice through system changes

Phase 1: Knowledge Development

The first phase in the ethical decision-making competency is developing core knowledge in both ethical theories and principles and the ethical issues common to specific patient populations or clinical settings. This dual knowledge enables the advanced practice nursing student to integrate philosophical concepts with contemporary clinical issues. In this initial stage of developing competence in ethical decision making, ethical conduct or comportment is formed and refined. The emphasis in this stage is on cognitive mastery, in which the APN learns the theories, principles, codes, paradigm cases, and relevant laws that influence ethical decision making. With this knowledge, the APN begins to compare current practices in the clinical setting with the ethical standards described in the literature.

Phase 1 is the beginning of the APN's personal journey toward developing a distinct and individualized ethical framework. The work of this phase includes developing sensitivity to the moral dimensions of clinical practice. A helpful initial step in building moral sensitivity is values clarification, where students clarify the personal and professional values that inform their care (Uustal, 1987). Values clarification uncovers personal values that may have been internalized and not openly acknowledged.

Another key aspect of this phase is developing the ability to distinguish a true ethical dilemma from a situation of moral distress or other clinically problematic situation. This requires a general understanding of ethical theories, principles, and standards that help the APN define and discern the essential elements of an ethical dilemma. Novice APNs should be able to recognize a moral problem as an ethical infringement and seek clarification and illumination of the concern. The APN identifies ethical issues and formulates the concerns about which others are uneasy. This step earns credibility and enables the APN to gain self-confidence by bringing the issue to the awareness and attention of others. If the issue remains a moral concern after clarification, the APN should pursue resolution and may seek additional help if needed.

Formal education in ethical theories and concepts should be included in graduate education programs for APNs. While some beginning graduate students will have had significant exposure to ethical issues in their undergraduate programs, most have not. Graduate education builds upon the ethical foundation of professional practice emphasized at the undergraduate level. Moreover, the graduate nursing student brings a knowledge of ethical issues that is blended with clinical experience. The American Association of Colleges of Nursing (1996) proposed that graduate nursing programs provide ethics education and experience for graduate students to understand and analyze the role of personal and professional values in systems of health care. Exposure to ethical theories, principles, and concepts also allows the APN to develop the language necessary to articulate ethical concerns in an interdisciplinary environment. It is important, however, that knowledge development extend beyond classroom discussions. Clinical practicum experiences also need to explicitly build in discussions of ethical dimensions of practice rather than assume such discussions will naturally occur. In one recent study of the clinical experiences in managed care settings of graduate students from four graduate programs, only four (of 20) students identified having experience with an ethical dilemma, and only two (of 22) preceptors noted any exposure to ethical dilemmas for students (Howard & Steinberg, 2002). The authors concluded that this apparent void in clinical education may have been a function of limited recognition of ethical decision-making processes by both APN students and preceptors, an even more compelling commentary on the need for Phase 1 activity in graduate curricula.

As noted, the core knowledge of ethical theories should be supplemented with an understanding of issues central to the patient populations with whom the APN works. As

APNs assume positions in specific clinical areas or with particular patient populations, it is incumbent upon them to gain an understanding of the applicable laws, standards, and regulations, as well as relevant paradigm cases in their specialty. This information may be garnered from current literature in the field, continuing education programs, or discussions with interdisciplinary colleagues. Information on legal and policy guidelines should be offered during graduate practicum experiences in the area of clinical concentration.

While Phase 1 is the building block for the other phases of this competency, it is also an ongoing process. APNs will gain core knowledge in graduate education, but as societal issues change and new technologies emerge, new dilemmas and ethical problems emerge. The ability to be a leader in creating ethical environments involves a commitment to lifelong learning about ethical issues, of which professional education is just the beginning.

Phase 2: Knowledge Application

The second phase of the core competency is applying the knowledge developed in the first level to the practice arena. Phase 2 continues the APN's journey in assessing real ethical problems and being actively involved in the process of resolving ethical dilemmas. As the APN acquires core ethical decision-making knowledge, the responsibility to take moral action becomes more compelling. Rather than retrospectively analyzing ethical dilemmas, the APN takes moral action, which implies that the APN recognizes, pursues, and responds to ethical issues. Moral action requires dedication to work until a resolution is achieved or options are exhausted and courage to pursue emotionally charged and complex ethical problems. Often, the inequities toward or infringements on other persons are enough to motivate moral action, and a timely response can change the course in present, as well as future, situations. Therefore the importance of moral action should not be underestimated as a core APN skill, and it should be recognized, fostered, and valued by others.

Although the core knowledge of ethical concepts such as respect for persons, truthfulness, and beneficence provide the foundation for moral reasoning, the practical application of these concepts enables the APN to evolve the practical wisdom of moral reasoning. It is the experience in the practice setting and the courage of the APN to openly discuss sensitive issues that enable the APN to assume an active role in dispute resolution. The success and speed with which the APN gains these behavioral skills is related to the presence of mentors in the clinical setting and the willingness of the APN to become immersed in ethical discussions.

Institutional resources such as ethics committees and institutional review boards provide valuable opportunities for APNs to participate in the discussion of ethical issues. Typically, hospital ethics committees serve three functions: policy formation, case review, and education (Spencer, 1997). As a member of the ethics committee, the APN exchanges ideas with colleagues and gains an understanding of ethical dilemmas from a variety of perspectives. In addition, the APN is informed of current legislation, regulations, and hospital policies that have ethical implications. This is an extremely valuable experience that can accelerate the development of ethical decision-making skills.

Unfortunately, the majority of APNs do not have the opportunity to serve on an interdisciplinary ethics committee, and in some cases, may have few professional colleagues available to mentor and develop the skills of ethical decision making. Thus the APN must advance this phase by actively seeking opportunities to engage in ethical dialogue with professional colleagues. Professional organizations offer workshops in which case studies are discussed and analyzed. This format is helpful to the inexperienced APN who needs guidance in applying knowledge to clinical cases.

Ideally, students should be given the opportunity to be actively involved in the ethical decision-making process with a clinical case during their graduate clinical experiences. Debriefing the situation with their preceptor can be a powerful learning experience, and such structured clinical experiences can greatly assist the student in moving to Phase 2 of this competency. At a minimum, students should have the opportunity to observe this process in action in their clinical work with advanced practice nursing preceptors. Clearly, preceptors who are themselves comfortable and skilled in the ethical decision-making competency are required for students to have this experience. If an APN graduate has not had such experiences, she or he will need to develop these behavioral skills in the clinical setting.

Phase 3: Creating an Ethical Environment

The quality of the ethical environment is a critical factor in whether ethical problems are productively addressed. In a recent study of NPs, the participants' perceptions of the ethical environment was the strongest predictor of ethical conflict in practice; the more ethical the environment, the lower was the ethical conflict (Ulrich, Soeken, & Miller, 2003). The APN's level of influence needs to extend beyond the individual patient encounter to create a climate in which ethical concerns are routinely addressed.

As the APN becomes more skilled in the application of ethical knowledge, the third phase of competence begins to develop. Role modeling and mentoring others regarding ethical decision making and creating an ethical environment are leadership behaviors seen in the practice of the mature APN. Once the APN transforms ethical knowledge into moral action, the role of mentoring others emerges. Often, other nurses and members of the health-care team remain silent about ethical issues. In a mentoring capacity, the APN helps colleagues deal with moral uncertainty and develop the ability to voice ethical concerns. In this way, the APN supports and empowers other team members to develop confidence in raising ethical concerns and fosters an environment in which diverse views are expressed and problems are moved toward resolution. The experienced APN also initiates informal learning opportunities for nurses and other professional colleagues. Ethics rounds and case review are two ways to engage colleagues in the discussion of moral issues.

The roots of interdisciplinary conflict in the clinical setting are often based on preconceived stereotypes of the moral viewpoints of other disciplines and perceptions of the moral superiority of one's own discipline (Shannon, 1997). The APN can help professionals from other disciplines understand the perspectives and socialization of nurses. In addition, the APN models successful negotiation with other disciplines. Teaching and mentoring activities of the mature APN often focus on other professional colleagues, to proactively prepare them to openly communicate with patients about ethical concerns. Often, the more experienced APN has developed professional working relationships with colleagues that are based on trust and mutual respect. One way for APNs to maintain the respect of professional colleagues is to acquire ethical knowledge and expertise in their area.

This important role of the APN also encompasses aspects of coaching and teaching patients and families in ethical decision making. It is not sufficient for the APN to simply provide information to patients and families facing difficult moral choices and expect them to arrive at a comfortable decision. The ethical competency is linked closely with the ability to mobilize patients and the APN's colleagues so that those who need help move through the necessary steps to reach resolution.

APNs should strive to develop environments that encourage patients and caregivers to express diverse views and raise questions about the ethical elements of clinical care.

Thoughtful ethical decision making arises from an environment that supports and values the critical exchange of ideas and promotes collaboration among members of the health care team, patients, and families. A collaborative practice environment, in turn, supports shared decision making, shared accountability, and group participation; and it fosters relationships based on equality and mutuality (Pike, 1991). Clearly, resolutions that originate from collaborative processes are more satisfactory, generate more creative solutions, and strengthen relationships (Spielman, 1993). The APN is integral to the development and preservation of a collaborative climate that inspires and empowers individuals to respond to moral dilemmas.

The nature of health-care delivery in both inpatient and outpatient settings creates a climate in which many workers feel overwhelmed, stressed, and discouraged by the lack of time to care for patients and their increased acuity levels. Over time, such climates can actually cause nurses and others to become accustomed and insensitive to the structures and the dilemmas around them (Chambliss, 1996). Combined with a sense of powerlessness, these factors can result in nurses retreating from a stance of moral agency. An ethically sensitive environment is one in which providers are encouraged to acknowledge when they feel overwhelmed and seek help when they need it (Scott, Aiken, Mechanic, & Moravcsik, 1995). The ANA's revised *Code of Ethics for Nurses* (ANA, 2001) affirms the importance of nurses contributing to an ethically sensitive health-care environment, as well as preserving personal integrity. Indeed, one new provision of the *Code of Ethics* states, "The nurse owes the same duties to self as to others, including the responsibility to preserve integrity and safety . . . " (p. 4). Only when care providers recognize and attend to their personal needs will they be better able to detect and nurture the needs of others.

As APNs become more competent and capable in ethical reasoning, they are able to anticipate situations in which moral conflicts will occur and recognize the more subtle presentations of moral dilemmas. The ability to look beyond the immediate situation and foresee potential issues directs the APN down a path of preventive ethics.

PREVENTIVE ETHICS

Ethical decision-making skills enable the APN to focus on identifying the values in conflict and developing a course of action suitable to the parties in dispute. This approach, however, concentrates on the resolution of current and ongoing issues rather than preventing the recurrence of moral dilemmas (Forrow, Arnold, & Parker, 1993). An additional important role of the APN is to extend the concept of ethical decision making beyond problem solving in individual cases and to move toward a paradigm of preventive ethics. Preventive ethics is derived from the model of preventive medicine (Forrow et al., 1993). An ethical environment fosters early identification of issues and anticipation of possible dilemmas. The ability to predict areas of conflict and develop plans in a proactive, rather than reactive, manner will avert some potentially difficult dilemmas (Benner, 1991; Forrow et al., 1993). When value conflicts arise, resolution is more difficult because one value must be chosen over another. Preventive ethics emphasizes that all important values should be reviewed and examined prior to the conflict so that situations in which values may differ can be anticipated (Forrow et al., 1993). In other words, the goals of the health-care team should be articulated as clearly as possible to avoid potential misinterpretations. For example, a certified registered nurse anesthetist should have an understanding of a terminally ill patient's values regarding aggressive treatment should a cardiopulmonary arrest occur during surgery. However, the certified registered nurse anesthetist's moral and legal obligations should be openly discussed so that the patient and professional appreciate and recognize each other's values and moral and legal positions.

The concept of preventive ethics can be modeled after the paradigm of palliative care. When a patient is first diagnosed with a terminal condition, efforts often focus on a potential cure or at least a delay of rapid decline. However, caregivers recognize that palliative care and symptom management will become a focus of care in the future. The responsibility of caregivers is to discuss the potential need to change the goals of management as the patient's condition deteriorates. In this way, the patient, family, and caregivers anticipate and acknowledge that changes in the patient's condition that will alter the goals of care are expected and will be addressed. Modeling this preventive approach in ethical deliberations encourages the early identification of values and beliefs that may influence treatment decisions and allows time to resolve impending issues before problems arise. In much the same way, early anticipation of potential complications in patient trajectories can lead to proactive discussions of ethical issues and restructuring of the care environment to anticipate and avoid ethical conflict.

In addition to the early examination and ongoing dialogue regarding values, a conscientious inspection of other factors that influence the evolution of moral dilemmas is required. The roles and responsibilities of all parties must be clearly defined to expose any existing power imbalance. During this process, issues of powerlessness and collaborative practice surface as areas in which the APN can influence change. By providing knowledge, promoting a positive self-image, and preparing others for participation in decision making, the APN empowers individuals. The skill of the APN is used not to resolve moral dilemmas single-handedly but to mentor others to assume a position of moral accountability and engage in shared decision making. This process of enhancing others' autonomy and providing opportunities for involvement in reaching resolution is a key concept in preventive ethics (Forrow et al., 1993). Although many ethical issues will develop with little warning, the practice of preventive ethics will improve the delivery of morally responsible, innovative, and humanistic patient care.

Preventive ethics environments are enhanced by a process of ongoing, rather than episodic, ethical inquiry. This approach to moral reflection sanctions open discussions of values and divergent views and is realized through reciprocal information exchange between members of the health-care team and the patient. Throughout this process, the APN incorporates the skills, ethical expertise, and clinical background on issues necessary to facilitate dialogue, mediate disputes, analyze options, and design optimal solutions. Therefore the ethical decision-making skills of the APN move the resolution of moral dilemmas beyond individual cases toward the cultivation of an environment in which the moral integrity of individuals is respected. Development and preservation of this ethical environment is the key contribution of the APN.

ACQUIRING AND DEVELOPING ETHICAL DECISION-MAKING COMPETENCE

The skills needed to identify, articulate, and address ethical dilemmas are complex and diverse. Particular strategies, such as those used in values clarification, negotiation, and mediation, provide a foundation for the practice aspects of ethical decision making. The APN must understand the theoretical elements of biomedical ethics and be aware of paradigm cases and relevant law to interpret moral issues in the health-care setting. Effective and compassionate communication skills undergird this competency.

Developing an Educational Foundation

As noted, education in ethical theories, principles, rules, and moral concepts provides the foundation for developing skills in ethical reasoning. Through graduate education, the APN studies models of ethical decision making and is introduced to the importance of understanding value systems. Because the APN will apply the theoretical principles in actual encounters with patients, it is imperative that consideration of the contextual factors in specific situations be strengthened. A portion of graduate ethics education should involve discussion of typical issues encountered by APNs, rather than issues that receive extensive media attention yet occur infrequently. Howard and Steinberg (2002) maintained that graduate curricula to prepare APNs to deal with managed care ethics needed to go beyond traditional ethical issues to encompass resource allocation decisions, individual versus population-based responsibilities, building trust in the APN-patient relationship, professionalism and patient advocacy, and managing tensions between business ethics and professional ethics.

Continuing education programs are also effective and necessary forums in which current information can be provided in a rapidly changing health-care environment. Ethical issues are dynamic and re-emerge in altered forms. As technology changes and new dilemmas confront practitioners, the APN must be prepared to anticipate conditions that erode an ethical environment. Knowledge and skills in all phases of developing this competency depend on the application of current ethical knowledge in the clinical setting. Ethical reasoning and clinical judgments share a common process, and each serves to teach and inform the other (Dreyfus et al., 1996; Leavitt, 1996; Solomon et al., 1991). Therefore the importance of clinical practice cannot be overemphasized.

OVERVIEW OF ETHICAL THEORIES

Although ethical decision making in health care is extensively discussed in the bioethics literature, two dominant models are most often applied in the clinical setting. The first model of decision making is a principle-based model (Box 11-1) in which ethical decision making is guided by theories, principles, and rules (Beauchamp & Childress, 2001). In

---

BOX 11-1 • PRINCIPLES AND RULES IMPORTANT TO PROFESSIONAL NURSING PRACTICE

Principle of Respect for Autonomy	The duty to respect others' personal liberty and individual values, beliefs, and choices
Principle of Nonmaleficence	The duty not to inflict harm or evil
Principle of Beneficence	The duty to do good and prevent or remove harm
Principle of Formal Justice	The duty to treat equals equally and treat those who are unequal according to their needs
Rule of Veracity	The duty to tell the truth and not to deceive others
Rule of Fidelity	The duty to honor commitments
Rule of Confidentiality	The duty not to disclose information shared in an intimate and trusted manner
Rule of Privacy	The duty to respect limited access to a person

Definitions adapted from Beauchamp, T. L., Childress, J. F. (2001). *Principles of biomedical ethics* (5th ed.). New York: Oxford University Press.

cases of conflict, the principles or rules in contention are balanced and interpreted with the contextual elements of the situation. However, the final decision and moral justification for actions are based on an appeal to principles. In this way, the principles are both binding and tolerant of the particularities of specific cases (Beauchamp & Childress, 2001; Childress, 1994).

The principles of respect for persons, autonomy, beneficence, nonmaleficence, and justice are commonly applied in the analysis of ethical issues in nursing. The ANA's *Code of Ethics for Nurses* (2001) endorses the principle of respect for persons and underscores the profession's commitment to serving individuals, families, and groups or communities. The emphasis on respect for persons throughout the *Code* implies that it is not only a philosophical value of nursing but also a binding principle within the profession.

Although ethical principles and rules are the cornerstone of most ethical decisions, the principle-based approach has been criticized as too formalistic for many clinicians and as lacking in moral substance (Clouser & Gert, 1990). Other critics argue that a principle-based approach conceals the particular person and relationships and reduces the resolution of a clinical case to simply balancing principles (Gudorf, 1994). Consequently, when conflicts among principles occur, the description of the principle is inadequate to provide guidance for moral action (Clouser & Gert, 1990; Childress, 1994).

The second approach to ethical decision making is the casuistic model, in which current cases are compared with paradigm cases (Beauchamp & Childress, 2001; Jonsen & Toulmin, 1988; Toulmin, 1994). The strength of this approach is that a dilemma is examined in a context-specific manner and then compared with an analogous earlier case. The fundamental philosophical assumption of this model is that ethics emerges from human moral experiences. The casuists approach dilemmas from an inductive position and work from the specific case to generalizations, rather than from generalizations to specific cases (Beauchamp & Childress, 2001; Gaul, 1995).

Some concerns arise when a casuistic model for ethical decision making is evaluated. As a moral dilemma arises, the selection of the paradigm case may differ among the decision makers, and thus the interpretation of the appropriate course of action will vary. In nursing, there are few paradigm cases of ethical issues on which to construct a decision-making process. Furthermore, other than the reliance on previous cases, casuists have no mechanisms to justify their actions. The possibility that previous cases were reasoned in a faulty or inaccurate manner may not be fully considered or evaluated (Beauchamp & Childress, 2001). In spite of these concerns, the case-based moral reasoning employed in casuistry appeals to clinicians because it mimics clinical reasoning, in which providers often appeal to earlier similar cases to make clinical judgments. Artnak and Dimmitt (1996) applied the casuistic model to an analysis of a complex case, concluding that the use of this approach allowed more full consideration of the contextual particulars of the case and a systematic approach for organizing and analyzing the facts of the case.

More recently, there has been great interest in narrative approaches to ethical deliberation (Charon, 1994; Nelson, 1997). Narrative ethics emphasizes particular stories as vehicles for discerning the meaning and values embedded in ethical decision making. The argument is that all knowing is bound up in a narrative tradition and that "all participants in an ethical deliberation—the medical ethicist, the health professionals, the patient, and the patient's family—require that which only narrative knowledge can give: the coherence, the resonance, and the singular meaning of particular human events" (Charon, 1994, p. 261). Narrative ethics begins with a patient's story and has some similarities with casuistry in its inductive, particularistic approach. There are a number of formulations of narrative ethics, each making claims about the importance of narrative to moral justification and challenging the dominant mode of ethical justification, namely appeal to principles (Arras,

1997). Critics of this approach have argued that while narrative is a necessary element in ethical analysis, it cannot supplant principle- or theory-based ethics (Arras, 1997; Childress, 1997). There is growing recognition that careful consideration of patient's stories can enlarge and enrich ethical deliberations; in commenting on narrative versus principle-based approaches, Childress (1997) noted, "We need both in any adequate ethics" (p. 268). As with casuistry, narrative-based approaches appeal to nurses, who find much of the meaning in their work in entering into the stories of their patient's lives. A more thorough discussion of narrative ethics is beyond the scope of this chapter, but the reader is referred to the references cited for more detail on this approach.

Other theories, such as utilitarianism, Kantianism, virtue-based theory, and care-based theory, provide alternative processes for moral reflection and argument (Beauchamp & Childress, 2001). In particular, the ethics of care has emerged as relevant to nursing (Cooper, 1989). The care perspective constructs moral problems as issues surrounding the intrinsic needs and corresponding responsibilities that occur within relationships (Cooper, 1989; Gilligan, 1982). Moral reasoning involves empathy and emphasizes responsibilities rather than rights. The response of the individual to a moral dilemma emerges from the affiliate relationship and the norms of friendship, care, and love (Beauchamp & Childress, 2001; Cooper, 1991). Viens (1995) found that NPs she interviewed used a moral reasoning process that mirrored Gilligan's model in the major themes of caring and responsibility.

Although every ethical theory has some limitations and problems, an understanding of contemporary approaches to ethics and bioethics is a central feature in achieving a moral resolution. In the clinical setting, ethical decision making most often reflects a blend of the various theories rather than the application of a single theory (Aronheim, Moreno, & Zuckerman, 2000).

PROFESSIONAL CODES AND GUIDELINES

Frequently the ANA's *Code of Ethics for Nurses* (2001) is used in undergraduate and graduate education to introduce the moral beliefs of the nursing profession. The *Code* serves a worthy function by describing the profession's philosophy and the general ethical obligations of the professional nurse. However, the *Code* describes broad guidelines that more reflect the profession's conscience than provide specific directions for particular clinical situations. In this sense, the *Code* provides a framework that delineates the nurse's overriding moral obligations to the patient, family, community, and profession but offers little specific help in balancing competing demands from the institution and other health-care professionals.

Professional organizations delineate standards of performance that reflect the responsibilities, obligations, duties, and rights of the members. These standards serve as guidelines for professional behavior and define desired conduct. Although the general principles are relatively stable, professional organizations often reflect on contemporary issues and assume a proactive posture on pivotal concerns. For example, the American Association of Critical-Care Nurses (2000) issued a position statement on maintaining patient-focused care in environments with nursing shortages and fiscal constraints. APNs must be familiar with the profession's position on topics relevant to the area of practice. Some degree of involvement with professional and specialty organizations is necessary to strengthen the APN's voice in guiding the profession's moral accountability to the public.

PERSONAL AND PROFESSIONAL VALUES

During graduate education, the APN should be introduced to the concept of value systems and undergo a process of values clarification. Individuals' interpretations and positions on issues are a reflection of their underlying value system. Value systems are enduring beliefs that guide life choices and decisions in conflict resolution (Uustal, 1987; Ludwick & Silva, 2000). Viens (1995) found that values were an essential feature of the everyday practice of the 10 primary care NPs she interviewed. Values of caring, responsibility, trust, justice, honesty, sanctity/quality of life, empathy, and religious beliefs were articulated by study participants. "Values were ideals that motivated the nurse practitioners as persons and as nurses. Values, therefore, played a part in the NP role, and this nursing role in turn played a part in defining values....the relationship between the environment, the NP role, and values was interlinked" (Viens, 1995, p. 280). An awareness of personal values generates more consistent choices and behaviors and can also assist APNs to be aware of the boundaries of their personal and professional values so they can recognize when their own positions may be unduly influencing patient and family decision making (Mahon, Deatrick, McKnight, & Mohr, 2000). Values clarification enables students to define and analyze their personal and professional beliefs, attitudes, and value systems (Saulo & Wagener, 1996). Uustal (1987) developed a number of interesting exercises in values clarification.

One effective approach to values education is to teach the concepts and skills of values clarification as part of an interdisciplinary course. This process enables health professional students to appreciate and articulate the personal and professional values that influence their behavior and to recognize and respect the values of other team members, patients, and families. Such education expands the health-care team's awareness of each other's professional beliefs and can also facilitate the decision making of patients and surrogates in the clinical setting. Careful examination of the patient's values enhances treatment decision making and clarifies the motivations underlying the individual's expressed wishes and treatment preferences for the health-care team (Doukas & Gorenflo, 1993; Doukas & McCullough, 1991).

Values awareness should include an understanding of the complex interplay between cultural values and ethical decision making (Buryska, 2001; Long, 2000; Ludwig & Silva, 2000; Wright, Cohen, & Caroselli, 1997). When patient/family decisions contradict traditional Western medical practice, health-care providers may resort to coercive or paternalistic measures to influence patient's choices to be more consistent with the provider's values. APNs and other health-care providers must understand the assumptions they make based on their own cultural values and biases and how these assumptions may influence their recommendations of particular treatments. As health-care professionals gain an understanding of factors that guide a person's decisions, treatment plans that reflect the patient's value preferences are more easily developed. For example, a patient from a Southeast Asian culture may show respect to authority figures by obeying the APN's treatment suggestions, even if he or she disagrees with the plan. In this situation, the APN could assure the patient that questions about the plan of care are welcomed and are not disrespectful (Wright et al., 1997).

By the same token, claims made in the name of religious and cultural beliefs are not absolute (Orr & Genesen, 1997; Buryska, 2001). Buryska (2001) offers a number of helpful guidelines for clinicians to consider in assessing the defensibility of patient and family claims made in the name of cultural or religious considerations. For example, he maintains that spiritual or cultural claims grounded in an identifiable and established community are more defensible than those that are idiosyncratic to the person making the claim. While it is critical for caregivers to respond with respectful dialogue, support, and compassionate care, patient/family demands for treatment must be considered in relation to other claims that also have ethical weight: the professional integrity of providers, legal considerations, economic realities, and issues of distributive justice.

PROFESSIONAL BOUNDARIES

In their professional capacity, APNs have access to personal and private information about their patients. The atmosphere of intimacy in the nurse-patient relationship coupled with the need to touch the patient during a physical examination sets up a power differential that accentuates the patient's vulnerability. Boundaries must be established that acknowledge the appropriate and necessary use of this patient information to meet the patient's needs and provide care. It is the responsibility of the APN to establish and maintain the professional boundaries of the therapeutic relationship and uphold the patient's needs and rights.

Boundary violations, in which the APN or another health-care professional either inadvertently or purposely breaches the limits and expectations of the relationship, may profoundly alter the foundation of a therapeutic relationship. Such transgressions may be subtle, such as the APN sharing excessive personal information, or blatant, as in sexually seductive behavior. Regardless of the magnitude of the violation, the behavior must be confronted immediately, and the culpable individual must be removed from interaction with the patient. Other members of the health-care team should strive to restore the patient's integrity and trust, involving the help of others as necessary (National Council of State Boards of Nursing, Inc., 1996).

Developing Skills in Ethical Decision Making

As noted, acquiring the skills and competence to facilitate the resolution of moral dilemmas is an evolutionary process. Because ethical decision making is not exclusively based on theoretical knowledge, moral reasoning must be tempered with clinical reality. As APNs gain the necessary knowledge and skills in ethical decision making, their involvement should intensify and become more extensive. *Once an advanced nursing role is assumed, the APN accepts the responsibility to be a full participant in the resolution of moral dilemmas rather than simply an interested observer or one of many parties in conflict.*

A number of decision-making frameworks have been proposed in the literature (Noland, 1999; Fry, 1994; Savage & Milton, 1989; Taylor, 1997). One procedural framework nurses can use in ethical decision making is to adapt the nursing process as a framework to organize and guide the gathering of morally relevant information (Box 11-2). This framework enables the APN to systematically organize the facts and contextual particularities of a dilemma. Although a framework provides structure and suggests a method of examining and studying the ethical issues, the essential component to resolution of ethical dilemmas is moral action. Simply knowing the right course of action does not guarantee that a person has the motivation or courage to act (Rest, 1986). Successful resolution of moral issues requires a blend of knowledge, conviction, emotions, beliefs, and individual character (van Hooft, 1990).

PROBLEM IDENTIFICATION

Ethical dilemmas and situations of moral distress are often first recognized by the intense emotional reactions they elicit. Emotions are present in all clinical settings, but when personal or professional values are questioned or trespassed, the instinctive response is to react with anger or frustration. Although this is a helpful gauge to awaken awareness that something may be amiss ethically, too often the individual becomes entangled in the emotions and is unable to move toward an awareness of the consequences for others. It is frequently this point at which the differing parties become polarized and embedded in a

---

BOX 11-2 • USE OF THE NURSING PROCESS IN ETHICAL DECISION MAKING

STEP	DESCRIPTION
1: Assessment	Problem identification
	Information gathering
	Medical facts
	Nursing facts
	Values, rights, and obligations of parties
	Other relevant factors
	Culture
	Religion
	Relationships
	Other contextual features
2: Plan	Strategies for resolution
	Collaboration
	Compromise
	Accommodation
	Coercion
	Avoidance
3: Implementation	Initiate a moral action
4: Evaluation	Process
	Outcome

---

particular viewpoint. A difficult but important step in problem identification is to allow and encourage the individuals in conflict to openly express their emotions. This action demonstrates that the perspectives and the emotional responses to the issue are legitimate and meaningful (Fisher & Ury, 1981). As a facilitator, the APN should recognize, understand, and acknowledge the emotions of all parties.

Many conflicts that arise in the clinical setting generate powerful emotional responses yet may not be ethical issues. Ethical issues involve some form of controversy concerning moral values and/or fundamental duties or obligations (Ahronheim, Moreno, & Zuckerman, 2000). It is essential that the APN distinguish and separate moral dilemmas from other issues such as administrative concerns, communication problems, or lack of clinical knowledge. With moral distress, it is not uncommon that staff may be reacting without a complete or accurate picture of the situation; once the facts are clear, the problem's resolution may become evident (Hamric, 2000). For example, less experienced staff may call an APN to resolve a dilemma in pain management. The less experienced nurse's interpretation is that the physician ordered an inadequate dose of an analgesic to manage the patient's symptoms. The nurse requested an increased dosage for the patient, but the physician refused. The APN may determine that the severity of the disease process requires the addition of another analgesic to enhance the effects of the original medication ordered. The issue encountered was not a moral issue but instead reflected problems with nurse-physician communication and the lack of knowledge regarding appropriate pharmacological management.

INFORMATION GATHERING

Once the ethical problem is identified, the APN implements a process to gather and examine the morally relevant facts. Generally, information such as the medical and nursing clinical situation; the values, rights, and obligations of the patient and others; legal factors; and cultural and religious factors should be gathered when the decision-making process is initiated. However, these facts are insufficient if they are not tempered with the contextual features of each case. Identifying the cause of the problem and determining why, where, and when it occurred, as well as whom or what was affected, will help clarify the nature of the problem (Beare, 1989). Only after the unique conditions of the case are considered can an ethically acceptable solution be identified.

Strategies for Resolution of Ethical Conflict

Moral discussions and deliberation can take the form of a debate that degenerates into an assault. One party presents an argument, the other party disputes it, the original party defends, and the second party attacks (Zaner, 1988). Breaking this cycle of destructive interactions is central to arriving at solutions that are resourceful and constructive. Resolutions are most effective when the parties in dispute create the solution.

When the APN is directly involved in a conflict situation, the skills of negotiation are most useful in moving toward a satisfactory settlement. However, in cases in which resolution is not easily achieved, it is best to solicit help from a member of the ethics committee or another professional colleague not involved in the case. The challenge in most cases of ethical disputes is to have all involved listen to each other's perspectives to understand the basis of the disagreement and to work together to create a collaborative solution (Saulo & Wagener, 1996). In many cases, the APN must serve as a facilitator for the parties in dispute and apply the strategies involved in mediation. The key difference between these roles is the level of active involvement in deciding the goals and strategies of resolving the dilemma. As a negotiating party, the APN suggests solutions and identifies acceptable plans (Beare, 1989). In the role of a mediator, the APN guides the process but does not offer opinions or solutions (Ostermeyer, 1991). The process and steps used in negotiation and mediation overlap in many ways, and in both approaches the parties in conflict discover and determine the acceptable solutions (Beare, 1989; Dubler & Marcus, 1994; Ostermeyer, 1991).

The objective of successful negotiation and mediation in ethical disputes is to achieve an integrity-preserving solution that is satisfactory to all parties. In reality, however, that is not always possible. The issues of time, cost, available resources, level of moral certainty, and the perceived value of the relationship play important roles in the strategy used and likelihood of reaching a desired outcome (Spielman, 1993). These issues are addressed later in the section "Barriers to Ethical Practice and Potential Solutions." The following strategies for negotiation are useful when the APN is facilitating resolution between two parties and when the professional or personal values of the APN collide with the values of others.

COLLABORATION

Collaboration is the preferred strategy for achieving a moral resolution. This section focuses on identifying and cultivating the elements necessary for collaboration regarding ethical problems. A full description of collaboration and additional methods to foster a collaborative environment are presented in Chapter 10.

The first step in the process of collaboration is to help the disputing parties agree on the issue in conflict and to understand both the cognitive and the emotional perspectives of each party. As noted earlier, because emotions maintain a significant position in moral dilemmas, it is important to provide an environment in which the parties can release unexpressed emotions without being judged. This first step toward moral resolution is particularly difficult, because people in power are often less interested in and less likely to acknowledge the perspectives of those with lesser power (Welton, 1991; Hamric, 2000). To eliminate this power imbalance, the responsibility and accountability of all parties in the negotiation process must be openly acknowledged and agreed upon. One strategy to move other parties toward a collaborative approach is for the APN to be the first to acknowledge her or his understanding of the issue. In this way the APN establishes the ground rules of open communication and mutual respect that frame the process in a collaborative and shared model of decision making.

The second step toward successful collaborative moral resolution is to engage all involved parties in active interactions and consensus building (Krouse & Roberts, 1989). Information presented should be questioned, analyzed, and examined. It is important to focus on the *interests* of each party rather than the *positions*. Asking the questions "why?" and "why not?" can identify interests of the involved individuals (Fisher & Ury, 1981). From this stage of active communication and interaction, the process of consensus building begins.

The third step in negotiating or mediating a moral resolution involves formulating a decision and developing a plan of action. The objective of both negotiation and mediation is to generate options and solutions that are consistent with all parties' principles and achieve an outcome that is mutually satisfying (Dubler & Marcus, 1994; Ostermeyer, 1991; Ury, 1993). Although this may initially seem unlikely, particularly if individuals are attached to their own positions, the APN can facilitate progression through complex situations by using communication skills such as reframing, identifying shared interests and needs, and examining the differences (Fisher & Ury, 1981; Smeltzer, 1991).

Although implementation of a collaborative process for the resolution of moral dilemmas is most desired, other approaches to manage conflict may be employed. The choice to employ another strategy for resolution may be deliberate or inadvertent, and there are distinct advantages and disadvantages with other methods. However, an environment in which collaborative conflict resolution is consistently avoided may be negating the importance of resolving ethical issues in a morally sensitive manner. The APN should recognize this pattern and work toward developing an environment that supports collaborative decision making.

COMPROMISE

When both parties possess a high level of moral certainty in their positions and are committed to preserving the relationship, they may choose to bargain and to have each party relinquish some control over the decision. This can be a time-consuming strategy because each party must determine what are acceptable tradeoffs. Problems are resolved through compromise when both parties are willing to waive some components of their moral position and embrace a position of cooperation (Spielman, 1993). For example, a chronically ill patient with dilated cardiomyopathy may refuse in-hospital management of the heart failure but agree to a short-term solution, such as a trial of intravenous therapy at home.

The clinical context in primary care settings often requires collaboration or compromise as an approach to moral resolution. In these situations the patient and APN maintain high degrees of commitment to the relationship. In addition, most encounters are nonemergent, and thus time is available for engaging in compromise and collaboration.

ACCOMMODATION

In some cases, one party will accommodate and simply agree to support the other's position. Accommodation frequently occurs when the issue is trivial, time is limited, or only one party holds a high level of commitment to preserving the relationship with the other participant (Spielman, 1993). In situations of a significant power imbalance between nurses and physicians, nurses may resort to this approach. Accommodation is sometimes employed as a tactic in negotiation. The concession is made to dissipate friction and additionally to imply that a reciprocal action is expected in future negotiations with the other party. However, accommodation is an inappropriate strategy when it is used routinely to gain acceptance or merely to avoid conflict.

COERCION

A coercive and controlling approach may be used when time is short, such as in an emergency, or when the party has little commitment to the relationship. This approach is often aggressive and competitive and reflects a high degree of commitment to a particular moral position (Spielman, 1993). Because control of the decision is assumed by one party and the differing perspectives are discounted, this approach damages the self-esteem of the other party and may result in a sense of powerlessness and moral outrage (Pike, 1991).

Although a coercive approach is aggressive and often undesirable in resolving ethical conflict, it is sometimes necessary. For example, when a child whose parents are Jehovah's Witnesses must emergently receive a blood transfusion and the parents refuse to give consent for the treatment, legal approval is sought. Time, in this case, is limited, and the caregivers are convinced of the moral rightness of their views, just as the parents are convinced of their moral position. Because the child's well-being depends on prompt action, the caregivers are limited to a coercive approach for resolution. In this case, the law usually compels the parents to permit treatment of the minor child.

AVOIDANCE

Participants may avoid, ignore, or deny the dilemma when the moral issue is perceived as trivial or, conversely, is deeply felt by one party and highly charged emotionally. Avoidance is also seen when time is short (Spielman, 1993). If a decision is unnecessary, it may be appropriate for a participant to withdraw from the process of decision making. However, this strategy is often employed when the participant abdicates moral accountability. The APN should consciously monitor avoidance behaviors and pursue the rationale for this approach. It is likely that the individual who practices this technique regularly avoids conflict and would benefit from additional knowledge, support, and role modeling of more effective approaches to conflict management.

There is an additional dynamic that may be operating in environments where avoidance is the norm in dealing with ethical conflict. In a report of three studies of nurses in acute care settings, Chambliss (1996) identified a phenomenon he called *routinization of the world*. He noted that over time, nurses became accustomed and desensitized to the hospital world. This acceptance was at times accompanied by a qualitative transformation in the nurses' thinking, which was often not recognized. The routine blunted the nurses' moral sensitivity and moral agency, so that moral difficulties were not recognized; nurses commented, "You just get used to it." Chambliss noted that nurses were aware of problems but often did not see them as "ethics problems," and neither did those in authority. The great ethical danger in such an environment is not that nurses would make the wrong choice when faced with an important decision, but rather that they would never realize that they are facing a decision at all. APNs must be alert for signs of routinization of the moral world in the environments where they practice. Individuals who consistently evade moral dilemmas may benefit from values clarification exercises to help them explore deeply held values and to learn ways to deal with them more productively. In addition, identifying and addressing features of the system that blunt or dismiss the moral sensitivity of any care provider is a critical part of advanced practice nursing leadership in the moral arena.

EVALUATION OF THE ETHICAL DECISION-MAKING COMPETENCY

The evaluation of ethical decision making should focus on two areas: the process and the outcome. Process evaluation is important because it provides an overview of the moral disagreement, the interpersonal skills employed, the interactions between both parties in conflict, and the problems encountered during the phases of resolution. Whether the APN was the facilitator or a party in conflict, a deliberate and reflective evaluation of the process of resolution should occur (Olczak, Grosch, & Duffy, 1991). It is useful for the APN to assess the type of issue, the interrelational and situational variables, the conceptual shifts that occurred during the process, and the strategies used by both parties during the negotiation phase (Olczak et al., 1991). As the APN reflects on the process, attention should be given to how similar situations could be anticipated and resolved in the future. Deliberate and consistent review of the process will help the APN assess various approaches to the resolution of ethical dilemmas and identify the onset of moral conflict earlier.

Evaluation of the outcome is also critical because it acknowledges creative solutions and celebrates moral action. Components of the outcome evaluation include the short-term and long-term consequences of the action taken and the satisfaction of all parties with the chosen solution (Olczak et al., 1991). Unfortunately, a successful process does not always result in a satisfactory outcome. Occasionally, the outcome reveals the need for changes within the institution or health-care system. The APN may choose to become involved in advancing these identified changes or identifying appropriate resources to pursue the desired objectives. The goal of the outcome evaluation is to minimize the risks of a similar event by identifying predictable patterns and thereby averting recurrent and future dilemmas.

Although evaluation of the ethical problem is an important step in preventing future dilemmas and building ethically sensitive environments, in some situations tension and uneasiness will remain. In true ethical dilemmas, even the best process may still result in a course of action that is not seen positively by all participants. It is important for the APN to acknowledge that many issues leave a "moral residue" that continues to trouble participants involved in the conflict. Part of the outcome evaluation must address the reality of these lingering feelings and the related tensions they create.

BARRIERS TO ETHICAL PRACTICE AND POTENTIAL SOLUTIONS

A number of factors influence how moral issues are addressed and resolved in the clinical setting. Some barriers, once identified, can be corrected and eliminated. Other issues that impede the resolution of ethical issues may require attention at the institutional, state, or national level. Regardless of the nature of the barrier, the APN must identify and respond to the barriers that inhibit the development of a morally responsive environment.

Intraprofessional Barriers

The APN often relies on other nurses and caregivers to recognize ethical issues and initiate dialogue with professional colleagues. In some situations, nurses are uncertain, fearful, insecure, unable to articulate their moral concern, or incapable of taking moral action (Pike, 1991). Nurses who do not feel secure with their ethical knowledge may dismiss an issue as insignificant or discount and minimize their perceptions of the dilemma. Unfortunately, too many ethical issues are "swept under the rug" because of this moral uncertainty and inaction. It is far better for nurses to raise a concern that may be viewed as insignificant than to wait for the problem to erupt with chaos and conflict. It is often the case that others are also concerned about the issue but have not voiced their perspective for fear of having their viewpoint invalidated.

Conflict between the nurse's personal values and the professional values of nursing may be a source of moral distress. As noted, the ANA *Code of Ethics for Nurses* (2001) elucidates the professional values of nursing, and professional nurses are accountable for practicing in a way that is congruent with the *Code*. In some cases, a nurse's personal values may conflict with the professional values, and the nurse may feel confused and distressed when faced with choosing a response. For example, an emergency room NP may be faced with providing care for a criminal injured in a gunfight that killed innocent bystanders. Although it is disturbing and difficult to provide care for an individual who has caused harm to others, the NP's personal views should not interfere with the quality of the care provided. The process of values clarification is helpful in preparing nurses for this situation. Once personal values are realized, the nurse can more easily anticipate situations in which such conflicts will arise and either avoid becoming part of the problem or develop a defined strategy to deal with the issue.

Perceptions of powerlessness influence how active nurses become in the resolution of ethical dilemmas (Erlen & Frost, 1991; Gaul, 1995). Powerlessness can be both an intraprofessional and an interprofessional barrier. Power issues between the APN and bedside nurse may evolve because the bedside nurse views the APN as having enhanced decision-making authority and a more direct line of communication to the physician. A sense of powerlessness suggests that the bedside nurse feels incapable or ineffective in changing the situation or correcting the problem. Certainly, in some cases, the sense of powerlessness is a reality. For example, nurses may not be able to change a managed care organization's perspective on the approved length of stay for a specific diagnosis-related group (DRG). However, all problems can be dissected into smaller parts, and the APN can work on more manageable components of the issue.

Feelings of powerlessness can result in individuals feeling vulnerable and defenseless. The APN's role encompasses empowering the professional staff and patients to overcome and avoid the destructive feelings of vulnerability (Copp, 1986). One of the most effective strategies for empowering others is that of role modeling and teaching from a stance of mutual respect and professional accountability. Fostering respect and collegiality among all members of the nursing staff and holding nurses accountable for their actions are potent antidotes to powerlessness. Through role modeling, APNs demonstrate critical thinking as they identify and clarify moral problems and guide others through the process. Including ethical aspects of a patient's case in multidisciplinary rounds, scheduling debriefing sessions after a particularly difficult case, or using simulation activities in which caregivers role play different scenarios are three additional strategies the APN can propose to cultivate skills in critical reflection and the ability to consider alternate interpretations of a situation. Such activities provide both education and support for other nurses in examining ethical issues and working toward collaborative problem solving.

Nurses must be able to express diverse views without fearing ridicule or rejection from peers. An environment that supports ethical reasoning and judgment will foster action.

Interprofessional Barriers

Nurses and physicians define, perceive, analyze, and reason through ethical problems from distinct and sometimes opposing perspectives (Shannon, 1997). Although the roles are complementary, these differing approaches may create conflict between a nurse and a physician, further separating and isolating the perspectives. The physician may be unaware of the nurse's differing opinion or may not recognize this difference as a conflict (Gramelspracher, Howell, & Young, 1986). Conflicts are intensified when the physician does not agree with the nurse that certain details and specifics of the situation are important or simply does not feel accountable to resolve the conflict with the nurse (Gramelspracher et al., 1986). A recent study indicated that physicians and nurses dealt with the same ethical problems and used similar moral reasoning but that differences were related to professional roles, the kinds of responsibilities each group had in the situation, and the resulting different questions each group raised (Oberle & Hughes, 2001). The APN must first deal with the interprofessional communication problems between the nurse and physician before seeking resolution of ethical problems.

Although open communication is a necessary component of a collaborative environment, it is not sufficient. Physicians and other members of the health care team must understand the nurse's role and responsibilities and vice versa. In the traditional hospital setting, some physicians may still view the nurse as subordinate and functioning primarily to carry out their orders (Gramelspracher et al., 1986). In some cases, physicians perceive their authority as threatened when nurses expand their education and assume more autonomous roles as APNs (Haddad, 1991). They may also feel threatened by the level of expertise that the APN demonstrates in her or his clinical area. However, respect may increase as the physician realizes the APN's competence and accountability and recognizes that physician and nurse roles are very complementary in improving patient care.

Successful collaboration between nurses and physicians is grounded in communication, cooperation, competence, respect, accountability, and trust (Baggs & Schmitt, 1988; see Chapter 10). These factors may be influenced negatively or positively by the professional relationship that exists between the physician and the APN. Important questions in understanding this relationship include the following: For whom does the APN work—the physician, the department, the institution? Who pays the APN's salary? Are APNs able to bill for their services, or are they paid from physician or institutional billings? These factors certainly influence the issue of power in the relationship. What role did the physician have in hiring the APN? Was the physician professionally invested in working with APNs initially, or did the institution mandate that physicians work with APNs? Has the physician had experience working with an APN, and what was the nature of the experience? Obviously, a physician who actively seeks to work with an APN is more likely to have a successful and collaborative interaction. However, even in this case, the intention may not necessarily be to improve patient care by adding another discipline's expertise, but rather to make the physician's job easier by bringing an APN on the team. Do the physician and APN work as a team or as two independent agents? What is the level of interaction between APN and physician: constant, side-by-side interaction, or once a day or once a week? Other factors also influence this professional relationship and issues of control within the relationship. It is more difficult to separate malpractice liabilities when the APN and physician are working together, collaboratively and complementarily, or in an employer-employee relationship, than when the two are entirely independent. The patient's perceptions and expectations of "who's in charge," "whom do I call with problems," and "who has the final say"; the APN's role in the patient's care; and the APN's interaction with the physician will all influence the interaction between physician and APN. If the patient sees early on that the APN has a role and the physician recognizes and reinforces that role, then in fact the APN will have a more significant and clinically important role. Conversely, if the physician does not refer APN-specific issues to the APN but attempts to handle them herself or himself, or does not define for the patient the importance of the APN's role, the patient is unlikely to see the APN as important to his or her health care. Thus in a somewhat circular manner, the physician then can influence the patient's perception of the APN's role. The patient's perception of the APN's role and influence in his or her care will in turn influence the professional interaction, balance of power, and level of collaborative behavior between physician and APN. All of these factors will either enhance or constrain the quality of ethical decision making that occurs.

Again, open communication, cooperation, demonstrated competence, accountability for both role and actions, and developing trust by both the physician and the APN will facilitate overcoming these barriers to successful collaboration. Time and ongoing interactions in this relatively new (for many physicians) arena will also aid in improving the professional relationship. Physicians and APNs need to engage in moral discourse to understand and support the ethical burden each professional carries (Oberle & Hughes, 2001; Shannon, 1997). Two encouraging indications of increased interdisciplinary activity include the work of the multidisciplinary Tavistock Group, who proposed a set of five ethical principles to guide all health professionals who deliver and affect health care (Smith, Hiatt, & Berwick, 1999). In addition, an interdisciplinary task force convened by the American College of Cardiology is reviewing and evaluating the roles of nurses, physician assistants, and NPs on cardiac care teams. The intent of this group is to identify elements of effective teams that may yield insights into how to improve collaborative programs.

Patient/Provider Barriers

Health-care providers, employees of the health-care institution, and patients and families make up the multicultural clinical settings in which most APNs practice. Nurses are taught to respect the patient's cultural values and beliefs and to avoid imposing traditional Western customs and values in a paternalistic manner. As noted earlier, APNs may encounter a conflict when they are confronted with a cultural practice that they regard as harmful (Kikuchi, 1996). For example, parents may inform an NP in a pediatric outpatient setting that because of cultural and religious reasons, they do not want their child immunized. In this case, the NP is faced with a cultural belief that places both the child and community at risk (Kikuchi, 1996). The NP wants to preserve the parent's rights and preferences but is concerned about the child's best interests and the potential harm to other children, should they be exposed to an illness from a nonimmunized child. Issues that result from cultural diversity are difficult to resolve without help from others more familiar with the specific cultural practices and beliefs. Occasionally, contact with the language department of a local university can direct the APN to helpful resources. In troubling cases, when the risk of harm is great, the APN should consult with clergy and other resources to help identify some reasonable options that preserve the rights and dignity of the patient and family without harming others.

The absence of an advance directive may be a barrier to upholding the patient's wishes regarding end-of-life care. Advance directives are legal documents that support the rights of patients to determine in advance their wishes for future end-of-life treatment. There are two types of advance directives, the living will and the durable power of attorney for health care (DPAHC) or health-care proxy. The DPAHC is the more flexible and legally binding advance directive, and all patients should be encouraged to have one. It allows the patient to appoint an individual who will make health-care treatment choices for the patient in the event the patient becomes incapacitated. For patients who have executed an advance directive, the APN should discuss with the patient and family how the advance directive would guide end-of-life decision making. If no advance directive is executed, the decision maker for the incapacitated patient is determined according to state statute, and an estranged relative may be assigned this responsibility. APNs in primary care settings have a particular responsibility to encourage patients and families to consider the DPAHC before an emergency renders the patient incapable of stating his or her wishes.

Another barrier to ethical practice that challenges many APNs is the issue of patient noncompliance. Patients may choose not to be actively involved in their care or in improving their well-being. A patient's actions may be entirely contradictory to the APN's instructions, which raises numerous ethical questions. Once the underlying reason for noncompliance is explored, the APN has several choices. Certainly, the first response is to determine whether the reason for the noncompliance can be rectified, such as by obtaining financial support to assist in purchasing medications. However, if the patient simply chooses to ignore the agreed-upon plan of care, the APN may be faced with terminating the patient-provider relationship, maintaining the relationship with less optimal objectives for care, or continuing to try to persuade the patient to comply with the best treatment plan. Often, the APN spends a disproportionate amount of time with noncompliant patients, attending to preventable exacerbations of their illness or in follow-up conversations attempting to convince these patients to follow the recommended treatment plans. These patients are unsettling to the APN because other patients, who are more amenable to the plan of care, receive less time than the noncompliant patients do. There are no easy solutions to managing the noncompliant patient. In many cases, patients do not intentionally choose to ignore the provider's recommendations. Other factors, such as impaired thinking and concentration, financial issues, emotional disorders, and having other priorities, conflict with the patient's ability to follow the prescribed treatment plan. Members of the health-care team often view patient compliance as a direct responsibility of the APN, and APNs may feel pressure from the team when efforts to enhance patient compliance are unsuccessful. In these cases, the APN should solicit help from other resources, such as social workers or home health nurses, to uncover the causes of noncompliance.

In some cases, the health-care team, including the APN, has one perspective based on common values and beliefs. When the team presents a unified perspective that challenges the patient's and family's values, feelings of intimidation surface, and the patient and family may become silent. Rather than first trying to elicit the patient's and family's perspectives, the health-care team often states the plan of care and goal of treatment without a clear understanding of the patient's wishes. The process of intimidation is subtle and unintentional. The health-care team does not strive to repress the patient's autonomy. However, the act of presenting information in a clear, direct, and straightforward manner can be interpreted as the only right way to manage the patient's condition. This practice is often seen in fast-paced environments with significant time constraints on providers.

It is often easier for patients and families to express diverse views when someone first solicits their position and genuinely listens to their perspectives. The APN can help patients and families overcome feelings of intimidation by asking what they think should be done, clarifying any misconceptions, and accepting their understanding and interpretation of the situation. Unconditional acceptance can break down barriers and lead to communication that is open and honest and facilitates shared decision making. This is not to suggest that providers must always agree with or act on the patients' and families' interpretations. Instead, listening carefully to another's perspective engenders trust and indicates respect. This creates an atmosphere in which the positions of the providers and family can more easily be aligned with a common goal of balancing best interests with patient autonomy. In a recent study of families of ICU patients, Ahrens, Yancey, and Kollef (2003) found that 42 of 43 families receiving support and enhanced communication from a clinical nurse specialist (CNS)–physician team were able to make decisions to withhold or withdraw care at the end of life. The authors noted, "This finding underscores the importance of intentional and well-designed communication and support systems for families making medical and moral decisions" (p. 322).

Organizational/Environmental Barriers

It is the unfortunate reality in many health-care settings that time is so limited that the benefits of collaboration or compromise are seldom realized. To overcome this barrier, the APN may need to resolve the dilemma in stages, with the most central issue addressed first. The APN also needs to enlist the aid of administrative and physician colleagues in recognizing the ongoing consequences of lack of time for team deliberations. For example, if a patient is not receiving adequate pain management because the bedside nurse is concerned about hastening death, the CNS should first focus on relieving the patient's pain. Once the immediate need is addressed, the CNS can help the nurse identify nonpharmacological interventions to promote comfort and educate the nurse about the dosage and timing of medications to prevent wide fluctuations in pain management. At this point, the administrative leadership may need to be approached about supporting ongoing staff education. An additional strategy such as arranging for the nurse to rotate to a hospice unit represents a preventive approach to avert similar dilemmas in the future.

The issues of continuity of care and knowing the patient and family are significant problems in acute care settings. Many institutions continue to push for shorter lengths of stay and more streamlined and "efficient" management of patients. In primary care settings, similar pressures to see more patients in less time can decrease the APN's time for individualized problem solving for patients and families. Typically, these environments do not embrace the concept of "knowing the patient" (Radwin, 1996). Tanner, Benner, Chesla, and Gordon (1993) found that knowing the patient was central to expert clinical judgment and facilitated patient and family advocacy. Whittemore (2000) argued that resolving ethical dilemmas requires knowing the patient as a person to be able to recognize the salient aspects of the situation that are important for resolution. However, care in too many acute care settings is based on knowing the expected response to illness and rapid and episodic treatment of a select population of patients. In other words, individualized care is not standard practice. Although this philosophy has numerous financial advantages, often the patient and family lose the necessary individualized attention that can greatly enhance their recovery. APNs struggle in this environment to better meet the needs of patients and families. In fact, some nurses have moved into APN roles specifically because they desire to spend more time with patients. Certainly, the APN must advocate for providing individualized care to patients and families; however, this position may be difficult and risky when it contradicts the objectives of the institution or third-party payors. Despite institutional or third-party payor goals, the APN is morally obligated to work toward improving the work environment if current conditions are not in the patient's best interests. Fortunately, many institutions are willing to make some concessions in the delivery of patient care if there are clear outcome data that support a change in practice.

It would also be wise for the APN to identify resources both within and outside the institution to assist with the process of resolution. Internal resources may include chaplain staff, liaison psychiatrists, ethics committees and their members, and ethics consultation services. Resources outside the institution include the ANA's Center on Ethics and Human Rights (www.nursingworld.org/ethics), ethics groups within national specialty organizations, and ethics centers in universities or large health-care institutions. The recognition of a moral dilemma does not commit the APN to individually conducting and managing the process of resolution. APNs should engage appropriate resources to address the identified needs and work toward agreement. However, in many situations, such as in rural clinics, resources within the organization are not available. Without another professional colleague to help decipher the problem, the APN is sometimes left with little more than intuition. Guidelines from professional organizations regarding the APN's moral obligations (see "Additional Resources," "Websites with Ethics Policy Statements or Guidelines," and "Ethics and Legal Search Sites" provided at the end of the chapter) are helpful in providing some direction for action. APNs practicing in isolation should network with colleagues (the Internet has greatly facilitated networking at a distance) and should establish contact with resources such as community religious leaders or ethicists in nearby institutions for providing direction in ethical reasoning.

Nursing's ethical obligations to maintain a competent and caring relationship with patients and their families can be challenged with the implementation of managed care structures. Taylor (2001) identified six challenges for nurse case managers, which apply to all APNs: fidelity to the unique needs of individual patients, competing loyalties, resolving role conflict, owning responsibilities to underserved populations, identifying personal biases, and balancing care for others with appropriate self-care. As the new health-care system alters nurses' roles, several strategies have been proposed to help nurses realize their ethical responsibilities (Erlen & Mellors, 1995). In addition to personal reflection and values clarification, nurses should assess their competence to provide effective care and address any deficiencies that are exposed. Because patients have shorter hospital stays in a managed care environment, open communication and collaboration with the health-care team, patients, and families are essential behaviors for optimal planning. Additionally, APNs should maintain and affirm patient's rights by questioning and challenging changes in the health-care system that negatively affect the quality of care delivered. Finally, there is a need to consistently review patient outcomes and quality of nursing care provided (Erlen & Mellors, 1995). These strategies empower the nurse to act on smaller and more manageable parts of the problem.

CONCLUSIONS

The changing health-care environment has placed extraordinary demands on nurses in all care settings. The limitations of time, reimbursement, and resources conflict with nursing's moral imperatives of involvement, connection, and commitment. Ethical decision-making skills are a core competency for the APN and reflect both the art and science of nursing. The APN is in a key position to assume a more decisive role in managing the resolution of moral issues and helping to create ethically responsive health-care environments. Ethical decision-making skills together with clinical expertise and leadership empower the APN to critically analyze and direct the decision-making process. The identification of patterns in the presentation of moral issues enables the APN to engage in preventive strategies to improve the ethical climate in patient care environments. Preparation for this competency begins in graduate education, but it continues throughout the APN's career.

REFERENCES

Ahrens, T., Yancey, V., & Kollef, M. (2003). Improving family communications at the end of life: Implications for length of stay in the intensive care unit and resource use. *American Journal of Critical Care, 12,* 317-323.

Ahronheim, J. C., Moreno, J., & Zuckerman, C. (2000). *Ethics in clinical practice* (2nd ed.). Gaithersburg, MD: Aspen.

American Academy of Pediatrics, Committee on Bioethics. (1996). Ethics and the care of critically ill infants and children (RE9624). *Pediatrics, 98,* 149-152.

American Association of Colleges of Nursing. (1996). *The essentials of master's education for advanced practice nursing.* Washington, DC: Author.

American Association of Critical-Case Nurses. (2000). *Maintaining patient-focused care in an environment of nursing staff shortages and financial constraints* [Position Statement]. Aliso Viejo, CA: Author.

American Nurses Association. (2001). *Code of ethics for nurses with interpretive statements.* Washington, DC: Author.

American Nurses Association. (1994). *Position statement on active euthanasia.* Washington, DC: Author.

Arras, J.D. (1997). Nice story, but so what? In H. L. Nelson (Ed.), *Stories and their limits: Narrative approaches to bioethics* (pp. 65-88). New York: Routledge.

Artnak, K., & Dimmit, J. H. (1996).Choosing a framework for ethical analysis in advanced practice settings: The case for casuistry. *Archives of Psychiatric Nursing, 10,* 16-23.

Baggs, J. G., & Schmitt, M. H. (1988). Collaboration between nurses and physicians. *Image: The Journal of Nursing Scholarship, 20,* 145-149.

Beare, P. G. (1989). The essentials of win-win negotiation for the clinical nurse specialist. *Clinical Nurse Specialist, 13,* 138-141.

Beauchamp, T. L., & Childress, J. F. (2001). *Principles of biomedical ethics* (5th ed.). New York: Oxford University Press.

Benner, P. (1991). The role of experience, narrative and community in skilled ethical comportment. *Advances in Nursing Science, 14,* 1-21.

Brown, K. (2003, March). Moral distress is common in critical care nursing. *AACN News, 20,* 5.

Buryska, J. F. (2001). Assessing the ethical weight of cultural, religious and spiritual claims in the clinical context. *Journal of Medical Ethics, 27,* 118-122.

Calkins, M. E. (1993). Ethical issues in the elderly ESRD patient. *ANNA Journal, 20,* 569-571.

Chambliss, D. F. (1996). *Beyond caring: Hospitals, nurses, and the social organization of ethics.* Chicago: University of Chicago Press.

Charon, R. (1994). Narrative contributions to medical ethics. In E. R. DuBose, R. Hamel, & L. J. O'Connell (Eds.), *A matter of principles?* (pp. 260-283). Valley Forge, PA: Trinity Press International.

Chervenak, F. A., & McCullough, L. B. (1995). The threat of the new managed practice of medicine to patients' autonomy. *Journal of Clinical Ethics, 6,* 320-323.

Childress, J. F. (1994). Principles-oriented bioethics: An analysis and assessment from within. In E. R. DuBose, R. Hamel, & L. J. O'Connell (Eds.), *A matter of principles?* (pp. 72-98). Valley Forge, PA: Trinity Press International.

Childress, J. F. (1997), Narrative(s) versus norm(s): A misplaced debate in bioethics. In H.L. Nelson (Ed.), *Stories and their limits: narrative approaches to bioethics* (pp. 252-271). New York: Routledge.

Clouser, K. D. & Gert, B. A critique of principlism. *Journal of Medicine and Philosophy,15,* 219-236.

Collins, F. S. & Mansoura, M. K. (2001). The Human Genome Project: Revealing the shared inheritance of all humankind. *Cancer, 91*(Suppl, 1), 221-225.

Cooper, M. C. (1989). Gilligan's different voice: A perspective for nursing. *Journal of Professional Nursing, 5,* 10-16.

Cooper, M. C. (1991). Principle-oriented ethics and the ethic of care: A creative tension. *Advances in Nursing Science, 14,* 22-31.

Copp, L. A. (1986). The nurse as advocate for vulnerable persons. *Journal of Advanced Nursing, 11,* 255-263.

Corley, M. C. (1995). Moral distress of critical care nurses. *American Journal of Critical Care, 4,* 280-285.

Corley, M. C. (2002). Nurse moral distress: A proposed theory and research agenda. *Nursing Ethics, 9,* 636-650.

Cruzan v. Missouri Department of Health, et al., 110 S. Ct. 2841 (1990).

Doukas D. J., & Gorenflo, D. W. (1993). Analyzing the values history: An evaluation of patient medical values and advance directives. *Journal of Clinical Ethics, 4,* 41-45.

Doukas, D. J., & McCullough, L. B. (1991). The values history: The evaluation of the patient's values and advance directives. *Journal of Family Practice, 32,* 145-153.

Dreyfus, H. L., Dreyfus, S. E., & Benner, P. (1996). Implications of the phenomenology of expertise for teaching and learning everyday skillful ethical comportment. In P. Benner, C. A. Tanner, & C. A. Chesla (Eds.), *Expertise in nursing practice: Caring, clinical judgment and ethics* (pp. 258-279). New York: Springer-Verlag.

Dubler, N. N., & Marcus, L. J. (1994). *Mediating bioethical disputes.* New York: United Hospital Fund.

Dwyer, M. L. (1998). Genetic research and ethical challenges: Implications for nursing practice. *AACN Clinical Issues, 9,* 600-605.

Eisenberg, L. (1999). The social imperatives of medical research. In T. L. Beauchamp & L. Walters (Eds.), *Contemporary issues in bioethics* (5th ed., pp. 449-456). London: Wadsworth.

Erlen, J. A., & Frost, B. (1991). Nurses' perceptions of powerlessness in influencing ethical decisions. *Western Journal of Nursing Research, 13,* 397-407.

Erlen, J. A., & Mellors, M. P. (1995). Managed care and the nurse's ethical obligations to patients. *Orthopaedic Nursing, 14,* 42-45.

Ewigman, B. G., Crane, J. D., Frigoletto, F. D., LeFevre, M. L., Bain, R. P., & McNellis, D. (1993). Effect of perinatal ultrasound screening on perinatal outcome; Radius Study Group. *New England Journal of Medicine 329*, 821-827.

Fisher, R., & Ury, W. (1981). *Getting to yes*. New York: Viking Penguin.

Forrow, L., Arnold, R. M., & Parker, L. S. (1993). Preventive ethics: Expanding the horizons of clinical ethics. *Journal of Clinical Ethics, 4*, 287-294.

Fowler, M. D. (1999). Relic or resource? The Code for Nurses. *American Journal of Nursing, 99*, 56-58.

Fry, S.T. (1994). *Ethics in nursing practice*. Geneva: International Council of Nurses.

Gaul, A. L. (1995). Casuistry, care, compassion and ethics data analysis. *Advances in Nursing Science, 17*, 47-57.

Gilligan, C. (1982). *In a different voice*. Cambridge, MA: Harvard University Press.

Grady, C. (1991). Ethical issues in clinical trials. *Seminars in Oncology Nursing, 7*, 288-296.

Gramelspracher, G. P., Howell, J. D., & Young, M. J. (1986). Perceptions of ethical problems by nurses and physicians. *Archives of Internal Medicine, 146*, 577-578.

Gudorf, C. E. (1994). A feminist critique of biomedical principlism. In E. R. DuBose, R. Hamel, & L. J. O'Connell (Eds.), *A matter of principles?* (pp. 164-181). Valley Forge, PA: Trinity Press International.

Haddad, A. M. (1991). The nurse/physician relationship and ethical decision making. *AORN Journal, 53*, 151-154, 156.

Hall, J. K. (1996). Assisted suicide: Nurse practitioners as providers? *Nurse Practitioner 21*, 63-66, 71.

Hamric, A. B. (2001) Reflections on being in the middle. *Nursing Outlook, 49*, 254-257.

Hamric, A. B. (2000). Moral distress in everyday ethics. *Nursing Outlook, 48*, 199-201.

Hebert, P. C., Levin, A. V., & Robertson, G. (2001). Bioethics for clinicians: Disclosure of medical error. *Canadian Medical Journal, 164*(4), 1-12.

Hopkinson, I., & Mackay, J. (2002). The clinical impact of the Human Genome Project: Inherited variants in cancer care. *Annals of Oncology, 13* (Suppl. 4), 105-107.

Howard, E. P., & Steinberg, S. (2002). Evaluations of clinical learning in a managed care environment. *Nursing Forum, 37*, 12-20.

Jameton, A. (1984). *Nursing practice: The ethical issues*. Englewood Cliff, NJ: Prentice Hall.

Jameton, A. (1993). Dilemmas of moral distress: Moral responsibility and nursing practice. *AWHONN's Clinical Issues in Perinatal and Women's Health Nursing, 4*, 542-551.

Jonsen, A. R., & Toulmin, S. (1988). *The abuse of casuistry: A history of moral reasoning*. Berkeley: University of California Press.

Juretschke, L. J. (2001). Ethical dilemmas and the nurse practitioner in the NICU. *Neonatal Network, 20*, 33-38.

Kikuchi, J. F. (1996). Multicultural ethics in nursing education: A potential threat to responsible practice. *Journal of Professional Nursing, 12*, 159-165.

Kopelman, L. M., Irons, T. G., & Kopelman, A. E. (1988). Neonatologists judge the "Baby Doe" regulations. *New England Journal of Medicine, 318*, 677-683.

Krouse, H. J., & Roberts, S. J. (1989). Nurse-patient interactive styles: Power, control, and satisfaction. *Western Journal of Nursing Research, 11*, 717-725.

LaMear-Tucker, D., & Friedson, J. (1997). Resolving moral conflict: The critical care nurse's role. *Critical Care Nurse, 17*, 55-63.

Leavitt, F. J. (1996). Educating nurses for their future role in bioethics. *Nursing Ethics, 3*, 39.

Long, S. O. (2000). Living poorly or dying well: Cultural decisions about life-supporting treatment for American and Japanese patients. *Journal of Clinical Ethics, 11*, 236-237.

Ludwig, R., & Silva, M. C. (2000). Nursing around the world: Cultural values and ethical conflicts. *Online Journal of Issues in Nursing*. Retrieved September 1, 2003, from http://www.nursing-world.org/ojin/ethicol/ethics_4.htm

Mahon, M. M., Deatrick, J. A., McKnight, H. J., & Mohr, W. K. (2000). Discontinuing treatment in children with chronic, critical illnesses. *Nurse Practitioner Forum, 11*, 6-14.

Meaney, M. (2002). Moral distress: I just can't take it anymore! *The Case Manager, 13*, 32-33.

National Council of State Boards of Nursing, Inc. (1996). *Professional boundaries: A nurse's guide to the importance of appropriate professional boundaries*. Chicago: Author.

Nelson, H. L. (Ed.). (1997). *Stories and their limits: Narrative approaches to bioethics*. New York: Routledge.

Noland, L. (1999). Ethical issues in nursing practice. In J. Lancaster (Ed.), *Nursing issues in Leading and managing change* (pp. 337-364). St. Louis: Mosby.

Oberle, K. R. & Hughes, D. (2001). Doctors' and nurses' perceptions of ethical problems in end-of-life decisions. *Journal of Advanced Nursing, 33*, 707-715.

O'Connor, K. F. (1996). Ethical/moral experiences of oncology nurses. *Oncology Nursing Forum, 23*, 787–794.

Oddi, L. F., & Cassidy, V. R. (1998). The message of SUPPORT: Change is long overdue. *Journal of Professional nursing, 14*, 165-174.

Olczak, P. V., Grosch, J. W., & Duffy, K. G. (1991). Toward a synthesis: The art with the science of community mediation. In K. G. Duffy, J. W. Grosch, & P. V. Olczak (Eds.), *Community mediation* (pp. 329-343). New York: The Guilford Press.

Omery, A., Henneman, E., Billet, B., Luna-Raines, M., & Brown-Saltzman, K. (1995). Ethical issues in hospital-based nursing practice. *Journal of Cardiovascular Nursing, 9*, 43-53.

Omnibus Budget Reconciliation Act of 1990, PL, 101-508, 42 U.S.C. § 4206.

Orr, R. D., & Genesen, L. B. (1997). Requests for "inappropriate" treatment based on religious beliefs. *Journal of Medical Ethics, 23*, 142-147.

Ostermeyer, M. (1991). Conducting the mediation. In K. G. Duffy, J. W. Grosch, & P. V. Olczak (Eds.),

Community mediation (pp. 91-104). New York: The Guilford Press.

Pike, A. W. (1991). Moral outrage and moral discourse in nurse-physician collaboration. *Journal of Professional Nursing, 7,* 351-362.

Purtilo, R. (1999). *Ethical dimensions in the health professions* (3rd ed.). Philadelphia: W. B. Saunders.

Radwin, L. E. (1996). "Knowing the patient": A review of research on an emerging concept. *Journal of Advanced Nursing, 23,* 1142-1146.

Rest, J. R. (1986). *Moral development: Advances in research and theory.* New York: Praeger.

Rowdin, M. A. (1995). Conflicts in managed care. *New England Journal of Medicine, 332,* 604-607.

Sadler, G. R., Lantz, J. M., Fullerton, J. T., & Dault, Y. (1999). Nurses' unique roles in randomized clinical trials. *Journal of Professional Nursing, 15,* 106-115.

Saulo, M., & Wagener, R. J. (1996). How good case managers make tough choices: Ethics and mediation. *Journal of Care Management, 2,* 10-16, 35-38, 42.

Savage, T. A. & Milton, C. B. (1989). Ethical decision-making models for nurses. *Chart, 86,* 2-5.

Scanlon, C. (1994). Survey yields significant results. *American Nurses Association Center for Ethics and Human Rights Communique, 3*(4).

Schlenk, J. S. (1997). Advance directives: Role of nurse practitioners. *Journal of the American Academy of Nurse Practitioners, 9,* 317-321.

Scott, R. A., Aiken, L. H., Mechanic, D., & Moravcsik, J. (1995). Organizational aspects of caring. *The Milbank Quarterly, 73,* 77-95.

Shannon, S. E. (1997). The roots of interdisciplinary conflict around ethical issues. *Critical Care Nursing Clinics of North America, 9,* 13-28.

Smeltzer, C. H. (1991). The art of negotiation: An everyday experience. *Journal of Nursing Administration, 21,* 26-30.

Smith, R., Hiatt, H., & Berwick, D. (1999). Shared ethical principles for everybody in health care: A working draft from the Tavistock group. *British Medical Journal, 318,* 248-251.

Solomon, M. Z., Jennings, B., Guilfoy, V., Jackson, R., O'Donnell, L., Wolf, S. M., et al. (1991). Toward an expanded vision of clinical ethics education: From individual to the institution. *Kennedy Institute of Ethics Journal, 1,* 225-245.

Solomon, M. Z., O'Donnell, L., Jennings, B., Guilfoy, V., Wolf, S. M., Nolan, K., et al. (1993). Decisions near the end of life: Professional views on life-sustaining treatments. *American Journal of Public Health, 83,* 14-23.

Spencer, E. M. (1997). A new role for institutional ethics committees: Organizational ethics. *Journal of Clinical Ethics, 8,* 372-376.

Spielman, B. J. (1993). Conflict in medical ethics cases: Seeking patterns of resolution. *Journal of Clinical Ethics, 4,* 212-218.

SUPPORT Principal Investigators. (1995). A controlled trial to improve care for seriously ill hospitalized patients: The Study to Understand Prognosis and Preferences for Outcomes and Risks of Treatments (SUPPORT). *JAMA: The Journal of the American Medical Association, 274,* 1591-1598.

Tanner, C. A., Benner, P., Chesla, C., & Gordon, D. R. (1993). The phenomenology of knowing the patient. *Image: The Journal of Nursing Scholarship, 25,* 273-280.

Taylor, C. (1997). Ethical perspectives. In M. M. Burke & M .B. Walsh (Eds.), *Gerontologic nursing: Care of the elderly* (2nd ed., pp.584-600). St. Louis, MO: Mosby.

Taylor, C. (2001). Ethical issues in case management. In E. L. Cohen & T. G. Cesta (Eds.), *Nursing Case Management* (pp. 369-386). St. Louis, MO: Mosby.

Tiedje, L. B. (1999). Moral distress in perinatal nursing. *Journal of Perinatal and Neonatal Nursing, 14,* 36-43.

Toulmin, S. (1994). Casuistry and clinical ethics. In E. R. DuBose, R. Hamel, & L. J. O'Connell (Eds.), *A matter of principles?* (pp. 310-318). Valley Forge, PA: Trinity Press International.

Turner, L. N., Marquis, K., & Burman, M. E. (1996). Rural nurse practitioners: Perceptions of ethical dilemmas. *Journal of the American Academy of Nurse Practitioners, 8,* 269-274.

United States Child Abuse Prevention and Treatment Amendments of 1984, 42 USCS § 5101.

Ury, W. (1993). *Getting past no.* New York: Bantam Books.

Uustal, D. (1987). Values: The cornerstone of nursing's moral art. In M. D. Fowler & J. Levine-Ariff (Eds.), *Ethics at the bedside* (pp. 136-153). Philadelphia: J. B. Lippincott.

van Hooft, S. (1990). Moral education for nursing decisions. *Journal of Advanced Nursing, 15,* 210-215.

Viens, D. C. (1994). Moral dilemmas experienced by nurse practitioners. *Nurse Practitioner Forum, 5,* 209-214.

Viens, D. C. (1995). The moral reasoning of nurse practitioners. *Journal of the American Academy of Nurse Practitioners, 7,* 277-285.

Waltman, P. A. & Schenk, L. K. (1999). Neonatal ethical decision making: Where does the NNP fit in? *Neonatal Network, 18,* 27-32.

Welton, G. L. (1991). Parties in conflict: Their characteristics and perceptions. In K. G. Duffy, J. W. Grosch, & P. V. Olczak (Eds.), *Community mediation* (pp. 105-118). New York: The Guilford Press.

Whittemore, R. (2000). Consequences of not "knowing the patient". *Clinical Nurse Specialist, 14,* 75-81.

Williams, J. K., & Lea, D. H. (1995). Applying new genetic technologies: Assessment and ethical considerations. *Nurse Practitioner, 20,* 16, 21-26.

Winters, G., Glass, E., & Sakurai, C. (1993). Ethical issues in oncology nursing practice: An overview of topics and strategies. *Oncology Nursing Forum, 20*(Suppl. 10), 21-34.

Wright, F., Cohen, S., & Caroselli, C. (1997). Diverse decisions: How culture affects ethical decision making. *Critical Care Nursing Clinics of North America, 9,* 63-74.

Zaner, R. M. (1988). *Ethics and the clinical encounter.* Englewood Cliffs, NJ: Prentice-Hall.

Additional Resources

American Hospital Association. (1994). *Values in conflict: Resolving ethical issues in health care.* Chicago: Author.

American Medical Association, Council on Ethical and Judicial Affairs. (1996). *Code of medical ethics: Current opinions with annotations.* Chicago: Author.

American Nurses Association. (1985). *Code for nurses with interpretive statements.* Kansas City, MO: Author.

American Society for Bioethics and Humanities. (1998). *Core competencies for health care ethics consultation.* Glenview, IL: Author.

Campbell, M. L. (1998). *Foregoing life-sustaining therapy.* Aliso Viejo, CA: American Association of Critical-Care Nurses.

Davis, A. J., Aroskar, M. A., Liaschenko, J., & Drought, T. S. (1997). *Ethical dilemmas and nursing practice* (4th ed.). Stamford, CT: Appleton & Lange.

Encyclopedia of bioethics. (1995). New York: Simon & Schuster Macmillan.

Fry, S. T. & Veatch, R. M. (2000). *Case studies in nursing ethics* (2nd ed.). Boston: Jones & Bartlett.

Hoffman, D. E., Boyle, P., & Levenson, S. A. (1995). *Handbook for nursing home ethics committees.* Washington, DC: American Association of Homes and Services for the Aging.

Joint Commission for Accreditation of Healthcare Organizations. (1997). *Accreditation manual for hospitals: Standards on patient rights and organization ethics.* Oakbrook, IL: Author.

Kennedy Institute of Ethics. (2003). *New titles in bioethics.* Washington, DC: Georgetown University Press.

National Institutes of Health Office of Extramural Research, Office for Protection from Research Risks. (1993). *Protecting human research subjects: Institutional review board guidebook.* Washington, DC: National Institutes of Health.

President's Commission for the Study of Ethical Problems in Medicine and Biomedical and Behavioral Research. (1983). *Deciding to forego life-sustaining treatment.* Washington, DC: Author.

President's Commission for the Study of Ethical Problems in Medicine and Biomedical and Behavioral Research. (1983). *Making health care decisions.* Washington, DC: Author.

President's Commission for the Study of Ethical Problems in Medicine and Biomedical and Behavioral Research. (1983). *Screening and counseling for genetic conditions.* Washington, DC: Author.

Ross, J. W., Bayley, C. M., & Pugh, D. (Eds.). (1986). *Handbook for hospital ethics committees.* Chicago: American Hospital Association.

Task-Force to Improve the Care of Terminally-Ill Oregonians. (1998). *The Oregon Death with Dignity Act: A guidebook for health care providers.* Portland OR: Oregon Health Sciences University Center for Ethics in Health Care.

Websites with Ethics Policy Statements or Guidelines

American Academy of Neurology, Practice Statements: http://www.aan.com/resources.html

American Academy of Pediatrics, Policy Statements: http://www.aap.org/policy

American Association of Nurse-Anesthetists (AANA): http://www.aana.com

American College of Nurse-Midwives: http://www.acnm.org/

American College of Medical Genetics, Policy Statements: http://www.faseb.org/genetics/acmg

American College of Physicians, Center for Ethics and Professionalism: http://www.acponline.org/ ethics

American College of Surgeons, Statements: http://www.facs.org

American Medical Association, Council on Ethical and Judicial Affairs: http://www.ama-assn.org

American Nurse's Association, Center for Ethics and Human Rights: http://www.ana.org/ethics/elinks.htm

American Society for Law, Medicine and Ethics: http://www.aslme.org

American Society for Reproductive Medicine: http://www.asrm.org

American Society of Anesthesiologists, Policy Statements: http://www.asahq.org/standards

American Society for Transplantation, Policy Statements: http://www.a-s-t.org/index.html

Americans for Better Care of the Dying: http://www.abcd-caring.org

Center to Improve the Care of the Dying: http://www.gwu.edu/~cicd

Institute of Medicine, National Academy of Sciences: http://www4.nas.edu/IOM/IOMHome.nsf

Midwest Bioethics Center: http://www.midbio.org

National Bioethics Advisory Commission: http://www.georgetown.edu/research/nrcbl/nbac/

National Catholic Bioethics Center: http://www.ncbcenter.org

National Hospice Organization: http://www.nho.org

National Human Genome Research Institute: http://www.nhgri.nih.gov

National Institutes of Health Resources on Bioethics: http://www.nih.gov/sigs/bioethics

National Institutes of Health, Office for Protection from Research Risks: http://www.grants.nih.gov/grants/oprr/oprr.htm

Project on Death in America: http://www.soros.org/death.html

Society for Critical Care Medicine: http://www.sccm.org

United Network for Organ Sharing, Policy Statements: http://www.unos.org

University of Pennsylvania Center for Bioethics: http://www.med.upenn.edu/~bioethic

Ethics and Legal Search Sites

Bioethicsline database on Internet Grateful Med (literature search): http://www.igm.nlm.nih.gov

Legal Information Institute: http://www.law. cornell.edu

Medical College of Wisconsin Center for the Study of Bioethics, Bioethics Online Service (literature search): http://www.mcw.edu/bioethics

National Reference Center for Bioethics Literature: http://www.georgetown.edu/research/nrcbl

State laws on the Internet: http://www.legalonline.com

U.S. National Library of Medicine and the National Institutes of Health: http://www.nlm.nih.gov/medlineplus.bioethics

Advanced Practice Roles: The Operational Definitions of Advanced Practice Nursing

CHAPTER 12

The Clinical Nurse Specialist

PATRICIA S. A. SPARACINO

INTRODUCTION

The clinical nurse specialist (CNS) role was created to retain expert nurses in clinical practice, to provide direct care to complex patients, and to improve patient care through the development of staff nurses' clinical skills and judgment. Historically the context of CNS role development and implementation has been in hospital settings, but over time CNSs have expanded practice to multiple nonhospital settings. The dimensions of the CNS role were conceptualized as expert clinician, consultant, educator, and researcher. Integrating these dimensions is difficult but essential to sustain the role's integrity, yet differentiating between the components is necessary to keep responsibilities clear and contributions distinct. Within these four dimensions of the role there are competencies, including, but not limited to, direct clinical practice, consultation, expert coaching and guidance, research, clinical and professional leadership, collaboration, and ethical decision making (American Nurses Association [ANA], 1986; Hamric, 1989a; Hamric, 2000; see Chapter 2). The impact and influence of the CNS is most clearly felt within these three spheres: patients or clients, nursing personnel, and organizations or networks (National Association of Clinical Nurse Specialists [NACNS], 1998, 2004). CNS competencies and spheres of influence are discussed in detail later in this chapter.

The first CNSs were specialists in psychiatry and mental health; they pioneered the role (see Chapter 1). The historical development of the CNS role in the United States has been described previously (Hamric, 1983b, 1989a; Hoeffer & Murphy, 1984; Sparacino, 1990) (see Chapter 1). The nurse specialist or CNS role also exists in other countries, such as Canada, the United Kingdom, Australia, Japan, and China. However, both the definition and implementation in each country are influenced by culture, education, standards, and practice differences that are not discussed in this chapter.

The evolution of the CNS role has not been logical or linear. The role's effectiveness is derived from its flexibility, yet the role's versatility has made it vulnerable to restructuring and retitling. The role was implemented before the existence of a coherent educational curriculum, criteria for certification, consistent use of capabilities, agreement about regulatory control, or implementation of third-party reimbursement. In the past decade these forces have reshaped and influenced contemporary CNS practice. Much has been expected of CNSs, and only recently has their impact been tied to improving patient outcomes, efficient use of resources, cost efficiency, and revenue generation (NACNS, 1998, 2004; see Chapter 25).

The intent of the CNS role has always been to improve patient care and influence others. Successful CNSs deliver high-quality care that can be measured in terms of cost-effectiveness, patient outcomes, and improvements in nursing practice. The CNS's clinical reasoning is not limited to the consideration of physiological and psychological variables, but extends beyond the boundaries of clinical practice to incorporate education, research, social policy, organizational factors, and political change. Historically CNSs focused primarily on direct patient care and consideration of the systems context in which care was given. The current emphasis on health-care reform and the restructuring of health-care reimbursement has added cost containment and care-efficient strategies to CNS responsibilities. Health-care policy and restructuring of health-care delivery has influenced the shift in emphasis from extraordinary to ordinary, from costly to more cost-efficient, and from curative to preventive. CNSs have been integral to this effort, designing and implementing practice guidelines and innovative practice models, evaluating the cost efficiency and fiscal impact of technology, and assessing its impact on patient care, the quality of care given, and the protection of continuity of care and patient satisfaction.

PROFILE OF THE ROLE

Role Definition

The nursing profession, specialty organizations, and nurse authors have developed and refined the definition of the CNS role. In 1976, the ANA provided an operational definition of the CNS (ANA, Congress of Nursing Practice, 1976). In 1980, the ANA published *Nursing: A Social Policy Statement.* This document was the first to differentiate between the specialist prepared at the graduate level and the nurse with a baccalaureate degree who is a specialist in nursing practice but "a generalist in providing the full range of nursing practice." It promulgated the classic CNS definition: a registered nurse "who, through study and supervised practice at the graduate level (master's or doctorate), has become expert in a defined area of knowledge and practice in a selected clinical area of nursing" (ANA, 1980, p. 23). In 1983, Hamric further developed the definition by making the distinction between the direct care functions (e.g., expert practitioner, role model, and patient advocate) and indirect care functions (e.g., change agent, consultant/resource person, clinical teacher, supervisor, researcher, liaison, and innovator) (Hamric, 1983b). In 1986, the ANA's Council of Clinical Nurse Specialists expanded the established definition to delineate the multifaceted dimensions of the role, including expert clinical practice, education, consultation, research, and administration components, and to define the flexible boundaries as determined by the needs of complex patient populations, evolving nursing specialties, and the needs of the health-care market. In 1989, Hamric proposed a three-dimensional model (Figure 12-1) to delineate the role's defining characteristics and the relationships between primary criteria for the role (e.g., graduate study in the specialty, certification, and focus of practice on the patient/client/family), the four

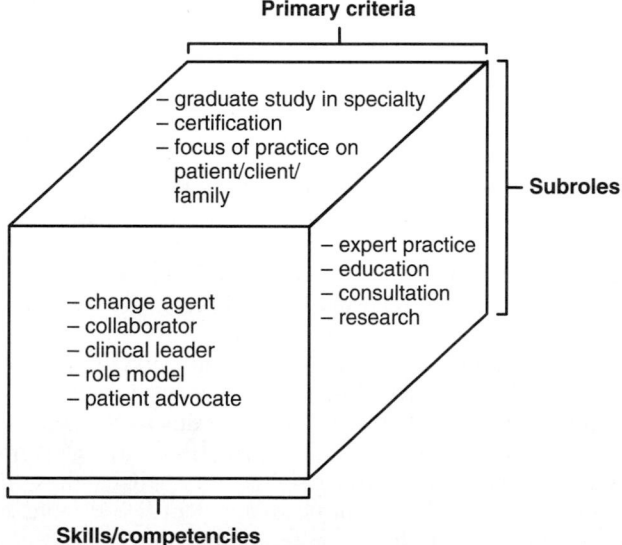

FIGURE 12-1 • Variables influencing CNS role expression. (From Hamric, A. B. [1989a]. History and overview of the CNS role. In A. B. Hamric & J. A. Spross [Eds.], *The clinical nurse specialist in theory and practice* [2nd ed.]. Philadelphia: W.B. Saunders.)

dimensions (clinical expert, consultant, educator, and researcher), and skills or competencies (e.g., change agent, collaborator, clinical leader, role model, patient advocate) (Hamric, 1989a). The current definition of the CNS role builds on its definitional evolution: A CNS is prepared at the master's or doctorate level as a clinical nurse specialist and is an expert clinician in a specialized area of nursing practice. The specialty may be a population (e.g., pediatrics, women's health), a setting (e.g., critical care), a disease or medical subspecialty (e.g., oncology, cardiovascular disease), a type of care (e.g., rehabilitation, psychiatric), or a type of problem (e.g., wounds, pain) (NACNS, 1994, 2004). Regardless of setting or specialty CNSs demonstrate the seven essential competencies proposed by Hamric: direct clinical practice, expert coaching and guidance, consultation, research, clinical and professional leadership, collaboration, and ethical decision making (Hamric, 1996, 2000; see Chapter 3). The NACNS (2004) further elucidates CNS competencies, describing CNS competencies particular to each sphere of influence.

For nearly two decades, nursing leaders have discussed the feasibility of singular titling for advanced practice nurses (APNs) (Cronenwett, 1995; Hamric 1983; Soehren & Schumann, 1994; Sparacino & Durand, 1986; Spross & Hamric, 1983), analyzing the commonalities and differences between the CNS and the nurse practitioner (NP) roles (Fenton & Brykczynski, 1993; Keane & Richmond, 1993; Lincoln, 2000; Williams & Valdivieso, 1994). The singular titling proposal attempted to address educational, regulatory, and other related issues with some uniformity and efficiency. Although the proposal for singular titling generated significant debate and opposition, APN designation became widely accepted as a generic term that includes the CNS, NP, certified nurse-midwife, and certified registered nurse anesthetist. Even though a common designation would be practical, the debate about whether the CNS and NP roles should (Moller & Haber, 1996) or should not be merged (Lincoln, 2000; Mick & Ackerman, 2002; Moller & Haber, 1996; NACNS, 2004) continues to focus on the differences between the roles. Although the CNS and NP roles share many overlapping similarities, the differences are attributed to distinct differences in ideology, role, and practice (Lincoln, 2000; Mick & Ackerman, 2002). The issues of merging or blending the roles are further addressed in Chapters 3 and 15.

Distribution

Determining how many CNSs are practicing in the United States has been an elusive goal. Most CNSs are members of specialty nursing organizations rather than general professional organizations. Some specialty nursing organizations use the generic APN category for reporting CNSs, NPs, CNSs that have dual training as NPs, and other APN roles. The ANA's database from 1980 listed 19,070 nurses who identified themselves as CNSs, but only 5245 of that number were prepared at the graduate level (ANA, 1985). In 2000, the Health Resources and Service Administration's (HRSA's) survey estimated that there were 54,374 master's-prepared CNSs, or 27.7% of registered nurses prepared for advanced practice. In addition, 14,643 CNSs had dual training as NPs, but they were more likely to be functioning as NPs (Sprately, Johnson, Sochalski, Fritz, & Spencer, 2000).

When CNSs gather for a professional meeting, there can be as many specialties represented as there are nurses. As patient needs are identified and organizational priorities are marketed, specialty appellations proliferate and roles emerge. When an APN role is assigned to an emerging specialty, it is critical not only that the role be appropriate for the population and setting but, more important, that direct care be a significant part of the role (Spross & Heaney, 2000). A nursing specialty may not evolve into an advanced practice nursing role if there is not standardization of graduate level educational preparation and APN competencies (Hanson & Hamric, 2003; see Chapter 19).

Education

The knowledge, skills, and clinical experience acquired in the graduate program should prepare a CNS to practice at an advanced level, regardless of setting or patient population. The goal of graduate level education is to prepare a nurse to think critically and abstractly, to assess care situations at an advanced level, and to use and integrate research into clinical practice (National Council of State Boards of Nursing [NCSBN], 2002b). The publication of *The Essentials of Master's Education for Advanced Practice Nursing* (American Association of Colleges of Nursing [AACN], 1996) provided a blueprint for graduate nursing programs, recommending a core curriculum common to all master's students and additional core content and clinical specialty courses for students preparing for advanced practice. The recommended core curriculum includes theory, research, ethics, health policy, and professional role development. The recommended advanced practice core curriculum includes advanced physical assessment, advanced pharmacology, physiology, and pathophysiology. The NACNS (2004) has further described 13 core content areas necessary for developing CNS competencies:

- Theoretical foundations for CNS practice
- Phenomena of concern
- Design and development of innovative nursing interventions
- Clinical inquiry/critical thinking using advanced knowledge
- Technology, products, and devices
- Teaching and coaching
- Influencing change
- Systems thinking
- Leadership for multidisciplinary collaboration
- Consultation theory
- Measurement
- Outcome evaluation methods
- Evidence-based practice and research utilization

A critical and integral part of a CNS's educational preparation is clinical practice, with sufficient opportunities to master knowledge, to apply the knowledge and skills, and to begin the transition from competence to expertise in a selected area of clinical practice. The clinical practice content should be divided into two components: practica that refine skills and increase clinical competency, and a residency that integrates the advanced practice element with consultation, education, and clinical leadership to provide depth and breadth of experience. Both the NACNS (2004) and the NCSBN (2002a) recommend 500 hours of clinical practice. The NACNS further specifies that the student's experience be "consistent with the conceptual framework of the three spheres of influence" (NACNS, 2004, p. 53). In addition, the NCSBN indicates that clinical experience should be directly related to the graduate student's specialty and supervision be provided by a person licensed for the same APN role (NCSBN, 2002b, 2002c).

THE CNS ROLE: DIMENSIONS, COMPETENCIES, AND SPHERES OF INFLUENCE

As noted earlier, the classic structure or dimensions of the CNS role are expert clinician, consultant, change agent (leader), educator, and researcher. Integrating these dimensions is difficult but necessary, yet maintaining distinction between the elements is important to keep role responsibilities clear (Sparacino & Cooper, 1990). Competencies are knowledge and skills. A CNS must master the direct clinical practice, expert coaching and guidance, consultation, and research core competencies to accomplish and integrate the CNS role dimensions. The clinical and professional leadership, collaboration, and ethical decision-making competencies are common threads that weave throughout the core competencies. What the CNS does (e.g., the four dimensions) and how the CNS performs the role (e.g., competencies) can have a substantial impact on the practice setting (e.g., spheres of influence). Practice in each sphere of influence (patients/clients, nurses, and organizations/networks) (NACNS, 1998, 2004), in combination with mastery of CNS competencies, is essential to be a successful CNS.

CNSs have been challenged to maintain patient care as the focus while successfully integrating the essential role dimensions, competencies, and multiple clinical and organizational responsibilities. Various texts (Gawlinski & Kern, 1994; Hamric & Spross, 1989; Hamric, Sprass, & Hanson, 1996, 2000; Shea, Pelletier, Poster, Stuart, & Verhey, 1999; Sparacino, Cooper, & Minarik, 1990; Wolbert Burgess, 1997) and the professional journal *Clinical Nurse Specialist* offer many practical suggestions for successfully implementing the CNS role. Rather than repeating those recommendations, this section emphasizes key elements and pragmatic implementation of the competencies, with examples of CNS impact within the spheres of influence.

CNS Competencies

DIRECT CLINICAL PRACTICE

Clinical practice is the heart of CNS practice. Skills (clinical, communication, and relational) and knowledge (theoretical, practical, and particular) are essential, but practical wisdom is a hallmark of advanced practice nursing (Oberle & Allen, 2001). The genesis of the CNS role was specialization and expert clinical practice with responsibility for direct care of patients. Many authors have described strategies for successfully implementing the expert clinician dimension, building on the foundations laid by earlier authors (Felder, 1983; Koetters, 1989; Sparacino & Cooper, 1990). Each strategy is dependent on the individual CNS, particular practice setting, and prevailing health-care environment.

Direct care or direct clinical practice refers to CNS activities and responsibilities that occur within the patient-nurse interface (see Chapter 5). For many years, the CNS's direct clinical practice was embedded in the interdisciplinary care of the hospital setting and was not linked to patient outcomes or resource utilization (Hamric, 1995). Thus there were few tangible or useful data to justify the role when health-care systems that were restructuring looked at the bottom line. However, most of the patients currently cared for in settings where CNSs practice (hospital, home care, or community) are sicker and frailer and in need of specialized, expert care. Questions that students might ask include the following: What patient is a CNS most likely to care for directly? What sort of care does a CNS give? How does a CNS decide to allocate time for direct care or guide other nurses delivering that care? How do the CNS direct care responsibilities differ from those of staff nurses and of other APNs? Does the specialist nurse enhance or de-skill the general nurse?

A CNS is most likely to care directly for a patient whose diagnosis or care is complex, unique, or problematic. A CNS's clinical expertise and specialty influence the patient population to whom care is given. Examples of complex or problematic patients include an infant with very low birth weight, a frail older person with multiple hospital readmissions, a young adult with a hereditary risk for early onset dementia, a child with complex congenital heart disease, a young pregnant woman with a transplanted organ, or a man with a diagnosis of bipolar disorder who has survived a suicide attempt but who requires prolonged physical rehabilitation. Examples of unique situations are the care of a patient with the rarely used Eloesser flap for treatment of a tuberculous empyema; the evaluation and implementation of a new intervention, such as using teletechnology to assess the efficacy of preventive interventions for pressure ulcers; or the introduction of an experimental chemotherapy.

Direct clinical practice is also a means by which the CNS can assess the quality of care for a specific patient population; it provides a qualitative assessment that enhances the interpretation of quantitative data and directs changes in care processes. For example, when a field nurse notes that older home care patients are not consistently taking medications, a CNS's clinical expertise and involvement with the direct care of the same patients can provide a more detailed and complex assessment. The result of a CNS's assessment may be that the older patients are cognitively impaired and therefore unable to remember to take their medications; the medication regimen is too complex, causing the patient to miss doses; or the medicines prescribed are too expensive and not covered by supplemental insurance or Medicaid, leading to doses that are halved or skipped and prescriptions that are not filled. Outcomes of the CNS's evaluation might include integrating advanced assessment skills such as cognitive screening into the admission assessment of all older patients, identifying therapeutic alternatives such as a simpler or more economical medication regimen to improve treatment adherence, or other creative interventions to promote health and quality of life.

The type of care a CNS gives is either regular or episodic (Koetters, 1989). Examples of regular care are providing nursing care for all patients with newly diagnosed diabetes in a community clinic, providing psychotherapy, medication management and other specialized nursing care for patients requiring mental health care, delivering total patient care for the first patients in a fetal surgery program, or visiting all patients with congestive heart failure in a home care agency who have had more than one hospital readmission within 60 days of the initial hospitalization. Episodic care helps a CNS assess and intervene in a particular problem. Examples of episodic care include planning and coordinating a patient's complex hospital discharge, facilitating a support group for patients with primary pulmonary hypertension, or providing total patient care (having the same responsibilities as a staff nurse) to determine the feasibility of proposed changes in patient care or other system changes. Involvement in regular or episodic care enables CNSs to identify problems that interfere with care and require CNS intervention. Examples include lack of staff knowledge, need for clinical policies or procedures, and the need for conflict mediation among team members. For each clinical situation, a CNS takes a comprehensive approach and uses a high level of discriminative judgment, advanced knowledge, and expert skill, including expertise in the technical and humanistic aspects of care. Although clinical expertise is the cornerstone of CNS practice, a CNS will not be successful because of knowledge or technical expertise alone.

The advantages of a CNS providing regular and consistent direct patient care are that it provides the CNS the opportunity to demonstrate clinical competency, maintain clinical expertise, meet direct care requirements for recertification, identify staff learning needs, role model important clinical behaviors, evaluate resource utilization, and ensure CNS visibility and accessibility. If certain clinical skills, particularly psychomotor ones such as administering chemotherapy and troubleshooting ventricular assist devices are not used periodically, CNSs become less proficient over time. Regular clinical practice helps a CNS to maintain the expertise and clinical competence needed to practice and to develop the skills of other nurses. In addition to maintaining and refining clinical skills, direct clinical practice is imperative at two particular points: during a CNS's orientation to establish credibility and prior to and occasionally throughout the implementation of organizational change to assess the impact of changes on patient care. CNSs must weigh the benefits and costs of different ways to implement the direct care competency. Advantages such as developing credibility with staff or maintaining one's skills are evaluated against potential disadvantages such as competing demands, time pressures, and other factors. In addition to episodic involvement with particular patients, a critical care CNS could schedule 8 hours of staff nursing per month, using the time to maintain clinical skills, assess staff needs and the quality of teamwork and communication, and identify challenges in the delivery of care. This level of involvement assists the CNS in understanding the conditions under which nurses are expected to implement standards of care and ensure quality.

A CNS's clinical practice interventions may be continuous or time limited but should result in improvements in clinical outcomes, patient/family satisfaction, resource allocation, staff knowledge and skills, health-care team collaboration, and organizational efficiency. A CNS intervention may be as simple as assisting a patient and family to navigate a hospital's bureaucratic maze; a successful outcome usually occurs because the CNS knows how and when to break the rules, bypass organizational or philosophical roadblocks, and focus on the patient and family.

A CNS is also engaged in clinical practice, for example, when a CNS delegates care to a staff nurse but still guides this direct care. A CNS's goal is always to improve the direct care skills and knowledge of the staff nurse. Another type of clinical practice is when a CNS selects a patient population in which there are recurrent problems or themes, poor outcomes, or recidivism and then collaborates with other members of the health-care team to develop and implement standards of care, critical pathways, clinical procedures, or quality or performance improvement plans. Implementation and adherence should be evaluated in order to compare outcomes; refine critical pathways, algorithms, or guidelines; improve clinical management; and further promote consistent adherence. A pathway or guideline is rarely self-sustaining and requires a key person who continuously champions its dependable implementation if it is to be successful and achieve its intended outcome. A CNS is often the primary coordinator of such an effort.

Another type of clinical practice provided by the CNS is related to system responsibilities for evaluating technology and its impact on patients and resources. Technological advances have made significant changes in health-care delivery. However, such advances, coupled with the emphasis on cost containment, increased competition, changing and greater consumer expectations, and capped budgets, create conflicting demands and priorities. Technology has provided objective criteria with which to make clinical judgments (e.g., medication titration based on hemodynamic indices), devices with which to remotely assess a patient (e.g., telemonitoring of vital signs and weights), and interventional alternatives with which to treat disease (e.g., fiberoptic, robotic, and virtual reality surgery). Yet technology warrants close scrutiny, for with technology comes a responsibility to evaluate the fiscal impact, quality, environmental impact, risk versus benefit, and patient response.

CONSULTATION

There are classic articles describing the essential components of consultation (see Chapter 7; Hamric, 1983b) and strategies for ensuring the success of a CNS as a consultant (Gurka, 1991; Noll, 1987; Sparacino & Cooper, 1990; Sneed, 1991). The CNS is a content expert and so assists in suggesting a wide range of alternative approaches or solutions to clinical or systems problems, whether internal or external to the practice setting.

The CNS is a resource consultant and provides pertinent information that enables nurses and others to make decisions based on a range of relevant and appropriate alternatives. The CNS is a process consultant and facilitates change so that decisions can be made for particular and future situations (Sparacino & Cooper, 1990). Process activities and outcome achievement are two critical and measurable elements of the CNS consultation competency. Documentation of consultations and linking the consultation to outcomes is important. An example of this connection is described by Gurka (1991), who used four consultative process activities (the fact-finder, educator, informational expert, and advocate modes) from Lippitt and Lippitt's Consultation Model and measured three major outcomes (prevention of complications, maintenance or development of standards of care, and improvement in staff nurses' clinical judgment skills).

A CNS can be an internal and external consultant. Internal consultation is part of a CNS's job description and includes assisting with staff and organizational development in one's own practice setting, especially the creative use of resources and alternative strategies to bypass perceived system obstacles. A CNS may recognize that a request for internal consultation requires the collaboration of multiple consultants, with more than one CNS and other disciplines participating; a CNS often initiates the plan, mobilizes the resources, defuses the politics, and facilitates the resolution. For example, a geropsychiatric CNS may consult with a nursing unit or nursing home about psychological issues associated with caring for an elderly population (Kennedy, Covington, Evans, & Williams, 2000), or an oncology CNS who rarely cares for patients with brain tumors may consult a neurology CNS for assistance in developing a care plan that addresses existing neurological deficits and that ensures effective monitoring of potential complications. Another example is a neurologist who consults with a cardiovascular surgery CNS for assistance in preparing a patient, admitted with a brain abscess and a previously undiagnosed congenital cardiac anomaly, for urgent cardiac surgery.

Unless consultation is a CNS's primary responsibility (e.g., a psychiatric consultation liaison CNS), there may be a problem if a CNS's time is used more for consultations than direct care; the impact on patient care is less visible, unless the content and process of consultations are well documented and the outcomes are measured. External consultation assists the nursing profession, a specialty organization, other health providers, and health systems external to the practice setting with approaches or solutions for specific problems. External consultation may require ongoing, intensive support to effect significant change (Rantz et al., 2001). Skill as a CNS consultant cannot be assumed although it is an expectation. Each CNS's consultative skill and the need to use this competency varies. See Chapter 7 for further discussion of the consultation competency.

EXPERT COACHING AND GUIDANCE

There are many descriptions in the literature of the essential components of the CNS educator role and of expert coaching and guidance skills (Sparacino & Cooper, 1990; Spross, Clarke, & Beauregard, 2000; see Chapter 6). Expert coaching and guidance depends on the interaction of technical, clinical, and interpersonal competence and self reflection (Spross et al., 2000; see Chapter 6), but it is influenced also by scholarly inquiry and research utilization. A CNS's teaching and coaching function is both formal and informal. A CNS teaches staff nurses, patients and families, graduate nursing students, clinical nurse specialists, health professionals, and consumer groups.

A CNS is a role model for staff nurses, demonstrating the practical integration of theory and evidence-based practice. By maintaining a focus on continuously improving clinical practice and integrating new knowledge into practice, a CNS influences the further development of the proficient and expert nurse and enhances the staff nurse's accountability and autonomy. A CNS is not effective when she or he is or is perceived to be territorial, omnipotent, or omniscient. Often a CNS's time is better used by teaching others the why, what, and how of common patient care interventions than being constrained by repeatedly providing the same patient interventions. Developing standards for patient education and providing resources to ensure that patient education is consistent across populations are also important educational activities of the CNS (read more about health literacy and patient coaching in Chapter 6). As a staff nurse applies the new knowledge and skills taught by a CNS, the CNS can move on to new or more complex responsibilities. A staff nurse can become the role model for the skill mastered or the knowledge gained, and so the influence of the CNS continues to improve patient care. This growth cycle is never complete. Whenever there is a major staff turnover or a CNS enters a new practice setting, the cycle must begin anew.

A CNS's expert coaching and guidance skills are pivotal in providing or influencing patient and family education. Teaching or coaching complements the care given to a patient and family by other nurses and health professionals. CNSs continually look for better ways to teach patients and families, using diverse combinations of cognitive, educational, and behavioral strategies to improve patient education and adherence to interventions. However, a CNS may not be able to teach every patient and family and so must assess whom to teach. For example, a CNS could delegate routine preoperative teaching for a cardiac surgical patient to the practice case manager or presurgical program educator. A CNS could therefore allocate more time to teach high-risk, complex, unusual, or "difficult" patients; for example, an octogenarian who is undecided about an aortic valve replacement or a young adult with a bicuspid aortic valve and leukemia, requiring intravenous chemotherapy, who has endocarditis. A CNS may demonstrate how to facilitate difficult conversations with patients and their families; for example, supporting the parents of a newborn who died, working with a patient and family members on end-of-life decisions, or translating what a physician has said into lay terms.

The restructuring of health-care systems has meant that patients must be more accountable for the care of their health. While many patients are more aware of the need to be better informed and educated about health risk determinants, preventive self-care, treatment options, and risks in addition to the benefits of treatments, their health-care behaviors are influenced by a variety of personal, psychological, and sociocultural factors. A patient is not always able or willing to adopt lifestyle changes or to adhere to health-care recommendations, thus a CNS uses a variety of considerations to determine which patient (or types of populations of patients) are more appropriate for the CNS to teach, such as a prenatal patient with poor social support living in an economically depressed community, an African American woman at risk of contracting human immunodeficiency virus (HIV), or a teen who is newly diagnosed with type I diabetes. In addition, many consumers seek health care from nontraditional providers (Eisenberg et al., 1998). CNSs often elicit this information and help patients and providers integrate conventional and integrative therapies into care plans.

A CNS has a professional responsibility to serve as an educator for graduate nursing students and, when the opportunity arises, as a mentor. By working with graduate nursing students in the classroom or in the clinical setting, a CNS shares knowledge, demonstrates the level of advanced practice nursing to which a student can aspire, and role models the integration of practical and scientific knowledge into expert clinical practice. A CNS can provide opportunities for a graduate nursing student to do a clinical practicum or residency; the reward of working with an excellent student is being able to do more, to extend one's influence more broadly, and to make advanced practice expertise more widely available. A graduate student's presence benefits the practice setting as well; in addition to providing patient care the student completes projects (e.g., writing patient education materials or clinical procedures) or tasks (e.g., a research literature review to support a proposed change in clinical practice) that benefit the practice setting.

A CNS has many opportunities to educate other health-care providers and consumer groups—usually more than one can reasonably fulfill. When considering whether to accept an opportunity, a CNS must examine the focus (within the specific area of specialty), the size of the audience or the numbers that can be reached, visibility (internal or external to the agency), and potential for cost savings or revenue for the agency. Usually, the focus should be within a CNS's specialty area. Sometimes such requests are opportunities to stretch and extend one's area of expertise, and the CNS chooses to accept such requests. When the content is outside a CNS's specialty, however, the CNS has to prepare extensively to compensate for inexperience and risks overcommitment. In any case, a CNS must carefully balance obligations for teaching within her or his practice setting with teaching outside of the practice setting or the immediate community. The more a CNS is pulled away from the needs of the practice setting, the greater is her or his risk of becoming an invisible and therefore unnecessary health-care provider.

RESEARCH

Historically the CNS role included a research subrole (Hamric, 1983b, 1989a; McGuire & Harwood, 1989; Sparacino & Cooper, 1990). The current emphasis on evidence-based practice, or implementation of relevant, credible research findings, is consistent with historic and contemporary CNS role implementation. The research competency as both an educated and scientific process intended to improve nursing practice, and it ranges from scholarly inquiry to research utilization and research conduct. All CNSs must demonstrate the research competency and have specific, ongoing accountability for monitoring and improving their own practice as well as the practice of other nurses (NACNS, 1998, 2004). CNSs operationalize the competency in a variety of ways, depending on experience, expertise, circumstances, setting, and resources.

There are three specific research competencies, and there are basic and advanced levels of activity for each of the competencies. The three research competencies are interpretation and use of research, evaluation of practice, and participation in collaborative research (McGuire & Harwood, 2000). These three research competencies are described in detail in Chapters 8; the discussion below illustrates the ways in which CNSs operationalize the competencies.

Interpretation and Use of Research Since the late 20th century, "evidence-based practice" has been the mantra of quality care practice and research. The term *evidence-based practice* is frequently used more loosely than its fundamental meaning: rules of evidence or evidence hierarchies. Instead, evidence-based practice is popularly used as an umbrella term for research utilization, research-based practice, or outcomes research (Jennings, 2000; see Chapter 8). Knowledge is the basis for practice, and yet, too frequently, routine practice may not be based on research findings. The foundation of improved quality of care and patient outcomes is analysis of research-based evidence and consensus-dependent practice changes to ensure best practice and achieve quality patient care. When research is systematically evaluated for its applicability, informed decisions about providing patient care and achieving good patient outcomes are made, and credible nursing practice is documented (McPheeters & Lohr, 1999). Inherent in the CNS role is the analysis and evaluation of the appropriateness of the research and the application of research findings to clinical practice. A CNS is the ideal clinician to assess the contextual factors that are barriers and facilitators to change and to develop, implement, and evaluate evidence-based practice. Evidence-based practice is realized in clinical procedures, administrative policies, educational materials for patients and staff, and clinical pathways. A CNS's involvement in the development of clinical pathways and procedures means that a CNS can ensure that evidence informs clinical processes and standards. There are multiple examples of evidence-based practice in the literature, and the number for which a CNS is acknowledged or is an author is significant.

The Center for Advanced Nursing Practice (Soukup, 2000) is an example of a collective effort on the part of APNs to operationalize the interpretation and use of research. The Center's purposes are to advance scholarship-based practice, to develop a practice model that includes four interactive phases (evidence triggered, evidence supported, evidence observed, and evidence based), and to promulgate evidence-based practice across the care continuum. Representative initiatives supported by the Center include improving chest pain management by linking staff at tertiary care institutions with those in rural settings (Rasmussen & Barnason, 2000), a mental health prevention intervention (Adams, 2000), an interdisciplinary approach to a total knee replacement program (Seemann, 2000), and selection and implementation of a transparent dressing for central vascular access devices (Woods, Nass, & Deisch, 2000).

Evaluation of Practice. At the most basic level, this competency requires a CNS to evaluate his or her own practice across spheres of influence. Several writers have written about CNS evaluation from a variety of perspectives, including self-evaluation, staff evaluation, and peer review (Cooper & Sparacino, 1990; Girouard, 1996; Girouard & Spross, 1983, 1988; Hamric, 1983a, 1989b). CNSs may document the numbers of patients seen, types and frequencies of interventions, and outcomes achieved; educational activities for staff, including individual coaching, in-service, orientation, and continuing education; and system initiatives such as quality improvement activities and interdisciplinary rounds. CNSs may elicit information on communication and collaboration from nursing and interdisciplinary colleagues to evaluate one's ability and effectiveness in exercising influence. CNSs may use these data for self-assessment to determine whether the activities are consistent with personal, professional, and institutional goals; to prepare quarterly reports; or to assemble a portfolio for one's annual evaluation. Tracking such data prospectively or retrospectively enables CNSs to identify generic recurring events that may require an intervention at the staff or system level as well as make midcourse corrections if schedule demands require a shift in goals or a realigning of expectations.

Studies of the impact of CNSs on patient and family outcomes accumulated slowly in the early days of CNS practice. However, the evidence is mounting and the positive impact on patient outcome is irrefutable. Students and practicing CNSs need to stay up-to-date on this research. Such studies can guide individual CNSs and groups of CNSs on the kinds of information they can collect to document CNS activities and their effects on patient and family outcomes. Classic studies include evaluation of the impact of CNS interventions on low birth weight infants and hospitalized elderly (Brooten et al., 1986; Neidlinger, Kennedy, & Scroggins, 1978). More recent studies have also shown the impact of CNS interventions on patients who received transitional care services from a CNS and were discharged from the hospital earlier than the norm (Brooten et al., 2002). Patients with congestive heart failure whose care was managed by CNSs had significantly shorter lengths of hospital stay and lower hospital expenses than those patients receiving usual care (Topp, Tucker, & Weber, 1998). As these topics suggest, CNSs can identify relevant structure, process, and outcome variables that can be used to assess the CNSs contributions to quality patient care. See Chapters 8 and 25 for further discussion of evaluation strategies.

Evaluation of practice often includes outcomes management. One component of outcomes management is the aggregation and analysis of data regarding care efficiency and cost-effectiveness, the results of which guide systematic and continuous process and performance improvement. Examples include the use of an outcome-driven clinical pathway developed by a multidisciplinary team to improve patient outcomes and reduce cost of care (Patton & Schaerf, 1995); initiation of an evidence-based, falls-prevention program in an acute care setting (Stetler, Corrigan, Sander-Buscemi, & Burns, 1999); and creation and implementation of a new central venous catheter procedure based on focused integrative review framework, application of research findings to practice, and an evidence-based practice construct (Newell-Stokes, Broughton, Guiliano, & Stetler, 2001).

CNSs have developed and implemented structured interventions, using an outcomes approach, to improve pain management. The results were improved patient satisfaction with pain management during hospitalization, consistency in patients' ability to identify a perceived level of acceptable pain, significant increase in staff nurses' knowledge of pain management, and more consistent pain management practice patterns by staff nurses (Barnason, Merboth, Pozehl, & Tietjen, et al., 1998). The evaluation of a CNS-directed outcomes management program for patients undergoing total hip and total knee arthroplasty demonstrated reduced length of hospital stay and hospital costs and a significant reduction in complications (Wammack & Mabrey, 1998; Wheeler, 2000).

Practice evaluation must be integrated into one's daily work. While researchers have begun to determine the types of interventions most often used by APNs, most of the work has been done in the evaluation of primary care or as part of programs evaluating the interventions of CNSs and NPs providing transitional care to discharged patients (Brooten et al., 1986; Brooten et al., 2002). Further study is needed to detail and substantiate which CNS competencies are most critical to improving clinical processes and patient outcomes. (See Chapter 25 for additional research evidence of APN impact.)

Participation in Collaborative Research. Before becoming involved in research, a CNS must assess whether there is readiness and receptiveness in the practice setting, whether there is administration support, and whether research activities are a realistic performance goal at a given time. Most often the practical level of involvement is collaborative nursing and interdisciplinary research (McGuire & Harwood, 2000). By being a member of a research team, a CNS is in the unique position to contribute to the generation of clinically based knowledge, to create a link between practical application and theoretical design, and to bridge the gap between how nursing *should* be practiced and *actually* is practiced. A CNS is the clinical expert, understands the clinical issues, and has access to patients; a nurse researcher is the research expert, knows research methodology, and has access to the resources that support the research. More CNSs and nurse researchers should conduct research that documents the impact of advanced practice nursing managed care, and other health-care changes on the quality of patient care. Interdisciplinary research offers opportunities for collaboration, but working together may reveal obstacles to collaborative research such as unexpected assumptions and divergent goals (O'Connell, 2001). The outcomes may be disappointing, recommendations misguided, and money misspent. For example, the SUPPORT study, a major effort to understand palliative care in intensive care units, was criticized for failing to involve CNSs in the design and conduct of the study or in the discussion of its results (Oddi & Cassidy, 1998).

As noted evaluating outcomes of practice to assess and improve the quality of care is an important element of the research competency (McGuire & Harwood, 2000; see also

Chapter 8). As CNSs become more experienced, they often want to participate in designing and conducting nursing research. Some CNSs pursue doctoral studies so that they use research skills more knowledgeably in their APN role. The CNS challenge is to facilitate evidence-based patient care interventions that are effective and cost-effective with all populations. One CNS-initiated performance improvement project evaluated the effect of antiplatelet drugs on the medical and surgical management of cardiac patients in general and the impact of clopidogrel bisulfate (Plavix) (Bristol-Meyers Squibb Co., New York, N.Y.) on patients undergoing cardiac surgery in particular; the project resulted in an evidence-based clinical practice guideline and improved blood use outcomes (Ley, 2001).

Recently nurse-sensitive indicators have been defined that capture nursing-unique contributions to patient outcomes. Assuming responsibility for identifying nursing-sensitive and multidisciplinary quality indicators (Duffy, 2002) and using outcome data to improve patient care delivery are prime opportunities for a CNS to assess patient care strategies and community systems, analyze interdisciplinary communication and collaboration, coordinate care, and monitor patient and system progress. Collaboration between CNSs and nurse researchers can facilitate quality improvement, strengthen the evidence base for nursing care, and enhance CNSs research skills. For example, there is a multisite project that uses outcomes and benchmarks for evidence-based practice and CNSs and other APNs as facilitators called the Nursing Improving Care for Healthsystem Elders (NICHE) project (Fulmer et al., 2002). The cooperative and collective data are used for benchmarking purposes against comparable institutions, evaluating unique data against the collective, and providing an evidence base for continuous performance improvement. The collaboration of a CNS and nurse researchers can provide research consultation for practice settings that want to implement practice changes to improve care and have the database to guide a quality improvement initiative but who do not have such expertise on staff. The University of Missouri-Columbia Minimum Data Set (MDS) and Nursing Home Quality Research Team, in collaboration with a gerontological CNS, work together with nursing home facilities to use the MDS-derived quality indicators to implement quality improvement efforts (Popejoy et al., 2000).

Whatever the model, a CNS is a key player in developing and implementing relevant nursing-sensitive and multidisciplinary quality indicators for measuring patient and system outcomes. In addition to applying research findings to clinical practice, CNSs must use research to influence public policy. It would be ideal to anticipate public policy needs in sufficient time to conduct research to influence the regulatory process. Although such foresight and the necessary time to conduct prospective research that might have policy implications are rare, that does not mean research results cannot be used to provide the substantive and objective facts that are more powerful and meaningful than impassioned pleas. The research literature is extensive, and professional, state, and national agencies have extensive data banks. This research must be used wisely, translating the findings to commonly understood and generally applicable language (Hamric, 1998).

CLINICAL AND PROFESSIONAL LEADERSHIP

The leadership competency is one of the three common threads that weave throughout the core competencies; the two other common threads are collaboration and ethical decision making. There are different types of leadership (e.g., clinical, interdisciplinary, entrepreneurial, organizational) and different attributes of leadership (e.g., vision, sense of timing, self-confidence, willingness to collaborate) (Hanson & Malone, 2000; see Chapter 9). Leadership is integral to the role because a CNS has responsibility for clinical innovation and change within the patient care system. A CNS has significant formal and informal impact and influence; a CNS must be visionary yet practical. Through a CNS's clinical leadership and influence, change strategies are implemented and nursing practice and patient care improve. A CNS is the link between a variety of disciplines and resources and asserts clinical and professional leadership in the practice setting or health-care system, in health-care policy and delivery decisions, and in the administration of direct care programs. A CNS identifies the need for practice changes and leads the development and implementation of clinical procedures, practice guidelines, and clinical pathways; designs and directs quality and performance improvement initiatives; chairs interdisciplinary committees or manages clinical projects; and influences or guides institutional health-care policy decisions. Clinical and professional leadership competencies are integrated with the other CNS competencies to support the overall purpose and goals of an organization. Most health-care organizations are a bureaucratic maze; a CNS works with, and advocates for, staff, patients, and families to help them comprehend the complexities and wend their way through the system. A CNS can serve as an advocate or "shuttle diplomat" between administrators and clinical staff, helping both groups understand the vagaries and particulars of organizational change, listening and supporting when appropriate, and explaining decisions when needed (Brown, 1989). As leaders, CNSs also help members of one discipline understand the perspectives and priorities of members of another discipline and often negotiate agreements that align these perspectives. Such mediation benefits patients and promotes communication, creating an environment that fosters collaboration as discussed in the next section.

COLLABORATION

Collaboration is the second common thread, and it is an essential competency, particularly because there are so many people with whom a CNS regularly works and interacts (see Chapter 10). A CNS collaborates with nurses, physicians, other health-care providers, and patients and their families. A CNS builds collaborative relationships with patients and families and provides an interface between patient, family members, and physician. Many patients have health-care needs that are so complex that no one health-care professional can manage them all. CNSs have a good understanding of the knowledge and skills of other team members and are active participants in interdisciplinary teams and rounds. A CNS is in the unique position to assist a patient and family members to determine their needs; help them to ask questions and assess treatment options; and facilitate timely referrals to other disciplines to ensure a positive outcome. Throughout her or his interactions with patients and colleagues, a CNS models for others the communication and collaboration skills that help teams mature.

A CNS is a nurse attending, a teacher, and a role model for nursing staff. CNSs are often leaders in identifying potential or actual conflicts. CNS advocacy often prevents adversarial situations and their negative sequelae. A CNS must be skilled in helping team members address and negotiate conflicts to optimize patient care. The outcome of CNS-coordinated collaboration is empowerment of nurses and recognition of the nurse as a critical member of the health-care team (Boyle, 1996). This results in team building, synergism, and integrative solutions. CNSs and physicians also collaborate, although some practice settings and working relationships are more conducive to partnership than others. When boundary issues and the pragmatic considerations of jobs and income are put aside, the differences in physician and CNS practice are complementary, afford integrative solutions, and further strengthen collaboration (Minarik & Sparacino, 1990). The outcome is high-quality and cost-efficient patient care (Baggs et al., 1999). Integrated care management, especially in controlling capitated risk in current health-care delivery systems, is best achieved by a collaborative team approach (Moss, Steiner, Mahnke, & Cohen, 1998).

Collaboration between a CNS and other health-care professionals contributes the necessary expertise to provide effective and efficient health care. CNSs can integrate the insights of many individuals with different perspectives, each providing theoretical and applied knowledge. Collaboration is an essential competency, but it is the well-earned result of clinical competence, effective communication, mutual trust, the valuing of complementary knowledge and skills, collegiality, and a favorable organizational structure (Hanson & Spross, 1996; Hanson, Spross, & Carr, 2000; Hughes & Mackenzie, 1990; Steele, 1986; see Chapter 10).

ETHICAL DECISION MAKING

Ethical decision making is a specific APN competency; it is also a common thread running through all core competencies. A CNS has significant influence on the negotiation of moral dilemmas, direction of patient care, access to care, and allocation of resources. CNSs consider numerous factors when making ethical decisions, including professional and religious codes, cultural values, bioethical principles, and ethical theories (Reigle, 1996; Reigle & Boyle, 2000; see Chapter 11). CNSs play critical roles in preventive and applied ethics. In promoting preventive ethics, a CNS is responsible for anticipating ethical conflicts when possible, teaching ethical theories, helping staff and patients clarify values, serving as a role model in discussions with patients about treatment preferences and options, demonstrating critical thinking in the analysis of moral dilemmas, and enhancing others' autonomy (Forrow, Arnold, & Parker, 1993).

CNSs have similar responsibilities when applying ethical decision-making skills to patient and organizational issues. They can articulate moral dilemmas. They can interpret and mediate patient, family, and team members' perspectives to ensure as complete a discussion as possible. They recognize the need for consultation with an ethics committee and often initiate the consult. When necessary, CNSs validate staff nurses' concerns and help nurses present their concerns to other team members, ensuring that the nursing perspective is considered when ethical issues are discussed. When CNSs are excluded from interdisciplinary processes involving ethical decisions, opportunities for effective nursing care are minimized and outcomes such as timely and appropriate end-of-life care are compromised (Oddi & Cassidy, 1998). As CNSs facilitate optimal care for frailer and sicker patients who require technological support but have inadequate financial resources, the ethical challenge is to balance the expectations for quality care with the limitations of managed care (Donagrandi & Eddy, 2000).

Spheres of Influence

Having described CNS competencies, it is apparent that there are three spheres of CNS influence: patient/clients, nursing personnel, and organizations or networks (NACNS, 1998, 2004). CNSs influence the patient/client sphere through activities such as assessment; diagnosis, planning, and outcome identification; interventions; and evaluation. CNSs influence nursing personnel by identifying and defining problems and opportunities in delivering care, nurse-specific outcomes, and collaborative practice; developing innovative solutions; and evaluating the effect of solutions. The organization/network sphere of influence includes identifying problems and opportunities, identifying resource management needs and developing innovative solutions, and evaluating the quality and cost-effectiveness of patient care technologies and care processes (NACNS, 1998, 2004).

The delineation of spheres of influence is theoretically intended to avoid the overlap of competencies and the perception of role ambiguity by distinguishing CNSs from other APNs (NACNS, 1998). Each sphere of influence requires various CNS competencies, so what a CNS does (e.g., dimensions) and how a CNS performs the role (e.g., competencies) affect the practice setting through the effective use of influence (e.g., spheres of influence). Understanding each sphere of influence and mastering CNS competencies are essential for a CNS to be successful.

EXEMPLAR OF CNS PRACTICE

Exemplar 12-1 illustrates how a CNS (the author) used the CNS competencies and spheres of influence to care for a complex and critically ill patient, her distraught but divided family, a concerned but overwhelmed physician, and a large group of caring but inexperienced nursing staff.

EXEMPLAR 12-1

Mrs. H. was an 82-year-old woman who was brought by paramedics to the emergency department with acute abdominal pain and severe pulmonary congestion. She was the matriarch of a large, supportive family who had differing opinions about the degree of her prehospital independence and state of health. For several weeks before admission, she had been experiencing dyspnea on exertion and was unable to walk more than a few steps. These symptoms progressively worsened. She was having severe respiratory distress at rest, was unable to walk more than a few steps without stopping to rest, and slept elevated on three pillows. Mrs. H. had worked her entire life until about 20 years ago, when she retired. Her husband had died at a young age. She had three children and a large extended family.

Her medical history included insulin-dependent diabetes mellitus, hypertension, atrial fibrillation, coronary artery disease, critical aortic stenosis, congestive heart failure (American Heart Association class IV), mild chronic obstructive pulmonary disease, chronic renal insufficiency, chronic urinary tract infections, and obesity. Pertinent findings on admission included the following:
1. *Physical examination:* alert and oriented but somnolent, coarse rales to midlung bilaterally, respiratory rate 26 to 34 and labored, accessory muscle use, 3 bilateral pitting edema to the knees, jugular venous distention
2. *Chest x-ray:* mild cardiac enlargement, bilateral interstitial pulmonary edema, calcification of the aortic valve, and a left pleural effusion
3. *Cardiac echo and catheterization:* severe aortic calcification not amenable to balloon valvuloplasty, peak aortic gradient 66 mm Hg, cardiac output 7.67 L/min, aortic valvular area 0.7 cm^2; no ejection fraction was recorded
4. *Laboratory:* white blood cell count 11.9/μl, hemoglobin 8.2 gm/dl, hematocrit 25.1%, sodium 126 mEq/L, fasting blood glucose 237 mg/dl, blood urea nitrogen 51 mg/dl, creatinine 1.9 mg/dl; urinalysis: yeast present

Mrs. H. stated that she could not go on as she was presently living and requested surgery. There was extensive discussion with the family, surgeon, and me about surgery, with the emphasis that the risks outweighed the benefits. The patient participated little in the discussion, only interjecting periodically that she wanted an operation to fix her aortic valve. Several days after hospital admission, Mrs. H. had surgery for an aortic valve replacement, using a

Continued

EXEMPLAR 12-1—cont'd

tissue valve. Her postoperative course was complicated by reoperation for bleeding and she needed pharmacological and pacer support for hypotension, complete heart block, and low urine output. The remainder of her 6-month hospital stay included reintubation and prolonged failure to wean from the ventilator, with a subsequent tracheotomy; ventricular ectopy and atrial fibrillation; drainage from her sternal wound and sepsis; and renal failure requiring dialysis. She was in the critical care unit for most of the 6 months because of ventilator dependency until, after one of many family conferences, she was extubated and transferred to an acute care unit, where she died about a week later.

Mrs. H.'s care was also confounded by various extended family dynamics. One son and one daughter shared unofficial power of attorney for health care. The son was very vocal about his preferences for his mother's future care, while the daughter, who had many personal crises, deferred to her two sons (Mrs. H's grandsons). Another daughter had financial power of attorney, but she felt culturally powerless to influence decisions because she was the youngest sibling. A nephew was an active participant in family conferences, and he opined that everything should be done.

Commentary

This was a difficult and challenging case, and it required using each of the CNS competencies and affecting each sphere of influence. There were numerous factors to consider in this case, and there were both successes and failures. Because of the nature of the CNS role, as well as the complexity of the case, it is nearly impossible to discuss each competency or influence separately. Rather, this section discusses key issues, interventions, successes, and failures, and the reader is referred to Table 12-1 to observe the overlapping nature of competencies and influence. The principal issues and interventions were the following:

1. Mrs. H. specifically stated that she did not want to continue to live as a "cardiac cripple" and demanded the surgery, despite the risks being clearly outlined. Her family did not want her to have the surgery but supported her decision. Her physician and I spent several hours with Mrs. H. and her family discussing the risks versus benefits of the surgery. In addition, her physician and I, together and independently, spent significant time with other physicians and nurses discussing the conflict between the patient's right to request treatment and the questionable chance for her survival or recovery. Specifically, could this elderly patient with multiple co-morbidities demand cardiac surgery, and at what level of risk could her surgeon conscionably refuse to perform the surgery? The key ethical principle we considered was the patient's autonomy, her preferences, and her freedom to act on her choice. We tried to clarify the sources of conflict and reviewed the primary ethical principles and theories involved in the decision making and consent process. After numerous discussions over several days, the surgery was done.

2. Mrs. H. had multiple nursing care needs postoperatively. Because of her multisystem failure, she

   - Had numerous episodes of hemodynamic instability as a result of the stress of hemodialysis on a depressed myocardium
   - Required a tracheotomy because of respiratory failure
   - Had complex dressing changes to her open sternal wound
   - Had difficulty communicating about the adequacy of pain control and comfort because of a variable level of consciousness, the fact that English was her second language, and her tracheotomy
   - Developed breakdown of the skin over her sacrum and was placed on a special bed to reduce pressure and prevent further breakdown

TABLE 12-1 OVERLAPPING COMPETENCIES AND INFLUENCE

KEY ISSUES	CORE COMPETENCIES				COMMON COMPETENCIES			SPHERES OF INFLUENCE		
	Clinical Practice	Consultation	Expert Teaching And Coaching	Scholarly or Scientific Inquiry	Clinical and Professional Leadership	Collaboration	Ethical Decision Making	Patients/Clients	Nurses	Organization
1. Preoperative surgical consent		✓		✓		✓	✓	✓	✓	
2. Postoperative nursing care	✓		✓					✓	✓	✓
3. Family discord	✓	✓ ✓				✓ ✓		✓	✓ ✓	
4. Overwhelmed nurses		✓	✓		✓		✓		✓	
5. Ethical dilemmas										
6. Appropriateness of cardiac surgery in the octogenarian		✓	✓	✓ ✓	✓		✓		✓	✓
7. Patient's limited ability to communicate	✓					✓		✓		

The amount of direct care I provided depended on whether Mrs. H. was in the critical care unit (experienced nurses) or the surgical floor (transitional care from critical care to acute care, where there were nurses with less experience). For example, sometimes I simply assessed the adequacy or appropriateness of a procedure performed by a staff nurse (e.g., sternal wound care or tracheotomy care) or determined if a new product was indicated (e.g., to protect the sacral wound). Other times I performed a procedure, such as tracheotomy care, to demonstrate appropriate technique or to assess the patient's response to the procedure. Often my involvement was, as Brown (Chapter 5) described, adjacent to the patient-nurse interface (e.g., working with the nurses to reevaluate her care, revise her nursing care plan, and influence the direction of care) rather than direct patient care.

3. The patient's family was large and divided in their opinions, so I facilitated many family conferences, sometimes just with family members and other times with the physician or other nursing staff, depending on the issue and the family's requests. The discussion in each of the many family conferences tended to stray from the meeting's intended purpose, and participants often became distracted by concerns about smaller but more tangible issues, such as Mrs. H.'s sacral wound instead of her ventilator dependency; the need to look for long-term placement, despite the grandson's lack of follow-through; unrealistic expectations for Mrs. H.'s recovery, such as the argument that she was a candidate for dialysis in an ambulatory care center, despite her bedbound status; and, as the poor chance for recovery became clearer, the family's clearly stated message of "you did the surgery—you cure her," forgetting the extensive preoperative discussion about the high risks and potential for a poor outcome.

4. The nursing staff felt overwhelmed with the extensive physical care combined with the various ethical issues involved. I, too, felt overwhelmed and wondered whether I was remaining objective but supportive. I therefore asked for a consultation with my psychiatric liaison CNS colleague; she provided support to me and to the nursing staff in private consultations as well as to the various health-care providers in the many interdisciplinary care planning conferences.

5. Because of the various ethical issues involved, the physician and I asked for a consultation with representatives of the hospital's Ethics Committee. Ethical principles and theories discussed included the following:

- Autonomy, related to Mrs. H.'s preferences and her freedom to act on a choice
- Beneficence, in relation to the right of the surgeon to refuse to perform a high-risk operation when the alternative of medical management had even higher risks and a poorer prognosis for the patient
- The theory of utilitarianism, in relation to the issues of rationing health care by age and allocation of resources (the relationship of the influence of resource allocation decisions on clinical judgment was also explored)

6. Ironically, Mrs. H's earlier request that she did not want to become ventilator dependent was "lost" and confounded subsequent medical and nursing decisions because of her inability to communicate for much of the postoperative period. Mrs. H. was awake and appeared alert when, many months later, the family made the decision to take her off the ventilator, transfer her to the surgical floor, and institute a "do not resuscitate" order. After discussion with the CNS and physician, the family agreed to a fenestrated tracheotomy tube so that Mrs. H. would have some chance for limited communication during her remaining life.

7. Throughout Mrs. H.'s hospitalization, the nursing staff had numerous questions about the conflict between the reasons for and the reasons against surgery in someone who was 82 years old. Specifically, they asked whether cardiac surgery in an elderly and ill patient was appropriate. I conducted an extensive literature search, discussed the findings with the surgeon to corroborate my conclusions and his opinion about a patient's right to autonomy and risks versus benefits, and then provided in-services for the nursing staff to discuss the results and practical application to Mrs. H.'s care.

There were various successes and failures in this case. The noteworthy successes included the excellent care that Mrs. H. and her family received from each provider; the knowledge (e.g., ethical principles, appropriateness of cardiac surgery in the elderly) and skills (e.g., tracheotomy care, complex sternal wound care, appropriate use of specialty beds) that many nurses acquired in the 6 months of caring for Mrs. H.; the collaboration between the CNSs (cardiovascular surgery CNS and psychiatric liaison CNS), nurses, physicians, and Ethics Committee consultants; and the fact that the dilemmas of caring for such a complex patient were supported by the medical center's mission and vision. There were failures from which valuable lessons for the future were learned, such as the physician's—and CNS's—dilemma of considering surgical risk versus benefit in this elderly patient with multiple co-morbidities and the need for earlier intervention to assist the family in reaching consensus about long-term treatment options and in understanding the emotional and financial impact of prolonging Mrs. H.'s inevitable death.

ISSUES AND CHALLENGES

Patient care has always been and will continue to be the very essence of the CNS role. A CNS's flexibility is well suited to adapt to systems changes while keeping the patient as the central focus. However, a CNS's ability to maintain a focus on patient care has been threatened by the changing demands of the health-care environment. A number of issues currently challenge the CNS role. These issues include but are not limited to educational preparation; factors influencing the evolution of CNS practice, such as role valuation, CNS position within an organization, and forced changes in role focus and titling; and legal and regulatory challenges, including credentialing, certification, and second licensure.

Educational Preparation

The dilemma in defining appropriate CNS education has been identifying and reaching consensus on a core body of knowledge for practice. All agree that basic CNS preparation requires a master's degree in nursing. Various efforts by the ANA's Council of Clinical Nurse Specialists and subsequently its Council for Advanced Practice Nursing, NACNS, and AACN have worked toward standardizing a curriculum. The AACN's *The Essentials of Master's Education for Advanced Practice Nursing* (AACN, 1996) has provided a blueprint for APN education, and the NACNS (1998, 2004) has made recommendations about inclusion of core CNS competencies (see p. 419, this chapter). The intent of developing a core curriculum is not homogenization but standardization. Without a common basis or standards for the educational preparation of a CNS, it is difficult to define consistent standards of practice and provide uniform certification at the advanced level. Nonetheless, graduate preparation of the CNS varies substantially, and the operative variable seems to be individual institutional educational philosophy that influences faculty philosophy and program emphasis. Recommendations have not been uniformly accepted or consistently implemented, and there is wide variability in the required minimum number of course credits and clinical hours. The minimum number of clinical hours will soon have to be one common element in graduate programs, however, because most certification exams require a minimum of 500 clinical hours and by 2006 the American Nurses Credentialing Center will require applicants for certification exams to have completed at least 500 clinical hours in their graduate program (Gerard & Walker, 2003). Over time these efforts should ensure standardization of CNS curricula and practicum requirements.

The development of a core curriculum must be specific enough to ensure a base of knowledge common to all CNSs, with the knowledge of the specialty area of nursing built onto the base of the core curriculum, yet a core curriculum must be flexible and forward thinking enough to respond to the rapidly changing health-care environment and move advanced practice nursing into the future. A core curriculum would include but not be limited to nursing and related theories, health assessment, research, and related topics such as ethics, legislative issues, economic concepts and health policy, and legal concepts. The curriculum would also incorporate the sciences of the selected specialty, diagnostic reasoning, disease and symptom management, critical thinking, supervised clinical practice, and a clinical residency specific to the specialty (Fenton & Brykczynski, 1993; Sparacino, 1994; AACN, 1996; Rasch & Frauman, 1996). The NACNS recommends additional content, including: "(1) differential diagnosis and treatment of symptoms, functional problems, or risk behaviors with nondisease-based etiologies, (2) a scientific base for the deliberate selection and use of specific nursing interventions, (3) clinical inquiry, (4) evaluation and measurement methodologies, (5) selection, design, and use of technology/products/services, and (6) change/influence theory" (NACNS, 1998, p. 11).

Much of the debate about curricular design has centered on the similarities and differences in the core curriculum of graduate nursing programs preparing CNSs and NPs and the advantages and disadvantages of combined education. There are various ways in which a framework could be developed for a core curriculum, especially when the curriculum combines the common areas of CNS and NP knowledge, domains, competencies, and practice (Fenton & Brykczynski, 1993). Opposition to combined education includes content differences (primary care, physical assessment, history taking) and different goals of care. Support for combined education cites the preparation of flexible clinicians who will be better prepared for broader practice opportunities or less conventional practice settings (Stark, 2000). (See Chapter 15 for a more complete discussion of these issues and further exploration of the blended CNS/NP role.)

When CNS master's programs were eliminated in the 1990s to make room for more NP programs, many in the CNS community questioned the lack of common sense and vision inherent in these decisions. The National Advisory Council on Nurse Education and Practice (NACNEP), however, issued a report in 1999 supporting the appropriate use of federal funds to support CNS graduate education. Included in the NACNEP report are policy issues, goals, and related policy options. Two of the goals are to clarify the CNS role in the changing health-care system and to ensure a place for the CNS within the health-care delivery system (Minarik, 2000; NACNEP, 1999). The enrollment and graduation numbers fluctuate, in part because of survey methods and responses, but also in part because of the nursing shortage, reactions to predictions about the influence of managed care's impact on hospital and health care, and employer interest. From 2000 to 2001, the percentage of CNSs who graduated increased by 15.2% and combined CNS/NPs by 79.1%, compared with a decline by 4.9% in NPs who graduated (AACN, 2002). The change from 2001 to 2002 saw a 1% decrease for CNS graduates, a decline by 6.7% in NPs who graduated, and a 7.9% reduction in CNS/NPs (Berlin, Stennett, & Bednash, 2003), yet between 1997 and 2001 the number of CNS-only programs increased by 28% (Walker et al., 2003). Adult medical-surgical nursing has remained the most popular area of specialization, but in the past several years there has been a reordering of other specialty interests: community health, pediatrics, gerontology, and psychiatric/mental health (Walker et al., 2003). Beginning in fall 2003, the NACNS and AACN/NONPF initiated a joint data collection effort, focused on identifying types of CNS-specific data and questions about education issues (AACN, 2003).

Factors Influencing the Evolution of CNS Practice

ROLE VALUATION

During the late 1980s and early 1990s, many administrators eliminated CNS roles for cost reasons. When CNSs and administrators do not understand the CNS role, disparate and arbitrary implementation and utilization dissipate its impact. Critics suggested that the positions were eliminated in part because few CNSs and administrators had linked CNS activities to patient outcomes or institutional outcomes, such as reduced staff nurse turnover, loss prevention, or increased revenue. Other critics thought that merging the CNS and NP roles would ensure job security. This issue is addressed in Chapters 3 and 15.

Although job security is never guaranteed, the proactive CNS designs and implements an evaluation plan as described earlier in this chapter. CNS effectiveness is measured or evaluated in various ways, such as appraisal of competencies or activities including self-evaluation and database analysis of consults and interventions, administrative and peer review, and program and outcomes evaluation (Cooper & Sparacino, 1990; Girouard, 1996; Hamric, 1983a, 1989b; Sample, 1983). The most compelling argument for the value of the CNS role will result when CNS effectiveness is evaluated in a way that focuses on patient care and visibility; that links structure and process variables; and that estimates CNS impact on cost, quality, and patient outcomes (Barnason et al., 1998; Broussard, 1996; Girouard, 1996; Mathew, Gutsch, Hackney, & Munsat, 1994; McAlpine, 1997; Smith & Waltman, 1994; Topp et al., 1998; Wammack & Mabrey, 1998). Evaluation strategies are usually planned with the nurse administrator. Routine evaluation is at least annual, with periodic interim reports. When a practice setting experiences a reorganization or financial exigency, a CNS may be asked to provide more detail about activities and outcomes.

ORGANIZATIONAL PLACEMENT

The constant threat of organizational redesign and other critical elements, including organizational structure and climate, administrative justification, and forced changes in role focus and role titling, can significantly affect a CNS's practice. A classic but recurring debate is whether a CNS should be in a staff or a line position (Prouty, 1983; Baird & Prouty, 1989). In a staff position, a CNS is freed from more administrative responsibilities and allowed to focus on patient care delivery and related issues, and the less threatening consultative capacity. The disadvantage of such a position is a lack of formal authority, such that power is referent or exercised by virtue of clinical expertise and knowledge. The advantage for a CNS in a line position is formal authority, but the distinct disadvantage is that administrative responsibilities may dominate her or his activities and erode the time available for clinical issues and patient care.

CNS ROLE DIGRESSIONS

When positions for CNSs were eliminated during the cost containment efforts of the 1990s, the merits of merging CNS and NP education were debated. While the profession was debating the issues, CNSs had to make decisions about their livelihood. Many CNSs went back to school to acquire NP education or accepted other leadership positions. As of 2004, many organizations have reintroduced the CNS role and it seems likely to remain an important APN position. Even so, the retrenchment that occurred in the 1990s has had a lingering effect. Because readers will still hear some discussion about a merged NP/CNS role (versus a blended CNS/NP role) and because experienced CNSs may decide to redirect their professional lives for reasons of personal growth or organizational change, it is worth describing some of the professional paths that experienced CNSs sometimes choose.

CNS or NP? Some CNSs have felt the need to acquire additional history-taking and physical assessment skills as well as prescriptive authority for job security. The basis for this challenge has been that CNSs have been increasingly pulled from the bedside to address competing demands and other organizational needs. Those who disagree with this proposal argue that an acute care NP's (ACNP's) primary emphasis is on patient care, limited to the particular practice setting and to the exclusion of a CNS's flexibility to care for patients across the continuum of care. In addition, the ACNP has fewer opportunities to participate in the other areas of usual CNS influence, such as staff education and development, nurse mentorship, leadership, consultation, research, and outcomes management. A CNS's decision to learn additional physical assessment skills may be based on clinical and practical concerns. For example, such skills may enable the CNS to provide better patient care in a CNS job or the CNS may make a deliberate decision to prepare for another APN role (NP or blended role). The CNS may believe that such preparation is needed to ensure job security in a changing environment. It may be that a state requires such preparation in order to be licensed as an APN. When a CNS makes this decision, it should be based on an assessment of personal, clinical, institutional, and statutory factors. Despite the many pendulum swings in popularity, the CNS role has not disappeared but has endured. In fact, graduate nursing programs have recently reinstated CNS preparation (Walker et al., 2003). Catholic University made a deliberative decision to prepare psychiatric–mental health APNs as community mental health CNSs. Their reasons were based on the community's need for APNs who could provide direct care to individual patients, including the performance of comprehensive assessments and provision of biological and behavioral interventions, as well as program planning, development, and evaluation (White, 2000). The need for CNSs who can care for patients, develop staff nurses, build interdisciplinary teams, and implement evidence-based practices and other systems changes is not going away.

CNS or APN Case Manager? The minimum educational requirement endorsed by the Case Management Society of America for a nurse case manager is a baccalaureate degree. However, the literature suggests that a CNS, with her or his expert clinical and consultant competencies, is better qualified to undertake the responsibilities of patient and quality measurement and research, financial analysis, provider education, and development and implementation of interdisciplinary practice improvements (Houston & Luquire, 1997; Weiss, 1998; see Chapter 18). In addition, case management involves many CNS responsibilities, such as patient care, collaboration with a multidisciplinary team, clinical system orchestration, administration of the interface between a patient and the health-care system, and involvement with, if not direction of, resource management and clinical system development. CNS implementation and facilitation of interdisciplinary rounds, broadening of the focus from discharge planning to early detection of problems, improved outcomes, and enhanced communication is another example of several integrated CNS competencies (Halm et al., 2003). In another example, CNS case managers identified older patients with multisystem failure who could become "outliers" and implemented cost-effective patient management strategies to reduce hospital length of stay and hospital costs (Cisar & Mitchell, 2001). In yet another example, CNS case managers developed a community-based multiple sclerosis clinic and served as clinical coordinators; the goals of the clinic were to coordinate services, mobilize individuals' personal and community resources, and reduce health-care costs (Taggart, Park, Banner, & Hart, 2000).

If a CNS is used exclusively as a (resource) utilization case manager, however, a CNS's impact and influence on direct patient care and coaching of nurses are neglected. Mahn and Spross (1996) first proposed nurse case management as an advanced practice role, different from the CNS role (see Chapter 18). An APN case manager's responsibilities are unit-, setting-, or population-based and involve direct care activities such as assessment and surveillance, as well as coaching, coordination of care, resource management, and clinical, financial, and outcome analyses for a particular patient population. Advanced educational preparation and clinical expertise lend credibility to a case manager's ability to develop, implement, and evaluate an outcomes management program.

Depending on the scope of case management responsibilities, case management may simply be an extension of existing CNS responsibilities, but in other settings it is a completely different APN role, as described in Chapter 18. I urge CNSs to avoid adding to the proliferation of job titles that seem designed to obscure the core responsibilities of advanced practice nursing. If a position encompasses the CNS dimensions, CNS competencies, and CNS spheres of influence, then the CNS title should be used. To continually introduce alternative but similar titles is confusing and erodes the profession's ability to define, assess, and document the impact of CNSs.

Legislative and Regulatory Challenges

Although progress has been made in overcoming the barriers imposed by state statutes and administrative dicta, financial changes in the current health-care market have created new challenges for APNs in general and CNSs in particular (Safriet, 1998). Legislative and regulatory barriers for a CNS are similar to those encountered by other APNs: restrictions on scope of practice, withholding of authority to prescribe drugs, and reimbursement. Statutory requirements for physician supervision or formalized APN-physician collaboration should be eliminated; APNs' prescriptive authority should be defined and controlled by Boards of Nursing regulations; and there should be a change in state and federal reimbursement and valuation of services provided (Safriet, 1992). While one legislative approach favors fewer references to specific titles, emphasizing similarities rather than the uniqueness of the various APN roles, another legislative approach advocates the statutory and regulatory recognition of the different contributions and scope of practice of each role, such as the CNS (Davidson et al., 2001). Some CNSs may not need or desire to prescribe drugs or may not have sufficient opportunity to prescribe often enough to do so safely. Nonetheless, CNS advocates should support legal efforts to obtain CNS prescriptive authority for those who can or must prescribe.

The current debate and divisive conflict about who will regulate CNS and APN practice is emanating primarily from within the nursing profession. The struggle centers on the retention of control by the nursing profession over scope of practice, interstate regulatory barriers, and standardization of APN practice. The NCSBN and NACNS have yet to reach agreement on all issues (see also Chapter 22). A brief summary of their opinions on credentialing and certification and secondary licensure follows.

CERTIFICATION, CREDENTIALING, AND LICENSING

As specialty practice becomes better defined, APN roles are more widely recognized, evidence-based practice guidelines are better accepted and used, and the quality and outcomes of patient care become more critical, issues of APN certification, credentialing, and licensing should become less controversial and contentious. Consensus and resolution of conflicting views on APN certification and credentialing are essential if the profession is to retain control over licensing and credentialing of APNs and ensure the protection of the public. The following paragraphs outline the differing perspectives of the NCSBN and the NACNS on CNS credentialing and licensing. Because they are evolving, readers will want to consult the publications of these national organizations for updated information.

NCSBN. The NCSBN Regulation of Advanced Practice Nursing position paper examines a number of issues, including APN education programs, certification, and responsibilities. The NCSBN's rationale for control over the APN licensing process is that a board of nursing cannot cede regulatory authority for certification examination content and scoring to private groups because the lack of quality control would have public safety implications. A certification examination is meant for regulatory purposes and measurement of job-related, entry-level knowledge and skills, at a minimum competence level. Thus APN licensure would be based on examination of broad, general categories such as medical-surgical or primary care nursing, or of developmental categories such as pediatric or adult practice. Specialty practice certification is considered "value-added" and is separate from licensure (NCSBN, 2002b).

NACNS. The NACNS is concerned about the extent of NCSBN regulation, for CNSs in particular, and considers state-level certification as overly restrictive (Lyons, 2002). The essence of CNS practice is expertise in the direct care of a specialty population (NACNS, 2003b). Many nursing specialties do not have certification examinations, however, because of the prohibitive test development and administration costs for a small number of APNs. Therefore a certification examination requirement for secondary licensure creates an obstacle for a CNS when a certification examination does not exist. Requiring a generalist certification examination is a less-than-satisfactory substitute because it cannot measure specialty practice competencies (NACNS, 2003a). The NACNS brought their concerns about these regulatory credentialing barriers to the Federal Trade Commission on June 11, 2003, raising concerns about the NCSBN's undue control over regulatory processes and the conflict between regulatory control and monetary gain from the sale of testing products.

SECONDARY LICENSURE

Some states require a CNS to obtain secondary licensure to practice as an APN. The criteria governing eligibility for this license varies. While a goal of regulatory control of a profession is to protect the public's safety, licensing regulations should enable and strengthen CNS practice, reduce practice and reimbursement barriers, and enhance public access to nursing care by an APN (Hanson & Hamric, 2003).

NCSBN. A final draft of the model language of the Advanced Practice Registered Nurse (APRN) Compact was approved in August 2002 (NCSBN, 2002a). An interstate compact addresses the more general licensure issues that hinder interstate practice by nurses and APNs, making mobility between two or more states possible, while keeping a state-based licensure and disciplinary arrangement. The NCSBN APRN Compact includes recognition of the CNS and other APNs only to the extent of an individual state's recognition of the role and title. The multistate privilege does not include prescriptive authority. The intent of the NCSBN APRN Compact is to ensure quality and consistency in the regulation of advanced practice nursing.

NACNS. The NACNS's position is the registered nurse license is the regulatory sanction for CNS practice. A CNS does not need a second license because CNS practice is within the scope of registered nurse licensure and does not extend into the medical domain, unlike NP practice. Secondary licensure is considered overregulation by members of the NACNS (NACNS, 2003b). However, a CNS who wants APN titling or who wants or needs prescriptive authority would have to meet all of the regulatory requirements of APN practice.

CONCLUSION

The CNS role survives. Its popularity has waxed and waned over the years but is again growing in this current climate of nursing shortages. CNSs have been recognized for their contributions to creating a healthy work environment (Disch Walton, & Barnsteiner, 2001) and improving patient outcomes. Although the health-care market and its future remain uncertain, it is imperative to sustain efforts to advance the CNS position and its influence. CNSs have weathered many challenges during the past several decades, including forced changes in role responsibilities and title, increased responsibility for directing other health-care providers, and constant organizational redesign oblivious to the CNS's diverse contributions. These threats to the CNS role and developmental changes in the health-care system, however, have also created exciting opportunities.

A CNS plays an indispensable, collaborative role in any health-care delivery system by ensuring a comprehensive focus on quality nursing care and extensive documentation to facilitate and measure quality patient outcomes. Various permutations of health-care reform in the past decade have provided CNSs with a singular opportunity to quantify what has always been the role's purpose: linking advanced practice nurse interventions and influence to patient outcomes and resource utilization. The impact of CNSs has been evident in patient and family outcomes, evidence-based practice, quality care outcomes, care efficiency, and cost-effectiveness.

This chapter chronicles a CNS's competencies and spheres of influence. Like other APNs, CNSs embody unique talents and skills, and the central focus of every CNS remains the patient. Now that a CNS's influence and impact can be measured, CNSs are well-positioned to improve patient outcomes, cost efficiency, and performance improvement by engaging in a variety of activities across spheres of influence. With the emphasis on evidence-based practice and improvement of the quality of patient care, CNSs will thrive as they integrate new knowledge into practice and influence and implement practice guidelines and innovative practice models.

See Box 12-1 for a list of Internet resources for the CNS.

BOX 12-1 • A SELECTION OF RESOURCES FOR THE CNS

American Association of Critical-Care Nurses	www.aacn.org
American Association of Colleges of Nursing	www.aacn.nche.edu
American Nurses Association	www.nursingworld.org
American Nurses Association (1996).	www.nursingworld.org/gova/rxauth.htm
Prescriptive authority chart.	
American Nurses Association (2000).	nursingworld.org/gova/charts/dea.htm
Prescriptive authority chart: Drug schedules.	
American Nurses Credentialing Center	www.nursingworld.org
Oncology Nursing Society	www.ons.org
National Association of Clinical Nurse Specialists	www.nacns.org
National Council of State Boards of Nursing	www.ncsbn.org
National Guideline Clearing House	www.guideline.gov

REFERENCES

Adams, P. (2000). Insight: A mental health prevention intervention. *Nursing Clinics of North America, 35,* 329-338.

American Association of Colleges of Nursing. (1996). *The essentials of master's education for advanced practice nursing.* Washington, DC: AACN.

American Association of Colleges of Nursing. (2003). *AACN and NACNS join forces to create a new data source for clinical nurse specialist education programs.* Retrieved July 20, 2003, from http://www.aacn.nche.edu/Media/NewsReleases/2003CNLEducation.htm

American Association of Colleges of Nursing. (2002). *Enrollment and graduations in baccalaureate and graduate programs in nursing.* Washington, DC: Author.

American Nurses Association. (1980). *Nursing: A social policy statement.* Kansas City, MO: Author.

American Nurses Association. (1985). *Facts about nursing 84–85* (p. 27). Kansas City, MO: Author.

American Nurses Association. (1986). *The role of the clinical nurse specialist.* Kansas City, MO: Author.

American Nurses Association, Congress of Nursing Practice. (1976). Description of practice: clinical nurse specialist. In *The scope of nursing practice.* Kansas City, MO: Author.

Baggs, J. G., Schmitt, M. H., Mushlin, A. I., Mitchell, P. H., Eldredge, D. H., Oakes, D., et al. (1999). Association between nurse-physician collaboration and patient outcomes in three intensive care units. *Critical Care Medicine, 27,* 1991-1998.

Baird, S. B., & Prouty, M. P. (1989). Administratively enhancing CNS contributions. In A. B. Hamric & J. A. Spross (Eds.), *The clinical nurse specialist in theory and practice* (2nd ed., pp. 261-284). Philadelphia: W. B. Saunders.

Barnason, S., Merboth, M., Pozehl, B., & Tietjen, M. J. (1998). Utilizing an outcome approach to improve pain management by nurses: A pilot study. *Clinical Nurse Specialist, 12,* 28-36.

Berlin, L. E., Stennett, J., & Bednash, G. D. (2003). *Enrollment and graduations in baccalaureate and graduate programs in nursing.* Washington, DC: American Association of Colleges of Nursing.

Boyle, D., M. (1996). The clinical nurse specialist. In A. B. Hamric, J. A. Spross, & C. M. Hanson (Eds.), *Advanced nursing practice: An integrative approach* (pp. 299-336). Philadelphia: W. B. Saunders.

Brooten, D., Kumer, S., Brown, L. P., Butts, P., Finkler, S. A., Bakewell-Sachs, S., et al. (1986). A randomized clinical trial of early hospital discharge and home follow-up of very-low-birth-weight infants. *New England Journal of Medicine, 315,* 934-939.

Brooten, D., Naylor, M. D., York, R., Brown, L. P., Munro, B. H., Hollingsworth, A. O., et al. (2002). Lessons learned from testing the Quality Cost Model of Advanced Practice Nursing (APN) Transitional Care. *Journal of Nursing Scholarship, 34,* 369-375.

Broussard, B. S. (1996). The role of the perinatal home care clinical nurse specialist. *Home Healthcare Nurse, 14,* 855-860.

Brown, S. J. (1989). Supportive supervision of the CNS. In A. B. Hamric & J. A. Spross (Eds.), *The clinical nurse specialist in theory and practice* (2nd ed., pp. 285-298). Philadelphia: W.B. Saunders.

Cisar, N. S., & Mitchell, A. (2001). Development of a program to manage costly outliers. *Clinical Nurse Specialist, 15,* 25-33.

Cooper, D. M., & Sparacino, P. S. A. (1990). Acquiring, implementing, and evaluating the clinical nurse specialist role. In P. S. A. Sparacino, D. M. Cooper, & P. A. Minarik (Eds.), *The clinical nurse specialist: Implementation and impact* (pp. 41-75). Norwalk, CT: Appleton & Lange.

Cronenwett, L. R. (1995). Molding the future of advanced practice nursing. *Nursing Outlook, 43,* 112-118.

Davidson, S. B., Beardsley, K., Busch, A. H., Garner, A., Heresa, S., Hodges, N. D., et al. (2001). Statutory and regulatory recognition for clinical nurse specialists in Oregon. *Clinical Nurse Specialist, 15,* 276-279.

Disch, J., Walton, M., & Barnsteiner, J. (2001). The role of the clinical nurse specialist in creating a healthy work environment. *AACN Clinical Issues, 12,* 345-355.

Donagrandi, M. A., & Eddy, M. (2000). Ethics of case management: Implications for advanced practice nursing. *Clinical Nurse Specialist, 14,* 241-246.

Duffy, J. R. (2002). The clinical leadership role of the CNS in the identification of nursing-sensitive and multidisciplinary quality indicator sets. *Clinical Nurse Specialist, 16,* 70-76.

Eisenberg, D. M., Davis, R. B., Ettner, S. L., Appel, S. Wilkey, S., Van Rompay, M., et al. (1998). Trends in alternative medicine use in the United States, 1990-1997: Results of a follow-up national survey. *Journal of the American Medical Association, 18,* 1569-1575.

Felder, L. (1983). Direct patient care and independent practice. In A. B. Hamric & J. Spross (Eds.), *The clinical nurse specialist in theory and practice* (pp. 59-72). New York: Grune & Stratton.

Fenton, M. V., & Brykcyznski, K. A. (1993). Qualitative distinctions and similarities in the practice of clinical nurse specialists and nurse practitioners. *Journal of Professional Nursing, 9,* 313-326.

Forrow, L., Arnold, R. M., & Parker, L. S. (1993). Preventive ethics: Expanding the horizons of clinical ethics. *Journal of Clinical Ethics, 4,* 287-294.

Fulmer, T., Mezey, M., Bottrell, M., Abraham, I., Sazant, J., Grossman, S., et al. (2002). Nurses Improving Care for Healthsystem Elders (NICHE): Using outcomes and benchmarks for evidence-based practice. *Geriatric Nursing, 23,* 121-127.

Gawlinksi, A., & Kern, L. S. (Eds.). (1994). *The clinical nurse specialist role in critical care.* Philadelphia: W. B. Saunders.

Gerard, P., & Walker, J. (2003). Charting a course for your future: A directory of clinical nurse specialist programs in the United States. *Clinical Nurse Specialist, 17,* 211-220.

Girouard, S. A. (1996). Evaluating advanced nursing practice. In A. B. Hamric, J. A. Spross, & C. M. Hanson (Eds.), *Advanced nursing practice: An integrative approach* (pp. 569-600). Philadelphia: W. B. Saunders.

Gurka, A. M. (1991). Process and outcome components of clinical nurse specialist consultation. *Dimensions of Critical Care Nursing, 10,* 169-175.

Halm, M. A., Gagner, S., Goering, M., Sabo, J., Smith, M., & Zaccagnini, M. (2003). Interdisciplinary rounds: Impact on patient, families, and staff. *Clinical Nurse Specialist, 17,* 133-142.

Hamric, A. B. (1983a). A model for developing evaluation strategies. In A. B. Hamric & J. A. Spross (Eds.), *The clinical nurse specialist in theory and practice* (pp. 187-206). New York: Grune & Stratton.

Hamric, A. B. (1983b). Role development and functions. In A. B. Hamric & J. Spross (Eds.), *The clinical nurse specialist in theory and practice* (pp. 39-56). New York: Grune & Stratton.

Hamric, A. B. (1989a). History and overview of the CNS role. In A. B. Hamric & J. A. Spross (Eds.), *The clinical nurse specialist in theory and practice* (2nd ed., pp. 3-18). Philadelphia: W. B. Saunders.

Hamric, A. B. (1989b). A model for CNS evaluation. In A. B. Hamric & J. A. Spross (Eds.), *The clinical nurse specialist in theory and practice* (2nd ed., pp. 83-104). Philadelphia: W. B. Saunders.

Hamric, A. B. (1995). Creating our future: Challenges and opportunities for the clinical nurse specialist. *Oncology Nursing Forum, 22,* 547-553.

Hamric, A. B. (1996). A definition of advanced nursing practice. In A. B. Hamric, J. A. Spross, & C. M. Hanson (Eds.), *Advanced nursing practice: An integrative approach* (pp. 42-56). Philadelphia: W. B. Saunders.

Hamric, A. B. (1998). Using research to influence the regulatory process. *Advanced Practice Nursing Quarterly, 4,* 44-50.

Hamric, A. B. (2000). A definition of advanced nursing practice. In A. B. Hamric, J. A. Spross, & C. M. Hanson (Eds.), *Advanced nursing practice: An integrative approach* (2nd ed., pp. 53-73). Philadelphia: W. B. Saunders.

Hamric, A. B. & Spross, J. A. (Eds.). (1989). *The clinical nurse specialist in theory and practice* (2nd ed.). Philadelphia: W. B. Saunders.

Hamric, A. B., Spross, J. A., & Hanson, C. M. (Eds.). (1996). *Advanced nursing practice: An integrative approach.* Philadelphia: W. B. Saunders.

Hamric, A. B., Spross, J. A., & Hanson, C. M. (Eds.). (2000). *Advanced nursing practice: An integrative approach* (2nd ed.). Philadelphia: W. B. Saunders.

Hanson, C. M., & Hamric, A. B. (2003). Reflections on the continuing evolution of advanced practice nursing. *Nursing Outlook, 19,* 262-268.

Hanson, C. M., & Malone, B. L. (2000). Leadership: Empowerment, change agency, and activism. In A. B. Hamric, J. A. Spross, & C. M. Hanson (Eds.), *Advanced nursing practice: An integrative approach* (2nd ed., pp. 279-313). Philadelphia: W. B. Saunders.

Hanson, C. M., & Spross, J. A. (1996). Collaboration. In A. B. Hamric, J. A. Spross, & C. M. Hanson (Eds.), *Advanced nursing practice: An integrative approach* (pp. 229-248). Philadelphia: W. B. Saunders.

Hanson, C. M., Spross, J. A., & Carr, D. B. (2000). Collaboration. In A. B. Hamric, J. A. Spross, & C. M. Hanson (Eds.), *Advanced nursing practice: An integrative approach* (2nd ed., pp. 315-347). Philadelphia: W. B. Saunders.

Hoeffer, B., & Murphy, S. A. (1984). Specialization in nursing practice. In *Issues in professional nursing practice* (pp. 1-10). Kansas City, MO: American Nurses Association.

Houston, S., & Luquire, R. (1997). Advanced practice nurse as outcomes manager. *Advanced Practice Nursing Quarterly, 3,* 1-9.

Hughes, A., & Mackenzie, C. (1990). Components necessary in a successful nurse practitioner-physician collaborative practice. *Journal of the American Academy of Nurse Practitioners, 2,* 54–57.

Jennings, B. M. (2000). Evidence-based practice: The road best traveled? *Research in Nursing & Health, 23,* 343-345.

Keane, A., & Richmond, T. S. (1993). Tertiary nurse practitioners. *Image: The Journal of Nursing Scholarship, 25,* 281-284.

Kennedy, B., Covington, K., Evans, T., & Williams, C. A. (2000). Mental health consultation in a nursing home. *Clinical Nurse Specialist, 14,* 261-266.

Koetters, T. L. (1989). Clinical practice and direct patient care. In A. B. Hamric & J. A. Spross (Eds.), *The clinical nurse specialist in theory and practice* (2nd ed., pp. 107-124). Philadelphia: W. B. Saunders.

Ley, S. J. (2001). Quality care outcomes in cardiac surgery: The role of evidence-based practice. *AACN Clinical Issues, 12,* 606-617.

Lincoln, P. E. (2000). Comparing CNS and NP role activities: A replication. *Clinical Nurse Specialist, 14,* 269-277.

Lyons, B. L. (2002). The regulation of clinical nurse specialist practice: Issues and current developments. *Clinical Nurse Specialist, 16,* 239-241.

Mahn, V. A., & Spross, J. A. (1996). Nurse case management as an advanced practice role. In A. B. Hamric, J. A. Spross, & C. M. Hanson (Eds.), *Advanced nursing practice: An integrative approach* (pp. 445-465). Philadelphia: W. B. Saunders.

Mathew, L. J., Gutsch, H. M., Hackney, N. W., & Munsat, E. M. (1994). Promoting quality and cost-effective care to geropsychiatric patients. *Issues in Mental Health Nursing, 15,* 169-185.

McAlpine, L. A. (1997). Process and outcome measures for the multidisciplinary collaborative projects of a critical care CNS. *Clinical Nurse Specialist, 11,* 134-138.

McGuire, D. B., & Harwood, K. V. (1989). The CNS as researcher. In A. B. Hamric & J. A. Spross (Eds.), *The clinical nurse specialist in theory and practice* (2nd ed., pp. 169-204). Philadelphia: W. B. Saunders.

McGuire, D. B., & Harwood, K. V. (2000). Research. In A. B. Hamric, J. A. Spross, & C. M. Hanson, (Eds.), *Advanced nursing practice: An integrative approach* (2nd ed., pp. 245-278). Philadelphia: W. B. Saunders.

McPheeters, M., & Lohr, K. N. (1999). Evidence-based practice and nursing: Commentary. *Outcomes Management for Nursing Practice, 3,* 99-101.

Mick, D. J., & Ackerman, M. H. (2002). Deconstructing the myth of the advanced practice blended role: Support for role divergence. *Heart & Lung, 31,* 393-398.

Minarik, P. A. (2000). Report recommends federal funding for CNS preparation. *Clinical Nurse Specialist, 14,* 82-83.

Minarik, P. A., & Sparacino, P. S. A. (1990). Clinical nurse specialist collaboration in a university medical center. In P. S. A. Sparacino, D. M. Cooper, & P. A Minarik (Eds.), *The clinical nurse specialist: Implementation and impact* (pp. 231-260). East Norwalk, CT: Appleton & Lange.

Moller, M. D., & Haber, J. (1996). Advanced practice psychiatric nursing: The need for a blended role. *Online Journal of Issues in Nursing, 1,* 6. Retrieved May 4, 2004, http://nursingworld.org/ojin/tpc1_7.htm

Moss, J. K., Steiner, K., Mahnke, K., & Cohen, R. (1998). A model to manage capitated risk. *Nursing Economics, 16,* 65–68.

National Advisory Council on Nurse Education and Practice (1999). *Federal support for the preparation of the clinical nurse specialist workforce through Title VIII: A report to the Secretary of Health and Human Services.* (HRSA Publication 99-40). Washington, DC: Division of Nursing, Bureau of Health Professions Health Resources and Services Administration, U.S. Department of Health and Human Services.

National Association of Clinical Nurse Specialists. (1998). *Statement on clinical nurse specialist practice and education.* Glenview, IL: Author.

National Association of Clinical Nurse Specialists. (2003a). Response of the NACNS to the NCSBN proposed revision to the uniform advanced practice registered nurse licensure/authority to practice requirements (March 2002). *Clinical Nurse Specialist, 17,* 59-65.

National Association of Clinical Nurse Specialists. (2003b). Regulatory credentialing of clinical nurse specialists. *Clinical Nurse Specialist, 17,* 163-169.

National Association of Clinical Nurse Specialists. (2004). *Statement on clinical nurse specialist practice and education.* Harrisburg, PA: Author.

National Council of State Boards of Nursing. (1998). *Interstate compact for a mutual recognition model of nursing.* Chicago: Author.

National Council of State Boards of Nursing. (2002a). *Advanced practice registered nurse compact.* Retrieved January 26, 2003, from www.ncsbn.org/pdfs/APRNCompact.pdf

National Council of State Boards of Nursing. (2002b). Regulation of advanced practice nursing: 2002 National Council of State Boards of Nursing Position Paper. *Retrieved July 20, 2003, from. (www.ncsbn.org/public/regulations/res/APRN_Position_Paper2002.pdf)*

National Council of State Boards of Nursing (2002c). *Requirements for accrediting agencies and criteria for APRN certification programs.* Retrieved April 24, 2004, from http://www.ncsbn.org/pdfs/APRN_approved_criteria_requirements_04.pdf

Neidlinger, S., Kennedy, L., & Scroggins, K. (1987). Effective and cost efficient discharge planning for hospitalized elders. *Nursing Economics, 5,* 225-230.

Newell-Stokes, V., Broughton, S., Guiliano, K. K., & Stetler, C. B. (2001). Developing an evidence-based procedure: Maintenance of central venous catheters. *Clinical Nurse Specialist, 15*, 199-204.

Noll, M. (1987). Internal consultation as a framework for clinical nurse specialist practice. *Clinical Nurse Specialist, 1*, 46-50.

Oberle, K., & Allen, M. (2001). The nature of advanced practice nursing. *Nursing Outlook, 49*, 148-153.

O'Connell, K. A. (2001). Barriers to interdisciplinary research. *Journal of Professional Nursing, 17*, 53-154.

Oddi, L. F., & Cassidy, V. R. (1998). The message of SUPPORT: Change is long overdue. *Journal of Professional Nursing, 14*, 165-174.

Patton, M. D., & Schaerf, R. (1995). Thoracotomy, critical pathway, and clinical outcomes. *Cancer Practice, 3*, 286-294.

Popejoy, L. L., Rantz, M. J., Conn, V., Wipke-Tevis, D., Grando, V. T., & Porter, R. (2000). Improving quality of care in nursing facilities: Gerontological clinical nurse specialist as research nurse consultant. *Journal of Gerontological Nursing, 26*, 6-13.

Prouty, M. P. (1983). Contributions and organizational role of the CNS: An administrator's viewpoint. In A. B. Hamric & J. Spross (Eds.), *The clinical nurse specialist in theory and practice*. New York: Grune & Stratton.

Rantz, M. J., Popejoy, L., Petroshki, P. F., Madsen, R. W., Mehr, D. R., Zwygart-Stauffacher, M., et al. (2001). Randomized clinical trial of a quality improvement intervention in nursing homes. *Gerontologist, 41*, 525-538.

Rasch, R. F., & Frauman, A. C. (1996). Advanced practice in nursing: Conceptual issues. *Journal of Professional Nursing, 12*, 141-146.

Rasmussen, D., & Barnason, S. (2000). Chest pain management: Liking tertiary and rural settings. *Nursing Clinics of North America, 35*, 321-328.

Reigle, J. (1996). Ethical decision-making skills. In A. B. Hamric, J. A. Spross, & C. M. Hanson (Eds.), *Advanced nursing practice: An integrative approach* (pp. 273–295). Philadelphia: W. B. Saunders.

Reigle, J., & Boyle, R. J. (2000). Ethical decision-making skills. In A. B. Hamric, J. A. Spross, & C. M. Hanson (Eds.), *Advanced nursing practice: An integrative approach* (2nd ed., pp. 349-378). Philadelphia: W. B. Saunders.

Safriet, B. J. (1992). Health care dollars and regulatory sense: The role of advanced practice nursing. *Yale Journal on Regulation, 9*, 149-220.

Safriet, B. J. (1998). Still spending dollars, still searching for sense: Advanced practice nursing in an era of regulatory and economic turmoil. *Advanced Practice Nursing Quarterly, 4*, 24-33.

Sample, S. A. (1983). Justifying and structuring the CNS role in the nursing department. In A.B. Hamric & J. Spross (Eds.), *The clinical nurse specialist in theory and practice* (pp. 117-128). New York: Grune & Stratton.

Seemann, S. (2000). Interdisciplinary approach to a total knee replacement program. *Nursing Clinics of North America, 35*, 405-415.

Shea, C.A., Pelletier, L.R., Poster, E.C., Stuart, G.W. & Verhey, M.P. (Eds.) (1999). *Advanced practice nursing in psychiatric and mental health care*. Philadelphia: Elsevier/Mosby.

Smith, J. E., & Waltman, N. L. (1994). Oncology clinical nurse specialists' perceptions of their influence on patient outcomes. *Oncology Nursing Forum, 21*, 887-893.

Sneed, N. V. (1991). Power: Its use and potential for misuse by nurse consultants. *Clinical Nurse Specialist, 5*, 58-62.

Soehren, P. M., & Schumann, L. L. (1994). Enhanced role opportunities available to the CNS/Nurse Practitioner. *Clinical Nurse Specialist, 8*, 123-127.

Soukup, M. (2000). The Center for Advanced Nursing Practice evidence-based practice model. *Nursing Clinics of North America, 35*, 301-309.

Sparacino, P. S. A. (1990). A historical perspective on the development of the clinical nurse specialist role. In P. S. A. Sparacino, D. M. Cooper, & P. A. Minarik (Eds.), *The clinical nurse specialist: implementation and impact* (pp. 3-10). East Norwalk, CT: Appleton & Lange.

Sparacino, P. S. A. (1994). Issues and future trends for the critical care clinical nurse specialist. In A. Gawlinski & L. S. Kern (Eds.), *The clinical nurse specialist role in critical care* (pp. 293-307). Philadelphia: W. B. Saunders.

Sparacino, P. S. A., & Cooper, D. M. (1990). The role components. In P. S. A. Sparacino, D. M. Cooper, & P. A. Minarik (Eds.), *The clinical nurse specialist: Implementation and impact* (pp. 11-40). Norwalk, CT: Appleton & Lange.

Sparacino, P. S. A., Cooper, D. M., & Minarik, P. A. (Eds.). (1990). *The clinical nurse specialist: Implementation and impact*. Norwalk, CT: Appleton & Lange.

Sparacino, P. S. A., & Durand, B. A. (1986). Editorial on specialization in advanced nursing practice. *Momentum, 4*, 2-3.

Sprately, E., Johnson, A., Sochalski, J., Fritz, M., & Spencer, W. (2000). *The registered nurse population: Findings from the national sample survey of registered nurses—March 2000*. Retrieved April 24, 2004, from http://bhpr.hrsa.gov/healthworkforce/rnsurvey/rnss1.htm

Spross, J., Clarke, E. B., & Beauregard, J. (2000). Expert coaching and guidance. In A. B. Hamric, J. A. Spross, & C. M. Hanson (Eds.), *Advanced nursing practice: An integrative approach* (2nd ed., pp. 183-215). Philadelphia: W. B. Saunders.

Spross, J., & Hamric, A. B. (1983). A model for future clinical nurse specialist practice. In A. B. Hamric & J. Spross (Eds.), *The clinical nurse specialist in theory and practice* (pp. 291-306). New York: Grune & Stratton.

Spross, J. A., & Heaney, C. A. (2000). Shaping advanced nursing practice in the new millennium. *Seminars in Oncology Nursing, 16,* 12-24.

Stark, S. W. (2000). Point of view: The case for combined education for the NP and CNS. *Journal of the American Academy of Nurse Practitioners, 12,* 85-87.

Steele, J. E. (Ed.). (1986). *Issues in collaborative practice.* Orlando: Grune & Stratton.

Stetler, C. B., Corrigan, B., Sander-Buscemi, K., & Burns, M. (1999). Integration of evidence into practice and the change process: Fall prevention program as a model. *Outcomes Management for Nursing Practice, 3,* 102-111.

Taggart, H. M., Park, M., Banner, J., & Hart, M. (2000). Case management model for a community-based multiple sclerosis clinic. *Clinical Nurse Specialist, 14,* 199-204

Topp, R., Tucker, D., & Weber, C. (1998). Effect of a clinical case manager/clinical nurse specialist on patients hospitalized with congestive heart failure. *Nursing Case Management, 3,* 140-147.

Walker, J., Gerard, P.S., Bayler, E. W., Coeling, H., Clark, A. P., Dayhoff, N., et al. (2003). A description of clinical nurse specialist programs in the United States. *Clinical Nurse Specialist, 17,* 50-57.

Wammack, L., & Mabrey, J. D. (1998). Outcomes assessment of total hip and total knee arthroplasty: Critical pathways, variance analysis, and continuous quality improvement. *Clinical Nurse Specialist, 12,* 122-129.

Weiss, M. E. (1998). Case management as a tool for clinical integration. *Advanced Practice Nursing Quarterly, 4,* 9-15.

Wheeler, E. C. (2000). The CNS's impact on process and outcome of patients with total knee replacement. *Clinical Nurse Specialist, 14,* 159-169.

White, J. H. (2000). Developing a CNS role to meet the mental health needs of the underserved. *Clinical Nurse Specialist, 14,* 141-149.

Williams, C. A., & Valdivieso, G. C. (1994). Advanced practice models: A comparison of clinical nurse specialist and nurse practitioner activities. *Clinical Nurse Specialist, 8,* 311-318.

Wolbert Burgess, A. (1997). *Advanced Practice Psychiatric Nursing.* Englewood Cliffs, NJ: Prentice Hall.

Woods, S. S., Nass, J., & Deisch, P. (2000). Selection and implementation of a transparent dressing for central vascular access devices. *Nursing Clinics of North America, 35,* 385-394.

CHAPTER 13

The Primary Care Nurse Practitioner

ANN REID ANDERSON

INTRODUCTION

This chapter provides an overview of the primary care nurse practitioner (NP) role. The primary care NP provides care for patients in several specialties and in multiple community-based settings. With today's emphasis on primary health care within cost containment systems, the advanced practice nurse (APN) role has gained widespread attention. This chapter explores the evolution of primary care NP roles and settings over time and as the NP role relates to the Institute of Medicine (IOM) definition of primary care. APN competencies of direct clinical practice, expert coaching and guidance, consultation, leadership, research and ethical decision making as operationalized in primary care NP practice are described. Exemplars of pediatric and family NPs practicing in urban and rural settings are provided to demonstrate the integration of NP competencies in diverse primary care settings. Finally, information about functional role preparation, transition to professional practice, and key issues for primary care NPs are presented.

PROFILE OF THE PRIMARY CARE NP ROLE

The first primary care NP role, that of the pediatric NP, focused on the care of children and was conceived to increase access to pediatric primary care (Ford & Silver, 1967; see Chapter 1). Since then, a variety of primary care NP roles have evolved, emphasizing care to specific populations such as families, adults, the elderly, and women. In general, these roles have evolved over time as the ability of nurses in advanced practice to address the needs of varied populations has been recognized. Primary care NPs can increase access to care for underserved populations (Clawson & Osterweis, 1993) and have been acknowledged as cost-effective providers of quality primary care (Brown & Grimes, 1993; Cook & Nolan, 1996; Kane et al., 1991; Kornbilt, Senderoff, Davis-Eriksen, & Zenk, 1990; Mabrook & Dale, 1998; Mundinger et al., 2000).

Policymakers at both the state and federal levels have cited the difficulty in obtaining accurate information on NPs in the workforce (National Advisory Council on Nurse Education and Practice [NACNEP], 2002; Virginia General Assembly, 1999). Overlapping of specialty areas, blended and dual NP practice roles, and varied titling by states make it difficult to determine the number of primary care NPs in the nation. A survey of NP programs nationwide conducted by the National Organization of Nurse Practitioner Faculties (NONPF) and the American Association of Colleges of Nursing (AACN) assessed the numbers of APNs available to enter the workforce (Berlin, Stennett, & Bednash, 2003). NP data from this survey are summarized in Tables 13-1 and 13-2.

There were 4963 graduates from master's-level nursing programs in primary care specialties from August 1, 2001, to July 31, 2002. Primary care specialties account for approximately 81% of all NP graduates. This number may be higher because graduates with dual preparation, such as those from combined NP/CNS (clinical nurse specialist) programs, are not reported. The overwhelming majority of primary care NP graduates were from family NP programs (3,212, or 54%) followed by adult NP (844, or 13.8%; see Table 3-1). Data from Table 13-2 indicate that, at this time, few NPs are prepared at the certificate level: master's level preparation for NP practice predominates, accounting for 93.7% of NP graduates (Berlin et al., 2003).

The author would like to thank Diane L. Hanna, MS, RNC, FNP, for her significant contributions to earlier editions of this chapter and her husband, Phil Anderson, for his editorial and technical assistance with this chapter.

TABLE 13-1	MASTER'S-LEVEL NURSE PRACTITIONERS: NP GRADUATES BY PRIMARY CARE SPECIALTY FROM ALL PROGRAMS (AUGUST 2001-JULY 2002)

	NO. OF GRADUATES	%
Family NP	3212	54
Adult NP	844	13.8
Pediatric NP	532	8.7
Gerontological NP	125	4.1
Women's health NP	250	2.0

From Berlin, L. E., Stennett, J., & Bednash, G. D. (2003). *2002-2003 Enrollment and graduations in baccalaureate and graduate programs in nursing.* Washington, DC: American Association of Colleges of Nursing.
NOTE: Data for NPs in dual track and combined NP/CNS programs do not specify specialty.

TABLE 13-2	STUDENTS COMPLETING NP PROGRAMS BY TYPE OF PROGRAM (AUGUST 2001-JULY 2002)

	NO. OF STUDENTS	%
Master's	6128	93.7%
Post-master's	795	6.0%
Certificate	19	0.3%

From Berlin, L. E., Stennett, J., & Bednash, G. D. (2003). *2002-2003 Enrollment and graduations in baccalaureate and graduate programs in nursing.* Washington DC: American Association of Colleges of Nursing.

The National Sample Survey of Registered Nurses in 2000 (Table 13-3) estimated the number of NPs at 102,829 as compared with 70,993 NPs in 1996 (Health Resources Services Administration [HRSA] (Spratley, Johnson, Sochalski, Fritz, & Spencer, 2000). In 2000, approximately 64% (58,512) of nurses with NP education and employed in nursing used the title nurse practitioner. Ambulatory care was the most frequently cited (41%) practice location for primary care NPs. Other sites included hospital (29%), community health (16%), student health (6%), occupational health (2%), and nursing education (0.5%). While the overall number of NPs continues to grow and the number of master's level NP programs expands, it is difficult to predict whether the growth will occur in the primary care setting or in other settings. The lack of NP faculty is a growing concern (Spratley, et al., 2000). *Healthy People 2010* reported that competing interests in the market, including physicians, nonphysician providers, and the insurance industry, make it difficult to predict the future role of primary care NPs (U.S. Department of Health and Human Services, 2000). However, national trends for the next two decades that project increasing population growth, increasing numbers of elderly people, and aging "baby boomers," and marked increase in cultural diversity within communities ensure the need for a growing primary care NP workforce (Showstack, Rothman, & Hassmiller, 2004b).

TABLE 13-3	REGISTERED NURSES WITH FORMAL PREPARATION TO PRACTICE AS NP	

	1996	2000
RNs with formal preparation as NP	71,000	102,829
% of RNs with preparation as NP employed in nursing	90%	89%
% of RNs with title of NP	58%	64%

From Spratley, E., Johnson, A., Sochalski, J., Fritz, M., Spencer, W. (2000). *The registered nurse population: Findings from the National Sample Survey of Registered Nurses.* Washington, DC: U.S. Department of Health and Human Services, Health Resources and Service Administration, Bureau of Health Professions, Division of Nursing.

Between 1992 and 1997, there was a striking increase in the number of institutions offering master's-level NP programs: from fewer than 100 nationwide to more than 250. This trend was sparked by discussions of major federal health reforms and a renewed interest in primary care. The result was a fourfold increase in the number of NPs graduating annually, with further increases anticipated in the future (Cooper, Laud, & Dietrich, 1998). This increase in primary care NP programs has stabilized as new NP roles have evolved, especially the role of the acute care NP (see Chapter 14). Moreover, more nurses are choosing the CNS as their APN role (Berlin et al., 2003). Nursing shortage issues across the country add to the complexity of the problem as APNs are recruited to fill hospital-based positions. The major NP member organizations, national certifying bodies, and the Department of Health and Human Services, Division of Nursing, continue to work together to determine the supply and demand for NP primary care providers across all settings and populations.

PRIMARY CARE NP PRACTICE

What do family, adult, pediatric, obstetric/gynecological, gerontological, and other primary care NPs have in common? The answer to this question lies in a more in-depth analysis of the terms "primary care" and "nurse practitioner." Definitions of primary care have evolved over time. As part of a 2-year study on the future of primary care, the IOM updated the definition of primary care (1996). The definition was intended to help health professionals, policymakers, educators, and the public confront the rapid changes under way in health care as primary care is re-emphasized in the United States. Although this "updated" definition is almost 10 years old, it remains the best working definition available:

*Primary care is the provision of **integrated, accessible health-care services** by clinicians who are **accountable** for addressing a large **majority of personal health-care needs,** developing a **sustained partnership** with **patients,** and practicing in the **context of family and community.***

The words in bold were defined by the IOM to clarify the nature of services, those involved in the delivery of care, and the nature of the relationship between clinician and patient. Box 13-1 summarizes the defining characteristics of the key terms, which are explained in detail in the IOM report (1996). Barbara Starfield, MD, MPH, and member of the American Academy of Family Physicians, reiterated the need for an integrated approach to primary care in the United States. "Every effort must be made to sustain the primary care field, including family physicians, general internists, pediatricians, nurse practitioners and, in some instances, obstetricians-gynecologists. Once we are ready to transform into an integrated system we must have in place the substrate and foundation of a primary care system" (Starfield, 2003). The inclusion of NPs in this statement is good news for primary care NPs, who are becoming recognized as valid, reimbursable primary care providers (PCPs) of record in many states. New work is being done to revitalize primary care as an integral part of our health-care system. A core concept of this renaissance of primary care includes the reconstruction of current health-care systems. Choice of provider, including primary care nurse practitioners, will be based on achieving desired outcomes (Showstock, Lurie, Larson, Rothman, & Hassmiller, 2004a).

The IOM definition of primary care encompasses much of the essence of advanced practice nursing with its emphasis on accountability, a holistic approach to patient care, inclusion of health promotion and disease prevention activities, and description of

---

BOX 13-1 • IOM TERMS USED TO DEFINE PRIMARY CARE

Integrated
- Comprehensive, coordinated care throughout the life cycle
- Focused on particular needs of patients
- Clinician continuity
- Effective communication of information
- Record continuity

Accessibility
- Ease with which care is attained
- Elimination of geographic, cultural, language, reimbursement, and administrative barriers

Clinician
- Uses recognized scientific knowledge base
- Authority to direct the delivery of care

Accountable
- Clinician and system accountability for services provided

Majority of personal health care needs
- Competency to manage majority of health problems
- Use of consultation or referral as needed

Sustained partnership
- Relationship between patient and clinician over time

Context of family and community
- Understanding of the circumstances and facts surrounding the patient (socioeconomic status, family dynamics, work issues)
- Awareness of public health trends
- Need for specific health promotion and disease prevention strategies

---

From Institute of Medicine. (1996). *Primary care: America's health in a new era.* Washington, DC: National Academy Press.

a patient-clinician relationship "predicated on the development of mutual trust, respect, and responsibility" (IOM, 1996, p. 37). A primary care NP certainly brings these attributes and activities to the primary care setting. The APN's use of *professional caring* with patients as *partners* in health care sets nursing's contributions to primary care apart from other providers' practice (Green-Hernandez, 1997). In Chapter 5, the use of a holistic framework and the forming of partnerships with patients are identified as two of the major characteristics of the APN style of care.

By engaging in the *nursing* process in the primary care setting (i.e., data collection, assessment, planning, implementation, and evaluation) with defined advanced practice skills and competencies, an NP can effectively provide primary care. The population of patients for which the NP is prepared to provide care (e.g., families, adults, children, women, the elderly) serves to differentiate the types of primary care NPs practice. The American Nurses Association (ANA) document concerning the scope and standards of primary care NP practice also reflects the integration of primary care delivery and the nursing process in this APN role (ANA, 1996).

The concept of *integrated, accessible health-care services* described by the IOM also underscores the importance of a team approach in primary care delivery, with collaboration between the professionals providing health services. Traditional medical models of care delivery have emphasized the diagnosis and treatment of disease (i.e., curing) although latest Accreditation Council for Graduate Medical Education (ACGME) competencies include criteria for collaboration and cultural competence (ACGME, 1999). Nursing models of care have emphasized developmental and systems theories in considering human responses to illness (i.e., caring over time). Using a holistic approach to assessment and treatment, the primary care NP addresses illness, promotes health, and prevents disease. Interpersonal skills, patient and family education, and coaching and guidance are critical elements of practice. APNs integrate elements of care from nursing and medical models in a collaborative approach to clinical practice that enhances the comprehensiveness and quality of care rendered. Many of the skills and competencies in primary care NP practice are based on the knowledge and skills needed to manage common acute and chronic health problems encountered in primary care settings. By employing expert clinical reasoning and utilizing diverse management approaches (see Chapter 5), the NP renders appropriate cost-effective primary care.

APN COMPETENCIES IN PRIMARY CARE NP PRACTICE

Primary care NP practice meets the criteria for advanced practice nursing as described in Chapter 3: graduate nursing education, national certification, and practice focused on the patient/family. Primary care NPs develop skills and competencies in their practices that build on a foundation of basic nursing education. NP competencies are *continually* developed through clinical experience and ongoing professional education. In Chapter 3, the synergistic impact of graduate education and clinical practice experience on APN development is described, and a set of core competencies in each APN role are identified. An overview of each of the APN competencies in primary care NP practice follows.

Primary care services encompass the entire life span of patients. Primary care NPs may be broadly prepared to care for patients at any stage of life (e.g., family NPs) or may have a particular population focus in their practice (e.g., pediatric NPs). No matter what the focus, primary care NPs are involved in the management of health and illness status using the nursing process.

Advanced patient history-taking and physical assessment skills are critical tools for primary care NPs during the data collection stage of the nursing process. Effective communication skills and the ability to establish partnerships with patients enhance the NP's ability to obtain a comprehensive history. A working knowledge of cultural diversity provides an important foundation for this process. Particular attention is paid to personal health habits, stressors, genetics, and an assessment of health risk factors to identify appropriate health promotion and disease prevention strategies.

Evaluating the subjective and objective data collected requires critical thinking and diagnostic reasoning skills on the part of the primary care NP. These aspects of clinical decision making are required not only in the identification of problems but in the further evaluation and management of health needs of primary care clients. Specific health promotion needs based on stages of physical and psychosocial development may be assessed. Much of primary care NP practice involves the diagnosis and management of acute, self-limiting, minor illnesses and stable chronic diseases. However, primary care practice requires an ability to recognize signs and symptoms of complex and unstable health problems requiring medical or other consultation. It also calls for the recognition of emergency situations and initiation of effective emergency care.

Following the initial assessment phase of the nursing process, primary care NPs may plan for care in the form of additional diagnostic studies, specific therapeutic measures, and coaching and guidance strategies. Clinical practice guidelines such as those cited on the websites for the Agency for Healthcare Research and Quality (AHRQ) (www.ahrq.gov/clinic/cpgonline.htm) and the National Guideline Clearinghouse (www.guideline.gov/) can help guide the clinician in planning for appropriate intervention (AHRQ, 2003). The efficacy and safety of therapy over time as well as the client's health goals, risk factors, and illness experience are also considered as plans are developed.

Further diagnostic tests (e.g., laboratory, radiography, or other diagnostic studies) may be required to more accurately assess the patient's health status. Age-specific screening examinations may be recommended as a part of clinical preventive service guidelines (AHRQ, 2004). Specific therapeutic measures may encompass both pharmacological and nonpharmacological therapies. If pharmacological therapy is initiated, the NP determines the appropriate treatment and counsels the patient about drug regimens and side effects (Yocum, Busby, Conway-Welch, & Viens, 1999).

Many of the primary care NP's therapeutic recommendations may be nonpharmacological (e.g., specific dietary or activity recommendations, stress management strategies). In fact, primary care NPs are more likely to use nonpharmacological therapies than are traditional medical practitioners (Moody, Smith, & Glenn, 1999). Patient education and counseling strategies in the management of health and illness status include anticipatory guidance related to normal growth and development for patients and families as well as potential changes they may experience in terms of specific health problems. Additional coaching and guidance competencies utilized in NP practice are discussed in the following section.

Once plans of care are developed and implemented, the primary care NP uses expected outcome criteria to evaluate the effectiveness of interventions. Scheduling phone or office follow-up visits to appropriately monitor clients is an important aspect of ongoing evaluation. When outcome criteria are not achieved, the plan of care is revised accordingly, and further consultation may be indicated (NONPF, 2002). Careful documentation of all services provided is the basis for professional reimbursement. Outcome data for groups of patients are a critical measure of practice safety and efficacy. These data are closely monitored by the payors of health care and help to validate professional practice. The Health Plan Employer Data and Information Set (HEDIS) is one example of performance measures used to evaluate primary care practice (Buppert, 1999; see Chapter 25).

Direct Clinical Practice

As with other advanced practice roles, direct clinical practice is the heart and soul of the work of the primary care NP. What is different is that NPs are likely to spend a greater proportion of their time in direct care activities than CNSs or APN CMs. Brown (in Chapter 5) defines direct clinical practice as the "activities and functions APNs perform within the patient-nurse interface" (p. 142). The work of the primary care NP unfolds around the premise that individuals seek care for a broad range of health-care concerns over time and across the life span. Relationships evolve over time, which facilitates a sense of mutual respect and trust. Within that relationship, a deep understanding of the patient's life and the meaning of the illness or health issue at hand develops. Knowing patients and their family members, their jobs and careers, and their challenges in raising children and caring for aging parents is part of walking with patients through the transitions of life. Spross et al. (2000) describe these transitions as "paradigms for life and living" (p. 191), and it is during these times that the APN can provide support and guidance. Exemplars follow that illustrate the central competency of direct clinical practice, as well as the core competencies of

Carol is a primary care APN working in a university-affiliated internal medicine practice. She has practiced in this setting for 9 years with six internists and a variety of specialists from the University Medical Center. While her focus is primary care, she has access to several subspecialists for consultation purposes. For Carol, scheduling patients occurs in several ways. Telephone triage nurses screen patient calls of an acute nature. The triage nurse makes a brief telephone assessment of their symptoms and then schedules the patient to see either Carol or a physician, depending on availability. Visits are typically 20 minutes for acute and follow-up visits. Educational and counseling visits are usually 40 minutes. Follow-up visits are also scheduled with the APN as appropriate. Physicians refer patients to the APN for follow-up of chronic medical problems such as hypertension, diabetes, asthma. Assessment of additional problems, counseling, education, and medication management may occur during these visits. Patients are also free to self-schedule appointments with Carol or another APN. Some patients utilize Carol's services on an intermittent basis, and others receive the majority of their primary care from her.

Table 13-4 provides a sampling of patients that Carol may see in her primary care practice during an 8-hour day and illustrates the range of competencies used throughout a typical day. The case of JD (Patient 3) illustrates the core competency of direct clinical practice and coaching and guidance.

JD is a 46-year-old female real estate agent whose presenting symptoms included a series of elevated blood pressure readings taken at local health screenings. She had not been seen in more than a year, but isolated systolic blood pressures in the 150 range are noted in her chart. While catching up on the year's events with JD, Carol learns that the patient's father recently died after a lengthy illness. JD kept long vigils at her father's hospital bedside while working long, demanding hours. She reports an increase in her caffeine and fast food intake during this time. The latter resulted in a 20-pound weight gain, which was documented in the chart. JD's BMI was 26 at her previous visit. Further discussion revealed that the patient had a fasting lipid profile done independently 6 months ago. Total cholesterol was 296 mg/dl, HDL-cholesterol 34 mg/dl, LDL-cholesterol 162 mg/dl, and trigycerides 400 mg/dl. Current medications include fexofenadine (Allegra), a steroid nasal spray, and oral contraceptives. The latter is prescribed by her gynecologist for menstrual cycle regulation.

Review of symptoms is negative for headache, shortness of breath, chest pain, and peripheral edema. On physical exam, JD's blood pressure was 130/90, and readings at previous visits were 150/90, 140/90, 146/90. The remainder of her exam is normal, with the exception of the 20-lb weight gain. During the interview and exam, the patient is tearful and articulate about her grief as well as the multitude of health problems she faces. She clearly understands the interconnectedness of the issues but is overwhelmed by them. Carol begins the discussion with the acknowledgment of JD's loss and the reality of her grief. They are tearful together as Carol briefly recounts the protracted illness and death of her own father. This acknowledgment seems to be a source of comfort to JD and a starting place to discuss the journey of grief. Carol gradually guides the discussion back to JD's current health issues. The role of stress, diet, weight gain, and oral contraceptives in the development of hypertension and dyslipidemia are reviewed. JD is encouraged to set two goals around self-care and risk reduction. She agrees to meet with her gynecologist to discuss the appropriateness of oral contraceptives in light of elevated blood pressure and cholesterol values. She reports that she has already resumed participation in a church-sponsored weight loss program in which she has been successful in the past. She is attending church again on a regular basis and finds comfort in the fellowship and spirituality there. Carol affirms these choices as healthy and adaptive. She recommends community support groups that may be appropriate in the future. Carol stresses the need for self-care and suggests activities such as connecting with friends, yoga, exercise classes, massage therapy, and reading. Finally, the patient is scheduled for follow-up with her primary care physician, with whom she has had a long-term relationship, for fasting labs and blood pressure evaluation. The APN informs the patient that she has a close working relationship with JD's primary care physician and she would be happy to meet again with JD as needed.

After direct care responsibilities, the remainder of the day is spent completing documentation, returning phone calls, reviewing labs, writing letters, refilling prescriptions, and authorizing referrals. The telephone triage nurse consults with Carol on several patient calls, and appropriate disposition is discussed. Carol's final call of the day is to a nurse practitioner student to arrange a start date for her adult health practicum.

HDL, High-density lipoprotein; *LDL,* low-density lipoprotein.

expert coaching and guidance, consultation, and collaboration. Leadership, research, and ethical decision-making skills will also be discussed as they relate to primary care.

Each day is as varied as the next. Some days are filled with episodic visits, and some days are spent more on health-care maintenance and education. This day, in particular, is the day of an experienced APN nurse practitioner. The complexity of care and the NP's familiarity with patients are cultivated over a series of encounters. While the hallmark of the primary care NP's practice is the breadth of health issues encountered, the privilege of relationships occurs over time. This enables the NP to tailor evidence-based interventions to the individual and sustain a holistic practice. Characteristics of direct clinical practice and strategies for enacting them are outlined by Brown in Chapter 5. Expert clinical thinking and skillful performance are cultivated through repeatedly evaluating similar sets of health and illness scenarios and formulating plans of care based on patient expectations, standards of care, experience, clinical judgment and current research. APNs continuously synthesize knowledge and experience so that over time they acquire practical wisdom, which Oberle and Allen (2001) define as "knowing when a particular action ought to be taken" (p. 151).

Experienced APNs incorporate this practical wisdom into their decision making, taking actions that they may have been unlikely to take as a novice practitioner. Practical wisdom involves knowing what to do and when. When is a patient ready to begin home glucose monitoring? When is it time to suggest respite care or home health? When is the right time to address sexuality issues with a preteen or teen? When is the right time to address an issue head on, and when is it time to back off from confronting difficult issues? For example in the case of SD (Patient 4) (see Table 13-4) on the typical day schedule, it was not beneficial to launch into a lengthy discussion of the risks of uncontrolled hypertension. SD simply did not believe that he had high blood pressure because he had not received that diagnosis from his trusted former primary care physician. It was not clear to the APN whether this strongly held belief was related to a health literacy, an educational, or a trust issue so the APN chose to try a simple contract with the patient to improve short-term adherence while enlisting the support of family for a more detailed assessment of the barriers to self-care.

Often, an assessment of the chief complaint unearths a multitude of issues, as in the case of JD (Patient 3), presented earlier in Exemplar 13-1. The skilled practitioner helps the patient sift and sort through the issues, establish priorities, and understand the interconnectedness of these priorities. Practical wisdom guides the practitioner to use expert clinical thinking and skillful performance to develop a plan of care that makes sense to the patient.

Table 13-4 illustrates the variety of health issues seen by a primary care NP in a typical day. Understanding the acute and potentially serious nature of GJ's (pneumonia and bronchospasm led to swift evaluation, treatment, and a plan for close follow-up within 24 hours). Knowing the complexity of glycemic control enabled the APN to approach LB's (Patient 11) hyperglycemia both pharmacologically and socially. When DT (Patient 5) exhibited presenting symptoms of upper respiratory infection (URI) the APN distinguished between symptoms of a viral infection and one of bacterial etiology. The experienced practitioner knew when otitis media with effusion would not clear with another round of antibiotics and knew when to refer the patients to an ear, nose, and throat (ENT) specialist, as in the case of JM (Patient 6). The expert clinical thinker listened carefully to the story of MW's (Patient 7) knee pain, combined the data with careful physical examination, and suspected that there was more to the story than periodic episodes of gout.

Partnerships with patients and families develop over time. This relationship should be therapeutic regardless of whether it is the first encounter or the hundredth. As partnerships deepen, the relationship becomes an even more important clinical tool. For example, FB and LB (Patients 10 and 11) are an elderly mother and mentally handicapped

TABLE 13-4	TYPICAL DAY FOR CAROL: A PRIMARY CARE NURSE PRACTITIONER				
PATIENT	AGE	SEX	CHIEF COMPLAINT	COMPLEXITY	COMPETENCY
1 GJ	50	F	Acute bronchitis Lupus Hypertension	Moderate	Direct clinical practice Expert coaching and guidance
2 TY	35	F	Back pain Carpal tunnel syndrome Situational stress	Moderate	Direct clinical practice Expert coaching and guidance Collaboration
3 JD	46	F	Hypertension Weight gain Grief reaction	Moderate	Direct clinical practice Expert coaching and guidance Collaboration
4 SD	87	M	Hypertension follow-up	Low	Direct clinical practice Expert coaching and guidance
5 DT	40	M	Viral URI	Low	Direct clinical practice Expert coaching and guidance

6 JM	50	M	Sinusitis
			Bilateral otitis media
			  with effusion
				Moderate	Direct clinical practice
					Expert coaching and
					  practice guidance
					Research skills
					Consultation

7 MW	35	M	Knee pain Psoriasis	Moderate	Direct clinical practice Expert coaching and guidance Consultation

8 KL	17	F	Contraception/annual
			  exam
			Chlamydia
				Moderate	Direct clinical practice
					Expert coaching and
					  guidance

9 MN	37	F	Depression Annual exam	Moderate	Direct clinical practice Expert coaching and guidance
10 FB	82	F	Hypertension Reflux Skin avulsions	Moderate	Direct clinical practice Expert coaching and guidance Collaboration
11 LB	55	F	Type 2 diabetes Hypertension Obesity Asthma Mental retardation	High	Direct clinical practice Expert coaching and guidance Consultation Ethical decision making
12 JP	39	M	Hypertension New onset type 2 diabetes Diabetes teaching	Moderate	Direct clinical practice Expert coaching and guidance Research skills Collaboration
13 PM	22	M	HIV screening	Moderate	Direct clinical practice Ethical decision making Expert coaching and guidance
14 LR	38	F	Orthostatic hypertension Dehydration Gastroenteritis	High	Direct clinical practice Consultation

daughter in Carol's practice (see Table 13-4). When the issue of transitioning to assisted living from their apartment surfaced, Carol drew on a relationship of trust developed over several years to approach the challenge cooperatively with LB and FB. Carol explored the losses entailed by the move and the meaning of the change for both of them. Acknowledging the grief associated with this major life change and identifying positive meanings helped them accept this transition.

Patients are more likely to comply with medical recommendations if they feel that they are given a part in the decisions about their care. The primary care NP worked to form a partnership with SD (Patient 4) as a means of improving his compliance with his antihypertensive medication. A partnership with KL (Patient 8) will be essential as they face the issues of young adulthood together.

The development of a holistic perspective is another characteristic of direct clinical practice. Understanding the relationship among poor ergonomics in the workplace, the responsibility to take care of a handicapped child, and the development of chronic pain reflects the NP's holistic view of symptoms and etiology and the implications for treatment in the case of TY (Patient 2). Issues of independence and dependence play into the success of caring for mother and daughter FB (Patient 10) and LB (Patient 11). Understanding functional and cognitive abilities is critical in the management of LB's diabetes.

In practice, APN core competencies (see Chapter 3) are often executed simultaneously to achieve the best outcome. However, for purposes of didactic discussion, specific competencies are discussed within the individual exemplars for clarity. The exemplars reflect the extent to which the core competencies enhance direct clinical practice: the core of primary care.

Expert Coaching and Guidance

The nature of the relationship of the primary care NP and the patient creates a strong foundation for the coaching and guidance competency (see Chapter 6). JD's (Patient 3) situation illustrates the application of the coaching competency. The primary care NP considers the reciprocal effects of grief on health and health on grief and realizes that JD is experiencing transitions arising from her recent loss and new health problems. The role of the APN is to coach and instruct about these health/illness transitions as well as monitor JD's response to appropriate treatment and lifestyle modifications.

Patient teaching is also a function of the coaching role. This occurs in every patient encounter when NPs routinely review medications and individualize self-care recommendations. NPs participate in or lead health information classes in areas such as diabetes, women's health, and prepared childbirth, in which groups of patients are coached regarding common health issues.

Adult and women's health NPs frequently encounter women experiencing perimenopause and menopause. The associated physiological and emotional changes are influenced by a woman's roles, lifestyle, and co-existing medical and psychological issues. This profoundly unique and personal journey may be complex. The following exemplar illustrates the coaching competency as described by Spross in Chapter 6. It also shows how the NP incorporates complementary therapies into the plan of care in response to a patient request. The use of research findings to direct evidence-based care is another core competency illustrated.

Primary care NPs weave multiple competencies throughout their practice. These competencies enable the APN to achieve positive results in caring for patients. APNs would

EXEMPLAR 13-2

EXPERT COACHING AND GUIDANCE

ML is a 42-year-old female who scheduled a visit with Janet, a primary care NP, to discuss peri-menopause issues. During this visit Janet determines that ML has no significant past medical history and that her health-care maintenance is up to date. ML initially reports feelings of anxiety related to her mother's recent diagnosis of coronary artery disease. Janet listens to her story, including the experience of her mother's recent myocardial infarction at age 65. Janet then guides the discussion back to the patient, who describes feeling worried and frightened, with periods of shortness of breath, palpitations, and insomnia. She denies chest pain but sometimes has diaphoresis. Her blood pressure, blood glucose level, cholesterol level, and weight are normal. She has never smoked and usually handles stress well. She has been able to exercise vigorously without symptoms. She reveals that she is afraid about her mother's condition but also worries that she may have heart disease herself. Janet reassures ML that her risk is low and describes why her mother has a higher risk. Janet concludes that ML has situational anxiety and agrees that it is reasonable to try to treat her symptoms, and, if they do not improve, further evaluation can be done. Janet briefly describes her practice as "integrative," meaning that she uses the best of mainstream as well as complementary therapies (Robins, 1999). Janet discusses the use of an anxiolytic medication on a short-term basis but also reviews breathing exercises and aromatherapy. She explains to ML that particular breathing exercises will help calm her sympathetic nervous system, allowing her to feel more relaxed. Janet reviews some research to indicate that lavender essential oil can help decrease stress and improve insomnia. After teaching ML diaphragmatic breathing, Janet gives her a handout on the use of aromatherapy oils as well as a resource for breath work (Weil, 1995) and aromatherapy (Robins, 1998; Worwood, 1991). A follow-up visit is scheduled for 1 week later. During that visit ML states that she feels better. She has used a few doses of the medication, which helped her and did not cause any side effects, and she thanks Janet for the information on breathing and aromatherapy. During the visit Janet teaches her a brief guided imagery exercise to combine with breathing and aromatherapy (Dossey, 1995).One month later, ML returns and reports that the complementary therapies have helped her feel more in control of her mind and body and had been easy to incorporate into her daily routine. Her mother had heart surgery and is doing well.

Three months pass, and ML returns, reporting disturbed sleep, constant fatigue, and significant pain in her neck, shoulders, hips, and thighs. These new symptoms have led to a recurrence of anxiety. She continued to experience some benefit from breath work and aromatherapy but used the remainder of the previously prescribed anxiolytic medication to help her sleep. ML indicates that she does not want to continue the use of this medication. After physical exam and appropriate diagnostic evaluation, ML is diagnosed with fibromyalgia. Janet spends time explaining fibromyalgia and treatment options, which include a balanced daily routine, focused on stress management, diet, and exercise. Janet helps her structure a treatment plan including referral for Tai Chi classes, which have been shown to improve fibromyalgia symptoms (Keel, 1998). Additionally, Janet adds a low dose tricyclic antidepressant at bedtime to help her sleep. A few weeks later, ML returns for an office visit and reports an overall reduction of her symptoms of about 50%. The NP and ML decide to continue the current treatment plan, and a 3-month follow-up visit is scheduled.

One year later, ML returns and complains that she feels depressed. Her mother recently died, and she has not been coping well. She is crying frequently, cannot concentrate, and is losing interest in her life. Janet refers her for psychotherapy, stops the low dose tricyclic antidepressant, and suggests the addition of an SSRI to help manage symptoms of depression. ML is warned that stopping the tricyclic antidepressant may result in an exacerbation of her fibromyalgia-related pain. She is encouraged to call Janet if this occurs. Janet also suggests that ML use her aromatherapy resources to select oils that may help with depression, including geranium, neroli, and chamomile. Focusing on her Tai Chi practice may also help (Jin, 1992). When Janet follows up with ML 2 weeks later, she is starting to improve;1 month later, she is feeling more like her old self. Janet speaks with ML on the phone every few months about various issues. ML explains that she values Janet's opinion, feels comfortable with her, and appreciates all her teaching about health and healing.

EXEMPLAR 13-2

EXPERT COACHING AND GUIDANCE—cont'd

About 18 months later, ML, now 45, reports hot flashes once or twice a day, cycle changes, and increasing premenstrual symptoms such as agitation and mood swings. These changes have caused her fibromyalgia to flare, and she is having more pain in her neck and hips during the day. Her cycles are now 21 days apart, and the amount of bleeding has decreased. She has continued to work with breathing and aromatherapy. She has not been doing Tai Chi or other exercise in the last 2 or 3 months. Janet informs her that it sounds like perimenopause, which can start up to 10 years before menopause begins. Janet discusses the hormonal changes and offers suggestions to help decrease hot flashes, including adding a serving of soy to ML's daily diet (nuts, tofu, tempeh, soy milk), ensuring adequate daily water intake (6 to 8 glasses), minimizing spicy foods, and adding a supplement containing calcium and magnesium and a daily B-complex vitamin to help with PMS and fatigue. In addition Janet recommends she resume regular exercise (Northrup, 2001). Within 4 weeks ML is feeling better.

The next year, ML arrives for her annual exam. She has not had a period in 6 months. She is also having severe hot flashes and intense night sweats. She would like to discuss hormone replacement therapy (HRT). Janet explains the risks and benefits, including new research that HRT is used for short-term management of severe vasomotor symptoms. Janet and ML decide on a 6-month trial of HRT, at which time they will reassess the need for therapy. Bone densitometry is scheduled because ML's mother and aunt had osteoporosis. Finally, Janet offers some resources for exploring the impact of postmenopause and the concomitant decrease in hormones on ML's cardiovascular health (Sinatra, 2000). A discussion ensues about ML's mother's illness and the ongoing need for risk reduction as well as the grief she feels since the death of her mother from heart disease. When ML returns for follow-up 1-month later, she is feeling much better. To express her appreciation for Janet's attentive and compassionate care, ML brings flowers and a beautiful card to the NP expressing how much she values their relationship. (See *References and Additional Readings* for complementary therapy references.)

PMS, Premenstrual syndrome; *SSRI,* selective serotonin reuptake inhibitor.

like to fill their days with successful, fulfilling patient encounters as described earlier, but this sometimes is not the case. Some patients exhibit ambivalence and inconsistency in their approach to their health, and despite mobilizing all of one's competencies, a positive outcome may be elusive. For example, patients with type 2 diabetes often struggle with not only the reality of the illness but in assuming self-care for its management. NPs need to develop skill in understanding and handling such situations, not only to facilitate patient care but also to manage their own feelings of frustration or failure when patients are unable to make lifestyle changes that promote health and reduce the risk of complications.

Although there is a clear genetic component associated with type 2 diabetes, the success of treatment is directly related to the ability of the patient to make a long-term commitment to significant lifestyle changes. These include losing weight and incorporating permanent changes in patterns of diet and exercise into the patient's lifestyle. Therapeutic success also depends on the patient's acceptance of the disease and his or her willingness to enter into a coaching relationship with the NP that fosters and supports the needed changes. Not all patients have the capacity for change, as in the case of LB (Patient 11). While cooperative and pleasant, LB's capacity for lifestyle modifications is limited by her mental handicap. More discouraging, however, is the subset of seemingly capable patients who are not ready to take an active role in their care: it is hard to understand why a patient seems to "choose" illness over health. Sometimes patients are simply not ready to make changes because they understand that such lifestyle changes will

[1]The author gratefully acknowledges Jo Wheeler Robbins, PhD, RN, for assistance with this exemplar.

increase the complexity of their lives, routines, or relationships. Other times, patients may reject recommendations as a way of maintaining control. Such patients present a particular challenge for APNs and all health-care providers. Their reluctance to make the lifestyle changes that would minimize complications or their failure to adhere to recommendations and treatment plans are a source of frustration to providers. There are times when, despite the best efforts to offer a coaching relationship or to match a particular patient with a provider who can be an effective coach, the APN's efforts are rebuffed. The following exemplar describes the frustration of this real situation.

There are a multitude of issues that could be explored in this exemplar: individual response to chronic illness, the role of denial in chronic illness, and nonadherence, to

 EXEMPLAR 13-3

HB is a 35-year-old male whom Paul, the primary care NP, has known for several years. HB was initially referred by his primary care physician (PCP) for diabetes education. He was diagnosed with diabetes a few years earlier by a physician in another state and was not on medication when he first visited the practice. His glycemic control eroded over the next several years despite triple drug oral therapy. He made no significant changes in his diet and did not exercise regularly despite participation in a diabetes education program. Paul would periodically see HB for episodic issues and would take the opportunity to check on the status of his diabetes. HB would always say that he felt fine; thus he did not need to check his blood sugars. During these visits, Paul would search for barriers to adherence, assess for symptoms of depression, and offer support and encouragement for HB to take a more proactive approach in the care of his diabetes. Approximately 1 year elapsed during which Paul did not see HB. His HbA1c level continued to rise, and his physician determined that the addition of insulin was necessary to improve glycemic control. Several more months elapsed before HB finally made an appointment with Paul for insulin teaching. During that visit HB admitted that he was not performing home glucose monitoring because sticking himself was too painful. He voiced serious reservation about daily insulin injections but felt pressured by his physician to keep the appointment. Paul could not determine any other mitigating factor except fear of pain and an apparent inability to grasp the seriousness of the issue. HB reluctantly agreed to proceed with the teaching program but refused to inject himself. He conceded that he might permit his wife to administer the insulin and agreed to bring her in for an educational session. When Paul realized that teaching was not going to happen during the visit, the focus shifted to assessing current stressors or other barriers to accepting his diabetes. HB reported that he is happily married and feels successful and satisfied in his work. He does not discuss his diabetes with his wife, family, or co-workers. Because HB generally feels well, he has difficulty accepting the fact that his diabetes control has deteriorated. He has no history of depression, anxiety, or substance abuse. He was not interested in any counseling to explore his issues with diabetes. He eventually agreed to ask his wife to learn how to give his insulin. Paul encouraged follow-up and tried to be positive and supportive so that HB would return. Paul followed up with a reminder note 2 weeks later. A month elapsed, and HB had not scheduled any follow-up.

Paul consults with the PCP and shares his concern about the lack of follow up and proactive behaviors HB demonstrates in the care of his diabetes. The PCP is equally puzzled about HB's adherence issues. The NP is unable to elicit from HB any insight as to his unwillingness to adopt the self-care skills and lifestyle changes required for effective disease management. Eventually, HB and his wife return for instructions on insulin use. HB still vigorously refuses to inject or perform home glucose monitoring, although his wife is willing to perform these tasks. She learns to inject insulin and perform finger sticks and is willing to perform these tasks for her husband. He agrees to the plan, and a schedule for bedtime insulin was prepared. Paul then negotiates with HB the minimum number of times each week he is willing to perform home glucose monitoring, and a schedule for this is also suggested. HB agreed to send or call in blood sugar results in 2 weeks, with follow up in 1 month. Paul receives no results, and a follow-up appointment was not made.

HbA1$_c$, Hemoglobin A1$_c$.

name a few. In direct clinical practice and in consultation, the APN uses a variety of strategies to ensure a successful encounter. Numerous strategies outlined in Chapters 5, 6, and 7 can be used to create a successful and satisfying encounter. However, the NP must be prepared for the frustration and disappointment that comes when, despite the best of efforts, the desired outcome is not achieved. What does, however, distinguish the APN from other nurses and practitioners is the tenacity to continue to use diverse approaches to problem solving, to look for other explanations, and to continue to develop the partnership with the patient. Time is another tool for the primary care NP. As in the case of HB, the primary care NP will be available to him on his journey with diabetes, either through a direct encounter about his diabetes or by way of another primary care issue over time. Each encounter may supply a piece of the puzzle about his nonadherence and an opportunity for HB to become an active participant in his care. A collaborative and supportive relationship with other primary care providers will sustain the APN in times of frustration. Tenacity and commitment will also sustain the primary care NP as she or he journeys with a reluctant HB through his transition, diabetes. In this situation, the fact that the patient continued to return to the NP for monitoring and care and that he did bring his wife to learn more about the illness were, for the NP, modest indicators of success.

Consultation

Consultative relationships are critical to primary care NP practice. Relationships with other NPs, physicians, nurses and other health-care providers ensure that patients have access to comprehensive care. The direct clinical practice exemplar illustrates different consultative relationships. Throughout the day, Carol informally consults with the primary care physicians in the practice about problematic cases or clarification of a treatment plan. She sees the patients of all of the PCPs in the practice and updates them if a new problem is identified or if a specific concern needs to be addressed in follow-up. This informal consultation style is a frequent part of the daily rhythm of the practice and includes elements of the collaboration competency. NPs in smaller or solo practices would not have easy access to this consultation style and would have to seek a style that suited their practice (see Chapter 7).

Formal consultations with specialists are also initiated for complex medical problems. JM (Patient 6) was referred to an ENT specialist for evaluation of his bilateral otitis media with effusion. The case of MW (Patient 7) involved consultation with the PCP and the rheumatologist (see Exemplar 13-4). Carol regularly provides consultation to the clinic nurses, who are the first line of communication with patients. Their assessments of patient problems and the patients' responses to treatment are valuable information for the NP.

EXEMPLAR 13-4

MW is a 35-year-old male (Patient 7) whose presenting symptoms include a protracted case of right knee pain. He was diagnosed with gout by his PCP, and after several flare-ups over the last 7 years, he was prescribed allopurinol. MW remained on the allopurinol until 1 month ago, at which time he had acute onset of right knee pain and swelling. He was initially treated with colchicine, with minimal improvement in his symptoms. His PCP changed his medication to indomethacin, with some improvement in his symptoms. MW was scheduled for follow-up with Carol, the primary care NP, at the request of the PCP. On physical exam, MW was pleasant

Continued

EXEMPLAR 13-4—cont'd

though discouraged by the lack of resolution of his symptoms. His right knee was mildly swollen and without warmth or erythema. He had pain on full flexion and full extension. There was no evidence of instability or meniscal or ligamentous involvement. Carol also noted several large psoriatic plaques on the extensor surfaces of his forearms and legs. MW was diagnosed with psoriasis 10 years ago. The first episode of gout was 5 years ago. He noted that the gout flares up in the winter months, which often disrupts his vacation plans. MW owns a landscaping business and maintains a brisk commercial business in the spring, fall, and summer. He usually schedules vacation in January to meet friends in the Florida Keys. This is now the second year in a row that his vacation plans have been thwarted by gout symptoms. In the course of further discussion, MW commented that he had also had painful swelling of his right index finger about 1 year ago and that the x-ray had shown some arthritis. Hand symptoms had not recurred. Carol reviewed the chart and read a radiology report indicating degenerative changes in the PIP joint of the right second digit. Physical exam of the right hand shows enlargement of the PIP joint of the right second digit. MW also reported two episodes of bilateral ankle pain that were never evaluated. A sedimentation rate and uric acid were ordered as well as a two-view x-ray of his right knee. MW is advised to stay on the indomethacin until test results are received. Labs and x-rays are within normal limits. Later that week Carol discussed the case with MW's PCP, and they decided to refer MW to a rheumatologist for further evaluation of possible psoriatic arthritis. The PCP agreed with the plan, and Carol called the patient and discussed the test results and the recommendation for a specialty evaluation. MW agreed and was transferred to the referral coordinator to set up the rheumatology appointment and obtain insurance preauthorization.

PCP, Primary care physician; *PIP,* proximal interphalangeal.

Other APNs in the outpatient and inpatient setting can provide consultations in their specialty areas. For example, the primary care NP might initiate a consultation with a psychiatric clinical nurse specialist to evaluate the depression of a hospitalized patient. A referral for consultation with a certified nurse midwife for preconception counseling provides valuable information to the woman ready to start a family. Newly diagnosed patients with type 2 diabetes benefit from consultation with a CNS whose specialty is diabetes management, and the expertise of home health nurses is critical in discharge planning. Community-based nursing professionals offer valuable insights into family issues and the home environment that can affect patient health. Community health nurses have a wealth of knowledge regarding other community resources and insurance coverage for home care services. NPs often initiate consultations with physical therapists, occupational therapists, speech therapists, and social workers based on a home health nurse's evaluation.

Research

Clinical practice in this "age of information" offers exciting opportunities and challenges for the primary care NP. Health-care knowledge resources in electronic form, especially on the Internet, are increasingly available. However, current information systems are not always easily integrated into clinical practice and contain content of varying quality (Hersh, 1999; Stange, 1996). Health-care informatics have facilitated the development of clinical practice guidelines based on current research and the consensus of clinical experts (Fonteyn, 1998; Pearson, 1998). Today's primary care NPs must be able to retrieve evidence-based information and appraise important practice innovations for their relevance and appropriateness to practice (Brown, 1999; Tsafrir et al., 1998; Worrall, 1999).

Evidence-based clinical practice guidelines can be used to improve primary care. With the advent of managed care systems, practice guidelines have also been used to reduce costs, standardize practice, and decrease medical liability. NPs can evaluate clinical practice guidelines and work to adopt those that will ensure that best practices are used in primary care delivery. AHRQ, the Health Plan Employer Data Information (HEDIS), the National Guideline Clearinghouse (NGC), and the National Quality Measures Clearinghouse are reliable resources for evidence-based clinical guidelines and performance measures that are available on the Internet (see Box 13-2). These guidelines can be modified to meet the needs of the local patient population (Bergman, 1999) and also used in conjunction with agency outcome and performance measures to provide feedback to clinicians on the extent to which best practices are used (see Chapter 25).

As experts in preventive and patient-centered care, primary care NPs should take an active role in clinical practice research, the development of clinical practice guidelines, and review of outcome and performance measures. Stange (1996) cited opportunities for interdisciplinary collaboration in primary care research and the creation of primary care research centers. These activities require a mastery of basic research skills, as discussed in Chapter 8.

Collaboration and Leadership

Each of the competencies in primary care NP practice discussed so far requires the development of collaborative relationships and leadership skills with patients and other health-care professionals. Direct clinical practice in primary care with expert coaching and guidance has a collaborative relationship between patient and NP at its core. The IOM definition of primary care (1996) implies the use of professional collaboration to deliver "integrated" and "accessible" care. Effective collaboration results in more comprehensive, patient-focused care (Hughes & Turner, 1996) that promotes high-quality, cost-effective outcomes (Brita-Rossi et al., 1996; Stichler, 1995). Expert coaching and guidance also require the establishment of a collaborative relationship between patient and provider. Professional consultation and research entail collaborative relationships between a variety of health-care providers with common goals and purposes (Conger & Craig, 1998; Weinstein, McCormack, Brown, & Rosenthal, 1998).

On a broader level, primary care NPs engaged in clinical and professional leadership must also utilize effective collaborative skills to assist groups and organizations to envision preferred futures, achieve consensus, and implement change. The essence of primary care is the sustained continuity of health care for the patient and family. As the long-term member of the team that provides continuity and stability in the care and management of patients over long periods of time, primary care NPs often emerge as leaders in primary care teams in health-care settings. Furthermore, the primary care NP's role as a leader in the community through membership on boards of health and education and as an influential policymaker cannot be underestimated (see Chapters 9 and 10).

Ethical Decision Making

The primary care NP may encounter patient care concerns that raise ethical issues. Examples include reproductive issues, informed consent, and conflicting health-care goals among family members. NPs have opportunities to engage in preventive ethics by initiating discussions about advance directives and organ donation with patients in a relaxed and thoughtful manner before they become pressing issues. In addition, NPs identify and address ethical conflicts that arise when clinical goals conflict with institutional goals (Ulrich, Soeken, & Miller, 2003).

Primary care NPs are accountable first and foremost to their patients, with patient confidentiality honored at all times. This professional value has recently become the focus of more intense government regulation and scrutiny with the implementation of HIPAA regulations (see Chapters 20 and 22). Primary care NPs must be vigilant in their protection of confidential patient information in whatever form it takes. In an era of managed care, the primary care clinician's accountability to the health-care system in which she or he practices may create tension, especially where the use of resources for patient care is concerned. Primary care NPs must always be ethically accountable for their actions, especially where financial incentives related to resource utilization are involved (Abel, 1994; Aroskar, 1998; Coolican & Swanson, 1998; IOM, 1996; see Chapter 11).

EXEMPLARS OF PRIMARY CARE NP PRACTICE IN URBAN AND RURAL SETTINGS

The role of the primary care NP in the interface of direct clinical practice has been discussed in earlier exemplars. However, the influence and skill of the primary care NP can extend beyond that basic relationship to assist in meeting the primary care needs of a particular community. The following two exemplars illustrate NPs engaged in the delivery of primary care to underserved populations in two very different settings, a low-income urban community and a rural health center. In community-based practices such as these, the importance of community assessment has been recognized as a way for primary care practitioners to more effectively meet the needs of the population they serve (Abraham & Fallon, 1997; Association of Academic Health Centers, 2002; Courtney, 1995; NONPF, 2003; Reece, 1998). A community needs assessment can identify existing and potential health problems as well as health promotion needs (Reece, 1998). Once these needs are identified, collaboration with other health-care professionals, educators, and community leaders can provide a critical link in empowering individuals, families, and communities to improve their health status.

EXEMPLAR 13-5

URBAN PEDIATRIC NP PRACTICE

Jane is a pediatric NP caring for children in a low-income urban community. This community once thrived as part of a major industrial center but was devastated by factory closings and a declining local economy. Recent health status indicators for this urban area reveal increasing rates of teen pregnancy. There is growing concern in the community about substance abuse, school drop-out rates, and community violence.

This setting is a challenging one, but Jane feels that, by working with children and families through the community Child Health Clinic, she might be able to help them deal with the risks that poverty introduces to their health. The clinic is a public-private venture jointly funded by the local health department, the community hospital, and various charitable organizations in the greater metropolitan area. It serves as a source of primary care to many of the community's children, whose health care is subsidized by Medicaid and who are now enrolled in a statewide managed care program. The clinic also provides services to non-Medicaid recipients using a sliding-scale fee. Jane sees a variety of infants, children, and adolescents who come to the clinic for both well-child visits and acute/episodic health problems. Her care entails thorough health assessments by history-taking, physical assessment, and appropriate diagnostic

EXEMPLAR 13-5

URBAN PEDIATRIC NP PRACTICE — cont'd

studies or screening examinations. She then recommends appropriate interventions (both pharmacological and nonpharmacological) for the child. These are in keeping with established clinical guidelines used in the clinic. Much of Jane's time is spent discussing with parents normal childhood growth and development as well as effective parenting skills, nutritional needs, immunizations, and age-specific injury prevention guidelines. If the child is ill, Jane describes ways to monitor the child's health status. Jane's days take on a busy pace as she sees children for regularly scheduled well-child visits and manages a variety of episodic health problems during the clinic's walk-in hours.

At times, Jane may consult with the clinic pediatrician about acute health problems or abnormal health screening findings. For children and families with complex health problems, she may also consult with other members of the clinic team for further evaluation and management. Public health nurses are available for home assessment and case management services, and the clinic social worker provides additional outreach services. A nutritionist and eligibility worker from the Women, Infants, and Children's nutrition program are on-site to address nutritional needs in depth.

Jane also engages with this community outside the walls of the clinic. Involvement with community activities enhances her credibility and acceptance among this low-income population. On occasion she is asked to assist with health screening examinations for the local Head Start program. Recently there has been growing concern about unmet needs for child health services in the greater urban area. Inappropriate use of local emergency rooms for episodic health care and a rising incidence of asthma and lead poisoning have contributed to a renewed commitment to pediatric primary care. Jane works closely with the school nurses to follow high-risk children and to provide back up for emergency situations. As a respected primary care provider for an underserved community, Jane has been asked to serve on a local Child Health Task Force. She will work with other health-care providers and community leaders to identify ways to more effectively use public and private resources in addressing children's health needs. Together, they hope to promote a healthier future for the community at large.

EXEMPLAR 13-6

With 3 years of experience as a family nurse practioner (FNP) at the Mountain Breeze Rural Health Center, Mary realized how much she had developed as a primary care provider. She had worked as a public health nurse for 10 years in this coal-mining and industrial community of Appalachia and was familiar with its poverty and limited access to health care. In fact, the mountains themselves, with their narrow winding roads, posed one of the major barriers to care in this area—transportation.

Before the longtime local family physician retired, Mary had been able to pursue her NP education through a master's degree program offered by the state university satellite program on the community college campus 40 miles away. The 1-hour commute to school seemed long, but that trip was short compared with the additional 300 miles she would have had to travel if teleconferencing with faculty on the main campus were not available. Mary was the recipient of a state scholarship for her graduate education, and in return she agreed to practice in a medically underserved area of the state that had been her home during her entire life.

Anticipating the loss of their beloved physician, the community had worked hard to support the establishment of a rural health center in the area. Mary was well known to the local citizens as a public health nurse, and they readily accepted her in her new role as an FNP. The nearest hospital, 30 miles away, had recently been engaged in the development of rural health networks and provided physician coverage in the center 3 days per week. The retiring family physician had been an important professional asset for Mary in her first year after graduation, as she made the transition to her new role. Now, on the 3 days per week that physicians were on-site to collaborate, she could be sure that patients requiring more complex medical management were scheduled.

Continued

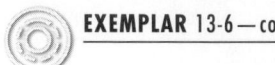

These days also provided an opportunity to review and discuss other patient management issues and to develop skills and knowledge related to the medical issues in her practice.

Mary's days at the center were always full but never predictable. As an FNP, she provided care for a wide range of episodic health concerns for patients across their life spans. She cared for many adults with chronic health problems such as diabetes and hypertension. She devoted much of her effort to working with patients and their families on improved nutritional status and other health promotion strategies. One of her diabetic patients had recently started insulin therapy. After teaching him how to monitor his glucose at home, she was able to adjust his initial insulin therapy over the phone. The phone proved to be a valuable tool for her practice because many families had no regular source of transportation to the clinic. As the only female primary care provider in the area, Mary found much of her time devoted to women's health care. Women found it easy to share their concerns with her, and Mary frequently discussed family health problems with them during these visits. She also followed many children from infancy through childhood for well-child and episodic visits.

One afternoon a week, Mary left the clinic and made rounds to visit patients in the local nursing home. She worked closely with the staff there to identify ways to assist this elderly population in maintaining as much independence as possible. She also enjoyed occasional trips to the local high school to assist with sports physicals. From time to time she was invited to be a speaker at the employee health seminars held at the nearby packaging plant.

Her work was rewarding, and there were many challenges ahead. She had recently discussed the area's low childhood immunization rates with local leaders. They were now developing a proposal for a mobile health unit to increase access to immunizations and other primary preventive services to remote sections of the tri-county area. Mary was asked to portray some of this Appalachian community's health needs to a contingent of state and federal legislators visiting the area. She hoped to make a compelling case for a mobile health unit so that funding for the project could be secured.

EDUCATIONAL PREPARATION OF PRIMARY CARE NPs

On the basis of the exemplars, it is clear that the scope of primary care NP practice requires competency in managing a broad range of clinical problems. Students in graduate primary care NP education programs must acquire a solid foundation of knowledge in primary care skills in order to facilitate autonomous clinical practice. They must understand the professional accountability that is assumed when undertaking this APN role and demonstrate a commitment to continuous professional growth and development. Skills as a team member are also essential to the primary care NP because the role calls for collaboration with a variety of health professionals and support staff

For students to be prepared for collaborative practice, interdisciplinary approaches to education should be undertaken (Felten Cady, Metzler, & Burton, 1997). In the classroom, clinical content can be effectively presented by NPs, physicians, and other members of the primary care team to facilitate understanding of the perspective and expertise that each brings to patient care. Clinical experiences for students are also enhanced by an interdisciplinary approach. By seeing firsthand how collaborative approaches to patient care can facilitate cost-effective, comprehensive care, students will be better prepared for interdependent primary care practice.

The National Task Force on Quality Nurse Practitioner Education (2002) and NONPF (2000, 2002) advocate a strong curriculum that provides an in-depth clinical knowledge base and skill level based on the NP specialty and scope of practice. In addition to basic role and clinical competencies developed in primary care NP programs, an understanding of other professional practice issues related to advanced practice nursing is critical. NPs must be familiar with statutes and regulations governing practice in their state as well as appropriate licensing, professional credentialing, and clinical privileging procedures. A clear understanding of one's professional scope of practice is directly related to professional regulation and reimbursement issues. Résumé and portfolio development and interview and contract negotiating skills are important tools for securing a rewarding clinical practice position (see Chapter 21). Familiarity with risk management procedures and appropriate professional liability coverage is required to protect oneself from costly malpractice litigation. Finally, changes in the health-care environment for NP practice require higher levels of understanding about the practice setting's billing and reimbursement policies and procedures, and privacy regulations. This awareness is essential for the development of economically sound primary care practice (see Chapters 20 and 22).

The emphasis on cost-effective care will continue as health-care markets expand. Reimbursement will be more closely tied to clinical productivity. NPs must have an understanding of the link between cost-efficient practices and clinical decision-making skills to be able to establish appropriate priorities in clinical care. In busy practice settings, the use of telephone triage and management skills is another tool in addressing both acute and chronic health problems (Greenberg & Schultz, 2002). The NP may require additional guidance and experience to develop telephone interview and follow-up skills. An ongoing emphasis on clinical preventive services for health promotion and disease prevention promotes cost-effective care (Ryan, 1993). The NP must learn ways to incorporate these services into routine patient visits and seize teachable moments with clients for effective health education. An "ethic of caring" must continue to undergird NP education and practice in order to bridge the gap between cost-containment strategies reducing quantity of services and those concerns related to quality of services (Abel, 1994; Cary, Goldberg, & McDaniel, 2003).

Market forces and health policy debates continue to create rapid change in primary care delivery systems. The primary care NP must understand the forces that are driving change and the ways they may shape practice in the future. Furthermore, student APNs should begin to develop an understanding of how they can influence health policy to ensure that high-quality health-care services are made accessible, affordable, and available to all.

TRANSITION TO PRIMARY CARE NP PRACTICE

With so many professional practice issues to consider, as well as the need for well-developed APN competencies, it is no surprise that newly prepared primary care NPs may feel overwhelmed as they face the realities of advanced practice. The initial year of NP practice is an important transitional year that provides the critical foundation for developing professional expertise and delivering high-quality health care. Brown and Olshansky (1997) have studied the experiences of new NP graduates during their first year of primary care practice. From their data collection and analysis, the authors constructed a theoretical model representing the transition to the primary care NP role. Their research has important implications for the primary care NP's first year of clinical practice. First, the new graduate may experience a considerable amount of anxiety and general sense of disequilibrium. The first 6 months of practice is a time for redefinition of one's professional self and a time of being "in limbo." The new practitioner, professional mentors, and others must maintain realistic expectations for practice knowledge, skills, and performance in the practice setting. As Brown and Olshansky noted, "the vital contribution of the first year of clinical practice experience and skill repetition to expanding knowledge and strengthening practice skills cannot be overemphasized" (1997, p. 51).

ISSUES FOR THE FUTURE OF PRIMARY CARE NPs

While nurse practitioners have made great strides over the past several years in establishing stable independent and collaborative practices, there is still work to be done (Mundinger et al., 2000; Sears Maxwell, & Townsend, 2003). Negotiating the evolving health-care marketplace and moving from an "invisible" provider status in many managed care systems to recognized members of provider panels are two major challenges facing primary care NPs today. NPs have long been recognized as providers of cost-effective, high-quality care. These attributes are in keeping with managed care's emphasis on prevention and cost savings. However, access to primary care NPs has been increasingly controlled by organized health agencies in the private sector. Many managed care plans do not extend contracts to NPs directly. Instead, physicians who hire them are responsible for NP performance and compensation. This invisible provider status makes it difficult for health-care consumers to gain direct access to NP care, and it is equally challenging to evaluate the impact of NP services on costs and outcomes in capitated systems of care (Cohen, Mason, Arsenie, Sargese, & Needham, 1998; Kendig, 2002; Yurkowski, 1997).

Managed care organization executives have reported a high degree of satisfaction with NPs serving as primary care providers and recognize their value in providing expert coaching and guidance (Mason, Cohen, O'Donnell, Baxter, & Chase, 2002). However, NPs must continue to educate administrators, payors, and patients about their role in primary care delivery. The development of sound marketing strategies that clearly define NP care and its benefits are essential in negotiating with managed care plans and other stakeholders (Kendig, 2002; Kennedy, 2003; Pakis, 1997. Kendig, a practicing primary care NP, suggests three important strategies for defining NP care: "Maintain your nursing identity. Remember that true collaboration is the key. I always try to focus on my unique skill set as an advanced practice *nurse*, rather than demonstrating how my practice is similar to physician practice" (2002, p. 271). Identifying a "professional niche" that contributes to decreased costs and improved outcomes may be of particular benefit in marketing efforts (see Chapter 21). To be successful in today's health care marketplace, NPs must also have a proficient understanding of accounting, finance, economics, and reimbursement practices (Bourne, 2001; Wing, 1998; see Chapter 20). Whether reimbursed by Medicare, Medicaid, indemnity insurers, or managed care organizations, the primary care NP must be familiar with the reimbursement policies of third-party payors including documentation and billing guidelines (Buppert, 2004).

The development of more formal contracting, credentialing, and privileging processes for NPs in a variety of health systems is likely as the health-care system evolves. The primary care NP must be familiar with organizational credentialing measures and complete them. It is likely that NPs will need to provide data on the outcomes of care they have provided. The HEDIS, with specific performance measures for primary care, has been developed by the National Committee for Quality Assurance, a nonprofit organization that accredits health plans. An understanding of HEDIS measures and how HEDIS scores will affect clinicians is critical to the future of all primary care providers (HEDIS, 2004 see Chapters 23 and 25).

Practice opportunities and perceived differences in NP scope of practice are largely related to state regulations and the practice environments they create (Cooper et al., 1998; Mason et al., 2002; Safriet, 2002; Sekscenski, Sansom, Bazell, Salmon, & Mullan, 1994). NPs must continue to address restrictions on their scope of practice, prescriptive authority, and eligibility for reimbursement that create barriers to professional practice. The committed efforts of NP leaders at state and national levels, combined with support from nursing organizations to educate policymakers and effect change in these areas, have been commendable. However, much remains to be done to remove remaining legal and regulatory restrictions to practice (see Chapter 22). Furthermore, ongoing professional vigilance is necessary to protect the gains of the past. Professional unity with APNs, coalition building, and strong leadership at state and national levels are critical to achieve these goals. NPs in primary care practice must be willing to invest in these organizations and activities to protect and promote their professional futures.

Global issues, such as bioterrorism and international political and economic unrest, are forces that also affect the future practice of primary care (Persell et al., 2001). Primary care NPS will serve as front line responders; this will require a more in-depth understanding and awareness of biological and chemical agents and the appropriate treatments needed to serve these patients and families.

The advent of telehealth technologies offers exciting possibilities for primary care nurse practitioners to expand the breadth and scope of their education and practice. With these developments come new professional challenges related to interstate licensure and professional reimbursement for telehealth services (Connors, 2002; Jenkins & White, 2001; Sharp, 1996, 1997; Williamson & Hutcherson, 1998). NPs (as well as patients) will have untold opportunities available to them via the Internet, cable television, and other evolving modalities. NPs will need to become familiar with the new sources of electronic health-care information available to their patients and counsel them about reliable resources to use. Useful URLs for primary care NPs are found in Box 13-2.

BOX 13-2 • USEFUL URLS FOR PRIMARY CARE

Association of Colleges of Graduate Medical Education	www.agcme.org	Medical Education Competencies
Agency for Healthcare Research and Quality	www.ahrq.gov/clinic	Clinical Practice Guidelines
National Quality Measures Clearinghouse	http://www.qualitymeasures.ahrq.gov/	
Preventive Services	http://www.ahrq.gov/clinic/prevenix.htm	Age Specific Screening Examination Recommendations
National Guideline Clearinghouse	http://www.guideline.gov/	
National Advisory Council on Nurse Education and Practice (NACNEP)	www.bhpr.gov/nursing/nacnep	APNs in the Workforce Data
National Organization of Nurse Practitioner Faculties (NONFP)	www.nonpf.com	APN Competencies APN Education Data APNs in the Workforce Data
American Association of Colleges of Nursing (AACN)	www.aacn.nche.edu	APNs in the Workforce Data
National Sample Survey of Registered Nurses	www.bhpr.hrsa.gov/nursing	RNs in the workforce data
Health Plan Employer Data Information (HEDIS)	www.ncqa.org/Programs/HEDIS	Performance measures for primary care practice
Robert Wood Johnson Foundation	www.rwjf.org	Health policy
Division of Nursing, Bureau of Health Professions, Health Resources and Services Administration, Department of Health and Human Services	www.bhpr.hrsa.gov/nursing	
Health Insurance and Portability and Accountability Act (HIPAA)	www.hrsa.gov/website.htm	

CONCLUSION

Primary care NPs have been recognized as pioneers in NP practice. This APN role was conceived to enhance access to cost-effective health-care practice for underserved populations. The cost, quality, and competence benefits of primary care NPs have been well validated since the role's inception in the mid-1960s. As the nation moves toward prepaid, managed systems of care with an emphasis on primary care and health promotion, the NP becomes an ideal provider of primary care for all patient populations.

The APN core competencies for primary care NP practice have been described to provide a comprehensive overview of this advanced practice role. As with other APN roles, the continued professional development of NPs will lead to greater proficiency in each of the competencies over time. The traditional period from student to professional primary care NP provides an important time to expand knowledge and strengthen clinical practice.

The health-care system, no doubt, will continue to evolve with marketplace and policy reforms as well as emerging communication technologies shaping its future. NPs should and will assume a critical role in the primary care workforce of the future. Both professional unity and interdisciplinary collegiality must undergird their efforts as they take an active role in developing health policy and care delivery systems that respond to the holistic primary care needs of their patients and families.

REFERENCES

Abel, E. (1994). Productivity versus quality of care: Ethical implications for clinical practice during health care reform. *Nurse Practitioner Forum, 5,* 238-242.

Abraham, T., & Fallon, P. J. (1997). Clinical exemplar. Caring for the community: Development of the advanced practice nurse role. *Clinical Nurse Specialist, 11,* 224-230.

Accreditation Council for Graduate Medical Education. (1999). Competencies. Retrieved May 8, 2004, from http://www.acgme.org/outcome/comp/comphome.asp

Agency for Healthcare Research and Quality. (2003). *Clinical information.* Retrieved September 25 2003, from http://www.ahrq.gov/clinic

Agency for Healthcare Research and Quality. (2004). *Preventive services.* Retrieved May 9, 2004, from http://www.ahrq.gov/clinic/prevenix.htm

American Association of Colleges of Nursing and the National Organization of Nurse Practitioner Faculties. (2003). *2002-2003 Enrollment and graduations in baccalaureate and graduate programs in nursing.* Washington, DC: American Association of Colleges of Nursing.

American Nurses Association. (1996). *The scope and standards of practice of advanced practice registered nursing.* Washington, DC: Author.

Aroskar, M. A. (1998). Ethical working relationships in patient care: Challenges and possibilities. *Nursing Clinics of North America, 33,* 313-324.

Association of Academic Health Centers (2002). *Partnerships for training.* Retrieved May 9, 2004, from http://www.pftweb.org

Bergman, D. A. (1999). Evidence-based guidelines and critical pathways for quality improvement. *Pediatrics, 103*(1SupplE), 225-232.

Berlin, L.E. Stennett, J. & Bednash, G. D. (2003). *2002-2003 Enrollment and graduations in baccalaureate and graduate programs in nursing.* Washington, DC: American Association of Colleges of Nursing.

Bourne, H. (2001). *A great deal: Compensation negotiation for nurse practitioners & physician assistants.* Arcata, CA: Open Spaces.

Brita-Rossi, P., Adduci, P., Kaufman, J., Lipson, S. J., Totte, C., & Wasserman, K. (1996). Improving the process of care: The cost-quality value of interdisciplinary collaboration. *Journal of Nursing Care Quarterly, 10,* 10-16.

Brown, S. J. (1999). *Knowledge for health care practice: A guide to using research evidence.* Philadelphia: WB Saunders.

Brown, M. A., & Olshansky, E. F. (1997). From limbo to legitimacy: A theoretical model of the transition to the primary care nurse practitioner role. *Nursing Research, 46,* 46-51.

Brown, S. A., & Grimes, D. E. (1993). *Nurse practitioners and certified nurse midwives: A meta analysis of process of care, clinical outcomes, and cost-effectiveness of nurses in primary care roles* (#NP-85). Washington, DC: American Nurses Association.

Buppert, C. (1999). HEDIS for the primary care provider: Getting an "A" on the managed care report card. *Nurse Practitioner, 24,* 84, 86, 88-89, 92-94, 97-99.

Buppert, C. (2000). *The primary care provider's guide to compensation and quality* (1st ed). Gaithersberg, MD: Aspen.

Buppert, C. (2004). *Nurse practitioner's business practice and legal guide*. Boston: Jones and Bartlett.

Cary, A. H., Goldberg, B., & McDaniel, S. (2003). Consumer views of primary care: An action agenda. *American Journal for Nurse Practitioners, 10*(7), 9-23.

Clawson, D. K., & Osterweis, M. (Eds.). (1993). *The roles of physician assistants and nurse practitioners in primary care*. Washington, DC: Association of Academic Health Centers.

Cohen, S. S., Mason, D. J., Arsenie, L. S., Sargese, S. M., & Needham, D. (1998). Focus groups reveal perils and promise of managed care for nurse practitioners. *Nurse Practitioner, 23*, 48, 54, 57-60 passim.

Conger, M., & Craig, C. (1998). Advanced nurse practice: A model for collaboration. *Nursing Case Management, 3*, 120-127.

Connors, H.R. (2002). Telehealth technologies enhance children's health care. *Journal of Professional Nursing, 18*, 311-312.

Cook, T., & Nolan, W. (1996). A nurse practitioner-led, collaborative, out-patient practice: A case study in outcomes management. *Seminars for Nurse Managers, 4*, 154-162.

Coolican, M. B., & Swanson, A. (1998). Primary health-care physicians: Vital roles in organ and tissue donation. *Connecticut Medicine, 62*, 149-153.

Cooper, R. A., Henderson, T., & Dietrich, C. L. (1998). Roles of nonphysician clinicians as autonomous providers of patient care. *Journal of the American Medical Association, 280*, 795-802.

Cooper, R. A., Laud, P., & Dietrich, C. L. (1998). Current and projected workforce of nonphysician clinicians. *Journal of the American Medical Association, 280*, 788-794.

Courtney, R. (1995). Community partnership primary care: A new paradigm for primary care. *Public Health Nursing, 12*, 366-373.

*Dossey, B. (1995). Using imagery to help your patient heal. *American Journal of Nursing, 95*, 40-47.

Felten, S., Cady, N., Metzler, M. H., & Burton, S. (1997). Implementation of collaborative practice through interdisciplinary rounds on a general surgery service. *Nursing Case Management, 2*, 122-126.

Fonteyn, M. (1998). The Agency for Health Care Policy and Research guidelines: Implications for home health care providers. *American Association of Colleges of Nursing Clinical Issues, 9*, 338-354.

Ford, L. C., & Silver, H. K. (1967). The expanded role of the nurse in childcare. *Nursing Outlook, 15*, 43-45.

Greenberg, M. E., & Schuetz, C. (2002). Telephone nursing client experiences and perceptions. *Nursing Economics, 20*, 181-187.

Green-Hernandez, C. (1997). Application of caring theory in primary care: A challenge for advanced practice. *Nursing Administration Quarterly, 21*, 77-82.

HEDIS 2004 (2004). *What's in it and why it matters* (Vol.1). Retrieved September 25, 2003, from http://www.ncqa.org/programs/HEDIS

Hersh, W. (1999). "A world of knowledge at your fingertips." The promise, reality, and future directions of on-line information retrieval. *Academic Medicine, 74*, 240-243.

Hughes, A. M., & Turner, L. C. (1996). Nurse-physician collaboration: Historical review and impact today. *Canadian Association of Critical Care Nurses, 7*, 24-28.

Institute of Medicine. (1996). *Primary care: America's health in a new era*. Washington, DC: National Academy Press.

Jenkins, R.L., & White, P. (2001). Telehealth: Advancing nursing practice. *Nursing Outlook, 49*(2), 100-105.

*Jin, P. (1992). Efficacy of Tai Chi, brisk walking, meditation, and reading in reducing mental and emotional stress. *Journal of Psychosomatic Research, 36*, 361-370.

Kane, R. L., Garrard, J., Buchanan, J. L., Rosenfeld, A., Skay, C., & McDermott, S. (1991). Improving primary care in nursing homes. *Journal of the American Geriatrics Society, 39*, 359-367.

*Keel, P., Bodoky, C., Gerhard, U., & Muller, W. (1998). Comparison of integrated group therapy and group relaxation training for fibromyalgia. *The Clinical Journal of Pain, 14*, 232-238.

Kendig, S. (2002). Managing managed care: A nurse practitioner response to barriers to direct third-party reimbursement. In D. J. Mason, J. K. Leavitt, & M. W. Chaffee (Eds.) *Policy and politics in nursing and health care* (4th ed., pp. 265-272). Philadelphia: Elsevier Science

Kennedy, B. L. (2003). Negotiation: Getting what you need. In J. J. Fitzpatrick, A. Glasgow, & J. N. Young (Eds.). *Managing your practice: A guide for advanced practice nurses*. New York: Springer.

Kornblit, P., Senderoff, J., Davis-Ericksen, M., & Zenk, J. (1990). Anticoagulant therapy: Patient management and evaluation of an outpatient clinic. *Nurse Practitioner, 15*, 21-26, 29, 32.

Mabrook, A. F., & Dale, B. (1998). Can nurse practitioners offer a quality service? *Journal of Accident and Emergency Medicine, 15*, 266-268.

Mason, D. J., Cohen, S. S., O'Donnell, J. P., Baxter, K., & Chase, A. B. (2002). Managed care organizations' arrangements with nurse practitioners. *Nursing Economics, 15*, 306-314.

Moody, N. B., Smith, P. L., & Glenn, L. L. (1999). Client characteristics and practice patterns of nurse practitioners and physicians. *Nurse Practitioner, 24*, 94-96, 99-100, 102-103.

Mundinger, M. O., Kane, R. L., Lenz, E. R., Totlen, A. M., Tsai, W., Cleary, P. D., et al. (2000). Primary care outcomes in patients treated by nurse practitioners or physicians: A randomized trial.

---

*Indicates complementary therapy reference.

Journal of the American Medical Association, 283, 59-68.

National Advisory Council on Nurse Education and Practice. (2002). *Nurse practitioner workforce report executive summary.* Washington, DC: Author.

National Committee for Quality Assurance. (2003).*The health plan employer data and information set (HEDIS®).* Retrieved September, 25, 2003, from http://www.ncqa.org/Programs/HEDIS

National Organization of Nurse Practitioner Faculties. (1995). *Advanced practice nursing: Nurse practitioner curriculum guidelines and program standards for nurse practitioner education.* Washington, DC: Author.

National Organization of Nurse Practitioner Faculties. (2000). *Domains and competencies of N.P. practice. An updating and revision of 1995 advanced nursing practice: Curriculum guidelines and program standards for N.P. education.* Washington, DC: Author.

National Organization of Nurse Practitioner Faculties and the American Association of College of Nursing. (2002, April). *Nurse practitioner primary care competencies in specialty areas: Adult, family, gerontological, pediatric, and women's health.* Washington, DC: Author.

National Organization of Nurse Practitioner Faculties. (2003). *Community health in family nurse practitioner education.* Washington, DC: Author.

National Task Force on Quality Nurse Practitioner Education. (2002). *Criteria for evaluation of nurse practitioner programs.* Washington, DC: Author.

*Northrup, C. (2001). *The wisdom of menopause.* New York: Bantam.

Oberle, K., & Allen, M. (2001) The nature of advanced practice nursing. *Nursing Outlook, 49,* 148-153.

Pakis, S. (1997). Managing the marketing function for advanced nurse practitioners in a managed care environment. *Seminars for Nurse Managers, 5,* 149-153.

Pearson, K. C. (1998). The role of evidence-based medicine and clinical practice guidelines in treatment decisions. *Clinical Therapeutics, 20*(SupplC), C80-C85.

Persell, D. J., Arangie, P., Young, C., Stokes, E. N., Payne, W. C., Skorga, P., et al. (2001). Preparing for bioterrorism. *Nurse Practitioner, 26,* 12-29.

Reece, S. M. (1998). Community analysis for health planning: Strategies for primary care practitioners. *Nurse Practitioner, 23,* 46-59.

Ryan, S. A. (1993). Nurse practitioners: Educational issues, practice styles, and service barriers. In M. Osterweis & S. Garfinkel (Eds.), *The roles of physician assistants and nurse practitioners in primary care* (pp. 41-49). Washington, DC: Association of Academic Health Centers.

Safriet, B. J. (2002). Closing the gap between can and may in health care providers' scopes of practice: A primer for policymakers. *Yale Journal of Regulation, 19,* 301-334.

Sears, L., Maxwell, W., & Townsend, C. (2003). Urgent-care visits to a geriatric primary care clinic. *American Journal for Nurse Practitioners, 7,* 15-18.

Sekscenski, E. S., Sansom, S., Bazell, C., Salmon, M. E., & Mullan, F. (1994). State practice environments and the supply of physician assistants, nurse practitioners, and certified nurse-midwives. *New England Journal of Medicine, 331,* 1266-1271.

Sharp, N. (1996). Nurse practitioners, telemedicine, and the Federal Communications Commission. *Nurse Practitioner, 21,* 9-100.

Sharp, N. (1997). Medicare reimbursement: For NPs, CNSs, MDs, and telehealth. *Nurse Practitioner, 22,* 143-146.

Showstack, J., Lurie, N., Larson, E. B., Rothman, A. A., & Hassmiller, S. B. (2004a). Primary care, the next renaissance. In J. Showstack, A. A., Rothman, & S. B. Hassmiller (Eds.), *The future of primary care.* San Francisco: Jossey-Bass.

Showstack, J., Rothman, A. A., & Hassmiller, S. B. (2004b). *The future of primary care.* San Francisco: Jossey-Bass.

*Sinatra, S. (2000). Alternative medicine for the conventional cardiologist. *Heart Disease, 2,* 16-30.

Spratley, E., Johnson, A., Solchaski, J., Fritz, M., & Spencer, W. (2000). *The registered nurse population: Findings from the National Sample Survey of Registered Nurses.* Washington, DC: U.S. Department of Health and Human Services, Health Resources and Service Administration, Bureau of Health Professions, Division of Nursing.

Spross, J. A., Clarke, E. B., & Beauregard, J. (2000). Expert coaching and guidance. In A. B. Hamric, J A. Spross, C. M. Hanson (Eds.), *Advanced nursing practice: An integrative approach* (2nd ed., pp. 186-215). Philadelphia: W.B. Saunders.

Stange, K. C. (1996). Primary care research: Barriers and opportunities. *Journal of Family Practice, 42,* 192-198.

Starfield, B. (2003). Press release from the American Academy of Family Physicians. March 20, 2003.

Stichler, J. F. (1995). Professional interdependence: The art of collaboration. *Advanced Practice Nursing Quarterly, 1,* 53-61.

Tsafrir, J., & Grinberg, M. (1998). Who needs evidence-based health care? *Bulletin of the Medical Library Association, 86,* 40-45.

Ulrich, C.M., Soeken, K.L., & Miller, N. (2003). Ethical conflict associated with managed care: Views of nurse practitioners. *Nursing Research, 52,* 168-175.

U.S. Department of Health and Human Services. (2000). *Healthy people 2010* (2nd ed.). Washington, DC: U.S. Government Printing Office.

Virginia General Assembly. (1999) *Directing the Joint Commission on Health Care to study the need to collect workforce data on nurse practitioners, clinical*

---

*Indicates complementary therapy reference.

nurse specialists, registered nurses, licensed practical nurses, and certified nurse aides (House Joint Resolution No. 682).

*Weil, A. (1999). *Breathing: The master key to self-healing* [cassette recording]. Boulder: Sounds True.

Weinstein, M. E., McCormack, B., Brown, M. E., & Rosenthal, D. S. (1998). Build consensus and develop collaborative practice guidelines. *Nursing Management, 29,* 48-52.

Williamson, S. H., & Hutcherson, C. (1998). Mutual recognition: Response to the regulatory implications of a changing health care environment. *Advanced Practice Nursing Quarterly, 4,* 86-93.

Wilson, R., & Hubert, J. (2002). Resurfacing the care in nursing by telephone: Lessons from ambulatory oncology. *Nursing Outlook, 50,* 160-164.

Wing, D. M. (1998). The business management preceptorship within the nurse practitioner program. *Journal of Professional Nursing, 14,* 150-156.

Worrall, G. (1999). Clinical practice guidelines: Questions family physicians should ask themselves. *Comprehensive Therapy, 25,* 46-49.

*Worwood, V.A. (1991). *The complete book of essential oils and aromatherapy.* San Rafael, CA: New World Library.

Yocum, C. Busby, L., Conway-Welch, C., & Viens, D. (1999). *Curriculum guidelines for family nurse practitioners seeking prescriptive authority to manage pharmacotherapeutics in primary care.* Washington, DC: National Organization of Nurse Practitioner Faculties.

Yurkowski, W. (1997). The use of nonphysician providers in managed care settings. *Journal of the American Medical Association, 277,* 1095.

Additional Readings

Arcangelo, V., Fitzgerald, M., Carroll, D., & Plumb, J. D. (1996). Collaborative care between nurse practitioners and primary care physicians. *Primary Care, 23,* 103-113.

*Barbour, C. (2000). Use of complementary and alternative treatments by individuals with fibromyalgia syndrome. *Journal of the American Academy of Nurse Practitioners, 12,* 311-316.

Bumenthal, M., Busse, W.R., Goldber, A., Gruenwalk, J., Hall, T., Riggins, C.W., et al. (Eds.). (1998). *The complete Commission E monographs.* Austin, TX: American Botanical Council.

Cooper, R. A. (1997). The growing independence of nonphysician clinicians in clinical practice. *Journal of the American Medical Association, 277,* 1092-1093.

Dossey, B. (1997). *Core curriculum for holistic nursing.* Gaithersburg, MD: Aspen Publishers.

Dossey, B., Keegan, L., Guzzetta, C., & Kolkmeier, L. (1995). *Holistic nursing: A handbook for practice.* Gaithersburg, MD: Aspen Publishers.

Duke, J. (1997). *The green pharmacy.* Emmaus, PA: Rodale.

Engebretson, J. (1996). Comparison of nurses and alternative healers. *Image, 28,* 95-99.

Gordon, J. S. (1996). Alternative medicine and the family physician. *American Family Physician, 54,* 2218-2224.

Hollinger-Smith, L. (1998). Partners in collaboration. *Journal of Professional Nursing, 14,* 344-349.

Leveille, S. G., Wagner, E. H., Davis, C., Grothaus, L., Wallace, J., LoGerfo, M., et al. (1998). Preventing disability and managing chronic illness in frail older adults: A randomized trial of a community-based partnership with primary care. *Journal of the American Geriatrics Society, 46,* 1191-1198.

McCain, N.L., & Smith, J.C. (1994). Stress and coping in the context of psychoneuroimmunology: A holistic framework for nursing practice and research. *Archives of Psychiatric Nursing, VIII,* 221-227.

*Robins, J. (1998). The science and art of aromatherapy. *Journal of Holistic Nursing, 17,* 18-33.

*Robins, J. (1999). Synthesizing reductionism and holism: Integrative advanced health care practice. *National Academies of Practice Forum, 1,* 197-202.

Schumacher, K., & Meleis, A. (1994). Transitions: A central concept in nursing. *Image: The Journal of Nursing Scholarship, 26,* 119-127.

*Spencer, J., & Jacobs, J. (1999). *Complementary/alternative medicine: An evidence-based approach.* St Louis: Mosby.

Wells-Federman, C.L., Stuart, E.M., Deckro, J.P., Mandle, C.L., Baim, M., & Medich, C. (1995). The mind-body connection: The psychophysiology of many traditional nursing interventions. *Clinical Nurse Specialist, 9,* 59-66.

Youngkin, E.Q., & Israel, D.S. (1996). A review and critique of common herbal alternative therapies. *Nurse Practitioner, 21*(10), 30-62.

---

*Indicates complementary therapy reference.

CHAPTER 14

The Acute Care Nurse Practitioner

MARILYN HRAVNAK • RUTH M. KLEINPELL • KATHY S. MAGDIC •
JANE GUTTENDORF

Continued

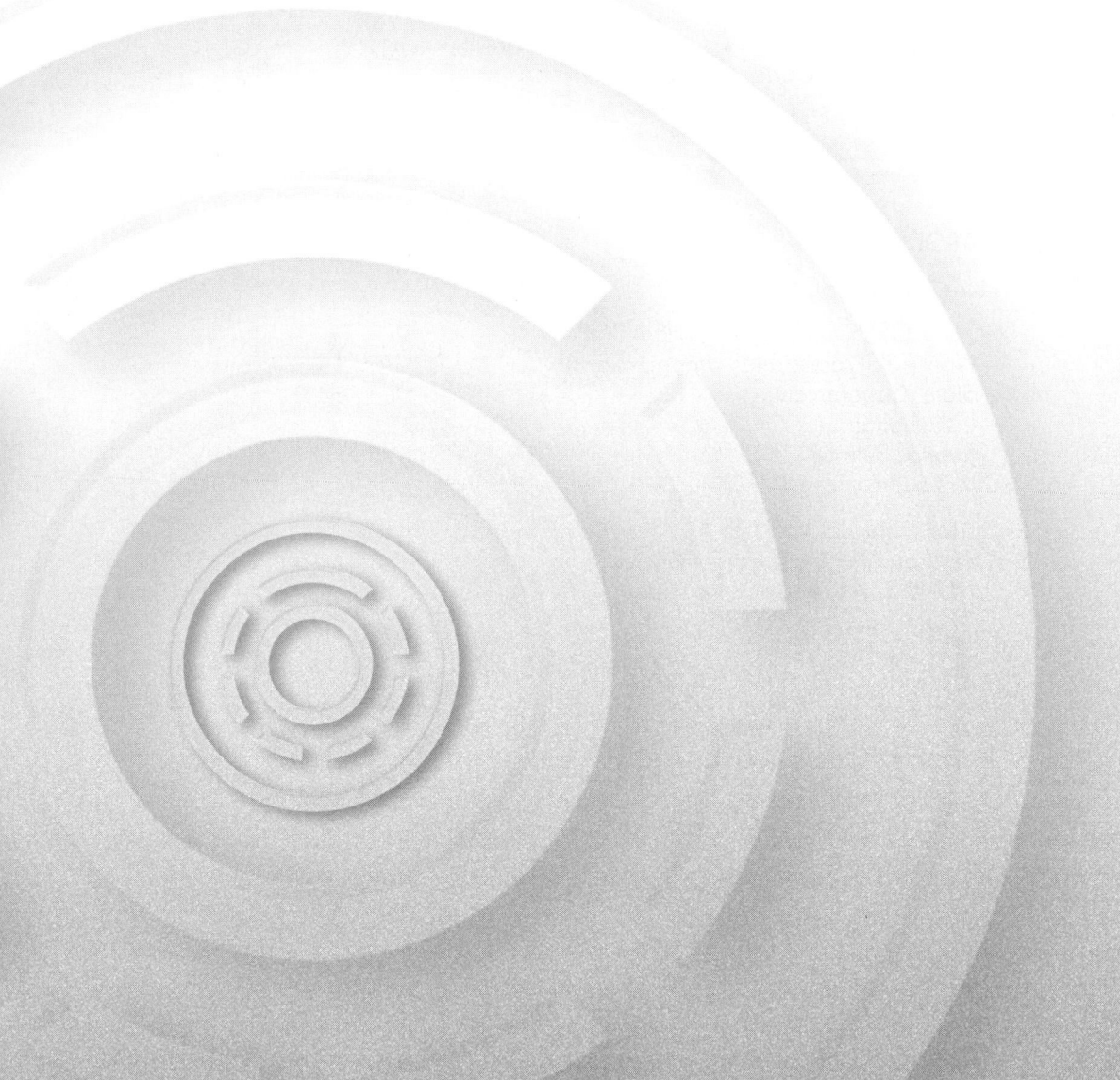

INTRODUCTION

As changes in health care have occurred, the acute care nurse practitioner (ACNP) has emerged to diagnose and manage disease and to promote the health of acute and critically ill patients with episodic and chronic health problems across the continuum of acute care services. The ACNP provides comprehensive care in a collaborative model with physicians, staff nurses, and other health-care providers, as well as with adult patients and their families. The ACNP shares common functions and skills with the other nurse practitioner (NP) subspecialties but also requires and applies unique knowledge and skills in caring for this very complex and vulnerable patient population. Although all ACNPs share specialty role attributes, there may be intrarole variability based on the nature of the care delivery system or location in which they practice (private practice group versus hospital employee, intensive care unit versus hospital ward or ambulatory care facility), or physiological specialty (cardiac, pulmonary, orthopedic, oncology, etc.). This chapter presents an overview of the ACNP role, scope of practice, competencies, educational preparation, reimbursement, and future challenges.

HISTORY OF THE ACNP ROLE

Although the role of nurse practitioners (NPs) in primary care has been well documented since the 1960s (see Chapter 13), the newer role of the ACNP in secondary and tertiary care has not been as extensively described or studied. Whereas neonatal NPs (NNPs) first began caring for acutely and critically ill infants in secondary and tertiary care settings in the 1970s because of cutbacks in pediatric residencies coupled with the increasing acuity and complexity of neonatal patients (Lott, Polak, Kenyon, & Kenner, 1996), changes in the delivery of acute and critical care of adults in the 1970s and 1980s similarly predated the ACNP role. Advances in medical care increased patient longevity, which in turn produced a larger pool of elderly, fragile patients with multiple co-morbidities who were more apt to require hospitalization when experiencing acute illness or exacerbation of chronic illness. Simultaneously, an explosion in health-care science resulted in the greater availability of technological monitoring and life support, further advancing the complexity of patient care and the need for health-care providers specially trained in supporting these patients. Conversely, at the very time when the acuity and the need for technological support of inpatients were increasing, a paradigm shift emerged among health systems of care toward primary care, with less focus on acute and specialty care. This paradigm shift resulted in less emphasis on the preparation of physician specialists and a decrease in medical trainee coverage for both infant and adult patients (Daly & Gent, 1997; Ingersoll, 1995; Keane, Richmond, & Kaiser, 1994; Parrinello, 1995). Silver and McAtee (1988) proposed to address the shortage of physicians, residents, and fellows in specialty practices by using NPs in the hospital setting. The goal of this proposal was to provide high-quality acute care in the face of physician reductions, particularly in teaching hospitals. ACNPs were to be educated to identify health risks and health promotion needs and to manage acute and chronic illness in collaboration with and under the supervision of a physician (e.g., intensivist, internist, or cardiologist). Silver and McAtee (1988) envisioned that these NPs would develop clinical decision-making skills and technical skills in order to admit patients to the hospital,

We thank Julie Fletcher Cuneo, ACNP-BC, and Kathryn Fletcher Cuneo for assistance with manuscript preparation.

complete the history and physical examination, assess patients' clinical status, and manage subsequent changes in their clinical condition. ACNPs would also write medical orders, perform a variety of diagnostic and therapeutic tests, order and interpret laboratory studies, and counsel patients and their families in collaboration with physicians. In 1992, Knickman, Lipkin, Finkler, Thompson, and Kiel published a study aimed at examining care models to address the hospital resident shortage and assessed the potential of using "midlevel providers" to compensate for reduced availability of residents. They conducted a time-and-motion study of internal medicine residents at two large urban New York City hospitals and utilized the data to develop two models of care. In the traditional model, in which the physician is the primary medical manager, 46% of the resident's time was spent in activities only a physician could perform. When the services of a midlevel provider were added to the model, the time requirement for physician-only tasks decreased to 20%.

All of the previous factors have been instrumental in the movement of the NP into the acute care setting to fill perceived gaps in health-care delivery (Keane & Richmond, 1993). Initially, primary care NPs (family NPs and adult NPs) were recruited to care for adult patients in hospital-based settings, with on-the-job training to provide secondary and tertiary care skills. By the late 1980s, NPs were increasingly utilized to care for critically ill adults within tertiary care centers (Barber & Burke, 1999). It became apparent that a new NP specialty was emerging—one that required educational preparation specifically designed to meet the needs of complex and vulnerable adult patients who were acutely and critically ill and to ensure consistency in the knowledge, training, and quality of care provided by NP graduates in this new specialty.

Master's-level graduate ACNP programs began to emerge in the late 1980s. Currently, there are over 65 ACNP programs in existence (Kleinpell & Hravnak, 2002). A national certification exam for ACNPs was developed jointly by the American Nurses Association (ANA) and the American Association of Critical-Care Nurses (AACN-a) in 1995. Between the initial exam offering in 1995 and June 30, 2003, 3340 persons have taken and passed this certification examination (L. Skinner, personal communication, September 5, 2003). Research studies demonstrate that the care that ACNPs provide is effective, is of high quality, is cost-effective, and results in patient satisfaction (Hoffman, Tasota, Scharfenberg, Zullo, & Donahoe, 2003; Piano & Zerwic-Johnson, 1998; Prescott & Driscoll, 1980; Russell, VorderBruegge, & Burns, 2002; Scharfenberg, Hoffman, Tasota, Happ, & Donahoe, 2003).

SCOPE OF PRACTICE FOR THE ACNP

The scope of practice and specialty competencies for the ACNP, as the newest fully-evolved NP subspecialty, are emerging based on a variety of influences. The scope of ACNP practice is influenced on five levels: national (professional organizations), state (government), health-care institution, service related, and individual (Figure 14-1). In common with other advanced practice nurses (APNs), the ACNP's scope of practice is broadly set forth in statements by professional nursing organizations, which delineate the scope of practice of ACNPs across the nation in the broadest sense. State governments, as regulatory agencies, further delineate the scope of practice in statutes such as nurse practice acts or title-protection statutes. However, because ACNPs frequently provide their services within health-care delivery systems such as hospitals, subacute care facilities, nursing homes, and clinics, their scope may be further defined by policies within these institutions, organizations, and health-care entities and even by the needs of a clinically specialized patient population. Lastly, each individual ACNP will further define her or his scope based

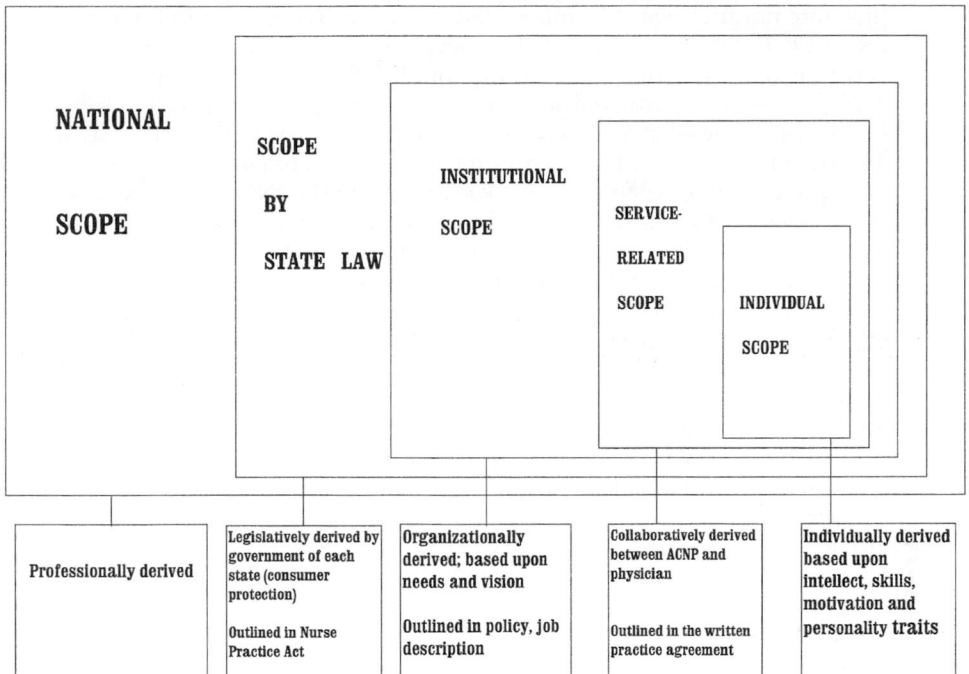

NATIONAL

SCOPE

SCOPE

BY

STATE LAW

INSTITUTIONAL

SCOPE

SERVICE-

RELATED

SCOPE

INDIVIDUAL

SCOPE

| Professionally derived | Legislatively derived by government of each state (consumer protection)

Outlined in Nurse Practice Act | Organizationally derived; based upon needs and vision

Outlined in policy, job description | Collaboratively derived between ACNP and physician

Outlined in the written practice agreement | Individually derived based upon intellect, skills, motivation and personality traits |

FIGURE 14-1 • The Scope of ACNP Practice. (From Hravnak, M., Rosenzweig, P., Rust, D., & Magdic, K. [1998b]. Scope of practice, credentialing, and privileging. In R. Kleinpell & M. Piano [Eds.], *Practice issues for the acute care nurse practitioner* [pp. 41-46]. New York: Springer.)

on her or his own talents, strengths, and attributes. How ACNP practice is configured at each of these levels is described in the following sections.

National (Professional Organizations)

At the national level, the competencies and domains of general NP practice are outlined by the National Organization of Nurse Practitioner Faculties (NONPF) within the document *Domains and Competencies of Nurse Practitioner Practice* (NONPF, 2000). The NONPF examined the domains of NP practice based on a study conducted by Karen Brykczynski (1989), which identified the domains of practice of a skilled primary care nurse practitioner using Benner's model of nursing practice (Benner, 1984). Brykczynski subsequently modified Benner's domains to describe primary care NP practice. The NONPF utilized Brykczynski's domains of NP practice with further modifications based on research by Hanson (1986), Monninger (1987), and NONPF members. The finally evolved domains of NP practice upon which the competencies of skilled primary care NPs were based (and ultimately curriculum content was delineated by the NONPF) are as follows: Management of Client Health/Illness, Monitoring and Ensuring the Quality of Health-Care Practice, Organizational and Role Competencies, the Healing Role of the Nurse, and the Teaching-Coaching Function of the Nurse. One of Benner's domains of nursing practice, Management of Rapidly Changing Situations, was not found to describe the practice of experienced primary care NPs according to Brykczynski's data and was therefore not included. The initial 1990 document (NONPF, 1990) was revised in 1995 (NONPF, 1995) and 2000 (NONPF, 2000). The newer versions have been broadened to accept general practice competencies of all NPs regardless of specialty setting. The NONPF has also partnered with the American Association of Colleges of Nursing (AACN-b) to develop more specific competencies for the primary care NP subspecialties. The final report, *Nurse Practitioner Primary Care Competencies in Specialty Areas: Adult, Family, Gerontological, Pediatric and Women's Health* (NONPF/AACN-b, 2002), identifies the national, consensus-based entry-level competencies that describe each of the primary care NP subspecialty areas, utilizing information and data from previously developed core and specialty competencies, role delineation studies, and other existing literature as the basis for their work. The specialty competencies for the ACNP have not yet been developed by national consensus. It is likely that many of the ACNP competencies will fall within the domain of the Management of Rapidly Changing Situations, in contrast to the other NP specialties. In the meantime, it is reasonable and in fact essential that practicing ACNPs and educators look to the core competencies described in the document *Domains and Competencies of Nurse Practitioner Practice* as the common basis for all NP practice and education, including that of ACNPs.

Two documents developed by professional nursing organizations at the national level provide further insight into the ACNP specialist's scope of practice. The first is the *Standards of Clinical Practice and Scope of Practice for the Acute Care Nurse Practitioner*, developed collaboratively by the American Nurses Association (ANA) and the American Association of Critical-Care Nurses (AACN-a). In this publication, "scope of practice" defines the ACNP as a provider of advanced nursing care across the continuum of acute care services to patients who are acutely and critically ill, using a collaborative model. The focus of care is restorative, with the short-term goal being patient stabilization, provision of physical and psychological care, and minimization of complications. The long-term goal is restoration of the patient's maximal health potential (with concurrent evaluation of risk factors in achieving this outcome) (ANA and AACN-a, 1995). The practice environment for the ACNP is "any setting in which patient care requirements include complex monitoring and therapies, high-intensity nursing interventions, or continuous nursing vigilance within the full range of high-acuity care" (ANA and AACN-a, 1995, p. 12). The "standards of clinical practice" and "standards of professional performance," along with measurement criteria examples for the ACNP as specified in this document, are summarized in Box 14-1. These standards describe a competent level of care and professional performance common to all ACNPs practicing in any acute care setting by which the quality of ACNP practice can be judged (ANA and AACN-a, 1995). Some common themes in the standards of ACNP clinical practice and professional performance that distinguish the practice of ACNPs from other NP specialties are the dynamic nature of the patient's health and illness status, the vulnerability of the patient population, the need for continuous assessment and adjustment of the management plan in the face of rapidly changing patient conditions, and the complexity of the monitoring and therapeutics. Additional themes include the collaborative nature of the practice and the interactive relationship between the ACNP and the health-care system.

A second resource that does not define scope of practice but does specify the knowledge necessary to perform within the specialty scope is the ACNP national certification examination. Although this examination was initially developed and administered jointly by the ANA and AACN-a, it is now administered solely by the American Nurses Credentialing Center (ANCC) of the ANA. The purpose of national certification is to provide documentation for the public that a licensed professional has demonstrated mastery of knowledge and skills to practice the profession (Hravnak & Baldessari, 1997; Kristeller, 1995) and

---

BOX 14-1 • STANDARDS OF CLINICAL PRACTICE AND PROFESSIONAL PERFORMANCE FOR THE ACUTE CARE NURSE PRACTITIONER

STANDARDS OF ACNP CLINICAL PRACTICE

Standard I: Assessment

The ACNP collects patient data.

Measurement criteria example: The data collection process is continuous, in acknowledgement of the dynamic nature of acute illness.

Standard II: Diagnosis

The ACNP analyzes the assessment data in determining diagnoses.

Measurement criteria example: Diagnoses are re-evaluated as new or additional assessment data become available.

Standard III: Outcome Identification

The ACNP identifies expected outcomes individualized to the patient.

Measurement criteria example: Expected outcomes are modified based on changes in the patient condition.

Standard IV: Planning

The ACNP develops a plan of care that prescribes interventions to attain expected outcomes.

Measurement criteria example: The plan is individualized, recognizes the dynamic nature of the patient's illness, and reflects the patient's needs across a full continuum of acute care services.

Standard V: Implementation

The ACNP implements the interventions identified in the multidisciplinary plan of care.

Measurement criteria example: Interventions are prescribed consistent with the established multidisciplinary plan of care.

Standard VI: Evaluation

The ACNP evaluates the patient's progress toward attainment of expected outcomes.

Measurement criteria example: Evaluation is systematic and ongoing.

STANDARDS OF ACNP PROFESSIONAL PERFORMANCE

Standard I: Quality of Care

The ACNP systematically evaluates the quality and effectiveness of acute care nursing practice.

Measurement criteria example: The ACNP formulates recommendations to improve clinical practice based on data obtained from quality of care activities.

Standard II: Systems Management

The ACNP facilitates the use of organizational resources in caring for the patient.

Measurement criteria example: The ACNP analyzes organizational system enhancements and barriers that have an impact on patient care.

Standard III: Performance Appraisal

The ACNP evaluates his/her clinical practice in relation to professional practice standards and relevant statutes and regulations.

Measurement criteria example: The ACNP analyzes the use of procedures, the incidence and types of complications, the impact on patients, and the uses of these data to evaluate patients.

Standard IV: Education

The ACNP acquires and maintains current knowledge in advanced practice nursing.

Measurement criteria example: The ACNP is accountable for engaging in educational activities directed at improving clinical outcomes and professional performance.

Standard V: Collegiality

The ACNP contributes to the professional development of peers, colleagues, and others.

Measurement criteria example: The ACNP actively seeks and participates in opportunities to share skills and clinical observations with colleagues and other care providers.

Standard VI: Ethics

The ACNP's decisions and actions on behalf of patients are determined in an ethical manner.

Measurement criteria example: The ACNP contributes to the creation of an individual and systems response to resolve ethical dilemmas.

Standard VII: Collaboration

The ACNP collaborates with the patient, significant others, and other health-care providers in patient care.

Measurement criteria example: The ACNP makes referrals, including provision for continuity of care, as needed.

Standard VIII: Research

The ACNP uses research findings in practice.

Measurement criteria example: The ACNP uses interventions substantiated by relevant research as appropriate to the patient's needs and practice environment.

Continued

BOX 14-1 • STANDARDS OF CLINICAL PRACTICE AND PROFESSIONAL PERFORMANCE FOR THE ACUTE CARE NURSE PRACTITIONER — cont'd

STANDARDS OF ACNP CLINICAL PRACTICE — cont'd	STANDARDS OF ACNP PROFESSIONAL PERFORMANCE — cont'd
	Standard IX: Resource Utilization The ACNP considers factors related to safety, effectiveness, and cost in planning and delivering care. *Measurement criteria example:* The ACNP assists multidisciplinary team members, patients, and families in selecting therapies that integrate perspectives of cost and quality/benefits.

Adapted from American Nurses Association. (2003). *Nursing: Scope and standards of practice.* Washington, DC: American Nurses Publishing.

---

serves as a primary criterion for APN practice (see Chapter 3). Additionally, Medicare regulations stipulate completion of a national certification examination as a requirement for NPs to obtain reimbursement. The first Acute Care Nurse Practitioner Certification Examination was administered in December 1995 (ANA and AACN-a, 1995). ACNP certification eligibility criteria include completion of a master's degree or higher in nursing and preparation as an ACNP in a master's-level nursing program or a formal postgraduate ACNP program within a school of nursing granting graduate-level academic credit. Eligibility criteria and the test content outline provide guidance to faculty developing ACNP educational programs in the absence of subspecialty-specific curriculum guidelines. Examination topics include system-specific health problems, common problems in acute care, ethics and scope of practice, and health promotion and disease prevention (ANCC, 1999). It is evident that the content of a certification examination should not "drive" educational standards or curriculum development. Rather, the state of clinical practice should determine the knowledge, skills, and competencies necessary for safe and effective practice, which in turn provides the basis for educational preparation. However, it should be noted that the topics and content outline for the ACNP specialty examination have been validated by role delineation studies conducted by ANA/ANCC. Successfully passing the ACNP certification exam entitles the ACNP to use the credentials "APRN-BC" or attachment of the "BC" component to the designation approved by the state in which they practice (Smolenski, 2002), Recertification is a mechanism that provides evidence that the individual reaffirms this mastery over time.

The scope of practice for ACNPs (from the standpoint of core competencies and specialty content) is therefore described to some degree according to national consensus in the aforementioned documents. However, detailed ACNP specialty competencies have not yet been derived consensually at the national level, although they have been described in the literature and by some research and will be summarized later in the chapter.

State (Government)

Each state's government provides the second mechanism whereby the professional scope of practice for the ACNP is defined. The nurse practice statute for each state governs NP practice. NP practice regulations are intended to define practice within a specific state, and these regulations vary from state to state (Cummings, 1997; Hall, 1993; Pearson, 2003).

Licensure is granted by the state, is required to practice a profession, guarantees a safe level of practice, and is generally not specialty specific (Hravnak & Baldisseri; 1997). In all states, APN regulation for practice is based on basic nursing licensure. However, many states also have varied additional rules and regulations that delineate additional requirements and define and limit who can use a specific advanced practice nursing title with protection (see Chapter 22). Many states do not differentiate between NP practice specialties (family, adult, pediatric, acute care), nor do they provide a list of skills, tasks, or procedures permissible within the specialty scope. When a particular state's practice act is examined to determine what an ACNP can and cannot do within her or his scope within that state, it is best to interpret the act as broadly as possible (assume "can" unless "cannot" is described) and assign plain and ordinary meanings to the words used in the statutes. When there is doubt regarding the interpretation of the nurse practice act for application in a specific employment situation, such as an acute care facility or practice plan, it may be helpful to seek the opinion of the employer's legal counsel for clarification (Hravnak, Rosenzweig, Rust, & Magdic, 1998b).

Institutional

As noted previously, the majority of ACNPs provide patient care within health-care institutions, either exclusively or as a component (both inpatient and outpatient) of their practice. Institutions may further delineate the ACNP's scope of practice within that facility by identifying the patient population the ACNP serves and the process for collaboration with other health-care providers in the institution (Parrinello, 1995). This further specification of the ACNP's practice scope may be set forth in job descriptions, in hospital policy, or through the health-care agency's credentialing and privileging process.

An employer is responsible for the acts of its employee while the employee performs on behalf of the employer. However, an employer cannot be held responsible for an employee should the employee step beyond the bounds the employer sets forth (Cummings, 1997). Hospitals bear a legal responsibility to protect their clientele and hold some degree of vicarious liability for the actions of both physician and nonphysician providers serving their patient population, even when they are not employees of the hospital. Employers and hospitals therefore have the right to further delineate a specific health-care provider's scope of practice within the employment situation in order to document initial training as well as ongoing provider competence in the application of specific skills to their clientele. This "scope of employment" may not exceed the scope of practice specified by the state's nurse practice act but may be curtailed based on the needs and mission of the employer. The institutional "scope of employment" may take the form of a job description, hospital policy, or both (Cummings, 1997; Hravnak et al., 1998b). In settings where the ACNP role is being newly introduced, a job description may not exist. Depending on the practice setting, the responsibility for developing the job description may be undertaken by the ACNP or performed jointly with the employer, but it is imperative that the ACNP have input into the process. In general, the job description should include ACNP responsibilities as they relate to patient care, collaborative relationships, professional conduct, and professional development. An example of a previously published job description from the University of Pittsburgh Medical Center (Burkholder & Dudjak, 1994) is provided in Box 14-2. Performance standards included in job descriptions delineate the responsibilities for which the ACNP is accountable and provide a template by which both the ACNP and

BOX 14-2 • SAMPLE ACNP JOB DESCRIPTION

UNIVERSITY OF PITTSBURGH MEDICAL CENTER
Job Title: Certified Registered Nurse Practitioner
Department: Clinical Administration
Reports to: Clinical Administrator

FUNCTION
The certified registered nurse practitioner (CRNP) functions as a member of the medical care management team. The CRNP diagnoses medical conditions, plans and implements interventions, and evaluates patient responses under the direction of and in collaboration with a physician supervisor or designated attending physician.*

QUALIFICATIONS
1. Licensure as a professional nurse in the Commonwealth of Pennsylvania.
2. Certification as a nurse practitioner by the Commonwealth of Pennsylvania (CRNP) or completion of submission of all required materials.
3. Certification by the American Nurses Credentialing Center as a nurse practitioner (preferred).
4. Minimum of 2 years' nursing experience.
5. Master's degree in nursing.
6. Advanced cardiac life support certification preferred.

Qualifications are reviewed annually and clinical privileges authorized through the Medical Staff credentialing process.

SCOPE
Clinical privileges for individual CRNPs are recommended by the supervising physician to the Allied Health Credentialing Committee through the Medical Staff approval process. CRNPs may engage in activities that normally constitute the practice of nursing without credentialing, provided they have the preparation, knowledge, and experience necessary to properly execute the practice. Medical diagnostic, therapeutic, and management functions will be instituted under medical supervision using protocols or guidelines developed by the individual services/programs.

RESPONSIBILITIES
The CRNP is responsible for
1. *Assembling* a complete medical database, including health history of chief complaint and physical examination upon patient admission of selected patients, and *documenting* the findings in the patient record.
2. *Assessing* selected patients using physically and technologically derived data, including the evaluation of diagnostic test results, and *documenting* this assessment in the patient record.
3. Under the direction of, and in consultation/collaboration with, the physician preceptor, or designee, *diagnosing* medical conditions and *planning* medical therapeutics and interventions based on the medical database. *Documenting and communicating* the diagnosis and plan to other members of the health-care team.
4. Under the direction of, and in consultation/collaboration with, the physician preceptor, or designee, *ordering* medical consultations, therapies, and interventions including, but not limited to, medications, diagnostic tests, respiratory care (including ventilator management, nutrition, fluid and electrolyte support), and blood and blood products. *Documenting* these orders and directives in the patient record and *communicating* them to other members of the health-care team.
5. *Performing* invasive diagnostic and therapeutic procedures based on the needs of the specific patient population as determined collaboratively by the CRNP, physician preceptor, and service or unit medical director and approved by the Allied Health Credentialing Committee of the medical staff. *Documenting* the procedures and the patient responses and results in the patient record.
6. *Evaluating and analyzing* patients' responses to disease processes and therapeutic interventions, and *determining* the effectiveness of care and the need to alter the plan of care.
7. *Presenting* selected patient's assessments, diagnoses, and plans of care during medical team rounds.
8. *Providing* information and support to patients and families. *Facilitating* communication between patients and family members and members of the health-care team.
9. *Collaborating* with nurses and nurse managers to implement and evaluate holistic patient care delivery.
10. *Serving* as a resource to members of the health-care team to facilitate patient delivery by using an in-depth pathophysiological and psychosocial knowledge base.

*The terminology related to "Physician Supervision" was based on the language in the Nurse Practice Act in Pennsylvania at the time of the source publication. It should be noted that this job description serves as a guide only and would need adaptation for use based on state regulatory language at a given time.

BOX 14-2 • SAMPLE ACNP JOB DESCRIPTION* — cont'd

11. *Participating* in activities that contribute to the education of other health-care professionals, including *presenting and publishing.*
12. *Acting* as a role model and, in selected cases, *precepting* nurses and other advanced practice nurses, including other nurse practitioners.
13. *Participating* in medical and nursing research projects, including *presenting and publishing* the findings.
14. *Promoting and practicing* economical and effective health care.
15. *Demonstrating* behavior that models the UPMC's service vision/philosophy.
16. *Teaching and promoting* practices to improve or maintain health to patients and family members, and others within and outside the UPMC.
17. *Participating in or initiating* activities necessary for annual reappointment and privileging. *Documenting* evidence of continuing competency in the areas of medical diagnoses, therapeutics, invasive procedures, and management, as well as required certification(s).
18. *Participating* in activities that enhance professional development with role as an advanced practice nurse, such as
    a. *serving* on UPMC committees related to CRNP utilization, including regularly updating medical management protocols;
    b. *reading* professional journals and texts to maintain currency on the latest clinical, professional and legislative trends and *sharing* the knowledge gained with other members of the health-care team;
    c. *attending* continuing education programs; and
    d. *participating* in professional organizations.
19. *Serving* on departmental and interdisciplinary committees.
20. *Performing* other duties as determined collaboratively by the physician preceptor, the CRNP, and the clinical administrator that are within the scope of practice of CRNPs and the policies of the UPMC.

From Burkholder, J., & Dudjak, L. (1994). The midlevel practitioner role: One medical center's experience. *AACN Clinical Issues in Critical Care Nursing, 5,* 372-374; reprinted with permission.

the employer can evaluate performance (Hravnak et al., 1998b). Once the job description is in place, a plan for conducting an ongoing performance evaluation should be outlined.

When providing care within a health-care institution, the ACNP will also need to undergo the process of provider credentialing and privileging by the institution, whether the ACNP is an employee of the hospital or an employee of a hospital-affiliated or private practice plan (see Chapter 22). Credentialing is the process whereby the employer is legally responsible for verifying the education, qualifications, and skills of the prospective employee. Health-care institutions are bound to verify the professional and technical competence of licensed providers (physician and nonphysician) caring for patients in the facility, as mandated by the Joint Commission of the Accreditation of Healthcare Organizations and the National Practitioner Data Bank (Kristeller, 1995). The ACNP is required to provide proof of licensure, certification, educational preparation, (generally) malpractice insurance, and skill performance (training, numbers performed, proof of competency) (Hravnak & Baldessari, 1997). Credentialing is necessary in order for the ACNP to provide care to patients within the institution, although the ACNP may or may not hold a medical staff appointment.

Once an individual is credentialed, a determination is made regarding the clinical privileges that may be granted. Privileging is a process whereby the institution determines which medical procedures may be performed and which conditions may be treated by both physician and nonphysician providers (Kristeller, 1995). Although a credentialed provider may be permitted by statute to perform certain acts or skills, the hospital is not bound to grant this provider the privilege to practice those acts or skills on its clientele. (For example, licensed physicians may bear the credentials to deliver babies or perform gastroscopies but may not be extended the privilege to do so within the institution.) The clinical privileges of the ACNP are partly based on the ACNP's professional license, certification, and inherent scope of practice (as previously discussed), documented training, experience, competence, and health status. The ACNP who has received educational preparation for performing invasive diagnostic procedures such as insertion of central line catheters, lumbar puncture, chest tube placement, and intubation can request that these privileges be a part of the "institutional" scope of practice if he or she can provide proof of training and competency. An ACNP may periodically request new privileges based on evolving mastery of skills, further training, and changes in services needed by the patient population and institution (Hravnak & Baldessari, 1997). It is important to understand that, although an ACNP may be qualified to perform certain procedures, privileges to perform these acts may not necessarily be granted or renewed (usually on a biannual basis) if the patient population the ACNP serves does not require these skills or if ongoing application and competency in the skill during the renewal period cannot be documented.

In states where physician collaboration is a requirement or in cases when the health-care organization has collaborative guidelines, the ACNP's institutional scope of practice and clinical privileges may be determined collaboratively by the physician and ACNP and set forth in a written agreement, which then provides the source document on which the hospital makes privileging decisions. (This subject is discussed in more detail later in this chapter.)

Service Related

The functions of the ACNP are also adjusted according to the needs of the specialty patient population served or of the care delivery team (i.e., service) in the organization with which the ACNP is affiliated. This service-related scope outlines the clinical functions and tasks that may be administered by the ACNP specific to the service team with which the ACNP works and the needs of the specialty patient population that she or he serves (Burkholder & Dudjak, 1994; Hravnak et al., 1998b). For example: An ACNP working with a cardiology service may initiate treatment for ischemia or infarction; an ACNP working with an oncology service may perform bone marrow aspirations or order antibiotics for suspected opportunistic infection; an ACNP on a renal medicine service may write orders for hemodialysis and insert central venous dialysis catheters; an ACNP with the cardiovascular surgery service may harvest the vein grafts for coronary artery bypass surgery; and the ACNP in the medical intensive care unit (MICU) may intubate and place arterial and central venous catheters (Hravnak et al., 1998b). Service-related scope therefore may vary among ACNPs affiliated with various services or specialties within the same institution, even among those who function under the same generic job description. The service-related scope outlines a more detailed and specific description of the types of activities the ACNP will perform as a member of the practice. In many cases, these specific activities are reflected in the written agreement, which in turn provides the basis for the request for clinical privileges. The level of communication or degree of supervision between the ACNP and the physician that is required before the performance of a specific function might also be outlined. This is particularly important to provide for patient safety as the ACNP moves from novice to expert in the performance of complex technical tasks, such as invasive procedures. An ACNP with novice skills in central line insertion may require direct supervision for a specified period of time or number of successful attempts. However, as the ACNP approaches expert status, the level of supervision may be changed to that of none required. Eventually, as the ACNP's expertise continues to advance, the ACNP may supervise medical trainees or novice ACNPs in these skills. In this case, the written agreement will also need to be modified. In some cases, the written agreement may be used to communicate the ACNP's scope of employment to other members of the health-care team, such as staff nurses and pharmacists.

Written agreements, often formatted as a checklist, are frequently helpful because the detail included in a written agreement usually cannot be spelled out in a job description. Job descriptions, by their very nature, tend to be global in nature in order to cover ACNPs working in a variety of settings within the institution. When negotiating the written agreement, both the ACNP and the physician need to ensure that no function is in conflict with the individual state's nurse practice act and the policies of the particular institution.

Individual

The final determinant of scope of practice is role individualization by each ACNP. Prior experience, specialization, interest, motivation, self-esteem, personal ethics, personality traits, and communication style affect the employment opportunities, clinical specialties, skills, practice arrangements, and the degree of autonomy the ACNP will seek out and/or apply in her or his uniquely personal enactment of the role (Hravnak et al., 1998b).

COMPETENCIES OF THE ACNP ROLE

APN and NP Core Competencies

The central and core competencies for the APN, as explained in Chapter 3, form the foundation of ACNP practice. The central competency for APNs is direct clinical practice. The six core competencies are coaching/guidance, consultation, research skills, clinical and professional leadership, collaboration, and ethical decision-making skills. The ways in which ACNPs enact these central and core competencies are consistent with other APN specialties, as discussed in Chapters 5 through 11. In addition, all NP specialties share common entry-level competencies as outlined in the *Domains and Competencies of Nurse Practitioner Practice* (NONPF, 2000). In accordance with the domains and competencies as outlined in this document, all NPs actively contribute to the management of patient health and illness status, the nurse-client relationship, the teaching-coaching function, professional role, the managing and negotiating of health-care delivery systems, the monitoring and ensuring of the quality of health-care practice, and demonstration of cultural competency. These core competencies of NP practice are essential behaviors for all the NP specialties, including ACNPs. Although the ACNP may need to utilize specialty skills and knowledge in the care of acutely and critically ill adults, ACNPs have the following factors in common with the other NP subspecialties: (1) a generalist nursing foundation, (2) a health promotion basis to their practice, and (3) the development and appreciation of diagnostic reasoning skills.

ACNP Specialty Competencies

In addition to the core NP competencies, each of the NP subspecialties has unique competencies that differentiate their practice. The primary care NP specialties have prepared consensus-based primary care competencies as outlined in the *Nurse Practitioner Primary Care Competencies in Specialty Areas: Adult, Family, Gerontological, Pediatric, and Women's Health* (NONPF/AACN-b, 2002). As noted previously, ACNP specialty competencies have not been developed by national consensus. Work on defining ACNP specialty competencies is currently under way through the National Organization of Nurse Practitioner Faculties. Therefore the ACNP specialty competencies about to be discussed are those that have been related in the literature and organized by the authors within the model for competencies described in this text.

ACNP SPECIALTY CENTRAL COMPETENCY: DIRECT CLINICAL PRACTICE

Specialty competencies for the ACNP supplement the generic NP core competencies and emphasize care competencies specifically related to the health problems of acutely and critically ill adults. Most ACNPs practice in acute and critical care settings, which include subacute care, emergency care, and intensive care settings. However, a growing number of ACNPs are practicing in specialty-based practice settings, including clinics, medical rehabilitation, home care, long-term care, sports medicine, holistic medicine, occupational medicine, employee health, mental health services, and medical flight programs, among others (Kleinpell-Nowell, 1999, 2001). The ACNP is prepared to provide direct care in acute care settings for patients who are acutely and critically ill and whose conditions are complex. Direct clinical practice, the central competency of ACNP practice, is the function that consumes the greatest percentage of ACNP practice time (Kleinpell-Nowell, 1999, 2001). Prior clinical nursing expertise is essential for the ACNP role, since even the novice ACNP cares for acutely and critically ill patients who may precipitously manifest life-threatening conditions that mandate an immediate response. These situations demand a strong clinical practice foundation.

The specialty practice of ACNPs consists of both short-term goals of care (stabilize patients, minimize complications, provide physical and psychological care) and long-term goals (restore maximal health potential, evaluate risk factors) (ANA and AACN-a, 1995). ACNPs achieve these specialty practice goals through the performance of cognitive skills common to all APNs, such as patient assessment, critical thinking, diagnostic reasoning, case management, and prescription of therapeutic interventions (Clochesy, Daly, Idemoto, Steel, & Fitzpatrick, 1994; Keane & Richmond, 1993; see Chapter 5). Assessing and intervening in complex, urgent, or emergency situations is a key component of ACNP specialty competencies (Kleinpell & Hravnak, 2002).

The central competencies of direct clinical practice as they apply to ACNP specialty practice can be broadly characterized as those related to (1) diagnosing and managing disease and (2) the promotion and protection of health.

ACNP CENTRAL COMPETENCY: DIRECT CLINICAL PRACTICE—DIAGNOSING AND MANAGING DISEASE

The broad subject headings for the specialty competencies that ACNPs utilize in the diagnosis and management of disease competencies (Box 14-3) include the following: demonstrates knowledge of advanced pathophysiology, completes a health history, conducts physical exams, rapidly assesses unstable and complex health problems, implements diag-

BOX 14-3 • ACNP SPECIALTY CENTRAL COMPETENCIES FOR DIRECT CLINICAL PRACTICE: DIAGNOSING AND MANAGING DISEASE

1. *Demonstrates knowledge of advanced pathophysiology in the following areas:*
   Neurology
   Cardiology
   Pulmonary
   Gastrointestinal
   Genitourinary
   Fluid balance
   Acid/base balance
2. *Completes a health history*
3. *Conducts a focused or compete physical examination*
4. *Rapidly assesses unstable and complex health problems*
5. *Demonstrates the ability to appropriately order and interpret the following:*
   Arterial blood gases
   Venous blood and serum analysis
   Cardiac enzymes
   Coagulation measures
   Liver function tests
   Urinalysis/culture
   X-rays—abdominal/chest/routine
   12-lead electrocardiogram (ECG)
   Hemodynamic monitoring parameters
   Spirometry and peak flow assessment
   Holter monitoring
   Standardized scales to measure cognitive, affective, and psychiatric symptoms
6. *Implements diagnostic strategies and therapeutic interventions to stabilize health problems*
7. *Institutes measures for health promotion and health protection*
8. *Demonstrates technical skill and knowledge of the indication/contraindication and complications associated with the following interventions:*

Cardiovascular:	Arterial puncture/cannulation/line removal
	Central venous line insertion
	Peripherally inserted central catheter (PICC)
	IABP management
	Pulmonary artery catheter: insertion/manipulation/removal/management
	Resuscitation management
	Vasoactive drugs: initiation/management
Pulmonary:	Artificial airway management
	Artificial airway—insertion/removal
	Oxygen therapy and delivery devices
	Chest tube—insertion/management/removal
	Needle thoracentesis
	Mechanical ventilation: initiation/maintenance/weaning
Neurological:	Lumbar puncture
Gastrointestinal:	Nasogastric/intestinal tube—insertion/removal
	G-tube: reinsertion/management/removal
	Paracentesis
	Enteral and parenteral nutritional support: initiation/management
Renal:	Peritoneal dialyses: management/removal of catheter
	Bladder suprapubic aspiration
Muskuloskeletal/integument:	Cutaneous suturing
	Wound management/irrigation/packing/debridement
	Apply local anesthesia
	Incision and drainage of superficial abscesses
Hematological:	Blood component therapy—initiates/manages
Infectious disease:	Perform pan cultures

Continued

BOX 14-3 • ACNP SPECIALTY CENTRAL COMPETENCIES FOR DIRECT CLINICAL PRACTICE: DIAGNOSING AND MANAGING DISEASE — cont'd

Specialty: Reduction and splinting of simple dislocations
                      Flexible sigmoidoscopy
                      Aspiration of synovial fluid
                      Bone marrow aspiration
                      Harvest saphenous vein grafts
                      Perform stress tests
                      Cricothyrotomies
                      Nerve blocks
                      Bronchoscopy
                      Diagnostic cardiac catheterization
                      First assistant at surgery
  9. *Modifies the plan of care based on a client's changing condition and response to interventions*
 10. *Collaborates with other care providers*
 11. *Discharge planning initiation*

Adapted from Shah, H., & Sullivan, D. T. (1998). Evaluation of the acute care nurse practitioner's role. In R. Kleinpell & M. Piano (Eds.), *Practice issues for the acute care nurse practitioner* (pp. 111–143). New York: Springer-Verlag; and from Kleinpell, R. M, & Hravnak, M. (2002). The acute care nurse practitioner. In M. K. Crabtree & R. Pruitt (Eds.), *Advanced nursing practice: Building curriculum for quality nurse practitioner education.* Washington, DC: National Organization of Nurse Practitioner Faculties.

nostic strategies and therapeutic interventions to stabilize health-care problems, demonstrates technical competence with procedures, modifies the plan of care based on a client's changing condition and response to interventions, and collaborates with other care providers to facilitate positive outcomes (Kleinpell & Hravnak, 2002; NONPF, 2000; Shah, Bruttomesso, Sullivan, & Lattanzio, 1997; Shah & Sullivan, 1998). In addition to these basic competencies, the varied practice settings of individual ACNPs across the continuum of acute care delivery services, and associated variance in some of the competencies that they perform, are reflected in the literature (Barkley & Rogers, 2001). Such specialty areas include, but are not limited to, acute and critical care neurology (Sarkissian & Wennberg, 1999), pulmonology (Burns, 1998), transplantation (Martin, 1999; Reel, 1999), perioperative care (Fox, Shira, & Wadlund, 2000), emergency care (Cole & Catalano, 1998), pain management services (Barkley & Whitney, 2001), and cardiac surgery (Hicks, 1998). Individual elements of the ACNP role differ depending on these varied practice settings and on the specialty patient populations served, but the basic elements necessary to function as a generalist ACNP remain. Kleinpell-Nowell (2001) reported results of a 5-year longitudinal study of 545 ACNP respondents (certified between 1996 and 1998) in the second year after certification. The results indicated that the majority of ACNPs practice in urban (47%), inner city (21%), and suburban (21%) settings, with only 11% practicing in small towns or rural settings. The majority practice in teaching hospitals (45%) or with physician groups (25%), whereas fewer practice in community or general acute care hospitals (9%) or clinics (3%). Respondents to the survey indicated that, in addition to their principal role responsibility of direct patient care, a number of them were also involved in teaching (65%), research (38%), department projects (34%), program development (30%), administrative responsibilities (31%), and quality assurance projects (29%). Rosenfeld, McEvoy, & Glassman (2003) corroborate Kleinpell-Nowell's finding that although ACNPs assume responsibilities beyond their predominant activity of direct patient care, the amount of time spent in other activities is much less. They surveyed 61 ACNPs practicing in two urban teaching hospitals and found that ACNPs spent the majority (55%) of their time in direct care activities (most notably patient examination and assessment; development, implementation, and evaluation of a treatment plan; and performing procedures), a lesser amount of time (31%) on indirect activities (predominantly consultation and collaboration, including rounds, and discharge planning), and only 14% of their time in education, research, and administrative activities.

The performance of patient procedures, which is at times invasive, also constitutes a portion of ACNP's direct clinical practice. Technical procedures most commonly performed by respondents to Kleinpell-Nowell's survey (2001) as well as 750 ACNPs certified from 1998 to 2000 (Kleinpell & Hravnak, 2002) are listed in the composite survey results in Table 14-1. The literature corroborates ACNP technical skill performance, such as endotracheal intubation, central line placement, pulmonary artery line placement, needle thoracotomies, chest tube insertion and removal, and cricothyrotomies for the trauma critical care focus (Keough, Jennrich, Holm, & Marshall, 1996); nerve blocks, joint needle aspiration, diagnostic peritoneal lavage, needle decompression of the chest, lumbar puncture, chest tube insertion, cricothyrotomy and tracheostomy, suturing of lacerations and wounds and splinting of injuries for the emergency care focus (Cole & Ramirez, 1997, 2000); endotracheal and nasotracheal intubation, chest tube insertion and removal, arterial puncture, and insertion of central lines for the critical care focus (Hravnak et al., 1995; Watts, 1997; Watts, Hanson, Burke, Gallagher, & Foster, 1996). An imperative understanding is that procedural skill performance is not limited to the task itself but includes knowledge of the indications, contraindications, complications, and skill in managing complications. When performing a procedural skill to derive physiological data, such as mean arterial pressure, pulmonary artery pressures, or lumbar cerebrospinal fluid pressure, the ACNP must be able to utilize this information skillfully for patient evaluation. ACNPs are also compelled to collect their individual practice data related to procedure performance, including number and type of complications, and utilize these data to document ongoing skill competence and facilitate patient safety.

CENTRAL COMPETENCY: DIRECT CLINICAL PRACTICE—PROMOTING AND PROTECTING HEALTH AND PREVENTING DISEASE

In addition to disease diagnosis and management, ACNPs also provide services to promote and protect health and prevent disease. These services include providing anticipatory guidance and counseling to patients and their families. Inevitably, some of the methods ACNPs use to implement health promotion/protection and disease prevention vary from those used by NPs in the primary care specialties. These variations in application are related to the prioritization of needs during acute and critical illness, and in some practice models, the episodic nature of the relationship between the ACNP and the patient/family is limited to a single acute illness event.

However, ACNPs are skilled in a unique form of health promotion/protection and disease prevention: recognizing and modifying health risk factors associated with an inpatient stay. These risks are inherent to patients experiencing an acute and critical illness requiring hospitalization, and the systems and structures of "institutionalized" care (Hravnak, 1998). The ACNP is qualified to identify the additional health problems for which the acutely and critically ill are at risk and to implement strategies to minimize or prevent that risk. This area forms a distinctive health promotion and health protection aspect of ACNP practice. As direct care providers, ACNPs have extensive and continuous knowledge of patients and their changing conditions. They also have the ability to activate strategies and systems to implement primary, secondary, or tertiary prevention initiatives related to these unique risk factors.

TABLE 14-1 SURVEY RESULTS FROM 1295 ACUTE CARE NURSE PRACTITIONERS REPORTING TASKS PERFORMED* (PERCENT ACNP RESPONDENTS PERFORMING PROCEDURE)

DIRECT PATIENT CARE

Task	%
Discuss care with family	95%
Order/interpret laboratory tests	90%
Initiate discharge planning	88%
Perform cultures	85%
Place nasogastric feeding tubes	84%
Initiate/adjust intravenous lines	82%
Interpret 12-lead electrocardiogram	81%
Interpret x-rays	81%
Initiate specialty consultation	79%
Examine/clean wounds	77%
Adjust nutritional support	65%
Perform defibrillation	64%
Institute blood replacement therapies	60%
Perform wound packing	60%
Apply local anesthesia	58%
Perform wound debridement	57%
Initiate vasoactive drug infusions	54%
Manage resuscitation	52%
Manage patients receiving mechanical ventilation	49%
Suture superficial lacerations	48%
Initiate/adjust intravenous therapy	43%
Perform cardioversion	42%
Perform incision/drainage	40%
Adjust temporary pacemakers	37%
Manipulate pulmonary artery catheter	33%
Insert arterial catheters	32%
Insert central venous catheters peripherally	29%
Remove intracardiac catheters	29%
Insert central venous catheters from a central site	18%
Adjust cardiac assist device	17%
Perform lumbar punctures	16%
Insert pulmonary artery catheters	16%
Perform endotracheal intubation	15%
Perform needle thoracentesis	11%
Insert chest tube	9%
Perform research	6%
Intra-aortic balloon pump removal	6%
Apply cast/mold brace	5%
Remove pacemaker wires	5%
Assist in operating room	5%
Perform paracentesis	5%
Pull arterial sheaths	3%
Perform bone marrow aspiration	3%
Shunt taps	3%
Harvest saphenous vein grafts	3%
Initiate thrombolytic therapy	3%
Perform stress tests	3%

INDIRECT PATIENT CARE

Task	%
Give nursing service	78%
Initiate QA/QI study	53%
Case manage inpatients	24%
Perform research	6%

*As reported by 545 ACNPs certified from 1996 to 1998, participating in a 5-year longitudinal survey of ACNPs and by 750 ACNPs certified from 1998 to 2000, surveyed in November 2000: data from Kleinpell-Nowell, R. (1999). Longitudinal survey of acute care nurse practitioners: Year 1. *AACN Clinical Issues, 10*, 515-520; 2000 study data from: Kleinpell, R. M. & Hravnak, M. (2002). The acute care nurse practitioner. In M. K. Crabtree & R. Pruitt (Eds.), *Advanced nursing practice: Building curriculum for quality nurse practitioner education.* Washington, DC: National Organization of Nurse Practitioner Faculties.

Some of the risk factors imposed by an inpatient stay are physiological in nature, including immobility, decreased nutritional intake, fluid and electrolyte imbalance, altered immunocompetence, impairment of self-care ability, existing or developing co-morbid disease states, and risk associated with invasive diagnostic and therapeutic interventions. Other risks have a psychological foundation: These include the psychological consequences of alterations in the patient's physical abilities and alteration of his or her environment, sleep deprivation, communication impairment, alteration of self-image, role reversal, financial challenges, knowledge deficits, and the consequences of medication administration, including but not limited to delirium and depression. Families are also influenced by many of these risks and require ANCP services. Additionally, risk factors related to hospitalization itself and the multiplicity of caregivers include the following: discontinuity of care, polypharmacy, system inefficiency and redundancy, miscommunication with families, and miscommunication among caregivers (Hravnak, 1998). The ACNP is competent to assess patients for these unique risks and implement interventions to prevent their occurrence or minimize their consequences.

ACNP SPECIALTY CORE COMPETENCIES

The ACNP also performs the APN core competencies described in Chapter 3, with specialization unique to her or his role. Providing expert guidance and teaching of patients, families, and other health-care providers is a core competency that is an essential part of ACNP care. In the primary care area, the plan of care may be mutually determined and fully implemented between the NP and patient/family dyad. In contrast, the process of assessment and diagnosis, care planning, implementation and evaluation in the acute care setting, while still centering on the ACNP and patient/family dyad, will likely include a number of other individuals, including but not limited to physicians, other nurses, respiratory therapists, dieticians, pharmacists, physical and occupational therapists, social workers, and clergy. In this complex setting the ACNP's ability to plan, interpret, and explain the plan of care while educating others about disease processes is a valued aspect of the ACNP role. Often, critical illness can require many complex treatments, and ACNPs are able to provide teaching to families, nursing staff, and other members of the health-care team to facilitate knowledge of indicated care. The core competency of coaching and teaching is played out at the highest levels when ACNPs prepare patients for discharge after serious illness or when they assist and prepare family members to care for loved ones who have undergone catastrophic or debilitating health problems (Rhodes & Carlson, 2001). At times, patients (particularly the poor and uninsured) may not have a consistent primary care provider in the outpatient setting. In this case, the ACNP becomes an important source for health information and health promotion/protection interventions during the inpatient encounter. Some patients may be more receptive to health teaching that occurs in close proximity to an acute health event (such as diet and exercise information after an acute myocardial infarction). ACNPs also provide coaching for both experienced and inexperienced nurses in complex care settings.

ACNPs often provide consultation; utilize, promote, and conduct research; and provide clinical and professional leadership. These core competencies represent additional components of the APN role. ACNPs may find that their involvement with these particular competencies fluctuates as a result of the focus of an individual ACNP role. The consultative activities of the ACNP may take the form of a formal medical consultation. Sometimes consultative services by the ACNP are delivered in more informal exchanges regarding the patient's condition and plan of care with other health-care providers. This aspect of the ACNP's practice is invaluable in the teaching hospital setting. In this environment, attending physicians and medical trainees rotate on and off the service, and staffing patterns may result in inconsistencies in the bedside nursing caregiver. As the consistent member of the health-care provider team, the ACNP is able to utilize consultative skills to keep the team informed of the patient's condition and changing plan of care across the entire length of stay. Research competencies may also vary among ACNP providers. All ACNPs utilize research to deliver evidence-based medical and nursing care, whereas a smaller number of ACNPs may actively participate in or lead research initiatives.

All ACNPs provide some form of professional and clinical leadership in their provider role; as mentors and role models for staff nurses; by providing administrative responsibilities in the health-care agency; and by acting as care facilitators and change agents within the health-care system. ACNPs act to coordinate care delivery in the health-care system, and several studies have demonstrated that this aspect of ACNP practice reduces inpatient length of stay (Burns & Earven, 2002; Russell et al., 2002). Acting as a change agent to promote a positive healing environment and espousing assertiveness and conflict negotiation skills are beneficial qualities for ACNPs. ACNPs also work to facilitate both individual practice and health-care system change through their participation in quality assurance or continuous quality improvement (CQI) initiatives (Rundio, 2001a; Stetler, Effken, Frigon, Tiernan, & Zwingman-Bagley, 1998). Participating in the planning and implementation of system-wide cost-containing or cost-effectiveness initiatives is also an aspect of the ACNP role. The range of opportunities to create system change in the ACNP role is infinite. With their other APN colleagues, all ACNPs bear responsibility for providing leadership to advance health-care policy that affects not only their practice but also the quality of care for patients and families in the acute and critical care environment (Riley-Bryan & Barkley, 2001).

Collaboration is one of the most frequently practiced core competencies of ACNPs. Collaborative practice in the clinical setting means "cooperatively working together, sharing responsibility for solving problems and making decisions to formulate and carry out plans for patient care" (Baggs & Schmitt, 1988, p. 145; see also Chapter 10). In the acute care setting, patient care delivery is always a collaborative effort of the multiple members of the multidisciplinary health-care team. Therefore the ability to collaborate successfully is one of the critical components of the ACNP role.

In a collaborative practice model, the emphasis is on patient outcomes. Each professional should be responsible for providing the care for which she or he is best prepared. A collaborative practice model in acute care focuses on the idea that each patient needs the services of different types of providers simultaneously (King & Baggs, 1998). It has been suggested that the dyad of APN and physician forms the core of collaborative practice in acute care (Buchanan, 1996; King & Baggs, 1998; Martin & Coniglio, 1996; Norsen Opladen, & Quinn, 1995; Shapiro & Rosenberg, 2002). The advantage to this model is the ongoing continuity and coordination of care (Norsen et al., 1995). To formulate a collaborative dyad between the ACNP and physician, each partner must achieve full professional status. This means that each partner has completed basic and postgraduate education, which, in turn, allows him or her to take advantage of and use the full scope of practice of each of the partners. In turn, this assumption refutes the resident replacement model that has been put forth by some as a role for APNs (King & Baggs, 1998).

Although there has been much support for collaborative practice between nurses and physicians, barriers still exist. Unfortunately, these barriers are created between those for whom collaborative practice should be the focus—other nurses and physicians. Incomplete understanding of the ACNP role may lead to concern among both physicians and nurses that, perhaps, ACNPs are inappropriately adopting or selling out to the medical model and trying to practice like "mini-doctors" (King & Baggs, 1998). However, there is growing recognition that the ACNP role promotes a collaborative model of care (Kleinpell, 1999; Kleinpell & Hravnak, 2002).

The final core competency comprises ethical decision making. ACNPs often find themselves acting as advocates for patients in care dilemmas. The age of the patient population (Miller, 2001), the routine application of life-sustaining interventions (Penas & Barkley, 2001), aggressive resuscitation, and a patient population that often includes victims of violence or abuse (Greenberg, 1996) frequently place ACNPs and their patients in ethical emergencies. Because ACNPs are often involved in planning and implementing end-of-life care, ethical decision-making skills are an essential component of ACNP practice (Rundio, 2001a). In helping to facilitate ethical decision making, ACNPs can be instrumental in resolving moral issues (see Chapter 11).

The APN core competencies form the essential elements of the ACNP specialist's role. In addition, ACNP specialty competencies that are being developed outline the knowledge base and scope of practice of the ACNP and the unique aspects of ACNP practice.

PROFILE OF THE ACNP ROLE

The majority of ACNPs practice in acute and critical care settings and in ever-expanding specialty-area practice sites (Kleinpell, 1998; Kleinpell-Nowell, 2001). ACNPs have transitioned into a variety of role implementation models. One ACNP role implementation model focuses on episodic management of patients in a single clinical specialty unit, one model involves following a caseload of hospitalized patients throughout their hospitalization, and another focuses on managing patients across the entire continuum of acute care services, from hospitalization to home.

The ACNP model focusing on episodic care of patients on a particular clinical inpatient unit provides the earliest model of ACNP practice (Kleinpell, 1998; Lott et al., 1996). Under this model the ACNP, in collaboration with an intensivist, might manage the care of a patient admitted to an intensive care unit with an acutely unstable medical or surgical condition. Once the patient is stabilized, the patient is transferred to another clinical unit under the care of another provider. ACNP roles such as these have been described in a variety of specialty clinical units. Under this model, confining their practice to episodic care at a defined level of acute care allows ACNPs the opportunity to develop their skill and knowledge about specific conditions in a delineated setting. However, the limitation of this model is that it does not allow for continuity of care across the continuum.

In another model of role implementation, the ACNP directly manages the care of a caseload of patients throughout their entire hospitalization, providing individualized ongoing care with continuity to the patient and family (Cintron, Bigas, Linates, Aranda, & Hernandez, 1983; Dahle, Smith, Ingersoll, & Wilson, 1998). The goal of this model is to facilitate and coordinate a patient's hospital stay in order to provide high-quality and cost-effective care (Clochesy et al., 1994). In this model the ACNP will, in collaboration with a physician, admit the patient to the hospital, complete the admission history and physical examination, assess the patient's initial clinical status, order and interpret diagnostic and therapeutic tests, perform procedures, evaluate and adjust the plan of care, and prepare the patient for discharge. In this model the ACNP will provide care continuously for patients as they move from high-acuity to lower-acuity inpatient care units, facilitate patients' movement through the health-care system, and plan for and implement discharge.

In another model of care, the ACNP delivers comprehensive specialty care to a group of patients across the entire continuum of care services. For example, an ACNP member of a heart failure care team may oversee patient management during hospitalization, provide postdischarge clinic follow-up, and ultimately manage home-based infusion therapy. With the growth of specialty-based practice, the number of ACNPs working in this type of model of care is increasing.

Although ACNPs might require some variation in skill sets depending on the model within which their role is implemented, there are strong commonalties that exist. As with other APN roles, all ACNPs are proficient in advanced physical assessment, clinical decision making (diagnostic reasoning), ordering and interpreting laboratory studies and procedures, and collaborating in the development and implementation of a treatment plan that includes prescribing medication. Diagnostic reasoning and advanced therapeutic interventions, consultation, and referral to other physicians, nurses, and providers are intrinsic components of this role as described by the ANA and AACN-a (1995). The ACNP role is one of evidenced-based practice as it relates to the basic sciences. Specifically, ACNPs should be able to demonstrate knowledge of pathophysiology for their decision making when ordering and interpreting diagnostic tests and in making treatment decisions.

The ACNP diagnoses the origin of a complex medical problem that develops in an acutely or critically ill patient utilizing diagnostic reasoning (see Chapter 5). The skills inherent in effective diagnostic reasoning include the fundamental skills of the ACNP role: history taking, physical examination skills, pattern recognition, the ability to analyze and synthesize data, and the ability to generate a working diagnosis. Failure to diagnose because of a lack of understanding of the disease process can lead to progression of the primary disease condition and the development of complications, or both. Incorrect diagnosis may lead to inappropriate or suboptimal therapy or unnecessary toxicity secondary to the side effects of treatment (Kassirer, 1989; Szaflarski, 1997). A number of factors affect the quality of diagnostic reasoning when applied to the acutely ill (Box 14-4), and add complexity to the diagnostic process. All of these factors challenge the ACNP's ability to accurately and expeditiously diagnose an acutely or critically ill patient's ever-changing physical condition.

Another inherent portion of the ACNP practice profile is the performance of technical skills, as indicated in the earlier discussion of ACNP Central Competencies for Direct Clinical Practice. The patient needs within a specialty practice ultimately influence the

---

BOX 14-4 • FACTORS AFFECTING QUALITY OF DIAGNOSTIC REASONING IN ACUTE CARE

PATIENT FACTORS
- Increasing level of patient acuity
- Multisystem disease
- Poor historians
- Altered mental status
- Unavailability of significant others

CLINICIAN FACTORS
- Clinical experience
- Knowledge of disease
- Knowledge of complex diagnostic technologies
- Incomplete history database as a result of unavailable medical records or diagnostic tests results
- Increasing workload
- Demands for cost-effective diagnostic evaluation

Adapted from Szaflarski, N. L. (1997). Diagnostic reasoning in acute and critical care. *AACN Clinical Issues, 8,* 291-302.

type and level of therapeutic and diagnostic psychomotor skills that an individual ACNP performs (Kleinpell & Hravnak, 2002).

Differences and Commonalties with Other APN Roles and Physician Assistant Role

The ACNP role differs from other APNs with regard to the type of patient care problems encountered, the acuity of the patient's condition, the need for rapid and continuous assessment, planning and intervention, and the setting in which the care is delivered (Lott et al., 1996). For example, the clinical nurse specialist (CNS) enacts the APN role through three spheres of influence: at the patient level, in direct care; at the nurse level, as with staff development; and at the institutional level, providing oversight for care. In comparison, the ACNP utilizes clinical assessment skills to assess complex and acutely ill patients through health history taking, physical and mental status examination, performing procedures, and risk appraisal for complications. Both the ACNP and CNS roles are targeted to a patient-centered approach to care, but the continuous on-unit presence of the ACNP at the bedside of patients often differentiates the role of the ACNP from the CNS role. CNSs have responsibilities for staff education and system change that consume a larger percentage of their roles than do ACNPs. Conversely, CNSs are generally not involved in carrying out many of the procedures and interventions that characterize the ACNP role. Institutional variations in role implementation for CNSs and ACNPs sometime lack clear-cut differentiation in role responsibilities (Lott et al., 1996). Yet, it is acknowledged that the CNS and NP roles are distinct, with distinct practice foci (Mick & Ackerman, 2002).

Table 14-2 can assist the reader in conceptualizing where the main focus of ACNP practice falls within the health-care continuum and where there might be differences or overlap with the primary care NP role. Within the table are examples of management strategies for common patient health-care problems encountered in the traditional primary, secondary, and tertiary health-care settings (Hravnak et al., 1995; Kleinpell & Hravnak, 2002). With diabetes care, for example, ACNP practice predominantly involves strategies directed toward management of the patient during an acute exacerbation of his or her diabetes (e.g., diabetic ketoacidosis). Because of the severity of symptoms, the patient must be admitted to the hospital, where he or she can be continuously monitored and where management strategies may change from hour to hour (tertiary care). During this same hospitalization the patient may need to have an infected foot ulcer treated with intravenous antibiotics (secondary care). Once the crisis is over, the ACNP may provide teaching on routine foot care (primary care), as well as diabetic diet and glucose monitoring. At this point the patient may be referred back to his or her primary care provider for further follow-up and management. In comparison, the primary care NP's practice predominantly involves strategies directed toward management of the patient's diabetes when it is stable (primary care). This would include ongoing surveillance of the patient's self-management of his or her diabetes along with education on diabetic risk factors and assessment of signs of disease progression and complications. The primary care NP may also assess when the patient's diabetes is not well controlled and requires adjustment of insulin or oral hypoglycemic agents (secondary care). At the point when the patient is not responding or becomes acutely ill, the primary care NP will recognize the need for the patient to be referred to a setting where continuous monitoring and management is provided (tertiary care). Using this example helps educators and clinicians understand that there is a natural overlap in some areas of knowledge and practice between acute care and primary care NPs. However, each NP specialty also has its own distinct focus. The knowledge base and practice of the ACNP cannot be limited to only unstable conditions requiring complex technological diagnostic and management strategies. Rather, ACNPs must be prepared to manage all the health-care problems of patients under their care. This includes not only the acute illness or exacerbation of chronic illness that requires acute care services but also the patient's co-morbidities. For example, the hospitalized diabetic patient previously discussed may also have stable hypertension, stable asthma, osteoarthritis, and an episode of vaginitis. The ACNP must simultaneously manage the stable co-morbid health conditions of the hospitalized patient to maintain quiescence. The stable co-morbidities may be managed with traditional primary care approaches applied in the hospital setting, whereas management of the exacerbating or acute illness requires the application of secondary and tertiary care interventions. Thus the scope of the ACNP's practice must include knowledge of health-care problems and interventions that span the entire health-care delivery continuum.

APNs, including ACNPs, are different from physician assistants (PAs). The PA role is under the jurisdiction of physician licensure, which is supervisory rather than collaborative and does not allow for independent functions. Although some of the care provided by PAs is similar to that provided by ACNPs, there are differences in philosophy, education, scope of practice, and patient approach between the APN and the PA (Daffurn, 1998; Lott et al., 1996; Mittman, Cawley, & Fenn, 2002). Although there is some overlap between the ACNP and PA in the central competency of direct clinical practice in terms

---

TABLE 14-2 PATIENT CARE PROBLEMS AND MANAGEMENT INTERVENTIONS TRADITIONALLY ASSOCIATED WITH HEALTH-CARE DELIVERY SETTINGS

DELIVERY SETTING	HEALTH PROBLEM AND INTERVENTIONS		
	DIABETES	HYPERTENSION	PNEUMONIA
Tertiary care management (ICU setting)	Diabetic ketoacidosis management Fluid replacement Electrolyte titration IV insulin	Continuous vasoactive drugs Arterial pressure monitoring Evaluation/management of possible CVA	Mechanical ventilation and artificial airway Pulmonary toilet Culture assessment Sepsis management Continuous monitoring
Secondary care management (in-patient ward)	Diabetic exacerbation management Sliding scale insulin administration and monitoring Hydration Etiology workup	Hypertensive crisis management Additional antihypertensives Adjunct therapy as needed	IV Antibiotics Oxygen therapy Advanced assessment CXR, arterial blood gases, SpO_2
Primary care management (outpatient setting)	Initial Dx or stable management Oral antihyperglycemics or subcutaneous insulin Diet Prevention/assessment associated complications Foot care Risk factor management	Diet Oral agents Lifestyle changes Prevention/assessment associated complications Risk factor management	Oral or intramuscular antibiotics

CVA, Cerebrovascular accident; *CXR,* chest x-ray; *Dx,* diagnosis; *ICU,* intensive care unit; *SpO$_2$,* peripheral arterial oxygen saturation.
Adapted from Hravnak, M., Kobert, S. N., Risco, K. G., Baldisseri, M., Hoffman, L. A., Clochesy, et al. (1995). Acute care nurse practitioner curriculum: Content and development process. *American Journal of Critical Care 4,* 179-188.

of the management of disease, the ACNP's direct clinical practice competencies also provide for the promotion and protection of health. A further differentiation is that ACNP practice also incorporates additional APN core competencies.

ACNP Collaboration with Physician Hospitalists

The hospitalist is a physician specialist in inpatient medicine who is responsible for managing the care of hospitalized patients in the same manner that a primary care physician is responsible for managing her or his outpatients. Physicians first described this emerging role in 1996 as a consequence of the explosive growth of the primary care and internist role secondary to managed care. Hospitalist specialists have a central role in hospitals in Great Britain and Canada, but until recently such a specialist has been a scarce commodity in the United States (Wachter, 1999; Wachter & Goldman, 1996). However, this physician role is now being incorporated in academic teaching centers and community settings. The physician hospitalist role has been based in internal medicine, and the ACNP recently has been added as a member of this health-care team. A primary care physician refers the patient to the hospitalist team for management during the acute care admission. This team provides care for the patient during hospitalization and refers the patient back to the primary care provider at the time of discharge. The goal of this service is to provide seamless, cost-effective care. This can be an advantage for a primary care physician with busy office hours who may have limited time to make hospital visits and may not be sufficiently familiar with acute care management. The specific role of the ACNP, as a member of the hospitalist team, is similar to the roles previously described, including obtaining an admission history and physical exam, performing daily physical exams, rounds with the physician, developing a treatment plan, reviewing laboratory studies and x-rays, and performing procedures. Furthermore, coordinating patient care management when many consultants are involved in decision making is a significant part of the role, as is consultation with the case managers to effectively facilitate discharge planning (Wachter & Goldman, 1996).

Outcome Studies Related to ACNP Practice

Measuring outcomes of practice (see Chapters 1 and 25) is an acknowledged component of establishing the value of any APN role (Kleinpell & Weiner, 1999). Most of the studies assessing outcomes of ACNP practice have only been published in the last several years. Positive outcomes of ACNP care have been demonstrated in subacute transitional and rehabilitation care (von Sternberg et al., 1997; Weinberg, Liljestrand, & Moore, 1983), emergency care (Buchanan & Powers, 1997; Cole & Catalano, 1998; Cooper, Lindsey, Kinn, & Swann, 2002; Rhee & Dermyer, 1995), surgical services (Hylka & Beschle, 1995), inpatient medical services (Genet et al., 1995; Howie & Erickson, 2002), cardiovascular care (Dahle et al., 1998; Gawlinski, McCloy, & Jesurum 2001; Paul, 2000), neuroscience care (Russell et al., 2002), respiratory care (Burns & Earven, 2002; Hoffman et al., 2002), gerontology care (Miller, 1997), epilepsy care (Sarkissian & Wennberg, 1999), perioperative care (Hylka & Beschle, 1995), trauma services (Spisso, O'Callaghan, McKennan, & Holcroft, 1990), and intensive care (Hoffman et al., 2003; Scharfenberg et al., 2003). These studies have demonstrated a positive impact of ACNP care, including decreased costs, decreased hospital length of stay, decreased use of laboratory tests, lower rates of urinary tract infections and skin breakdown, time savings for house physicians, similar care outcomes compared with those in physician practice, patient and family satisfaction, and an increased role in discussing patient outcomes with nurses and families, among others.

While these studies exploring ACNP effectiveness have been conducted in several types of care settings, continued research on the impact of ACNP practice is needed to establish more fully the outcomes of the ACNP role (Kleinpell, 2001; Kleinpell, 2002). In reviewing ACNP research, Piano and Zerwic-Johnson (1998) concluded that methodological flaws, including lack of randomization and appropriate control of comparison groups and insufficient sample size, limit the interpretations of some studies (Piano & Zerwic-Johnson, 1998). The majority of the studies on utilization and outcomes of ACNPs have focused on comparing ACNP care to physician care, reducing costs, or discussing the impact of ACNP care on a focused area of care. No study has fully evaluated the impact of ACNPs; it would be useful to study a variety of outcomes associated with patient care managed by ACNPs (Howie & Erickson, 2002). If ACNPs are to delineate the impact of their care and justify their existence, it is imperative that their worth be supported by careful research (see Chapter 25).

ACNP ROLE IMPLEMENTATION EXAMPLES

The following practice Exemplar 14-1 describes the ACNP practicing in a cardiothoracic intensive care unit. Additional vignettes illustrate the ACNP in other role implementation models.

 EXEMPLAR 14-1

In the cardiothoracic intensive care unit (CTICU), an ACNP named Marie functions collaboratively with the critical care provider team consisting of the ACNP, an attending physician (intensivist), one or two critical care medicine fellows, and other members of the delivery team including bedside nurses and respiratory therapists. The team works in collaboration with the surgeons, surgical fellows and residents on the cardiac, thoracic, transplant, vascular, and trauma services.

The day begins with a report from the team members providing care during the previous night, highlighting changes in patient condition and providing information on new patients. Next, Marie participates in dynamic patient-focused rounds during which each patient is examined at the bedside and interviewed when possible. A wealth of other data is reviewed, including vital signs, hemodynamic data (pulmonary artery pressures, CVP, cardiac outputs), ventilator settings, and results of previous weaning trials, chest radiographs and diagnostic testing, laboratory and culture data, and a complete list of medications, continuous infusions, and fluid balances. Based on the clinical exam and review of data, and with input from members of the provider and delivery team, a comprehensive plan of care is devised for the patient. Marie assumes varying roles during these patient-focused rounds (e.g., presenting and reviewing data, doing the physical exam, writing orders, calling consultants). During this time, Marie is making note of issues to be addressed later, treatment outcomes to follow up, planned procedures, culture and diagnostic test results to review, family conferences, and expected admissions and discharges. Once rounds are complete, Marie will begin to address some of the specific issues on her work list.

Marie begins by seeing the four patients who are to be transferred out of the ICU that morning. She briefly examines each patient and reviews their data to ensure that the patient's responses to interventions are appropriate. She verifies that these patients have been weaned from their vasoactive medicines and removes their chest tubes. Marie reviews each patient's H & P and restarts home medications that are appropriate to the patient's cardiac conditions and co-morbidities as needed. She writes transfer orders and collaborates with the bedside nurse to ensure that all patient care issues have been addressed in the orders. One patient has a history of active smoking, and Marie discusses with the patient the relationship between smoking and heart disease, as well as smoking cessation strategies. One patient needs to maintain a central intravenous access on the hospital ward. Marie converts the 14-gauge introducer in the patient's right internal jugular vein to a triple lumen catheter utilizing re-wire technique. One patient has developed an arrhythmia with some hemodynamic instability, and Marie initiates appropriate treatment, cancels the patient's transfer to the floor, and informs the intensivist of the change in condition. One patient is being transferred to a subacute-care facility. Marie collaborates with the unit case manager to finalize transfer plans, speaks with the patient's family prior to discharge, and speaks with the receiving team in the subacute-care facility to ensure continuity of care.

During the course of the day Marie might perform other invasive procedures, such as inserting arterial lines, central venous lines, dialysis catheters, chest tubes, and nasoduodenal feeding tubes and performing thoracentesis, endotracheal intubation, and removal of intra-aortic balloons.

Marie will continuously monitor the patients on the unit throughout the day and provide problem-focused care in response to changing patient needs and condition. She will be contacted by the nurse providing bedside care for the patient to address patient problems such as hypotension, hypertension, low cardiac output, low urine output, bleeding, low oxygen saturations, fever, difficulty with ventilation or ventilator changes, agitation and delirium, mental status changes, inadequate pain management, arrhythmia, electrolyte abnormalities, and problems with lines or catheters. She will see patients multiple times throughout the day in response to these concerns, each time assessing possible causes, performing directed physical exams, formulating a treatment plan, and reassessing clinical findings to evaluate response to therapy. Some treatments Marie initiates independently, whereas other more complex situations may require her to consult with the intensivist and/or surgeon to review the management options. Marie will provide consultative services to the cardiologists, who visit their patients daily.

During the day, Marie participates in the care of patients newly admitted following surgery as well. As patients arrive from the operating room, Marie receives a brief report from the anesthesiologist and surgical fellow. She reviews the chart, examines the patient, and reviews initial laboratory results, electocardiograph results, and chest radiograph results. She reviews the plan of care with the critical care nurse and respiratory therapist. She documents a progress note and writes orders, then returns frequently to reassess the patient's status and make adjustments to the plan. One postoperative patient is bleeding severely. Marie alerts the surgeon, orders and reviews a mini-coagulation screen, and ensures that the patient is being rewarmed. She orders blood products to correct the abnormality and monitors the patient to determine whether this therapy is effective or whether the patient will have to return to the operating room for mediastinal exploration.

At the end of the day, the team rounds again, seeing the new patients, evaluating the progress of and plans for other patients, and developing a plan for the next 12-hour period. The dynamic environment of the ICU and the ICU care team members requires the ACNP to frequently assess and reassess patient condition, remain flexible and responsive to subtle changes and carefully organize and manage time.

As a permanent member of the critical care team, Marie provides needed continuity to care. She is available to interact with social service, case managers, physical and occupational therapists, and nutritional consultants. She is able to participate in discharge planning. She is readily available to the nursing staff for questions or problem-solving. She participates in the CTICU's CQI activities. She participates in research protocols, screens patients for eligibility criteria, and educates others concerning the research initiatives. The ACNP plays an important role in communication with patients and families, and has a unique opportunity for teaching and reinforcing teaching.

As the CTICU ACNP, Marie manages the patient from admission to discharge from the unit. Health promotion and protection assessment and intervention are integral, but in different areas than one might expect in the primary care setting. For example, in the CTICU, Marie addresses stress ulcer prophylaxis, preventing complications from immobility, promoting skin integrity, and nutritional support.

ACNP, Acute care nurse practitioner; *CQI*, continuous quality improvement; *CVP*, central venous pressure; *H & P*, history and physical examination; *ICU*, intensive care unit.

Role Vignettes in Other Clinical Practice Settings

In addition to the exemplar of the unit-based ACNP role presented here, the following vignettes illustrate ACNP role implementation as part of global specialty clinical services and across the spectrum of acute care services.

SPECIALTY CLINICAL SERVICES

The ACNP might participate as a member of a specific clinical specialty or consult service practicing within an acute care setting. Examples might include an ACNP working as part of an internal medicine team, trauma service, surgical service, acute stroke team, renal medicine team, pulmonary medicine service, electrophysiology service, interventional cardiology service, preadmission surgical service, and oncology service.

Bone Marrow Transplantation Services. The ACNP working as a member of the bone marrow transplantation service has an autonomous role while functioning as a part of a collaborative practice model; the team is composed of a resident, a fellow, an attending physician, and the ACNP. The ACNP provides the continuity of care for the service by being the only consistent member of the academic health-care team where physicians rotate between clinical and research activities. The ACNP carries a caseload of patients and follows them through their hospital stay until discharge. Role responsibilities include preliminary rounding daily on each patient, performing physical examinations, interpreting laboratory tests (electrolytes and x-rays), performing marrow aspirations, and consulting specialists (e.g., in gastroenterology, infectious disease, pulmonary medicine) to assist in patient management. On the basis of the information gathered, the ACNP collaborates with the other provider team members during daily rounds to develop the daily and long-term treatment plan. In addition, the ACNP provides teaching to the house staff and nursing staff and incorporates health teaching and health promotion/protection (especially risk associated with immunosuppression) activities into her or his practice.

Diagnostic and Interventional Services. In preadmission surgical services, the major clinical functions of an ACNP include history taking and physical examinations; performing pre-procedure evaluations; providing patient and family education; obtaining and interpreting laboratory, electrocardiographical, and radiological data; identifying at-risk individuals in need of preadmission discharge planning; initiating contacts with social services; and discharge planning and making management recommendations for patients in the surgical holding area. The ACNP consults with the anesthesiologist and surgeon regarding patient health problems that may affect or preclude anesthesia delivery of surgery. ACNPs may provide services similar to these in the cardiac catheterization suite or the gastrointestinal procedure lab.

ACROSS A SPECTRUM OF CLINICAL SETTINGS

Alternatively, an ACNP may function as part of a team that provides care in continuity across a spectrum of clinical encounters or settings.

Heart Failure Services. In this example, a team of three ACNPs on the heart failure service in a university medical center collaborate with each other and with the physician provider team members to provide care for their patients in order to optimize continuity of care. Each ACNP has a caseload of patients for whom she or he assumes responsibility in the outpatient area. They see each patient in clinic on a regular basis, examine patients, and make adjustments to the treatment plan. They perform follow-up by phone contact on a weekly basis, helping patients to assess their symptoms, follow daily weights, discuss dietary changes, and adjust oral mediations as needed. Based on this discussion, the ACNP may have the patient come in to the outpatient clinic for further clinical assessment and treatment (e.g., a dose of intravenous diuretic, adjustment of continuous inotropic medication infusions). When a patient requires admission to the hospital for an acute exacerbation of heart failure, one ACNP (each ACNP team member provides in-hospital coverage on a weekly rotating basis) along with the physician manage the patient in the hospital setting. They are familiar with the patient's problems and treatment plan, can provide continuity, have established a trusting relationship with the patient and the care delivery team, and can readily facilitate discharge planning and follow-up when the patient is ready for discharge to home.

Orthopedic Services. The role of the ACNP working with patients with orthopedic problems has been reported to include responsibilities shared among several team members. This team provides coverage for the emergency room, orthopedic clinic, and the orthopedic service. The orthopedic ACNP works closely with the attending physicians, staff nurses, and residents to coordinate care from preadmission testing to discharge. Each of the ACNPs carries a caseload of hospitalized patients and outpatients undergoing short procedures. This role may include perioperative management as first assistant in the operating room (Gates, 1993).

EDUCATIONAL PREPARATION OF THE ACNP

Both patient safety and professional integrity demand that the ACNP be well prepared to function competently and efficiently in managing the illness and promoting the health of acutely and critically ill adults. ACNPs are registered nurses who are prepared at the master's level of graduate nursing education.

The majority of ACNP educational programs require prior clinical nursing experience, although these requirements vary widely between programs (Kleinpell & Hravnak, 2002). The expertise needed to provide care to this complex and vulnerable patient population relies heavily on critical thinking skills and the ability to assess and manage rapidly changing situations, attributes that are generally associated with the expert rather than the novice nurse. With this in mind, some practicing ACNP clinicians have, based on their own experiences, recommended that program applicants have 3 to 5 or more years of clinical nursing experience in acute care before entering the ACNP program (Kleinpell-Nowell 2001).

The ACNP curriculum is based on four components: the graduate core, the advanced practice core, the NP specialty curricula, and the ACNP subspecialty curricula. The graduate and advanced practice nursing core curricula are based on the recommendations of the American Association of Colleges of Nursing (AACN-b) in *The Essentials of Master's Education for Advanced Practice Nursing* (1996). The graduate core consists of cognate core courses such as research, health-care policy, cultural diversity, and theoretical foundations. The advanced practice core consists of advanced health and physical assessment, physiology, pathophysiology, and pharmacology. The advanced practice core is taught in conjunction with, or simultaneous to, the graduate nursing core.

The core for nurse practitioner education, regardless of NP subspecialty, is recommended by the National Organization of Nurse Practitioner Faculties. These recommendations were released by the NONPF in 1990 (NONPF, 1990) and subsequently revised and updated in 1995 (NONPF, 1995) and 2000 (NONPF, 2000). The NONPF curricular recommendations do not provide lists of physiological, pathophysiological, or health-promoting topics. Rather, they delineate the domains of NP practice and list the entry-level competencies that NP students should be expected to achieve on graduation from the academic program and entry into the profession. Therefore the NP specialty core should provide both didactic and clinical preparation to prepare NPs to develop entry-level competencies in the following domains of NP practice: I. Management of Client Health/Illness Status; II. The NP/Patient Relationship; III. The Teaching/Coaching Function; IV. Professional Role; V. Managing and Negotiating Health-Care Delivery Systems; VI. Monitoring and Ensuring the Quality of Health-Care Practice; VII. Cultural Competence. There is not a prescription for credit requirements to achieve these competencies, but the NONPF does recommend a minimum of 500 clinical hours, with more hours recommended for programs that prepare specialists to provide care to multiple age groups or across multiple care settings. Clinical practica are vital for ACNP students, because they provide opportunities not only for improving competencies in direct clinical practice but also in the other core competencies, with a particular emphasis on collaboration (Hollinger-Smith & Murphy, 1998). In curriculum data collected by NONPF and AACN-b (2001), 41 ACNP programs reported a range of clinical hours from 480 to 1112, with a mean of 669. This variability may reflect broad inconsistencies in program structure, objectives, and outcome competencies.

A number of publications have addressed ACNP educational preparation and curricular recommendations (Clochesy & Daly, 1997; Clochesy et al., 1994; Hravnak et al., 1995; Hravnak, Rosenzweig, & Baldisseri, 1996; Keough et al., 1996; King & Ackerman, 1995; Kleinpell & Hravnak, 2002; Piano, Kleinpell, & Johnson, 1996; Schwertz, Piano, Kleinpell, & Johnson, 1997; Shah, Sullivan, Lattanzio, & Bruttomesso, 1993; Watts et al., 1996). All single-track ACNP programs focus solely on the care of adults, and the only national certification examination for ACNPs delineates that same focus. Therefore the ACNP specialty content should focus on knowledge and skills essential to diagnose and manage the episodic and chronic problems commonly experienced by acutely and critically ill adults, while performing health promotion/protection and disease prevention activities within the context of the continuum of the acute care delivery system. As illustrated within the conceptual model of care services presented in Table 14-2, the ACNP must diagnose and manage not only the acute health problems associated with the patient's chief complaint but also quiescent stable co-morbid health conditions. Because ACNPs must be prepared to manage health problems across the full continuum of acute care services, their didactic information and clinical experiences should provide for this broad focus. Likewise, the program should provide didactic and clinical preparation in the competencies delineated in Box 14-3. In contrast to the other NP subspecialties, the program should also focus on the ability of the ACNP to safely and competently perform within the nursing domain of the Management of Rapidly Changing Situations in the context of functioning as a primary provider of care. Consensus regarding the set of technical skills recommended for inclusion in ACNP programs has not yet been achieved. Debate centers on determining (1) which technical skills, especially invasive procedures, constitute the common denominator for ACNP education regardless of the future employment setting or specialty patient populations and (2) the degree of educational and technical training that is required prior to supervised skill performance in the clinical setting. ACNP educators and clinicians will need to determine the minimum common technical skill set required for the entry-level ACNP. This is an important topic, because peer review panels generally require documentation of training for privileges to be granted to perform technical procedures.

REIMBURSEMENT FOR ACNPs

Gaining third-party reimbursement for NP services continues to be a challenge, one that is not unique to ACNPs. An ACNP providing care for patients at the ambulatory boundary of the acute care health services continuum faces the same challenges as her or his primary care NP counterpart. These challenges include issues such as gaining admission to provider panels and determining whether a service will be covered and whether to bill directly or as "incident to" physician services. Regulations related to payment for services delivered to hospitalized patients present an additional challenge to ACNPs, one that many physician colleagues and administrators are navigating as well. It is important that ACNPs take an active role in becoming knowledgeable about billing mechanisms and the policy issues that affect reimbursement decisions related to ACNP services (Hravnak et al., 1998a; Rundio, 2001b). In many cases, the ability of ACNPs to gain third-party payment will affect decisions to hire or retain ACNPs in the practice plan over time. There are several reasons that ACNPs should secure direct reimbursement for their services, including recognition of their professional worth as a result of produced income and tangible recognition of their professional standing, which leads to professional satisfaction and peer recognition. Direct reimbursement will also bring visibility to the quantity and type of care for which ACNPs are compensated through documentation and monitoring of billed services in the National Claims History File established by the Center for Medicare and Medicaid Services (CMS) (Richmond et al., 2000). Through the evaluation of services billed by ACNPs at the national level, it will be possible to develop an aggregate profile of ACNP practice with respect to billable direct patient care activities (Richmond, Thompson, & Sullivan-Marx, 2000).

Almost every encounter between an ACNP and a patient is associated with a private or public payor, although not every payor will pay every ACNP for every service (Buppert, 1998). The five major types of payors under which ACNP services can be billed are Medicare, Medicaid, indemnity-type insurance, managed care organizations, and businesses that contract for certain services. Each type of payor operates under a separate body of regulations and has its own reimbursement policies and fee for service; descriptions of a variety of third-party providers, as well as other issues surrounding reimbursement for NP services, are described in greater detail elsewhere within this book (see Chapters 20 and 23). In this chapter, the authors will concentrate on reimbursement for ACNPs within the Medicare framework. Medicare has served as the gold standard for reimbursement of NP services by most third-party payors. Each insurance company may have its own unique variation, but if an ACNP gains an understanding of Medicare, he or she will be better equipped to understand the policies of other companies.

MEDICARE

At about the same time Medicare legislation was being enacted in the 1960s, the role of the NP was evolving, but in the area of pediatrics, not geriatrics. Historically, the primary mechanism by which NPs caring for older adults were reimbursed by Medicare in the office setting was referred to as billing "incident to" physician services (Richmond et al., 2000). Hospital-affiliated offices, clinics, and emergency departments were not acceptable for "incident to" billing. Only physicians could bill for services provided to hospitalized patients or in hospital-affiliated settings. As health care evolved, NPs began to care for patients of all ages and in diverse practice sites. However, because of the wording of the Medicare regulations, NPs could receive direct reimbursement for their services only when they were provided in certain geographic locations (in skilled nursing facilities or in federally designated rural medically underserved areas). NPs practicing in urban and suburban hospital settings were not included in these designated locations. Therefore, as the role of the ACNP practicing in the inpatient setting emerged, no reimbursement mechanism for these services existed under Medicare. Eventually, NPs and their employers began seeking legislation that would include NPs in the evolving reimbursement system as well as finding ways to arrange for payment within the existing system (Towers, 1999). Facilitated by a grass roots effort of NPs and their supporters, the Balanced Budget Act of 1997 included language that granted direct reimbursement to NPs, CNSs, and PAs regardless of the location in which the services were provided. This historic piece of legislation eliminated the geographical barriers, thus allowing for reimbursement in any setting, including hospitals.

Medicare Reimbursement for ACNPs in the Office/Nonhospital Clinic Setting

Although ACNPs typically provide services to hospitalized patients or to patients in hospital-affiliated offices and clinics, a portion of their practice may occur in the nonhospital-affiliated office or clinic setting as described previously in the discussion of ACNP role implementation models. In the office or clinic, ACNPs may either bill directly (at 85% of the physician fee schedule) or "incident to" (at 100% of the physician fee schedule). This decision depends on who is providing the Evaluation and Management (E/M) service. "Incident to" payment (the part of Medicare law that provides for coverage of services and supplies furnished incident to the professional services of a physician) is made to the physician as if he or she provided the service (Abood & Keepnews, 2000). Direct billing means that the ACNP provides an E/M service and submits the bill under his or her own provider number. "Incident to" means that the ACNP provides the service and submits the bill under the physician's provider number *if* certain requirements are met. A recent update to the Medicare Carriers Manual, which is discussed later, addresses those instances in which both the ACNP and the physician participate (share) in the E/M service. If the shared visit meets the "incident to" requirements, then it can be billed as "incident to." If the shared visit does not meet the "incident to" requirements, then the work of both the physician and the ACNP may be combined but must be billed under the ACNP's provider number (Center for Medicare and Medicaid Services, 2003a). It is important to note that the "incident to" billing option applies only to Medicare and, consistent with Medicare regulations prior to 1997, applies only to nonhospital-affiliated outpatient settings. There is still no "incident to" billing option for hospitalized patients. Also consistent with the prior regulations, Medicare considers emergency departments and hospital-affiliated clinics to be a part of the hospital, so that ACNPs working in these practice settings may not use "incident to" billing (Richmond et al., 2000). For more information regarding "incident to" billing, the reader is referred to the Medicare Carriers Manual of the Center for Medicare and Medicaid Services, Part 3 Claims Process, Transmittal 1764 (Center for Medicare and Medicaid Services, 2003a).

Hospital Inpatient/Hospital Outpatient/Emergency Department Reimbursement for ACNPs

Hospitals and emergency departments are common practice sites for ACNPs. The high patient acuity necessitates a close collaborative relationship with physician colleagues. It is not uncommon for both the ACNP and the physician to provide services to the hospitalized patient on the same day. ACNPs may bill Medicare as long as their services are not already covered by Medicare Part A payment to hospitals (see Chapter 23). As long as the ACNP's salary is secured from an individual professional practice plan, charges for services can be submitted to Medicare Part B. On October 25, 2002, CMS issued a Change Request (CR) 2321. This request updated Medicare Carriers Manual §15501 guidelines for E/M services. It provides guidelines for billing and reimbursement of E/M services provided by both the physician and the NP when they are in the same group practice and the physician provides any face-to-face portion of the E/M encounter in the hospital or hospital-affiliated setting (Center for Medicare and Medicaid Services, 2003b).

The key issues regarding shared/split E/M services are as follows:

- If the ACNP provides a medically necessary service and there is no face-to-face encounter with the physician, the service must be billed under the ACNP's provider number. Face-to-face encounter means that the physician must perform some portion of the E/M service and provide supporting documentation. Simply reviewing the chart and making a note does not constitute a face-to-face encounter.
- If both the ACNP and the physician provide portions of the E/M service on the same day, at the same or different times, they may combine those services and bill at the level supported by their combined documentation. The provider number used may be either the ACNP's or the physician's. The decision as to which number to use usually depends on which will provide the higher reimbursement amount.

The employment requirement for shared/split E/M services is important. Either the physician should employ the ACNP or both of them should be employed by the same entity (Center for Medicare and Medicaid Services, 2003b).

The preceding discussion also applies to billing for hospital outpatient visits in a hospital-affiliated office or clinic.

Critical Care Reimbursement for ACNPs

Reimbursement for critical care services can occur in any location where critical care services are performed, including intensive care units, emergency departments, and general medical-surgical floors (Vachani, DeLong, & Manaker, 2003). Critical care services are billed according to time based Current Procedural Terminology (CPT) codes. The first 30 to 74 minutes of critical care services on a given calendar date are billed under one specific CPT code. For each additional 30 minutes, a second code is used. If the total time spent providing critical care services is less than 30 minutes, then other E/M codes must be used (American Medical Association, 2002).

CHALLENGES FOR THE ACNP ROLE

The role of the ACNP is continuing to evolve and gain recognition. The increased need for ACNPs to directly manage patient care in an expanding health-care arena will continue to provide unique practice opportunities. Simultaneously, ACNPs will continue to face challenges to practice that will need to be resolved in order to firmly establish the role. Practicing ACNPs continue to report that physicians and hospital administrators are unfamiliar with the role and the differences between the primary care NP specialties and the ACNP. Additionally, some physicians feel threatened by the role. Misperceptions about the role and labeling of the role as a physician extender have stemmed from the perception that ACNPs are replacements for house staff and function as "resident replacements." Indeed, one of the earliest publications on the ACNP fueled this perception (Silver & McAtee, 1988). Many of these perceived threats and misperceptions can be addressed through education. ACNPs can use both formal and informal opportunities to educate the professional public about the purpose and practice of ACNPs, providing clear and concrete examples of their utilization and efficacy. It is extremely important for ACNPs to frame their practice within the nursing paradigm, one that uses the admitting history and physical examination to put forth a plan of care that includes the patient's holistic problems as well as the medical diagnosis; to address these nursing and medical problems throughout the hospital stay; to utilize interventions that not only diagnose and manage disease but also promote and protect health; to frame the discharge summary so that patients have a continuum of nursing as well as medical care as they return to the community; and to apply all the ACNP role competencies, not only those related to direct clinical care, to their practice.

Changing employment trends have also affected ACNP practice (Geier, 2000; Kleinpell & Hravnak, 2002). Originally, ACNPs were predominantly hired into tertiary medical center settings. ACNPs now report increased employment with physician practice groups, MCOs, independent subacute care facilities and even individual contractual relationships, yet these opportunities also bring the challenges of negotiating legal contracts, multiorganizational credentialing and privileging, group practice and managed care organization policies, and reimbursement issues (Kleinpell & Hravnak, 2002).

ACNPs need to continue to develop strong collaborative relationships with physicians to provide optimal patient care. Collaboration is the cornerstone of successful interdisciplinary practice. ACNP practice enhances the quality of care with a unique focus on collaborative patient care management (Shapiro & Rosenberg, 2002). Working to negotiate a collaborative practice partnership can be a challenge. In working to establish collegial relationships and by sharing successful practice models, ACNPs can promote enhanced collaborative relationships (see Chapter 21).

Exposure to the comprehensive care that ACNPs provide and education of the healthcare team regarding the role will lead to continued role recognition and role acceptance. Waiting for potential employers or the public to have a passive or situational exposure to the role is an inactive means of marketing the role (Hravnak & Magdic, 1997). Furthermore, ACNPs should recognize that, because the role is still relatively new, active marketing must include describing role capabilities and role effectiveness in terms of outcome data relative to a population served by the ACNP. Resistance to the role has been reported from physicians and other health-care professionals (Kleinpell, 1997). Such resistance primarily stems from uncertainty of the functions of the ACNP role and perceived blurring of professional boundaries (van Soeren & Micevski, 2001). Educating administrators and nurses can facilitate acceptance of the role, which will in turn provide an opportunity for independent contracting for ACNP professional services. Awareness of worth in terms of billable revenue and the care that ACNPS are able to provide is imperative for successful contract negotiations and marketing purposes.

In the future, ACNPs may practice in multiple settings with individually negotiated contracts. Managing episodes of acute illness or exacerbation of chronic illness in home health care, subacute care, and outpatient settings might be directed by the ACNP, as is already the case in some areas. These areas are natural extensions of acute care services and encompass the scope of ACNP practice, the stabilization of acute and chronic disease. Myriad opportunities relative to acute and chronic therapeutic management exist—for example, the management of renal dialysis or ventilator-dependent patients.

Cost reduction within acute care services will continue. Currently, collaborative teams composed of a physician, resident, and ACNP are popular in many practice settings. In the future, certain patient populations may be managed by teams composed of several ACNPs with one physician, as in the heart failure service vignette described earlier and in other examples in the literature (McMullen, Alexander, Bourgeois, & Goodman, 2001; Shapiro & Rosenberg, 2002).

Monitoring the outcomes of ACNP practice remains essential. While a growing number of utilization and outcome-based studies of ACNP practice have been conducted and published, the need to demonstrate the impact of ACNP care in a growing number of practice arenas remains. The emphasis on continuous quality improvement will continue to mandate the need for ACNPs to become proactive and involved in measuring the impact of their care.

As the ACNP role continues to evolve, it will be the responsibility of ACNP nurse leaders to encourage standardization of education for the ACNP in order to reduce the wide variability in ACNP program structure, requirements, lengths, and outcomes. Although some degree of variability between programs is desirable and enriching, too much variance results in lack of educational quality consistency, and poorly prepared graduates entering the job market (which in turn promotes negative perceptions of the role by employers and the public). Consensus development of clinical competencies that provide consistency in education and training will help to promote standardization. Utilizing accepted standards for educational program certification that are NP specific will ensure quality.

With all ACNPs holding master's degrees, and some holding doctoral degrees, there is an increased potential to apply scientific knowledge to clinical practice and to establish and uphold evidence-based practice. Collaboration with public policymakers to influence legislation issues related to the ACNP role or, on a larger scope, health policy issues is an imperative for all ACNPs (AACN-a, 1995; see Chapters 22 and 23). In the evolving health-care arena, ACNPs practice is rapidly expanding, and holds unlimited potential.

ACNPs must accept the challenge to continually improve and advance themselves and their profession. In order to provide safe, high-quality, efficient care, the ACNP must persistently pursue ongoing education to be knowledgeable about recent advances in health care and judicious in the application of research findings. ACNPs should not only read the literature but also publish on both clinical and role topics. Sharing their clinical expertise and experiences can benefit their peers as those peers seek to develop and enhance their roles. It is important that ACNPs be involved in their NP professional and clinical specialty organizations so that the issues unique to ACNP practice gain recognition by the leaders of the national organizations and also to ensure that ACNPs can have a voice in the legislative and political decision-making process.

CONCLUSION

The ACNP role provides an opportunity for NPs to have a significant impact on patient outcomes at a dynamic time in the history of health-care delivery. As the role continues to evolve along with the market and as health-care systems respond to economic change, opportunities to further develop the ACNP role will arise. Future development of the ACNP role should be based on the evaluation of the need for the role, understanding the scope of the role, assessment of the practice or organization, and the service needs of the patient population (Irvine et al., 2000). Because the ACNP role is still evolving, participation in national organizations to develop consensus regarding role components, program curriculum, marketing, and evaluation of the role is necessary to ensure that the preparation and practice of ACNPs is safe, effective, and fully represented. ACNPs must be strong activists in efforts to gain full recognition of the role within their proper scope of practice across acute care settings.

REFERENCES

Abood, S., & Keepnews, D. (2000). *Understanding payment for advanced practice nursing services: Medicare reimbursement. (Vol 1)*. Washington DC: American Nurses Publishing.

American Association of Colleges of Nursing. (1996). *The essentials of master's education for advanced practice nursing*. Washington, DC: Author.

American Association of Critical-Care Nurses. (1995). *Advanced nursing practice: Facts and strategies for regulation, reimbursement and prescriptive authority*. Washington, DC: Author.

American Medical Association. (2002). *Current procedural terminology: CPT 2003. Standard edition*. Chicago: Author.

American Nurses Association and American Association of Critical-Care Nurses. (1995). *Standards of clinical practice and scope of practice for acute care nurse practitioner*. Washington, DC: American Nurses Publishing.

American Nurses Credentialing Center. (1999). *Nurse practitioner board certification examination catalog*. Washington, DC: Author.

Baggs, J. G., & Schmitt, M. H. (1988). Collaboration between nurses and physicians. *Image: The Journal of Nursing Scholarship, 20,* 145-149.

Barber, P. M., & Burke, M. (1999). Advanced practice nursing in managed care. In M. D. Mezy & D. O. McGivern (Eds.), *Nurses, nurse practitioners* (pp. 203-218). New York: Springer.

Barkley, T.W., & Rogers, J.E. (2001). Dynamic roles and scope of the acute care nurse practitioner. *Nurse Practitioner Forum, 12,* 115-120.

Barkley, T.W., & Whitney, F. (2001). The acute care nurse practitioner's role in pain and pain management. *Nurse Practitioner Forum, 12,* 166-174.

Benner, P.E. (1984). *From novice to expert: Excellence and power in clinical nursing practice*. Menlo Park, CA: Addison-Wesley.

Brykczynski, K.A. (1989). An interpretive study describing the clinical judgment of nurse practitioners. *Scholarly Inquiry for Nursing Practice, 3,* 75-104.

Buchanan, L. (1996). The acute care nurse practitioner in collaborative practice. *Journal of the American Academy of Nurse Practitioners, 8,* 13-16, 17-20.

Buchanan, L., & Powers, R. D. (1997). Establishing an NP-staffed minor emergency area. *Nurse Practitioner, 22,* 175-178, 183, 187.

Buppert, C. (1998). Reimbursement for nurse practitioner services. *The Nurse Practitioner 23,* 67-81.

Burkholder, J. S., & Dudjak, L. A. (1994). The midlevel practitioner role: One medical center's experience. *AACN Clinical Issues in Critical Care Nursing, 5,* 369-403.

Burns, S. M. (1998). An evolving critical care acute care nurse practitioner role: the pulmonary acute care nurse practitioner and the management of patients requiring prolonged ventilation. In R. Kleinpell & M. Piano (Eds.), *Practice issues for the acute care nurse practitioner* (pp. 160-170). New York: Springer.

Burns, S. M., & Earven, S. (2002). Improving outcomes for mechanically ventilated medical intensive care unit patients using advanced practice nurses: A 6-year experience. *Critical Care Nursing Clinics of North America, 14,* 231-243.

Center for Medicare and Medicaid Services. (2003a). *Medicare Carriers Manual, Claim Processing, Part 3, Transmittal 1764.* Section 2050.0-2050.3. Retrieved September 10, 2003, from http://www.cms.hhs.gov/manuals/pm_trans/R1764B3.pdf

Center for Medicare and Medicaid Services. (2003b). *Medicare Carriers Manual, Claim Processing, Part 3, Transmittal 1776.* Section 15501. Retrieved September 10, 2003, from http://www.cms.hhs.gov/manuals/pm_trans/R1776B3.pdf

Cintron, G., Bigas, C., Linates, E., Aranda, J. M., & Hernandez, E. (1983). Nurse practitioner role in a chronic congestive heart failure clinic: In-hospital time, costs, and patient satisfaction. *Heart and Lung, 12,* 237-240.

Clochesy, J., & Daly, B. (1997). Educational standards for acute care nurse practitioners. In B. Daly (Ed.), *The acute care nurse practitioner* (pp. 57-80). New York: Springer.

Clochesy, J., Daly, B. J., Idemoto, B. K., Steel, J., & Fitzpatrick, J. J. (1994). Preparing advanced practice nurses for acute care. *American Journal of Critical Care, 3,* 255-259.

Cole, F. L., & Catalano, J. M. (1998). The acute care nurse practitioner in the emergency department setting. In R. Kleinpell & M. Piano (Eds.), *Practice issues for the acute care nurse practitioner* (pp. 144-159). New York: Springer.

Cole, F. L., & Ramirez, E. (1997). The emergency nurse practitioner: An educational model. *Journal of Emergency Nursing, 23,* 112-115.

Cole, F. L., & Ramirez, E. (2000). Activities and procedures performed by nurse practitioners in emergency care settings. *Journal of Emergency Nursing, 26,* 455-463.

Cooper, M. A., Lindsey, G. M., Kinn, S., & Swann I. J. (2002). Evaluating emergency nurse practitioner services: A randomized controlled trial. *Journal of Advanced Nursing, 40,* 721-730.

Cummings, C. M. (1997). Scope of employment vs. scope of practice. *Advance for Nurse Practitioners, 5,* 17.

Daffurn, K. (1998). Roles of acute care nurse practitioners, physician assistants, and resident physicians in acute care settings. *American Journal of Critical Care, 7,* 253-4.

Dahle, K. L., Smith, J. S., Ingersoll, G. L., & Wilson, J. R. (1998). Impact of a nurse practitioner on the cost of managing inpatients with heart failure. *American Journal of Cardiology, 82,* 686-688, A-8.

Daly, B., & Gent, C. (1997). Influence of the health care environment. In B. Daly (Ed.), *The acute care nurse practitioner* (pp. 29-56). Washington, DC: American Nurses Publishing.

Fox, V. J., Schira, M., & Wadlund, D. (2000). The pioneer spirit in perioperative advanced practice—two practice examples. *AORN Journal, 72,* 241-248, 250-253.

Gates, S. J. (1993). Continuity of care: The orthopaedic nurse practitioner in tertiary care. *Orthopaedic Nursing, 12,* 48-50, 66.

Gawlinski, A., McCloy, K., & Jesurum, J. (2001). Measuring outcomes in cardiovascular APN practice. In R. Kleinpell (Ed.), *Outcome assessment in advanced practice nursing* (pp. 131-187). New York: Springer.

Geier, W. (2000). The evolving role of the acute care nurse practitioner. *Nurse Practitioner, 25,* 126-129.

Genet, C. A., Brennan, P. F., Ibbotson-Wolff, S., Phelps, C., Rosenthal, G., & Landefeld, G. S. (1995). Nurse practitioners in a teaching hospital. *Nurse Practitioner, 9,* 47-54.

Greenberg, E.M. (1996). Violence and the older adult: The role of the acute care nurse practitioner. *Critical Care Nursing Quarterly, 19,* 76-84.

Hall, J. K. (1993). How to analyze nurse practitioner licensure laws. *Nurse Practitioner, 18,* 31–34.

Hanson, C. M. (1986). Desired competencies for nurse practitioners: A delphi study of master's level curriculum priorities. *Dissertation Abstracts International, 47,* 4276A. (UMI No. 87-06868)

Hicks, G. L. (1998). Cardiac surgery and the acute care nurse practitioner—"the perfect link." *Heart & Lung, 27,* 283-284.

Hollinger-Smith, L., & Murphy, M. P. (1998). Implementing a residency program for the acute care nurse practitioner. *MEDSURG Nursing, 7,* 28-33, 36-38.

Hoffman, L. A., Tasota, F. J., Scharfenberg, C., Zullo, T. G., & Donahoe, M. P. (2002). Management of ventilator-dependent patients: 5-month comparison of acute care nurse practitioner (ACNP) versus physician in training (PIT). *American Journal of Respiratory and Critical Care Medicine, 165,* A388.

Hoffman, L. A., Tasota, F. J., Scharfenberg, C., Zullo, T. G., & Donahoe, M. P. (2003). Management of

patients in the Intensive Care Unit: Comparison via work sampling analysis of an acute care nurse practitioner and physicians in training. *American Journal of Critical Care, 12,* 436-443.

Howie, J. N., & Erickson, M. (2002). Acute care nurse practitioners: Creating and implementing a model of care for an inpatient general medical service. *American Journal of Critical Care, 11,* 448-458.

Hravnak, M. (1998). Is there a health promotion and protection foundation to the practice of acute care nurse practitioners? *AACN Clinical Issues, 9,* 283-289.

Hravnak, M., & Baldiserri, M. (1997). Credentialing and privileging: Insight into the process for acute care nurse practitioners. *AACN Clinical Issues, 8,* 108-115.

Hravnak, M., Kobert, S. N., Risco, K. G., Baldisseri, M., Hoffman, L. A., Clochesy, J. M., et al. (1995). Acute care nurse practitioner curriculum: Content and development process. *American Journal of Critical Care 4,* 179-188.

Hravnak, M., & Magdic, K. (1997). Marketing the acute care nurse practitioner. *Clinical Excellence for the Nurse Practitioner, 1,* 9-13.

Hravnak, M., Rosenzweig, M. Q., & Baldisseri, M. (1996). Current questions with regard to acute care nurse practitioner preparation and role implementation. *AACN Clinical Issues, 7,* 289-299.

Hravnak, M., Rosenzweig, P., Rust, D., & Magdic, K. (1998a). Reimbursement, liability and insurance. In R. Kleinpell & M. Piano (Eds.), *Practice issues for the acute care nurse practitioner* (pp. 27-40). New York: Springer.

Hravnak, M., Rosenzweig, P., Rust, D., & Magdic, K. (1998b). Scope of practice, credentialing, and privileging. In R. Kleinpell & M. Piano (Eds.), *Practice issues for the acute care nurse practitioner* (pp. 41-46). New York: Springer.

Hylka, S. C., & Beschle, J. C. (1995). Nurse practitioners, cost savings, and improved patient care in the department of surgery. *Nursing Economics, 13,* 349-354.

Ingersoll, G. (1995). Evaluation of the advanced practice nurse role in acute care and specialty care. *Critical Care Nursing Clinics of North America, 7,* 25-33.

Irvine, D., Sidani, S., Porter, H., O-Brien-Pallas, L., Simpson, B., McGillis Hall, L. (2000). Organizational factors influencing nurse practitioners' role in acute care settings. *Canadian Journal of Nursing Leadership, 13,* 28-35.

Kassirer, J. P. (1989). Diagnostic reasoning. *Annals of Internal Medicine, 110,* 893-900.

Keane, A., & Richmond, T. (1993). Tertiary NPs. *Image: The Journal of Nursing Scholarship, 25,* 281-284.

Keane, A., Richmond, T., & Kaiser, L. (1994). Critical care nurse practitioners: Evolution of the advanced practice nursing role. *American Journal of Critical Care, 3,* 232-237.

Keough, V., Jennrich, J., Holm, K., & Marshall, W. (1996). A collaborative program for advanced practice in trauma/critical care nursing. *Critical Care Nurse, 16*(2), 120-127.

King, K., & Baggs, J. (1998). Collaboration: The essence of acute care nurse practitioner practice. In R. Kleinpell & M. Piano (Eds.), *Practice issues for the acute care nurse practitioner* (pp. 67-78). New York: Springer.

King, K. B., & Ackerman, M. H. (1995). An educational model for the acute care nurse practitioner. *Critical Care Nursing Clinics of North America, 7*, 1-7.

Kleinpell, R. M. (1997). Acute care nurse practitioner: Roles and practice profiles. *AACN Clinical Issues 8*, 156–162.

Kleinpell, R. M. (1998). Acute care nurse practitioner: Reports from the practice settings profiles. In R. Kleinpell & M. Piano (Eds.), *Practice issues for the acute care nurse practitioner* (pp. 1-9). New York: Springer.

Kleinpell, R. M. (1999). Evolving role descriptions of the acute care nurse practitioner. *Critical Care Nurse Quarterly, 21*, 9-15.

Kleinpell, R. (2001). Measuring outcomes in advanced practice nursing. In Kleinpell, R. (Ed) *Outcome assessment in advanced practice nursing* (pp. 1-50), New York: Springer.

Kleinpell, R. (2002). The acute care nurse practitioner: An expanding career opportunity for critical care nurses. *Critical Care Nurse*, (Suppl. February) 12-16, 74.

Kleinpell, R. M., & Hravnak, M. (2002). The acute care nurse practitioner. In M. K. Crabtree & R. Pruitt (Eds.), *Advanced nursing practice: Building curriculum for quality nurse practitioner education* (pp. 113-126). Washington, DC: National Organization of Nurse Practitioner Faculties.

Kleinpell, R., & Weiner, T. (1999). Measuring advanced practice nursing outcomes. *AACN Clinical Issues 10*, 40-47.

Kleinpell-Nowell, R. (1999). Longitudinal survey of acute-care nurse practitioners: Year 1. *AACN Clinical Issues, 10*, 515-520.

Kleinpell-Nowell, R. (2001). Longitudinal survey of acute care nurse practitioner practice: Year 2. *AACN Clinical Issues, 12*, 447-452.

Knickman, J. R., Lipkin, M., Finkler, S. A., Thompson, W. G., & Kiel, J. (1992). The potential for using nonphysicians to compensate for the reduced availability of residents. *Academic Medicine, 67*, 429-438.

Kristeller, A. R. (1995). Medical staff: Privileging and credentialing. *New Jersey Medicine, 92*, 26-28.

Lott, J. W., Polak, J. D., Kenyon, T. B., & Kenner, C. A. (1996). Acute care nurse practitioner. In A. B. Hamric, J. A. Spross, & C. M. Hanson (Eds.), *Advanced practice nursing: An integrative approach* (pp. 351-373). Philadelphia: W. B. Saunders.

Martin, B., & Coniglio, J .U. (1996). The acute care nurse practitioner in collaborative practice. *AACN Clinical Issues, 7*, 309-314.

Martin, R. K. (1999). Organ transplantation: the role of the acute care nurse practitioner across the spectrum of care. *AACN Clinical Issues, 10*, 285-292.

McMullen, M., Alexander, M.K., Bourgeois, A., & Goodman, L. (2001). Evaluating a nurse practitioner service. *Dimensions of Critical Care Nursing, 20*, 30-34.

Mick, D. J., & Ackerman, M. H. (2002). Deconstructing the myth of the advanced practice blended role: Support for role divergence. *Heart & Lung, 31*, 393-398.

Miller, S. (1997). Impact of a gerontological nurse practitioner on the nursing home elderly in the acute care setting. *AACN Clinical Issues, 8*, 609-615.

Miller, S.K. (2001). Gerontology and geriatrics: Considerations for the acute care nurse practitioner. *Nurse Practitioner Forum, 12*, 155-160.

Mittman, D .E., Cawley, J. F., & Fenn, W. H. (2002). Physician assistants in the United States. *British Medical Journal, 325*, 485-487.

Monninger, M. E. (1987). A description of professional competencies of family nurse practitioners and congruence of goals of practice. *Dissertation Abstracts International, 47*, 2375-B. (UMI No. 86-18549)

National Organization of Nurse Practitioner Faculties (2000). *Domains and competencies of nurse practitioner practice.* Washington, DC: Author.

National Organization of Nurse Practitioner Faculties and American Association of Colleges of Nursing. (2001). *2000 survey of nurse practitioner educational programs.* Unpublished manuscript.

National Organization of Nurse Practitioner Faculties and the American Association of Colleges of Nursing (2002). *Nurse practitioner primary care competencies in specialty areas: Adult, family, gerontological, pediatric, and women's health.* Rockville, Maryland: United States Department of Health & Human Services Health Resources and Services Administration, Bureau of Health Professions, Division of Nursing.

National Organization of Nurse Practitioner Faculties. (1990). *Advanced nursing practice: Nurse practitioner curriculum guidelines.* Washington, DC: National Organization of Nurse Practitioner Faculties.

National Organization of Nurse Practitioner Faculties. (1995). *Advanced nursing practice: Curriculum guidelines and program standards for nurse practitioner education.* Washington, DC: National Organization of Nurse Practitioner Faculties.

National Organization of Nurse Practitioner Faculties. (2000). *Domains and competencies of nurse practitioner practice.* Washington, DC: National Organization of Nurse Practitioner Faculties.

Norsen, L., Opladen, J., & Quinn, J. (1995). Practice model: Collaborative practice. *Critical Care Nursing Clinics of North America, 7*, 43-52.

Parrinello, K. (1995). Advanced practice nursing: An administrative perspective. *Critical Care Nursing Clinics of North America, 7*, 9-16.

Paul, S. (2000). Impact of a nurse-managed heart failure clinic: A pilot study. *American Journal of Critical Care, 9,* 140-146.

Pearson, L. (2003). Fifteenth annual legislative update: How each state stands on legislative issues affecting advanced nursing practice. *The Nurse Practitioner, 28,* 26-58.

Penas, C. D., & Barkley, T. W. (2001). Ethical theory and principles of decision-making for the acute care nurse practitioner. *Nurse Practitioner Forum, 12,* 161-165.

Piano, M. R., Kleinpell, R., & Johnson, J. A. (1996). The acute care nurse practitioner and management of common health problems: A proposal. *American Journal of Critical Care, 5,* 289-292.

Piano, M. R., & Zerwic-Johnson, J. (1998). Demonstrating the effectiveness of the acute care nurse practitioner: Current and future research. In R. Kleinpell & M. Piano (Eds.), *Practice issues for the acute care nurse practitioner* (pp. 10-26). New York: Springer.

Prescott, P. A., & Driscoll, L. (1980). Evaluating nurse practitioner performance. *Nurse Practitioner, 5,* 28-29, 31-32.

Reel, V. K. (1999). Utilization of the acute care nurse practice in lung transplantation. *Clinical Excellence for Nurse Practitioners, 3,* 80-83.

Rhee, K. J., & Dermeyer, A. L. (1995). Patient satisfaction with a nurse practitioner in a university emergency service. *Annals of Emergency Medicine, 26,* 130-132.

Rhodes, R. S., & Carlson, J. H. (2001). Patient teaching tips for the acute care nurse practitioner. *Nurse Practitioner Forum, 12,* 86-91.

Richmond, T. S., Thompson, H. J., & Sullivan-Marx, E.M. (2000). Reimbursement for acute care nurse practitioner services. *American Journal of Critical Care, 9,* 52-61.

Riley-Bryan, K. D., & Barkley, T. W. (2001). Health policy concerns for the acute care nurse practitioner. *Nurse Practitioner Forum, 12,* 98-105.

Rosenfeld, P., McEvoy, M. D., & Glassman, K. (2003). Measuring practice patterns among acute care nurse practitioners. *Journal of Nursing Administration, 33,* 159-163.

Rundio, A. (2001a). Continuous quality improvement and problem solving techniques for the acute care nurse practitioner. *Nurse Practitioner Forum, 12,* 97-92.

Rundio, A. (2001b). Reimbursement hieroglyphics for the acute care nurse practitioner. *Nurse Practitioner Forum, 12,* 138-146.

Russell, D., VorderBruegge, M., & Burns, S. (2002). Effect of an outcomes-managed approach to care of neuroscience patients by acute care nurse practitioners. *American Journal of Critical Care, 11,* 353-362.

Sarkissian, S., & Wennberg, R. (1999). Effects of the acute care nurse practitioner role on epilepsy monitoring outcomes. *Outcomes Management for Nursing Practice, 3,* 161-166.

Scharfenberg, C., Hoffman, L. A., Tasota, F. J., Happ, M. B., & Donahoe, M. P. (2003). Advantages and disadvantages of an acute care nurse practitioner (ACNP) and physicians in training (PIT): Perceptions of ICU clinicians. *American Journal of Respiratory and Critical Care Medicine, 167,* A102.

Schwertz, D. W., Piano, M. R., Kleinpell, R., & Johnson, J. (1997). Teaching pharmacology to advanced practice nursing students: Issues and strategies. *AACN Clinical Issues, 8,* 132-146.

Shah, H., & Sullivan, D. T. (1998). Evaluation of the acute care nurse practitioner's role. In R. Kleinpell & M. Piano (Eds.), *Practice issues for the acute care nurse practitioner* (pp. 111-143). New York: Springer.

Shah, H. S., Bruttomesso, K. A., Sullivan, D. T., & Lattanzio, J. (1997). An evaluation of the role and practices of the acute-care nurse practitioner. *AACN Clinical Issues, 8,* 147-155.

Shah, H. S., Sullivan, D. T., Lattanzio, J., & Bruttomesso, K. (1993). Preparing acute care nurse practitioners at the University of Connecticut. *AACN Clinical Issues, 4,* 625-629.

Shapiro, D., & Rosenberg, N. (2002). Acute care nurse practitioner collaborative practice negotiation. *AACN Clinical Issues, 13,* 470-478.

Silver, H. K., & McAtee, P. (1988). Speaking out: Should nurses substitute for house staff? *American Journal of Nursing, 88,* 1671-1673.

Smolenski, M. C. (2002, July). Playing the credentials game. *Nursing Spectrum Career Fitness Online.* Retrieved April 30, 2004, from http://community.nursingspectrum.com/magazinearticles/article.cfm?aid_7126

Spisso, J., O'Callaghan, C., McKennan, M., & Holcroft, J. W. (1990). Improved quality of care and reduction of housestaff workload using trauma nurse practitioners. *Journal of Trauma, 30,* 660-663.

Stetler, C. B., Effken, J., Frigon, L., Tiernan, C., & Zwingman-Bagley, C. (1998). Utilization-focused evaluation of acute care nurse practitioner role. *Outcomes Management for Nursing Practice, 2,* 152-160.

Szaflarski, N. L. (1997). Diagnostic reasoning in acute and critical care. *AACN Clinical Issues, 8,* 291-302.

Towers, J. (1999). Corner on issues: Medicare reimbursement for nurse practitioners. *Journal of the American Academy of Nurse Practitioners, 11,* 289-292.

Vachani, A., DeLong, P., & Manaker, S. (2003). Documentation and coding of critical care professional services. *Clinical Pulmonary Medicine 10,* 85-92.

van Soeren, M. H., & Micevski, V. (2001). Success indicators and barriers to acute care nurse practitioner role implementation in four Ontario hospitals. *AACN Clinical Issues, 12,* 424-437.

von Sternberg, T., Hepburn, K., Cibuzar, P., Convery, L., Dokken, B., & Haefemeyer, J. (1997). Post-hospital sub-acute care: An example of a managed care model. *Journal of the American Geriatric Society, 45,* 87-91.

Wachter, R. M. (1999). An introduction to the hospitalist model. *Annals of Internal Medicine, 130*(4Pt2), 338-342.

Wachter, R. M., & Goldman, L. (1996). The emerging role of "hospitalists" in the American health care system. *New England Journal of Medicine, 335,* 514-517.

Watts, R. J. (1997). The critical-care nurse practitioner curriculum at the University of Pennsylvania: Update and revision. *AACN Clinical Issues, 8,* 116-122.

Watts, R. J., Hanson, M. J., Burke, K. G., Gallagher, S. M., & Foster, D. E. (1996). The critical care nurse practitioner: An advanced practice role for the critical care nurse. *Dimensions of Critical Care Nursing, 15,* 48-56.

Weinberg, R. M., Liljestrand, J. S., & Moore, S. (1983). Inpatient management by a nurse practitioner: Effectiveness in a rehabilitation setting. *Archives of Physical Medicine and Rehabilitation, 64,* 588-590.

CHAPTER 15

The Blended Role of the Clinical Nurse Specialist and the Nurse Practitioner

KAREN SKALLA • ANN B. HAMRIC • PAULA A. CARON

Continued

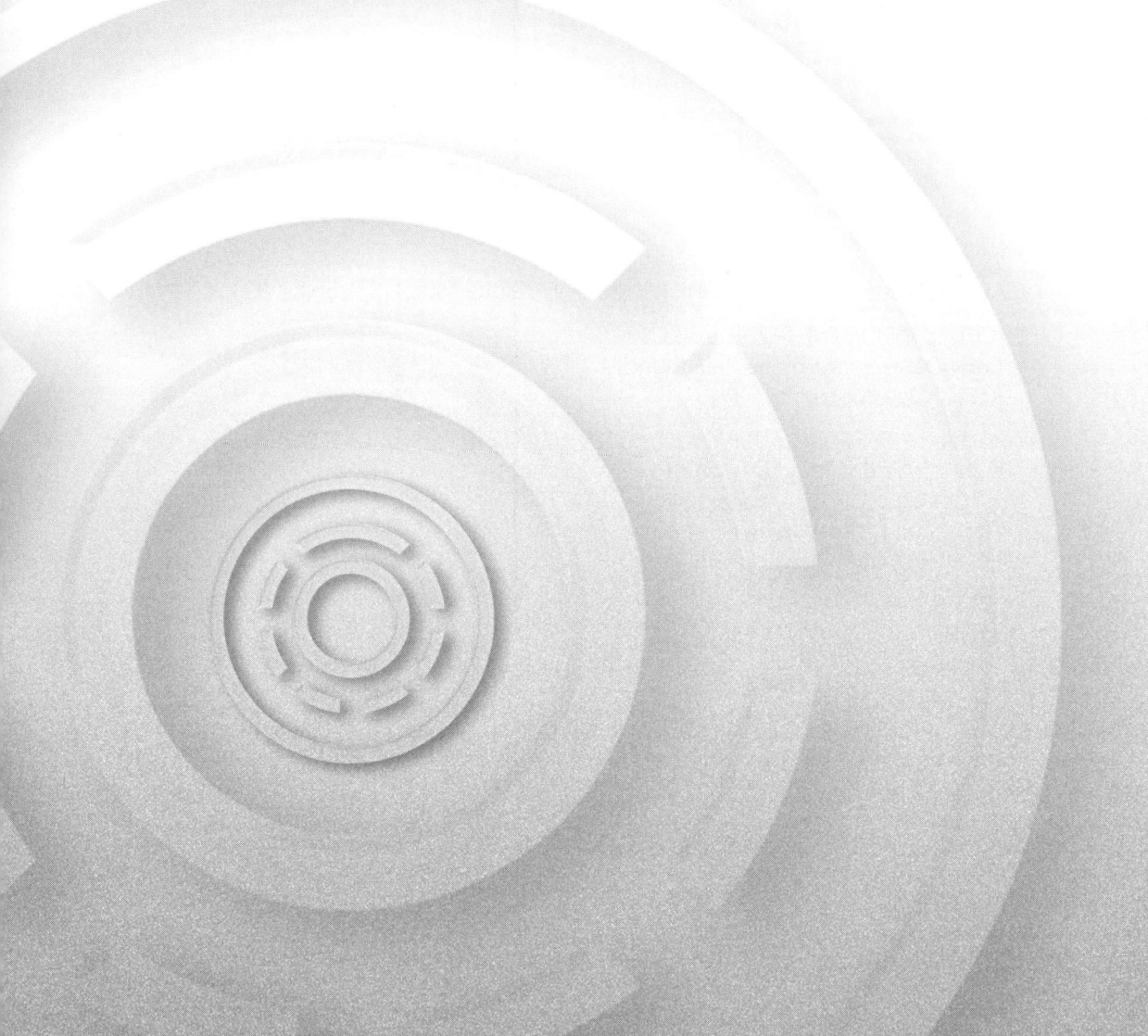

INTRODUCTION

Over the last two decades, there have been calls to merge the clinical nurse specialist (CNS) and nurse practitioner (NP) roles into one advanced practice nursing role (Anonymous, 2001; Cooper, 1990; Deane, 1997; Elder & Bullough, 1990; Finke, 2000; Hanson & Martin, 1990; Hockenberry-Eaton & Powell, 1991; Quaal, 1999; Shuren, 1996; Spross & Hamric, 1983; Wright, 1990; Wright, 1997). With few exceptions, most of these authors have argued for or against merging as a substitution for the individual CNS and NP roles, rather than as the creation of an additional advanced practice nursing role. However, the need for a new advanced practice nursing role, the blended CNS/NP, has emerged over time as a response to numerous changes in patient populations, the health professions workforce, and the health-care system. The authors of this chapter and the book's editors have argued that these trends indicate the need for blending CNS and NP skills into a new role, rather than completely merging these two valuable and distinct advanced practice nursing roles (Hamric, 2000; Shuren, 1996; Skalla & Hamric, 2000; Hanson & Hamric, 2003).

This chapter defines the blended CNS/NP, which we will refer to as the *blended role advanced practice nurse (APN)*. The evolution and current profile of this role are described. While the authors, two of whom are blended role APNs with primary care and specialty certifications, recognize that there are other possible "blendings," in this chapter the blended role of APNs prepared as CNSs in a specialty and as primary care NPs is profiled. Challenges in role development and implementation are discussed and illustrated by clinical case presentations and role exemplars. Current issues related to ongoing development of the blended role APN are addressed, and recommendations for strengthening and sustaining this role are made.[1]

The blended role APN is a graduate of a master's degree program in nursing that prepares students to fulfill two APN roles, usually those of CNS and primary care NP. The blended role APN is eligible for dual certification as a CNS in a specialty and as an NP. Blended role APNs demonstrate the core advanced practice nursing competencies through the provision of comprehensive primary and specialty care to a narrowly defined complex patient population. They have practices that cross settings from primary through tertiary care. Blended role practice includes elements of CNS and NP practices yet is a unique role that is distinct from the practice of these other APNs. The blended role preparation discussed here combines the strengths of two traditional roles: the primary health-care skills of NPs and the in-depth specialty and systems knowledge of CNSs. Dual preparation and certification expand the repertoire of knowledge and skills that blended role APNs can offer. One value of the blended role is in the ability of these practitioners to fulfill a variety of functions. They are "value added" because they bring primary care skills to the specialty setting and specialty skills to the primary care setting. The specialty practice of the CNS is necessary to understand complex chronic illness, as well as its impact on the patient and on society. This understanding enables the CNS to act in proactive ways to improve care within systems and across settings. The primary care training of the NP facilitates the delivery of primary care within the specialty and enables the practitioner to maintain continuity in delivering comprehensive care. Blended role APNs are particularly well prepared to provide care across settings that addresses the health-care

---

[1]Portions of this chapter appeared in the first edition of this book. The authors and editors gratefully acknowledge the work of Allison Weber Shuren, MSN, RN, CCRN, CPNP, for her important contribution (Shuren, 1996).

needs of the underserved, those with multiple chronic illnesses, and those with unusual and complex health problems (Sperhac & Strodtbeck, 2001). "These blended APNs are efficient, effective, and deliver care in seamless coordinated models that do not separate inpatient and outpatient care. These expert specialized nurses provide a full range of health-care services within a holistic. . . framework" (Sperhac & Strodtbeck, 2001, p. 126).

CALLS FOR MERGING CNS/NP ROLES: MERGING VERSUS BLENDING

Before the blended role APN is described, there is a need to clarify the distinction between the terms *blending* and *merging*. We see a difference between "blending" CNS and NP roles into a new configuration with a distinct title and "merging" all CNSs and NPs into one homogeneous product. The issues of merging roles and reconceptualizing advanced practice educational models have been and continue to be much debated topics among nursing leaders, educators, and APNs (Finke, 2000; Hunsberger et al., 1992; McCabe & Grover, 1999; Naegle & Krainovich-Miller, 2001; Sperhac & Strodtbeck, 2001; Verger, Trimarchi, & Barnsteiner, 2002). Numerous articles and editorials continue to address the pros and cons of merging CNS and NP roles (Anonymous, 2001; Deane, 1997; Finke, 2000; Mick & Ackerman, 2002; Page & Mackowiak, 1997; Redekopp, 1997; Wright, 1997). However, the authors of these articles rarely consider the issue of blending or dual preparation and credentialing as one response among many to better meet evolving patient care needs. Some authors believe that the debate is more theoretical and based on minimal research (Fenton & Brykczynski, 1993). Others suggest that the merger of the CNS and NP roles is inevitable and believe that merging the roles would be advantageous for health-care organizations, patient care, and graduate nursing education (Cooper, 1990; Elder & Bullough, 1990; McGivern, 1993; Quaal, 1999; Wright, 1990; Wright, 1997). Still others assert that the roles are distinctly different in scope of practice and setting and should be maintained as such (Beecroft, 1994; King & Ackerman, 1995; Lincoln, 2000; Page & Arena, 1994; Page & Mackowiak, 1997; Zimmer et al., 1990). The National Association of Clinical Nurse Specialists does not recommend either blending or merging CNS and NP roles (NACNS, 2004). The debate reflects the lack of consensus within the profession, as well as differing professional perspectives at the various times these articles were written. However, what is notable in these articles is the either-or tone asserting that either the roles must merge or they must stay distinct. *The contention here is that this is not an either-or debate*. No one role can "do it all" in advanced practice nursing. Patient needs, care delivery settings, and health-care specialties are too diverse and complex for any one role to master the knowledge base required. Blended role APNs *as well as* individual CNS and NP roles are needed to meet the health-care needs of diverse populations in diverse settings.

EVOLUTION OF THE BLENDED ROLE

Early Descriptions of the Blended Role

The development of an advanced practice nursing role that blends the practice of the CNS and NP cannot be traced to any particular event. Davitt and Jensen (1981) provided one of the earliest job descriptions in the literature that parallels the blended role APN described in this chapter. Historically, the CNS has been viewed as providing specialized nursing care for a specific patient population, staff development, and systems change in secondary and tertiary inpatient care settings. In contrast, NPs have been viewed as generalists who provide primary and preventative care and treat illnesses for a broad patient population in outpatient care settings. In the 1980s, some authors anticipated the need for an APN who possessed the assessment, diagnostic, and treatment skills of NPs and the direct care, staff coaching, and change agent skills of CNSs (Kitzman, 1983, 1989; Spross & Hamric, 1983). Spross and Hamric (1983) proposed one possible model describing future CNS practice in which CNSs would acquire and use competencies traditionally associated with NPs. This future APN would be educationally prepared in both CNS and NP roles, and his or her practice would combine the domains of service and scopes of practice of NPs and CNSs. This APN was seen as a practitioner who would be client based rather than setting based, providing care in primary, secondary, and tertiary settings to ensure continuity of services to a specialty-based patient population. Through independent and interdependent practice with physicians, the APN would deliver direct care, such as advanced clinical assessment; manage acute and chronic problems associated with a specific patient population; and provide ongoing guidance about potential diagnosis-specific problems as well as generic primary prevention education. The APN would also provide vital indirect patient care through expert clinical consultation, coordination and facilitation of patient services, and support for improved nursing practice (Spross & Hamric, 1983). Their description of this future role is consistent with the blended role described in this chapter. In 1990, Gleeson and colleagues reported a similar model of collaborative practice that suggests how and why a blended role APN, who is different from either a CNS or an NP, may be the most appropriate APN for a defined population (Gleeson et al., 1990).

Kitzman (1983, 1989) and others offered further evidence that some type of blending of APN roles seemed inevitable. Kitzman pointed out that CNSs and NPs have contributed significantly to the growth of each other's practice. CNSs have been credited with cultivating a climate within nursing that is open to expanded nursing practice (Kitzman, 1989), developing theory-based practice, and establishing the behavioral expectations of a nurse in advanced practice. NPs can take credit for expanding practice beyond traditional nursing boundaries; fostering lay recognition of APNs, which has promoted consumer acceptance of advanced practice nursing (Hanson & Martin, 1990); and developing collegial relationships with physicians (Kitzman, 1989). As early as 1983, Kitzman noted that the inpatient CNS and outpatient NP stereotypes were breaking down, because CNSs could be found in outpatient settings and NPs were working in inpatient settings (Kitzman, 1983). Her observations have been borne out by more recent descriptions of CNSs in outpatient settings who provide extensive primary and preventative services and assessment and management of illness related to their specialties (Brooten et al., 2002). Also, NPs have been and are currently practicing in tertiary care centers, managing acute and chronic illnesses for specific patient populations and improving nursing care through education, consultation, and research (Dale, 1991; Davitt & Jensen, 1981; Gleeson et al., 1990; Hunsberger et al., 1992; Keane & Richmond, 1993; Mick & Ackerman, 2000, 2002; Nemes, Barnaby, & Shamberger, 1992; Weinberg, Likestrand, & Moore, 1983). As the CNS and NP roles have expanded and matured, their practice settings have crossed (Deane, 1997). All of these factors have contributed to the current development of the blended role APN.

Recent Developments

There is evidence in the literature that there are APNs practicing in blended roles as we define the role here but who do not explicitly refer to their roles as blended role practice. One health-care system reorganized outpatient care to reduce the costs incurred by readmission of patients with heart disease to the hospital (Paladichuk, Brass-Mynderse, & Kaliangara, 1997). The clinic, staffed by one blended role APN and two NPs, saved 160 readmissions per year across two hospitals at a cost savings of $1.2 million. Paladichuk et al. (1997) reported that patients were very satisfied and more adherent to treatment because of their access to blended role APNs. Another example of the potential impact of APNs, including blended role APNs, is a study in which a comprehensive discharge plan and a home follow-up program were implemented for hospitalized elders (Naylor et al., 1999). The gerontological specialty background of the APNs enabled them to devise a program that reduced readmissions, lengthened the time between discharge and readmission, and decreased the costs of providing health care (Naylor et al, 1999; see also Chapter 25).

The evolution of certain advanced practice specialties such as psychiatric nursing and acute care has created a climate that can be seen as supporting the development of a blended role (Naegle & Krainovich-Miller, 2001; Tappen & Dunphy, 1998; Verger et al., 2002). For example, development of the psychiatric CNS/NP role illustrates the challenges in reshaping an existing advanced practice nursing role to respond to new patient needs and health-care trends. In a review of the literature on psychiatric advanced practice nursing and the creation of educational programs to prepare a blended role psychiatric APN, several factors that relate to blended role evolution in general become clear. First, there were emerging health-care trends and population needs: psychiatric care became more outpatient based, a trend toward primary care practitioners managing psychiatric medications evolved, patients drove the need for one-stop service for prescribing and counseling, and a need arose for more skill in differentiating psychiatric illnesses from co-existing medical problems (Scharer, Boyd, Williams, & Head, 2003). Leaders in the specialty recognized that psychiatric CNS practice was changing; but achieving a consensus on evolving core competencies, curriculum revisions, and certification criteria within the specialty was difficult. The pace with which practice changed and the initial curricular efforts to accommodate these changes led to some confusion regarding core competencies. Over time, leaders recognized that divisiveness within the specialty was confusing providers, payors, and patients, which resulted in fewer referrals to psychiatric nurses as the care of their patient population was absorbed into primary care. Finally, the health-care trend toward outpatient care had a tremendous impact—both directly, on the psychiatric patient population, and indirectly, through reimbursement for APN services (Edmands, Hoff, Kaylor, Mower, & Sorrell, 1999; Hoff & Edmands, 1998; McCabe & Grover, 1999). The psychiatric specialty responded by developing curricula that offer a blended role of psychiatric CNS and primary care NP (Naegle & Krainovich-Miller, 2001; Tappen & Dunphy, 1998; Scharer et al., 2003; Verger et al., 2002). While these programs are in the early stages of development and do not yet have standardized curricula, preliminary encouraging evaluation of blended psychiatric CNS/NP practice has been reported (Scharer et al, 2003).

HEALTH-CARE TRENDS DRIVING EVOLUTION OF THE BLENDED ROLE

Current development of the blended role has been driven by a variety of forces, chiefly changing population dynamics and cost containment initiatives. Patient needs and health-care system needs have contributed to the way in which this role is being implemented.

Changing Population Dynamics

The demographics of the United States population are changing. Baby boomers are aging, creating the need and demand for affordable primary care and chronic disease management across primary, acute, and long-term care settings (Tappen & Dunphy, 1998). Prosperity and subsequent medical advances have produced better health care, resulting in a population that is living longer with chronic disease (Lynn & Harrold, 1999). These forces have caused a shift in the focus of care from younger people with more acute care health needs to older people with more chronic disease issues (Porter-O'Grady, 1997). With these population shifts has come an increasing need to improve access to more complex long-term care in a way that primary care patient issues can also be monitored.

Clinically, these trends have created the need for a provider who has both primary NP and CNS skills. The system's complexity increasingly requires the skills of both the CNS and the NP to manage growing populations of specialty and chronically ill patients—for example, the patient with cancer, the patient with congestive heart failure, the geriatric patient, or the patient requiring palliative care. As increasing numbers of patients of all ages are living with multiple chronic illnesses, they require a type of provider who can assess, diagnose, and treat illnesses commonly seen in primary care while practicing in the specialty setting and who can assist these patients to navigate a complex care system. The same emphasis on wellness and prevention found in traditional primary care settings needs to be maintained for patients who are living longer with complex chronic illnesses. The dual preparation of the blended role allows the APN to maintain a holistic perspective—seeing patients and their families across settings, assisting in negotiating multiple life stages, monitoring chronic disease processes and treatments, and helping patients and families cope with the demands of the illness. To manage complex care needs over time and across settings, blended role APNs must also be able to manage and influence the systems within which they function.

Functionally, the blended role APN also requires skills of staff education, consultation, and leadership to improve nurses' and other providers' abilities to care for these patients. It is important to note that not all patients with complex care needs require a blended role APN; they may be better served by an advanced practice nursing case manager or an acute care NP (ACNP). In addition, some institutions may have need for a particular APN such as a CNS, if staff education and support need to be a primary component of the practice. The issue of which provider is appropriate depends on a variety of factors. However, certain patients with complex care needs require a blended role APN to deliver specialty primary care across settings. This point is illustrated in the literature by the account of a CNS who had used CNS-specific skills to initiate and maintain a chronic disease clinic (Paladichuk et al., 1997). She found she could not practice independently in diagnosis and treatment, so she returned to an NP program to gain those skills. The niche for the blended role may in fact lie with chronic disease management, where the combined skills of the blended role APN are critical to ensure holistic care and state-of-the-art symptom management for patients facing longer lives with chronic disease.

Health-Care Cost Containment

The rapid pace of change in today's health-care system from an illness-driven health-care industry to one emphasizing primary health care and prevention means that organizations and individuals must accommodate multiple, simultaneous changes. Cost containment continues to be a major driving force in health care. The need to keep health-care costs down necessitates that chronically ill patients be treated in outpatient rather than inpatient settings, at the same time that specialty inpatient services are being downsized or abandoned. This has resulted in the movement of specialty care to the outpatient setting

(Lesser & Ginsberg, 2001), creating a population of outpatients who are more acutely ill. At the same time, as noted previously, there are increasing numbers of individuals who are being treated for chronic disease and still need preventive and primary care.

Cost-effective health care that prevents disease and provides quality care to those who are acutely and chronically ill is the bottom line. Efforts to control costs and to forge a new balance between primary care and illness services are changing the availability and types of positions in health care. In primary care, the patient is viewed as part of the system from birth to death, moving along a continuum of health (Mayer, 1997). At any particular time, health-care practitioners are expected to identify where a particular patient's problem fits most appropriately on the health-care continuum, with respect to both care and cost. Blended role APNs are prepared to "match" patients to the right point on the continuum to maximize appropriate care that is cost-effective.

The blended role can address many of the clinical management challenges raised by cost containment efforts while demonstrating cost-effectiveness (Brooten et al., 2002). First, patients can get accessible, timely, and appropriate primary care. In addition, it is well recognized that chronic illness care is expensive. These patients require intense follow-up and, in some cases, multiple hospital admissions (for an example, see George et al., 1999). In general, their experiences in the health-care system have made these patients more sophisticated consumers. They have higher expectations of providers and health-care systems with respect to continuity of care, access to health-care providers, and decision-making power. Familiarity with both inpatient and outpatient systems allows blended role APNs to cross care settings to provide the continuity of care that promotes effective management of chronic illness. The blended role APN also coordinates complex services to ensure continuity of care for patients in need of specialized long-term follow-up. Routine follow-up, chronic illness monitoring, and management of specialty medical problems are done by blended role APNs in collaborative practices with physicians. Blended role practitioners can play a pivotal role in assisting the patient to navigate the health-care system by providing both direct care and care coordination. The APN's specialty expertise enables him or her to recognize critical turning points in a patient's illness course and prevent unnecessary use of health-care resources through early intervention and prevention. For example, a palliative care blended role APN may recognize that an ambulatory patient with cancer who presents with abdominal pain is having narcotic-related constipation and prescribe aggressive bowel management; whereas a primary care provider, without this specialized knowledge, might assume that the patient has a bowel obstruction and admit the patient to the hospital for emergency surgery.

Various other advanced practice nursing competencies are needed and valuable when cost containment efforts are undertaken. Health maintenance organizations (HMOs) have received a great deal of attention in the press, not all of it positive (Mayer, 1997). Blended role APNs can use their consultative and educational skills to improve system problems and market effective programs to counter negative press and promote quality health care. The effectiveness of cost containment initiatives depends, in large part, on educated consumers. Because blended role APNs have in-depth specialty knowledge and are involved with individual patients across settings, they have credibility with consumers. They integrate medical and nursing therapeutics to "bring everything together" in their educational activities and programs. Blended role skills are also suited to the tasks of demand management, case management (Paladichuk et al., 1997), disease management (see Chapter 18), and other processes aimed at containing health-care costs.

Access and Affordability

Access and affordability continue to be difficult issues (Lesser & Ginsberg, 2003). The number of underinsured persons has increased, adding to populations that are underserved such as those in rural areas and those in poor, urban settings. Rural populations, in particular, have difficulty accessing the specialized services of tertiary, academic medical centers; and fewer specialists are in these areas, which may mean delays in appointments for referrals and consultations. These patients are treated in a wide variety of settings, including hospitals, freestanding clinics, private offices, public clinics, rural outreach clinics, and other "mobile" settings.

Complex care provided by blended role APNs improves access not only for people in urban or suburban areas but also for rural populations that are currently underserved because of distance and costs. Health-care economics cannot support both specialists and primary care medical providers in these areas, but blended role APNs can enhance physician practice or provide a reasonable alternative to help bridge this gap and improve access to quality care.

Increasing Specialty Knowledge Base

There is an ever-increasing knowledge base to be mastered within specialties. For example, in the hematology/oncology department in which two of us (K.S. and P.C.) work, there are now 22 APNs—blended role APNs, CNSs, and NPs. The subspecialties represented by these APN roles include breast, gynecology, gastrointestinal, hematology, genitourinary, pulmonary, palliative care, surgery, and hemophilia. Some APNs are specialized by setting, for example, inpatient or outreach. Other specialties in nursing are evolving in a similar fashion, with developing subspecialty expertise (see Chapter 19). From a knowledge standpoint, the British Medical Journal (BMJ) Publishing Group Ltd. (2001) has noted that daily there are 30 kg of guidelines produced and more than 8000 articles published in 25,000 medical journals. This growing knowledge base points both to the necessity for formal CNS training in a specialty and NP skills so that blended role APNs are adequately prepared to care for these growing subspecialty populations.

Impact of Physician and Nursing Workforce Shortages

Cost containment continues to drive policymakers to reexamine provider training and workforce needs. There are greater demands for primary care physicians to manage overall patient care and reduce costly specialty care. In the early 1990s the Council on Graduate Medical Education advocated a decrease in specialty residency programs and a restructuring of medical training to attract more physicians to primary care. The goal was to have a more even distribution of physician expertise, with 50% of physicians being generalists and 50% being specialists (Kindig, Cultice, & Mullen, 1993). This goal has not been realized; more medical school graduates chose a nonprimary care specialty than family practice in 2003, a trend that has continued for more than 5 years (American Academy of Family Physicians, 2003). The need for more primary care providers is even greater, given the growth of the elderly population and the increase in the number of chronic conditions seen as individuals age (Wolff, Starfield, & Anderson, 2002). High-level specialists who focus on one body system (such as the cardiovascular system) may overlook patients' other chronic problems (such as chronic urinary tract infections or women's health issues). This situation is one important reason that blended role APNs, with their holistic focus and delivery of primary care in specialized settings, are such a timely innovation in the current health care system.

The other dynamic in relation to the physician workforce is the mandated decrease in residency hours. Since 2003, the Accreditation Council for Graduate Medical Education has required resident hours to be restricted to 80 hours of work per week, averaged over a month (Romano, 2003). This change has dramatically reduced available hospital resident coverage and has already left some institutions in a quandary as to how they will meet patient care needs. This change represents an opportunity for a number of APNs, notably ACNPs, certified registered nurse anesthetists, and blended role APNs. Blended role APNs with specialty expertise can assist with patient management in inpatient settings as well as deliver specialty care in primary care settings.

The current nursing shortage also represents an opportunity for blended role APNs. Compared with NPs for whom the emphasis of the role is on direct clinical practice, blended role APNs have explicit responsibility for developing, educating, and supporting nursing staff to be better able to care for patients with complex specialty care needs. In this capacity, blended role APNs can promote nursing retention and help staff better design unit systems to deal with staff shortages. As Hanson and Hamric (2003) note, new advanced practice nursing roles that involve support and mentoring of hospital nurses and that replenish nursing faculty ranks need to be encouraged: the blended role APN is such a role. One institution reported an 8% increase in its nursing retention rate since implementing the blended APN role (Whitcomb et al., 2002).

The blending of CNS and NP clinical, leadership, and system competencies makes the blended role APN's marketability quite high (Cronenwett, 1995). If current healthcare trends continue, one would expect that the number of blended role APNs will significantly increase in the future.

PROFILE OF THE BLENDED ROLE APN

The professions' understanding of and consensus about the blended role are evolving. As noted, many nurses who practice in this blended role may not identify themselves as such. Rather, they may identify themselves as either CNSs or NPs, although by education and role they function as both. The number of registered nurses (RNs) educated both as CNSs and NPs has increased dramatically, and 96% of these RNs are currently practicing. From 1996 (the first year data were available) to 2000, the number of RNs with dual preparation increased from 7,802 to 14,643, an 88% increase. (Spratley, Johnson, Sochalski, Fritz, & Spencer, 2001). These numbers do not necessarily indicate that all these nurses are working in blended role positions, however, and data on blended role positions are more difficult to obtain. Within the Oncology Nursing Society (ONS), for example, there is no specific designation for a blended role APN to be identified in the Society's demographic database. Similar information was sought from the specialties of gastroenterology, pulmonary care, and critical care; however, this information was not available because it had not been collected in a way that would provide an estimate of blended role providers. A sampling of demographics published by several state boards of nursing revealed the same problem. It is very important that this role be described, documented, and monitored within general and specialty professional organizations so that accurate numbers of blended role APNs can be monitored over time.

Several key characteristics define the blended role, such as setting, education, and competencies. The competencies include both those that are core to advanced practice nursing and those that make the blended role distinct from either the NP or the CNS role.

Settings

Blended role APNs are able to both deliver limited primary care in the specialty setting and bring specialist skills to the primary care setting. At this time, blended role APNs function primarily in outpatient specialty settings but incorporate a component of inpatient care that varies, depending on patient care needs and institutional demands. Practice settings for blended role APNs range from hospitals to private practice, from intensive care units to the home setting, and from rural outreach clinics to tertiary care centers. Patient care needs dictate both the settings and the focus of practice. Regardless, crossing settings to provide continuity of care is a key distinguishing characteristic of the blended role APN.

The diversity of settings illustrates the range of practice demands placed on the blended role APN. Despite the challenges, many settings in which the skills of the blended role APN have positively affected patient care have been identified. For example, blended role APNs can be found staffing congestive heart failure clinics in the acute care setting (Paul, 1997), delivering comprehensive care in an outpatient oncology clinic (Jacobs & Kreamer, 1997) and a breastfeeding clinic (Gibbins, Green, Scott, & MacDonell, 2000), managing patients in an abdominal organ transport program (Martin, 1999), managing symptoms in a palliative care research program, managing complex care needs of elderly patients in a life-care community, or functioning in rural oncology outreach settings (Shuren, 1996). Functions of the blended role APN in these various settings include highly technical tasks, delivery of basic primary care and specialty care, staff and patient education, research, and system improvements.

Blended role APNs collaborate with a variety of providers and support staff in these various practice settings as they manage their complex patient populations. These health-care providers may include allied health-care professionals, physicians, clinical assistants (e.g., nursing assistants, physical therapy assistants), laboratory personnel, and technicians. Additionally, other patients, families, and peers assist the blended role APN in delivering care. An example of this collaborative network is as follows. The blended role APN might begin by consulting a dietitian regarding the nutritional status of a patient with cancer who is losing weight. This would be followed by collaboration with the oncologist regarding modification of the chemotherapy for that patient's disease. The APN might then teach the nursing staff about certain aspects of the patient's chemotherapy administration. Finally, the blended role provider may participate in a family meeting with a social worker to plan the patient's transfer home. The circle would be complete when the patient returns to the clinic for follow-up with the blended role APN regarding pain issues, and medications or interventions would be prescribed accordingly. This scenario illustrates the strength of the role: a blended role APN has the skills to manage patients with complex care needs by providing specialty care across practice settings, thereby facilitating the patients' passage through the health-care system.

Education

A primary feature of the blended role APN is educational preparation in two APN roles, usually a primary care NP and a CNS specialty (possibilities for other types of blended roles are discussed later in the chapter). While there are many possible ways to prepare for a blended role, preparation generally begins with specialist training in a master's degree CNS program. Master's preparation is followed by a post-master's certificate program integrating core CNS skills with the clinical skills of an NP, usually after acquiring some experience in the CNS role. In our experience, this trajectory is the most common. CNSs may be motivated to return for NP education by changes in their clinical populations, reorganization of nursing roles in their settings, changes in state regulations (Quaal, 1999), nursing workforce initiatives (Tappen & Dunphy, 1998), or other personal or professional goals. NPs may also return to graduate programs to gain CNS skills, but this path seems less common. Many programs have now been developed that offer tracks specifically for the blended role (Sperhac & Strodtbeck, 2001; Tappen & Dunphy, 1998; Scharer et al., 2003; Verger et al., 2002), so more students may be prepared in integrated graduate programs in the future. In addition, recent clinical doctoral programs have emerged for blended role APNs, a trend that is discussed later in the chapter. Regardless of the path a blended role APN student chooses, the result should be an APN who is prepared as *both a* CNS and an NP, eligible to sit for two examinations, and able to apply these skills across care environments with a specialty patient population in collaboration with specialists in other disciplines (Hoff & Edmands, 1998). By their nature, programs that prepare graduates for this role are longer.

Several criteria should be considered when programs for blended role education are chosen. The quality of faculty is critical. Instructors should have CNS and NP experience, preferably in a blended role. The availability of appropriate clinical sites is also critical. A site that already employs blended role APNs is ideal. These issues are challenging because there are few blended role APNs and there may not be appropriate clinical instruction. Experiences should be structured to first allow students to master both the specialty CNS and NP competencies and then to negotiate a clinical site that allows for or needs a blended role APN. Faculty, by necessity, must closely mentor the integration of the roles to ensure that students are adequately prepared and subsequently confident to implement the role. Based on evaluation of graduates of a blended psychiatric CNS/NP program, Scharer and colleagues (2003) noted the importance of including content on managing complex medical conditions and content and practice experiences related to CNS skills of system negotiation and consultation.

In addition, CNSs seeking to obtain NP certification should investigate both the quantity and nature of clinical time necessary to complete the program to ensure that clinical hours are sufficient to meet requirements to sit for certification. For example, the first author is an adult NP and an advanced oncology certified nurse. The adult NP exam through the American Nurses Association's American Nurses Credentialing Center (ANCC) requires that students complete 1500 hours, and the advanced oncology certified nurse exam requires 2000 hours (ONS, 2003). The ideal program will look at students individually, identify their weaknesses, and strengthen them to fulfill a blended role. Requirements for repeating previous work and courses are not useful, are expensive, and should be approached carefully. The CNS, as an expert in a specialty, may find the transition from expert to novice in an NP program stressful (see Chapter 5 for more discussion of this phenomenon), but the opportunity to bring primary care skills to the specialty setting is usually sufficient motivation to manage stress. Additionally, programs should be evaluated for proximity as well as cost. Lost wages from clinical practice should be considered in factoring educational costs. Negotiation with employers to share the cost and provide time for training can be undertaken by using the value-added aspects of blended practice as a rationale for funding. As new research providing outcomes data becomes available, this negotiation should become easier.

There are tremendous benefits from successful blended role education. Students gain a deliberative, thorough background and subsequently benefit their patients, their clinical sites, and ultimately future employers. This is demonstrated in the following exemplar.

EXEMPLAR 15-1

The advanced practice nursing curriculum at Rush University blends pediatric NP (PNP) and CNS content. The education program and the capstone project, an evidence-based protocol, demonstrate synthesis and application of the APN role components that are expected of the students near the completion of the program.

One blended role student developed and implemented a comprehensive program to address practice inconsistencies in the treatment of infants with diarrhea in an inner-city, hospital-based ambulatory clinic. During her clinical experiences, the student observed that information given by the pediatricians to parents of infants with diarrhea often differed from that given to them by the PNP. The student surveyed the pediatricians and the PNPs in the group practice about their recommendations to parents of children with diarrhea, compiled the data, conducted a literature search, and obtained the American Academy of Pediatrics guidelines for diarrhea management.

After she disseminated this information to the group for discussion, the group members reached consensus on a uniform approach to treating these infants. The student then developed a practice protocol that was later adopted by the primary care provider group. She also developed and delivered formal in-services for the clinic's professional and ancillary staff on the protocol and developed parent information sheets.

After implementing the practice changes, a formal evaluation was conducted on the education and protocol used in the treatment of children with diarrhea. In a subsequent accreditation visit by Joint Commission on Accreditation of Healthcare Organizations (JCAHO), the diarrhea program was highlighted as an example of effective quality improvement.[2]

Core Competencies: Framework for Practice

A framework for practice remains the biggest challenge facing blended role APNs. Practice has not yet been standardized across practice settings but is currently evolving with the role. It is critical to articulate blended role practice for several reasons. First, blended role APNs have a broad range of skills. Those skills must be identified in collaborative practice to clearly define the scope of practice for the blended role APN. Second, in order for blended role APNs to properly market themselves, both to potential employers and to the public, a framework for practice must be developed and communicated so that others may understand this role. Third, blended role APNs themselves must be educated to have an understanding of their unique role so they identify themselves as blended role APNs and track outcomes resulting from their practice.

Figure 15-1 provides a conceptualization of the blended role. It is important to understand this role as a distinctive practice with a distinctive title and not as a term for any APN with dual educational preparation as a CNS and NP. It is the practice of this framework of competencies that defines the blended role APN (Hanson & Hamric, 2003). The figure demonstrates that the core competencies common to all advanced nursing practice are at the center of blended role practice. Selected CNS and NP competencies combine with features unique to the blended role to shape this practice. As noted earlier,

[2]The authors gratefully acknowledge the contribution of Arlene Sperhac, PhD, RNC, PNP, Rush University College of Nursing, Chicago, for this exemplar.

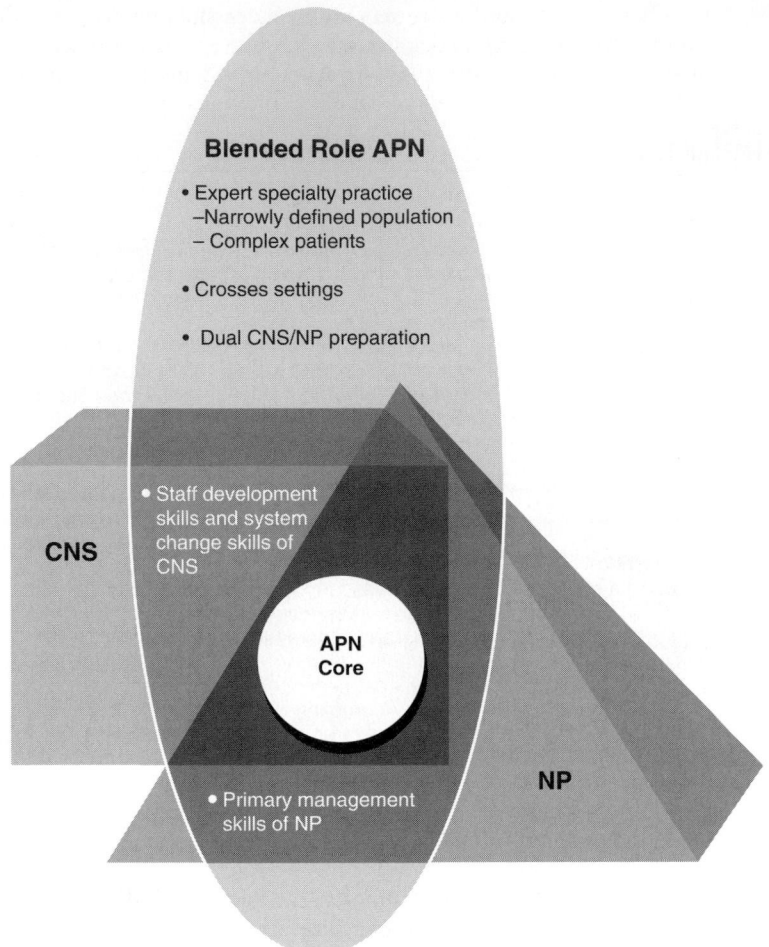

FIGURE 15-1 • Conceptual model of the blended role: framework and competencies.

expert specialty practice with a narrowly defined and complex patient population, crossing settings to deliver care, and dual CNS/NP educational preparation are three distinguishing characteristics of the blended role. This discussion of APN competencies illustrates the common APN core competencies (see Chapter 3 and Part II) as they are implemented in a blended role. As such, the following sections operationalize Figure 15-1 and illustrate the distinct ways in which blended role APNs practice.

EXPERT CLINICAL PRACTICE

Direct care of a narrowly defined population of patients with complex needs is the primary component of blended role practice. Patient care is holistic and delivered by the blended role APN as an individual or as a member of a formal team. Tasks associated with clinical responsibility vary depending on the practice setting and specialty. Expert clinical reasoning and skillful performance are used to provide basic wellness and preventive care, diagnosis and management of illness at the level of a primary care practitioner, and management of the sequela of chronic illnesses within specialty settings.

The blended role APN most often functions within a team to deliver care. Team members range from dyad models of physician–blended role APN in collaborative practice to group practices or hospital services. Team responsibilities may include patient rounds, case presentations at weekly team meetings, cross-coverage, and on-call duties. As integral members of health-care teams, blended role APNs must delineate the expanded scope of their practice and negotiate patient coverage during off time in collaboration with peers and physician colleagues. Criteria should be agreed on to identify the inpatients and outpatients whose care will be the APN's responsibility. A maximum caseload of patients must be determined to prevent overextension and to enable the APN to provide the range of services that she or he can offer. In addition, time and activities relating to ambulatory patient care should be stipulated. Specifically, the APN should have standard clinic schedule limitations on numbers of patients seen per clinic, guidelines for decision making, and protocols for staff who triage patient phone calls. Human and other resources, such as clinical assistants and computers to address clerical functions, need to be negotiated during the hiring process. Ignoring this aspect of providing care may mean that the APN performs these functions by default, compromising productivity, cost-effectiveness, and the role itself. Other personal and political consequences may ensue, such as job dissatisfaction and devaluation of the APN's contributions.

Emphasis on the direct care component of the blended role necessitates that a shift be made with respect to other role components to compensate for the time required to address direct patient care issues. For example, system responsibilities, including staff consultation, form a smaller component of blended role practice than that of the CNS role. Alternatively, there is less emphasis on the direct care component for a blended role APN than for an ACNP because of the blended role APN's emphasis on other role components. Within the direct care component, there is more emphasis on primary care for a primary care NP than for a blended role APN whose main focus is specialty care and whose secondary focus is primary care.

The holistic approach to direct care is particularly well suited to the skills of blended role APNs as they work with patients and staff. The dual knowledge base of specialty practice and primary care permits the blended role APN to provide comprehensive care for patients. As determined from interviews with recent graduates of psychiatric CNS/NP programs, this ability to practice holistically is a major source of job satisfaction (Scharer et al., 2003). The direct care management of blended role practice is shown in the following exemplar.

 EXEMPLAR 15-2

AB is a 79-year-old female who has Alzheimer's disease that was initially diagnosed 9 or 10 years ago when she moved into an apartment in a continuing care retirement community. She has been a resident in the health center's Alzheimer's unit for the last 3 years. Her level of dementia is considered to be moderate to severe, with language disturbance, severely impaired memory/recall, and dependence in all activities of daily living. Her days are filled with walking in the halls, singing, and occasional interchange with staff during therapeutic activities.

Continued

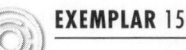

EXEMPLAR 15-2—cont'd

AB has had numerous falls without injury but, after an unwitnessed fall in the evening, was unwilling to stand and was holding onto her right hip/thigh. The registered nurse present was unable to examine the leg because of AB's agitation. The blended role APN who was on call that evening was contacted, and the situation was described. It seemed very likely from the description of the fall and the limited examination that AB had sustained a fracture. She had been lifted into bed and seemed comfortable if she was not moved. Knowing the risk of delirium inherent in sending a patient with dementia to the emergency department for evaluation, the blended role APN concluded that it was preferable to keep AB in familiar surroundings.

Consequently, she prescribed oral medications to treat the pain and ordered an x-ray examination of the hip with a mobile x-ray unit in the morning. The next day, together with AB's brother, the physician, and an orthopedic consult, the blended role APN determined a course of action/plan of care. The x-ray film confirmed a nondisplaced intertrochanteric fracture, and plans were made to admit AB to the acute care facility at 6:00 AM on the second day after the fracture for a multiple pinning procedure, with recovery in the evening and immediate transport back to the extended care facility. The orthopedic surgeon also understood that AB would begin physical therapy immediately after surgery so that she would not experience muscular atrophy resulting from immobility and would maintain baseline cognition.

Prior to admission, the blended role APN communicated with the hospital, providing great detail about AB, her dementia, and those interventions that could be used to calm her, such as singing if she became agitated while hospitalized. It was clearly communicated that AB should not receive psychotropics and should not be restrained. AB was readmitted to the long-term care unit at 9:00 AM the morning after surgery and began touch down weight-bearing on postoperative day 2. The staff was supported with education regarding the orthopedic procedure done and why she would resume activity so quickly. Her baseline cognition remained unchanged, and within 3 weeks she was walking with assistance and was singing in the halls.[3]

ETHICAL DECISION MAKING

Ethical decision-making skills (see Chapter 11) are part of the holistic approach to care provided by blended role APNs to assist patients through their illness process. Ethical decision making is necessary to help both patients and staff manage a range of issues, for example, advance directives, durable power of attorney for health care, or sedation at the end of life. One example of this is the first author's experience in a palliative care setting, assisting family members in making choices consistent with the patient's preferences for end-of-life care when the patient is terminally ill and unable to state those preferences. These skills may also be used at an organizational level by the blended role APN who is a member of an ethics committee to address institutional issues such as allocation of a drug that is in short supply. Caring for chronically ill patients facilitates formation of intricate partnerships with patients that help them with decision making, particularly when patients and family members are faced with the demands of a complex chronic illness.

EXPERT GUIDANCE AND COACHING OF PATIENTS, FAMILIES, AND OTHER CARE PROVIDERS

Blended role APNs, like all APNs, must be skilled coaches because they fulfill a variety of educational functions. Patients and families, communities, and professionals all benefit from their guidance and coaching. In addition, blended role APNs have the

---

[3]The authors gratefully acknowledge Brenda Jordan, MS, ARNP, CS, Kendall at Hanover, NH, for her assistance with this exemplar.

educational competencies to serve as formal educators for nurses and other care providers.

COACHING NURSING STAFF, OTHER PROVIDERS, AND STUDENTS

Because they work across settings and their scope of practice crosses both medicine and nursing, blended role APNs are in a strong position to influence the delivery of health care by educating providers across disciplines. Like other APNs, blended role APNs have opportunities to teach and role model for nurses and other clinicians. What may be unique for the blended role APN is the opportunity to teach and influence staff across settings—in acute, ambulatory, and home care. For example, blended role APNs engage in formal and informal teaching and role modeling of behavior for staff nurses, home care nurses, and ambulatory care nurses. Formal teaching includes classroom presentations and clinical mentoring of both graduate advanced practice nursing students and staff nurses. Blended role APNs may teach in formal educational institutions as guest lecturers or clinical instructors. They are frequently asked to assist in staff development through presentations at in-services and conferences, particularly for issues within their clinical specialty. Informally, education of peers and other providers occurs during consultation for specific patient issues as specialty knowledge is shared.

When they are caring for patients with complex needs, it is critical that blended role APNs communicate how to provide the best possible nursing care to the nurses who care for those patients on a daily basis. Conducting similar activities with medical students and residents may fall informally within the scope of practice, but the practitioner must evaluate whether to make it a formal part of her or his practice. The following exemplar illustrates this competency.

EXEMPLAR 15-3

A tertiary care medical center with a well-established oncology program established an outreach site at a community hospital 100 miles away. The physician/blended role advanced practice nurse (APN) team model in effect at the cancer center was implemented at the outreach clinic. Shortly after the clinic began treating patients, it became clear that the medical/surgical nursing staff in the community hospital were not comfortable treating patients who had previously had chemotherapy, those who were admitted with chemotherapy infusing, or those for whom chemotherapy precautions were necessary. Community hospital administrators asked the APN to address the situation and design an educational program to meet the nurses' needs.

Needs assessment, design, and implementation were enhanced by the APN's dual competencies of CNS and NP. The inpatient nursing staff were already familiar with the APN through her clinical visits to oncology inpatients. Using adult education principles and change theory, the APN developed a 4-hour program for the nurses to learn the basics of safe handling of chemotherapy and treatment of patients who would be receiving or had received chemotherapy in the past 48 hours. In collaboration with one of the clinic oncology nurses, the majority of the medical/surgical and critical care nurses at the community hospital were taught safe handling of antineoplastic drugs, patient assessment around chemotherapy administration, and precautions to observe after the chemotherapy had been administered. Vital components of the program that promoted greater acceptance were the APN's firsthand experience with administering the drugs that were being discussed and her daily experience assessing patients in the process of receiving chemotherapy and managing the accompanying side effects.

COACHING PATIENTS, FAMILIES, AND COMMUNITIES

In contemporary health care, the patient is expected to take an active role in health maintenance, and so patients must be effectively educated in order to be partners in their care. At a time when patients now need more information, providers have less time to provide it because of the reimbursement constraints imposed by the health-care system. Adding to the burden, medical advances have produced a wealth of knowledge about which patients, as well as providers, need to be informed. Blended role APNs are in an excellent position to offer both individual and programmatic patient education. Knowledge of both primary and specialty care enables them to identify the patient education needs for a defined patient population, critique existing material for applicability, and assist in development of programs and materials. While some portion of patient education is billable, funding group educational programs is frequently a challenge. Familiarity with the research process enables blended role APNs to identify and act on potential sources of grant funding for group education, while contacts made in their activities as educators and consultants help them pursue private or corporate sources of funding.

Information seeking on the Internet has become an integral part of patient education today. The Internet is used by both providers and patients to identify resources, referrals, and educational material. Much of this information can be overwhelming and misleading to patients. Blended role APNs, in utilizing their research and coaching competencies, can act as resources to filter and validate much of this information while providing the expertise to explain complex information in a way that patients can understand. The blended role APN has the opportunity to effectively educate patients with chronic illness about both specialty illness issues and wellness. Blended role APNs can focus on topics that explore how attention to primary care in the context of chronic illness improves the quality of life for chronically ill patients. Intensive and ongoing education of this population is critical to successful clinical management. In addition, blended role APNs integrate teaching and coaching activities into the direct clinical time they spend with patients. As pressures mount to see more patients in less time, this critical activity must be safeguarded.

Community or public education is also an important point of practice for blended role APNs. Their visibility across settings and their credibility as nurses make them ideal for educating groups and organizing specialty screening clinics and events. Their expert practice within the specialty gives them the added ability to offer diagnostic/screening services and make referrals to specialists based on the findings of the screening.

CONSULTATION

Blended role APNs may find themselves in the role of consultant, although in blended practice this activity will likely play a smaller part than it would for a CNS (see Chapters 7 and 12). In a review of consultation in nursing, Berragan (1998) described internal and external consultation. Internal consultation occurs within the context of the practitioner's role. External consultation occurs when the practitioner is an independently practicing consultant. Although prepared to do both, the blended role APN primarily functions as an internal consultant. As practitioners across health care settings, these APNs are consulted on a variety of patient and family issues. Consultation usually focuses on specific patient problems such as symptom management but may address broader issues such as initiating and delivering palliative care. Consultation frequently occurs between blended role APNs and physicians or other nonspecialty providers over specific patient care issues with respect to diagnosis and treatment. In a study of psychiatric CNS/NPs, a process of cross-consultation was identified. Not only did the blended role APNs consult with physicians, but physicians and nonpsychiatric NPs consulted with the APNs. In primary care settings, physicians asked for help with psychiatric–mental health problems, and in the psychiatric setting, psychiatrists asked for assistance in managing medical problems (Scharer et al., 2003). This consultation with physicians is in contrast to the role of the CNS, who most frequently consults with nursing staff for nursing care or organizational issues. Opportunities for external consultation are uncommon but may occur depending on the practitioner. One example is a pulmonary blended role APN hired as an outside consultant to assist in the development of a ventilator weaning program at a local community hospital. Consultation can be a rich source of professional satisfaction and growth and represents an important vehicle for blended role APNs to establish credibility and promote visibility, particularly when the outcomes are successful.

RESEARCH SKILLS

All APNs are prepared by graduate education to utilize research in clinical practice, to collaborate with researchers, and to use evidence-based practice approaches (see Chapter 8). They have an important opportunity to identify clinically relevant research questions directly from their clinical practice.

A variety of opportunities exist for integrating research into blended role practice. As an expert clinician and problem solver, the blended role APN is well suited to identify research topics for investigation of complex patient problems and to then follow through in research utilization and dissemination. For example, many nationally developed clinical guidelines provide answers to clinical questions such as how best to manage pain or incontinence, which may take on added complexity when applied to a particular patient group. Blended role APNs promote continuity of care by utilizing and disseminating these guidelines as they manage patients whose chronic problems cross care settings. For example, a blended role APN in oncology used evidence-based clinical guidelines to help the staff develop a pain management plan for a terminally ill patient admitted to the hospital, then followed up with that patient in the ambulatory care setting to modify the plan as the patient's condition changed. In collaboration with staff, the blended role APN can identify areas of practice that are problematic and subsequently model evidence-based practice. When faced with a clinical question, the practitioner can locate current research to answer a pressing clinical question or collaborate with others to develop an approach to answering the question—whether it is a research-based practice guideline to improve practice or a pilot study to better understand the phenomenon (Redekopp, 1997). Involvement in professional activities provides a network of colleagues who may be consulted for assistance with applying evidence or identifying potential sources of research funding for projects. Furthermore, the blended role APN may professionally present or publish the findings in order for others to benefit from the experience.

In addition to research utilization and dissemination, the blended role APN may have the opportunity to collaborate in research efforts within institutions and in large multicenter cooperative studies. As front-line providers, blended role APNs are also in an excellent position to recruit patients for participation in studies.

LEADERSHIP: CLINICAL, PROFESSIONAL, AND SYSTEMS

The variety of activities fulfilled by blended role APNs gives them the broad skills necessary to be credible leaders. Diverse experiences help mold blended role APNs into expert practitioners, change agents, and negotiators who communicate effectively. Leadership activities can be conducted locally or nationally, through organizational committees or professional groups. APNs' organizational responsibilities vary, depending on how APNs are utilized within their organization. APNs may be asked to provide staff development programs in their area of specialty or participate in a committee that forms practice guidelines for a particular patient population. In working with a particular population, they identify systematic changes that affect the care of their patients. For example, a palliative care blended role APN may identify an urgent need for designated beds within his or her institution, since the population he or she works with increasingly needs inpatient placement. The APN identifies that this need has arisen because financial concerns have forced family members to work rather than provide care at home. The APN then works at the administrative levels necessary to effect the required changes.

Leadership within the health-care delivery system is critical to successful implementation of the blended role (see Chapter 20). This component develops over time with practice and experience. It includes management of patient care through the health-care continuum and so requires the practitioner to manage diverse systems of care in order to treat the patient. Skill at working the system is gained by utilizing familiar activities of the blended role APN: problem solving, negotiation, collaboration, and education. The complexity of the health-care delivery system demands creative management approaches to patient problems, while the complexity of the modern patient demands expert clinicians. Utilization of leadership in the political arena enables APNs to be particularly effective in legislative advocacy and lobbying for health-care reform. One way to do this is to assist legislators (Milstead, 1997; Hamric, 1998) by developing connections with them, providing fact sheets, statistics, and personal vignettes. One concrete example of this was the effort by a large group of blended role APNs in our (K.S. and P.C.) oncology department to write letters to their members of congress to address ambulatory payment classifications (Mortenson, Edwards, & Bowers, 1998), an issue that greatly affected APN reimbursement. They were able to speak as providers of direct care who understood the complexities of the financial interests of the government, insurers, and their institution, as well as the effect the legislation would have on their patients.

As nurses, blended role APNs are innately trusted by the public as patient advocates. As clinicians, they have the specialty expertise to identify problems, particularly related to their respective specialties, and the experience across care settings to identify creative solutions. Considerable impact on health-care systems is possible if APNs utilize their leadership skills in policy development and implementation. For example, the blended role perspective can be applied to lobby successfully for such things as increased coverage for specialty medications for Medicare patients. Blended role APNs can use their ability to bill various payors to lobby for needed resources for their patient populations.

COLLABORATION

Interdisciplinary care has received increased attention as a model of health-care delivery in health-care systems (Simpson, 1998). By virtue of working across settings and interacting with a number of providers and staff in different settings, APNs frequently enact the collaboration competency. Blended role APNs are in a position to communicate on behalf of patients and their families with many of their caregivers within the health-care system, reducing the burden on patients to reexplain to yet another person their history, needs, etc. This competency is integrated into blended role practice on many levels, as demonstrated by the variety of peers and providers with whom blended role APNs interact. Collaborative efforts facilitate patient care across settings, aid in problem solving, and provide many professional opportunities. Interdisciplinary care environments provide opportunities to develop true collaborative practice with physicians, because patients such as those with chronic illness are in need of integrated care from both medicine and nursing. In Chapter 10 the collaboration competency is discussed in detail.

The following exemplar demonstrates how a blended role APN collaborated with other advanced practice nursing providers to manage a variety of clinical and system issues in a particular patient case.

EXEMPLAR 15-4

Mr. P is an 84-year-old gentleman with newly diagnosed advanced esophageal cancer, macular degeneration, and very mild dementia. He is seen by the blended role oncology advanced practice nurse (APN) at his local community outreach clinic, part of the nearest comprehensive cancer center. During his assessment the APN finds that he lives alone in a bordering town and he is currently carrying out all of his activities of daily living independently. He has a family but they do not live locally and are not able to be directly involved in his care. His disease and treatment regimen are reviewed, and the oncologist offers radiation and concurrent chemotherapy at the regional cancer center. Knowing that he is at risk for confusion regarding this complex regimen because of his baseline mild dementia, that there is a high potential for development of problematic symptoms, and that his prognosis is poor, the oncology APN makes two referrals. The first referral is to a blended role oncology APN colleague at the regional cancer center to monitor him clinically and assist in his care at the larger institution. The second is to the blended role palliative care APN to obtain assistance with both symptom management and facilitating a plan for end-of-life care. All three APNs keep in constant communication by phone and e-mail. After his first dose of chemotherapy, the patient was seen and evaluated by the palliative care APN who recognized acute dehydration and was able to facilitate his admission in collaboration with the oncologist. After discharge, he continued to be followed up by the oncology APNs who subsequently discussed a dose reduction with the oncologist for safety reasons to avoid another admission. The palliative care APN meanwhile was able to work with Mr. P's daughter regarding plans for his continuing care once therapy ended. The communication between providers led to successful holistic management of this gentleman through radiation and medical oncology departments, across the inpatient setting for an admission for treatment of dehydration, and back to the outpatient setting in an assisted care facility. In this way, a safety net was created that was able to help him successfully complete his treatment, and with his family, to plan for his continuing care.[4]

Differentiating Blended Role Practice from Other APN Roles

What differentiates blended role practice from other advanced practice nursing roles? As shown in Figure 15-1, three characteristics distinguish the blended role APN. First, blended role APNs are educationally prepared differently than other practitioners, because they learn both CNS and NP roles and expectations. Second, because of this preparation, blended role clinical practice differs from that of the CNS and NP in that the blended role APN crosses settings while clinically managing a specialty population. These two characteristics have created the third, in that the blended role APN cares for a more narrowly defined complex patient population than other APNs, for example, pediatric patients, patients with cancer, geriatric patients with chronic disease, or adult patients with cardiac disease. This narrow focus is necessary to enable staff education and support, as well as system change activities characteristic of the blended role.

Hanson and Hamric (2003) attempted to clarify the blended role by listing practices that are not blended CNS/NP practice. "We would submit that the blended CNS/NP role is NOT: a CNS who has returned to school for an NP credential and is practicing as an NP . . .;

[4]The authors gratefully acknowledge the contribution of Constance Dahlin, RN, APRN, BC, PCM, Massachusetts General Hospital, Boston, MA for this exemplar.

a graduate of an educational program that has homogenized the distinctive features of the CNS and NP so that neither role is clearly taught . . . [or] a specialty NP that crosses settings but has a strictly patient-focused practice" (Hanson & Hamric, 2003, pp. 208-209).

The blended role APN differs the most from the APN case manager. Both are educationally prepared for the role of primary coordinator of care by virtue of their master's degrees so they share some role overlap (see Chapter 18). The APN case manager is accountable for clinical and fiscal outcomes. While the blended role APN cannot afford to be oblivious to fiscal outcomes, primary responsibility will fall to someone else. In the role of an APN case manager, there is greater emphasis on organization, coordination, and monitoring of patient care (Smith, 1994) and on system-level interventions to enhance quality of care and contain costs. The most notable difference in practice is evident in the level of direct tertiary clinical management of patients. Most advanced practice nursing case management models include elements of direct patient assessment and clinical decision making in ambulatory care settings but end there. Although APN case managers closely monitor established patients when they are admitted to the hospital, they typically relinquish direct patient management to the hospital-based team.

The blended role APN's scope of clinical practice differs from the ACNP's scope in the amount of outpatient follow-up that is incorporated into clinical responsibilities, as well as the CNS activities of staff support and systems change. Unlike the ACNP, who is responsible for a variety of acutely or critically ill patients and for limited ambulatory care activities (if any), the blended role APN is responsible for ongoing follow-up of a particular patient population across settings. The blended role APN has a greater focus on primary care than does the ACNP, having a greater opportunity to meet primary care needs as patients present for follow-up in outpatient clinics. For example, the blended role APN may discover that a breast cancer survivor has not had a colonoscopy as recommended by current guidelines for colon cancer screening and would follow up with the appropriate referral. A blended role APN who cares for a woman with chronic obstructive pulmonary disease (COPD) may treat her for a simple urinary tract infection while also seeing her for an exacerbation of COPD. As this practitioner cares for a patient with complex needs, the care delivered is "complete" in that the whole person must be addressed. The ACNP is more often treating a specific acute problem. Another difference in focus is illustrated by a descriptive report of the ACNP role (Kleinpell, 1998) in which mean time spent in the clinical practice component was reported to be 89%. Other activities of teaching, research, and staff education played a much smaller part in ACNP practice than they would in blended role APN.

The blended role APN also has responsibility for fulfilling CNS competencies in nursing and system spheres of influence (National Association of Clinical Nurse Specialists, 1998) in addition to the focus on primary care in a specialty setting. However, the time spent in these nondirect patient care activities is more limited than it would be for the CNS. The blended role APN is also distinguished from the CNS who completes a certificate NP program but returns to her or his current position, functioning strictly as a CNS without an expanded focus on direct and primary care. One example presented in the literature is the case of an NP and a CNS who worked collaboratively in building a pediatric diabetes program (Page & Mackowiak, 1997). They each needed a part of the other's role to meet the needs of their patient population.

It is challenging to clarify the role differences among NP, CNS, and blended role APN. One particular primary care setting was described by a critical care CNS who became a family NP as follows:

Without my knowledge of secondary care, hospital practice . . . it would be very difficult and uncomfortable [practicing in my new primary care role]. Additionally, it was quite helpful when two [patients with] acute myocardial infarctions, two hemorrhages, and one case of acute, severe respiratory distress presented in the office during my first seven months of practice. . . . the most frequent questions asked me [by patients] had to do with my experiences in critical care, cardiology, and trauma. Few questions were asked about my family practice experience. This seemed a little odd at first. However, the reason for the interest in secondary care experience soon became clear. Many patients in our practice have chronic disease like chronic obstructive pulmonary disease, coronary artery disease, and congestive heart failure that require hospitalization at times. They wanted to make sure I knew what to do when [it was my turn to make] rounds. (Crotty, 1998, pp. 19-20)

This family NP, although utilizing CNS specialty knowledge, is not practicing in a blended role because he is functioning as a primary care clinician in one clinical setting. There are CNSs and NPs currently in practice who identify their role as blended but who may not practice in a true blended role. The distinction is that the blended role APN utilizes the NP role and all dimensions of the CNS role in a specialty setting. Various examples of the blended role in different practice settings are beginning to appear in the literature; two such settings are a breastfeeding clinic (Gibbins et al., 2000) and an outpatient congestive heart failure clinic (Paul, 1997). The blended role APNs in these settings describe clinical responsibility for their specialty population across settings, the educational role with patients, families and staff, the research role of evaluating clinical outcomes, and the systems focus in managing system/organizational issues.

EVALUATION OF BLENDED ROLE PRACTICE

In addition to determination of the impact of the blended APN role on patient outcomes, evaluation is necessary for financial justification of the position and future development. Cost analysis should focus not only on dollars saved or earned by virtue of having a blended role APN but on clinical outcomes, so that value can be demonstrated. Initial research supports the validity of this role (Naylor et al., 1999). Models are being developed to test outcomes that are specific for advanced practice nursing and that support the need for blended role functions (Brooten et al., 2002). All APNs must support their practice by aggressive use of computer technology to track data in local and national databases to demonstrate accountability for their outcomes (see Chapter 25). A lack of specific historical measures upon which to base blended role practice evaluation has slowed research for the blended role; such measures are important to provide validity and illustrate the value of the role to health-care institutions.

The first step is identification or development of valid and reliable tools that can be used in a variety of settings. Many tools exist to standardize health-care data collection (see Chapter 25). While no evaluation tool currently captures the blended role, many contain useful measures of patient outcomes that could be used to demonstrate the impact of this practice. Blended role practice may have the added value of improving both processes of care and outcomes such as patient satisfaction, adherence to therapy, and improved health maintenance. These outcomes should be studied in settings where blended role APNs practice.

Donabedian's (1966) model of structure, process, and outcome components of evaluation supports the blended role because it captures many different aspects of care, both direct and indirect (see Chapter 25). Consultation with outcome managers (Fleschler & Luquire, 1998) in hospital quality improvement departments and outcome management programs can help the blended role APN address such issues as when to measure an outcome, to what level of analysis the research should be taken, and how to achieve appropriate scientific rigor (Carroll & Fay, 1997) for what is being studied. In order to conduct complete outcome studies, the issue of admission privileges for blended role APNs must be addressed. For example, tracking admission and readmission rates could be very useful for evaluating a practitioner's ability to manage a patient population clinically across settings and over time. However, because admission privileges for APNs are restricted, most often by state or institutional policy (Kinney, Hawkins, & Hudman, 1997), admission rates often cannot be accurately determined for an individual blended role APN. Thus while outcomes may well be improved by the continuity of care available through blended role practice, it is exceedingly difficult to conduct outcome studies that measure this continuity.

It is clear that comprehensive practice evaluation must be a priority for all APNs in order to describe their roles and measure their practice. Performance measures specific for blended role APNs must be developed. Efforts have begun for other nursing roles (Herman, 1998; Irvine, Sidani, & McGillis-Hall, 1998), including NP and CNS roles, that can be adapted to create models for blended role performance measures. Measures such as the Health Plan Employer Data and Information Set (HEDIS) (NCQA, 2003) which measure performance, are useful as tools both to address liability issues and to demonstrate a blended role APN's impact on the quality of care. (These issues are discussed more extensively in Chapter 25.)

CHALLENGES IN IMPLEMENTATION OF THE BLENDED ROLE

Many issues are raised in blending the CNS and NP roles that, if not addressed, can create confusion both inside and outside the profession. It is critical to focus on blended role APN definition and clarity, not the job title (see Chapter 3; Hamric & Hanson, 2003), to avoid confusion. The blended role is relatively new, so the degree of clarity that facilitates a consensus as to titling does not yet exist. This lack of clarity is the first hurdle to overcome to strengthen implementation of blended role practices. Examining the advantages and disadvantages of blending from the perspective of a variety of stakeholders can help address issues of role development and identity. Blending the CNS and NP roles affects not only individual practitioners but also the disciplines of both medicine and nursing. In addition, as noted earlier, health-care consumers have a stake in how this role evolves, and indeed, may affect future role implementation.

Titling

Difficulties with advanced practice nursing titling (Fitzpatrick, 1998) and a summary of efforts to build consensus around the meaning of advanced practice nursing (see Chapter 3) have been described. However, it must be acknowledged that if and when the term *advanced practice nurse* is accepted by the profession and policymakers as embracing a variety of advanced practice nursing positions, the issue of titling the blended role APN will remain difficult. Spross and Hamric (1983) proposed the advanced registered nurse practitioner (ARNP) title for the role described in this chapter. Since that time, the ARNP title has been increasingly used in state regulations to refer to the NP. Consequently, it has significant problems as a title and does not readily convey that the APN possesses blended role skills. The blended role is an advanced practice nursing role that is in need of a clear title in order to articulate the uniqueness of the role to both professionals and the public.

Some authors suggest designating blended role APNs as advanced NPs (Dunn, 1997). This idea has merit because it could distinguish the blended role from both the CNS and NP roles through the designation *advanced*, or through naming the specialty, such as *oncology NP*. For example, in 1994 the American Nurses Association and other organizations wrote a practice statement that made the psychiatric CNS eligible for NP certification and titling as a psychiatric NP (Caverly, 1996). This is not necessarily a blended role, but it does highlight the specialty skills of the APN. The difficulty with this title is the absence of any explicit CNS designation.

Some leaders have advocated using the generic title of *APN* for the blended role (Snyder & Mirr, 1995). This stance supports the merging of CNS and NP roles into one advanced practice nursing role. Combining the skills and competencies of the CNS and NP has been the focus of this chapter and is an important trend in the continuing evolution of advanced practice nursing. However, the title *APN* is more appropriately used as an umbrella term to describe all advanced practice roles, including CNS, certified nurse-midwife, certified registered nurse anesthetist, NP, ACNP, and APN case manager, as well as the blended CNS/NP role (see Chapter 3). Titles should reflect the actual practice and should be unique if the practice is unique. Because the blended role APN is a distinct advanced practice role, it needs a distinct title.

This leaves the possibilities of *blended role APN* and *CNS/NP*. In practice, the first author (KS) uses NP when introducing herself to patients because the public is more likely to be familiar with this term. When interacting with other health-care professionals, this author endeavors to explain and clarify the blended role by explaining the similarities and differences between her practice and the practices of CNSs and NPs. In professional identification, this author and most of her departmental colleagues use the credentials "MSN, ARNP" (New Hampshire's regulatory designation for the adult NP) to designate a blended role.

The alternative title of *CNS/NP* has not been widely explored, nor has it been used often in the literature. This title was seen in a recent article that used the designation *psychiatric CS/NP*, indicating both the specialty and the blending of CNS (with use of the initials CS for clinical specialist) and NP roles (Scharer et al., 2003). This possibility deserves to be considered, because it clarifies the specialty focus of the APN and explicitly denotes both CNS and NP roles merged into one practice. However, this option may be viewed as cumbersome and confusing to consumers. As the blended role is becoming more clearly definable as a distinct advanced practice nursing role, this lack of a consensus title represents an increasing problem in marketing (Maclaine, 1998). Employers may have some understanding of what role they need but not enough of an understanding to properly advertise and attract the appropriate candidates. As noted, examples of blended role practice were found with authors referring to themselves as *NPs*, or just *APNs* (Paul, 1997; Paladichuk, 1997). Nursing leaders, including those in practice and in education, need to come to consensus on the title and preparation for the blended role APN if it is to become a fully legitimate advanced practice nursing role.

Balancing NP and CNS Responsibilities in the Blended Role

Both CNSs and NPs come to blended role practice with special skills and a role identity developed through education, experience, and socialization. Therefore both will need to create a new identity as blended role APNs (Wright, 1997). This may present a challenge as the role itself evolves. Role identification and clarification require both a degree of tolerance for ambiguity and the determination to define a new role. In the quest to define this role, blended role APNs must be careful to maintain their nursing focus. Blended role APNs frequently work within a medical model in collaborative practice with physicians. It would be easy to adopt a medical model, but the greatest strength of the role is the nursing focus it brings to health care.

There are many issues to consider specific to the CNS component of the blended role. Historically, the clinical expertise of CNSs has been limited to the inpatient setting, where the critical roles of educator, consultant, and researcher have been relatively "invisible"—both publicly and politically. The public's interaction with a CNS is generally limited to management of a clinical issue in the inpatient setting. In response to a need for specialty nursing care in the outpatient setting, some CNSs have developed a practice in the outpatient setting. The public may have more contact with the few CNSs who work in collaborative practices, but the limitations of lack of prescriptive privileges in many states and inability to provide overall clinical management are frequently difficult to overcome. Blending the roles helps to address many of these issues while expanding the scope of advanced practice nursing across settings.

However, institutions that have converted their CNSs to blended role APNs must carefully consider the consequences for staff support. Provision of staff support is an important component of blended role practice. Shuren (1996) suggested that her outpatient activities enabled her to identify and resolve a problem with inpatient staff's patient education practices. However, the blended role APN is unable to provide staff support to the extent that a CNS can. The impact of blending in the inpatient setting has been to create a need for additional CNSs dedicated to staff support, because blended role providers primarily move across settings and are not as available for extended staff support. Because of their greater direct care management responsibilities, blended role providers spend significant time with outpatients and so are limited in the amount of time they have to provide support to staff. It is critical for institutions to recognize this; otherwise, the gains made in improving the care of chronically ill patients by blended role APNs will be offset by patient readmissions caused by a lack of staff education, increased staff turnover, and/or poor nursing care resulting from lack of support by a CNS (Page & Arena, 1994). Therefore the development of the blended role must progress with concurrent support of CNS positions.

Several issues of particular concern to the NP component of the blended role have been identified in the literature (Wright, 1997), but few are currently relevant. NPs stand to strengthen their credibility with the specialty focus and added competencies acquired with CNS preparation. In addition, because NPs have been accused of losing their nursing roots by training within a medical model, blending strengthens their alliance with the nursing profession. As cost control efforts continue, the real concern should be focused on the inevitable time when NPs and blended role APNs both become increasingly subject to the demands of the system to see more patients in less time, as is currently the case for physicians. This needs to be addressed by NPs and blended role APNs at both the institutional and national levels to advocate that critical nursing functions remain a part of patient care. Research documenting outcomes of successful educational programs will assist in this effort (see George et al., 1999 and Chapter 25).

Incorporating all of the competencies described previously with these characteristics means that blended role APNs are continually challenged by issues of balance and emphasis on role components in their practice. Individual blended role APNs must be clear about their roles and scopes of practice in order to continue to meet patient needs and avoid becoming subject to the restructuring of positions as institutions struggle with a dynamic health-care system.

Impact on Physicians

The blended CNS/NP role clearly affects physicians. Within primary care, the blended role APN can strengthen what the primary care physician has to offer. For example, the first author, as an oncology CNS, completed a clinical rotation with a primary care physician for her NP program. She was able to help educate that physician, also a new hospice director, about current pain management strategies. The blended role APN prepared in a specialty can expand the ability of a primary care practitioner to manage a wide range of chronic illnesses and the symptoms resulting from those illnesses. Alternatively, blended role APNs can ensure that primary care issues are addressed and appropriately managed in the specialty setting. Even though a medical specialist does not have primary care training, patients seen on a frequent basis use their physician specialist as a primary care provider (Rosenblatt, Hart, Baldwin, Chan, & Schneeweis, 1998). In the study by Rosenblatt and colleagues (1998), pulmonologists, oncologists, and gynecologists each had a substantial proportion of patients—27%, 21%, and 20%, respectively—for whom they provided care outside their specialty domain. In general, specialists provided out-of-domain care to patients with whom they had a majority-of-care relationship. This intuitively makes sense and points to a system of care that has not been explicitly addressed. Patients whose care is usually delivered by a specialist do not want to make another trip to a generalist if the specialist is willing to take care of the primary care problem. An example in the first author's institution is a blended role APN who performs routine Pap smears when indicated for patients seen by the oncologist with whom she collaborates. Though seldom acknowledged, this phenomenon of providing primary care for acute issues seems to be relatively common, because it is an efficient practice and patients appreciate such service. Over time, the blended role provider could become the primary provider of record for selected chronically ill populations. This system would promote continuity of care, ensuring that both specialty and primary care needs of chronically ill patients are met in a timely, efficient, and effective manner.

The blended role can be perceived to have both negative and positive effects on the medical profession. Some physicians have expressed a perceived loss of identity: if blended role APNs can do the tasks of a physician, then what is left for that physician to do? This can lead to the perception of being threatened and can result in conflict over issues related to competition. For example, the first author had a situation in which she was seeing a patient with cancer in the outpatient setting for arm pain and discovered a pathologic fracture. Appropriate referrals were made to orthopedics and radiation oncology, but the primary care physician believed in that case that he should have been the practitioner to see the patient for pain control and a sling. In response to this concern, it is important to note that clear role limitations have been established by state nurse practice acts as to what is and is not within nursing's scope of practice. Clear communication with local primary care physicians should take place in a collaborative fashion to determine how the blended role practitioner can best serve the patient within his or her community. The emphasis should be on the value-added complement to medical care that the blended role APN brings to patients and to the practice (see Chapter 3). In addition, the blended role APN's ability to function is different when the APN is providing primary care versus specialty care. For example, in the oncology specialty, blended role APNs licensed to function as primary care NPs can diagnose and treat primary care problems in the specialty setting. However, they are not licensed to initially diagnose and treat a disease within the specialty, nor can they bill for a specialty new patient visit. This limits their practice within specialty settings and therefore should reduce the perception of competition with oncologists.

Finally, role limitations are dictated by the credentialing and privileging system within many institutions. These limitations are important and should be utilized by experienced blended role APNs who may find themselves asked to stretch beyond their scope of practice because of their competence. Within specialty practice, these role limitations must be maintained because APNs are not physicians, and there are certain tasks that may not be within the scope of blended role nursing practice. These tasks may need to be formally defined for each specialty (e.g., the ACNP may perform more medical procedures), but they are also negotiated by each practitioner within the existing institution's privileging policy. The blended role APN, by definition more limited in specialty practice, can participate in that portion of patient care that is within her or his scope of practice, providing advanced nursing care (e.g., managing pain medication in terminal stages of cancer) and freeing the physician specialist to be a specialist. This can provide both practitioners with time to remain current and pursue professional interests.

Accountability Issues

By definition the blended role APN is both CNS and NP. Therefore to whom is the blended role APN directly accountable? It is an important question, for accountability entails both a reporting structure and a philosophical clinical practice alliance. Various possibilities should be considered thoroughly when this role is implemented. Historically, the CNS has been accountable to nursing, and this is a strong reason to implement the blended role position under the direction of nursing. The functions of educator, consultant, and researcher are likely to be most utilized by nursing. However, the clinical component of the position may be more logically aligned with medicine. Collaborative practice models and many NP positions are often structured with accountability to medicine or jointly to medicine and nursing. In addition, it could be argued that medicine has the most to learn about advanced practice nursing from the blended role APN, and so a greater impact on the system can be made by accountability to medicine. There is no one correct answer to this question. Each practitioner must assess the practice and strengths and weaknesses of the system and use her or his negotiation skills to establish an appropriate route of accountability for a given position and setting. It is critical, however, for the accountability structure to support a balanced practice so that both CNS and NP components are visible.

PROMOTING SUCCESSFUL ROLE DEVELOPMENT AND IMPLEMENTATION: STRATEGIES AND BARRIERS

The journey to the blended CNS/NP role can be long and painful. Discarding or modifying a former role socialization in favor of a new one can be uncomfortable, and transitioning from expert to novice to expert can be frustrating. Implementation of the blended APN role is a challenge. The practitioner faces a variety of issues that need to be addressed for success to be achieved. Recognition of the role's duality is the first issue to address because it presents many challenges. Duality creates the biggest challenge in meeting the demands of diverse role activities in a blended role position. Although diversity is a central component of role success, excellent time management skills are required to balance the demands that this diversity creates.

Several keys to success in APN development can be applied specifically to the blended role (Brown, 1998). First, as noted earlier, a clear scope of practice mutually agreed upon in a collaborative practice is critical for the blended role APN to function efficiently and avoid turf issues. Second, there must be consensus regarding schedule and workload. This consensus must be negotiated at the time the provider is hired and should be formally reviewed on a regular basis. Third, organizational support for the role must exist. The organization must value the blended role APN and provide support for a balanced role. Interdisciplinary networks for collaboration, consultation, and referral should be available for the practitioner to be most effective. These networks may not exist in some settings but can be established during role implementation or made available through Internet access and formal organizational affiliations for blended role APNs. Developing interdisciplinary and intradisciplinary relationships and lines of support are important to role success.

Fourth, one priceless asset in development of the successful blended role is peer support. Peer support is vital to assist in problem solving, provide collegial support, and collaborate in outcomes research. The blended role is among the newest APN roles to be developed. Therefore it is critically important that opportunities for sharing issues regarding development and implementation of the role be provided in order to facilitate problem solving. A setting without multiple peers is common, but developing a regional peer network through online discussions, formal meetings, and informal consultation should be integral to the practice of any blended role APN.

In addition to peer support, effective leadership can facilitate role development and support within the practice setting or institution. An effective leader who can mentor, advocate for academic time, negotiate hours and responsibilities, and encourage research development will ultimately foster development of the successful blended role practitioner. The following exemplar illustrates the power of organizational and peer support, and strong leadership.

 EXEMPLAR 15-5

Over the past 10 years at the authors' (K.S. and P.C.) tertiary academic medical center, the advanced practice nursing group in the cancer center has grown from 6 to 22 advanced practice nurses (APNs), most of whom are blended role practitioners. The APNs were accountable to the physicians with whom they worked on a daily basis, and ultimately, to the section chief (a physician). During that time, as new practitioners were added, it became clear that the group needed to meet on a regular basis to discuss department issues that affected them and to obtain peer support. Leadership among the APNs rotated on a yearly basis.

Out of that group, APNs developed careers over time that took on local, regional, and national recognition and accountability. The APN group realized that their clinical practice and career development needs were such that they needed one leader who could foster development of the group in terms of clinical practice, education, and research. They wanted these goals to be consistent with the goals of the institution. The group had enormous potential to add to the cancer center but needed a focus for integration and representation at administrative levels that were not yet accessible.

Over the course of a year, the group met with a facilitator to identify their vision, mission, and goals. A director-level position was created to serve as the focal point for launching this organized group and integrating the APNs into the section. This organizational change has meant the APNs now have direct accountability to a peer, rather than to a physician. As a result, over the past 2 years, the group has accomplished such tasks as recognition and support for protected academic time, re-engineering the review process so it is conducted by and supervised by peers, and collectively authoring many publications. Two retreats have been held, the second of which focused entirely on formation and development of the group's research agenda and resulted in the group's active contribution to a National Institutes of Health (NIH) core grant application for funding the cancer center.

Dealing with Role Strain

Specific barriers can be identified in development of the blended role. The challenge of role strain is of most concern. An important question to ask is, "Is the blended role APN trying to be everything to everyone?" The NP and CNS roles are each valuable roles in themselves. The blended role APN must give up a piece of each of these roles in the blending process in order to be successful. The risk for role strain leading to burnout is a serious one. APNs who try to be everything to everyone will soon find themselves with more responsibility than they can handle. They run the risk of doing an inferior job with too broad a scope of practice rather than doing a good job with a limited scope of practice. These risks are analogous to those experienced by CNSs in the 1980s (Hamric, 1989).

One example of how this issue arises is in the performance of medical procedures such as a lumbar puncture, paracentesis, or special surgical technique. When determining whether to include either a medical task or any other responsibility in blended role practice, the provider must decide whether doing the task will meet the ultimate goal of quality patient care. Careful consideration of several questions may be helpful in this evaluation process. Is the task within the state's nurse practice act, and is it legal? Is the task nursing or medical, and is this issue important? Will adequate training be provided for the APN to take on this new task or responsibility? How much time will be spent doing the task and how much will it benefit the specific patient population? What aspect of practice will the provider have to give up to make room for the added responsibility? What is the risk/benefit ratio of the task for the provider and/or the patient? What are the political ramifications of accepting or declining the responsibility? Investigation of these questions can be used to clarify limits on practice that are consistent with meeting the needs of both patients and the institution.

Successful development depends on two additional concepts. First, the diversity of skills defined by each role (Jacobs & Kreamer, 1997) is critical to successful implementation of the role. Second, successful time management is important for both professional success and personal satisfaction. As noted, success in the blended role requires balance and time management. Balance in this role may be difficult to achieve, but the balanced practice as described earlier must be maintained. For example, blended role APNs may be asked to participate in multiple educational programs in the settings where they practice. Over time, accepting too many of these commitments can lead to difficulty in managing competing priorities. Skilled negotiation with administrators and colleagues to balance activities such as patient care, research, patient and staff education, and improving system practices is critical. The goal is to avoid excessive emphasis on any one activity, and this presents a challenge, particularly because the clinical component generates revenue. However, a balance must be created in order to successfully maintain the diversity that the blended role offers and to maintain job satisfaction.

Educational Issues

Another potential challenge to blended role APNs is educational preparation and continuing education (Conger & Craig, 1998). In the current health-care system, one difficulty at times lies in attempting to match either a CNS or an NP to a position that may require the skill of both roles. While many blended role skills can be acquired on the job, acquisition of skills in this way requires competent preceptorship with collaborating practitioners who have the time to adequately impart those skills. A CNS functioning in a pulmonary clinic is an expert in pulmonary care but may lack the primary care skills to ensure comprehensive care. Similarly, an NP in the same setting may have the skills to provide good primary care but would require years of on-the-job training to function at the level of a CNS specialized in pulmonary care. The health-care system can no longer pay for the time required for those practitioners to acquire skills they lack on the job. It is becoming increasingly evident that both expert clinical skills of the NP and interpersonal, collaborative, research, and leadership skills of the CNS are needed to treat certain patients with complex care needs in today's dynamic health-care system (Wright, 1997). Both primary treatment and management of acute and chronic illness have increased in complexity and require more specialized training.

FORMAL EDUCATION

The increasing interest in preparing blended role APNs is evident in a recent report of enrollment in graduate education programs (Berlin, Stennett, & Bednash, 2003). As of Fall 2002, 43 programs offering combined NP and CNS preparation enrolled or graduated 1771 students, or 4% of total APN graduates (p. 51).Thirteen different clinical track titles in combined NP and CNS programs were listed; all included primary care NP preparation except for psychiatric and neonatal specialties.

As noted, graduate programs that offer a combined CNS/NP blended role curriculum should be longer to ensure sufficient preparation for both roles and may need to incorporate a year of extra education for graduates to be eligible to sit for both NP and specialty certifications. Generic programs that merge content and do not prepare students for the specific CNS and NP competencies needed for blended role practice are doing their students a disservice, and potential students should examine curricula carefully for evidence that both roles are taught. As Scharer and colleagues noted, "as new content and skills are added to accommodate the NP component of the role, it is essential that critical CS content and skills are not lost" (2003, p. 143).

One emerging recommendation for APN education with relevance for the blended role is the professional or clinical doctorate. A number of authors have advocated expanding education for advanced practice nursing to the doctoral level, in programs geared toward practice rather than the traditional research-oriented PhD (Fitzpatrick, 2003; Mundinger et al., 2000; Pearson, Borbasi, & Gott, 1997). Fitzpatrick (2003) noted that many other professional disciplines have moved toward expecting clinical doctorates for clinical teaching and expert clinical practice, specifically the PharmD for pharmacy and the PsychD for psychology. In fact, although they do not use the term, Mundinger and colleagues (2000) appear to be referring to the blended role APN in their discussion of "differentiated cross-site, full-scope practice" (p. 326). Given the expanded competency set necessary for blended role APN, the profession may need to give careful consideration to doctoral preparation for this evolving advanced practice nursing role (Hanson & Hamric, 2003).

The issues surrounding these proposals to move to a clinical doctorate for advanced practice nursing in general and the blended role in particular are beyond the scope of this chapter, and some believe the move is premature in the absence of consensus on curricula, degree name, and evidence to support the need for such educational preparation (Minnick & Halstead, 2002; Hanson & Hamric, 2003). In a call for a shared strategic vision to shape this initiative, a National Organization of Nurse Practitioner Faculty (NONPF) Task Force expressed support for the practice doctorate (NONPF, 2003). But these nursing leaders also detailed a number of challenges that are not yet resolved, commenting, "only time will tell if the practice doctorate is truly the future or just a fringe movement" (p. 6).

CONTINUING EDUCATION

Finding appropriate continuing education can also be a challenge for blended role APNs. The practitioner must take the responsibility to maintain continuing education (CE) in both specialty and primary care practices. For CE for blended role APNs, national meetings of primary care NP and specialty organizations are likely to provide the best opportunities for advanced practice nursing–related CE. APNs also have opportunities to pursue CE on the Internet and through journal subscriptions. Blended role APNs have the challenge of staying informed about clinical updates related to both roles. Some specialty organizations such as the ONS are likely to offer educational opportunities related to both roles. However, it will most likely be up to the individual practitioner to choose offerings from both specialty organizations and primary care organizations, depending on what is needed for their clinical practice.

This can be a challenge but should become easier as more blended role APNs are educated and begin practicing. CE is also an issue facing physician specialists. The amount of new information to process in order to keep current in their profession is growing beyond the ability of the specialists to manage, particularly within the current health-care system. The value of a blended role APN in this context is in augmenting the practice of the physician specialist, leaving time for both to pursue appropriate continuing education. One strategy to define a realistic practice is to negotiate regular protected time for professional activities, particularly those of education and research. This may be difficult to do and is most successful when it is negotiated at the time of hire.

A LOOK TO THE FUTURE

While this chapter has described the blending of primary care NP and CNS roles, other possibilities for blended roles exist. For example, a blended CNS/neonatal NP role has been described as a preferred role for a breastfeeding clinic in Canada (Gibbins et al., 2000). At the second author's (AH) institution, students have expressed an interest in blending ACNP and CNS roles. Evolving specialties such as wound, ostomy and continence nursing and transplant nursing may benefit from proactive development of blended role educational programs to develop the competencies needed to care for their complex patient populations. As the need for staff nurse support and skill in treating patients across systems continues to grow, we believe that interest in blended roles will also grow. The challenge as specialties and subspecialties proliferate is to define a cohesive understanding of blended role practice to guide education and role enactment. This chapter has described such an understanding, and evidence of this definition of the blended role APN is evident in the literature.

A Call for a Cohesive Deliberative Approach

The debate continues: Why blend the CNS and NP roles? The answer to this question lies in the present needs of patients with complex problems, the demands of the evolving health-care system, and in how the profession chooses to shape the future of advanced practice nursing.

Despite demands by the health-care system, nursing as a profession must maintain control over the development of the blended role. It is critical that the profession be deliberative and cohesive in its approach, rather than allow blended role practice to evolve haphazardly in ways not consistent with the blending of CNS and NP skills. The risk of losing control over development is that fragmentation and further confusion occur, which will weaken the public's understanding and support of advanced practice nursing. In addition, losing control over development could result in loss of the diverse components of the role that may not be billable but that make the role valuable to many settings. The blended role cannot be driven by medicine or by the need for providers (Deane, 1997), and it must not be driven by adjustment to a medical gap or surplus (Wright, 1997). Development must also not be driven by outside forces that may seek to diminish the ability of APNs to coalesce into a political force, which is so necessary to change restrictive state statutes (Caverly, 1996). Instead, the role must be driven by the need for quality patient-centered care delivered by nurses who bring a wide variety of special skills to patients across settings. The employment of blended role APNs is one practice alternative to augment the ranks of CNSs and NPs in expanding the profession's ability to deliver advanced nursing care to patients with complex needs.

CONCLUSION

"For APNs who embrace change, there are unlimited opportunities to actively participate in the redefinition of health care, the transformation of practice settings, and the creation of provider roles" (O'Malley & Cummings, 1995, p. 6). New models of education and increased clarity regarding definition and titling will be needed for the blended role APN to develop to its full potential. It is critical that blended role practitioners identify themselves as such, so that they can mentor APNs and students interested in blended role practice.

On a societal level, patient satisfaction and quality improvement are becoming increasingly important goals in a competitive health-care market. As consumers, patients are demanding high-quality care, while as taxpayers, they are demanding lower costs. In order to thrive, nursing must adjust to these trends. The blended role APN is one such promising adjustment. This new APN role has evolved to augment the NP and CNS roles to meet the needs of specialty populations who require complex coordinated care in a dynamic health-care system.

REFERENCES

American Academy of Family Physicians. (2003, March 20). *Medical student interest in primary care continues to decline.* Retrieved September 1, 2003, from http://www.aaf.org/x20098.xml

American Nurses Association. (1996). *Nursing's social policy statement.* Washington, DC: Author.

Anonymous. (2001). Nurse practitioners (NPs) and clinical nurse specialists (CNSs) regarding the blending of these two roles. *Clinical Nurse Specialist, 15,* 187.

Beecroft, P. C. (1994). CNS: Thriving or heading for extinction? *Clinical Nurse Specialist, 8,* 63.

Berlin, L. E., Stennett, J., & Bednash, G. D. (2003). *2002-2003 Enrollment and graduations in baccalaureate and graduate programs in nursing.* Washington, DC: American Association of Colleges of Nursing.

Berragan, L. (1998). Consultancy in nursing: Roles and opportunities. *Journal of Clinical Nursing, 7,* 139-143.

British Medical Journal (BMJ) Publishing Group, Ltd. (2001). *Barriers between research and practice* [Slides]. Retrieved May 18, 2003, from http://www.clinicalevidence.com

Brooten, D., Naylor, M. D., York, R., Brown, L. P., Munro, B. H., Hollingsworth, A. O., et al. (2002). Lessons learned from testing the Quality Cost Model of Advanced Practice Nursing (APN) Transitional Care. *Journal of Nursing Scholarship, 34,* 369-375.

Brown, S. J. (1998). A framework for advanced practice nursing. *Journal of Professional Nursing, 12,* 117-120.

Caverly, S. (1996). The role of the psychiatric nurse practitioner. *Advanced Practice Nursing, 31,* 449-463.

Conger, M., & Craig, C. (1998). Advanced nurse practice: A model for collaboration. *Nursing Case Management, 3,* 120-127.

Cooper, D. (1990). Today-assessments and intuitions: Tomorrow-projections. In P. S. A. Sparacino, D. M. Cooper, & P. A. Minarik (Eds.), *The clinical nurse specialist: Implementation and impact* (pp. 285-311). Norwalk, CT: Appleton & Lange.

Cronenwett, L. R. (1995). Molding the future of advanced practice nursing. *Nursing Outlook, 43,* 112-118.

Crotty, G. (1998). Clinical nurse specialist to nurse practitioner: Personal observations. *Tennessee Nurse,* 6(2), 19-20.

Dale, J. C. (1991). New role for pediatric nurse practitioners in an in-patient setting. *Journal of Pediatric Health Care, 5,* 336-337.

Davitt, P., & Jensen, L. (1981). The role of the acute care nurse practitioner in cardiac surgery. *Nursing Administration Quarterly, 3,* 16-19.

Deane, K. A. (1997). CNS and NP: Should the roles be merged? *Canadian Nurse, 93,* 24-30.

Donabedian, A. (1966). Evaluating the quality of medical care. *Milbank Quarterly, 44,* 166-206.

Dunn, L. (1997). A literature review of advanced clinical nursing practice in the United States of America. *Journal of Advanced Nursing, 25,* 814-819.

Edmands, M. S., Hoff, L. A., Kaylor, L., Mower, L., & Sorrell, S. (1999). Bridging gaps between mind, body, spirit: Healing the whole person. *Journal of Psychosocial Nursing, 37,* 35-42.

Elder, R. G., & Bullough, B. (1990). Nurse practitioner and clinical nurse specialists: Are the roles merging? *Clinical Nurse Specialist, 4,* 78-84.

Fenton, M. V., & Brykczynski, K. A. (1993). Qualitative distinctions and similarities in the practice of clinical nurse specialists and nurse practitioners. *Journal of Professional Nursing, 9,* 313-326.

Finke, D. (2000). Blending CNS and NP roles increases employment opportunities. *Journal of Emergency Nursing, 26,* 98.

Fitzpatrick, E. R. (1998). Analysis and synthesis of the role of the advanced practice nurse. *Clinical Nurse Specialist, 12,* 106-107.

Fitzpatrick, J. (2003). The case for the clinical doctorate in nursing. *Reflections on Nursing Leadership,* 29(1), 8-9, 37, 52.

Fleschler, R., & Luquire, R. (1998). Advanced practice role of the outcomes manager. *Outcomes Management for Nursing Practice, 2,* 54-56.

George, M. R., O'Dowd, L. C., Martin, I., Lindell, K. O., Whitney, F., Jones, M., et al. (1999). A comprehensive educational program improves clinical outcome measures in inner-city patients with asthma. *Archives of Internal Medicine, 159,* 1710-1716.

Gibbins, S. A., Green, P. E., Scott, P. A., & MacDonell, J. W. (2000). The role of the clinical nurse specialist/neonatal nurse practitioner in a breastfeeding clinic: A model of advanced practice. *Clinical Nurse Specialist, 14,* 56-59.

Gleeson, R. M., McIlvain-Simpson, G., Boos, M. L., Sweet, E., Trzcinski, K. M., Solberg, C. A., et al. (1990). Advanced practice nursing: A model of collaborative care. *MCN, The American Journal of Maternal Child Nursing , 15,* 9-12.

Hamric, A. B. (1989). History and overview of the CNS role. In A. B. Hamric & J. A. Spross (Eds.), *The clinical nurse specialist in theory and practice* (2nd ed., pp. 2-18). Philadelphia: W. B. Saunders.

Hamric, A. B. (1998). Using research to influence the regulatory process. *Advanced Practice Nursing Quarterly, 4,* 44-50.

Hamric, A. B. (2000). A definition of advanced nursing practice. In A. B. Hamric, J. A. Spross, & C. M. Hanson (Eds.), *Advanced nursing practice: An integrative approach* (2nd ed., pp. 53-73). Philadelphia: W. B. Saunders.

Hanson, C. M., & Hamric, A. B. (2003). Reflections on the continuing evolution of advanced practice nursing. *Nursing Outlook, 51,* 203-211.

Hanson, C., & Martin, L. L. (1990). The nurse practitioner and clinical nurse specialist: Should the roles be merged? *Journal of the American Academy of Nurse Practitioners, 2,* 2-9.

Herman, J. (1998). Documenting acute care nurse practitioner practice characteristics. *AACN Clinical Issues, 9,* 277-282.

Hockenberry-Eaton, M., & Powell, M. L. (1991). Merging advanced practice roles: The CNS and NP. *Journal of Pediatric Health Care, 5,* 158-159.

Hoff, L. A., & Edmands, M. S. (1998). Healing the mind-body and nursing specialty splits. *Journal of Psychosocial Nursing, 36,* 38-44.

Hunsberger, M., Mitchell, A., Blatz, P., Paes, B., Pinelli, J., Southwell, D., et al. (1992). Definition of an advanced nursing role in the NICU: The clinical nurse specialist/nurse practitioner. *Clinical Nurse Specialist, 6,* 91-96.

Irvine, D., Sidani, S., & McGillis-Hall, L. (1998). Linking outcomes to nurses' roles in health care. *Nursing Economics, 16,* 58-64, 87.

Jacobs, L. A., & Kreamer, K. M. (1997). The oncology clinical nurse specialist in a post-master's nurse practitioner program: A personal and professional journey. *Oncology Nursing Forum, 24,* 1387-1392.

Keane, A., & Richmond, T. (1993). Tertiary nurse practitioners. *Image: The Journal of Nursing Scholarship, 25,* 281-293.

Kindig, D., Cultice, J., & Mullen, F. (1993). The elusive generalist physician: Can we reach a 50% goal? *JAMA: The Journal of the American Medical Association, 270,* 1069-1073.

King, K. B., & Ackerman, M. H. (1995). An educational model for the acute care nurse practitioner. *Critical Care Nursing Clinics of North America, 7,* 1-8.

Kinney, A., Hawkins, R., & Hudman, K. S. (1997). A descriptive study of the role of the oncology nurse practitioner. *Oncology Nursing Forum, 24,* 811-820.

Kitzman, H. J. (1983). The CNS and the nurse practitioner. In A. B. Hamric & J. Spross (Eds.), *The clinical nurse specialist in theory and practice* (pp. 275-290). New York: Grune & Stratton.

Kitzman, H. J. (1989). The CNS and the nurse practitioner. In A. B. Hamric & J. A. Spross (Eds.), *The clinical nurse specialist in theory and practice* (2nd ed., pp. 379-394). Philadelphia: W. B. Saunders.

Kleinpell, R. M. (1998). Reports of role descriptions of acute care nurse practitioners. *AACN Clinical Issues, 9,* 290-295.

Lesser, C. S., & Ginsberg, P. B. (2001). Back to the future? New cost and access challenges emerge. Initial findings from HSC's recent site visits. *Issue Brief/Center for Studying Health System Change, 35,* 1-4.

Lesser, C. S., & Ginsberg, P. B. (2003). Health care cost and access problems intensify: Initial findings from HSC's recent site visits. *Issue Brief/Center for Studying Health System Change, 63,* 1-6.

Lincoln, P. E. (2000). Comparing CNS and NP role activities: A replication. *Clinical Nurse Specialist, 14,* 269-277.

Maclaine, K. (1998). Clarifying higher level roles in nursing practice. *Professional Nurse, 14,* 159-163.

Martin, R. K. (1999). The role of the transplant advanced practice nurse: A professional and personal evolution. *Critical Care Nursing Quarterly, 21,* 69-76.

Mayer, G. (1997). The impact of managed care on hospital nursing. *Best Practices and Benchmarking in Healthcare, 4,* 162-167.

McCabe, S., & Grover, S. (1999). Psychiatric nurse practitioner versus clinical nurse specialist: Moving from debate to action on the future of advanced psychiatric nursing. *Archives of Psychiatric Nursing, 13,* 111-116.

McGivern, D. O. (1993). The evolution to advanced nursing practice. In M. D. Mezey & D. O. McGivern (Eds.), *Nurses, nurse practitioners: Evolution to advanced practice* (pp. 3-30). New York: Springer.

Mick, D. J., & Ackerman, M. H. (2000). Advanced practice nursing role delineation in acute and critical care: Application of the Strong Model of Advanced Practice. *Heart & Lung, 29,* 210-221.

Mick, D. J., & Ackerman, M. H. (2002). Deconstructing the myth of the advanced practice blended role: Support for role divergence. *Heart & Lung, 31,* 393-398.

Milstead, J. A. (1997). Using advanced practice to shape public policy: Agenda setting. *Nursing Administration Quarterly, 21,* 12-18.

Minnick, A. F., & Halstead, L. A. (2002). A database agenda for doctoral nursing education reform. *Nursing Outlook, 50,* 24-29.

Mortenson, L. E., Edwards, J. J., & Bowers, M. L. (1998). APCs threaten hospital outpatient cancer programs, use of new agents, and supportive care drugs. *Oncology Issues, 13,* 25-29.

Mundinger, M. O., Cook, S. S., Lenz, E. R., Piacentini, K., Auerhahn, C., & Smith, J. (2000). Assuring quality and access in advanced practice nursing: A challenge to nurse educators. *Journal of Professional Nursing, 16,* 322-329.

Naegle, M. A., & Krainovich-Miller, B. (2001). Shaping the advanced practice psychiatric-mental health nursing role: A futuristic model. *Issues in Mental Health Nursing, 22,* 461-482.

National Association of Clinical Nurse Specialists. (2004). *Statement on clinical nurse specialist practice and education.* Harrisburg, PA: Author.

National Committee for Quality Assurance. (2003). *The Health Plan Employer Data and Information Set (HEDIS®).* Retrieved September 25, 2003, from http://www.ncqa.org/Programs/HEDIS/

National Organization of Nurse Practitioner Faculty Practice Doctorate Task Force. (2003). The practice doctorate in nursing: Future or fringe? [Electronic version]. *Topics in Advanced Practice Nursing eJournal, 3,* 1-9. Retrieved May 23, 2003, from http://www.medscape.com/viewarticle/453247

Naylor, M. D., Brooten, D., Campbell, R., Jacobsen, B. S., Mezey, M. D., Pauly, M. V., et al. (1999). Comprehensive discharge planning and home follow-up of hospitalized elders. *JAMA: The Journal of the American Medical Association, 281,* 613-620.

Nemes, J., Barnaby, K., & Shamberger, R. (1992). Experience with a nurse practitioner program in the surgical department of a children's hospital. *Journal of Pediatric Surgery, 27,* 1038-1042.

O'Malley, J., & Cummings, S. H. (1995). Change...more change... and change again. *Advanced Practice Nursing Quarterly, 1,* 1-6.

Oncology Nursing Society. (2003). *Eligibility criteria for initial and renewal of AOCN certification* [Internet]. Oncology Nursing Certification Corporation. Retrieved October 10, 2003, from http://www.oncc.org/?v2_group=0&g=1340&p=12308

Page, N. E., & Arena, D. M. (1994). Rethinking the merger of the clinical nurse specialist and the nurse practitioner roles. *Image: The Journal of Nursing Scholarship, 26,* 315-318.

Page, N. E., & Mackowiak, L. (1997). Role play: The clinical nurse specialist and nurse practitioner: Complementary roles. *Journal of the Society of Pediatric Nurses, 2,* 188-190.

Paladichuk, A., Brass-Mynderse, N., & Kaliangara, O. (1997). Chronic disease management: An outpatient approach. *Critical Care Nurse, 17,* 90-95.

Paul, S. (1997). Implementing an outpatient congestive heart failure clinic: The nurse practitioner role. *Heart & Lung, 26,* 486-491.

Pearson, A., Borbasi, S., & Gott, M. (1997). Doctoral education in nursing for practitioner knowledge and for academic knowledge: The University of Adelaide, Australia. *Image: The Journal of Nursing Scholarship, 29,* 365-368.

Porter-O'Grady, T. (1997). Over the horizon: The future and the advanced practice nurse. *Nursing Administration Quarterly, 21,* 1-11.

Quaal, S. J. (1999). Clinical nurse specialist: Role restructuring to advanced practice registered nurse. *Critical Care Nursing Quarterly, 21,* 37-49.

Redekopp, M. A. (1997). Clinical nurse specialist role confusion: The need for identity. *Clinical Nurse Specialist, 11*, 87-91.

Romano, M. (2003). Resident restrictions. Most teaching hospitals ready for work-hour rules. *Modern Healthcare, 33*, 10-11.

Rosenblatt, R. A., Hart, L. G., Baldwin, L. M., Chan, L., & Schneeweiss, R. (1998). The generalist role of specialty physicians: Is there a hidden system of primary care? *JAMA: The Journal of the American Medical Association, 279*, 1364-1370.

Scharer, K., Boyd, M., Williams, C. A., & Head, K. (2003). Blending specialist and practitioner roles in psychiatric nursing: Experiences of graduates. *Journal of the American Psychiatric Nurses Association, 9*, 136-144.

Shuren, A. (1996). The blended role of the clinical nurse specialist and nurse practitioner. In A. B. Hamric, J. A. Spross, & C. M. Hanson (Eds.), *Advanced nursing practice: An integrative approach* (pp. 375-394). Philadelphia: W. B. Saunders.

Skalla, K., & Hamric, A. B. (2000). The blended role of the clinical nurse specialist and nurse practitioner. In A. B. Hamric, J. A. Spross, & C. M. Hanson (Eds.), *Advanced nursing practice: An integrative approach* (2nd ed., pp.459-490). Philadelphia: W. B. Saunders.

Simpson, R. L. (1998). Bridging the nursing-physician gap: Technology's role in interdisciplinary practice. *Nursing Administration Quarterly, 22*, 87-90.

Smith, L. D. (1994). Continuity of care through nursing case management of the chronically ill child. *Clinical Nurse Specialist, 8*, 65-68.

Snyder, M., & Mirr, M. P. (Eds.). (1995). *Advanced practice nursing: Guide to professional development.* New York: Springer.

Sperhac, A. M., & Strodtbeck, F. (2001). Advanced practice in pediatric nursing: Blending roles. *Journal of Pediatric Nursing, 16*, 120-126.

Spratley, E., Johnson, A., Sochalski, J., Fritz, M., & Spencer, W. (2001, September). *The registered nurse population: Findings from the National Sample Survey of Registered Nurses.* Washington, DC: U. S. Department of Health and Human Services, Health Resources and Services Administration, Bureau of Health Professions Division of Nursing.

Spross, J., & Hamric, A. (1983). A model for future clinical specialist practice. In A. B. Hamric & J. Spross (Eds.), *The clinical nurse specialist in theory and practice.* New York: Grune & Stratton.

Tappen, R. M., & Dunphy, L. (1998). Blended role advanced practice in gerontological nursing. *The Florida Nurse, 46*(8), 21-22.

Verger, J., Trimarchi, T., & Barnsteiner, J. H. (2002). Challenges of advanced practice nursing in pediatric acute and critical care: Education to practice. *Critical Care Clinics of North America, 14*, 315-326.

Weinberg, R. M., Likestrand, J. S., & Moore, S. (1983). In-patient management by a nurse practitioner: Effectiveness in a rehabilitation setting. *Archives of Physical Medicine and Rehabilitation, 64*, 588-590.

Whitcomb, R., Wilson, S. Chang-Dawkins, S., Durand, J., Pitcher, D., Lauzon, C. et al. (2002). Advanced practice nursing: Acute model in progress. *Journal of Nursing Administration, 32*(3), 123-125.

Wolff, J. L., Starfield, B., & Anderson, G. (2002). Prevalence, expenditures, and complications of multiple chronic conditions in the elderly. *Archives of Internal Medicine, 162*, 2269-2276.

Wright, J. E. (1990). Joining forces for the good of our clients. *Clinical Nurse Specialist, 4*, 76-77.

Wright, K. B. (1997). Advanced practice nursing: Merging the clinical nurse specialist and nurse practitioner roles. *Gastroenterology Nursing, 20*, 57-60.

Zimmer, P., Brykczynski, K., Martin, A. C., Newberry, Y. G., Price, M. J., & Warren, B. (1990, April). *Advanced nursing practice: Nurse practitioner curriculum guidelines (Final Report: NONPF Education Committee).* Paper presented at the National Organization of Nurse Practitioner Faculties, Washington, DC.

CHAPTER 16

The Certified Nurse-Midwife

MARGARET W. DORROH • MAUREEN A. KELLEY

Continued

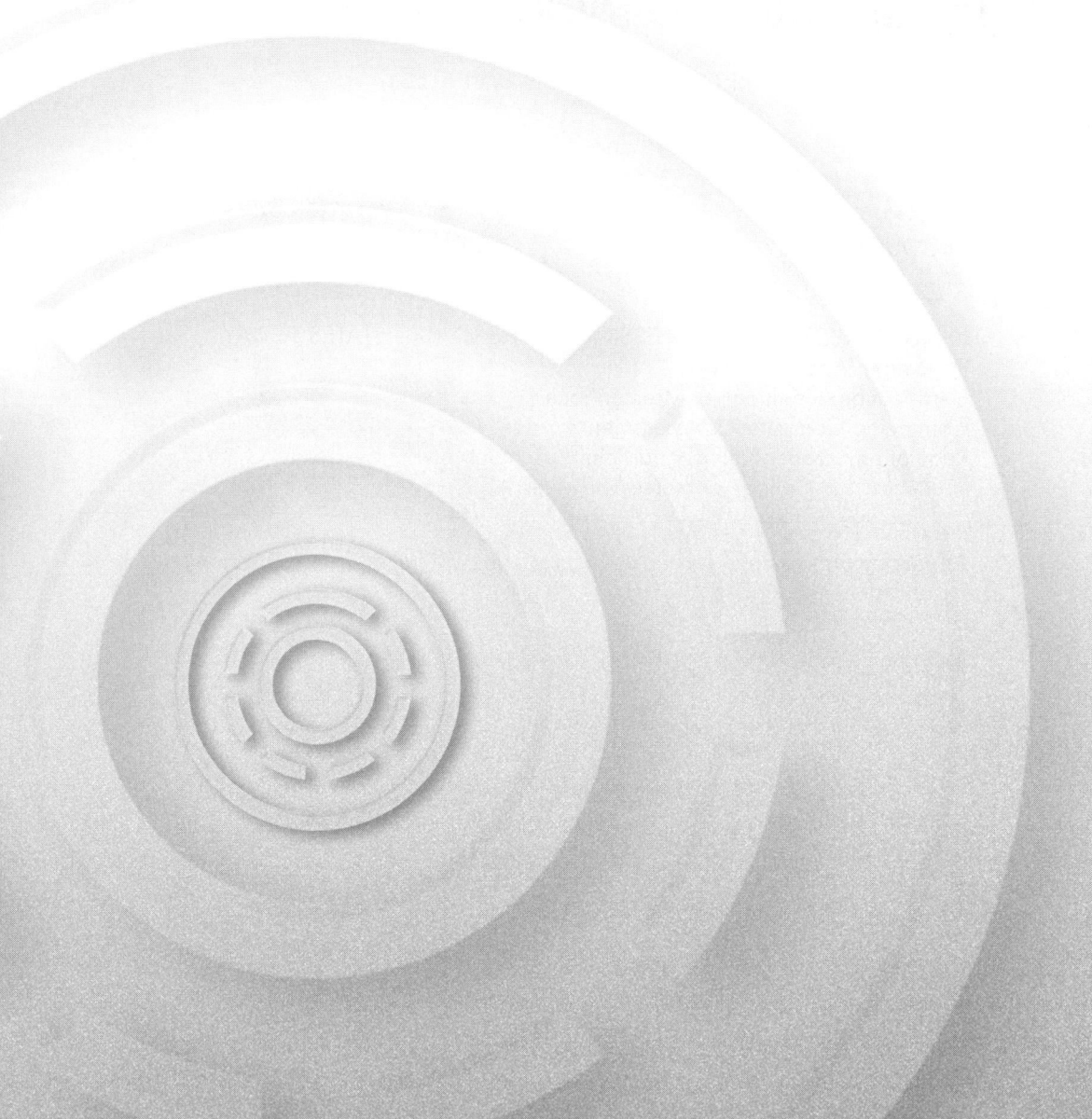

INTRODUCTION

Certified nurse-midwives (CNMs) are registered nurses who have graduated from a midwifery education program accredited by the American College of Nurse-Midwives (ACNM) Division of Accreditation and have passed a national certification examination administered by the ACNM Certification Council, Inc (ACNM, 1997h). The word *midwife* has universal recognition. Not all midwives are professionally educated; not all midwives are nurses. According to the definition in Chapter 3 and specifically with regard to master's preparation in nursing, not all nurse-midwives (NMs) are advanced practice nurses (APNs). The term *midwife* encompasses lay midwives, empirical midwives, "granny" midwives, professional midwives, and certified midwives. Some of these practitioners are legally recognized; some have had formal midwifery training. Few of these practitioners are nurses, and all are therefore excluded from the designation of APNs. In this chapter, the authors are discussing CNMs who are practicing in an advanced practice nursing role. For the purposes of this text, the terms *midwife*, NM, and CNM are used interchangeably to describe the advanced practice nursing midwifery role. When issues related to nonnurse midwives are addressed, an attempt will be made to make that clear.

Nurse-midwifery has its roots in nursing and has made many contributions that have paved the way for advanced practice nursing to flourish. These efforts have included the development of standards, core clinical competencies, and successful legislative and regulatory initiatives. Nurse-midwifery activities that have been instrumental in securing prescriptive authority and direct reimbursement by insurers for CNMs have also had an indirect and favorable impact on all APNs. The pioneering efforts of CNMs have helped to cultivate a clinical and political climate of acceptance not only for them but also for clinical nurse specialists (CNSs), certified registered nurse anesthetists, and nurse practitioners (NPs) as legitimate and visible providers of care across all settings.

Despite these contributions, there are tensions between the ACNM and advanced practice nursing. Organized nurse-midwifery has not been viewed as joining forces with the nursing profession's efforts to organize and align all advanced practice roles. Several factors may account for this. A high priority of the midwifery profession is increasing availability of and access to midwifery services. Much effort has gone into meeting the increasing demand for CNMs. Because the ACNM defines the CNM as an individual educated in the two disciplines of nursing and midwifery (ACNM, 1997i), new graduates are viewed as *beginning-level practitioners of midwifery*, not as APNs. Herein may lie one of the fundamental philosophical differences with the larger nursing profession. Paradoxically, availability and access are central arguments for health-care reform initiatives that promote advanced practice nursing roles. Legislation adds to the confusion. As of 2000, only 24 states had laws or regulations that recognized CNMs as APNs (Reed, 2000).

The purpose of this chapter is to describe nurse-midwifery practice so that the reader should appreciate why it can be seen as an advanced practice nursing role. As authors, we offer our own perspectives on the issues that prevent full integration of nurse-midwifery into advanced practice nursing. Nurses and CNMs alike have a stake in issues related to this level of professional practice. The reflections offered in this chapter are meant to foster dialogue, understanding, and wisdom as nurses and CNMs work to accomplish their goals related to practice. It is our hope that all in nursing will continue to work productively and collaboratively in activities that promote advanced practice nursing. While

We wish to acknowledge Dorroh and Norton for their important contribution to the first edition of this text (Dorroh & Norton, 1996).

remaining mindful and respectful of the rich history and groundwork laid by nurse-mid-wifery, we support all of the criteria for practice put forth in this text.

HISTORICAL PERSPECTIVE

Throughout time and in all cultures, the midwife has played a recognized role. In biblical times, the midwife assisted a woman in labor, helped with the delivery, and provided after-care for the mother and child. Novice midwives acquired knowledge and skill from apprenticeship with experienced midwives and through their own observation and expe-rience. Skilled midwives provided emergency medical or surgical assistance as needed and, in recognition of their importance, were exempted from injunctions against work on the Sabbath when they were performing their duties. Present-day midwives are granted the same privilege. This period in midwifery history is beautifully depicted in Anita Diamant's novel *The Red Tent* (1997).

In colonial times, midwives were an integral part of community life and were highly respected. By the early 1900s, a number of developments had considerably diminished that respect and led to an ebb in the practice of midwifery. The late 19th and early 20th centuries brought with them massive immigration. European immigrant midwives served these newly arrived immigrants. Likewise, African American women in the South were cared for by traditional African American midwives. An active campaign was waged to discredit these care providers, a campaign in which data that showed good care outcomes were ignored (Dawley, 2003). A key factor in moving birth from home to the hospital and in eliminating midwives was the medicalization of childbirth. In the early 1900s, the med-ical field had become highly competitive; attending labor and delivery was a means to physicians establishing a practice. Families pleased with the medical care provided at childbirth would return to the same physician for other care. This phenomenon, com-bined with women's low social status, made it difficult for midwives to compete against physicians. Physicians arrived on the childbearing scene rather late, but this accident of history continues to influence the regulation and practice of nurse-midwifery.

Although midwifery remained part of mainstream health care in many European, Asian, and African countries, the renaissance of midwifery in the United States was not to occur until the 1940s and 1950s. Strong nursing leaders and the childbirth education movement largely shaped the reappearance of midwifery as a nursing role (Dawley, 2003). Like other forms of advanced practice nursing that emerged much later, the resurgence of midwifery and the evolution of nurse-midwifery occurred in response to the need for care by the underserved. By the late 1960s, the contributions of nurse-midwifery were accepted and recognized. The profession was inundated with requests for CNMs and was criticized for not having enough CNMs trained to meet the needs of women in this country. This led to a proliferation of nurse-midwifery educational programs and the development of more nurse-midwifery practices. In an effort to provide even more practitioners, the ACNM explored and encouraged the devel-opment of educational programs to prepare and accredit nonnurse midwives. As these educa-tional progams evolved, the ACNM proposed changing its name to the American College of Midwives in an effort to be more inclusive of nonnurse midwives who achieved ACNM certi-fication. In a demonstration of allegiance to nursing, the ACNM membership voted over-whelmingly to retain *Nurse* in the name of the organization (Kraus, 1997b). However, in 2000, the official publication of the ACNM, the *Journal of Nurse-Midwifery*, changed its name to the *Journal of Midwifery and Women's Health* to ". . . more accurately reflect the evolution of contemporary midwifery . . ." (Shah, 2000). For additional historical background, the reader is directed to Chapter 1 by Keeling and Bigbee. Table 16-1 presents a timeline of key events that influenced the development of modern nurse-midwifery as described by Varney (1996).

TABLE 16-1	THE EVOLUTION OF NURSE-MIDWIFERY: A TIMELINE OF CRITICAL EVENTS	
YEAR	EVENT	SIGNIFICANCE
Colonial times to early 1900s	Midwives traveled to the colonies. They were respected in communities and trained in apprenticeships. Practices were often handed down from mother to daughter.	Midwifery had a strong basis in service to others. Went beyond an occupation—often seen as a "calling." The women who practiced midwifery tended to be rich in life experience if not in formal education.
Early 1900s	Midwifery was co-opted by organized medicine.	Decreased number and experience of practitioners effectively put midwives "in the closet."
1925	Frontier Nursing Service was founded in Hyden, Kentucky.	Imported British-trained midwives utilized the nursing model. Designed to meet the specific needs in an underserved area. Births took place in homes. Neonatal mortality rate 9.1/1000 births from 1925 to 1951 (not matched by United States at large until 1990s).
1931	The Maternity Center Association, in New York, opened the Lobenstine Clinic.	Provided care for immigrant families in upper Manhattan tenements.
1932	The first nurse-midwifery education program was developed at the Lobenstine Clinic.	Offered advanced preparation in midwifery to public health nurses. Acknowledged relationship of nursing and midwifery.
1941	The Tuskegee School of Nurse-Midwifery opened in Alabama.	Access to nurse-midwifery education for minorities.
1943	The Catholic Maternity Institute was founded in Santa Fe, New Mexico.	Many nurse-midwifery leaders came from this program.
Mid-1940s	The National Organization of Public Health Nurses (later absorbed into the American Nurses Association) was established for nurse-midwives.	Recognition of midwifery as having a foundation in nursing.
1955	The American College of Nurse-Midwives was founded.	Began formalizing standards for education, certification, and practice. The basic certificate program was the norm. Also provided a formal voice for nurse-midwives.
Early 1960s	A certified nurse-midwife pilot project was conducted in Madera County, California.	Continues to be used as "gold standard" in assessing nurse-midwifery care.
Late 1960s and 1970s	Nurse-midwifery services and educational programs (mostly certificates) proliferated; autonomous birth centers were developed.	Increased utilization of and demand for CNMs in a variety of settings.
1980s	Malpractice crisis arose.	Closed some practices and threatened closure at some programs until issue resolved.
1980s and 1990s	CNMs moved to graduate-level education.	Majority of programs now prepare students at master's level.
1990s	The milieu for health-care practice is changing; CNMs are moving toward primary care of women.	CNMs adapting to environment in which quality, access, and cost must all be addressed.

CNMs, Certified nurse-midwives.

THE NURSE-MIDWIFERY PROFESSION IN THE UNITED STATES TODAY

There are currently more than 6700 active and student members of the ACNM. Of that number, approximately 5700 are in clinical practice. Overall, 68% of CNMs hold master's degrees; 4% have doctorates. Approximately 1% of CNMs are men (Kovner & Burkhardt, 2001). In 2000, the most current year for which data are available, CNMs attended 298,060 births, which constitute 9.48% of the nation's vaginal births. This represents a 3.7% increase since 1990 (Declercq, 2003).

Education/Accreditation

The ACNM established a national mechanism for the accreditation of education programs in 1962. Because the organization wanted to have its process subject to peer review and recognition, it applied to the Department of Education for recognition as an accrediting agency. This recognition was granted in 1982 and has been maintained since that time. ACNM-accredited programs must receive preaccreditation status prior to enrollment of students, and once initial accreditation is granted, programs are revisited at least every 8 years.

Currently, 43 programs are accredited by or with preaccreditation status from the Division of Accreditation (DOA) of the ACNM. Four of these programs are postbaccalaureate certificate-level programs and 39 are master's programs (ACNM, 2003). The profession supports preparation of midwives at both the certificate level and the degree level. This position is based on two rationales. The first is that differences in preparation have not resulted in differences in certification test results (Fullerton & Severino, 1995). The second is the concern that "mandatory degree requirements would limit access to maternity and gynecological services for women who have been shown to benefit from midwifery care by denying [them] practice opportunities" (Carrington & Decker, 1997; Shah, 2002) Although the DOA supports different educational pathways, it mandates that all ACNM-accredited education programs either require a baccalaureate upon entrance or grant no less than a baccalaureate upon graduation (ACNM, 2003).

The accreditation process rests on two cornerstones. The first cornerstone is the Criteria for the Evaluation of Education Programs (ACNM, 1997g), which are currently under revision. These criteria specify the elements necessary to develop and maintain a nurse-midwifery program. Because they evaluate the specialty content of midwifery (i.e., content that addresses the *hallmarks and components of midwifery*, including but not limited to intrapartum care), these criteria apply regardless of the academic "house" in which the program resides (e.g., nursing, public health, allied health, medicine). In addition, the criteria apply regardless of the level at which the student is being prepared (baccalaureate, master's, doctoral, certificate) (Bellack, Graber, O' Neil, & Musham, 1998; Carr, 1999). This approach to education is not without difficulties, such as when state laws require a certain level of education to practice or to perform certain aspects of practice such as prescribing medication. The ACNM criteria are revised every 5 years in order to maintain currency. The criteria do require that a midwifery program be directed by a midwife, that midwifery faculty have at least 1 year of clinical nurse-midwifery experience prior to teaching, and that the faculty remain current in clinical practice.

The second cornerstone of the accreditation process is the *Core Competencies for Basic Midwifery Practice*, most recently revised in 2002 (ACNM, 2002). This document represents the delineation of the fundamental knowledge, skills, and behaviors expected of a new practitioner. It is divided into five major sections: (1) hallmarks, which speak to the underlying philosophy of the profession; (2) professional responsibilities, which delineate the nonclinical requirements of the professional midwife; (3) the midwifery management process, which is the clinical decision-making framework for practice; (4) the fundamentals of midwifery care; and (5) the components of clinical care. This document ensures equivalent preparation for all graduates of midwifery education programs accredited by the ACNM's DOA. It likewise contributes to the blueprint for the certification examination for CNMs (ACNM, 1997j).

Certification/Certification Maintenance

A national certification examination for entry into practice was instituted in 1971. The ACNM Certification Council, Inc. (ACC) develops and administers this examination. The examination has a multiple-choice format and is based on both the core competencies and a task analysis of currently practicing midwives that is periodically updated. Each year, approximately 400 students graduate from an ACNM-accredited program and take the certifying examination.

As of January 1, 1996, the certificate became a time-limited one, valid for 8 years from date of issue. Mechanisms for certification maintenance, administered by the ACC, include such options as certification maintenance modules, continuing education units, and retaking the certification examination. At this juncture, the time-limited certificate does not apply to midwives certified prior to 1996, and therefore the certification maintenance program is optional for this group. Instead, the continuing competency assessment mechanism, which was developed in 1987, may be used.

Continuing Competency Assessment

In 1987, the ACNM developed a continuing competency assessment mechanism for its members in clinical practice. The purpose of continuing competency assessment was to demonstrate that clinicians continued to maintain contemporary knowledge and meet a national standard for practice. This 5-year cycle requires that practicing midwives either acquire 50 contact hours of continuing education appropriate for midwifery practice or retake the certification examination. The ACNM Continuing Education Committee grants continuing education units for programs that meet the guidelines of the International Association for Continuing Education and Training. The ACNM initially "mandated" competency assessment but modified this position in 1995, placing the decision to mandate participation in the hands of state regulators or employers. The ACNM still sets the standard that all CNMs must demonstrate continuing competency, and a number of states and employers have adopted ACNM's continuing competency mechanism as evidence for meeting the requirement for licensure or employment (ACNM, 1997f). There is no requirement for ongoing clinical practice for either certification maintenance or continuing competency assessment.

Regulation, Credentialing, and Reimbursement

As with all health-care professions in the United States, CNM practice is regulated on a state-by-state basis. CNMs must comply with the legal requirements for the practice of nurse-midwifery in the jurisdiction in which they practice (the District of Columbia, the Virgin Islands, and Puerto Rico, as well as the 50 states). The practice of nurse-midwifery differs in the various jurisdictions because of legal, regulatory, and other influences. Such influences include statutes, rules and regulations, opinions of the state attorney general, court decisions, licensure, registration, and certification. This results in differences in such parameters as what state agency regulates midwifery practice, whether midwives have prescriptive authority, what educational degrees are required for practice, and what types of employers and practice arrangements are permitted. States may also have regulations about private insurance reimbursement and are required to set the Medicaid reimbursement schedule for CNMs. The effect that this variation in state law and regulation has on midwifery practice was examined by Declercq, Paine, Dejoseph, and Simmes (1998). They found that, when compared with states with low regulatory support for nurse-midwifery practice, states with high regulatory support had a nurse-midwifery workforce three times larger than that of other states, three times the number of midwife-attended births, and two times as many midwife-patient contacts.

The political climate affects nurse-midwifery practice and can promote or restrain the practice of CNMs. For example, the relative power of constituencies such as medical and nursing organizations and consumer groups and the relationships among them can shape legislation and patterns of referral to CNMs. Laws and other ordinances that regulate CNM practice should ensure that all practitioners are qualified to practice nurse-midwifery. The ACNM recently reaffirmed the autonomy with which the CNM practices. The ACNM's official clinical practice statement on independent nurse-midwifery practice is presented in Box 16-1.

In addition to state regulation, hospitals and health plans have established credentialing requirements for health-care professionals. These credentialing standards determine who may have hospital admitting privileges, who may be employed by health-care sys-

---

BOX 16-1 • CLINICAL PRACTICE STATEMENT ON INDEPENDENT MIDWIFERY PRACTICE

It is the position of the ACNM that midwifery practice is the independent management of women's health care, focusing particularly on pregnancy, childbirth, the postpartum period, care of the newborn, and the family planning and gynecologic needs of women. The practice occurs within a health-care system that provides for consultation, collaborative management or referral as indicated by the health status of the client.

Independent midwifery enables certified nurse-midwives (CNMs) and certified midwives (CMs) to utilize knowledge, skills, judgment and authority in the provision of primary women's health services while maintaining accountability for the management of patient care in accordance with the ACNM *Standards for the Practice of Nurse-Midwifery*.

The ACNM believes that independent practice is not defined by the place of employment, the employee-employer relationship, requirements for physician co-signature, or the method of reimbursement for services. Nor should *independent* be interpreted to mean *alone*, as there are clinical situations when any prudent practitioner would seek the assistance of another qualified practitioner.

The ACNM also believes that collaboration is the process whereby health-care professionals jointly manage care. The goal of collaboration is to share authority while providing quality care within each individual's professional scope of practice. Successful collaboration is a way of thinking and relating that requires knowledge, open communication, mutual respect, a commitment to providing quality care, trust, and the ability to share responsibility.

From the American College of Nurse-Midwives. (1997h). *Definition of a certified nurse-midwife/definition of midwifery practice.* Washington, DC: Author.

tems, and who may be listed on managed care provider panels. An optimum system would create a mechanism that is consistent with the profession's standards, recognize midwifery as distinct from other health-care professions, and recognize processes that permit CNMs to build upon entry-level competencies within their statutory scope of practice (Dower, Miller, O'Neil, & the Taskforce on Midwifery, 1999).

The Pew Health Professions Commission on the Future of Midwifery made a number of recommendations about the practice environment (Dower et al., 1999). These recommendations reflect the understanding that the professional and regulatory environments combine to have a significant impact on the ability of CNMs to be part of the health-care team. Table 16-2 contains a summary of these recommendations.

The American College of Nurse-Midwives

The growth and development of American nurse-midwifery was fostered by the ACNM, founded in 1955. The mission of the ACNM is to promote the health and well-being of women and infants within their families and communities through the development and support of professional midwifery. The organization establishes clinical standards, creates liaisons with state and federal agencies and members of Congress, administers and promotes continuing education programs, supports midwifery-relevant research and practice, and supports the accreditation mechanism.

The ACNM Philosophy (ACNM, 1989) (Box 16-2) and Code of Ethics, both of which are currently under revision, embody the spirit of the profession. The Code of Ethics (Ad Hoc Committee on Code of Ethics, 1990) aligns with the American Nurses Association's Code of Ethics. A CNM has professional moral obligations. The code identifies the obligations that guide the CNM in the practice of nurse-midwifery and clarifies what consumers, the public, other professionals, and prospective practitioners can expect of the profession. Nurse-midwifery exists for the good of women and their families; this good is safeguarded by practice that is consistent with the ACNM Philosophy (ACNM, 1989) and ACNM Standards for the Practice of Nurse-Midwifery (ACNM, 1993). The belief that pregnancy and childbirth are normal life processes is at the heart of nurse-midwifery practice. The CNM learns to be "with woman" (the original meaning of *midwife*) without having to "manage" pregnancy, labor, or delivery. The patience to allow normal processes to proceed at an unhurried pace is one of the hallmarks of nurse-midwifery. This is one of the key differences between nurse-midwifery and medical approaches to the care of women. Adherents to the medical model tend to intervene even when things are proceeding normally. In nurse-midwifery, when intervention is indicated, CNMs ensure that it is integrated into care in a way that preserves the dignity of the woman and her family. The Code of Ethics further describes expectations regarding practice competence, CNM-patient relationships, ethical responsibilities, collegial practice, and nondiscrimination. Responsibilities for conducting research in nurse-midwifery and for supporting community and political activities that promote access to health care are also delineated. CNMs take responsibility for implementing the Health Insurance Privacy and Portability Act (HIPAA) regulations in an understandable and usable format in their individual practices. Other essential documents, position papers, and fact sheets about ACNM can be found on its Internet website. The website can be accessed at either www.acnm.org or www.midwife.org. The site is also rich in information for consumers and the second Web address makes it accessible to the lay public.

TABLE 16-2   PRACTICE ENVIRONMENT RECOMMENDATION

PRACTICE	REGULATION & CREDENTIALING	EDUCATION	RESEARCH	POLICY
Four recommendations are offered to health-care system administrators and practitioners—including midwives and other professionals—to help ensure that practice structures are designed to provide the best health care possible by making the midwifery model of care readily available to women. 1. Midwives should be recognized as independent and collaborative practitioners with the rights and responsibilities regarding scope of practice authority and accountability that all independent professionals share. 2. Every health-care system should integrate midwifery services into the continuum of care for women by contracting with or employing midwives and informing women of their options.	RECOMMENDATIONS: 5. Stage legislatures should enact laws that base entry-to-practice standards on successful completion of accredited education programs, or the equivalent, and national certification; do not require midwives to be directed or supervised by other health-care professionals; and allow midwives to own or co-own health-care practices. 6. Hospitals, health systems, and public programs, including Medicare and Medicaid, should ensure that enrollees have access to midwives and the midwifery model of care by eliminating barriers to access and inequitable reimbursement rates that discriminate against midwives. 7. Health-care systems should develop hospital privileging and credentialing mechanisms	The following recommendations will challenge educators to continue to develop faculty, programs, curricula and recruitment policies to meet consumer demands in a changing health-care area. 8. Education programs should provide opportunities for interprofessional education and training experiences and allow for multiple points at which midwifery education can be entered. This requires proactive intra- and interprofessional collaboration between colleges, universities and education programs to develop affiliations and complementary curriculum pathways. 9. Midwifery education programs should include training in practice management and the impact of health-care policy and financing on midwifery practice, with	12. Midwifery research should be strengthened and funded in the following areas: • Demand for maternity care, demand for midwifery care, and numbers and distribution of midwives; • Analyses of how midwives complement and broaden the woman's choice of provider, setting, and model of care; • Cost benefit, cost effectiveness, and cost utility analyses, including the relationship between knowledge of economic/cost analyses and provider practices; • Midwifery practice and benchmarking data (among midwives) with a goal of developing appropriate productivity	14. A research and policy body, such as the Institute of Medicine, should be requested to study and offer guidance on significant aspects of the midwifery profession including • Workforce supply and demand; • Coordination of regulation by the states; • Funding of research, education, and training; and • Coordination among the federal agencies whose policies affect the practice of midwifery.

for midwives that are consistent with the profession's standards, recognize midwifery as distinct from other health-care professions, and recognize established processes that permit midwives to build upon their entry-level competencies within their statutory scope of practice.

3. When integrating midwifery services, health-care organizations should use productivity standards based on the midwifery model of care and measure the overall financial benefits of such care.

4. Midwives and physicians should ensure that their systems of consultation, collaboration and referral provide integrated and uninterrupted care to women. This requires active engagement and participation by members of both professions.

special attention to managed care.

10. The profession should recognize and acknowledge the benefits of teaching the midwifery model of care in a variety of education programs and affirm the value of competency-based education in all midwifery programs.

11. The midwifery profession should identify, develop and implement mechanisms to recruit student populations that more closely reflect the U.S. population and include cultural competence concepts in basic and continuing education programs.

standards;
• Descriptions and outcomes analyses of midwifery methods and processes;
• Analysis of midwifery practice outcomes, from preconception through infancy, using an evidence-based perspective;
• Normal pregnancy, normal labor and birth, healthy parent-infant relationships, and breastfeeding; and
• Satisfaction with maternity and midwifery care.

13. Federal and state agencies should broaden systematic data collection, which has traditionally focused on medicine and physicians, to include midwifery and midwives.

From Dower, C. M., Miller, J. E., O'Neil, E. H., & the Taskforce on Midwifery. (1999). *Charting a course for the 21st century: The future of midwifery* (pp. i–v). San Francisco: Pew Health Professions Commission and the UCSF Center for the Health Professions; reprinted with permission.

BOX 16-2 • ACNM PHILOSOPHY

Certified nurse-midwives believe that every individual has a right to safe, satisfying health care with respect for human dignity and cultural variations. ACNM further supports each person's right to self-determination, to complete information and to active participation in all aspects of care. ACNM members believe the normal process of pregnancy and birth can be enhanced through education, health care and supportive intervention.

Nurse-midwifery is focused on the needs of the individual and family for physical care, emotional and social support and active involvement of significant others according to cultural values and personal preferences. The practice of nurse-midwifery encourages continuity of care; emphasizes safe, competent clinical management; advocates non-intervention in normal processes; and promotes health education for women throughout the childbearing cycle. This practice may extend to include gynecological care of women throughout the life cycle. Such comprehensive health care is most effectively and efficiently provided by nurse-midwives in collaboration with other members of an interdependent health-care team.

ACNM assumes a leadership role in the development and promotion of high quality health care for women and infants both nationally and internationally. The profession of nurse-midwifery is committed to ensuring that certified nurse-midwives are provided with sound educational preparation, to expanding knowledge through research and to evaluating and revising care through quality assurance. The profession further ensures that its members adhere to the *Standards of Practice for Nurse Midwifery* in accordance with the *ACNM Philosophy*.

From the American College of Nurse Midwives. (1989). *Philosophy of the American Collegeof Nurse-Midwives.* Washington, DC: Author.

IMPLEMENTING APN COMPETENCIES

Nurse-midwifery is multifaceted, constantly evolving, and broader in scope than its pioneers first envisioned it. It is a dynamic discipline (Bergstrom, 1997) that should clearly reflect advanced practice nursing competencies. The direct care role (as described in Chapter 5) is integral to CNM practice and is well substantiated in the exemplar included later in this chapter. Patient-centered assessment and management are hallmarks of CNM prenatal care. CNMs have, in common with all APNs, the characteristics of using a holistic, research-based perspective that is evidence based. They use research methodologies and ethical decision making to support a caring, low technology approach to childbirth (see Table 16-3). The way that CNMs enact the competencies of collaboration and consultation has been used as a model for APN practice and is described more fully later in this chapter. CNMs have demonstrated leadership in the development of birthing centers and in efforts to remove legislative barriers restraining midwifery practice. It is informative to take a closer look at the competencies related to advocacy and patient education to further understand midwifery practice. These ACNM-defined competencies parallel the advanced practice core competencies of ethical decision making and coaching and guidance.

Advocacy and Client Education: Cornerstones of Nurse Midwifery Practice

Advocacy

Advocacy is central to nurse-midwifery practice. Client education and support of clients' rights and self-determination inform every aspect of nurse-midwifery care. These values have been challenged by the burgeoning growth of medical technology in the last two decades and the incursion of managed care in the 1990s. The availability of highly technical interventions for many aspects of childbearing—such as infertility, monitoring pregnancies, and delivery—conflicts with the traditionally low-tech, low-interventionist approach of CNMs.

Vulnerable populations (e.g., women who have not had access to early prenatal care or low-income women receiving care at a teaching hospital clinic) are more likely to be exposed to high-tech interventions. This presents CNMs with several challenges: to evaluate technologies to determine whether and how they can be incorporated into nurse-midwifery care, to incorporate such therapies into practice in ways that are consistent with nurse-midwifery's values, to explain technology in a way that empowers women to make informed decisions, and to provide equal access to the technology. Creativity is required to enact the midwifery model of care across many settings (ACNM, 1997b; Corry & Rooks, 1999). Interestingly, a recent survey of women from diverse educational backgrounds revealed that women selecting a midwife felt more knowledgeable about birth attendants and more in control of their decision to select a birth attendant (Galotti, Pierce, Reimer, & Luckner, 2000).

The advent of cost-containment strategies in health care has often restricted the choices that women can make for their personal health care. The ACNM is strongly supportive of legislation ensuring that consumers have access to the full spectrum of qualified health-care professionals and providers. To that end, women should be able to designate a CNM as their primary care provider (ACNM, 1998a).

Client Education

Client education is another cornerstone of nurse-midwifery practice and is integral to the CNM's advocacy role. CNMs best fulfill the role of advocate when they invest time, effort, and caring in establishing a partnership with the patient and provide her with the teaching, coaching and counseling that are characteristic of nurse-midwifery practice (see parallels to coaching and teaching in Chapter 6). Results of a study of 1181 women suggest that this emphasis on education explains some of the differences between CNMs' and obstetricians' care processes (Oakley et al., 1995). Although many processes were similar, CNMs emphasized educational/psychosocial care and restrained use of technology tailored to the individual, whereas the obstetricians' practice reflected routine use of state-of-the-art technology. An example is current publicity regarding elective cesarean deliveries for the convenience of patient or provider, the avoidance of pain, or legal concerns. CNMs attempt to sort out these data for their patients and help them critically evaluate such information. CNMs' emphasis on education enables women to participate knowledgeably and fully in their care. The value of a partnership that has been built over the course of the pregnancy becomes eminently clear during labor, when decisions have to be made. CNMs understand that a woman in the midst of labor may not be in the best position to make good, coherent decisions. The CNM and informed significant others can act in the patient's best interests at this time, because the woman's goals and her contingency plans for events that might interfere with them are jointly determined before labor begins.

Patient education, never an easy task, is made even more daunting by the rapidity with which new technologies are developed, tested, and offered to women. Many women make decisions about their care without adequate information and then suffer the consequences (Franklin, 1994). The CNM often represents a pregnant woman's best hope of receiving adequate information and assurance that she is not left bewildered and alone. CNMs bring the gifts of skill, knowledge, and love to a health-care setting that can be devoid of human warmth, all the more so as the technological aspects of care become more prevalent and more complex. There can be few more noble tasks than providing every woman a safer passage to motherhood and a better future for her children and family (Hsia, 1991).

THE CURRENT PRACTICE OF NURSE-MIDWIFERY

Scope of Practice

Originally, midwifery practice was limited to prenatal, intrapartum, postpartum, and newborn care. Today, although some CNMs limit their practice or are limited by their practice settings to pregnancy care alone, nurse-midwifery care has expanded to include the primary care of women, as well as preconception, gynecological, contraceptive, and infertility care. CNMs care for teenage women, women in their childbearing years, women in midlife, and elderly women. This expansion is due largely to consumer demand and the need for greater access to these services. Interestingly, in many other countries midwifery practice continues to be somewhat restricted to care related to childbirth only.

A general discussion of the scope of advanced practice nursing can be found in Chapter 22. "Scope of practice" refers to what CNMs are actually doing in practice, once the core competencies have been met. The ACNM (1997i) provides a guide for the evaluation and addition of other skills and procedures to nurse-midwifery practice. Thus procedures such as circumcision, vacuum extraction delivery, endometrial biopsy, colposcopy, and elective termination of pregnancy can be included in some CNMs' practice. The term *scope of practice* is also used to differentiate nurse-midwifery practice that is office based, in which no labor and delivery care is provided, from full-scope practice, which includes labor and delivery care. Both types of practice may or may not include the additional procedures previously mentioned.

The ACNM Core Competencies (ACNM, 2002) codify knowledge and practice expectations of the graduate CNM, serve as a guide for education programs, and represent basic CNM practice to other organizations, health-care professionals, and practice settings (Roberts, 1997; Roberts & Huser, 2002). Table 16-3 offers an overview of nurse-midwifery practice, including the knowledge needed and the processes used to provide care. Care of women at other developmental stages or with other health-care needs follows similar guidelines. Nurse-midwifery practice incorporates knowledge of the following: normal human physical and psychological development, anatomy and physiology, physiological and psychological deviations from normal, embryology and genetics, reproduction, sexuality, and pharmacology. CNMs recognize indicators of developmental changes throughout women's life cycles and can counsel women regarding health promotion measures specific to these changes. They recognize indicators of problems with sexuality and can counsel or initiate consultation or referral for problems outside the scope of nurse-midwifery practice. Like all APNs, CNMs are familiar with deviations from normal, risk factors, appropriate preventive measures, and interventions for selected pathology. Whatever a woman's developmental stage or health-care concern, CNMs are expected to teach and counsel patients regarding self-care practices, health promotion, nutritional issues, emotional concerns, and sexuality. Nurse-midwifery practice includes well-defined processes for interacting with physicians and other colleagues to ensure high-quality care. The core competencies, practice guidelines, and an agency's standards of care together with state regulations determine the scope of practice for a particular agency or practice setting.

Although nurse-midwifery practice overlaps with aspects of care provided by other health-care professionals, elements of CNM care are unique. CNMs adhere to the belief that the life processes they deal with are *normal*; therefore, the midwifery approach, at least initially, is noninterventive. When interventions are indicated, CNMs may not limit themselves to modern allopathic (medical) approaches and may advise patients to use traditional measures that women have found comforting and effective, such as acupressure, herbals, homeopathics, healing touch, bodywork, and nutritional interventions. These complementary interventions are most likely to be used for common discomforts of pregnancy, labor, premenstrual problems, or menopausal symptoms.

Nurse-Midwifery Management Processes

Regardless of practice setting, nurse-midwifery care encompasses four aspects of management: independent management, consultation, co-management (collaborative management), and referral (ACNM, 1997e). Implicit in these processes are timely action and documentation of the three aspects other than independent management (Avery, 1992; Keleher, 1998). The key differences among these aspects of management relate to accountability (see also Chapter 7).

INDEPENDENT MANAGEMENT

CNMs are responsible and accountable for the management decisions they make in caring for patients. CNMs provide independent management when they systematically obtain or update a complete and relevant database for assessment of the patient's health status. This includes the history, the physical examination results, and laboratory data. On the basis and interpretation of these findings, CNMs accurately identify problems and diagnoses and implement a plan of action. They delineate health-care goals and formulate and communicate a complete needs/problem list in collaboration with the woman. CNMs know when consultation, co-management, or referral is needed and initiate these interactions in a timely manner.

CONSULTATION

When CNMs identify problems or complications, they seek advice from another member of the health-care team, often a physician but not always an obstetrician. When they retain independent management responsibility for the patient while seeking advice, this is called *consultation* (ACNM, 1997d, 1997e). A consultation may center on an ongoing health problem (e.g., hypothyroidism), a nonobstetrical, time-limited problem that arises during pregnancy (e.g., bronchitis or food poisoning), or an obstetrical complication (e.g., size-date discrepancy). After consultation, the CNM and the woman discuss the recommendations, if any, and modify the plan of care accordingly. In the process of consultation, CNMs retain responsibility for decisions. If they seek consultation from another professional and the suggestions the other professional makes do not seem to be in the patient's best interests, the suggestions will not be used. Thus the process of consultation used by CNMs is consistent with the consultation process described in Chapter 7. It is fair to say that novice CNMs are likely to consult often and to use most of the recommendations they receive until they acquire more experience. Consulting is one way of continuing to learn. The experienced CNM is likely to have a tentative plan in mind when he or she consults with another health-care provider and to utilize consultation to verify the approach or to seek alternatives. It is important to emphasize that CNMs assume direct responsibility for implementing the plan of care in light of their independent management role.

CO-MANAGEMENT OR COLLABORATIVE CARE

One outcome of consultation may be the decision to shift to co-management or collaborative care. This usually occurs if part of the woman's care is related to an ongoing medical,

TABLE 16-3 OVERVIEW OF NURSE-MIDWIFERY PRACTICE

	GENERAL WOMEN'S HEALTH	PREGNANCY	INTRAPARTUM	POSTPARTUM	CARE OF THE NEWBORN
Knowledge needed	Bioethics Interpersonal communication Culture and community resources Counseling Normal reproductive biology Scientific bases of prescriptions to prevent or facilitate pregnancy	Genetics Physiology of normal pregnancy Embryology Pathophysiology Risks Clinical indicators for complications Pharmacokinetics of medications commonly used in pregnancy	Anatomy of normal and abnormal labor in all stages Anatomy of fetal skull and its landmarks Prescription of medications and solutions	Anatomy and physiology (A & P) of the puerperium involutional process Lactation and methods for facilitation or suppression Recognition of deviations from normal	A & P and indications of normal adaptation to extrauterine life Stabilization of the neonate
Assessment and diagnosis	History, physical, lab data, and health risks	Parameters and methods for assessing progress of pregnancy and fetal well-being	Progress of labor Maternal and fetal status	Emotional, psychosocial, and sexual factors	Neonatal physical assessment Neonatal gestational age assessment
Teaching	Health promotion Preventative self-care	Childbirth education Parenting Nutritional education	Reinforcing labor comfort measures taught in childbirth classes Hygiene	Anticipatory guidance re: self-care, infant care, family planning, family relationships	Infant care Nutritional needs of the infant
Comforting	Drug and nondrug measures for discomforts related to menstruation and menopause Information on coping with stress	Drug and nondrug measures for the discomforts of pregnancy	Sensitivity to emotional changes Hands-on care Drug and nondrug measures for pain Local and pudendal anesthesia administration	Managing discomforts of puerperium	Enhancing bonding
Supporting	Active listening	Assisting and supporting the woman in decision making	Physical and emotional support	Supporting woman in breastfeeding and self- and infant care	Support for the changes in family structure with a new member

| Treatment and management | Promotion of family-centered care | Monitoring progress of pregnancy | Monitoring progress of labor
Managing abnormal birth events
Placental expulsion
Repair of lacerations or episiotomy | Appropriate interventions for any deviation from normal | Facilitating adaptation of newborn to extrauterine life |
| Coordination and complex management | Collaboration, referral
Practice/business management
Promotion of the continuity of care
Consultation and co-management | Advocacy
Care jointly planned with woman
Developing a birth plan
Managing deviations from normal | Back-up plans for emergencies in place
Promotion of continuity of care | Providing for continuity of care for the woman and neonate | Resuscitation and emergency care when needed
Referrals as necessary |

gynecological, or obstetrical complication beyond the scope of the CNM's practice. In this situation, the CNM and physician *collaboratively treat* the patient, with the CNM defining and retaining accountability for nurse-midwifery aspects of care (ACNM, 1997e) (see Chapters 7 and 10 for further discussions of consultation and collaboration, respectively).

REFERRAL

When CNMs identify the need for comprehensive management and care that are outside the scope of nurse-midwifery practice, they direct the patient to a physician or another professional for treatment of the particular problem (ACNM, 1997d, 1997e). Referral involves the transfer of some or all of the care and some or all accountability to another provider. This management aspect is usually temporary, and, once the patient's condition returns to that which is within the CNM's scope of practice, the CNM resumes independent management or co-management. For example, the CNM would refer a woman to an internist for hospitalization for pneumonia, to a surgeon for appendicitis, or to an obstetrician for a cesarean delivery. Once the woman regains her health or recovers from surgery, she could return to the care of the CNM.

The details of these aspects of management are developed by individual CNMs in concert with obstetrical consultants/backups and the practice settings in which CNMs practice. In addition to providing these aspects of care, CNMs also serve as consultants to or co-managers with other providers, including physicians, advanced practice nursing colleagues, registered nurses, physical therapists, and mental health colleagues (Hunter & Lops, 1994).

Practice Settings

One soon learns that there are many different practice styles and roles in nurse-midwifery, from full-scope CNMs to office-based CNMs who are not on a call schedule and do not do deliveries. CNMs practice in urban, suburban, and rural areas in a variety of settings. They practice in tertiary and secondary hospitals, often as part of a group practice of CNMs or CNMs and obstetrician-gynecologists or family practice physicians. CNMs are employed by health maintenance organizations and neighborhood health centers. Many CNMs are in private practice, either self-employed or employed by physicians or other CNMs. In some settings, the CNM is the primary care provider; in others, the CNM may have a much more circumscribed practice (Kraus, 1997a; Miller, King, Lurie, & Choitz, 1997). The CNM's actual practice depends on the needs of the population being served, the CNM's willingness to undertake a variety of functions, the availability of educational resources for the many different functions a CNM performs in a specific setting, the particular needs and requests of patients, the availability of physician and CNM colleagues for backup and coverage, and other organizational variables (Ament, 1998).

Some of the settings in which CNMs provide labor and delivery care are patients' homes; autonomous birth centers; birth centers within hospitals; and traditional labor and delivery units of community, regional, and tertiary care hospitals. For patients, the choice of setting may be a matter of philosophy, comfort, convenience, degree of medical risk, or a combination of these factors. Each setting has its unique advantages and disadvantages, and the ACNM has published a position statement on practice settings (ACNM, 1997a).

Using the patient's home as the setting for birth seems in many ways ideal. What could be more family centered? The CNM is in a position to evaluate the patient's resources and help her prepare for childbirth and motherhood within her own setting. Any problems the patient might have will be more apparent if she is seen in her own home. Risks of iatrogenic complications or nosocomial infections are minimized. After the birth of the baby, the patient can rest or sleep in her own bed, comfort and nurse her baby at will, and enjoy the attention and support of her loved ones. Birth at home certainly makes inclusion of family members in the birth (if the mother desires it) a simpler matter than it would be in some other settings.

There are disadvantages to home birth as well. The patient's home may be too far from emergency services. It might be difficult to have the degree of privacy needed for the birth if the house is crowded. Depending on the mother's other responsibilities and support system, her ability to rest may be promoted or compromised. The CNM's resources may be spread too thin, for instance, when two patients are in labor at the same time on opposite sides of town. It can be difficult to get medical backup (either house calls or admitting privileges) for home births in some areas (Scupholme & Walsh, 1994).

The *autonomous birth center* offers solutions to some of the problems with home births. It usually has homelike, attractive birth rooms. Selected emergency equipment is available, which can save crucial seconds that, in a less controlled environment, might be spent searching for such items. The CNMs and patients are at one location, and more than one patient can be cared for at a time. The disadvantages of the autonomous birth center are similar to those of home birth. When an emergency exceeds the birth center's resources, the patient must be transported to a hospital for care. Another important factor is that the patient must get up and take her baby home in a relatively short time, because birth centers do not generally have the ability to keep patients for more than 24 hours.

The *birth center within the hospital* would seem to offer safety in emergencies as an advantage, but many believe that the simple proximity of epidural anesthesia, operating rooms, and other highly interventive technologies leads to their increased use. It is easy to lose sight of the "high-touch/low-tech" approach when one is located in the midst of multitudinous technical devices (Fullerton, 1994). However, being within the hospital setting does eliminate some of the problems CNMs have encountered in obtaining medical backup when it is needed.

Differences in Practice between Nurse-Midwives and Other Providers

The most significant difference between CNMs, obstetrical-gynecological (OB-GYN) NPs, and family NPs (FNPs) is the management of labor and delivery and the care of the newborn infant. OB-GYN NPs and FNPs do not provide independent care or co-management of care during labor and delivery. Some OB-GYN NPs and CNMs may have practices that are evenly divided between pregnancy-related and gynecological services. Others limit their practices to pregnancy-related care. FNP practices are usually more varied and include providing health care for men and children, as well as women.

The practices of maternal-child health CNSs and CNMs also overlap in many ways. Like FNPs or OB-GYN NPs, maternal-child health CNSs do not provide independent management of labor and delivery. However, they are likely to be involved with specific patients and programs related to mother-infant services. Brooten and colleagues' (1986) study of CNS interventions with premature infants is an example of such intervention. The maternal-child health CNS often has more preparation in the care of older infants and children than does the CNM. Unlike the CNM, OB-GYN NP, or FNP, the maternal-child health CNS is also likely to be responsible for some staff development related to mother-infant care. She or he is more likely to practice in a hospital or community health or public health agency.

There are midwives who are not nurses (Johnson & The Midwifery Research Project Group, 1998). In the United States, they are known as *professional midwives* (preferred term), *independent midwives, apprentice midwives, community midwives,* or *lay midwives*. They are most likely to practice within their communities, providing care to pregnant women and attending home births. Their practices are determined partly by the degree to which a particular jurisdiction regulates midwifery and partly by what the prevailing consumer demand and level of medical support are for this type of care. CNMs and midwives relate to each other differently depending on the perceived quality of care provided by both groups, the ability to recognize mutual interest in providing high-quality women's health care, and the consumer demand and medical support for each group within a particular community. The debate over nonnurse midwifery is discussed further in the "Professional Issues" section.

Research suggests that CNMs and obstetricians differ most prominently in the processes they use in providing care (Oakley et al., 1995). Many differences between CNMs and obstetricians can be explained by the differing values between medicine and nursing. CNMs approach the care of women, particularly during pregnancy, with the expectation that all will occur normally until proven otherwise.

Obstetricians are trained to diagnose and treat abnormalities and approach the care of women with the expectation that problems are likely to occur. Each professional group has expertise of value to the other. Successfully meeting the challenges of working together with obstetricians is as essential to providing nurse-midwifery care as are the core competencies for practice.

Summary

It should be evident from this discussion of nurse-midwifery care, scope of practice, management processes, and practice settings that CNMs have many opportunities to influence women's health care. Nurse-midwifery allows its practitioners to provide patient-focused care that is both autonomous and collaborative within or across a variety of settings (Crofts, 1994). It offers a woman the opportunity to obtain, throughout her life as well as during her childbearing years, accessible, understandable, high-quality care that will be safe, satisfying, and individualized to her and her family's needs and desires.

AN EXEMPLAR OF NURSE-MIDWIFERY PRACTICE

The day-to-day practice of midwifery is similar in all settings. In this section, the first author (MWD) describes the practice she established in an autonomous CNM-owned birth center to illustrate how the components of nurse-midwifery care are enacted in this setting.

EXEMPLAR 16-1

The patient education process begins before a patient is accepted into the practice. Orientation sessions are held to provide prospective patients with information to assist them in determining whether they want to have their baby in a birth center. These sessions, conducted by the certified nurse-midwife (CNM), are designed to provide both information and a tour of the physical facility. Prospective patients can see firsthand the comfort measures (such as the whirlpool tub) and the equipment on hand to handle normal deliveries and emergencies. Finances are discussed. The cost of care in the birth center is approximately half of that for obstetrical care in a hospital setting with a physician. Many insurers, Medicaid, and Medicare provide reimbursement; managed care entities have been slower to embrace this form of safe, satisfying, and cost-effective care.

In an autonomous setting such as this, clinical documentation must be meticulous, and an individualized health record ensures that accurate, consistent, and complete information is obtained. Thorough health and family histories are taken. The questions asked elicit information about the woman's physical health and her psychological well-being. How does she feel about being pregnant? What kind of support system does she have in place? What resources might she have that are not currently being called upon? Was the pregnancy planned or a surprise? What are her family circumstances? Is there a stable relationship? Are there other children? It is important to document both positive and negative influences that can have an impact on the patient's health and the health of her baby. Once the assessment is complete, risk factors that would prevent us from being able to accept a patient are reviewed; if we cannot accept a patient, we make a referral. If no risk factors are identified, we schedule the patient's first visit.

When patients are accepted into the practice, they are told that they are equal partners in their care. It is the goal of patient education to bring this to reality. To be active participants in their care, patients are taught to weigh themselves and do their own urine dipstick tests. They participate in charting the information, thus noting the progress of their pregnancy firsthand. The program of care for pregnant patients at our birth center includes 10 to 15 prenatal visits, childbirth classes, labor and delivery in the birth center, a home visit within 72 hours of birth, and two office follow-up visits for mother and baby—one at 1 week and the other at 6 weeks after birth.

Clinical hours are held daily. The CNMs in the practice share in doing patient visits, teaching classes, and on-call time. Other responsibilities include administration and facility maintenance. We see pregnant patients, postpartum patients with their babies, and gynecological patients. The amount of time scheduled for a visit is based on need. A first visit for a pregnant patient is an hour long. An established gynecological patient who is coming for her contraceptive injection requires only a few minutes, long enough to establish that she's having no problems.

A pregnant patient is given the CNM pager number and instructions on how and when to use it. When a patient is in active labor or her membranes have ruptured, she calls the CNM on duty. She is met at the birth center and examined. Most often when the woman arrives she is in active labor. We attribute this largely to the educational process that has taken place. On the rare occasion of false labor or very early labor, we are able to individualize care. If a patient lives far away, we may elect to observe progress for a number of hours. If the woman is sleep deprived, she and her labor may benefit from some sedation. We remain with our patients in the birth center during labor. There is a registered nurse (RN) on call for every delivery. If the CNM attending the patient is tiring from having been up for a long labor, or several labors, the RN can be called to come in early to care for the patient while the CNM rests. Sometimes, the RN is not needed until close to time for the birth.

The mother-to-be helps us to accommodate her wishes by preparing a birth plan. As her due date nears, one of her tasks (along with packing a bag to bring to the birth center and readying her home for a baby) is to write a birth plan, which will become a part of her record. This form allows her to tell us who she wants with her during labor, what she imagines labor will be like, what she *hopes* labor will be like, and what comfort measures would assist her during labor. We use this tool in several ways. We evaluate the effectiveness of our teaching by reading what the woman thinks labor will be like. Mention of fears not previously revealed gives us an opportunity to resolve any emotional factors that could hinder a successful labor. Knowing the person(s) the patient wants with her during labor informs us about her support system. The people present during labor are an important factor in enhancing the woman's experience of labor.

Continued

The list of comfort measures is mainly a reminder to us, although it is a key contribution from the patient. In the midst of labor, a woman may forget that she was looking forward to the whirlpool tub for relaxation and pain relief. A glance at the birth plan helps us try the things the patient has already identified as potentially helpful to her. The birth plan helps to emphasize to the patient that this is *her* labor, with its inherent responsibilities and rights. Her dignity and worth as a human being are underscored. We try to nourish the woman's self-esteem and strengths that help in labor, life, and motherhood. The stronger the woman is in every way, the better her outcome is going to be.

Patients are given plenty of written material to help with their recall of information covered in classes. (If a patient is unable to read, extra time is spent providing information verbally and making sure the patient understands it.) To help the patient assume responsibility for herself and her labor, she is expected to bring with her to the birth center food and beverages that she would like to have available during labor and certain supplies, such as perineal pads, bed pads, and diapers. Patients take their babies home dressed in their own clothes and wrapped in their own blankets. They take with them an instructional booklet that they were given in the postpartum class. The booklet describes mother and baby care for the first few days in detail. Because mothers and babies are discharged early, often in 4 to 6 hours, it is imperative that the mother be prepared to check the baby's temperature and respirations, to check her own uterus, and to be able to recognize signs of complications that require attention. These are all enumerated in the instructions, and there is room for notes and questions. Having a reference helps new moms feel more secure. If something needs attention, they can always call the nurse-midwife, but they usually find what they need to know in the booklet. It often confirms what they sensed—either that everything was okay or that they need to get in touch with the nurse-midwife. Thus new mothers start out having faith in their own perceptions regarding their infants reinforced.

Empowering our patients, enhancing their decision-making abilities, reinforcing the mind-body connection, and enhancing family life by helping women find their personal power are goals of CNM care at the birth center. When I think of the enormous effects of empowerment, two new moms come to mind.

M. L.'s case is proof positive of the benefits of teaching new mothers to trust their feelings and make decisions based on them. On the third or fourth day after delivery, M. L.'s baby ceased nursing well. He had been nursing vigorously and now was not. Nursing poorly is one of the signs listed in our booklet as requiring professional help. M. L. insisted to her husband that they had to go to the emergency room immediately. They lived a long distance from the birth center, and it had been decided earlier that, if there should be a problem that seemed serious, she should go to a nearby emergency room, rather than try to get to the CNM. Initially, doctors could find nothing wrong, but M. L. insisted they keep looking. As it turned out, the baby had a congenital heart defect that does not show up on clinical examination until 3 or 4 days after birth. M. L. said she was glad she had been given the information at the birth center; it gave her the confidence to trust her feelings that something was seriously wrong. The baby had heart surgery and is doing well.

A woman with confidence and trust in herself can do almost anything, as the case of S. J. shows. S. J. was 26 years old and came to the birth center soon after it opened to have her fourth child. She had a high school education and was home with her children, all of whom were under the age of 5. Her self-esteem was negligible. Her husband came to a few of the prenatal classes but was sullen and unsupportive. S. J. seemed to droop, but she was an excellent mother and was an attentive and fast learner at everything to do with childbirth, childrearing, and health in general. Her interest and enthusiasm grew as we reinforced her abilities and strengths. By the time she gave birth to her son, she seemed a different person from the withdrawn, self-effacing young woman we'd met 7 months earlier. Two years after this baby's birth, S. J. paid a visit to the birth center. "I just wanted to thank you," she said. "Before I came here, I never felt I was any good at anything. You told me I was a good mother, you noticed how well cared for my children were, and you encouraged me to learn all about birth and even let me borrow books and tapes. Well, I learned I was good—at a lot of things! You all showed me that. And I wanted you to know I'm in nursing school now because I want to be able to do what you do—not just take care of people physically, but help people grow."

The ability to have such a positive impact on others is very satisfying. However, it is clear that being a CNM does not entail "doing it all" for our patients. It is far more important, and healthier for all concerned, to teach our patients so that they are empowered to provide themselves and their families with the best possible care for every situation. We cannot be there for every health difficulty our patients may have, but we can give them the confidence to *know* when something is wrong and the knowledge of what to do in various situations. CNMs *give* from the core of their being. They listen, which is one of the crucial skills CNMs bring to their practice. The listening is more than an auditory experience. CNMs listen observantly to hear clearly. They communicate confidence in the care of their patients in everyday matters. They hear clearly, and their patients respond.

The rewards of our practice are many, but we have faced some challenges, too. On the rare occasions that things go wrong, we are scrutinized intensely. Vacation coverage is difficult to find. Other challenges include complying with regulations and legislation, finding appropriate resources for medical consultation and referral, and dealing with misperceptions of our practice within the larger health-care system. These issues are not unique to our practice, as the next section shows.

PROFESSIONAL ISSUES

Image

Although there is universal recognition of the term *midwife*, the word also conjures up a variety of images—some positive and others negative. Rather recently the term *midwife* has come into common usage as a metaphor for positive experiences of guidance, compassion, strength, or peace (Paine, 2000). After their first encounter with a CNM, many people comment that they are surprised at how "normal" and/or how "professional" she or he was, but most are unable to say just what they expected. Stereotypes that have been voiced about CNMs include "old, stooped, with stringy gray hair," "someone shuffling around in jeans and Birkenstocks," "someone practicing illegally," and "backward." These images are damaging and misleading. In contrast, actual experiences with CNMs are judged overwhelmingly positive. A commonly heard refrain from patients of CNMs is that every woman should have the privilege of being cared for by a CNM.

Part of the confusion about the image of the midwife stems from the different types of midwives that can be found in the United States. In addition to CNMs, there are direct-entry midwives, lay midwives, and granny midwives. A direct-entry midwife is someone who has completed formal academic midwifery preparation without a nursing background. These individuals tend to have baccalaureate degrees in areas other than nursing, and are more likely to practice in homes or birth centers. Lay midwives are typically associated with home birth practice and informal training or apprenticeship experience. A new type of this practitioner evolved in response to a counterculture movement in the 1960s. Over time, some members of this group developed training courses, ranging from weekend workshops to intense academic programs. An unfortunate result of this lack of standardization has been marked variation between practitioners, and thus difficulty in characterizing this practice as professional. Finally, granny midwives are women who attended births of women in communities throughout the southeastern United States from the founding of the country until the middle 20th century. The granny midwife was likewise apprentice trained and was responding to a need in her community (Rooks, 1997).

From this discussion, it is no wonder that the public image of the CNM is unclear. In addition to consumer confusion, there has been a fair amount of professional resistance to

CNMs from the medical community. This is not unlike their response to other APNs. Despite both the confusion and resistance, the ACNM is committed to ensuring that a positive image of the professional CNM emerges and seeks media opportunities to educate consumers about the role of the CNM. Even with these efforts, each CNM in clinical practice also spends a portion of the day explaining who he or she is and striving to both educate and improve the image of the midwife—one patient at a time.

Credentialing Nonnurses (Direct Entry Midwives)

In 1994, the ACNM made the difficult decision to develop a mechanism to accredit midwifery education programs that do not require a nursing credential (ACNM, 1998b). In addition, the certification body, the ACC, similarly decided to give graduates of these programs the same examination administered to graduates of nurse-midwifery education programs (Burst, 1995; Shah & Hsia, 1996). These decisions were based on political realities. The issues surrounding the nursing shortage played into the decision-making process.

First, an increasing number of states or hospitals were granting recognition to attend births to individuals whose credentials to practice were less than those established by the ACNM. Second, New York passed a midwifery practice act with the intent of having all midwives take the same examination. The assumption was made that, with equivalent educational criteria, a sound program could be developed for those who desired to practice midwifery without a nursing degree (Williams & Kelley, 1998). We were also well aware that the international midwifery community has been successful in educating both nurses and nonnurses as midwives within their education and practice structure (Rooks, 1997). The ultimate reason for the ACNM's decision was to advance a single standard for professional midwifery in this country.

Once that decision was made, the ACNM's DOA developed accreditation standards that included skills, knowledge, and competencies in health science that would be prerequisite to midwifery practice. In addition, each graduate must successfully complete college-level courses in biology, chemistry, microbiology, anatomy and physiology, human development, psychology, epidemiology/statistics, pathophysiology, and nutrition (Burst, 1995). The profession also supported research to examine the quality of education and practice of these early graduates. A pilot study at the State University of New York Health Science Center "confirmed that direct-entry students could acquire and demonstrate the basic health skills at a level equivalent to their RN classmates" (Fullerton, Shah, Holmes, Roe, & Campau, 1998, p. 105). A follow-up study (Fullerton, Shah, Schechter, & Muller, 2000) of the first two graduating classes in this program demonstrated that the direct-entry students' first-time pass rate on the ACC certification examination was equivalent to that of the registered nursing students in the program. In this program, once the nonnurse students had successfully completed the "basic health skills" section of their curriculum, nonnurse and nurse-midwifery students were educated together.

This decision by the ACNM has been met with mixed reactions. There are those who believe that these initiatives further obscure advanced practice nursing and make it even more difficult for APNs to attain some of the regulatory and legislative support they seek. However, the ACNM may be at the cutting edge of developing a transdisciplinary workforce, a legion of people with different backgrounds but the same core set of midwifery competencies. It is difficult to predict where such practitioners will fit into the current and future health-care system. Part of their ability to succeed will rest on the state regulatory agencies. In 16 states, midwifery, without a registered nursing credential, is regulated by a state agency. In 11 more states, the practice of midwifery by nonnurses is legal but unregulated. There are 15 states in which one must have a registered nursing credential to practice legally as a midwife (ACNM, 1999). If the demand for this type of practitioner grows, and states use the ACNM national standards, which demonstrate equivalent preparation, the public will be assured of well-qualified providers. Such a group of providers does seem consistent with projections regarding the type of workforce needed in the future (Dower et al., 1999).

Congruence/Incongruence of Midwifery Practice with Advanced Practice Nursing

In our opinion, the ACNM's commitments to expand the pool of available midwives and to include nonnurse midwives in a diverse midwifery workforce make it difficult for the organization to advocate master's-level preparation for all CNMs. In this sense, midwifery is diverging from the vision of advanced practice nursing advocated in this text. Several observations can be made, however, that suggest that the mainstreaming of nurse-midwifery within advanced practice nursing may be inevitable. Despite the fact that there are inconsistencies regarding the CNM role within advanced practice nursing, CNMs are developing in ways congruent with the vision that is bringing together CNSs, certified registered nurse anesthetists, NPs, and other APNs. The core competencies defined by the ACNM and their implementation are consistent with the core competencies of advanced practice described in Chapter 3. Most nurse-midwifery education is delivered in master's-level programs and within schools of nursing. Clinical and regulatory issues such as access to and availability of services, as well as second licensure for APNs, are likely to engage CNMs in collaborative efforts to promote the values and vision driving advanced practice. Some states already require a master's degree for licensing as an APN (including CNMs) and/or for prescriptive authority; others have established a date by which a master's degree will be required. These precedents could well affect federal funding for nurse-midwifery education. It is unlikely that CNMs will risk the legal privileges for which they fought so hard by resisting efforts to ensure a common definition of advanced practice nursing across state and federal laws and regulations. Appeals to the ACNM have been made by CNMs in states that have passed the requirement for a master's degree. The ACNM Board of Directors has responded by reaffirming support for certificate programs and referring members to other resources and offering specific strategic suggestions. Safriet (1992), an attorney, has argued that consistency in the definition of advanced practice nursing and in the criteria for being licensed as an APN is needed if APNs are to be able to practice with the autonomy that other professionals enjoy. In the current climate, however, it is difficult to anticipate how nurse-midwifery will address the regulatory complexity that is likely to result from the entry of nonnurses into midwifery. Whether the regulatory climate will be more or less open to innovative programs such as those contemplated by the ACNM is not clear.

These are the driving forces that are likely to carry CNMs and nurse-midwifery along in their currents or wake as APN roles are defined and regulated at federal and state levels. Failure to be involved or opposition to the changes will undermine nurse-midwifery's efforts to secure accessible health care for individuals and may well undo its historical legislative achievements, which have enabled CNMs to practice autonomously.

Collegial Relationships and Autonomy

It will come as no surprise to the reader that the factors that have been associated with job satisfaction are often the areas in which barriers to nurse-midwifery practice exist. These factors include working with competent personnel, having high-quality patient interactions, having the time to provide a preferred style of care, being involved with patients' care plans and decision making, having good interpersonal relationships with other CNMs and with backup physicians, having professional autonomy, experiencing feelings of personal worth, and participating in teamwork (Collins, 1990). Although CNMs can enjoy many of these rewards, as the earlier description of practice at the birth center shows, they often encounter difficulties in securing them, especially with regard to relationships with physicians, professional autonomy, and workload. For both the nurse-midwifery profession and individual CNMs, the goal is to pursue productive, collaborative relationships with all involved.

PHYSICIANS

Professional relationships between obstetrician-gynecologists and CNMs are addressed in a joint statement recently updated and agreed upon by the American College of Obstetricians and Gynecologists and the ACNM (Shah, 2002) (Box 16-3). Individual CNMs and individual physicians often get along and develop the kind of mature collaborative relationships described in Chapter 10. However, the current health-care environment, in which organizations and providers are scrambling to cut costs and services, is not conducive to building the kind of CNM-physician rapport that has made so many CNM-run practices successful. Barriers to effective working relationships between CNMs and physicians often arise within organizations. Although there may be individual members of organized medical groups with whom CNMs work well, the organizations themselves often spend time and money on efforts to restrict APNs' ability to practice autonomously. These efforts include lobbying against federal and state laws and regulations that are favorable to CNMs and other APNs. Chapter 21 describes the American Medical Association's public relations campaign to convince the public that APNs and other non-physician providers are quacks. The American Medical Association (1995) described "integrated" practice with APNs but declared the physician the "captain of the ship." Some state medical and nursing associations have found common ground on which to base organizational collaboration. However, CNMs who enjoy excellent collaborative

---

BOX 16-3 • OBSTETRICIAN-GYNECOLOGISTS AND CERTIFIED NURSE-MIDWIVES/CERTIFIED MIDWIVES

The American College of Obstetricians and Gynecologists (ACOG) and the American College of Nurse-Midwives (ACNM) recognize that in those circumstances in which obstetrician-gynecologists and certified nurse-midwives/certified midwives collaborate in the care of women, the quality of those practices is enhanced by a working relationship characterized by mutual respect and trust as well as professional responsibility and accountability. When obstetrician-gynecologists and certified nurse-midwives/certified midwives collaborate, they should concur on a clear mechanism for consultation, collaboration and referral based on the individual needs of each patient.

Recognizing the high level of responsibility that obstetrician-gynecologists and certified nurse-midwives/certified midwives assume when providing care to women, ACOG and ACNM affirm their commitment to promote appropriate standards for education and certification of their respective members, to support appropriate practice guidelines, and to facilitate communication and collegial relationships between obstetrician-gynecologists and certified nurse-midwives/certified midwives.

From the American College of Nurse-Midwives and American College of Obstetricians and Gynecologists. *Joint statement of practice relations between obstetrician-gynecologists and certified nurse-midwives/certified midwives*. Washington, DC: American College of Nurse-Midwives.

relationships with individual physicians should be alert to the activities of organized medical groups, both nationally and within their jurisdictions, so that they can protect their rights to practice nurse-midwifery and encourage their physician colleagues to speak out against limitations on CNM practice.

In hospitals and communities in which physicians continue to have (or are seen as having) power over who can and cannot practice, entrepreneurial CNMs may have more difficulty gaining clinical privileges or medical backup. Often, CNMs need to apply to a hospital's medical board if they wish to be able to attend laboring women in that hospital. A CNM who is the first APN to apply for these privileges in that hospital must be prepared to blaze a trail in everything, from attempting to change hospital bylaws and educating labor and delivery nursing staff regarding CNM practice, to obtaining a chart box in medical records, to negotiating for a locker in a changing room (Scoggin, 1997). However, more and more hospital credentialing committees have representatives from nursing who are supportive of CNMs and APNs.

Whether they need clinical privileges or not, CNMs must have physician consultation and medical backup. This requirement may be incorporated into a state practice act, but, even if it is not, clinical practice and ACNM standards demand it. For the CNM working in an agency, formal and informal structures to ensure physician availability are likely to be established. If the CNM is the first one to practice in the organization, these structures will have to be developed. Regardless of practice setting, CNMs need to have a physician with whom they can consult or to whom they can make a referral when needed. Entrepreneurial CNMs will find physicians who are quite willing to be available and welcome the opportunity to collaborate. However, a CNM may find herself or himself in the position of negotiating for such backup with physicians who are reluctant at best and actively hostile at worst. Many times, it is a matter of education, public relations (see Chapter 21), and consumer demand. Just seeing the care provided at a CNM-run birth center can diminish resistance and elicit support. A combination of interpersonal skills, business savvy, and marketing strategies can help CNMs overcome barriers that arise from lack of knowledge, lack of trust, and power imbalances.

BARRIERS TO PRACTICE

Legislative, Regulatory, and Financial Barriers

Last but not least, there continue to exist barriers to full-scope nurse-midwifery practice. Restrictions to practice can be found at the local, state, and federal levels. If interpersonal, marketing, and public relations efforts fail to secure admitting and clinical privileges for CNMs, legislation that ensures CNMs and other APNs access to these privileges will be needed (ACNM, 1997c). Inequitable reimbursement for services remains a problem for CNMs in many states. Legislation and regulations that mandate reimbursement equitable to the value of CNMs' work, practice costs, and malpractice expenses must be enacted. Nurse-midwifery care should be an option in managed care systems, but it may not be if APNs and consumers do not make their voices heard. CNMs must have prescriptive authority, and greater uniformity and consistency of regulations at the federal and state levels for prescribing and dispensing medications are needed. CNMs must be assured of a continuing source of professional liability insurance. Allocations for nurse-midwifery education from federal and state funding agencies are at risk in the current political climate, in which many politicians are seeking to minimize government initiatives that promote health and education. Medicare and Medicaid must ensure facility fee payment for birth centers.

Workload

When there is a full complement of CNMs to share the work of night call (e.g., being on call one or two nights a week), clinics, and other responsibilities, the unpredictable timing of labor and delivery and the erratic sleep patterns that result are manageable (Flanagan, 1993). For many CNMs, especially those in solo or independent practices, however, a full complement of staff is a luxury. To give their best to their patients and to stay healthy, CNMs with a heavy on-call schedule need to develop self-care strategies that enable them to balance work with personal responsibilities and relationships. The sabbatical has been proposed as one way to promote professional development while decreasing the demands of full-scope practice (Keleher, 1993). This is likely to work only in large, well-funded practices. In addition, finding other CNMs who can cover for vacation and sick time can become a minor crisis. The physical and emotional demands of "catching" babies, in addition to the long hours and periods of sleep deprivation, mean that nurse-midwifery is not for everyone. For those who love it, the satisfaction of watching pregnancy progress, the physical and mental demands of labor and delivery, the element of unpredictability in the timing of birth, and the joy of birth make nurse-midwifery fascinating, exciting, and personally rewarding (Lubic, 1997).

Malpractice Issues

Like their physician colleagues, CNMs are facing limited options in obtaining reasonable and comprehensive professional liability coverage. Malpractice premiums are extremely high and difficult for CNMs to obtain in their own right. At the same time, because of the burgeoning rates for their own malpractice policies, physicians are no longer able nor do they want to cover nurse-midwives under their umbrella policies. The American College of Nurse-Midwives (ACNM) offers strong support for CNMs in this area. They have worked diligently to provide support for programs that preserve the risk management goals of the midwifery profession. The ACNM uses its influence to enter into relationships with insurance entities that specifically include benefits to ACNM members. Readers are referred to the ACNM website (www.ACNM.org) to access current options for obtaining liability coverage. Insurance to cover liability has been, and will continue to be, a major barrier to CNMs that requires constant monitoring and innovative strategies.

CONCLUSION

In spite of the resistance from the established medical community, there is a growing demand and need for CNMs' unique services. CNMs are woman centered and family centered (VandeVusse, 1997). They have been thinking globally and acting locally long before it became trendy to do so. They are called to do what they do. As long as there are pregnant women who wish to give birth in an informed and caring fashion, there will be a need for CNMs. Indeed, there are those in the profession who feel that midwifery holds the key to contemporary obstetrical problems (Baldwin, 1999; Rooks, 1998).

Nurse-midwifery, advanced practice nursing, and the profession of nursing in general are at a critical juncture. Although nurse-midwifery is standing somewhat apart from advanced practice efforts, it seems clear that there is a need to recognize the interdependence of advanced practice nursing and nurse-midwifery. By examining the separate yet related courses being charted by the nursing profession (related to advanced practice nursing) and by CNMs (to meet demands for midwifery services), one can see that there is great potential for divisiveness at a time in our history when we need to be unified. The directions CNMs are pursuing may seem unfathomable to those outside nurse-midwifery. The authors have each been involved in political battles for the right to practice and have watched nurse-midwifery evolve in different regions of the United States. We believe there is vision and wisdom in the ACNM's initiatives that will benefit advanced practice nursing and APNs in the long run. However, there appear to be many forces driving the nursing profession toward requiring a master's degree for second licensing, and midwifery's opposition to this requirement is unlikely to be successful. Mounting such an opposition will drain energy away from CNMs and all APNs whose main goals are to improve access to health care and to provide that care. More important, it could undermine every hard-won political and legislative victory. All CNMs need to give serious consideration to the insights of Safriet (1992), who maintains that APNs will only be able to practice autonomously when there is a uniform definition of advanced practice nursing on which laws and regulations are based.

CNMs have often led the nursing profession into the future, and many of the initiatives mentioned in this chapter indicate that the profession continues to move forward. It may now be time for CNMs to join forces with the nursing profession, which is investing its energy and resources in preserving and expanding the climate for autonomous nursing practice that CNMs helped to create.

REFERENCES

Ad Hoc Committee on Code of Ethics. (1990). *Code of ethics for certified nurse-midwives.* Washington, DC: American College of Nurse-Midwives.

Ament, L. (1998). Reimbursement, employment, and hospital privilege data of certified nurse-midwifery services. *Journal of Nurse-Midwifery, 43,* 305-309.

American College of Nurse-Midwives. (1989). *Philosophy of the American College of Nurse-Midwives.* Washington, DC: Author.

American College of Nurse-Midwives. (1993). *Standards for the practice of nurse-midwifery.* Washington, DC: Author.

American College of Nurse-Midwives. (1997a). *ACNM statement on practice settings.* Washington, DC: Author.

American College of Nurse-Midwives. (1997b). *The appropriate use of technology in childbirth.* Washington, DC: Author.

American College of Nurse-Midwives. (1997c). *Barriers to midwifery practice.* Washington, DC: Author.

American College of Nurse-Midwives. (1997d). *Certified nurse-midwives and certified midwives as primary care providers/case managers.* Washington, DC: Author.

American College of Nurse-Midwives. (1997e). *Collaborative management in nurse-midwifery practice for medical, gynecological, and obstetrical conditions.* Washington, DC: Author.

American College of Nurse-Midwives. (1997f). *Continuing competency assessment.* Washington, DC: Author.

American College of Nurse-Midwives. (1997g). *Criteria for preaccreditation and accreditation of education programs in nurse-midwifery and midwifery.* Washington, DC: Author.

American College of Nurse-Midwives. (1997h). *Definition of a certified nurse-midwife/definition of midwifery practice.* Washington, DC: Author.

American College of Nurse-Midwives. (1997i). *Expansion of nurse-midwifery practice and skills beyond basic care competencies.* Washington, DC: Author.

American College of Nurse-Midwives. (1997j). *Midwifery education.* Washington, DC: Author.

American College of Nurse-Midwives. (1998a). *Healthcare/managed care reform.* Washington, DC: Author.

American College of Nurse-Midwives. (1998b). *Mandatory degree requirements for midwives.* Washington, DC: Author.

American College of Nurse-Midwives. (1999). *Nurse-midwifery today: A handbook of state laws & regulations.* Washington, DC: Author.

American College of Nurse-Midwives. (2002) *Core competencies for basic midwifery practice.* Washington, DC: Author.

American College of Nurse-Midwives. (2003). *Standards for the practice of nurse-midwifery.* Washington, DC: Author. Retrieved May 3, 2004, from http://www.midwife.org/prof/display.cfm?id=138

American Medical Association Board of Trustees. (1995). *Model guidelines for physician and nurse practicitioner integrated practice* (Report 6-A-95). Chicago: AMA.

Avery, M. D. (1992). Advanced nurse-midwifery practice. *Journal of Nurse-Midwifery, 37,* 150-154.

Baldwin, K. A. (1999). The midwifery solution to contemporary problems in American obstetrics. *Journal of Nurse-Midwifery, 44,* 75-79.

Bellack, J., Graber, D., O'Neil, E. H., & Musham, C. (1998). Curriculum trends in nurse-midwifery education: Views of program directors. *Journal of Nurse-Midwifery, 43,* 341-350.

Bergstrom, L. (1997). Midwifery as a discipline. *Journal of Nurse-Midwifery, 42,* 417-420.

Brooten, D., Kumar, S., Brown, L. P., Butts, P., Finkler, S. A., Bakewell-Sachs, S., et al. (1986). A randomized clinical trial of early hospital discharge and home follow-up of very-low-birth-weight infants. *New England Journal of Medicine, 315,* 934-939.

Burst, H. V. (1995). An update on the credentialing of midwives by the American College of Nurse-Midwives. *Journal of Nurse-Midwifery, 40,* 290-296.

Carr, K. C. (1999). Creating off-campus/distance learning courses for midwifery education: A brief introduction. *Journal of Nurse-Midwifery, 44,* 57-64.

Carrington, B. W., & Decker, B. (1997). A master's degree for entry-level ACNM certified-midwives: An option or necessity? *Journal of Nurse-Midwifery, 42,* 364-366.

Collins, C. (1990, May). CNM *job satisfaction: Luxury or necessity?* Presented at the ACNM Convention, Atlanta, GA.

Corry, M. P., & Rooks, J. (1999). Public education: Promoting the midwifery model of care in partnership with the Maternity Center Association. *Journal of Nurse-Midwifery, 44,* 47-56.

Crofts, A. J. (1994). Entrepreneurship—the realities of today. *Journal of Nurse-Midwifery, 39,* 39-42.

Dawley, K. (2003). Origins of nurse-midwifery in the United States and its expansion in the 1940s. *Journal of Midwifery and Women's Health, 48,* 86-95.

Declercq, E. (2003). Births attended by CNMs in the U.S. *Journal of Midwifery & Women's Health, 48,* 83-84.

Declercq, E. R., Paine, L. L., Dejoseph, J. F., & Simmes, D. (1998). State regulation, payment policies, and nurse-midwife services. *Health Affairs, 17,* 190-200.

Diamant, A. (1997). *The red tent.* New York: St. Martin's Press.

Dorroh, M. W., & Norton, S. F. (1996). The certified nurse-midwife. In A. B. Hamric, J. A. Spross, & C. M. Hanson (Eds.), *Advanced practice nursing: An integrative approach* (pp. 395-420). Philadelphia: W. B. Saunders.

Dower, C. M., Miller, J. E., O'Neil, E. H., & the Taskforce on Midwifery. (1999). *Charting a course for the 21st century: The future of midwifery.* San Francisco: Pew Health Professions Commission and the University of California, San Francisco, Center for the Health Professions.

Flanagan, J. (1993). Speaking up and talking out— barriers to nurse-midwifery practice. *Journal of Nurse-Midwifery, 38,* 246-251.

Franklin, M. (1994). The nurse-midwifery challenge. *Journal of Nurse-Midwifery, 39,* 110-111.

Fullerton, J. T. (1994). Reflections on nurse-midwifery role and functions. *Journal of Nurse-Midwifery, 39,* 107-109.

Fullerton, J. T., & Severino, R. (1995). Factors that predict performance on the national certification examination for nurse-midwives. *Journal of Nurse-Midwifery, 40,* 19-25.

Fullerton, J. T., Shah, M. A., Holmes, G., Roe, V., & Campau, N. (1998). Direct entry midwifery education: Evaluation of program innovations. *Journal of Nurse-Midwifery, 43,* 102-105.

Fullerton, J. T., Shah, M. A., Schechter, S., & Muller, J. H. (2000). Integrating qualified nurses and non-nurses in midwifery education: The two-year experience of an ACNM DOA accredited program. *Journal of Midwifery & Women's Health, 45:*45-54.

Galotti, K. M., Pierce, B., Reimer, R. L., & Luckner, A. E. (2000). Midwife or doctor: A study of pregnant women making delivery decisions. *Journal of Midwifery & Women's Health, 45,* 320-329.

Hsia, L. (1991). Midwives and the empowerment of women. *Journal of Nurse-Midwifery, 36,* 85-87.

Hunter, L. P., & Lops, V. R. (1994). Critical thinking and the nurse-midwifery management process. *Journal of Nurse-Midwifery, 39,* 43-46.

Johnson, P. G., & The Midwifery Research Project Group. (1998). Midwife and nurse-midwife: The effect of title on perception and confidence in services provided by professional midwives. *Journal of Nurse-Midwifery, 43,* 296-304.

Keleher, K. C. (1993). Sabbatical leaves for nurse-midwives in clinical practice. *Journal of Nurse-Midwifery, 38,* 165-167.

Keleher, K. C. (1998). Collaborative practice, characteristics, barriers, benefits, and implications for midwifery. *Journal of Nurse-Midwifery, 43,* 8-11.

Kovner, C. T. & Burkhardt, P. (2001). Findings from the American College of Nurse-Midwives annual membership survey, 1995-1999. *Journal of Midwifery & Women's Health, 46,* 24-29.

Kraus, N. (1997a). Practice profile of members of the American College of Nurse-Midwives: Findings of a direct mail survey. *Journal of Nurse-Midwifery, 42,* 355-363.

Kraus, N. (1997b). What's in a name: Defining the professions of midwifery. *Journal of Nurse-Midwifery, 42,* 69-70.

Lubic, R. W. (1997). Principles for a successful professional life. *Journal of Nurse-Midwifery, 42,* 53-58.

Miller, S., King, T., Lurie, P., & Choitz, P. (1997). Certified nurse-midwife and physician collaborative practice: Piloting a survey on the Internet. *Journal of Nurse-Midwifery, 42,* 308-315.

Nitzsche, R. E. (1995). 40 years old and still growing. *Quickening, 26,* 2.

Oakley, D., Murtland, T., Mayes, F., Hayashi, R., Petersen, B. A., Rorie, C., et al. (1995). Processes of care: Comparisons of certified nurse-midwives and obstetricians. *Journal of Nurse-Midwifery, 40,* 399-403.

Paine, L. L. (2000). Editorial: Midwife as metaphor. *Journal of Midwifery & Women's Health, 45,* 367.

Reed, A., & Roberts, J. E. (2000). State regulation of midwives: Issues and options. *Journal of Midwifery & Women's Health, 45,* 130-149.

Roberts, J. (1997). The core competencies for basic midwifery practice: Critical ACNM document revised. *Journal of Nurse-Midwifery, 42,* 371-372.

Roberts, J., & Huser, S. (2002). The evolution of midwifery as reflected in the 2002 revisions of the ACNMs core competencies. *Journal of Nurse-Midwifery & Women's Health, 47,* 301-302.

Rooks, J. P. (1997). *Midwifery and childbirth in America.* Philadelphia: Temple University Press.

Rooks, J. P. (1998). Unity in midwifery: Realities and alternative. *Journal of Nurse-Midwifery, 43,* 315-319.

Safriet, B. (1992). Health care dollars and regulatory sense: The role of advanced practice nursing. *Yale Journal of Regulation, 9,* 417-488.

Scoggin, J. (1997). The historical relationship of nurse-midwifery with medicine. *Journal of Nurse-Midwifery, 42,* 49-52.

Scupholme, A., & Walsh, L. (1994). Home-based services by nurse-midwives. *Journal of Nurse-Midwifery, 39,* 358-362.

Shah, M. A. (2000). Editorial: The Journal of Midwifery & Women's Health: Celebrating its heritage—forging its future. *Journal of Midwifery & Women's Health, 45,* 1-2.

Shah, M. A. (2002, May 27). *Professional visions...contemporary realities.* Presidential Address delivered at the 47th Annual Meeting of the American College of Nurse-Midwives, Atlanta, GA.

Shah, M. S., & Hsia, L. (1996). Direct entry midwifery education: History in the making. *Journal of Nurse-Midwifery, 41,* 351-353.

VandeVusse, L. (1997). Sculpting a nurse-midwifery philosophy: Ernestine Wiedenbach's influence. *Journal of Nurse-Midwifery, 42,* 43-48.

Varney, H. (1996). *Nurse-midwifery* (3rd ed.). Boston: Blackwell Scientific Publications.

Williams, D. R., & Kelley, M. A. (1998). Core competency-based education, certification and practice: The nurse-midwifery model. *Advanced Practice Nursing Quarterly, 4,* 63-71.

CHAPTER 17

The Certified Registered Nurse Anesthetist

MARGARET FAUT-CALLAHAN • MICHAEL J. KREMER

INTRODUCTION

As noted in Chapter 1, nurse anesthesia is the oldest organized specialty in nursing. Standardized postgraduate education, credentialing, and continuing education were all areas pioneered by certified registered nurse anesthetists (CRNAs). CRNAs were among the first nurse specialists to receive direct reimbursement for their services, and they have a history of activism in legislative and regulatory matters, such as prescriptive authority. This chapter discusses professional definitions of nurse anesthesia practice and issues important to the specialty. The American Association of Nurse Anesthetists (AANA) is described, and the model of professional competence for CRNAs is presented. Nurse anesthesia education, credentialing, certification, and recertification processes are all explored. A profile of current CRNA practice is presented, reimbursement mechanisms are delineated, and projections for future trends are proposed.

PROFESSIONAL DEFINITIONS

A CRNA is a registered nurse who is educationally prepared for and competent to engage in the practice of nurse anesthesia. CRNAs are both responsible and accountable to others for their individual professional practices. In addition, nurse anesthetists are capable of exercising independent professional judgment within their scopes of competence and licensure (Jordan, 1994).

Nurse anesthesia is not a medically delegated act (Jordan, 1994). The practice of anesthesia is not exclusively the practice of medicine or the practice of nursing. It has been said that, if anesthesia is administered by a nurse, it is the practice of nursing, whereas physician-administered anesthesia is the practice of medicine (Gunn, 1991).

Licensure for CRNAs and other advanced practice nurses (APNs) varies by state, as discussed elsewhere in this text (see Chapter 22). Statutory and accreditation (Joint Commission on Accreditation for Healthcare Organizations [JCAHO]) requirements do not mandate supervision of nurse anesthetists by anesthesiologists. CRNAs work in collaboration with providers from a variety of backgrounds: surgeons, dentists, podiatrists, and anesthesiologists. The degree to which CRNA practice is addressed in state nurse practice acts is not consistent. In some states (Florida, New Jersey, Illinois), proposed or enacted regulations for office-based surgery have attempted to mandate collaboration between anesthesiologists and nurse anesthetists in these settings. Legislated prescriptive authority variability affects CRNA practice. Debate continues as to whether CRNAs need prescriptive authority to work in most settings. Conventional wisdom holds that CRNAs do not require prescriptive authority protection because CRNAs are most commonly institutionally based and administer, but do not independently prescribe, medications. Federal law indicates that nurse anesthesia practice and related drug administration are not prescriptive but rather represent a request for anesthesia services. Choosing anesthesia techniques and selecting and ordering drugs by nurse anesthetists are not construed as prescriptive behavior by the federal courts (Blumenreich, Stallone, & Tobin, 1990).

Nurse anesthesia practice is, by historical and legal precedents, part of nursing practice. Two precedent-setting cases were *Frank v. Smith*, 175 Ky. 416, 194 S.W. 375 (1917) and *Chalmers-Francis v. Nelson*, 6 Cal. 2d 402, 57 P.2d (1936) (cited in Thatcher, 1953). The latter case involved Dagmar Nelson, a California nurse anesthetist. Legal challenges to Nelson's right to provide anesthesia came from local anesthesiologists, with resulting litigation eventually going to the California Supreme Court. The professional organization representing CRNAs at that time, the National Association of Nurse Anesthetists, filed an amicus curiae brief with the Supreme Court. The case was a watershed in deciding the legality of nurse-administered anesthesia (Bankert, 1989). Case law is replete with other examples of successful challenges by nurse anesthetists for their right to practice.

The question of which professional group CRNAs should be aligned with has been a topic explored legally, ethically, and educationally since the inception of the practice of nurse anesthesia. Some courts of law have held that nurse anesthesia is not the practice of medicine; rather, it is by virtue of nursing licensure that CRNAs are able to practice anesthesia legally. Other courts have found that anesthesiology cannot be easily classified within either the discipline of nursing or the discipline of medicine (Waugaman, 1991).

The roles of physicians and nurses in anesthesia overlap. The components of this overlap include a similar educational heritage, comparable socialization into the specialty, constant time and space in the operating room environment, and similar relationships and therapeutic interventions with patients. The noncurative nature of surgical anesthesia is more similar to the practice of nursing than to the practice of medicine (Faut, 1984).

Callahan (1995) reported that there was an 88% role overlap in the practice of nurse anesthetists and anesthesiologists as evaluated by experts in both fields. The findings of Callahan mirror those of Cromwell and Rosenbach (1988), health-care economists who extensively studied economics in anesthesiology and cost-effective anesthesia provider mixes. These investigators found that CRNAs were underutilized, close substitutes for anesthesiologists and that full utilization of CRNAs would result in significant savings in health-care expenditures. Nurse anesthetists frequently work with anesthesiologists. There is ongoing debate about the merits of the "anesthesia care team" (e.g., CRNAs practicing with anesthesiologists). Publications on this topic in the anesthesiology literature have at times advocated team anesthesia from both economic and safety perspectives (Abenstein & Warner, 1996; Schubert, Eckhout, Cooperider, & Kubel, 2001) implying that anesthesiologist involvement in anesthesia care improves outcomes, although existing outcomes research findings do not uniformly support this contention (Jordan, Kremer, & Crawforth, 2001; Kremer & Faut-Callahan, 2001).

In a recent study, surgical mortality rates and type of anesthesia provider were examined. Risk-adjusted mortality rates were analyzed for more than 400,000 Medicare-covered inpatients. Mortality rates for anesthesiologists working alone, CRNAs working alone, and anesthesia care teams were compared. Mortality rates for condition studied ranged from 0.11% to 1.2%. The observed and predicted values by type of provider were not statistically significantly different. The investigators found that hospitals without anesthesiologists had results similar to hospitals where anesthesiologists provided or directed anesthesia care (Pine, Holt, & Lou, 2003).

Acknowledging that the practices of nurse anesthetists and anesthesiologists are similar, the courts had to decide whether nurse anesthetists and anesthesiologists indeed compete in practice settings (*Oltz v. St. Peter's Community Hospital*, 861 F.2d 1440, 1443 [9th Cir. 1988]; cited in Bankert, 1989]). There is no other area of health care in which a provider can substitute for a physician, as does the CRNA in the provision of anesthesia services. Institutional credentialing may limit the ability of CRNAs to perform functions such as discharging patients from the facility or in components of prescription writing. However, strategies have been developed to overcome these barriers in various settings.

CRNA PRACTICE PROFILES

AANA membership increased steadily between 1992 and 2002, from 25,310 to 30,156 (Figure 17-1). The AANA conducts an annual practice profile survey. The response rate

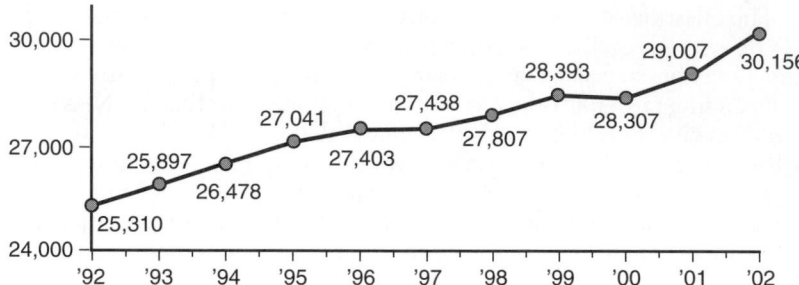

Membership 1992–2002

FIGURE 17-1 • AANA membership, 1992-2002. (From Rivera, L. [2003]. *Practice profile survey summary*. Unpublished document. American Association of Nurse Anesthetists, Park Ridge, IL; reproduced with permission.)

for the 2002 survey was 58% (Rivera, 2003). Practice data reported here are those reported in the 2002 AANA Practice Profile Survey.

The average AANA member age is 48 years old; 45% of members are male and 55% are female. CRNAs who report their practice as part time are predominantly female (87%). The median full-time CRNA income in 2002 was $113,000 (Figure 17-2). During calendar year 2002, 29% of CRNAs who responded to the AANA member survey administered more than 1000 anesthetics. An additional 56% of respondents provided more than 400 anesthetics annually (Rivera, 2003).

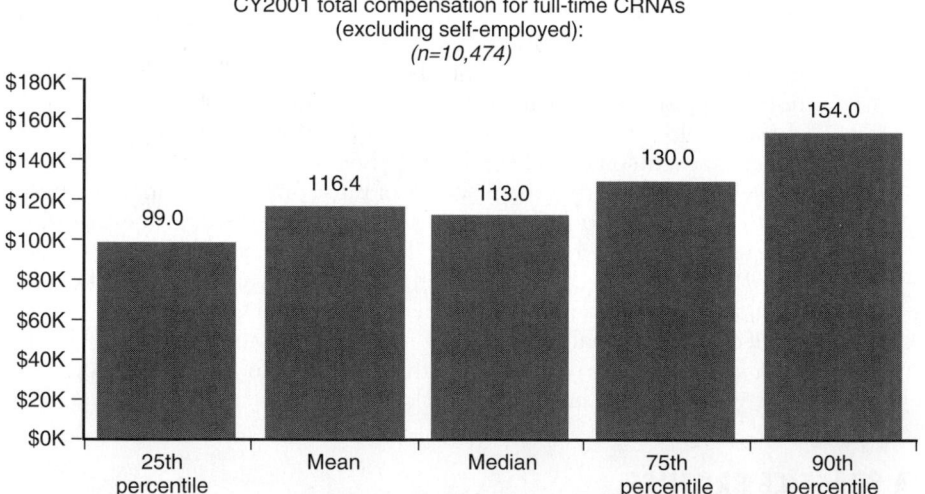

CY2001 total compensation for full-time CRNAs
(excluding self-employed):
(n=10,474)

FIGURE 17-2 • CRNA compensation for calendar year 2001. (From Rivera, L. [2003]. *Practice profile survey summary*. Unpublished document. American Association of Nurse Anesthetists, Park Ridge, IL; reproduced with permission.)

Regarding scope and settings of practice, 99% of CRNA respondents provided general anesthesia; 70% performed spinal anesthesia; 57% provided epidural blocks; and 32% reported that they inserted central venous access lines (Figure 17-3). Most respondents practiced in hospitals (84%); 8% worked in ambulatory surgical centers; 6% provided care in university hospitals; and 2% provided office-based anesthesia services (Rivera, 2003). Sixty-eight percent of 2001 survey respondents practiced with anesthesiologists; the remaining 32% collaborated with an operating surgeon, dentist, or podiatrist (Beutler, 2002).

The employment arrangements reported by CRNA survey respondents in 2002 were as follows: 50% were group employees; 33% worked for hospitals; 14% were independent contractors; 6% listed their employment setting as "other"; 6% were owners or partners in anesthesia practice groups; and 4% were employed by the military or federal government (Rivera, 2003).

With a continued focus on cost containment, hospitals endeavor to decrease their fixed costs, such as payroll. Surgical case volumes have remained constant or increased while reimbursement rates have fallen. An initial reaction to this trend was to decrease the number of available beds and licensed staff in acute care settings. However, to deal with current surgical patient volumes, some hospitals have found it necessary to aggressively recruit professional nursing staff and re-open previously closed units. Economic considerations such as decreased reimbursement have caused hospital employment for CRNAs and other APNs to be less common as cost shifting of these providers out of hospitals occurs. Therefore cost shifting may lead to managing caseloads with fewer practitioners who may be group employees or independent contractors. Most AANA members (89%) are employed in nonrural or urban areas, while 11% practice in rural areas (Rivera, 2003). These rural CRNAs significantly increase access to health care for rural citizens.

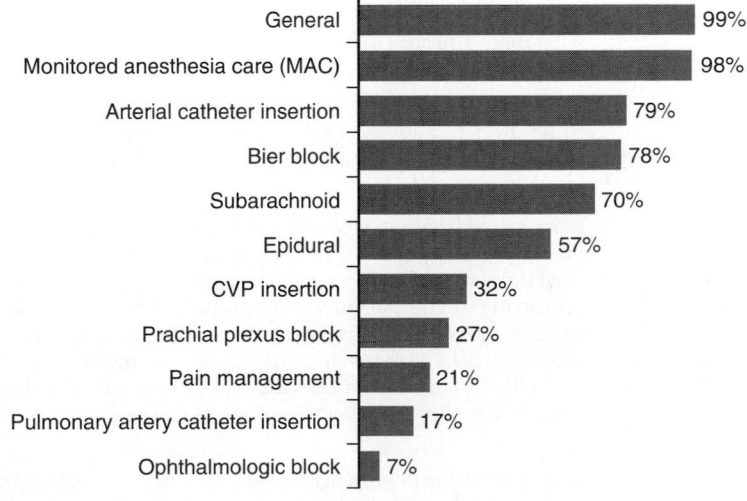

FIGURE 17-3 • Anesthesia techniques performed by CRNAs in 2002. (From Rivera, L. [2003]. *Practice profile survey summary.* Unpublished document. American Association of Nurse Anesthetists, Park Ridge, IL; reproduced with permission.)

Orkin (1998) reported on a survey of rural hospital administrators regarding their satisfaction with anesthesia outcomes in settings where most anesthesia was provided by CRNAs. There was strong satisfaction with anesthesia services provided by CRNAs reported by the administrators in this dataset. In downstate Illinois, 58 hospitals serving 300,000 citizens have anesthesia services solely provided by CRNAs. Research findings demonstrated similarly high hospital administrator satisfaction with anesthesia services provided by rural Illinois CRNAs (Stark & Kremer, 2001). In another study, morbidity and mortality rates for gallbladder surgery in one rural hospital, in which anesthesia was provided by the same CRNA for more than 25 years, were compared with gallbladder surgery morbidity and mortality rates in urban hospitals. When controls for significant variables such as patient acuity, there was no statistically significant difference in morbidity and mortality rates between the two groups (Callaghan, 1995).

Employment Factors

The CRNA Manpower Study from the National Center for Nursing Research (1991) projected a need for more than 35,000 CRNAs by the year 2010. The current average CRNA age of 48 years and an abundance of unfilled positions reflect the current high demand and continued need for CRNAs (Beutler, 2002). At the time of this writing, a national shortfall of some 4000 nurse anesthetists has been reported in the United States (Merwin & Stern, 2003). Downturns in the equities markets that have adversely affected retirement funds may delay retirement plans for some CRNAs. In addition to potentially delayed CRNA retirements, another factor that will benefit the nurse anesthesia workforce is a projected increase in nurse anesthesia program graduates to more than 1700 in 2004 (see Figure 17-6).

Anesthesiologists are also in high demand. One model indicates that a shortfall of these physicians will exist through 2005 (Schubert, Eckhout, & Trempert, 2003). Other trends in physician practice include unionization, an 80-hour workweek for house staff, and hospital employment. Moves such as these may lead to increased utilization of CRNAs as external entities examine safe, cost-effective anesthesia provider mixes.

Multiple variables affect anesthesia provider mixes in various settings. The term *provider mix* refers to the following variations in anesthesia practice: physicians may practice anesthesia without nurse anesthetists; in team anesthesia, physicians may collaborate with one or more CRNAs; or CRNAs may practice anesthesia collaborating with an operating surgeon, dentist, or podiatrist.

Team anesthesia is the predominant model within which CRNAs practice. Although some anesthesiologists may be ambivalent about nurse anesthesia, Dr. Robert Dripps, a pioneering academic anesthesiologist, had very positive beliefs about CRNAs.

It is apparent that the physician anesthesiologist offers greater depth of training than the nurse anesthetist, but this does not necessarily qualify the physician as a better anesthetist. By achieving the technical skills and the appropriate experience and knowledge, a conscientious nurse can easily surmount the gap in training. An anesthesiologist, acting as a technician, who fails to keep abreast of advances in medicine soon loses the advantage. In most large hospital departments, nurse and physician anesthetists and technicians work in harmony. . . . Considering the extensive national demands for anesthesia care, it is unlikely that all anesthetics will ever be given solely by physicians. As paralleled by the trend toward midwifery in obstetrics, there is and always will be a need for nurse anesthetists. (Dripps, 1977, p. 3)

Nurse anesthesia education and anesthesia practice have advanced tremendously in the time since these thoughts were recorded. Although medical anesthesiology residency programs take longer, educational requirements for the two provider groups are similar (Jordan, 1994; Kaye, Scibetta, & Grogono, 1999).

Another factor affecting employment is the anesthesia assistant. Programs at Emory and Case Western Universities prepare anesthesia assistants, who go directly from their undergraduate education in nonclinical disciplines to training as anesthesia assistants. Therefore the preparation for this role is different from that of physicians, nurses, or physician assistants. Practice privileges of anesthesia assistants, who are legally recognized in only five states at this writing, are linked to a sponsoring physician (visit the following websites for more information: www.aana.com and www.anesthesiology.emory.edu/PA_Program).

Access to Care

As stated earlier, nurse anesthetists are involved in the administration of 65% of the 26 million anesthetics given in this country each year. Furthermore, nurse anesthetists provide approximately 70% of anesthesia given in rural settings. CRNAs collaborate closely with other providers, such as surgeons and primary care practitioners, in all settings. Without the services of CRNAs in these communities, many small hospitals would close, leaving few alternatives for health care. Some rural CRNAs have completed additional training in the management of acute and chronic pain and offer services such as pain clinics so that patients do not have to travel to distant centers for treatment of pain (Quinlan, 2001).

CRNAs have traditionally been represented in other underserved population setting areas. Urban and county hospitals frequently employ CRNAs. Nurse anesthetists are actively involved in anesthesia care in settings such as the Maryland Institute for Emergency Medical Services, Chicago's Stroger/Cook County Hospital, and San Francisco General Hospital. Many CRNAs practice in the Veterans Administration hospital system, dealing with complex surgical patients. The military heavily relies on and actively recruits nurse anesthetists. A CRNA may be the only anesthesia provider on a Navy vessel. In such a situation, knowledge of regional anesthesia and the ability to practice independently enable the CRNA to capably respond to mass casualty situations, in which many trauma victims simultaneously require anesthesia.

Settings in Which CRNAs Practice

With most surgery currently conducted on a same-day admission or outpatient basis, patients may not meet their anesthetist until shortly before surgery. Multiple mechanisms, such as telephone interviews or preanesthesia clinics, can be used to conduct preanesthesia assessment and allow anesthesia providers to discuss care options, procedures, and risks with patients. Patients and health-care providers continue to readjust to this reimbursement-driven shift in services. Clinical information obtained through telephone interviews is confirmed when patients arrive; detailed physical assessment and establishing rapport also occur on the day of surgery.

Anesthesia services can facilitate diagnosis, as in the case of the "curare test" for myasthenia gravis. Anesthesia as a therapeutic modality is seen in the treatment of acute and chronic pain; it is also used in psychiatry for conducting interviews under the influence of ultra-short-acting intravenously administered barbiturates and for accelerated detoxification of opioid-dependent patients. However, the most common use of anesthesia resources is for the administration of surgical anesthesia.

Anesthesia services are frequently used in obstetrics, for providing analgesia and anesthesia to parturients. Regional anesthesia and applied pharmacology have greatly advanced obstetrical anesthesia, which in the past relied on systemic drugs that could cause neonatal depression. Epidural analgesia has become increasingly common for vaginal and cesarean delivery, often obviating the need for general anesthesia and its attendant risks (Bader & Datta, 1994). In addition to utilizing regional anesthesia in obstetrical and postpartum settings, CRNAs work collaboratively with other clinicians in these areas to manage intra- and postpartum pain with a variety of pharmacological and nonpharmacological modalities (Faut-Callahan & Paice, 1990).

International Practice

Nurse anesthesia practice exists in western Europe, portions of eastern Europe, Scandinavia, and parts of Africa and Asia. The International Federation of Nurse Anesthetists (IFNA) was chartered in 1989 with 11 founding member countries and has grown to 20 member countries representing more than 30,000 nurse anesthetists worldwide. The AANA, under the leadership of past president and IFNA executive director Ronald Caulk, CRNA, FAAN, has spearheaded this fledgling organization. The IFNA meets every 4 years to discuss issues related to practice and education. Although the practice of nurse anesthesia reaches around the globe, the scope of practice and educational processes for nurse anesthetists varies from one country to another (Kelly, 1994). CRNA volunteers participate in charitable surgical services throughout the third world through services such as Operation Smile and the Orbis Project. These volunteer surgeons, nurses, and CRNAs provide services such as cleft lip and palate repair for children in underserved areas. Through Health Volunteers Overseas, volunteers also provide anesthesia and surgical services in addition to teaching clinical anesthesia in third-world countries (M. Catchpole, personal communication, 1995).

A study by McAuliffe and Henry (1998) demonstrated that nurses were providing anesthesia services in more than 100 countries that comprise 60% of the member states of the World Health Organization. Data were collected from 96 countries, in all world regions, at four levels of development, and were analyzed for commonalities and differences. The authors found that the use of nurses to provide anesthesia was not related to a country's level of development. Nurses provided anesthesia in two thirds of developed, developing, and underdeveloped countries, working with and without anesthesiologists. Nurses in this sample performed all the critical tasks required in the administration of anesthesia. Nurse anesthetists worldwide are making significant contributions to health care.

SCOPE OF PRACTICE

Anesthesiology is the art and science of rendering a patient insensible to pain by administration of anesthetic agents and related drugs and procedures. Anesthesia and anesthesia-related care are those services that anesthesia professionals provide on request, assignment, or referral by the patient's physician (or other health-care professional authorized by law), most often to facilitate diagnostic, therapeutic, or surgical procedures. In other instances, the referral or request for consultation or assistance may be for management of pain associated with labor and delivery, management of acute and chronic ventilatory problems, or management of acute or chronic pain through the performance of selected diagnostic or therapeutic blocks or other forms of pain management (AANA, 2002a).

The scope of practice of the CRNA encompasses the professional functions, privileges, and responsibilities associated with nurse anesthesia practice. These activities are performed in collaboration with qualified and legally authorized professional health-care providers. CRNAs are prepared to recognize situations in which health-care requirements are beyond their individual competencies and to seek consultation or referral when such situations arise (AANA, 2002a). Anesthesia care is provided by CRNAs in four general categories: (1) preanesthetic evaluation and preparation; (2) anesthesia induction, maintenance, and emergence; (3) postanesthesia care; and (4) perianesthetic and clinical support functions. Parallels between nursing and nurse anesthesia can be seen. CRNAs perform preanesthetic assessments, plan appropriate anesthetic interventions, implement planned anesthetic care, and evaluate patients postoperatively to determine the efficacy of their interventions. CRNAs working alone routinely perform all of these aspects of clinical practice. When CRNAs and anesthesiologists work together in "team" anesthesia, a variety of factors, such as local anesthesia practice patterns, determine to what extent each practitioner is involved in specific anesthesia care areas.

Preoperative evaluation has become more complex with the increasing acuity of patients undergoing surgery. Thorough preanesthetic assessments, combined with specialty consultation as needed, are essential activities at which nurse anesthetists must be proficient. Other aspects of preanesthetic patient preparation are requesting indicated diagnostic studies; selecting, obtaining, ordering, or administering preanesthetic medications and fluids; and obtaining informed consent for anesthesia (AANA, 2002a).

Developing and implementing an anesthetic care plan is another aspect of CRNA practice. This care plan is formulated with input from the patient, the surgeon, and, in team anesthesia settings, the collaborating anesthesiologist. Similarly, the choice of administering regional or general anesthesia is not solely the province of any one of the aforementioned participants. Input from the patient, the surgeon, and the anesthetist is relevant in the important decision about which type of anesthetic to administer in a given situation. Compromise and flexibility may be necessary to achieve the goals of surgery and anesthesia without incident.

CRNAs select, obtain, or administer the anesthetics, adjuvant drugs, accessory drugs, and fluids necessary to manage the anesthesia, to maintain physiological homeostasis, and to correct abnormal responses to anesthesia or surgery (AANA, 2002a). When CRNAs perform these activities, they are recognized legally to be providing anesthesia services on request, not to be prescribing as defined by federal law. With the advent of legislated prescriptive authority for CRNAs and other APNs, these providers can prescribe legend and in some cases Schedules II through V controlled substances.

Monitoring is another vital area in which CRNAs participate. Nurse anesthetists select, apply, and insert appropriate noninvasive and invasive monitoring modalities for collecting and interpreting physiological data. These activities are all recognized components of anesthesia services performed on request by CRNAs and are not prescriptive. Criteria for the use of invasive monitors and who places them vary by institution and geographical region. Professional fees associated with the placement of devices such as pulmonary artery catheters at times leads to conflict over which practitioner (e.g., anesthetist or surgeon) will place invasive monitors and receive the associated reimbursement.

Nurse anesthesia practice also includes airway management by means of endotracheal intubation, mechanical ventilation, and pharmacological support, both within and outside the operating room. In some settings, CRNAs are the sole providers of this service. A combination of technical skills required for airway management, in which a variety of instruments and knowledge of respiratory anatomy and physiology and pharmacology are utilized, is important. For example, indiscriminate use of muscle relaxants in critically ill ventilator-dependent patients can occur (Loper, Butler, Nessly, & Wild, 1989), leading to undesirable outcomes such as posttraumatic stress syndrome. CRNAs need to remind clinicians caring for ventilator-dependent patients that sedative/amnestic drugs and analgesics need to be included when critically ill patients are mechanically ventilated. In addition, the role of the CRNA in helping patients and families to understand these procedures is important.

Nurse anesthetists manage emergence and recovery from anesthesia by selecting, obtaining, ordering, or administering medications, fluids, or ventilatory support in order to maintain homeostasis, to provide relief from pain and anesthesia side effects, and/or to prevent or manage complications (AANA, 2002a). These activities also fall within the scope of providing anesthesia services and are not prescriptive in the traditional sense (e.g., where a practitioner would write a prescription that a pharmacist would fill). Releasing or discharging patients from a postanesthesia care area can be performed by the CRNA. Conducting postanesthesia follow-up evaluation and providing care related to anesthetic side effects or complications are other CRNA functions.

Regional anesthesia is used by many CRNAs in the management of surgical anesthesia, labor pain, and postoperative pain. CRNAs are increasingly involved with pain management services. The use of epidural analgesic infusions and patient-controlled analgesia has greatly contributed to the effective treatment of preventable pain. Nurse anesthetists should have a role in the formulation of protocols and staff education when acute pain protocols are introduced.

Nurse anesthetists respond to emergency situations by providing airway management and by implementing basic and advanced life support techniques. CRNAs can provide leadership in these settings, away from the operating room, reinforcing the need for nationally promulgated standards of anesthesia care. One of these standards of care, for example, is the measurement of end-tidal carbon dioxide to rule out esophageal intubation (AANA, 2002a). Nurse anesthetists are bound by the standards of practice adopted by the profession as shown in Box 17-1.

Accountability

CRNAs are legally liable for the quality of the services they render. They make independent judgments and decisions as to the appropriateness of their professional services and the probable effects of those services on the patient. A CRNA who believes that the anesthesia care plan for a particular patient is inappropriate should seek consultation for more appropriate direction. CRNAs should be patient advocates and always seek resolution of these issues. If reasonable doubt continues, it is the responsibility of the CRNA to consider withdrawal from rendering the service, provided that the well-being of the patient is not jeopardized (AANA, 2002a).

Credentialing of CRNAs

CRNAs practice according to their expertise, state statutes or regulations, and local institutional policy. Institutional credentialing procedures may require additional evidence of clinical and didactic education in areas such as cardiothoracic or regional anesthesia.

BOX 17-1 • STANDARDS FOR NURSE ANESTHESIA PRACTICE

Introduction

These standards are intended to:

1. Assist the profession in evaluating the quality of care provided by its practitioners.
2. Provide a common base for practitioners to use in their development of a quality practice.
3. Assist the public in understanding what to expect from the practitioner.
4. Support and preserve the basic rights of the patient.

These standards apply to all anesthetizing locations. While the standards are intended to encourage high quality patient care, they cannot assure specific outcomes.

Standard I.

Perform a thorough and complete preanesthesia assessment.

Interpretation:
The responsibility for the care of the patient begins with the preanesthetic assessment. Except in emergency situations, the CRNA has an obligation to complete a thorough evaluation and determine that relevant tests have been obtained and reviewed.

Standard II.
Obtain informed consent for the planned anesthetic intervention from the patient or legal guardian.

Interpretation:
The CRNA shall obtain or verify that an informed consent has been obtained by a qualified provider. Discuss anesthetic options and risks with the patient and/or legal guardian in language the patient and/or legal guardian can understand. Document in the patient's medical record that informed consent was obtained.

Standard III.
Formulate a patient-specific plan for anesthesia care.

Interpretation:
The plan of care developed by the CRNA is based upon comprehensive patient assessment, problem analysis, anticipated surgical or therapeutic procedure, patient and surgeon preferences, and current anesthesia principles.

Standard IV.
Implement and adjust the anesthesia care plan based on the patient's physiological response.

Interpretation:
The CRNA shall induce and maintain anesthesia at required levels. The CRNA shall continuously assess the patient's response to the anesthetic and/or surgical intervention and intervene as required to maintain the patient in a satisfactory physiologic condition.

Standard V.
Monitor the patient's physiologic condition as appropriate for the type of anesthesia and specific patient needs.

A. **Monitor ventilation continuously.** Verify intubation of the trachea by auscultation, chest excursion, and confirmation of carbon dioxide in the expired gas. Continuously monitor end-tidal carbon dioxide during controlled or assisted ventilation. Use spirometry and ventilatory pressure monitors.
B. **Monitor oxygenation continuously** by clinical observation, pulse oximetry, and if indicated, arterial blood gas analysis.
C. **Monitor cardiovascular status continuously** via electrocardiogram and heart sounds. Record blood pressure and heart rate at least every five minutes.
D. **Monitor body temperature continuously** on all pediatric patients receiving general anesthesia and when indicated, on all other patients.
E. **Monitor neuromuscular function and status** when neuromuscular blocking agents are administered.
F. **Monitor and assess the patient's positioning** and protective measures.

Interpretation:
Continuous clinical observation and vigilance are the basis of safe anesthesia care. The standard applies to all patients receiving anesthesia care and may be exceeded at any time at the discretion of the CRNA. Unless otherwise stipulated in the standards, a means to monitor and evaluate the patient's status shall be immediately available for all patients. As new patient safety technologies evolve, integration into the current anesthesia practice shall be considered. The omission of any monitoring standards shall be documented and the reason stated on the patient's anesthesia record. The CRNA shall be in constant attendance of the patient until the responsibility for care has been accepted by another qualified health care provider.

Standard VI.
There shall be complete, accurate, and timely documentation of pertinent information on the patient's medical record.

Interpretation:
Document all anesthetic interventions and patient responses. Accurate documentation facilitates comprehensive patient care, provides information for retrospective review and research data, and establishes a medical-legal record.

Continued

BOX 17-1 • STANDARDS FOR NURSE ANESTHESIA PRACTICE—cont'd

Standard VII.
Transfer the responsibility for care of the patient to other qualified providers in a manner which assures continuity of care and patient safety.

Interpretation:
The CRNA shall assess the patient's status and determine when it is safe to transfer the responsibility of care to other qualified providers. The CRNA shall accurately report the patient's condition and all essential information to the provider assuming responsibility for the patient.

Standard VIII.
Adhere to appropriate safety precautions, as established within the institution, to minimize the risks of fire, explosion, electrical shock, and equipment malfunction. Document on the patient's medical record that the anesthesia machine and equipment were checked.

Interpretation
Prior to use, the CRNA shall inspect the anesthesia machine and monitors according to established guidelines. The CRNA shall check the readiness, availability, cleanliness, and working condition of all equipment to be utilized in the administration of the anesthesia care. When the patient is ventilated by an automatic mechanical ventilator, monitor the integrity of the breathing system with a device capable of detecting a disconnection by emitting an audible alarm. Monitor oxygen concentration continuously with an oxygen supply failure alarm system.

Standard IX.
Precautions shall be taken to minimize the risk of infection to the patient, the CRNA, and other health care providers.

Interpretation:
Written policies and procedures in infection control shall be developed for personnel and equipment.

Standard X.
Anesthesia care shall be assessed to assure its quality and contribution to positive patient outcomes.

Interpretation:
The CRNA shall participate in the ongoing review and evaluation of the quality and appropriateness of anesthesia care. Evaluation shall be performed based upon appropriate outcome criteria and reviewed on an ongoing basis. The CRNA shall participate in a continual process of self evaluation and strive to incorporate new techniques and knowledge into practice.

Standard XI.
The CRNA shall respect and maintain the basic rights of patients.

Interpretation:
The CRNA shall support and preserve the rights of patients to personal dignity and ethical norms of practice.

From the American Association of Nurse Anesthetists. (2002). *Scope and standards for nurse anesthesia practice*. Park Ridge, IL: Author; reproduced with permission.

State nurse practice acts and practice patterns in the anesthesia community contribute to variability in the scope of nurse anesthesia practice in different settings.

To be a nurse anesthetist, one must meet the following four requirements:

1. Graduation from an approved nursing school with current state registered nurse licensure
2. Graduation from a nurse anesthesia educational program accredited by the Council on Accreditation of Nurse Anesthesia Educational Programs or its predecessor
3. Successful completion of the certification examination administered by the Council on Certification of Nurse Anesthetists or its predecessor
4. Compliance with criteria for biennial recertification

These criteria are defined by the Council on Recertification of Nurse Anesthetists (AANA, 2002b).

Competence can be partially assured through institutional credentialing processes. A hospital may delineate procedures that the CRNA is authorized to perform by the authority of the governing board. Guidelines for granting CRNAs clinical privileges are found in the *Guidelines and Standards for Nurse Anesthesia Practice* (AANA, 2002a). Recommended clinical privileges for CRNAs are in the areas of preanesthetic preparation and evaluation; anesthesia induction, maintenance and emergence; postanesthetic care; and perianesthetic and clinical support functions.

ROLE DEVELOPMENT AND MEASURES OF CLINICAL COMPETENCE

The role of the nurse anesthetist encompasses many facets. Callahan (1994) described a competency-based model for nurse anesthesia practice that demonstrated areas in which nurse anesthetists must strive to achieve competence (Figure 17-4). The unifying themes of caring, collaboration, communication, and technology are defined in Box 17-2. Many of the characteristics of advanced practice nursing described in Chapter 3 are found in this model. Although the model is in its infancy and further research on its use is in progress, it depicts the many facets of the CRNA role. Munguia-Biddle, Maree, Klein, Callahan, and Gilles (1990) defined components of the model and suggested that the nurse anesthesia process is a problem-solving model that utilizes assessment, analysis,

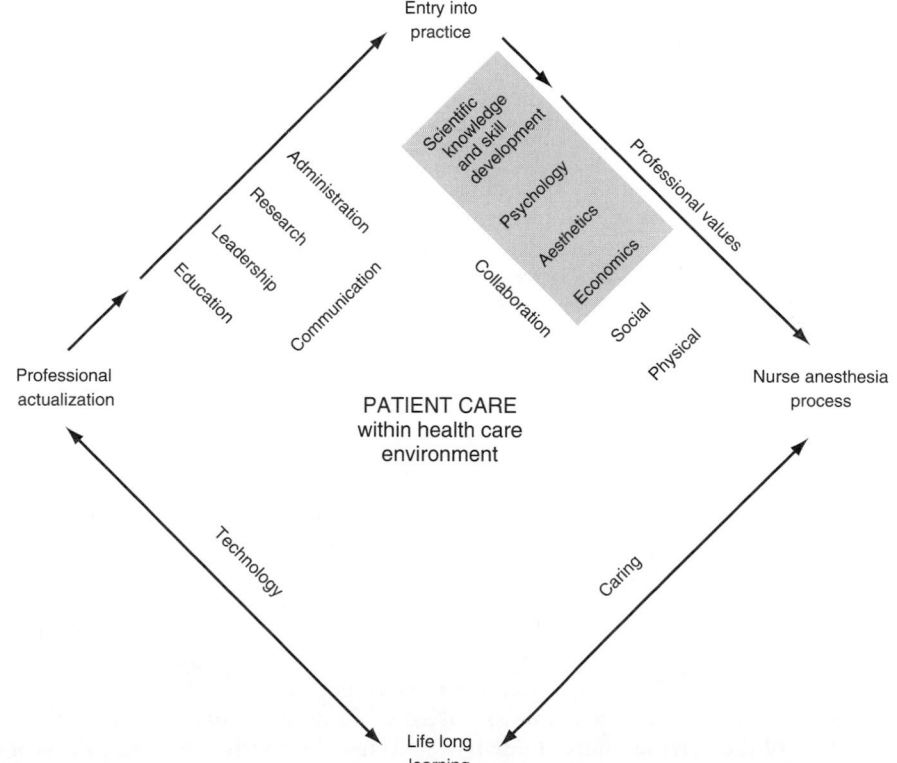

FIGURE 17-4 • Nurse anesthesia practice model. (From Munguia-Biddle, F., Maree, S., Klein, E., Callahan, L., & Gilles, B. [1990]. *Nurse anesthesiology competence evaluation: Mechanism for accountability.* Unpublished document, American Association of Nurse Anesthetists, Park Ridge, IL; reproduced with permission.)

BOX 17-2 • NURSE ANESTHESIA PRACTICE MODEL

The advanced practice of nursing in the specialty of nurse anesthesia has special attributes that speak to the strength and uniqueness of the CRNA role in the provision of anesthesia care in the health environment.

Caring for the patient as a holistic being is an important tenet of CRNA professional behavior. CRNAs strive to be altruistic human beings, believing that caring is essential to one's personal development.

Collaboration between the nurse anesthetist and other members of the health care team takes place in separate and joined activities and responsibilities that are directed at attaining mutual goals of excellence in patient care.

Communication is sharing information to achieve mutual understanding. Communication skills are a cornerstone of patient interviews, imparting information to other health professionals, documentation of practice, and participation as a contributory member in meeting society's health needs.

Technology denotes an area rich in technological advances and scientific content that requires strengthening and updating through the professional life. Practitioners have the ability to apply the nursing process to complex problems at a high level of competence.

From Munguia-Biddle, F., Maree, S., Klein, E., Callahan, L., & Gilles, B. (1990). *Nurse anesthesiology competence evaluation: Mechanism for accountability*. Unpublished document, American Association of Nurse Anesthetists, Park Ridge, IL; reproduced with permission.

planning, implementation, and evaluation in the complex decision making and actions that exemplify CRNA practice within the health-care environment. They further defined lifelong learning as a part of the nurse anesthesia process. This essential process function is in concert with the changing characteristics of nurse anesthesia practice.

Additional clarification of the components of the model can be found in Box 17-3 (p. 600). The nurse anesthesia process parallels the nursing process and emphasizes the importance of this approach to comprehensive anesthesia care following the model and its components. Two exemplars that describe CRNA practice are provided.

CRNA PRACTICE EXEMPLARS

Many of the observations of Dorroh and Norton (1996) and Dorroh and Kelley (Chapter 16) about the role of the certified nurse-midwife pertain to the CRNAs depicted in the following exemplars. There are many rewards associated with their practice, but there are also challenges. Surgical or anesthetic morbidity and mortality understandably result in close internal and some external scrutiny. CRNAs must be able to defend their actions in terms of congruence with standards of care and existing hospital policies. Vacation coverage can be difficult to find and expensive, given the current undersupply of CRNAs. Like certified nurse-midwives, CRNAs find that complying with regulations (e.g., Medicare/Medicaid) and other health policy legislation can be challenging. Fortunately, state and national professional associations are available for consultation on these issues. Like certified nurse-midwives, CRNAs deal with "misperceptions of our practice from within the larger health-care system" (Dorroh & Norton, 1996, p. 214). One of the ongoing challenges for CRNAs and other APNs is to have effective public relations and government relations strategies in place to minimize these misperceptions.

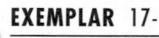

EXEMPLAR 17-1

David and Patty are hospital-employed certified registered nurse anesthetists (CRNAs) at a community hospital in central Illinois. David has practiced as a CRNA for 20 years, and Patty, for 22 years. Their practice includes a physician anesthesiologist, who is also hospital employed. The hospital has four operating rooms and an active obstetrics department, where labor epidurals are provided by the CRNAs and the anesthesiologist. All three anesthesia providers rotate taking call. They act as backups for each other if additional help is needed, such as caring for a patient with multiple trauma injuries.

The nurse anesthetists have deep ties with the community in which they practice. Because it is a town of 30,000, many people know each other. David and Patty are active in church and community groups. They are very cognizant of the perceptions of colleagues and area residents. They work with the same surgeons and obstetricians routinely. Competence, caring, and dependability are qualities that David and Patty convey; these attributes help solidify their roles as trusted advanced practice nurses (APNs) in the community.

Because the majority of their surgical cases are performed on an outpatient basis, preanesthetic assessment takes place in the outpatient unit, one floor below the surgical suite. One of the CRNAs or the anesthesiologist conducts a preoperative interview in a private room with each patient. This time is crucial for establishment of the necessary rapport between patients and anesthesia providers. The health history is obtained, and patients are asked for additional information as necessary. Anesthetic options are explained in easily understood language. The risks and benefits associated with each anesthetic option are described. Sometimes, surgeons indicate preferences for particular anesthetic techniques; however, the anesthesia provider ensures that patients are comfortable with the proposed anesthetic, its benefits, and potential risks.

On a typical day, several elective surgical cases are scheduled. Emergency cases may be scheduled at any time later in the day. Other clinical activities for David and Patty include the placement and management of labor epidurals, helping with venous access, emergency airway management, and acting as team leaders during cardiac arrests. The CRNAs are consulted on pain and ventilator management. They serve on the pharmacy and therapeutics committee because perioperatively administered medications constitute a large part of the hospital formulary. They are also members of the operating room committee. This committee has representation from operating room nursing, surgery, and anesthesia. Time and resource allocation are two of the priority areas for this committee. These clinical and leadership roles emphasize the following core APN competencies:

1. *Expert clinical practice:* The CRNAs must be highly competent because the other anesthesia providers are frequently busy when they are performing their duties. When taking call, the CRNAs, collaborating with the staff physicians and nurses, are responsible for expert anesthetic assessment, crisis management, decision making, implementation, and evaluation.
2. *Expert guidance and coaching of patients, families, and other care providers:* This core competency is evident in both the perioperative and obstetrical arenas. In the obstetrical arena, the CRNAs provide expert guidance and coaching to patients and their families regarding labor analgesia that they provide with labor epidurals. The guidelines used for implementation and management of labor epidurals were collectively developed by the anesthesia department, the staff obstetricians, and the labor and delivery unit nurses.
3. *Informal Consultation:* The CRNAs are consulted regarding pain management; treatment of postoperative/postprocedure nausea and vomiting, ventilator management, acquisition of new equipment for the operating room and intensive care units, oral intake guidelines for surgery and other diagnostic and therapeutic procedures, and sedation techniques.
4. *Research skills:* The CRNAs read anesthesia journals and visit anesthesia websites (e.g., www.aana.com; www.anesthesia-analgesia.org; and gasnet.med.yale.edu; see also Box 17-4) regularly. The rapid development of new technology and pharmacology in anesthesia mandates an ability to critique and utilize these developments to ensure evidence-based practice. CRNAs also collaborate in clinical research on anesthesia and pain management.

Continued

EXEMPLAR 17-1—cont'd

5. *Clinical and professional leadership:* This core competency is evident on multiple levels. The CRNAs are regarded as clinical leaders in the operating room. Their counsel on positioning, monitoring, and fluid management is important to surgeons and operating room nurses. Professional leadership opportunities exist both in the hospital and through local forums, as well as in state and national organizations. David and Patty have served on committees for their state professional organization and stay actively involved in developments affecting their national organization (e.g., writing letters to legislators).

6. *Collaboration:* Collaboration is key to nurse anesthesia practice. The CRNAs collaborate with surgeons, dentists, podiatrists, and the anesthesiologist in their department. There is significant mutual respect between the CRNAs and these clinicians. The long record of clinical competence, dependability, and affability that David and Patty exhibit helps maintain their positions as valued collaborators in their practice setting.

7. *Change agent skills:* The CRNAs bring their knowledge, skills, and abilities in perioperative monitoring, pain management, and airway management to their colleagues. One example of how David and Patty brought about change was to advise the hospital to purchase two anesthesia machines with computerized record-keeping capabilities. Rather than having to keep an anesthetic record by hand, this technology requires the anesthetist to enter only patient demographics, drugs and fluids administered, and other information deemed necessary for the case. A laser-printed anesthetic record is printed at the end of each case. The information entered into the computer can also be used for billing and continuous quality improvement.

On a typical day, Patty or David may deal with cases as diverse as an elective cesarean delivery, a hip pinning in an elderly patient, a closed reduction of a Colles' fracture in a 10-year-old, and placement of labor epidurals. The labor epidurals require monitoring for adequate analgesia and potential side effects. Each patient has unique requirements for anesthesia management; often, family members will have questions and need support from the anesthesia providers.

EXEMPLAR 17-2

Paul is a 38-year-old certified registered nurse anesthetist (CRNA) employed in a tertiary-level academic medical center. He has practiced in this setting for 10 years. He is a teaching associate in the department of anesthesiology in the school of medicine. His salary is derived from two sources: the medical center pays two thirds, and the physician practice group affiliated with the university pays one third. Paul could earn more working at the local health maintenance organization (HMO) or providing locum tenens anesthesia coverage. He stays at the university because his position there offers a wide scope of practice, challenging cases, complex procedures, a collegial atmosphere, and the opportunity to share his expertise with students.

Paul provides expert guidance and coaching to patients and families when he rotates through the preanesthesia evaluation clinic. When surgery is scheduled, patients and their families have scheduled appointments in this clinic, where an anesthesia provider obtains their health history, performs physical assessment, and develops an anesthesia care plan with the patient. Additional guidance and coaching occur during the postoperative period, when questions related to pain management and control of postoperative nausea and vomiting arise.

Expert guidance and coaching of other care providers occurs on several levels: with newly hired peers, with surgical and anesthesia house staff, and with perioperative nursing colleagues. Paul may be assigned to help orient a new CRNA, especially to areas where the CRNA may not have recently worked, such as in cardiovascular anesthesia. Surgical house staff may work with Paul during their anesthesia rotation. Surgeons frequently ask for advice regarding postoperative pain management. In some tertiary centers, Paul and his CRNA

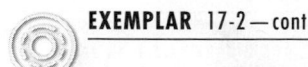

EXEMPLAR 17-2—cont'd

colleagues will be asked by the staff anesthesiologists to work as clinical preceptors with beginning anesthesiology residents, and with medical students completing their anesthesia clerkships. Paul works closely with perioperative nurses on issues such as patient positioning, sending laboratory specimens, obtaining medications, and assisting with issues related to operating room turnover times.

Consultation occurs with peers, attending physicians, and other colleagues such as operating room nurses and educators. Another CRNA may want to compare experiences with Paul regarding certain types of procedures. Paul is respected because of his experience in this health care system, and attending physicians will ask him what his experience has been with particular treatment regimens. Paul is also a member of the quality assurance committee in his department and is consulted about his knowledge of standard-of-care issues. Because Paul is known as a clinical expert in nurse anesthesia, nursing colleagues frequently consult with him on areas as diverse as conscious sedation and reimbursement for advanced practice nurses (APNs).

Because Paul works in an academic environment, he is constantly challenged to be aware of current anesthesiology literature. Case reports and clinical and basic research papers are discussed formally and informally with attending and resident physicians and nurses in the department. His department is involved in clinical and basic research. Although Paul has not been a primary investigator, he has helped collect data on numerous clinical studies and has been asked for his input on clinical research protocols. Part of the mission of Paul's department is to conduct research, and he feels strongly that he should be an informed user of applicable research findings in his practice.

Clinical and professional leadership come naturally to Paul and some of his colleagues at the medical center. The CRNAs are considered clinical leaders because they represent a clinical constant in their department; residents, fellows, and some attending physicians are transient. New attending physicians are usually told when working with an experienced CRNA that the CRNA is knowledgeable about the surgical procedures and anesthetic requirements, so that the attending physician can concentrate on resident education. Attending physicians are typically assigned to work with a resident or fellow in one operating room and will also provide coverage for a second room staffed by a CRNA.

In terms of professional leadership, Paul and his colleagues are often asked to plan continuing education meetings for their state nurse anesthesia association. The clinical and academic resources at their tertiary medical center allow these CRNAs access to high-quality speakers who draw from extensive clinical experiences. Some of Paul's colleagues hold elected or appointed offices within their state and national professional organizations. Another CRNA with whom Paul works is active in a state-level APN coalition.

Because CRNAs always collaborate with physicians when they practice, the academic medical center is similar to other practice settings with respect to professional relationships. Paul and his colleagues interface with surgeons, perioperative nurses, anesthesiologists, and technicians routinely. At this tertiary center, patients always have input regarding their anesthesia management, so Paul and his colleagues collaborate with patients to formulate individual anesthetic care plans.

As a highly motivated professional, Paul has well-developed change agent skills. He is well aware of the departmental hierarchy in which he works and has found niches within the department where he has been especially interested in practicing, such as cardiovascular anesthesia. Within this specialty area, Paul has been a change agent with regard to the standardization of the management of vasoactive drips. He had colleagues who did not routinely use infusion pumps for all their vasoactive drips, which occasionally resulted in drug overdoses. Another area in which he has been influential is in developing expertise with the management of airway access problems and sharing techniques he has learned with other clinicians in the department.

NURSE ANESTHESIA EDUCATION

Nurse anesthesia education occurs in diverse settings. This is demonstrated by the many academic units that house nurse anesthesia educational programs. Educators in nurse anesthesia are proud of the educational diversity of their graduates. However, the relative

---

BOX 17-3 • DEFINITION OF NURSE ANESTHESIA PRACTICE MODEL COMPONENTS

Professional Actualization

Professional actualization is a dynamic, ongoing endeavor to realize maximum development of professional potential.

Education provides an environment that allows for exploration and application of strategies to facilitate the preparation of future practitioners, thereby assuring continuance.

Leadership demonstrates the ability to define reality, set goals, communicate a vision, and influence the willing participation of others in purposeful action that is directed to goal achievement.

Research encourages active involvement in scientific inquiry as a consumer, participant, or contributor. It is the driving force of actualization that validates our role in the provision of anesthesia services, enhances growth for the nurse anesthetist and the profession, and leads to new knowledge and improved safety in patient care.

Administration provides the interface between people, groups, departments, organizations, professions, and society that enhances individual and collective professional growth.

Professional Values

A **profession** may be defined in terms of the domains of human endeavor valued by the members of the profession. Such are the following domains within the profession of nurse anesthesia practice.

Intellectual. Integral concepts within this domain are based on advanced knowledge in the fields of anatomy, physiology, pathophysiology, technology, and pharmacology as applied to anesthetic practice. The continued development of technical expertise and competence in practice are inherent in this area of concern.

Psychological. The professional nurse anesthetist is concerned with enhancement of the patient's coping skills in a time of possible physical and emotional disruption produced by the perioperative experience. Recognition of the needs of the practitioner are expressed as concern with issues such as communication, autonomy, counseling, and impairment or incompetence practice within the workplace and the profession as a whole.

Aesthetics. Spiritual growth and religious preferences are recognized and respected as inherent to full development of human potential within the patient and the nurse anesthetist. Ethical development and involvement within the political realm encompassing the nurse anesthetist as a member of society is held to be a continual and necessary growth process.

Economics. CRNAs place great value on the historical role of the nurse anesthesia profession in providing continuity of anesthesia care that supports an economically viable health care industry. The exploration of strategies leading to resolution of liability issues as well as mechanisms to increase feelings of potential job security are recognized as valuable to continued professional and personal growth and well-being.

Social. Valued concepts within this domain include enhancement and preservation of the professional role of nurse anesthetists in the societal health-care delivery system, legal and legislative responsibility for competent patient care, constant development of improved standards of care, patient education, and continued liaison with other health care providers.

Physical. Patient safety and the interface between technology and humankind or machines and the patient are of paramount concern. The appropriateness of physical work that considers the impact of schedules, stress, fatigue, and vigilance must be demonstrated in the clinical setting as important factors in securing the patient care environment.

From Munguia-Biddle, F., Maree, S., Klein, E., Callahan, L., & Gilles, B. (1990). *Nurse anesthesiology competence evaluation: Mechanism for accountability*. Unpublished document, American Association of Nurse Anesthetists, Park Ridge, IL; reproduced with permission.

value of this diversity has never been quantified in terms of an academic power base or educational credibility. This diversity exists because the nurse anesthesia educational community values various undergraduate degrees for entrance into nurse anesthesia programs and because of the initial difficulty nurse anesthesia educators experienced when they were trying to move certificate nurse anesthesia programs into schools of nursing.

Since 1998, all nurse anesthesia programs have been at the graduate level. However, this requirement does not dictate the movement of programs into one academic discipline. One reason for this may be that that, in the 1970s, nurse anesthesia programs established relationships with whichever academic unit was open to affiliating with a nurse anesthesia program. The first four graduate programs in nurse anesthesia all had different academic affiliations: medicine, nursing, allied health, and education. Programs that pioneered nurse anesthesia education at the graduate level established relationships with those departments in colleges and universities that were willing to take risks with the small numbers of students in nurse anesthesia programs. This diversified model of nurse anesthesia education has proliferated in the last 15 years, and many of these long-established programs would find it difficult to change their academic affiliations.

As described in Chapter 1, the Catholic Franciscan sisters offered one of the first organized nurse anesthesia courses at St. John's Hospital in Springfield, Illinois, in 1912. Although other nurse anesthesia programs opened in the early 20th century, curricula and clinical experiences were not standardized. At the first meeting of the National Association of Nurse Anesthetists, educational standards for the specialty were discussed by founding members. Nurse anesthesia educators agreed that the minimum length of academic programs in the specialty would be 6 months. Formal accreditation of nurse anesthesia programs began in 1952 (Bankert, 1989; Thatcher, 1953).

In the mid-1970s, more than 170 nurse anesthesia educational programs existed. Currently, 88 CRNA educational programs operate in the United States (Council on Accreditation of Nurse Anesthesia Educational Programs, 2003). Several new CRNA educational programs are on the horizon. A rapid decline in the numbers of nurse anesthesia programs occurred in the 1980s. This change was of great concern to the specialty. The closures were attributed variously to physician pressure, declining support, the inability of hospitals to continue support of small programs, and lack of a geographically accessible university with which a nurse anesthesia program could affiliate (Faut-Callahan, 1991). Those who argued that nurse anesthesia programs closed solely because of the graduate degree mandate offered little evidence to support that claim. One can surmise that if the requirement for graduate education were the only reason for program closures, those programs would have remained open until 1998, when the master's degree was required.

Despite the decline in the overall numbers of nurse anesthesia programs, many of which were certificate programs that had enrollments of fewer than five students, the level of educational programs changed dramatically (Figure 17-5). Through the 1990s, the overall number of CRNA graduates has leveled at approximately 950 annually (Figure 17-6). After an initial decline in graduates, the newer graduate programs increased their admissions. To accomplish this, programs had to increase the numbers of clinical training sites (Figure 17-6). The result has been a strengthened educational system, deeply entrenched in an academic model. The anticipated number of nurse anesthesia graduates in 2004 is 1700. There will be more than 900 clinical training sites by 2004.

Colleges of nursing are more frequently becoming the sites for nurse anesthesia programs as nurse anesthesia and other APN groups increasingly collaborate on legislative, policy, and educational matters. Agatha Hodgins' expressed desire for a separate professional organization and education process for nurse anesthesia has been partially supplanted by the rapprochement between nursing and nurse anesthesia (Mungia-Biddle et al., 1990). Coalitions of APNs have been effectively working together on the state and federal levels with health-care reform issues.

Nurse anesthesia educational curricula include time requirements for both didactic and clinical activities that reflect minimum standards for entry into practice. Academic

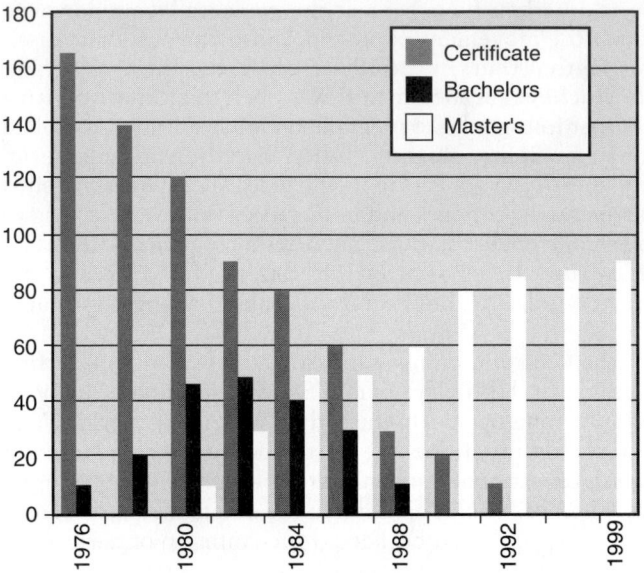

FIGURE 17-5 • Numbers and types of nurse anesthesia programs, 1976-1999. (From Council on Accreditation of Nurse Anesthesia Educational Programs, Park Ridge, IL [1999]; reprinted with permission.)

content areas are crucial to the preparation of practitioners for beginning-level competence in a highly demanding, rapidly changing specialty. Various colleges and schools that administratively house nurse anesthesia programs may have additional academic requirements. Nurse anesthesia programs in colleges of nursing include core graduate-level courses taken by all graduate-level nursing students. These courses include graduate-level nursing theory, nursing research, advanced physical assessment, and pharmacology.

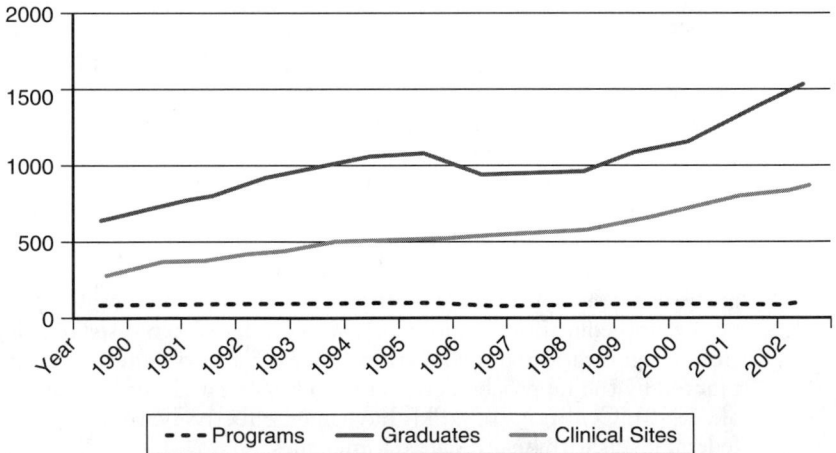

FIGURE 17-6 • Nurse anesthesia programs, graduates and clinical sites, 1990-2003. (From the Council on Accreditation of Nurse Anesthesia Educational Programs, Park Ridge, IL [2003]; reprinted with permission.)

The content areas and mandated time allocations for the nurse anesthesia core courses are listed in Table 17-1.

The clinical component requires that the student administer a minimum of 450 anesthetics. An external agency, the Council on Certification of Nurse Anesthetists, requires that students complete given numbers of surgical procedures and anesthetic techniques. For example, all students must administer at least 45 general anesthetics using a mask airway (versus endotracheal intubation), and provide care for patients across the lifespan. Similarly, graduates of nurse anesthesia programs must complete a required number of endotracheal intubations or thoracic surgical cases to be eligible to take the national certification examination.

Most programs exceed these minimum requirements. In addition, many require study in methods of scientific inquiry and statistics, as well as active participation in student-generated and faculty-sponsored research (AANA, 2002b).

The Council on Accreditation of Nurse Anesthesia Educational Programs accredits nurse anesthesia educational programs. Council members include CRNAs, physicians, and other members of the professional community. The Council on Accreditation conducts mandatory, on-site program reviews with a maximum accreditation period of 10 years. Nurse anesthesia educators and the Council on Accreditation have found that retaining a prescriptive curriculum in terms of hours and types of clinical experiences has helped the survival of educational programs. That is, when documented deviations from established standards for nurse anesthesia educational programs occur (e.g., physicians restricting clinical access), program directors can cite Council on Accreditation standards mandating these experiences.

Nurse anesthesia was the first nursing specialty to have mandatory certification. This process began in 1945, when the first certification examination in nurse anesthesia was given. The Council on Certification, like other AANA councils, is administratively independent of the AANA. The mission of the certification council is to certify nurse anesthesia graduates by examination, thus protecting the public and assuring patients of CRNA competency. The Council on Certification utilizes psychometricians, an academy of test item writers, and computer adaptive testing to assess beginning-level competence in nurse anesthesia graduates.

Another AANA council, the Council on Recertification, was developed in the late 1970s. The impetus for its development was the need to document for the public continued professional excellence for practicing CRNAs. The certification period for CRNAs is every 2 years and is renewable. Documentation of both anesthesia practice and continuing education activities is required for recertification. Continuing education programs must be approved by the council to meet requirements for recertification (AANA, 2002b).

These three councils, plus the Council for Public Interest in Anesthesia, endeavor to assure the public that the education and practice of CRNAs is more than adequate for the demands of the specialty. Nurse anesthesia education continues to evolve along with education in other advanced practice nursing areas.

TABLE 17-1	ACADEMIC COURSE REQUIREMENTS
TOPIC	**REQUIRED CONTACT HOURS**
Professional aspects of nurse anesthesia practice	45
Advanced anatomy, physiology, and pathophysiology	135
Chemistry and physics of anesthesia	45
Advanced pharmacology	90
Principles of anesthesia practice	90
Clinical and literature review conferences	45

AMERICAN ASSOCIATION OF NURSE ANESTHETISTS

Since its organization as the National Association of Nurse Anesthetists in 1931, the AANA has placed its responsibilities to the public above or at the same level as its responsibilities to its membership. The association has produced education and practice standards, implemented a certification process for nurse anesthetists (1945), and developed an accreditation program for nurse anesthetists (1952). It was a leader in forming multidisciplinary councils with public representation to fulfill the profession's autonomous credentialing functions (AANA, 1992b).

When founder Agatha Hodgins became ill, Gertrude Fife, who provided anesthesia for pioneering heart surgeon Claude Beck, assumed the burden of developing the young National Association of Nurse Anesthetists (Thatcher, 1953). The Association's name was changed to the American Association of Nurse Anesthetists in 1939. Helen Lamb, who served two terms as AANA president (1940-1942), worked exclusively with Dr. Evarts Graham, one of the first modern thoracic surgeons (Bankert, 1989). The first anesthesia administered for correction of tetralogy of Fallot was given by a nurse anesthetist, Olive Berger, at Johns Hopkins Hospital (Johns Hopkins Health System and Johns Hopkins University, 1999). Early CRNA leaders were involved in complex practice settings with surgeons who were also influential in their fields.

In addition to developing a professional identity for nurse anesthesia, early CRNA leaders developed curricular standards for nurse anesthesia educational programs. These standards included a minimum program length of 6 months and, later, institution of mandatory certification and recertification policies.

The AANA was among the first nursing specialty organizations. At a 1931 regional nurse anesthesia meeting, Agatha Hodgins put forth the essentials for a national organization of nurse anesthetists as she saw them:

Improvement of the present situation is in the hands of the nurse anesthetists themselves. If the work is to be properly safeguarded and hoped-for progress attained, it is necessary that remedies be applied to certain detrimental conditions now acknowledgedly existing. It would seem that the first step should be the awakening of deeper interest and the development of constructive leadership. Following in logical order would be: self-organization as a special division of hospital service . . . educational standards, post-graduate schools of anesthesia . . . required to conform to an accepted criteria of education; state registration, putting right the nurse anesthetist to practice her vocation beyond criticism; constant effort toward improving the quality of work by means of study and research, thus affording still greater protection to the patient; [and] dissemination of information gained through proper channels. (Thatcher, 1953, p. 183)

The division between nurse anesthesia and nursing service has occurred in many practice settings in which CRNAs are responsible to the hospital rather than to the nursing administration.

Early affiliation with the American Nurses Association did not occur, as noted earlier, because each organization had different ideas of what such an affiliation would entail (Gunn, 1991; Thatcher, 1953). With time, the breach between nursing and nurse anesthesia has narrowed considerably. Legislative and regulatory advances for APNs, such as direct reimbursement, prescriptive authority, and expanded scope of practice, have involved coalitions of APNs. As more nurse anesthesia programs have moved into schools of nursing, shared values have readily been identified by nurse anesthesia educators. These values include concepts such as ensuring access to primary and specialty care that can be provided by APNs for all citizens.

The AANA represents 95% of the practicing CRNAs in this country (Garde, 1998). This is an unusually high percentage of members for any professional organization. It is believed that this is because the AANA endeavors to be responsive to member concerns. The AANA allows multiple venues for direct member input rather than relying on a delegate system for member feedback to leadership (Foster & Garde, 1994).

The AANA has steadily grown, responding to member needs and legislative, regulatory, practice, and educational concerns. The organization has 10 major departments at its Park Ridge, Illinois, headquarters and in a Washington, DC, office (Figure 17-7). AANA affairs are handled by an elected board of directors in conjunction with AANA staff members. More than 20 committees and subcommittees conduct activities directed by the board. The AANA has one annual business meeting. Other national meetings that focus on areas such as education and government relations are held at various sites each year. Additionally, four autonomous councils function independently of the executive office. Councils in the areas of accreditation, certification, recertification, and public interest have been developed autonomously of the AANA to avoid potential conflicts of interest.

PROFESSIONAL ISSUES FOR CRNAs

Reimbursement for Nurse Anesthesia Clinical Services

In the early years of the 20th century and through the 1950s, CRNAs were usually paid employees of either the surgeon or the hospital for whom they worked. In rural areas,

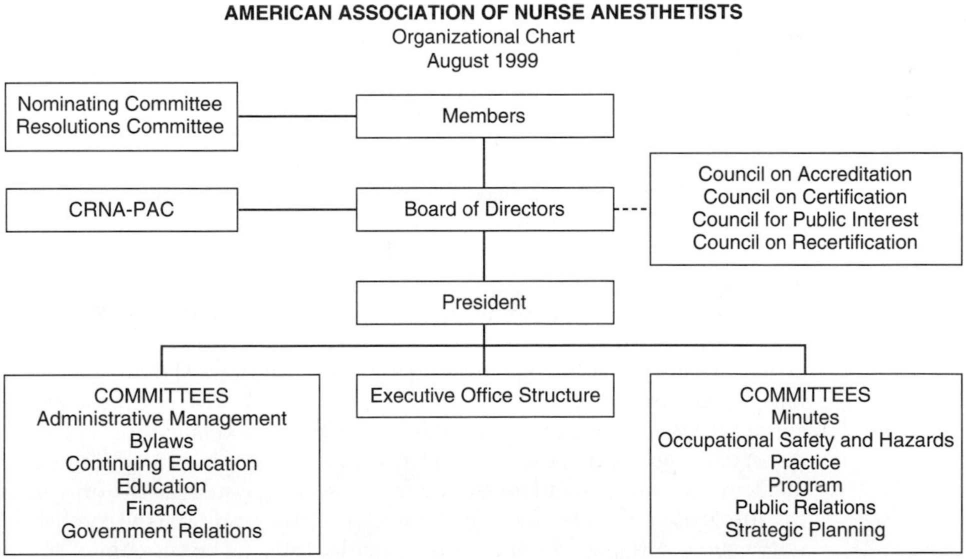

AMERICAN ASSOCIATION OF NURSE ANESTHETISTS
Organizational Chart
August 1999

FIGURE 17-7 • AANA organizational chart. (From American Association of Nurse Anesthetists; reprinted with permission.)

CRNAs often contracted with hospitals to provide services based on fee-for-service structures, that is, a set amount of compensation per case as opposed to a straight salary for hours worked (Simonson & Garde, 1994). With the advent of private payors such as Blue Cross/Blue Shield, only physician providers and hospitals were paid by the plan. Other health-care providers, such as CRNAs, psychologists, and physical therapists, would submit charges to the hospital or treating physician. The hospital or physician would then obtain reimbursement for services as "incident to" their own and pass the money on to the nonreimbursed provider (Simonson & Garde, 1994).

Because of escalating health-care costs in the 1970s and 1980s, Medicare instituted a prospective payment system in 1983. Although initially this legislation affected only Medicare Part A (hospital costs), it ultimately affected Medicare Part B (physician and nonphysician costs). Prospective payment system legislation mandated a fixed payment rate for all hospital care, covering Part A services paid to hospitals based on a patient's diagnosis-related classification group. This fixed rate was to cover all costs associated with hospital admission, including services provided by nonphysician health-care providers. CRNAs were in great jeopardy under this system because, in their effort to cut costs, hospitals had no incentive to hire CRNAs, because their cost would come directly from the hospital diagnosis-related classification group payment. Congress inadvertently created reimbursement disincentives for the use of CRNAs while bolstering incentives for the use of anesthesiologists. AANA lobbying efforts caused the Health Care Financing Administration (HCFA)—now the Centers for Medicare and Medicaid Services (CMS) to rewrite portions of this legislation, enabling all CRNAs to obtain direct Medicare reimbursement or to sign over their billing rights to their employer (Simonson & Garde, 1994).

Historically, anesthesia charges have been based on direct time involvement, either as a charge for simple time or as a charge based on a combination of time and the complexity of the anesthetic. The resource-based relative value scale, developed in the 1960s, is used to determine anesthesia charges based on the complexity of the surgical procedure. The result is charges for "base units," or surgical procedures described by anatomical or functional units. Additional "modifier units" can be added to base units for factors such as emergency procedures, extremes of age, or anesthetic risk. After base and modifier units have been added, time units are calculated at one unit per 15 minutes. The value of time units is determined by the payor (e.g., Medicare or Blue Cross/Blue Shield) and the market. One unit of anesthesia time may be billed from $15 to more than $70. The total of base, modifier, and time units determines the professional fee for the administration of anesthesia. Many third-party payors, such as Medicare and some Blue Cross insurers, completely ignore the practitioner's charges and base payments on their own fee schedules. These payments are often determined by what providers charge "on average" for their services (Simonson & Garde, 1994).

Attempts to control spiraling health-care costs and improve access to care have resulted in the previously mentioned proliferation of managed care contracts and a resurgence of interest in health maintenance organizations (HMOs). Fee-for-service reimbursement structures, as described earlier, may become things of the past as cost containment increasingly dominates health-care markets. All providers, including physicians, may eventually be salaried. Despite the trend of increased retrenchment, organized medicine continues to advocate the fee-for-service system as the only means to maintain the integrity of the physician-patient relationship and fights vigorously to maintain the status quo (Lester, 2003; Simonson & Garde, 1994). The economics of cost containment do not ensure APNs access to patients based on their cost-effectiveness. Because of the desire to maintain fee-for-service payment in some settings, the most cost-effective provider may not be the one chosen to participate in the system. Transitional mechanisms in vertical integration strategy (e.g., combining payors, provider, and a wide spectrum of services in the same network, such as physician-hospital organizations) still focus on physicians and hospitals as principal health-care resources. Some sources consider this a stopgap measure, not addressing all players, such as insurance providers, in the system. Cost-effectiveness and provider practice profiles are increasingly considered in managed care contracting, but there may be a reticence to disrupt traditional local practice patterns as managed care increasingly influences some markets (Kongstvedt, 1994).

Recently, the CMS presented revised (mostly lower) reimbursement amounts for CRNA services provided under Medicare. The overall change for all areas combined was a slight increase for a few surgical procedures; the majority of procedures have lower values (Lester, 2003).

The AANA was asked by the American Society of Anesthesiologists to join them in an effort to seek congressional help to reverse the CMS proposal and seek increases for all surgical procedures. Paradoxically, the American Society of Anesthesiologists actively opposed an AANA effort to change Medicare Part A supervision requirements and was not supportive of efforts to obtain reimbursement for medically directed CRNAs working with nurse anesthesia students (Lester, 2003). These experiences demonstrate ongoing efforts to decrease anesthesia reimbursement and indicate that complex policy initiatives are difficult to achieve unilaterally.

Impact of Cost Containment on CRNA Education and Practice

Historically, APNs and physician assistants have practiced collaboratively with physicians in HMOs, providing both primary and specialty care. HMO physicians acknowledge the continued role for APNs in HMOs and group practice arrangements (Bowser, 1994). A paradigm shift in acute care has occurred, wherein hospitals are no longer financial profit centers but are now recognized as cost centers. Critical pathways and other utilization review mechanisms are used to minimize the average length of hospital stay. The need for inpatient beds is less because early discharge, home health, and outpatient care services are increasingly the norm.

Increasingly, capitated payments are made to health-care providers. Under capitation, a per member per month allotment of money is paid to cover the health-care needs of a predefined population. Providers are expected to treat patients within this cost or incur a loss of income. Thus financial risk for health care has shifted from insurance companies to health-care providers. For example, a surgical inpatient who spends 2 hours of a 5-day hospitalization in the operating room finds that operating room costs comprise 35% to 40% of the entire hospitalization cost. Today's anesthesia providers have to keep pace with the huge growth in knowledge, medicolegal pressures, greater financial complexity, and new ethical dilemmas associated with managed care organizations (Kaye et al., 1999).

Some of the purported effects of cost containment on anesthesia practice include the need to demonstrate value by improving quality of care at a reduced cost, or by maintaining quality while reducing cost. Suggested strategies (Kaye et al., 1999) include the following:

1. Fostering more appropriate use of anesthesia drugs
2. Using anesthesia information management for pharmaceutical cost containment
3. Fast-tracking patients who need coronary artery bypass grafting and ambulatory surgical patients

Nurse anesthesia education programs have been affected by the restructuring of healthcare organizations. Traditional certificate programs were based in hospitals that paid for significant portions of overhead expenses. As hospitals have downsized or joined corporate entities, some remaining hospital-based, university-affiliated programs have had to develop alternative fiscal management strategies. CRNA educators must be able to demonstrate the value added to the organization by the nurse anesthesia program, its faculty, and its students.

CRNAs and APNs can play significant roles in the shift from inpatient acute care to outpatient and home health services. It seems likely for CRNAs that hospital employment will be less common as hospitals decrease their fixed costs, such as payroll, and wish to outsource services such as anesthesia to private groups. However, there is also a recent trend toward hospital employment of some specialty health-care providers. It is imperative that CRNAs and other APNs track these trends closely and negotiate for a place at the decision-making table.

Whether CRNAs will be self-employed, employed by CRNA groups, or employed by physician-CRNA groups will depend on local market dynamics. Independent contracting by CRNAs for their professional services will continue to increase. It will be imperative for CRNAs and other APNs to know their worth in terms of billable revenue and quality of care provided for contract negotiation and public relations purposes.

In the future, each CRNA may practice in multiple settings with individually negotiated contracts. Home health services such as parenteral infusion therapy and management of chronic pain might be directed by CRNAs, as is already the case in some areas. These settings are natural extensions of anesthesia, pharmacology, and clinical skills. Myriad opportunities will exist for CRNAs and other APNs to collaborate in the management of acute and chronic pain and the treatment of respiratory and nutritional disorders.

Continued Challenges for CRNAs

MEDICAL MALPRACTICE COVERAGE

The cost of medical malpractice insurance has increased steadily. The "hard market" began in 2000, after almost a decade of essentially flat prices. Rate increases have been precipitated in part by the growing size of claims, more frequent claims in some urban areas, and soaring defense costs. Losses are growing at a time when investment income, the cushion against losses, is declining, thus widening the gap between revenues (premiums) and claims. In addition, reinsurance, the insurance coverage for insurers, has become significantly more expensive, pushing up the costs for insurers. Among the other factors driving up prices is a reduced supply of available coverage as insurers exit the medical malpractice business because of the difficulties associated with profitability (Insurance Information Institute, 2004).

As a result of these market forces, the St. Paul Fire and Marine Casualty Insurance Company ceased providing medical malpractice coverage for CRNAs in 2001. The St. Paul Company was the largest provider of CRNA medical malpractice coverage. TIG, another medical malpractice carrier for CRNAs, also no longer provides this coverage. However, AANA Insurance, an AANA subsidiary, identified the C.N.A. Company as a medical malpractice underwriter for CRNAs. AANA Insurance has also identified other potential carriers.

Many CRNAs receive their medical malpractice coverage from employers, some of whom are self-insured. To date, malpractice premiums do not appear to have affected the robust salaries enjoyed by most CRNAs.

SUPERVISION

The CMS published a final rule concerning the federal Medicare and Medicaid physician supervision requirement for CRNAs (2001). The federal requirement had been that

CRNAs be supervised by a physician. This rule allowed states to "opt out" or be exempted from the federal supervision requirements (AANA, 2001).

For a state to "opt out" from the federal supervision requirement, the state's governor must send a letter to the CMS attesting to the following:

1. That the state governor has consulted with the state boards of medicine and nursing about issues related to access and to the quality of anesthesia services in the state
2. That it is in the best interests of state citizens to opt out of the current federal physician supervision requirement
3. That the opt out is consistent with state law

Many states do not require CRNAs to be physician supervised. Thirty-nine states do not have a physician supervision requirement for CRNAs in nursing or medical laws or regulations (AANA, 2001).

The CMS has indicated that the Agency for Healthcare Research and Quality (AHRQ) will "conduct a study of anesthesia outcomes in those states that choose to opt out of the CRNA supervision requirement compared to those states that have not" (AANA, 2001, p. 56764).

Whether or not a state opts out of the federal supervision requirement, individual facilities may still require CRNAs to be physician supervised. The CMS noted that states [have] "traditional domain in establishing professional licensure and scope of practice laws . . . it is not unusual to find differences in state law." States make decisions based upon their unique needs and specifications. The following states have opted out of the federal supervision requirement at this writing: Iowa, Nebraska, Idaho, Minnesota, New Hampshire, New Mexico and Kansas (AANA, 2001).

The CMS final rule change does not affect how nurse anesthetists currently practice or are reimbursed under Medicare Part B. Medicare conditions of payment under Part A for hospitals and ambulatory surgical centers were unchanged after November 13, 2001. The rule retains a physician supervision requirement for nurse anesthetists in order for hospitals and ambulatory surgical centers to receive Medicare Part A payment. The management of a patient's medical and surgical care continues to be the responsibility of a physician, although that physician may be a surgeon or internist. The rule does not require CRNAs to be under the supervision of anesthesiologists. Every state permits CRNAs to practice without anesthesiologist supervision. The JCAHO does not require anesthesiologist supervision (Blumenreich, 1995).

The CMS does not define supervision, and hospitals are not required to define supervision. Defining supervision can create complicated compliance issues that most hospitals would rather avoid (Blumenreich, 1997). The JCAHO does not define supervision or require such definition.

The responsibility of the operating or diagnostic physician does not change based on the anesthesia provider. Typically, the physician has the following responsibilities:

• Determination of whether a patient requires a surgical or diagnostic procedure
• Requesting that an anesthetic be administered
• Determination that the patient is an appropriate candidate for the planned procedure and anesthetic

The supervising physician is not required to have privileges to actually administer anesthesia. Surgeons are no more likely than anesthesiologists to be held liable for the actions of CRNAs (Cromwell, 1998; Foster, 1998). The courts have not found physicians and surgeons to be automatically liable for the actions of CRNAs, nor are these providers immune from liability when they work with anesthesiologists. CRNAs are accountable for their own actions. Courts typically do not look at the type of anesthesia provider, but at the amount of control the physician or surgeon exercises over the anesthesia provider (Blumenreich, 1998).

STUDENT SUPERVISION RULES

Another current issue affecting nurse anesthesia education is reimbursement inequity under Medicare and some private insurance plans. Compensation for cases performed by student nurse anesthetists is less than the reimbursement for resident anesthesiologists, producing an economic disincentive for the education of nurse anesthetists. This issue is being addressed by the AANA.

DOCTORAL EDUCATION

In the educational arena, there is continued debate about the preparation of CRNAs. Currently, the minimum length of nurse anesthesia programs is 24 months. However, because of the combination of didactic and clinical time requirements, many programs are 27 to 36 months long. Nurse anesthesia curricular requirements can overload the typical master's curriculum. Because of the time commitment and academic rigor necessary for this specialty area, there is increasing interest in a clinical doctorate as the exit degree in nurse anesthesia. The vision of nursing leader Dr. Luther Christman for nurses to be prepared with advanced degrees both in their discipline and in a basic science reflects the trend to propose preparation beyond the master's degree for entry into this and other advanced practice specialty areas (Christman, 1977). Doctoral programs in nurse anesthesia are being developed. Approximately 1% of practicing nurse anesthetists possess doctoral degrees in disciplines including education, nursing, physiology, and pharmacology.

The Council on Accreditation of Nurse Anesthesia Educational Programs has mandated doctoral preparation for nurse anesthesia program directors by 2014. Currently, 32 of the 87 program directors (37%) listed in the Council on Accreditation's *List of Recognized Educational Programs* (2002) have doctoral degrees. CRNAs continue to seek doctoral education, but the incentives for pursuing this type of education are quite different from those for a practice-oriented master's degree.

An AANA task force conducted a survey to investigate the feasibility of a doctorate for nurse anesthetists. Results of the survey showed that 65% of the respondents did not support the requirement of a doctorate for entry into practice; 60% of nurse anesthesia education programs stated it was not feasible to offer doctorates at their institutions because of insufficient faculty resources (Jordan & Shott, 1998).

There was no statistically significant relationship between year of graduation from an anesthesia program and doctorate entry support for all respondents. A significant association was found between planned retirement year and doctorate entry support for female respondents. However, respondents who believed that the AANA should promote doctoral programs tended to be more recent graduates (median graduation year, 1982) than those who did not agree with this (median graduation year, 1980) ($P = 0.044$) (Jordan & Shott, 1998).

The themes that emerged for faculty related to doctoral education were in four major areas. Adequate time for doctoral studies was an impediment for almost half the respondents (44%). Inadequate finances for doctoral education was identified as an area of difficulty by 27% of respondents, and 25% of responding CRNA faculty members had no interest in obtaining a doctorate (Jordan & Shott, 1998). The lack of interest in pursuing a doctorate could be related to time demands on program directors.

EVIDENCE-BASED PRACTICE

The influx of CRNAs with graduate degrees into the profession combined with expectations of consumers, legislators, and regulators provide opportunities to objectively assess clinical practices in terms of safety and economy. In this era of rapidly shifting resources and changing models of care, CRNAs must demonstrate quality and cost-effective patient care. Historically, quality of anesthesia care has been studied by measuring variables such as mortality and morbidity rates, length of stay, readmission, and cost. Methods have not been readily available to define quality in terms of the effect of care delivery on the health of patients. Combined administrative and health-related databases are essential, albeit limited, in elucidating the outcomes associated with nurse anesthesia practice. Development of methodologically sound research will require the preparation of more scholars in the specialty who have expertise in research design and measurement (Kremer & Faut-Callahan, 2001). Some recent publications, described in the following paragraphs, reveal trends in nurse anesthesia research.

In one study, investigators compared research reported in the *AANA Journal* from 1995 to 1996 (n = 38 studies), from 1985 to 1986 (n = 18), and from 1975 to 1976 (n = 14). The amount of research published in the *AANA Journal* has increased steadily, with a stable focus on clinical practice. In addition, there has been an increase in educational and safety-related research reported. Another 28 articles authored by CRNAs were found in other medical and nursing journals for the 1995-1996 period (Connelly, Schretenhaler, & Taunton, 2002).

By the 1990s, all studies contained at least one indicator of theoretical orientation. The most frequently represented sampling technique was utilization of convenience samples of hospitalized patients. There was minimal reporting on reliability and validity of data and the psychometric evaluation of research tools. The authors recommended increased emphasis on methodological studies, multisite studies, programs of research, collaboration among CRNAs, nurses in other specialties, and practitioners from other disciplines (Connelly et al., 2002).

Some recent papers published by CRNAs have evidence-based content. For example, Norred (2003) described the state of the science in antiemetic prophylaxis in an *AANA Journal* course for continuing education credit. Norred (2003) stated that postoperative nausea and vomiting (PONV) [is] a common problem with complex causes that may result in substantial complications, for example, wound dehiscence or unplanned hospital admission. The pathogenesis of postoperative nausea and vomiting and the array of drugs used for antiemetic purposes—corticosteroids, gastrointestinal prokinetics, neuroleptic butyrophenones, phenothiazines, and serotonin receptor antagonists—were reviewed. State-of-the-art anesthetic techniques to prevent postoperative nausea and vomiting were described. Mutimodal therapy with combined low-dose antiemetics affecting multiple receptors was suggested to prevent postoperative nausea and vomiting in high-risk patients such as nonsmokers, females with a previous history of nausea, and patients with high postoperative narcotic requirements (Norred, 2003).

Another group of investigators examined the anesthetic implications of morbid obesity, which is associated with multiple metabolic and mechanical abnormalities that increase morbidity and mortality after major abdominal surgery. Bariatric surgery has been performed with increasing frequency, and investigators sought to clarify the frequency of postoperative pulmonary complications in these patients. A retrospective chart review of 207 patients who underwent elective gastric bypass surgery was conducted. The rates of respiratory failure and total postoperative complications were 8% in patients with a body mass index of 43 or less and 14% in patients with a body mass index of greater than 43. The authors noted that "skillful anesthetic care allows patients with significant comorbid conditions to benefit from bariatric surgery with reasonable risk in terms of postoperative complications" (Blouw, Rudolph, Narr, & Sarr, 2003, p. 47).

Investigators have also examined the association between postoperative complications and the type of regional anesthesia used. Faas et al. (2002) examined the effects of spinal ($n = 113$) versus epidural ($n = 31$) anesthetic techniques on three common postoperative complications: pain, urinary retention, and mobility for patients undergoing inguinal herniorrhaphy. This study was also a retrospective chart review. Results demonstrated that pain was not significantly different between the two anesthetic groups ($P = 0.65$); however, subjects in the epidural anesthesia group were able to ambulate ($P = 0.008$) and void ($P = 0.02$) sooner than subjects in the spinal anesthesia group. In this sample, epidural anesthesia appeared to optimize recovery for patients who had undergone herniorrhaphy.

These studies demonstrate CRNA-authored research with tangible practice implications. These are valuable additions to the anesthesia literature and contain useful, data-based practice recommendations. Websites that are useful to CRNA practice can be found in Box 17-4.

With the challenges described, the future of nurse anesthesia is promising. More CRNAs hold graduate degrees, and there is potential for additional CRNA-conducted basic and applied research. Additional graduate education in nursing, the basic sciences, and business will better enable CRNAs to collaborate with other investigators in the arenas of clinical and bench research; practice, legislation, and policy formulation will also be enhanced by this additional educational preparation. A greater nurse anesthesia voice in policy formulation has already been heard, with CRNA members securing places on state boards of nursing and other governmental positions.

The tradition of strong leadership meeting challenges directly continues. Former AANA Executive Director John Garde, CRNA, MS, FAAN, said:

[T]he profession has an optimistic future. I point out with pride the commitment that AANA members have toward [the future of their profession]—a commitment that encompasses being outstanding anesthesia practitioners who belong to their Association. I am reminded, too, what each of you

---

BOX 17-4 • POPULAR ANESTHESIA WEBSITES

American Association of Nurse Anesthetists	www.aana.com
Anesthesiology—the journal of the American Society of Anesthesiologists	www.anesthesiology.org
Anesthesia & Analgesia	www.anesthesia-analgesia.org
Anesthesia & Intensive Care	www.aaic.net.au/home.html
Anesthesia Online	www.priory.co.uk/anes.html
Internet Journal of Anesthesiology	www.ispub.com/journals/ija.htm
Journal of Clinical Anesthesia	www.elsevier.com/locate/jcaonline
Journal of Cardiothoracic & Vascular Anesthesia	www.jcardioanesthesia.com
Pain (the journal for the International Association for the Study of Pain)	www.elsevier.nl/ inca/publicatiions/store/ 5/0/6/0/8/3/
Survey of Anesthesiology	www.gasnet.mail.yale.edu/periodicals/sa
International Trauma Anesthesia & Critical Care Society	www.trauma.itaccs.com/news.html.
GASNets—anesthesiology discussion list archives	www.gasnet.med.yale.edu/

brings every day to your patients. Dick Davidson, president of the American Hospital Association, said when asked about what will remain in health care 100 years from now, "There will always be personal contact and caring. We will always have hands touching patients. Everything we do is about human need. That's the constant over time." And, that is the legacy of the nurse anesthesia profession. (Garde, 1998, p. 15)

CONCLUSION

Nurse anesthesia, the earliest nursing specialty, was also the first nursing specialty to have standardized educational programs, a certification process, mandatory continuing education, and recertification. Nurse anesthetists have been involved in the development of anesthetic techniques along with physicians and engineers. Nurse anesthetists have been nursing leaders in obtaining third-party reimbursement for professional services and in coping with challenges such as the prospective payment system, managed care, and physician supervision.

Nurse anesthetists provide surgical and nonsurgical anesthesia services in a variety of settings both in the United States and in other parts of the world. CRNAs work in collaboration with physicians, as do other APNs, and are capable of providing the full spectrum of anesthesia services.

Activism in the state and federal legislative and regulatory arenas is a recognized CRNA activity. Increasing coalition building between nurse anesthetists, other APNs, and nursing educators is congruent with a shared nursing vision. This vision values health care for all Americans provided in a safe and cost-effective manner by APNs collaborating with other health-care professionals.

REFERENCES

Abenstein, J., & Warner, M. (1996). Anesthesia providers, patient outcomes, and costs. *Anesthesia & Analgesia, 82,* 1273-1283.

American Association of Nurse Anesthetists. (2001). *Fact sheet concerning state opt-outs and November 13, 2001 CMS rule.* Retrieved May 13, 2003, from http://www.aana.com/capcorner/factsheet_111301.asp

American Association of Nurse Anesthetists. (2002a). *Guidelines and standards for nurse anesthesia practice.* Park Ridge, IL: Author.

American Association of Nurse Anesthetists. (2002b). *Qualifications and capabilities of the CRNA.* Park Ridge, IL: Author.

Bader, A., & Datta, S. (1994). Obstetric anesthesia. In M. C. Rogers, J. Tinker, & B. Covino (Eds.), *Principles and practice of anesthesiology* (pp. 2065-2104). St. Louis, MO: C. V. Mosby.

Bankert, M. (1989). *Watchful care: A history of America's nurse anesthetists.* New York: Continuum.

Beutler, J. (2002). Report of the AANA executive director. *AANA News Bulletin, 56,* 7-11.

Blouw, E., Rudolph, A., Narr, B., & Sarr, M. (2003). The frequency of respiratory failure in patients with morbid obesity undergoing gastric bypass. *AANA Journal, 71,* 45-50.

Blumenreich, G. (1997). LeCroix case. *AANA Journal, 65,* 419-423.

Blumenreich, G. A. (1995). *Anesthesia and JCAHO.* Retrieved May 17, 2004, from http://www.aana.com/legal/legbrfs/1995/12lb95.asp

Blumenreich, G. A. (1998). *Do surgeons get sued when they work with anesthesiologists?* Retrieved May 17, 2004, from http://www.aana.com/legal/legbrfs/1998/04lb98.asp

Blumenreich, G. A., Stallone, D. R., & Tobin, M. H. (1990). *Federal drug laws and CRNAs.* Retrieved May 13, 2003, from http://www.aana.com/legal/legbrfs/1990/08lb90.asp

Bowser, R. (1994). *Lecture from HMO physician administrator in Managed Care Course in Health Systems Management.* Unpublished manuscript, Rush University, Chicago.

Callaghan, J. (1995). Twenty-five years of gallbladder surgery in a small rural hospital. *American Journal of Surgery, 169,* 313-315.

Callahan, L. (1994). Establishing measures of competence. In S. Foster & L. Jordan (Eds.), *Professional* aspects of nurse anesthesia practice (pp. 275-290). Philadelphia: F. A. Davis.

Callahan, L. (1995). *Development of a single blended anesthesia provider: An exploratory study.* Unpublished doctoral dissertation, Florida State University, Tallahassee.

Center for Medicare and Medicaid Services. (2001, November 13). Medicare and Medicaid physician supervision requirements for certified registered nurse anesthetists (CRNAs). *Federal Register* [01-28439], pp. 56762-56769.

Christman, L. (1977). Doctoral education: A shot in the arm for the nursing profession. *Health Services Manager, 10,* 6, 7.

Connelly, L., Schretenthaler, J., & Taunton, R. (2002). Nurse anesthesia research: A follow-up study. *AANA Journal, 70,* 463-469.

Council on Accreditation of Nurse Anesthesia Educational Programs. (2002). *List of recognized educational programs.* Park Ridge, IL: Author.

Council on Accreditation of Nurse Anesthesia Educational Programs. (2003). *Accredited nurse anesthesia programs.* Retrieved May 13, 2003, from http://www.aana.com/coa/accreditedprograms.asp

Cromwell, J. (1998, November 15). *Barriers to achieving the optimal workforce mix.* Paper presented at the AANA Fall Assembly of States, Colorado Springs, CO.

Cromwell, J., & Rosenbach, M. (1988). The economics of anesthesia delivery. *Health Affairs, 7,* 118-131.

Dorroh, M., & Norton, S. (1996). The certified nurse-midwife. In A. B. Hamric, J. A. Spross, & C. M. Hanson (Eds.), *Advanced nursing practice: An integrative approach* (pp. 395-420). Philadelphia: W. B. Saunders.

Dripps, R. (1977). Preface. In R. D. Dripps, J. E. Eckenhoff, & L. D. Vandam Dripps (Eds.), *Introduction to anesthesia* (5th ed., pp. 1-11). Philadelphia: W. B. Saunders.

Faas, C., Acosta, F., Campbell, M., O'Hagan C., Newton, S., & Zaglaniczny, K. (2002). The effects of spinal vs epidural anesthesia on three potential postoperative complications: Pain, urinary retention, and mobility following inguinal herniorrhaphy. *AANA Journal, 70,* 441-447.

Faut, M. (1984). *Doctoral education for nurse anesthesia practice.* Unpublished clinical defense paper, Rush University, Chicago.

Faut-Callahan, M. (1991). Graduate education for nurse anesthetists: Master's versus a clinical doctorate. In *National Commission on Nurse Anesthesia Education Report* (pp. 110-115). Park Ridge, IL: American Association of Nurse Anesthetists.

Faut-Callahan, M., & Paice, J. (1990). Post-operative pain control for the parturient. *Journal of Perinatal and Neonatal Nursing, 4,* 27-41.

Foster, S. (1998). *Comments of the American Association of Nurse Anesthetists on the proposed rule regarding the Medicare and Medicaid programs; hospital conditions of participation; provider and supplier approval.* Unpublished document, American Association of Nurse Anesthetists, Park Ridge, IL.

Foster, S., & Garde, J. (1994). The American Association of Nurse Anesthetists: The role of the professional organization. In S. Foster & L. Jordan (Eds.), *Professional aspects of nurse anesthesia practice* (pp. 35-48). Philadelphia: F. A. Davis.

Garde, J. (1998, November). Annual report of the executive director. *AANA News Bulletin,* pp. 14-16.

Gunn, I. (1991). The history of nurse anesthesia education: Highlights and influences. In *National Commission on Nurse Anesthesia Education Report* (pp. 33-41). Park Ridge, IL: American Association of Nurse Anesthetists.

Insurance Information Institute, Inc. (2004). *Medical malpractice.* Retrieved May 17, 2004 from http://www.iii.org/media/hottopics/insurance/medicalmal/

Johns Hopkins Health System and Johns Hopkins University. (1999). The Alan Mason Chesney Medical Archives of the Johns Hopkins Medical Institutions, The Olive Louise Berger Collection. Retrieved May 17, 2004, from http://www.medicalarchives.jhmi.edu/sgml/berger.html

Jordan, L. (1994). Qualifications and capabilities of the certified registered nurse anesthetist. In S. Foster & L. Jordan, (Eds.), *Professional aspects of nurse anesthesia practice* (pp. 3-10). Philadelphia: F. A. Davis.

Jordan, L., & Shott, S. (1998). Feasibility of a doctoral degree for nurse anesthetists. *AANA Journal, 66,* 287-298.

Jordan, L., Kremer, M., Crawforth, K. (2001). Data-driven practice improvement: The AANA Foundation Closed Malpractice Claims Study. *AANA Journal, 69,* 301-316.

Kaye, D., Scibetta, W., & Grogono, A. (1999). Anesthesia manpower and recruitment 1998: An update. *Advances in Anesthesia, 16,* 1-27.

Kelly, J. (1994). An international study of educational programs for nurses providing anesthesia care. *AANA Journal, 62,* 484-495.

Kongstvedt, P. (1994). *The managed care handbook* (2nd ed.). Gaithersburg, MD: Aspen.

Kremer, M., & Faut-Callahan, M. (2001). Outcome assessment in nurse anesthesia. In R. M. Kleinpell (Ed.), *Outcome assessment in advanced practice nursing* (pp. 227-260). New York: Springer.

Lester, R. (2003). President's message. *AANA News Bulletin,* 57, 2.

Loper, K., Butler, S., Nessly, M., & Wild, L. (1989). Paralyzed with pain: The need for education. *Pain, 37,* 315-316.

McAuliffe, M., & Henry, B. (1998). Survey of nurse anesthesia practice, education, and regulation in 96 countries. *AANA Journal, 66,* 273-286.

Merwin, E., & Stern, S. (2003, April 28). *Preliminary findings of the AANA Foundation Manpower Study.* Third-Year Assembly National Healthcare Policy and Advocacy Conference. Podium presentation. Washington, DC.

Munguia-Biddle, F., Maree, S., Klein, E., Callahan, L., & Gilles, B. (1990). *Nurse anesthesiology competence evaluation: Mechanism for accountability.* Unpublished document, American Association of Nurse Anesthetists, Park Ridge, IL.

National Center for Nursing Research. (1991). *CRNA manpower study.* Washington, DC: U. S. Department of Health and Human Services.

Norred, C. L. (2003). Antiemetic prophylaxis: Pharmacologic and therapeutics. *AANA Journal, 71,* 133-140.

Orkin, F. (1998). Rural realities. *Anesthesiology, 88,* 1597-1598.

Pine, M., Holt, K., & Lou, Y. (2003). Surgical mortality and type of anesthesia provider. *AANA Journal, 71,* 109-116.

Quinlan, D. (2001). Peer assistance—Part 2. In S. Foster &. M. Faut-Callahan, (Eds). *A professional study and resource guide for the CRNA.* Park Ridge, IL: AANA Publishing Inc. 476-477. Retrieved April 20, 2003, from http:www.aana.com/peer/foster/pain_management.asp

Rivera, L. (2003). *Practice profile survey summary.* Unpublished manuscript, American Association of Nurse Anesthetists, Park Ridge, IL.

Schubert, A., Eckhout, G., Cooperider, T., & Kubel, A. (2001). Evidence of a current and lasting national anesthesia personnel shortage. *Mayo Clinic Proceedings, 76,* 995-1010.

Schubert, A., Eckhout, G., & Trempert, K. (2003). An updated view of the national anesthesia personnel shortfall. *Anesthesia & Analgesia, 96,* 207-214.

Simonson, D., & Garde, J. (1994). Reimbursement for clinical services. In S. Foster & L. Jordan (Eds.), *Professional aspects of nurse anesthesia practice* (pp. 129-142). Philadelphia: F. A. Davis.

Stark, P., & Kremer, M. (2001, August 16). Poster Presentation: Rural Realities Revisited: Perioperative Care in Rural Illinois. AANA Annual Meeting, San Francisco, CA.

Thatcher, V. (1953). *History of anesthesia with emphasis on the nurse specialist.* Philadelphia: J. B. Lippincott.

Waugaman, W. (1991). Nurse anesthesia: The practice of nursing, medicine, or something else? *Nurse Anesthesia, 2,* 157-159.

CHAPTER 18

The Advanced Practice Nurse Case Manager

VICKY A. MAHN-DiNICOLA • DONNA J. ZAZWORSKY

Continued

APN CM COMPETENCIES
Consultation and Collaboration
Ethical Decision-Making Skills
Leadership, Empowerment, Change Agency, and Activism
Research

CRITICAL ELEMENTS OF THE APN CM PRACTICE ENVIRONMENT
Business Elements
Organizational Structures and Cultures
Shared Accountability for Managing Utilization
Productivity and Acuity
Indirect Costs
Reimbursements
Billing Methods
Marketing
Certification and Credentialing Requirements

CONCLUSION: LOOKING TOWARD THE FUTURE OF APN CM PRACTICE

INTRODUCTION

Over the last decade, the need to manage care more efficiently and effectively has informed almost every effort to reinvent the health-care system. Driven largely by economics, the delivery of cost-effective care through prudent use of resources and the elimination of redundant and unnecessary services was the predominant goal of the 1990s. This focus is expected to continue throughout the next several decades as the population ages and chronic disease continues to account for an increasing percentage of health-care resources. A variety of strategies to improve care and contain costs in the competitive health-care market have been implemented. These include utilization management, critical pathways, patient care guidelines, disease management and case management. Despite these resource management strategies, fiscal performance in the health-care marketplace has not improved significantly because patients or clients usually enter the health-care system when they are already sick and need costly intervention. In essence, the health-care system is a reactive system, rather than proactive system. Although a few dollars can be saved through prudent use of pharmaceuticals or diagnostics or by restricting access to care, the largest gain is thought to result from the prevention of costly health problems and better management of existing chronic diseases (Zitter, 1994).

According to recent statistics (Utilization Review Accreditation Commission [URAC], 2002), the number of people with chronic diseases is growing at an alarming rate. In 2000, 20 million more people had one or more chronic conditions than originally predicted in 1996. In 2002, 25% of the American population was living with multiple chronic conditions that accounted for more than 60% of our nation's medical care costs. The number of people with chronic diseases is projected to increase from 125 million in 2000 to 171 million by 2030.

In the new millennium, case managers (CMs), including nurse case managers (NCMs), will adopt more proactive and systematic approaches to managing care processes and outcomes for both acutely and chronically ill populations. Not only will there be a need to perform the traditional case management activities of assessing, planning, implementing, monitoring, and coordinating activities for individuals with immediate health-care needs, there will also be a need to develop system-focused and population-focused interventions for promoting wellness and facilitating healthy lifestyle choices in order to stave off chronic disease. *System-focused programs* are interventions directed at the health-care delivery system itself and include the use of research and predictive modeling, data management, and evaluation of clinical processes within a given care delivery system. *Population-focused programs* target specific patient groups and include interventions aimed at prevention, early identification, and management and coordination of chronic illness or acute disease and injury across the continuum. NCMs with both direct care and systems responsibilities will find themselves in a unique role to influence care on a larger scale. Not only will they be educating, supporting, coaching, and advocating for individual clients at risk, they will be designing programs and interventions for chronic disease management and other high-risk health problems so that those clients adopt behaviors known to reduce disease, limit chronicity or progression, and prevent complications. We believe that the advanced practice nurse (APN) CMs are ideal candidates for such positions. Whether an APN is functioning in a designated APN CM role or functioning in an NP or CNS role that incorporates the elements of CM practice into a new blended role, the APN will be instrumental in refining the definition, implementation, and evaluation of the NCM and APN CM roles. While it is not yet clear whether the APN CM role will become a sanctioned specialty under the

American Nursing Association's (ANA's) APN umbrella, it is clear that both the literature and graduate nursing curricula are promoting unique roles and responsibilities that are consistent with "advanced practice" in nursing case management.

This chapter begins with a conceptual overview of case management, NCM, and APN CM and then discusses current and emerging care management trends so that the reader can understand the care environments where opportunities exist for APN CM intervention. A variety of NCM models are presented. This chapter also reviews care management strategies, including health promotion and prevention, acute complication management, chronic disease management, and population health management. The role of the APN CM in each of these strategies is illustrated by way of exemplars drawn from our own practice experience of the authors. Finally, there is a comprehensive discussion about the competencies, skills and unique knowledge base required for successful practice as an APN CM.

OVERVIEW OF CASE MANAGEMENT, NURSE CASE MANAGEMENT, AND APN CASE MANAGEMENT

Case Management

Case management is a practice framework that has been implemented in a variety of public and private settings by nurses, social workers, rehabilitation specialists, and other health-care providers. Case management can be traced back to the early 1900s (Mahn & Zazworsky, 2000; see Chapter 1). In the 1970s, and 1980s, national reimbursement trends began to reshape American health care, and the current scope of CM practice emerged from those changes. To foster a common understanding of the evolving nature of case management, the interdisciplinary Case Management Society of America (CMSA) recently revised its 1995 definition of case management as "a collaborative process which assesses, plans, implements, coordinates, monitors and evaluates options and services to meet an individual's health needs through communications and available resources to promote quality, cost effective outcomes" (CMSA, 2002, p. 5). CMSA recognizes that CM is practiced by a variety of health-care professionals, so this definition is not discipline specific. An interdisciplinary definition is useful because it applies to a range of health-care systems and service settings. For example, some patient populations, such as indigent patients, may be best served by social work CMs, whereas rehabilitation counselors may best serve other populations, such as patients with head injuries, and nurses manage those with cancer, diabetes, and other chronic illnesses.

The 2002 definition mirrors the nursing process less directly than CMSA's earlier definition, which included problem identification, planning, monitoring, evaluation, and outcomes (CMSA, 1995) These activities are addressed to a greater degree within the new CMSA standards of care (CMSA, 2002). The new standards of care include objective measurement guidelines for each standard of care and emphasize evaluation and outcomes more than the previous standards. Although the new definition and standards incorporate the system, clinical, and fiscal aspects that are central to the case management process, the CMSA definition of case management still does not fully address the specialized clinical nursing expertise that seems essential to achieve optimal cost and quality outcomes in certain patients who require health promotion or illness management.

Nurse Case Management

The ANA definition of nursing case management has undergone similar evolution. In 1988 the ANA defined NCM as a health-care delivery process that aims to provide quality health care, enhance quality of life, diminish fragmentation, and contain costs (ANA, 1988) The more recent ANA definition (ANA, 2003) places greater emphasis on the nursing process and adds a new element called "interaction," which implies the elements of "advocacy" and "communication" that are included in the CMSA 2002 definition. The current ANA definition defines nursing case management as the following:

A dynamic and systematic collaborative approach to providing and coordinating health care services to a defined population. It is a participative process to identify and facilitate options and services for meeting individual's health needs, while decreasing the fragmentation and duplication of care and enhancing quality, cost effective clinical outcomes. The framework for nursing case management includes five components: assessment, planning, implementation, evaluation and interaction. (ANA, 2003a, p. 10)

The ANA definition speaks to the specific delivery system problems and patient concerns that have shaped nurse case management, problems that are reflected in the literature on nurse case management. The primary reasons for using NCMs are to improve patient care, increase patient satisfaction, prevent complications, control costs, and enhance quality of care by decreasing fragmentation, limiting duplication of services, providing surveillance and ensuring accountability (Doell Smith, 1994). NCM interventions are based on holism, scientific and experiential knowledge, and partnership with the patient. Acute, primary, and community care settings have all implemented innovative NCM programs as a way to promote quality outcomes in a cost-effective manner. Although NCMs traditionally practiced in environments linked to the hospital setting, new avenues for nurse case management have emerged. For example, NCMs may practice telephone case management by following the client's progress over time and ensuring timely and appropriate utilization of health-care benefits (Bushnell, 1992; Friedman, Gleeson, Kent, Foris, & Rodriguez, 1998). Sponsored by the payor, provider, or employer, NCMs establish relationships with clients and monitor their health status based on telephone interviews. Depending on the client's responses, the NCM determines whether interventions are needed. Referrals to local resources are initiated when necessary, and in general, the telephone NCM serves as an advocate for the client, maintaining an ongoing "telephonic" relationship with the client over time, with the incentive of lowering health-care costs (see the discussion on telehealth later in this chapter). NCMs also practice in physician offices and clinics and utilize Internet technologies to educate patients and facilitate appropriate utilization of evidence-based health-care resources. Such approaches are now becoming more structured and are evolving into disease management and telemedicine programs, which incorporate evidence-based practices into the care management routines for designated clinical populations.

APN Case Management

Contemporary nurse case management reflects a natural evolution from nursing's history of client advocacy, social service, and public health. It is widely understood that nurse practitioners (NPs), certified nurse-midwives (CNMs), and clinical nurse specialists

(CNSs) also provide care that is congruent with case management concepts; their care can improve health-care access, coordination, and continuity across settings (Brooten et al., 1991, 2001; Brooten, Youngblut, Deatrick, Naylor, & York, 2003; Newman, 1990; Office of Technology Assessment, 1986). APN case management has also been viewed as a way of enhancing the visibility of advanced nursing practice (Cooper, 1990; Hamric, 1992; Mahn & Spross, 1996). Although the APN CM is still viewed by many as an evolving advanced practice role (see Chapter 1) and has yet to be formally recognized by the ANA as advanced nursing practice, many arguments have been made for having nurse case management done by APNs (Connors, 1993; Fralic, 1992; Hamric, 1992). Chin and Papenhausen (2002) suggested that NPs, particularly those employed in primary care settings, use strategies that are consistent with population-focused case management techniques. According to Chin and Papenhausen, such strategies require a degree of clinical expertise and exemplary communication and collaboration skills that are more likely to be found in nurses prepared at a graduate nursing level. They further suggest that the master's-prepared nurse is more likely to function successfully in unstructured practice settings, such as the community or home environments, or in new or innovative disease or case management programs in which they are responsible for creating their own structure and practice routines. A graduate curriculum designed to prepare the APN CM has not been broadly adopted; however, it is clear that the APN CM must be master's prepared and must have expert knowledge and certification in a clinical specialty, the skills to establish mutually agreeable goals between the client and other members of the health-care team, and the ability to establish an intervention schema that will help clients reach their health goals.

The scope of influence of the APN CM differs from that of other APN roles in that the APN CM is expected to influence care at a systems level through establishing more effective care delivery or clinical practices, disease management strategies, health promotion, disease prevention, and complication management programs for given clinical populations. The APN CM's scope of influence occurs at multiple points across the continuum of health-care services. Finally, the APN CM is accountable for evaluating the effectiveness of the case management intervention, both at the level of an individual patient/client and at a system-wide and population-based level. Although the APN CM role has a component of outcome management responsibilities, this role differs from an outcomes manager role in that APN CMs retain a direct care component in their practices and are directly engaged in patient and client intervention. In contrast, outcomes managers typically have no direct practice component to their role and have greater responsibility for monitoring and analyzing clinical and financial information about a given product line or target population. Based on the previous discussion, the following definitions of an NCM and an APN CM guide this discussion of APN case management.

> *Nurse Case Manager:* An NCM is an experienced, bachelor's-prepared registered nurse (RN) who is accountable for managing a defined group of patients/clients in order to optimize clinical and cost outcomes. Outcomes are achieved through clinical practice and partnership and collaboration with patients and other members of the interdisciplinary team. The NCM is responsible for matching the patient's/client's care needs to the most appropriate level of service based on predefined guidelines, clinical protocols, and payor-based criteria in order to achieve optimal clinical outcomes in the most resource-efficient manner.
>
> *APN Case Manager:* An APN CM has graduate preparation in nursing with established expertise in a clinical specialty. The APN CM is accountable for managing high-risk, clinically complex, or resource-intensive clients/patients within her or his specialty in order to optimize clinical, functional, and cost outcomes. The APN CM

also establishes programs and system improvements within a continuum of health-care services in order to improve care rendered to her or his "at-risk" populations. The APN CM is accountable for evaluating resultant cost, quality, and process of care outcomes for those they serve.

AN OVERVIEW OF THE HEALTH-CARE MARKETPLACE

Shifts in health policymaking and health-care marketplace dynamics exert extensive and almost immediate influence on case management delivery systems (see Chapters 20 and 23). Thus APN CMs are likely to be directly involved in implementing or managing changes in health-care delivery that arise from these shifts. This section provides a brief overview of forces that drive changes in the health-care marketplace and therefore affect APN CMs, with a particular emphasis on managed care models and reimbursement trends. In addition, economic and clinical risk assessments as part of case and disease management strategies are presented.

Government Programs, Health-Care Initiatives, and the Public Health Sector

Federal and state mandates and health-care priorities often dictate the focus of an agency's health-care initiatives, which can change with a new administration or national crisis. Examples include the faith-based initiatives (some of which are health-related) that have characterized President George W. Bush's administration and the emphasis on training health-care professionals to respond to bioterrorism in the wake of the terrorist attack in the United States on September 11, 2001. Similarly, changes in benefits and services in Medicare, Medicaid, and other federal and state health-care programs are often operationalized by APN CMs. For example, the APN CM may be involved in the implementation of a policy change that involves planning, coordination, and public and professional communications regarding the appropriate use of smallpox vaccine in military and civilian populations. A challenge for the APN CM is to stay abreast of national, state, and local government programs; to understand the various health-care initiatives and reforms that may have an impact on the populations the APN CM serves; and to anticipate and respond to changes in ways that best serve his or her clients. A few examples of public health services that the APN CM may become involved with are immunization programs for children and adults; nutritional services for women, infants, children, and the elderly; community water fluoridation; smoking cessation campaigns; domestic violence identification and prevention; control of communicable diseases; and maintaining and monitoring vital statistics. In addition, the APN CM may face complex political issues surrounding many public health initiatives, as fewer dollars are available to care for the uninsured and underinsured. Exemplar 18-6 demonstrates an APN CM's impact on local and city government through her efforts to support a program for the multiple sclerosis (MS) population of her community.

APN CM practice is also influenced by the decisions about health-care plans and workers' compensation benefits that employers offer to their employees. An awareness of employers' responsibilities for covered benefits and services is relevant to APN CM practice in that the APN CM may see a patient who has both an injury covered by workers' compensation and a co-existing health problem, such as diabetes. The APN CM must be aware of these fine points to ensure that care is properly billed. In some cases, large employers become self-insured to reduce costs or they form cooperatives to share in cost savings. The APN CM has opportunities to deliver APN services to an employer group through services such as health promotion programs, disease management, and acute complications management.

Managed Care Models and Reimbursement Trends

The APN CM often must make decisions based on the reimbursement structure that exists between the client's payor and providers. Because the ways in which an institution is reimbursed for care influences APN case management, a brief overview of different reimbursement structures is presented here (see Chapter 20 for more detail on APN reimbursement). *Managed care* is an integrated network that combines the financing and delivery of health-care services to covered individuals. Generally, the managed care organization (MCO) serves as the payor and contracts with health-care organizations, physicians, and other clinicians to furnish health-care services to plan members. In managed care, financial incentives encourage members to use providers associated with the plan and to follow procedures that help the plan to control costs. Financial incentives also encourage providers to control expenditures. For example, shared risk pools may be established whereby unused portions of designated moneys for specialty services would be distributed among primary care providers. Thus, managed care is a system of controlled resource use and coordination of care that may be applied to *all* clients within a delivery system in order to optimize quality and cost-effective care (see Chapter 20).

In *indemnity plans*, often understood as "fee-for-service" plans, the member pays a premium for health-care coverage and has a wide selection of providers and health-care settings. Typically, the provider or health-care facility will bill the expenses to the insurance company, and a percentage of the charges will be reimbursed (within reasonable limits) for the geographic region. This payor structure may encourage the provider and health-care facility to increase admissions and length of stay (LOS); resource consumption generally goes up because the majority of charges will be reimbursed. Indemnity plans are costly to the member and are decreasing in availability. Regions in the United States that are heavily saturated with managed care may have as little as 3% to 5% of their health-care market covered by indemnity insurance (S. Johnson, personal communication, 1999). A modification of indemnity insurance that preserves the client's ability to choose a provider within a cost-containment framework is the preferred provider organization (PPO). This system contracts with providers at a discounted fee-for-service rate.

Since the mid-1980s, Medicare reimbursements have been structured by *diagnosis-related group* (DRG) pricing (see Chapter 23). Reimbursement is fixed for each retrospectively assigned DRG based on the final listing of diagnoses and procedures found in the patient's medical record following discharge. Frequently, DRG reimbursement fails to cover the health-care organization's expenses, particularly for complicated or extended stays. Under this reimbursement structure, the health care facility has incentives to increase admissions; however, they are at risk for absorbing the costs when LOS or resource utilization exceeds reimbursable amounts. Thus APN CMs working within a DRG-based reimbursement structure have a greater need to reduce LOS and resource consumption for their sponsoring organizations. As a result, the APN CM must be in a position to assist the patient to adjust to shorter hospital stays and to find alternative methods to facilitate recuperation, such as skilled nursing facilities (SNFs) and home health care (HHC).

As managed care has begun to dominate the health-care market in both commercial and Medicare sectors, two other methods of reimbursement have emerged. *Per diem reimbursement* means the health-care organization receives a fixed dollar amount for services provided, such as hospital bed days, home care visits, or SNF days. This reimbursement structure encourages the facility to increase admissions and utilize resources sparingly. However, for each day the patient stays, the institution receives more dollars. Thus, under this structure, the APN CM may be far less concerned with decreasing LOS than she or he might be under other structures. In fact, the APN CM must recognize that in many case types, such as total joint replacement procedures, the majority of costs are incurred the first day of admission. Subsequent days of care are less expensive for hospitals because fewer costly resources are used. In order for the hospital to cover its costs for such a procedure under a fixed per diem structure, a longer length of stay is desirable. To complicate this payment structure, the health-care organization may have risk pools built into the contract, which provide economic incentives when costs or hospital bed days fall under certain targets. Each contract between payor and provider may be different, and APN CMs must stay informed about managed care contractual agreements made by their sponsoring organizations.

Capitated reimbursement structures place the greatest amount of fiscal risk on the health-care facility. Unlike the three structures described previously, capitated reimbursement structures offer incentives to avoid hospital admissions and service utilization altogether. In capitated structures, the health-care organization receives a fixed amount per member per month regardless of which members are utilizing service. Thus the fewer members who require services, the more profit the health-care organization can realize. When members require hospitalization, the APN CM has incentives to move the patient out as quickly as possible and limit resource consumption. Health-care organizations may have numerous capitated agreements with payors within their communities. In addition, the degree of financial risk may vary among contracts. Some capitated contracts may be for "global risk," which means that the health-care organization has agreed to accept full economic responsibility for all contracted services for a population of covered lives. This may include accountability for resource management (e.g., service authorization, utilization management, and case management services). In contrast, "partial risk" means that the MCO (payor) may retain accountability for resource management. Under the terms of some contracts, selected services such as case management may be "carved out" as a separate contract with separate reimbursement structures. For example, in the mid-1990s The Carondelet Health Care Network had a partial risk contract with a Medicaid-based managed care plan for hospital, physician, and ancillary services. A carved-out contract for community case management services was arranged in a fee-for-service reimbursement structure. The MCO would refer and authorize visits for high-risk clients to the case management program. When the contract with the health-care system was renegotiated, it changed into a global risk structure, and case management was included in the monthly capitation reimbursement.

APN CMs must be able to recognize the discrepancies among multiple reimbursement structures that affect decision making for the clients for whom they are responsible. To complicate the matter even further, the APN CM must also be aware that financial incentives among hospitals, providers, and payors are often far from aligned. For example, an agreement may exist between a hospital and a payor to provide services under a capitated agreement. However, if the patient's physician is reimbursed under a traditional fee-for-service structure, it may be difficult to motivate the physician to reduce admissions or LOS. In addition, there may be few economic incentives for the physician to limit use of medically prescribed resources, which account for most health-care expenses. APN CMs may then find themselves in a situation of conflict between the medical providers and the health-care organization. Likewise, APN CMs may find themselves in a situation of conflict between the needs of the patient and the payor. In these situations, they need to be able to influence decisions made by other stakeholders through their expertise in clinical assessment and articulation of the patient's needs in order to secure the most appropriate health-care settings and services.

PROFILE OF APN CM PRACTICE

APN case management is still evolving, and it can be difficult to precisely define what makes an NCM an "advanced practice nurse" or to distinguish APN CMs from other APNs who incorporate aspects of case management into their practice. It is therefore difficult to estimate the numbers of APN CMs in practice.

Evidence suggests that traditional APNs (specifically NPs and CNSs) incorporate NCM competencies and skills into their practices and that many NCMs who have a master's degree exhibit competencies and skills that are congruent with advanced nursing practice. Rosenfeld, McEvoy, & Glassman (2003) conducted a study of workforce trends and practice patterns of acute care nurse practitioners (ACNPs) working in academic health sciences centers. Their data indicated that ACNPs routinely performed discharge planning and case management tasks. On the basis of numerous studies of the APN Transitional Care Model, which employed NPs and CNSs, Brooten et al. (2002) concluded that outcomes of APN interventions such as discharge planning and follow-up largely depend on the APNs' skills in assessment, teaching, counseling, communication, collaboration, health behaviors, negotiating systems, and condition-specific knowledge of patient problems within a specified population. Furthermore, some evidence suggests that APNs may not achieve mastery of these skills through formal education programs but that additional, advanced competencies related to information technology and the complexities of interfacing with the insurance industry are required for successful APN practice (Hopkins, Mundinger, Lenz, Lin, & Clark, 2002). NPs and CNSs are seeking to expand their knowledge of health-care system issues and case management strategies, as demonstrated by their increasing attendance in preparatory courses in case management certification and other continuing education workshops for case management professionals (D. Zazworsky, personal communication, September 9, 2003). It would appear therefore that there is a convergence of roles, tasks, and competencies that characterize APN case management as we and others had projected (Mahn & Spross, 1996; Mahn & Zazworsky, 2000). To understand the APN CM role, one must first place it in the larger context of nursing case management.

APN CM Employment Patterns

NCMs are employed in hospitals, home care, behavioral health settings, managed care organizations, health insurance companies, clinics, physician offices, long-term care agencies, public health organizations, schools, rehabilitation agencies, occupational health settings, and independent case management companies. Employment patterns of the APN CM have changed over the past 4 years. In 1999, Pace University conducted a survey of 69 hospitals, home health-care agencies, managed care companies, and long-term care facilities. Administrators and managers at the study facilities were interviewed. Of the 69 facilities, 52 (75%) employed NCMs. Interviewees identified clinical experience as the single most important qualification for the nurse case management role, followed by experience in home care and utilization management. Seventy-seven percent of the facilities hired NCMs with a bachelor of science degree, although three facility administrators (5%) said that an advanced degree was an important qualification to perform successfully in the current case management role, and 31 (53%) agreed that case managers should be educated at the master's level. Most relevant was the finding that 39 facilities (67%) reported that their case managers were involved with the management of outcome data. Another 19 facilities (32%) reported that their case managers were not involved in data management, simply because they do not possess the technology to store and report outcome data (Falter, Cesta, Concert, & Mason, 1999). A more recent review of the marketplace conducted on behalf of the American Case Management Association (ACMA) revealed that 52% of 437 hospitals surveyed in 2002 hired one or more NCMs prepared at the master's level (ACMA, 2003). In this survey, 14% of the hospitals reported that their NCMs were prepared as either NPs (8%) or CNSs (6%). Finally, more hospital NCMs are performing functions relevant to outcomes management: 77% of NCMs surveyed in the ACMA survey were involved in some type of benchmarking or outcome measurement activity within the course of their roles. Taken together, these reports suggest the NCM is an evolving APN role (see Chapter 19) and that information technology, data management, and outcomes management are important competencies.

A Shift Toward Data and Outcomes Management

The previously summarized findings suggest that health-care organizations are beginning to see the link between the case management role and outcomes data management. As noted earlier, a fundamental distinction between the NCM and the outcomes manager role is the clinical practice component, which is a core competency of both NCM and APN CM. Regulatory bodies such as the Centers for Medicare and Medicaid Services (CMS) and the Joint Commission for the Accreditation of Healthcare Organizations (JCAHO) have begun to require that institutions use outcome data to demonstrate that they meet accrediting standards. Sources of outcome data such as the Minimum Data Set (MDS) for Long Term Care, the OASIS (Outcome ASsessment Information Set) Data Set for Home Care, and the collection of Core Measures for Hospitals are being used by regulators and accreditors to assess whether standards are met. These mandates require that health-care agencies adopt the necessary technology to support data collection, analysis, and report preparation. With this rise in technology, there will be a greater demand for case managers not only to manage the care of patients but also to manage and interpret data and to serve as change agents for their organizations in order to improve quality and cost performance. This increased emphasis on sophisticated data management provides a strong argument for NCMs who are prepared at the graduate level for both advanced clinical practice *and* data and outcome management skills. For APN CMs, the data and outcome management component of APN CM practice is an expansion of the APN research competency and a bigger component of APN CM practice than for any other APN role.

Types of Nurse Case Management

Nurse case management models may be focused on health or illness. Although community and acute care models differ in terms of practice setting, target populations, and span of accountability, the success of NCM relies on the nurse's clinical knowledge and expertise. Some classic examples of populations for which NCM has been used include acute care populations such as cardiovascular surgical patients (Mahn, 1993), the chronically mentally ill (Bryson, Naqvi, Callahan, & Fontenot, 1990); HIV-positive women (Riley, 1992); perinatal clients (Ladden, 1991); clients in rural settings (Parker et al., 1990); trauma patients (Daleiden, 1993); and community health centers for health assessment, counseling, education, and screening (Ethridge, 1991). For a comprehensive review of case management models and best practice care coordination demonstration projects within the past 5 to 10 years, the reader is referred to Chen, Brown, Archibald, Aliotta, and Fox, 2000.

The NCM model that a health-care agency chooses depends on the agency's goals and the creativity of the NCMs. Furthermore, a health-care agency may elect to implement multiple case management models simultaneously. Common organizational goals that justify the use of NCM include reducing lengths of acute care stay, readmissions, resource use, and costs; increasing access to services and market share; and becoming a recognized center of excellence for a particular product line (Zander, 1993). Table 18-1 illustrates the span of accountability and common functions for six types of NCMs. The reader should note that functions appearing in bold type represent APN CM functions.

Increasingly, one finds that NCMs and APN CMs are sharing direct and indirect fiscal risk with their sponsoring organizations. In some organizations, continued employment of the NCM or APN CM is contingent on the person's ability to demonstrate a cost savings of at least her or his annual salary, in addition to the demonstration of measurable outcomes that improve patient function; patient, provider, and payor satisfaction; and other clinical and fiscal outcomes. The methods used by both NCMs and APN CMs to accomplish such outcomes rely on advocacy for access, holistic assessment, partnership with patients and families over time, interventions related to health promotion and self-care skills, and coordination of care across settings (Smith, 1993). Box 18-1 illustrates activities common to NCMs and APN CMs, regardless of their clinical specialty or practice setting. Health-care organizations that provide nurse case management resources to their clients, patients, or plan members must be cognizant of the potential for role confusion, redundancy, and duplication when multiple models of NCM are used within the health-care network. All NCM services must be clearly defined and well integrated into the health-care environment. Patients, families, and other members of the health-care team may become confused when faced with multiple staff members who have the title "case manager."

Characteristics and Functions that Distinguish NCM from APN CM Practice

The distinguishing features between the NCM and the APN CM have yet to be sufficiently supported by research or endorsed by professional nursing organizations. Nevertheless, we believe that even though APN CMs and NCMs share common activities as outlined in Box 18-1, the two roles can be distinguished through advanced education, skills and competencies, span of accountability, and scope of practice.

ADVANCED EDUCATION

Perhaps the characteristic that most readily distinguishes the NCM from the APN CM is an advanced degree in nursing with a clinical specialty. Regardless of years of experience, expertise, or certification as an NCM, one cannot be considered as an APN CM without a formal advanced education beyond a 4-year bachelor's degree in nursing science. Fralic (1992) observed that the successful NCM is able to operate in an unstructured environment and has a high tolerance for ambiguity, uncertainty, and change. The NCM is "required to bring innovation, enthusiasm, and confidence to the role" (p. 14). APN graduate education fosters these qualities through its emphasis on role socialization,

TABLE 18-1	SPAN OF ACCOUNTABILITY AND COMMON FUNCTIONS ASSOCIATED WITH SIX COMMON NCM MODELS		
NCM TYPE	TYPICAL SETTING	SPAN OF ACCOUNTABILITY	COMMON FUNCTIONS
Utilization resource manager	Hospital Clinic	Patients assigned within a geographically defined unit or department *(Typically carries a case load of 20-30 patients)*	• Daily chart review for LOS and medical appropriateness • Ensure payor-based criteria are met (e.g., Interqual or Milliman & Roberts) • DC planning • Referral and authorization procurement • Claims monitoring • Collaboration with nursing, medicine, social work, payor • Minimal patient contact
Staff nurse case manager	Hospital Clinic Primary care Physician office	Patients assigned within a geographically defined unit or department *(Typically carries a case load of 8-12 patients)*	• Direct patient care during a shift • 24-hour care planning • Patient/family education • DC planning in collaboration with other care members • Daily review of pathway/guidelines • May participate in pathway, guideline, or protocol development • May participate in quality improvement initiatives (e.g., quality committees, CQI teams)
Telephone nurse case manager	Payor office (e.g., HMO, insurance company) Hospital Clinic	Caseload may be organized by physician groups, clinical specialty, or payor *(Typically carries an active case load of 150-200 clients)*	• Intake/triage • Identify and prioritize client problems • Referral, coordination, and authorization for services • Periodic follow-up phone contact with patient or family depending on need • Evaluation of patient's adherence to prescribed or recommended health-care behaviors following disease management guidelines or protocols • Patient/family education • May participate in the development of disease management guidelines and protocols • May have additional utilization management responsibilities depending on employer

Continued

TABLE 18-1 SPAN OF ACCOUNTABILITY AND COMMON FUNCTIONS ASSOCIATED WITH SIX COMMON NCM MODELS—cont'd

NCM TYPE	TYPICAL SETTING	SPAN OF ACCOUNTABILITY	COMMON FUNCTIONS
Clinical nurse case manager	Hospital Ambulatory care setting Home care	Patients assigned by case type, product line, or physician service; crosses geographical boundaries to follow patient throughout an episode of care (*Typically carries a case load of 8-20 patients*)	• Limited day-to-day bedside care • Comprehensive assessment (e.g., admission, preoperative, periodic, postdischarge) • Patient/family teaching • 24-hour accountability • Daily assessment of patient status and response to treatments • Facilitation of care plan through multidisciplinary collaboration • Coordination of DC plan • **Staff education and expert consultation** • **Oversight of pathway, guideline, and protocol development, implementation, and aggregate evaluation** • **Evaluation of clinical and financial outcomes for aggregate population** • **Facilitate, coordinate, and lead process improvement initiatives within the care delivery system** • **Influence nursing practice and health-care policy through publications, lecturing, and consultation in academic and practice environments**
Community nurse case manager	Hospital Home Physician office SNF Community centers Industry	Predefined geographic region within community or by client case type if specialized; follows clients across multiple settings and over time (*Typically carries an active case load of 30-40 clients*)	• Comprehensive assessment upon referral • Evaluate client's level of risk and appropriateness of referral • Identify and prioritize client problems • Establish mutually agreed upon goals with client and care team • Coordinate needed resources • Collaborate with client to determine frequency of follow-up contacts to evaluate client's status (e.g., face-to-face visits and telephone follow-up) • Patient/family education

- Ongoing evaluation to establish interventions most appropriate to client's disease trajectory
- **Oversight of disease management, guideline development, implementation, and evaluation**
- **Evaluation of clinical and financial outcomes related to aggregate population**
- **Facilitate, coordinate, and lead process improvement initiatives within local care delivery system**
- **Influence nursing practice and health-care policy through publications, lectures, and consultation in academic and practice environments**

Outcomes manager	Hospital Clinic Payor	Population focus, typically organized around a clinical product line or case type; responsible for monitoring data collection activities and analysis of clinical, financial, humanistic, quality, and organizational outcomes resulting from the health-care delivery system *(Typically no direct patient caseload unless role is blended with one of the other five NCM roles)*	- **Identify clinical, financial, and other quality indicators appropriate for assigned aggregate population** - **Conduct and/or supervise data collection activities required to conduct outcome studies and evaluations** - **Utilize and/or manage data information systems and tools used for tracking clinical and financial outcomes** - **Analyze and evaluate outcomes and processes of care related to assigned aggregate population** - **Facilitate, coordinate, and lead process improvement initiatives within local care delivery system** - **Influence nursing and medical practice through diffusion of evidence-based practice knowledge across multiple points of service within the health-care organization**

CQI, Continuous quality improvement; *DC,* discharge; *HMO,* health maintenance organization; *LOS,* length of stay; *SNF,* skilled nursing facility.

BOX 18-1 • ACTIVITIES COMMON TO NCMs AND APN CMs

- Collaboration with administrative, management, and clinical staff who are responsible for specified patient groups
- Assessment, planning, implementation, coordination, referral, and evaluation of patients and families in assigned target populations
- Provision of internal consultation to other disciplines and departments with the goal of managing care of patients and families expeditiously
- Participation in the development of documentation systems and tools (i.e., critical pathways or practice guidelines) to monitor clinical and fiscal outcomes
- Collecting, analyzing, and sharing of data and information in order to influence process improvements and support integration of core systems and processes within the care environment
- Development of partnerships with physicians in order to achieve clinical and fiscal outcomes
- Teaching and coaching other caregivers on the health-care team regarding clinical, fiscal, and system processes related to patient care management
- Role modeling of professional nursing practice

---

self-learning, and self-direction, as well as content on change theories. In addition, advanced clinical and leadership skills help students to develop these characteristics. Just as role socialization and mentoring are critical to the development of the CNS (Hamric & Taylor, 1989; see also Chapter 4), students in APN CM curricula must experience the NCM role during clinical and mentoring experiences with practicing APNs who perform advanced practice nurse care management. Given the APN CM role's similarity to the traditional CNS role, it is reasonable to assume that a developmental process exists in which the APN CM experiences the phases of role development as described by Hamric and Taylor (1989) (see also Chapter 4).

There is still considerable debate about whether specialized graduate level NCM programs are needed or whether CNS and NP programs should just increase their level of case management instruction (Falter et al., 1999). Evidence suggests that some schools of nursing offer specialized nursing degrees in "care management," "outcome management," or "case management." One such program is the Pacific Lutheran University School of Nursing. This master's-level curriculum prepares nurses for roles as a "care and outcomes manager" for a clinical specialty. This program prepares the nurse as a CNS and provides extensive coursework in outcomes research, nursing informatics, resource management, and a clinical practicum that appears to emphasize experiential skills in managing and negotiating health-care delivery systems (see www.plu.edu/~nurs/programs/gradcom.html). The authors of this chapter believe that this role is most congruent with APN CM because it retains the elements of clinical practice required for APN practice while encompassing elements of case management, outcome evaluation, and systems.

Johns Hopkins University School of Nursing master's-level NP and CNS curricula also have evolved to include specific coursework requirements on case management, outcome management, and system effectiveness (see www.son.jhmi.edu/academic_programs/masters/hlthsys/dual.asp). Nurses who graduate from this program may elect to practice as traditional NPs or CNSs; however, those whose primary role responsibility is case management would be considered APN CMs.

Finally, the Lienhard School of Nursing at Pace University, in Pleasantville, New York, revised its core master's curriculum in 1998 to include case management concepts, which were seen as common to all APN roles. This program prepares APN CMs with the option of tailoring their clinical focus to one of three advanced practice nursing roles: adult CNS, psychiatric–mental health CNS, and family NP. The curriculum includes courses in economics, quality, systems, and roles (see appserv.pace.edu/ execute/page.cfm?doc_id=2128). Clinical course work prepares students for certification in their APN role and prepares them to perform case management roles in a variety of health-care settings. As with graduates from the Hopkins program, CNSs or NPs who function primarily as case managers would be considered APN CMs.

A common component in all three of the preceding academic programs is systems management. The need for a systems focus in both graduate- and doctoral-level nursing curricula may be shaping the way of the future. For example, the University of Arizona in Tucson, Arizona, reshaped the graduate-level case management curriculum in 1998-1999 to provide an option for systems case management, which emphasizes outcome and population management as opposed to direct care of the individual (J. Verran, personal communication, September 15, 2003). Because this role does not include a direct practice component, it would not meet the criteria for APN CM practice as defined in this text. As health-care complexity and technology advances, it is likely that both clinical and nonclinical nursing roles prepared at the master's level will fulfill the needs for system management.

DIFFERENTIATING NCM FROM APN CM

Research indicates that there are patients who require the advanced skills and competencies of the APN CM (see Chapter 25). Using work by Calkin (1984) and Connors (1993), Mahn and Spross (1996) recommended some approaches for differentiating basic nurse case management from APN case management (see Chapter 2 for a description of Calkin's model). Calkin (1984) differentiated among levels of nursing practice based on education, experience, complexity, and the range of problems a nurse at a particular level could assess and manage effectively. Connors (1993) suggested that managing patients' health-care needs could be conceptualized as a continuum anchored by care coordination on one end and case management on the other. She asserted that every patient needs care coordination but not all patients need case management. Mahn and Spross (1996) proposed that NCM and APN NCM could be differentiated along similar dimensions. NCMs are more likely to coordinate care and provide case management for the less complex and more predictable cases, frequently guided by standards, clinical pathways, and other evidence-based guidelines. APN CMs manage more complex cases, and APN CM practice is not limited to the illness side of the continuum. APN CMs may be actively engaged in program development and clinical practice associated with health promotion and prevention strategies, as noted earlier.

Case management by APNs is characterized by greater complexity of clinical decision making and greater skill in managing constraints of care related to organizational bureaucracy than is basic NCM. Unlike NCMs, APN CMs have greater autonomy; they can perform more extensive assessments and initiate a variety of treatments, which may include ordering laboratory tests; prescribing; and, if they are licensed as an NP or CNS, being able to perform certain treatments and procedures. Because APN CMs are recognized as clinical experts based on experience and advanced education, their span of influence typically extends across multiple points of service within their work settings.

Accountability for more complex clinical and fiscal outcome evaluation and program analysis further differentiates the APN CM from the NCM. In contrast, basic NCM may best describe the processes used to achieve clinical and fiscal outcomes when clinical situations are simple, common, time limited, or predictable, or require few and inexpensive resources, and that such outcomes are typically monitored with established documentation systems and other variance analysis tools that include critical pathways, standards of care, practice guidelines, and disease management protocols.

In contrast, patients or subpopulations with novel or uncommon diagnoses and whose care is complex, resource intensive, or unpredictable are likely to need an APN, not only because they require a higher level of clinical expertise and system savvy in order to negotiate the health-care delivery system, but also because the outcome evaluation plan, which is likely to be complex, must be established, executed, and monitored in a competent manner. This may involve the use of computer technology and information management skills in order to perform baseline evaluations and to design suitable metrics and indicators to monitor clinical and fiscal outcomes. While both the NCM and the APN CM may be accountable for the outcomes achieved, accountability for the design and implementation of the outcome evaluation plan is more likely to be the responsibility of the APN CM (see Chapter 25).

Research is needed to validate the differences between basic and advanced nurse case management. At this stage in the evolution of NCM and APN CM, most health-care agencies do distinguish between the type of employees who are needed to conduct daily tasks associated with care coordination, utilization management, and discharge planning (NCM) and the type of employees needed to manage high-risk specialty populations by providing direct care, program oversight, and outcome management (APN CM). The titles and roles to describe such positions, and the qualifications to fill them, currently lack consistency across health-care agencies and academic programs. However, as experience with APN CM and care management strategies accumulates, the profession will be in a better position to articulate the specialty role of the APN CM, as well as to determine what mix of APNs and experts-by-experience is needed to ensure that clinical, fiscal, and system goals are met.

CASE MANAGEMENT STRATEGIES

To understand the ways in which APN CMs implement APN competencies, readers must understand the variety of case management strategies for populations that have emerged. Several case management strategies are discussed in this section so that the APN CM student or practitioner can better understand the leverage points and opportunities for managing the needs of the clinical populations in a variety of different health-care settings.

Health Promotion and Disease Prevention

Health promotion, health protection, and disease prevention concepts and activities are common to all APN roles and directly relate to a primary goal of NCM: to reduce costs associated with utilization of health-care services, hospitalization, and premature disability. For example, as the APN CM partners with the patient and family to provide health education, their knowledge increases and health attitudes and behaviors are more likely to change, resulting in increased adherence to a more healthy lifestyle. The APN CM who is approaching this strategy from a program perspective may first perform a risk assessment of the target population to understand any cultural barriers that may exist and identify the health behaviors most in need of intervention before a successful health promotion or disease prevention intervention can be deployed. The APN CM should seek assistance from doctorally prepared nurse scientists or other researchers if the APN CM lacks the expertise required to select or design the appropriate risk assessment tool and conduct the assessment. In addition, the APN CM should understand the sponsoring organization's agenda for implementing a health promotion or disease prevention program, such as decreased absenteeism, reduced workers' compensation claims, or lower health-care insurance premiums, in order to ensure that appropriate baseline measures can be obtained. Only then will a useful "return on investment" analysis be possible once the program outcomes have been evaluated. Health promotion and disease prevention strategies can be implemented in a variety of settings; strategies may be aimed at preventing costly debilitation associated with chronic disease such as diabetes or heart disease or preventing obesity and sedentary lifestyle choices in healthy children and adolescents. Exemplar 18-1 illustrates an APN CM's use of a healthy promotion and prevention strategy.

EXEMPLAR 18-1

Susan was an APN CM working as an independent case management consultant, hired to address the higher-than-average teacher absenteeism rates in a local school district. The school board decided to start an employee wellness program, and Susan was charged with assessing the health-care needs of the teacher population and designing an overall plan that would ultimately reduce absenteeism and increase employee satisfaction. The APN CM selected a computerized health risk appraisal (HRA) to assess the needs of the population and administered the appraisal to employees during monthly staff meetings. Over the course of several months, the appraisal was completed and a wellness program was established, which offered discounted wellness physicals by local APNs and other providers and a series of health education programs geared toward weight reduction, smoking cessation, stress reduction, and teen-age parenting skills. The APN CM collaborated with a benefits specialist to modify the employee benefit package to cover the costs of screening for lipids, Pap smears, and annual mammograms for female employees over the age of 40. The APN CM conducted an impact analysis of the program after 12 months, which revealed a 71% (396/558) employee participation rate and a 22% reduction in employee absenteeism. The reduced absenteeism resulted in a total direct cost savings of $43,876 attributed to reduced utilization of substitute teachers. A postintervention employee survey revealed that 92% (364/396) of employees who had used the wellness benefit were either extremely satisfied or somewhat satisfied with their experience, and 42% (166/396) reported making at least one healthy lifestyle change (e.g., smoking cessation, exercise program, weight reduction, wearing a seat belt) within the past 12 months as a result of attending the educational programs provided during monthly staff meetings.

Acute Care Complication Management

APN CMs employed in acute care settings are actively engaged in acute care complication management to prevent costly, often life-threatening adverse events that are associated with the usual disease trajectory or medical error. The strategy used by the APN CM is prevention and early detection of clinical complications (also called *surveillance*; see Chapter 5), as in the case of a patient who has undergone coronary artery bypass grafting (CABG) surgery and developed lower lung atelectasis, which, if untreated, could result in pneumonia. The APN CM might address this issue by establishing a plan to increase out of bed activity for the patient, as well as provide education and coaching to the nursing staff on the importance of frequent ambulation in the postsurgical cardiac patient.

The APN could also conduct a baseline assessment of the clinical population to identify adverse outcomes and potential complications. The APN CM can use *International Classification of Diseases, Ninth Revision* (ICD-9) diagnosis and procedure codes to identify complications of care identified through the medical records coding process. For complications that occurred but were not coded in medical records, the APN CM should consult an ICD-9 Code Book located in the medical records department and review diagnosis codes in the 900 series. Some complications, however, such as nausea and vomiting or unmanaged pain, do not have ICD-9 codes and require careful review of the medical record. The APN CM may collaborate with Quality Management staff to coordinate the necessary data collection needed to secure such information. Once complication types and frequency are determined, the APN CM should look for patterns in the data that explain potential causal links or other related factors. Sorting complication occurrence by nursing unit, day of week, time of day, medical provider, admission source, patient age, or other co-morbid factors are useful methods for identifying variables that may contribute to complications. Only after such variables are known can the APN CM devise an effective intervention plan to reduce complications. Another method of identifying complication patterns within the acute care setting is the review of patients with an LOS beyond two standard deviations from the mean. Generally, extended acute care admissions are due to an unanticipated complication or a preventable event.

In addition to hospital performance data, a review of evidence-based literature is useful to identify common complications of care that a population is likely to experience and to determine strategies for prevention and early detection. It is here that the APN CM is likely to find opportunities to improve nursing and medical management of the target population. APN CMs who have established themselves as trusted and credible clinical experts with medical staff are in a unique position to communicate "best practices" to physicians and collaborate in the implementation, monitoring, and evaluation of practice changes. Some examples include best practices regarding the use of appropriate antibiotics in the treatment of pneumonia patients or the avoidance of calcium channel blockers in patients with an evolving cerebrovascular accident (CVA); evaluation of such practices would examine both quality and cost outcomes. Exemplar 18-2 illustrates this aspect of APN CM practice.

EXEMPLAR 18-2

Bob is an APN CM/CNS for the cardiac surgical population at a large community hospital in southeast Ohio. Bob follows cardiac surgical patients from preadmission through discharge, including selected posthospital home follow-up for high-risk patients. Bob provides preadmission assessment and teaching to all cardiac surgical patients who are admitted to his hospital and sees approximately 8 to 12 patients daily. In addition to his clinical role, Bob is the team leader for the Open Heart Surgery Quality Improvement Team and teaches advanced cardiac life support courses in the hospital's critical care department. At a recent cardiac committee meeting, it was reported that readmission rates of the cardiac surgical patients had increased from 4% to 16% over the past 3 months. Using a control chart, Bob trended out readmission rates for his population for the past 16 months and noted a special cause signal, which began approximately 4 months ago. Unable to identify any particular explanation for this phenomenon, he reviewed all records for patients readmitted within 60 days of discharge following any open-heart procedures. Sorting the population by coded admitting diagnosis, Bob discovered that 12% of the patients were readmitted with gastrointestinal-related complaints, 30% were readmitted with pulmonary conditions, and 42% were readmitted with febrile conditions. The remaining readmissions were due to a variety of complaints ranging from syncope to hiccups. Concerned with the patients who were readmitted with the febrile conditions, Bob reviewed the records and determined that all patients readmitted with a febrile condition had undergone a coronary artery bypass procedure, rather than valve repair. Furthermore, all cases were re-admitted within 4 to 7 days following discharge. Suspecting a possible nosocomial infection common to CABG patients only, Bob reviewed the admission notes to find that all patients had leg incisions that were red and inflamed upon admission. In collaboration with one of the cardiac surgeons and the infection control specialist, a closer review or the records revealed that all re-admitted patients had been operated on by three of the eight cardiac surgeons in practice at the hospital and that all three surgeons utilized the same type of sutures for leg incisions, which had not been utilized by the other five surgeons. The suture company was notified, and a recall was initiated when it was determined that a specific batch of sutures was contaminated and was the origin of infection in the CABG patients who were re-admitted. No medical malpractice claims were incurred for any of the patients who required readmission for debridement and treatment of their infected graft sites. Following the recall of the contaminated sutures, readmission rates returned to their expected rates.

Once the opportunities for improvement have been identified, the APN CM can implement an action plan to reduce complications. Some interventions may require direct assessment by APN CMs of patients at risk for such complications. Other interventions may involve establishing clinical protocols that can be used by all staff to prevent or rapidly identify complications and initiate treatment. Still other interventions may require more systemic change, such as a change in product purchasing or policies and procedures that affect the use of medications and medical devices. Interventions are likely to be interdisciplinary and will require the APN CM to facilitate change across multiple departments and nursing units. Finally, the APN CM is usually responsible for demonstrating outcomes resulting from the improvement strategies. For more details on strategies to facilitate quality improvement and outcome evaluation, see Chapter 25.

Chronic Care Management

There are many opportunities for the APN CM to practice within the community and in primary care settings, providing care to high-risk clients with preexisting conditions, chronic disease, or terminal disease. Since the majority of health-care resources are used in the treatment of chronic disease, this area will be a case management priority for the foreseeable future. As with acute care complication management, review of evidence-based literature enables APN CMs to identify opportunities to reduce resource utilization and improve quality outcomes for specific populations with chronic conditions. Evidence-based guidelines exist for conditions such as asthma, diabetes, hypertension, and depression. For example, APN CMs can improve patient and organizational outcomes by ensuring that all patients with diabetes mellitus receive the following annually: eye examinations with pupil dilation to assess for retinopathy, physical examination including peripheral vascular exam, hemoglobin A1C to assess for metabolic control of the disease, cholesterol screening, and influenza vaccination. Many patients with chronic diseases require life coaching and counseling interventions, rather than curative care, to assist them with developing effective self-management strategies. In addition, chronic care management also requires the APN CM to be knowledgeable about financial aid programs, end of life planning, and other ethical implications of chronic illness.

Disease Management

Disease management is a broader care delivery strategy that evolved from the concept of chronic care management. Disease management is generally defined as a comprehensive approach to care across an integrated health-care delivery system and involves improving care coordination and controlling costs through the application of appropriate tools (e.g., guidelines, protocols, and information systems) specifically designed for the population in question (Institute of Medicine, 2001). The goal of disease management is to address the illness or condition with maximal effectiveness and efficiency regardless of treatment settings or avenues of reimbursement. Also described as "proactive case management" (Zalta et al., 1994), the concept and philosophy of APN CM is congruent with the principles of disease management because the APN CM "is accountable for cost-benefit and acuity management across the entire continuum" (Ward & Rieve, 1997, p. 256). However, an argument can be made that case management is a distinct strategy within the larger strategy of disease management. In this view, disease management may be seen as an organized process in which health providers from many disciplines collaborate across settings to ensure the appropriate management of a particular disease or population of patients (Zazworsky, 2002a). Although APN CMs may be instrumental in coordinating the efforts of a team developing such programs, they may simultaneously focus their case management practice within a specific point of care in the continuum. Thus, APN CMs collaborate with other providers to improve health-care processes.

For example, one APN CM may work in the area of health promotion and disease prevention, assessing the population and developing longitudinal interventions to prevent costly debilitation associated with chronic disease in patients at risk. Another APN CM may practice in acute care and focus on complication management to achieve desired outcomes associated with hospital care. Finally, there are opportunities for the APN CM to practice within the community, following high-risk clients with preexisting conditions, chronic disease, or terminal illness. At any point on the continuum, the APN CM may collaborate with physicians, NPs, and other providers to promote optimal treatment decisions and reduce costly variations among practitioners and health-care delivery processes. The APN CM must have a working knowledge of all disease management system components, including the people, the tools, and the evaluation methods.

Eichert and Patterson (1997) described the key elements of disease management as follows:

1. Clinical management through the use of risk assessments and evidence-based guidelines
2. Behavior change using applicable theories and practices for the particular population being managed for a specified disease
3. Outcomes measurement that reflects behavior change, cost savings, and quality of clinical practice
4. Financial management that demonstrates costs of care across the continuum

In essence, the APN CM facilitates the development and implementation of a systematic approach to disease management that incorporates these elements for one or more points on the continuum of care. In addition to a direct practice role, managing patients within a defined population (e.g., patients with chronic low back pain, diabetes, multiple sclerosis, or heart failure), the APN assumes a leadership role in establishing evidence-based practice guidelines and identifying appropriate patient interventions, such as telephone case management, selection of educational media for small group education/activities, and home visits. The intent of these interventions is to augment physician/NP visits and redirect care to less costly outpatient environments (Plocher, 1996). For a more comprehensive review of disease management, the reader is referred to *Disease Management: A Systems Approach to Improving Patient Outcomes* (Todd & Nash, 1997).

TOOLS OF DISEASE MANAGEMENT

APN CMs must be able to select the most effective Disease Management (DM) tool to guide decision making and influence clinical practice. Three common disease management tools are as follows:

Care guidelines: Care guidelines are established based on formal research or substantial clinical evidence. The information within the guideline is what should be done most of the time in the management of a particular disease or population of patients. Variances in practice are to be expected and should be documented because they may teach health-care providers something new.

Critical pathways: Critical pathways are elements of practice or key decision points that are time ordered and presumed to influence clinical or economic outcomes. They have an interdisciplinary focus and are designed to promote standardization of care; however, variations are expected. It is probably not necessary to collect variance data on a routine basis unless a particular process or outcome is under focus review.

Protocols: Protocols are standards of practice, such as advanced cardiac life support protocols. They are things that should be done nearly all the time. Minimal variation should occur, and collection of variances need not occur once the process is stabilized within the organization.

DISEASE MANAGEMENT OUTCOMES

The success of a disease management program is reflected in the following evaluation areas:

Return on investment (ROI): How much did it cost to implement the program versus how much did the organization save during the period of time that the program was being evaluated?

Changes in utilization patterns: Have admissions, readmission rates, or bed-days/1,000 covered lives decreased significantly?

Clinical outcomes: Are desired health-care goals being achieved? For example, is the diabetic patient staying within a desired range of glucose control as evidenced by the hemoglobin A1C blood test?

Satisfaction of the patients, providers, and plans: Are patients more satisfied with their personal health, providers, health-care services, and treatment plans? Are the providers satisfied with their patients' health status and support services? Are health plan administrators satisfied with the program? Did the disease management program demonstrate value for future marketing?

Telehealth

The field of telehealth is an additional care management strategy used in both case and disease management. Telehealth is the removal of time and distance barriers to deliver health-care services or related activities (ANA, 1997). Some of the technologies used in telehealth include telephones, computers, interactive video transmissions, direct links to health-care instruments, and transmission of images and teleconferencing by telephone or video. The term *telemedicine* refers to the delivery of medical care, using telehealth technology, such as teleradiology, telepsychiatry, teleophthalmology, and telepathology. In addition, telenursing may be applied to nursing specialties, such as primary NP care, home care, school nursing, psychiatric nursing, and case management. With the expanding applications of technology, telehealth may quickly become a bigger part of APN CM practice than other APN roles, and the APN CM must be familiar with its applications in various practice settings and populations.

Telehealth can be used to improve access to health-care providers. For example, an asthmatic child can go to a school nurse in a rural or urban school and be seen, through a telemedicine visit, by a physician or an NP who is located 100 miles away. Through a computerized peak flow meter, the provider can assess the child's asthmatic severity and treat accordingly. Telehealth has also been demonstrated as an efficient and cost effective modality in home health care. In one plan, home health providers were able to increase their caseload by three to four times using telehealth visits (Tweed, 1998). The APN CM may be instrumental in identifying the specific patients who could benefit from telehealth technology. In addition, the APN CM can lead efforts to adopt telehealth technology and promote acceptance of such innovations by physicians, nursing, support staff, and patients (see Exemplar 18-3).

Employers and payors are also using telehealth as a care management strategy. One example of how telehealth is being used in the health-care marketplace is Health Dialog. This company uses a variety of health-care professionals, including nurses, dieticians, and respiratory therapists, to provide around-the-clock health coaching on a wide variety of acute and chronic diseases to individual members. In addition, the service offers providers and employers with decision support tools, which assist them to better understand practice variation, enhancing evidence-based clinical practice and identifying members at risk for disease. The service uses proprietary risk analysis models to identify, stratify, and segment the member population. Finally, the telehealth staff collaborates with individual providers and case managers in order to refer members to appropriate services and promote a more seamless experience for their members with complex care needs (see www.healthdialog.com).

EXEMPLAR 18-3

An APN CM working in a community health center received a referral from a local hospital to follow a 17-year-old Hispanic male who had been hospitalized for a gunshot wound to his head. The young man was bedbound, had a tracheostomy and percutaneous endogastric (PEG) feeding tube. Unfortunately he was not eligible for Medicaid because he had not completed his immigration status. The APN CM accepted the referral and began coordinating primary care at the clinic. On the initial home visit, the APN CM and clinic physician were surprised to see that the patient was alert and oriented. The patient's mother was the primary caregiver managing the tracheostomy, tube feedings, medication administration, and wound care. Although the mother demonstrated a high level of complex caregiving skills, she called

EXEMPLAR 18-3—cont'd

the APN CM almost daily to ask questions about drainage from the various tubes and wound, breathing patterns, and medication administration. The APN CM was able to obtain charity care from a home health agency for respiratory and nutrition management oversight. However, with the nature and regularity of calls, the APN CM recognized that this would be a prime opportunity to utilize telehealth technology in her caregiving. The APN CM contacted the telemedicine program at the local university and coordinated placement of a home telemedicine unit.

The home telehealth connection offered a sense of security for the patient and his mother. It allowed the APN CM to visually assess the patient and provide education regarding caregiver techniques in feeding, wound care, and medication administration. For example, when the APN CM received a phone call from the mother reporting that the patient was bleeding around the tracheotomy tube, the APN CM contacted the physician and immediately set up a telehealth visit. The providers were able to see that the patient was not in any obvious distress and had just been fitted with a tracheotomy tube that allowed him to talk with a forced effort. As a result of this increased effort, the patient was experiencing some irritation around the tube, which presented as a minimal amount of serosanguinous drainage. The physician was able to explain to both patient and mother what was happening and then instructed the patient to reduce his talking effort and build up slowly.

Population-Based Health Management

Whereas disease management focuses on diseases, complications, and specific treatments and interventions such as pharmaceuticals, laboratory tests, and educational tactics, population-based health management considers the entire range of health risk for a population. According to Peterson and Kane (1997), the objectives of population-based health management include the following:

- Optimizing functional health and well-being
- Minimizing health risk factors
- Preventing specific diseases in at-risk populations
- Facilitating the early diagnosis of disease
- Maximizing clinical effectiveness and efficiency
- Avoiding preventable disease-related complications
- Eliminating or minimizing ineffective or unnecessary care
- Measuring outcomes and providing continuous assessment and improvement

Population-based health management is a continuum-of-care model with broad application to case management strategies. Lamb and Zazworsky (2002a) applied a population-based management model when they integrated primary and specialty care services, disease management strategies, and a variety of community support systems to establish a community-wide program for the management of diabetes for the uninsured population of southern Arizona. APN CMs working in a managed care or nonprofit ambulatory care environment may find the following discussion useful when designing programs that will span an entire continuum of health-care services. Lamb and Zazworsky's model emphasizes a focus on risk assessment and risk stratification, the utilization of appropriate medical and self-care treatment according to risk, and the ability to monitor and track changes in risk status and outcomes. Figure 18-1 illustrates their model, adapted from the original model developed by Hasting Healthcare Group (cited in Peterson and Kane, 1997). This

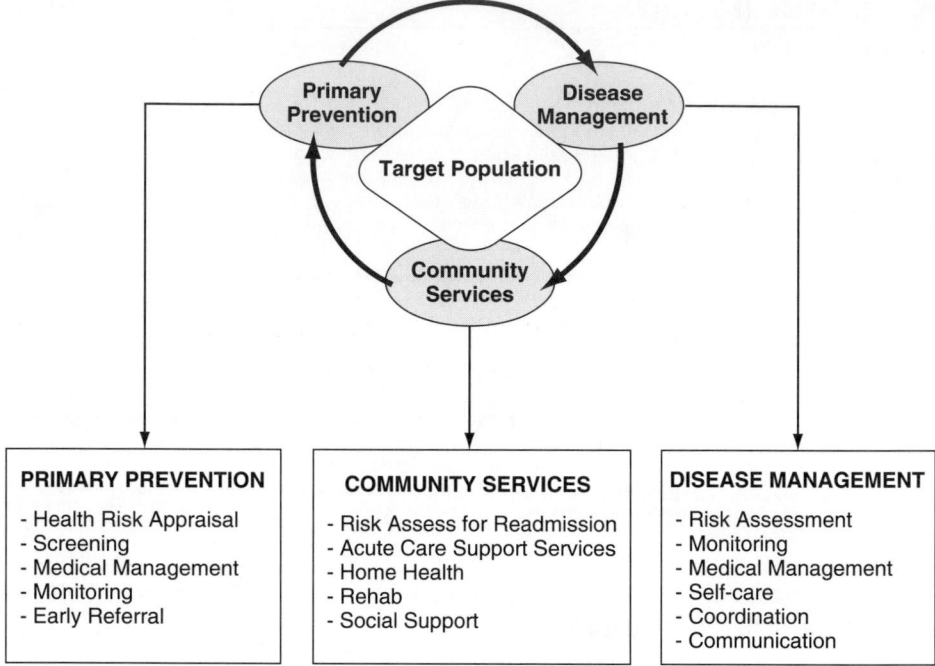

FIGURE 18-1 • Population-based health management for chronic illness.(From Lamb, G., & Zazworsky, D. [1999, January]. Disease Management [slide presentation]. Presentation conducted at the Carondelet Health Network Executive Team Meeting: Tucson, Arizona.)

model illustrates the linkages among primary prevention, disease management, and community services as applied to a chronic illness population.

TOOLS FOR RISK ASSESSMENT AND EVALUATION

To implement cost-effective, population-based health management strategies, APN CMs must understand methodologies that can identify population members who are at greatest risk for illness or disease and would be most likely to benefit from case management. It is critical to target the high-utilization/expenditure groups within a larger population for early interventions to prevent complications or treat them promptly (Eichert, Wong, & Smith, 1997). Numerous methods to determine these groups exist. These include the use of the payor's claims data to identify those clients with various co-morbidities, diagnoses, or procedures; software applications that can search historical claims data on patients/members with selected diagnoses; and applications that analyze Current Procedural Terminology (CPT) codes and identify those clients who are actually underutilizing effective health-care services (Mahn, 1999; Rieve, 1999). For example, if a patient/member with a diagnosis of diabetes type 2 is being managed according to the American Association of Diabetes guidelines, he or she would be expected to have CPT codes in his or her claims data for fasting blood sugars and hemoglobin A1c blood tests within the last 6 months. If the codes were missing, it would trigger the software to identify the patient/member for case management follow-up.

Other risk assessment tools are available to identify high-risk populations. The Short Form (SF)-36 or SF-12 health status profiles originally were used to identify patients/members most at risk for a decline in health status (Ware, Snow, Kosinski, &

Gandek, 1993). Originally developed by the Rand Corporation, this tool and others like it have evolved into a full range of health-care assessment technologies designed to complement disease and population health management strategies. They may be administered in any setting and can be used to assess changes in physical and emotional functioning over time. Normative values for a wide range of disease types have been established through Quality Metrics (see www.qualitymetric.com/) and can be useful as a comparison benchmark. The Probability for Repeated Admissions (PRA+) is another tool that is frequently used to identify patients/members who are most likely to become heavy users of health-care services (Boult, Pacala, & Boult, 1995). This questionnaire can be used to risk-stratify new health plan enrollees. For example, based on the questionnaire results, low-to-moderate-risk members may be referred to a telephone case management program, and high-risk members may be referred to a home case management program for long-term follow-up. Another tool that has been successfully used to predict risk for hospital and emergency department visits in an elderly population is the Community Assessment Risk Screen (CARS) developed and tested by Shelton, Sager, and Schraeder, (2000) at Carle Clinic in Urbana, Illinois.

The Knowledge-Behavior-Status (K-B-S) scale, part of the Omaha Documentation System (Martin & Scheet, 1992), is a useful tool for baseline assessment and ongoing evaluation of patient behavior and knowledge changes that are the focus of NCM. This system allows the APN CM to assess and objectively communicate patients' levels of knowledge regarding their disease process, their behavior associated with managing their disease, and their health status. Changes over time can be quantified, and conclusions may be drawn about the effectiveness of case management interventions. This approach also may be used to evaluate aggregate population outcomes. Mean changes in K-B-S scores over time are quantifiable measures of outcomes associated with case management intervention. In addition, a quality improvement system must be established to ensure that all clinicians using the Omaha system do so with an acceptable degree of interrater reliability.

The Self Management Goal Support Tool (Bodenheimer, Lorig, Holman, & Grumbach, 2002) has been key in the successful promotion of self-management behaviors. Developed and promoted through a number of chronic care collaborative initiatives, for example, the Bureau of Primary Health Care and Robert Wood Johnson Foundation (see www.improvingchroniccare.org, www.QualityHealthCare.org, and www.healthdisparities.net), the self-management tool is based on the readiness model (Prochaska et. al, 1992; Prochaska & DiClemente, 1999), which helps patients identify the problems that they are ready to work on in order to achieve their self-care goals. The self-management plan (template available at www.improvingchroniccare.org), sometimes referred to as a Wellness Plan, is short and concise and describes realistic goals that are identified and negotiated with the patient. Typically, the patient writes one or two goals with defined time frames for each goal. Other components of a self-management plan include barrier identification and reduction, identifying the level of confidence the patient has in achieving the goal, and a date for a review of their goal. The APN CM utilizes these plans to target patient needs and build readiness in self-management skills. Wellness plans may not be pertinent when patients are in an acute episode of their disease process. In a crisis situation, patients tend to be more dependent and require specific direction and coordination.

Finally, the Patient and Family Case Management Plan (CMP) is a guide that outlines the overall course of a patient's self-management process (Cesta & Tahan, 2003). It addresses the patient and family's role within a multidisciplinary team approach and includes elements such as care providers, testing and treatments, education topics, self-management skills, and prevention activities. This type of tool is useful in hospital settings or when working in the community with patients who have chronic illnesses such as diabetes or congestive heart failure. Exemplar 18-4 illustrates an APN CM's population-based approach to case management.

Sara was an APN CM hired by a nonprofit community organization whose primary mission was to serve the low-income and uninsured in southern Arizona. Over 2½ years, Sara applied a population-based management approach to a clinic population that had a 12% to 14% rate of patients with diabetes, which was twice the national norm. The program consisted of three major strategies: primary prevention, disease management, and community services.

The primary prevention strategy had three major components. The first involved a community risk appraisal that was designed for early detection of diabetes in members of the population who were least likely to obtain primary care services. Because the southern Arizona residents are primarily Mexican, a Promotora model consistent with their cultural beliefs about health was developed. The Promotora model relies on lay community health workers who have been trained to offer basic health education and social service support to members in their community. Promotoras distributed diabetes health risk appraisals to the general public at health fairs, community events, church gatherings, and other community activities. Once the appraisals were returned to the clinic and scored, the Promotora contacted respondents to begin appropriate referrals. The second component involved the administration of the diabetes risk appraisal to members who were registering at the clinic for the first time. Members who self-reported a known diabetic condition were rapidly identified and placed on diabetes protocols. Members with prediabetic conditions were screened by the primary care provider promptly, and if appropriate, placed on prediabetes protocols, which included nutrition and exercise education and appropriate referrals to a dietician. The third primary prevention component involved a grant-funded mobile podiatry unit that traveled to senior centers within the community and identified patients with podiatric symptoms requiring more immediate treatment or diabetic screening. Sara provided direct care to clients and expert guidance and coaching for patients and staff for this component of the program, seeing patients in the clinic and overseeing both paid and volunteer staff who administered and scored the screening tool. In addition, she utilized her research skills and competencies in data and information management to evaluate the reliability and validity of the screening tools as well as the overall program.

Disease management, the second major strategy, relied heavily on Sara's collaborative skills and competencies to work with physicians, dietitians, certified diabetic educators (CDEs) and other providers in implementing evidence-based guidelines and flow sheets to document the process of care for the diabetic population. The successful diffusion of guidelines required Sara to conduct staff meetings to educate personnel on the benefits of the tools, as well as many one-on-one feedback sessions with physician providers who initially resisted complying with the new documentation requirements. Sara used their feedback to modify the documents to make them user-friendly to ensure consistent and reliable data collection. She also assisted the medical director to initiate a monthly Diabetes Day Group Visit, in which 8 to 10 patients with diabetes attended a scheduled group educational meeting conducted by the CDE and nutritionist. During the Group Visit, they were also evaluated by the ophthalmologist (retinopathy examination), the podiatrist, and their primary care provider. In addition, she established a monthly Diabetes Health Care Team Conference, during which providers met to discuss cases and formulate a multidisciplinary plan for the complex cases. This team also served as the forum for CQI, a process that Sara facilitated using her skills and competencies in the PDSA (Plan-Do-Study-Act) process. One important outcome of the CQI process for Sara's team was the implementation of an "on-site" HbA1c finger stick during a primary care visit, which dramatically reduced time and financial barriers encountered by diabetics because medications could be adjusted during the same visit, rather than requiring a repeat visit to the clinic to follow up on the lab results.

The third strategy of the program involved referrals and triage for patients who required immediate medical interventions, as well as follow-up on patients whose ongoing care needs were being met in other settings within the community, including acute care hospital, home care, and rehabilitation. In some cases, Sara served in a consultative and collaborative role with other providers within the community to coordinate care for clinic patients in her caseload. Finally, Sara provided direct care when she accompanied the Promotora on home visits for patients who were initially entering the program or who were "stuck" and had not adhered to their care regimen.

This exemplar is based on actual practice by Donna Zazworsky at St. Elizabeth of Hungary Clinic in Tucson, Arizona, and is used with permission to advance the practice of the APN CM role.

In summary, the APN CM must be knowledgeable about the advantages and dis-advantages of various assessment tools and surveying techniques. For example, the SF-36 or PRA+ may be more cost-effective to administer via a mailed survey; however, the reliability of these instruments decreases when administered in this fashion. Administering these tools via telephone survey increases the reliability, whereas a face-to-face interview with the client yields maximal reliability. Although the methodologies associated with obtaining claims data or administering risk assessment surveys are beyond the scope of this chapter, these approaches are quickly becoming industry standards and are currently mandated by the CMS for senior risk members. They can be effective tools to identify case management leverage points within the total risk population.

APN CM COMPETENCIES

APNs have been valued for their specialized knowledge and their training in complex decision making (Madden & Reid Ponte, 1994). Parallels between traditional APN roles and the NCM role have been observed (Connors, 1993; Fralic, 1992; Hamric, 1992; Newman, cited in Smith, 1993). Hamric (1992) analyzed the nurse case management literature and suggested that the NCM role be viewed as an APN role. She exhorted APNs to "confront the challenge of case management forcefully and articulate their role to this practice modality" (Hamric, 1992, p. 13). Interestingly, NCM functions closely align with the traditional subroles of the CNS, clinical practice, consultation, education, and research (Hamric, 1989), and incorporate the CNS's change agent, management, and leadership skills (Gournic, 1989). The parallels between the APN CM role and the traditional CNS role are also reflected in the number of nurse case management articles published by CNSs (e.g., Cronin & Maklebust, 1989; Flynn & Kilgallen, 1993; Lynn-McHale, Fitzpatrick, & Shaller, 1993; Nugent, 1992; Sherman & Johnson, 1994; Strong, 1992; Trinidad, 1993; Wagner & Menke, 1992). Patient populations that have been cared for by CNSs include multisystem failure patients in critical care (Strong, 1991), long-term care patients (Schroer, 1991), trauma patients (Daleiden, 1993; Rotz, Yates, & Schare, 1994), pediatric patients with cardiac defects or chronic illness (Doell Smith, 1994; Gaedeke-Norris & Hill, 1991), and patients who have undergone coronary artery bypass graft (Tidwell, 1994). Jenkins and Sullivan-Marx (1994) proposed a primary care delivery model in which NPs would practice as NCMs.

Because the APN CM continues to evolve, this section focuses on how the APN competencies, described in this text (see Chapter 3), are currently operationalized in APN case management. We also discuss additional elements of the core competencies that APN CMs need to perform well in the role. Table 18-2 outlines the seven APN competencies as they pertain to the APN CM role. Particular emphasis is placed on the APN CM knowledge and skill component, which demonstrates how the APN CM is likely to be different from more established APN roles.

Direct Clinical Practice

A central competency of an APN CM is direct clinical practice as outlined in Chapter 6. In order for APN CMs to influence practice, it is critical for them to be viewed by other members of the health-care team as clinicians who are expert at physical assessment and who are able to anticipate physiological responses to illness, medications, treatments, and

TABLE 18-2   APN CM COMPETENCIES AND RELATED SKILLS AND FUNCTIONS

APN COMPETENCY	APN CM KNOWLEDGE/SKILL	APN CM FUNCTIONS
Direct Clinical Practice	• In-depth biopsychosocial assessment skills • Expert knowledge and skills related to clinical specialty area • Expert clinical reasoning • Anticipation of physiological responses to illness, medications, and treatments • Interpret lab and medical diagnostic information • Recognition of health impact of chronic disease in acute care crisis • Application of diverse health management approaches	• Case finding and referral screening • Conduct risk assessment and assign severity • Conduct physical, social, functional and cognitive health assessments • Domestic abuse screening • Establish client goals and time frames • Documentation in medical record • Coordinate interventions among providers • Client referral to appropriate resources • Monitor client's progress toward goals • Identify compliance barriers • Evaluate effects of interventions
Expert Coaching and Guidance	• Formation of effective client-nurse partnership • Behavioral Change Theory • Health Belief Model • Teaching-Learning theory • Nonjudgmental communication style	• Assess level of client readiness to modify lifestyle choices • Provide client, family, and caregiver teaching • Coach clients and families through developmental, health, and illness transitions • Educate other providers about clinical, fiscal, and system processes
Consultation	• Expertise in clinical practice area or specialty • Health Promotion and prevention • Acute complication management • Chronic Disease Management • Disease and Population Health management • Quality Improvement Theory	• Review of complex, high-risk clients • Conduct analysis of work flow and processes • Participation in work redesign efforts • Participation on quality improvement teams • Development of documentation tools • Consultant for information systems
Collaboration	• Communication and negotiation skills • Organizational culture and behavior • Conflict negotiation/resolution strategies • Affirmation of others	• Foster shared vision among clinical stakeholders • Support strategic decision making of management and leadership team • Participation on interdisciplinary teams
Ethical Decision Making	• Recognition and raising of ethical dilemmas • Understanding of organizational mission and purpose • Knowledge about how to activate ethics committee within organization	• Identification of options available to client • Evaluate risks and benefits of decision options • Balance provider, payor, and client goals • Maintain satisfaction of both internal and external customers
Leadership	• Demonstrates ability to influence others • Change agency/change theory • Knowledge of business and operations	• Organizational/systems assessment • Facilitate system-wide change • Develop or revise policies, procedures, guidelines, protocols, or processes of care

TABLE 18-2	APN CM COMPETENCIES AND RELATED SKILLS AND FUNCTIONS—cont'd	
APN COMPETENCY	APN CM KNOWLEDGE/SKILL	APN CM FUNCTIONS
Leadership—cont'd	• Organizational/community political awareness • Public speaking and publication skills • Grant-writing skills • Social Marketing Theory • Organizational theories	• Conduct needs of population and build support for new services/programs • Establish program objectives, interventions, and evaluation plan • Market program and build stakeholder buy-in through public speaking, publications, and political activism • Lead QI and other interdisciplinary teams
Research	• Evidence-based best practices • Research utilization and conduct • Knowledge dissemination theories • Quality Improvement Theories • Outcomes Management • Data Analysis and Information Management • Health-care finance; knowledge of billing codes and procedures • Diffusion of Innovation Theory	• Review, evaluate, and disseminate best practices literature and research • Defines indicators for program effectiveness • Design, prioritize, and facilitate information capture and data collection methodologies • Perform information queries and run reports • Analyze data and draw conclusions • Self-evaluate statistical process control and performance trends • Prepare, present, and disseminate findings

These competencies, skills, and functions have been revised from their previous forms in Mahn and Zazworsky (2000).

invasive interventions. Depending on their practice settings, they must be highly skilled at recognizing the impact of chronic disease on acute health-care crises. Thus, APN CMs must be able to conduct screening assessments and interpret laboratory and pathology findings and other medical diagnostic information. APN CMs discuss the findings with colleagues and patients in order to facilitate the plan of care. APN CMs who are credentialed in their jurisdiction as NPs or CNSs and whose activities are covered by their APN scope of practice may also perform other interventions, including prescribing medications, performing Pap tests, and removing chest tubes. In addition to assessment of physical issues, functional status, and symptom distress, the APN CM might be more likely than other APNs to perform more detailed assessment of environmental, organizational, psychosocial, sociocultural, spiritual, economic, ethical, and other contextual factors that affect individual patients and their health-care choices. Based on assessment data, APN CMs use diverse management approaches, including complementary and alternative medicine approaches, to meet the needs of their populations. A comprehensive, holistic, and integrated synthesis of assessment information is necessary for the APN CM to develop a successful care management plan. APN CMs are responsible for monitoring a client's progress toward his or her goals, evaluating the effects of their interventions, and linking the client with appropriate resources for ongoing management as warranted by the intensity and severity of the client's illness. Depending on the setting and the context of the client-nurse relationship, APN CMs may retain the client as a primary client or refer the care of the client to other care providers who better match the level of care required by the client and the available resources. When APN CMs refer a client to other providers, they typically remain sufficiently connected to the client to ensure that he or she remains "anchored" in the health-care system, with the APN CM coordinating and reevaluating care as needed. As a final note, APN CMs must have enough autonomy and control over their daily work and schedule to be able to shift back and forth between involvement with direct care and involvement with system issues in order to achieve desired outcomes for individual patients and their population.

Expert Coaching and Guidance

Expert coaching and guidance is perhaps the most critical competency for the APN CM because it is the hallmark of the service that she or he provides to patients, providers, and payors. The unique interpersonal process that nurses utilize is described throughout the CM literature. The NCM literature consistently advocates a relationship focus, which is necessary in order to coach and guide individuals toward more skillful living choices (Fralic, 1992; Lamb & Stempel, 1994; Newman, Lamb, & Michaels, 1989; Stempel, Carlson, & Michaels, 1996). This is consistent with the discussion of formation of partnerships with patients (see Chapters 5 and 6). Analysis of interviews with patients experiencing NCM suggested that the process used in NCM practice is one in which the NCM becomes a "trusted insider" to the client. As the process unfolds, patients integrate the nurse's teaching and coaching so that they become their own "insider experts," able to make judgments about their needs for care (Lamb & Stempel, 1994). Until the NCM becomes a "trusted insider," interventions to optimize wellness or foster self-care skills may have limited impact. Within the partnership context, patient and family values and health perceptions must be honored. Lamb and Stempel (1994) suggested that successful outcomes such as fewer days in the hospital and critical care unit, fewer readmissions, and reduced use of emergency room services are related to "monitoring and teaching activities of the nurse case managers, which occur in the context of a caring nurse-client relationship" (p. 9).

This understanding of how the nurse-client relationship contributes to the success of NCM interventions directly relates to the APN CM competencies of direct clinical practice and expert coaching, since so much of APN CM practice is about influencing personal choice and successful navigation through the health-care system (Newman, 1994). The APN CM must not assume responsibility for clients' health-care decisions but rather assist them to more actively participate in self-care behaviors. Although the ability to facilitate health-care behaviors and decisions may be based on the art of "connecting" with the patient, it is also a skill based on demonstrated research in the areas of patient education and behavioral change theories. Thus, responsibility for analyses of processes and outcomes of care, a core job responsibility in APN CM practice, gives these APNs a unique opportunity to apply and test middle-range theories to clinical practice.

The Health Belief Model (HBM) (Becker, 1974) is another model that is helpful to the coaching competency of the APN CM because key concepts such as individual perception, cues to action, and likeliness for action are used to guide and predict client behavior. *Individual perception* refers to whether a patient perceives the illness or health problem to be of a serious nature and his or her own perceived degree of susceptibility to the illness. The term *cues to action* refers to factors that affect clients' choices—who and what influences their health-care behaviors and decisions, and how. *Likeliness for action* refers to the *benefits and barriers* of adopting a new behavior identified by the client. It is important for the APN CM to distinguish between the benefits that she or he perceives for the client and the benefit that the client perceives. An assessment of barriers such as cost, time, distance, accessibility, language, culture, and physical ability must also be taken into consideration. Assessing barriers can assist the APN CM when establishing a plan of care with the client.

Consultation and Collaboration

APN CMs are expected to influence at both the system and individual levels. For example, APN CMs have consultative and collaborative skills that enable them to build the interdisciplinary consensus that is required to develop and implement care guidelines, protocols, standard order sets, critical pathways, decision algorithms, or comprehensive disease management programs. Despite the fact that the APN CM does not typically possess direct line authority for all the points of service and interdisciplinary providers that they must influence, their collaborative and consultative skills enable them to influence direct care and health-care delivery systems on multiple levels. The APN CM's accountability for clinical, fiscal, and organizational outcomes on a system-wide level significantly influences the expression of these particular competencies. This accountability is one key difference between the APN CM and other APNs and may be one of the reasons so many CNSs have moved into APN CM roles; case management positions directly link APNs to outcomes.

As a recognized clinical expert in a specialty, the APN CM functions as a clinical consultant in the development of population-specific strategies and process improvements within her or his health-care system. One of the advantages of being an APN CM is that one's practice influence can be exercised at multiple points along the continuum and is not limited to one department or point of service. For this reason, APN CMs are excellence consultants on work redesign and process improvements within and across clinical services or care settings (Baird, 1995). APN CMs often facilitate such system changes by collaboration with other stakeholders who exercise leadership on clinical, financial, and political issues that affect patient care and the care delivery system. The APN CM must identify the stakeholders and cultivate their interest in and commitment to designing, implementing, and evaluating changes aimed at improving care delivery. Prior to implementing a change, the APN CM fosters a shared vision with stakeholders, establishes mutually agreed-upon goals and accountabilities, and defines a process for evaluation, including responsibilities for data collection and analysis.

Another way in which APN CMs serve as consultants is through their participation in continuous quality improvement (CQI) teams and other quality improvement activities. Because APN CMs are members of a team that is accountable for treating, comforting, and administering care within specified time frames to meet both quality and economic targets, they can become champions for CQI within their areas of clinical accountability. Their involvement in providing direct care, analyzing the care delivery system for costly inefficiencies and inconveniences, and initiating process improvements makes APN CMs ideal consultants to other health-care associates who are charged with system reengineering or process improvement.

Ethical Decision-Making Skills

Embedded in the concept of partnership with patients and families is the APN CM's role as client advocate. If the organization is truly committed to quality and customer satisfaction, the barriers to effective advocacy are fewer. The APN CM's dual accountability for patient and organizational outcomes may give rise to ethical dilemmas with somewhat different features than those encountered by other APNs (Donagrandi & Eddy, 2000). For example, patient and organizational outcomes can come into conflict, and these conflicts are likely to be more visible because the costs of clinical decisions are monitored—a phenomenon that has been studied in NPs working in managed care (Ulrich, Soeken, & Miller, 2003). The APN CM must be able to articulate the risks and benefits of choices and decisions for both the patient and organization. Within the NCM process, APNs have opportunities to apply "preventive ethics" (see Chapter 11). For example, a well-designed critical pathway may indicate that a particular patient population can be discharged to home within a week of admission. However, if successful discharge depends on adequate social supports and a patient does not have these, the pathway and the data used to develop it can provide the justification for deviating from the pathway. Knowledge of fiscal variables and costs of services also enables the APN CM to articulate the costs of *not* pursuing a decision that is in the patient's best interests, in order to persuade others to do what is best for the patient. Finally, the APN CM must be able to anticipate situations in which her or his clinical decisions or those of other health-care professionals may conflict with the goals and concerns of other stakeholders, such as third-party payors. In these situations, the APN CM can reaffirm the value of other care providers without diminishing their contributions and interventions, while negotiating for options that are truly in the best interest of the patient. The APN CM's ability to influence others is more likely to result from her or his clinical expertise and ethical decision-making skills, rather than from an explicit position of authority. Exemplar 18-5 shows how one APN CM integrated these four competencies in the care of a patient with multiple sclerosis.

 EXEMPLAR 18-5

June was a 65-year-old female with a long-standing diagnosis of multiple sclerosis (MS). She lived alone in an apartment, and with Medicare and self-funding, she managed her symptoms and caregiving needs independently. She attended a weekly exercise program provided by Sue, an APN CM who specialized in MS. Sue invited June to participate in a special research program funded through Medicare that was designed to study the quality and cost-effectiveness of a nurse-managed community care delivery system. Those selected into the study group were partnered with an NCM. June decided to participate and was assigned to partner with Sue because of her multiple health problems and complex social issues. On the first home visit, Sue and June identified and prioritized the problems that June wanted to work on and developed a holistic plan of care that would support her needs.

June wanted an expert for her growing problems with bladder incontinence, leg spasticity, and caregiving needs. This was a delicate time to build a partnership, yet not foster dependency. Sue helped June identify her greatest concern related to her health and well-being as being able to live in her own home. Sue acknowledged June's need to be in control and began to negotiate the areas in which she would offer assistance, such as patient and caregiver education and coaching, coordination of local and national resources, and being a liaison with other health-care providers. At this point, Sue's emphasis was on her role as a facilitator and coach, rather than as a direct caregiver. The goal was not to take care of June but to have June learn how to manage her own care safely and to know when to seek further assistance.

During the first month Sue concentrated on June's bladder and caregiver issues. June's goal was to remain in her home and utilize part-time caregivers to assist her with activities of daily living and mobility. June was morbidly obese and relied on a wheelchair for 100% of her mobility. She required two caregivers to transfer her from the chair to the bed in the morning, one during the day and two in the evening. June was alone through the night, so safety became the third priority. Sue provided June with information about Lifeline, which June installed within the next week.

Concerns about June's caregivers (e.g., staff turnover and varying skill levels) prompted Sue to initiate a communication book and a daily checklist in which the caregivers could record

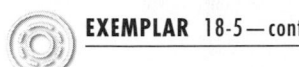

notes and activities on June's care, including medication times, daily exercises, deep breathing and coughing, and measuring urine output. These techniques enhanced caregiver continuity and consistency and helped Sue identify patterns to facilitate symptom management.

The next priority was gaining greater control over bladder management. Sue initiated a plan of care that included educating June about options for treating a neurogenic bladder (e.g., self-catheterization, intermittent catheterization per caregivers, and using a long-term indwelling catheter, and the pros and cons of each). June chose the long-term catheter, and Sue contacted June's primary care physician to arranged for a home health care (HHC) RN to monitor June for catheter problems until June could be evaluated by a urologist who specialized in MS. Sue was present for June's first home visit with the HHC RN in order to review the Foley catheter management plan and promote continuity of care. Sue recognized that although the HHC RN functioned independently, her patient would benefit from her continued clinical expertise, coordination of care, patient advocacy, and evaluation skills, while the HHC RN provided the skilled nursing needs. The relationship between the HHC RN and Sue was complementary, rather than competitive.

Sue employed a number of tools to help June learn and empower her in her self-care management. The *Patient Map and Self-Management Wellness Plan* reflected the initial plan and self-management areas on which June was ready to start working. June's actual case management care plan was more extensive and addressed other areas, including bladder, bowel, emotional, caregiving, respiratory, smoking cessation, physical activity, and nutrition issues. After June's initial plan, Sue and the HHC RN worked with the caregivers to build their confidence in managing the Foley catheter and troubleshoot problems. Because June was experiencing numerous problems related to bladder spasms, pain, and catheter leakage, Sue arranged a patient care conference with June's caregivers and the HHC RN. In this conference, Sue served as a facilitator and educator in order to resolve problems and negotiate action plans. Sue accompanied June to her urology visit to clarify short-term and long-range plans for managing her bladder problems. Although June had an indwelling Foley catheter, she was not ready to accept the long-term implications of a suprapubic catheter. In order to determine the extent of her bladder potential, the urologist recommended urodynamic testing to determine future treatment directions. Over the next 2 months, June underwent testing and treatment but was unable to achieve the level of independence that would accommodate her preferred living arrangement. After discussions with the urologist and caregivers, June decided to continue with the indwelling catheter. The next step for Sue was to help June become independent of HHC. This meant that key caregivers would need to be trained to insert and manage the Foley catheter, as well as obtain urine samples for culture and sensitivity. Sue coordinated the training with the urologist and office staff and served as a coach to the caregivers. Within a few weeks, the caregivers become confident in their abilities to identify and report symptoms of urinary tract infection and to collect urine samples accurately. The urologist also gained confidence in the caregivers' abilities and began to communicate directly with them as needed. HHC was discontinued after June's caregivers were successfully trained. Over the next 3 months, Sue's focus shifted from a direct clinical care role to consultant to June and her caregivers when certain problems arose and the caregivers were unsure of whom to call. At this point, Sue was performing reassessments at 6-month intervals to assure that the care plan was working.

Because Sue was a specialist in MS, she was able to network and establish relationships with physicians and other providers in the community who specialize in the treatment of MS. These relationships were beneficial to Sue's caseload and helped to create a team approach to care. It was not unusual for Sue to have the direct lines and extensions to physicians in order to discuss patient issues promptly when needed. Sue's focus was to assist her patients to build relationships with their physicians and other health-care providers. As a result, they learned how to communicate more effectively with their providers and become more confident in making health-care decisions on their own. Sue recognized that self-care management empowers patients so that they begin to trust themselves and that her relationship with her patients typically shifts from one of dependency to one of a coaching partnership when she has performed her role well.

The successful management of Sue's patients with MS also required a collaboration among physical therapists, exercise physiologists, speech therapists, occupational therapists, enterostomal therapists, nutritionists, behavioral health specialists, and social workers. Sue established relationships with June's team members and served as the liaison to communicate and coordinate expectations among providers, caregivers, and patients.

Leadership, Empowerment, Change Agency, and Activism

Leadership is a critical competency for APN CMs. Defined in terms of the APN CM role, leadership is simply "the art of influence." Influencing the choices patients make, the treatment and resource utilization decisions that providers make, or system-wide decisions of those in administrative roles, the APN CM will find his or her ability to influence closely tied to role effectiveness. In order to influence cost and quality outcomes, the APN CM must act as a change agent and develop systematic approaches to organize the new care processes that will be applied to a clinical population.

Implementing change strategies is central to the APN CM role. Social marketing theory has been used to guide change management when developing programs to influence care for a population. Social marketing is the design, implementation, and control of programs aimed at increasing the acceptability of a social idea, cause, or practice among members of a target group (Kotler & Zaltman, 1971). The first step in social marketing is planning. The objectives must be clearly defined and supported by a literature review and evidence. It is important for APN CMs to compare the demographics of their community with other communities that have been successful with a similar innovation and determine the level of community support required to initiate such a program. If the APN CM's community is comparable demographically, the APN CM then defines the proposed interventions based on a detailed analysis of the services that are needed. The third step is a thorough assessment of the target population, including demographics, frequency of the disease, and prior health-care utilization patterns. The results of this assessment will serve as crucial baseline data for program evaluation. The fourth step is determining an implementation plan. The implementation plan should include the resources needed, a description of projected improvements, explicit time frames, and actual performance measures (the evaluation plan) that will determine whether the program objectives were met. Pretest or evaluation instruments and marketing materials need to be developed (or selected from existing ones). Prior to full implementation, the instruments, marketing materials, and intervention/program are piloted. Based on the pilot results, the program, instruments, and marketing materials could be modified as necessary. Collaboration with interdisciplinary care providers, administrative leaders, insurance partners, and financial and informatics specialists throughout the process of program development and implementation is essential to ensure the program's success. Hospodar and Zazworsky (1997, 1999) described their use of social marketing theory to create a case management program as part of a national Medicare Demonstration Project called *The Community Nursing Organization* (see Chapter 21).

Finally, leadership in the APN CM role involves a degree of activism, through attendance at professional meetings, publications, grant writing, public speaking, professional networking on online news groups, use of radio or television media to educate the public (Zazworsky, 2002b), and participation in local, state, or national health-care policymaking (see Chapter 10). APN CMs are in a unique position to educate and inform the public, as well as private and elected policymakers and legislators about the unique needs of their populations. Exemplar 18-6 illustrates the impact that APN CMs can have on health-care policy and that they improve care for their clients.

Research

Research is an established APN competency that is congruent with APN CM practice. Because so much of advanced practice case management is data driven, this

EXEMPLAR 18-6

POLITICAL ACTIVISM

Donna Zazworsky is an APN CM with a clinical specialty in Multiple Sclerosis (MS). Originally funded through a demonstration grant, and later funded through independent funding, she and a physical therapist provided water exercise classes for anyone with MS at several local city pools during the months from April through September. From October through March, however, only one indoor facility in the community was acceptable for scheduling the classes, since most places kept their water temperature too high for people with MS. Donna identified the need for additional city pools to accommodate patients with special needs and became actively involved with the Therapeutic Recreation Program's Advisory Council under the city's Parks and Recreation Division. As a result, a community coalition was formed to investigate and to advise as to the feasibility of an indoor adaptive recreation center. It was recommended that the proposal go before the mayor and the city council to be considered as part of the city's master plan, which was soon going to the voters in an upcoming election. However, the chairman of the Therapeutic Recreation Advisory Council unexpectedly relocated to another state. Donna assumed the leadership for the initiative and began to make the project more visible to community leaders. She attended the mayor's open forum for citizens to voice their opinions on the upcoming bond election and presented a compelling testimony to the mayor and city council in support of putting the Parks and Recreations Bond on the ballot.

Donna began her presentation by introducing herself as the chairperson of the Community Coalition for the Adaptive Recreation Center and a member of the Parks and Recreation Advisory Council. She informed the audience that she was a registered nurse, listed her professional and academic credentials and affiliations, and went on to establish herself as an expert clinician who had, for the past 10 years, provided land and water exercise programs for hundreds of people with MS. Donna presented a briefing on the long-term exercise needs of wheelchair-bound citizens and those with chronic diseases such as MS and built her case for a centrally located, year-round indoor aquatic facility design specifically for seniors and people with disabilities. She concisely outlined a phased approach for the development of the aquatic facility and presented the requirements for dressing rooms, pool depth, water temperature, and modes of entry to accommodate various disabilities. At the conclusion of Donna's presentation, the bond was approved for the ballot, and Donna continued her advocacy for the program through letters and through special interest stories in local media outlets. Less than a year later, the bond was passed and plans moved forward to begin the architectural plans and community meetings.

competency will be discussed in terms of four distinct components: evidence-based practice, quality improvement, data and outcomes management, and research utilization and conduct. Each of these four components aligns with the framework for APN Research Competencies described in Chapter 9. Emphasis on the various research competencies will depend on the APN CMs role and employment setting.

RESEARCH COMPETENCY I: INTERPRETATION AND USE OF RESEARCH

Evidence-Based Practice. Evidence-based literature is a major tool in the identification of best practices, which guide professional decision making and contribute to desirable quality and cost outcomes (see Chapter 8). The APN CM should understand the strengths and limits of evidence-based practice, particularly for uncommon diseases for which adequate evidence of effective interventions is not available or feasible to collect.

APN CMs must be able to review and synthesize evidence and assist other health-care team members to draw meaningful conclusions and see potential applications to their own practices. Presenting such information to interdisciplinary providers should be done in a nonjudgmental manner and for the sole purpose of supporting quality improvement. Box 25-1 (see Chapter 25, p. 916) provides the reader with selected online sources of evidence-based practice literature that are particularly useful to APN CMs.

RESEARCH COMPETENCY II: EVALUATION OF PRACTICE

Quality Improvement. Nurse case management and quality improvement (QI) are linked in philosophy and process (Cesta, 1993). APN CMs must be able to lead interdisciplinary teams toward data-based conclusions and process improvements. Approaches to QI include CQI, TQI (Total Quality Improvement), TQM (Total Quality Management), PDCA Cycle (Plan-Do-Check-Act), and, more recently, Six Sigma Improvement. Many of these methodologies have evolved from the work of Dr. W. Edwards Deming and Dr. Joseph M. Juran, both considered to be forefathers in modern statistical process control theory (Landesberg, 1999). The reader is referred to the work of Marash, Berman, and Flynn (2003) for a comprehensive overview of these QI methodologies. Regardless of the type of QI approach an organization chooses to adopt, the APN CM should be competent in a variety of specific techniques, tools, and methodologies that are used to evaluate process performance and outcomes. Most approaches involve the use of various types of charts and analysis tools to examine findings and process linkages. Some charts are easy to learn, such as flow charts. Other charts, such as Pareto charts, run charts, process control charts, scatter diagrams, and cause-and-effect diagrams (also referred to as fishbone or Ishikawa diagrams), require specific training and expertise in statistical software. A variety of packages are available, including SAS (see www.sas.com/index.html), SPSS (see www.spss.com/), and QI Macros, an easy-to-use software program that works with Microsoft Excel and can be downloaded from the Internet at a reasonable cost (see www.qimacros.com/).

QI training typically includes techniques for analyzing how people and processes work. Root cause analysis is one popular approach to identifying underlying causes of problems and process failures within the health-care system. This approach may be particularly useful for examining adverse events and other patient safety issues. APN CMs should seek QI training through reading, continuing education, and participation in formal QI training programs if they have not learned these techniques as part of their APN training program. Ideally, training in QI principles should be included in the APN CM's orientation to a health-care organization, and if such programs are not in place, APN CMs are strongly encouraged to include formal QI training in their performance and learning objectives within the first year of hire. APN CMs can foster an organizational mindset, wherein data and information are used as tools to promote learning and improve care. A comprehensive introduction to QI charts and tools and the specific applications to case, disease, and population management may be found in *Advanced Case Management: Outcomes and Beyond* (Powell, 2000).

Data and Outcomes Management. More than other APNs, APN CMs must learn specific knowledge and skills for data collection and analysis (i.e. data management). Because these skills are a prerequisite for APN CM success in outcomes management, this element of the APN CM's research competency will be discussed in detail.

Outcomes management, as defined by Powell (2000), seeks to produce desirable outcomes in a clinical setting and is the application of outcomes research in practice. This definition implies the use of research and evidence-based best practices; however, it lacks any reference to the actual use of data or the act of measurement itself, which is at the heart of outcomes management. Therefore we propose the following definition of outcomes management: *the ability to manage data and information effectively in order to assess, plan, implement, and evaluate strategies to improve care processes and outcomes for individuals and populations*. This definition is congruent with the nursing process and describes the process used by APN CMs to evaluate program effectiveness and continuously improve performance.

While data analysis is mentioned as a specific skill for research competency II (see Chapter 9), little emphasis is placed on the actual manipulation of raw data, skills in querying information within a database containing clinical or financial information, or the ability to actually utilize an information system to collect data and trend performance because most APNs would not need this level of skill. However, for APN CMs, these skills are important because APN CMs are able to recognize meaningful patterns within clinical data sets and reports that they have generated themselves, rather than relying on reports that have already been prepared and summarized for them by nonclinical experts in information systems. Only after patterns in the data are observed do certain questions emerge about the meaning of such patterns, which often leads to further data inquiry. This process, often referred to as *data mining*, is a dynamic one that requires immediate access to raw data and rapid report turn-around time. To develop this skill, APN CMs should learn what types of information management systems are available at their organizations and request training in how to use these systems or, at the very least, become familiar with the types of data available from the systems so that they can effectively request information from designated experts who manage such systems. Information systems that are most likely to contain data needed for outcomes management include, but are not limited to, dedicated case or care management systems, medical records coding systems, billing and claims data, pharmacy, risk, quality, claims management systems, infection control, nursing acuity, and cost accounting systems.

Exemplar 18-7 illustrates this unique pattern-recognition skill when an APN CM is given a summary report describing volume, admitting source, LOS, average cost, readmission rates, and mortality rates for patients with congestive heart failure, versus a data spreadsheet containing the actual encounter level detail used to create the summary report.

EXEMPLAR 18-7

Figure 18-2 illustrates the "summary report," which provides useful administrative information, but the APN CM cannot identify clinically relevant patterns in the data that are opportunities for improvement. In addition, the APN CM is going to require additional information, including national comparison data or benchmarks to determine if the LOS, readmission rates, mortality rates, and charges are in alignment with other organizations similar to themselves. In contrast, raw data provided to the APN CM in a spreadsheet, such as the one illustrated in Figure 18-3, allows APN CMs to immerse themselves in the data in order to find unexpected pieces of information about the population that may not have been part of their original report request. Electronic source data most commonly available from health-care information systems are outlined in Box 18-2 and are discussed in greater detail in Chapter 25. With the use of Excel, the data can be sorted, filtered, grouped, and organized using spreadsheet functions to identify meaningful patterns in resource utilization, complications of care, variations in physician practice, and patient characteristics that affect severity of illness or intensity of service.

The APN CM used to sort patients using the following criteria: whether they were admitted through the emergency department (ED), admitting times (in ascending order), and time of arrival at ED (to see the distribution of arrivals) (Figure 18-3). Using this simple approach, she

Continued

EXEMPLAR 18-7 — Cont'd

was able to determine that the peak time of day in which admissions were occurring was between 1400 and 2200. When she used an Excel tool to sort the data by day of week (not shown), the APN CM noted that fewer patients were admitted over the weekend, with the largest spike occurring on Mondays. The APN CM inferred that patients delayed reporting symptoms until the doctor's office opened on Monday and that by the time physician's returned the calls on Monday the patients' symptoms had worsened, requiring more urgent medical intervention in the emergency department. The APN CM leveraged this information, along with additional data from patients admitted with chest pain who had similar utilization patterns, to build support for an ED-based "CHF and Chest Pain Clinic" at the hospital, staffed heaviest in the late afternoon and evening hours, which could accommodate this volume and more efficiently manage, treat, and triage patients with CHF and chest pain. A community-wide marketing plan was implemented to inform both the public and providers across the community of this service.

When analyzing patterns of acute care hospital utilization, the APN CM should evaluate patterns in LOS data in relation to other variables that influence LOS for a given population. These include the following:

- Admission volume (*larger population denominators tend to reflect shorter LOS*)
- Readmission rates (*evaluate readmissions for any condition, including conditions different than the index admission, within 15 and 31 days of discharge*)
- Percentage of patients discharged alive with an LOS of 1 to 2 days (*this reflects the percentage of patients that may not have been as acutely ill and therefore may have been admitted to the hospital unnecessarily*)
- Percentage of patients who are discharged to other places of care along the continuum other than home or death (*this reflects the degree to which patients are transitioned to alternative levels of care*)
- Complication rates or unexpected adverse medical outcomes (*this reflects quality of care and the degree of successful acute care complication management*)
- Severity of illness (*this reflects preexisting conditions, co-morbidities, and physiological variables of the population*)

The relative "goodness or badness" of LOS performance must be interpreted within the context of the health-care organization's reimbursement structure. For example, organizations that have exemplary average LOS (ALOS) performance but who have a higher proportion of patients that are readmitted within 15 days of discharge may actually have greater concerns with ineffective resource utilization than hospitals with slightly higher LOSs but lower readmission rates. In addition, competitive ALOS performance may be achieved as a result of aggressive transition planning to other points of care along the continuum. As long as the costs of providing care at these alternative care settings (e.g., SNF, acute rehabilitation, long-term care [LTC]) do not outweigh the minimal costs associated with a few more end-hospital days of bed, board, and recuperative nursing care, then the LOS is commendable. As soon as such aggressive transitional planning begins to cost the health-care system more than it would cost to have kept the patient in the acute care environment and does not offer significant advantages to the patient, the organization may well be satisfied with a slightly higher LOS performance versus such an arbitrary marker of success. Of course, LOS performance can also be affected by adverse medical outcomes and unexpected changes in the disease trajectory. For these situations the APN CM's skill in acute care complication management, which also involves the ability to see patterns in the data and apply best practice research, will be instrumental in determining the outcome.

Utilization Profile: CHF DRG 127
USA Memorial Hospital
Start month 1/2002   End month 6/2002

Total Volume	240
Mean LOS	5.6
Median LOS	5.0
Std. Deviation	3.83
Max LOS	21
Total Charges	$3,501,338.58
Total Costs	$949,625.00
Average Charge/Case	$14,588.88
Average Cost/Case	$3,956.77
31 day readmission rate	11.57%
Mortality rate	9.56%

Admission Source
      ER   80% (192/240)
      Physician office 17% (40/240)
      SNF   2%   (5/240)

FIGURE 18-2 • Sample data summary report for CHF.

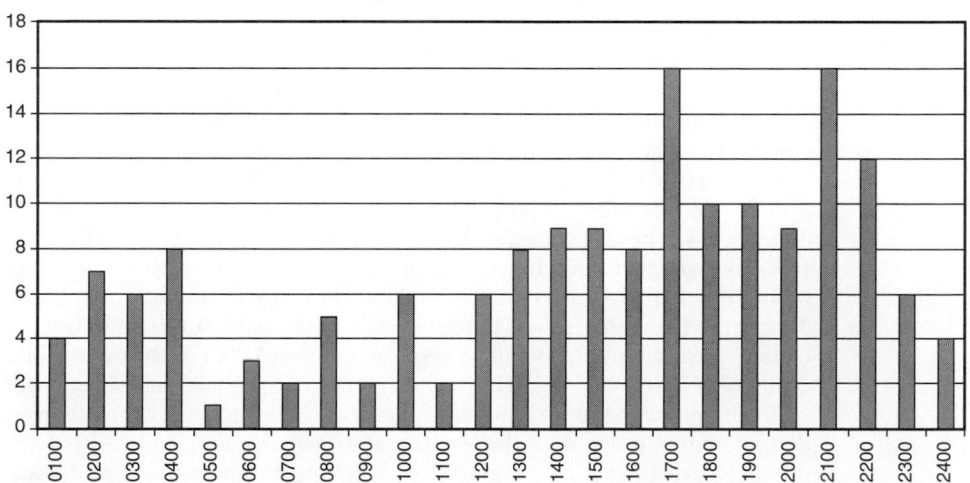

Arrival Time to ED for CHF Patients at USA Memorial Hospital
N = 169 patients admitted January - June 2002

FIGURE 18-3 • Histogram of admission times to emergency department. (Sample data reprinted with permission ACS MIDAS+, Tucson, Arizona.)

BOX 18-2 • DATA ELEMENTS TYPICALLY AVAILABLE FROM HOSPITAL INFORMATION SYSTEMS THAT ARE USEFUL FOR CASE MANAGEMENT EVALUATION

- Facility ID
- Account number
- Medical record number
- Social Security number
- Date of birth
- Gender
- Patient type
- Financial class
- Home zip code

- Admission date
- Admission time
- Reason for admission
- Admit status
- Emergency admit
- Discharge date
- Discharge time
- Discharge disposition
- Primary care physician

- Admitting physician
- Attending physician
- Total charges
- Total cost
- Insurance carrier
- Insurance type
- Insurance plan
- DRG
- DRG description

- Primary ICD-9 diagnosis
- Secondary ICD-9 diagonoses (15)
- Primary ICD-9 procedure
- Secondary ICD-9 procedures

Finally, the APN CM who is evaluating outcomes for a clinical population that is cared for at multiple points of service and over time must understand that the information needed to conduct such an analysis will reside in multiple data collection points and information systems. In order for the outcome management plan to be successful, the APN CM must bring the plan together into an organized framework. This is helpful not only in coordinating the data collection efforts needed to conduct a population-focused outcomes evaluation plan, but also for communicating the information needs to the various information systems staff who support and control information throughout the organization.

One way to effectively communicate a multiseries evaluation plan is by using a conceptual data plan wheel, illustrated in Figure 18-4. The wheel illustrates a conceptual data plan for a population with congestive heart failure (CHF) in an integrated delivery network. The central circle indicates that CHF is the focus of the performance evaluation plan. The wedges within the second circle identify points of service delivery (e.g., primary care) to CHF patients, specific care processes (e.g., risk assessment), and care focus (e.g., patient and family) that are being monitored. Key outcome measures for each of these aspects of service delivery are specified in the third circle. The sources of data for each measure that will be used to evaluate the care of CHF patients are indicated on the perimeter of the wheel. The CHF conceptual data plan addresses several processes and outcomes of interest to the multiple stakeholders across the care continuum. This particular "scorecard" format permits one to examine the impact of selected interventions on patient outcomes and resource utilization, and effectively illustrates that the information needed to carry out the data plan exists within multiple information systems and across multiple points of service that may not be readily available to the APN CM who is accountable for the evaluation plan. Because the information associated with each point of service is generally considered to be proprietary to that service, the combined efforts of the stakeholders themselves are necessary to ensure the availability of the information required to carry out the evaluation plan. Thus, the evaluation plan becomes a means to determine the organization's clinical effectiveness, cost effectiveness, and overall efficiency of managing the population for which the APN CM is responsible. Further detail on the APN's role in conducting an outcomes management plan is discussed in Chapter 25.

In summary, the model shown in Figure 18-5 ties together the seven traditional APN competencies, along with the additional knowledge and skills APN CMs need for care management (direct care and expert coaching competencies) and data and outcomes management (research competency) that are used in acute, chronic, and community care settings. The outer clockwise circle represents the complexities of the health-care system that the APN CM influences, and the inner circle represents the nursing processes and the client-nurse partnership that is at the core of all NCM interactions.

RESEARCH COMPETENCY III: PARTICIPATION IN COLLABORATIVE RESEARCH

As incumbents in an evolving APN role with significant focus on outcome evaluation, APN CMs may have more opportunities to participate in research that is interdisciplinary (Hartigan et al., 2003). Increasingly, APN CMs are engaged in national demonstration projects with rigorous evaluation components. Such programs typically involve federal funding or national endowments and generally require the presence of a nurse or physician researcher to guide the project; however, APN CMs may be actively involved with all phases of such as conceptualization, program design, program evaluation, analysis, and dissemination of results. APN CMs who practice in academic health centers are also likely to be involved in other types of research, such as clinical trials. For example, APNs

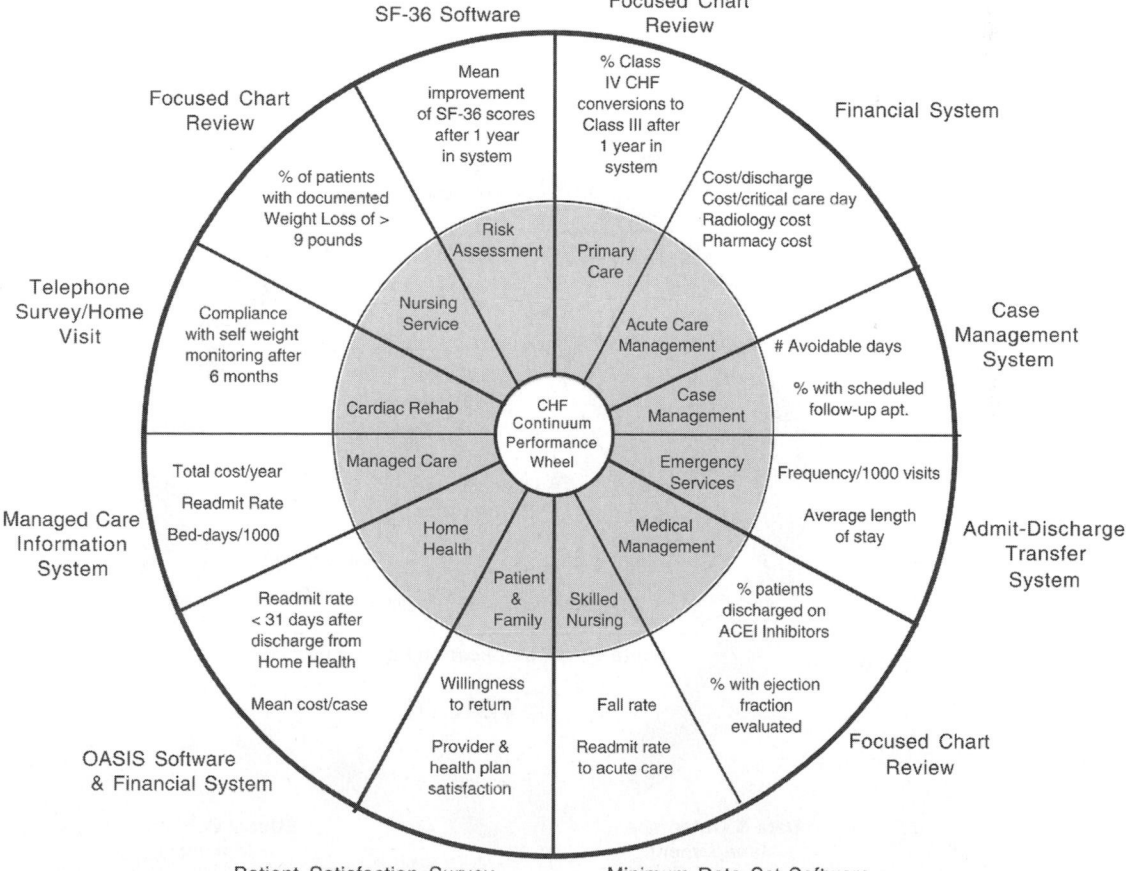

FIGURE 18-4 • Conceptual data plan for coordinating cross continuum outcomes data for patients with congestive heart failure. (Copyright 1998-2003 by ACS MIDAS+, Tucson, Arizona; reprinted with permission.)

were hired as "Advanced Practice Case Managers" to assist with prostate cancer clinical trials at the Preventative Medicine Research Institute in Sausalito, California. These APN CMs were responsible for recruiting and enrolling research participants into the study, clinical management of subjects' care, monitoring of clinical trial implementation, data collection, and facilitation of participant retention. In addition, they provided case management through telephone sessions and regularly scheduled visits with participants to evaluate their adherence to study requirements and to assess changes in their medication regimen or medical status (C. Jimenez-Raisin, personal communication, September 18, 2003).

CRITICAL ELEMENTS OF THE APN CM PRACTICE ENVIRONMENT

Whether employed in acute care, in the community, or as an independent contractor, the APN CM must address critical elements in order to achieve a successful practice. Success in the business decisions associated with case management programs as well as acquisition of APN competencies will determine the survival and success of APN CM clinical practice.

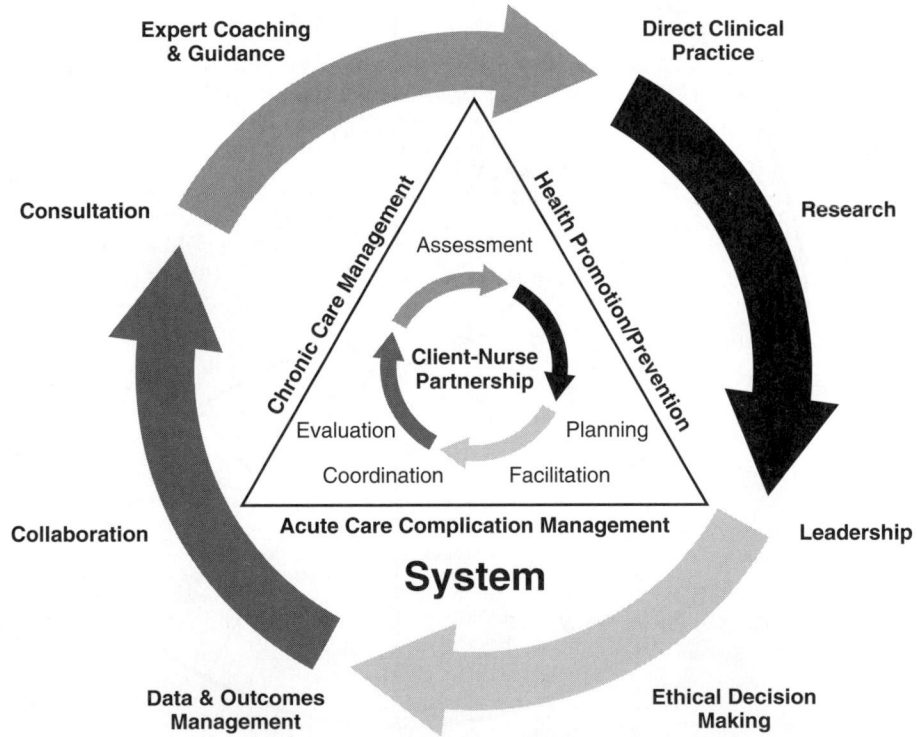

FIGURE 18-5 • Competencies and care management strategies of APN CM practice. (Copyright 1998-2003 by ACS MIDAS+, Tucson, Arizona; reprinted with permission.)

Business Elements

When examining the business of the APN CM, accountability must be defined from both the direct practice and the business perspectives (Porter-O'Grady, 1996). This means demonstrating value through quality, cost, and satisfaction in terms that are meaningful to patients, providers, and payors. These processes translate into the business functions of reimbursement structuring, cost-benefit analyzing, marketing, and contracting (see Chapter 21). The APN CM must work with the staff in finance, marketing, and contracting departments to determine how best to demonstrate that accountabilities for quality, cost, and satisfaction are being met.

Organizational Structures and Cultures

The APN CM typically practices in a hospital or integrated delivery network (IDN) setting through an acute care clinical model and/or community-based model. Because an APN CM's practice typically crosses many units, departments, and points of service within the organization, it is important to consider carefully the reporting structures that will best support APN CMs in their role. A wide variety of administrative structures exist for CMs. NCMs may be based in the following departments or settings: quality and performance improvement, utilization resource management, medical staff office, social work, home health, nursing, or even finance or information systems (IS). Many healthcare systems have redesigned their organizational structures to create independent case management departments that blend the functions of quality management, utilization resource management, discharge planning, social work, and performance improvement. Still other organizations have positioned their nurse case management resources to be more closely aligned with nursing or medical services. A recent survey conducted by the American Case Management Association (ACMA) indicated that there has been an increase from 9% to 18% of case managers reporting to the vice president of medical affairs within the last year, and approximately 24% of case managers report to the vice president of nursing or patient care services (ACMA, 2003). Regardless of the reporting structure, the APN CM should seek to work within a reporting structure that supports "whole-system" thinking and places a high value on innovation and process improvement. APN CMs should avoid reporting structures that constrain their practices to one unit or department's interests or seem to place a particular emphasis on task-oriented activities. Optimally, the organization and its administrators should recognize that the APN CM is in a unique position to promote excellence in clinical practice and system performance. To achieve such outcomes, the APN CM may at times require the formal and tacit authority that comes with the position and title of those to whom the APN CM reports. Those who lead APN CMs must be prepared to "take the heat" if necessary for changes that are perceived as coming from the APN CM. Although the APN CM will not need daily, or even weekly, supervision, she or he will need to be kept abreast of organizational issues that are likely to affect the practice and business environment. The APN CM should have routine debriefing sessions scheduled with her or his immediate supervisor to clarify goals and expected outcomes, identify any resource needs, discuss any barriers, and exchange information relating to pending contracts, changes in the product line, medical practice issues, or staff education needs. Ideally, APN CMs should have representation on the hospital quality oversight committee and any high-level meetings where decisions are made that affect their practice. Active membership on key medical committees and direct access to administrative decision makers are imperative. This is where

APN CMs have particular opportunities to integrate clinical expertise with communication, negotiation, and leadership skills to promote effective and efficient clinical processes. For those APN CMs who contract independently, becoming familiar with the organizational structure and culture and becoming a "trusted insider" to the organization will be critical to successful contracting and service delivery.

Shared Accountability for Managing Utilization

The APN CM is a member of the team who designs and produces reports on outcomes for administrators and clinicians at the organizational, departmental, and practice levels. For example, if a hospital working in cooperation with a managed care plan is striving to decrease inpatient admissions, bed-days per 1000 covered lives, and costs of delivering care, both APN CMs working in the hospital and those working in the community will share accountability with the product line administrators to achieve related goals and financial targets at the department and practice levels. APN CMs with the charge of specified clinical populations within the product line, such as CHF patients within a cardiovascular product line, may implement specific interventions, such as the implementation of a CHF admission protocol, standard order sets, or best practice guidelines, and then report to the cardiovascular product line director on the reduced numbers of unnecessary CHF admissions and critical care bed-days by payor. In contrast, a community based APN CM may give a report to the same cardiovascular product line director on the reduced CHF readmission rate by payor. Both clinical and community APN CMs would provide reports that translate the reductions into cost savings by payor. Below are come common formulas used by payors and providers to evaluate utilization. The formula is presented first, followed by an explanation.

Bed Days per 1,000 Covered Lives

Calculation:

$$X = \frac{\text{Sum of all inpatient days for a selected health plan}}{\text{Total count of members enrolled in the health-care plan}}$$

Example:

- 182 total inpatient days during the month of January
- 12,845 members enrolled in January
  - ✔ $182 \div 12{,}825 = 0.01417$
  - ✔ $0.01417 \times 1{,}000 = 14.17$ days in January per 1000*
  - ✔ 14.17×12 months = 170.04 days/1,000 (annualized)

*Note: This figure is generally reported as an annualized rate.

One of the most utilized markers of utilization of hospital services in managed care is bed-days per 1000 covered lives. This measure is widely used by executives to monitor "the big picture." As an industry standard, this measure gives health-care providers and managed care organizations the ability to compare utilization of inpatient days with a common denominator. Determination of whether bed-days are within acceptable ranges of performance may be based on comparative data or medical management guidelines, such as Milliman and Robertson, Inc. Health Care Management Guidelines (1999), which lists expected bed-day ranges for a wide variety of DRG and ICD-9 diagnosis codes in various managed care market environments. The calculation of bed-days is a function of both LOS and admission frequency. Therefore, if bed-days per 1000 covered lives are higher than desired, the APN CM will need to ascertain whether bed-days are higher as a result of excess hospital admissions or whether they are a result of a longer LOS. These are important data, because interventions to reduce admissions are very different from those needed to reduce LOS within the acute care environment.

Inpatient Admissions per 1,000 Covered Lives

Calculation:

$$X = \frac{\text{Total number of admissions}}{\text{Total count of members enrolled in the health-care plan}}$$

Example:

- 67 patients admitted during the month of January
- 12,845 members enrolled in January
  - ✔ 67 ÷ 12,825 = 0.00522
  - ✔ 0.00522 × 1,000 = 5.22 admits per 1,000 lives[*]
  - ✔ 5.22 × 12 months = 62.7 per 1,000 lives per year (annualized)

[*] Note: This figure is generally reported as an annualized rate.

Inpatient admissions are widely used by executives to monitor overall utilization of inpatient services. Similar to admissions per 1,000 covered lives, industry standards exist for various case types for both commercial and Medicare populations. This allows APN CMs to benchmark their organization's utilization against similar markets.

Cost per Patient Day

Calculation:

$$X = \frac{\text{Total direct costs}}{\text{Total patient days}}$$

Example:

- $286,342.21 direct costs assigned to a cardiac medical unit during the month of June
- 1908.9 patient days in June
  - ✔ $286,342.21 ÷ 1908.9 = $150.00/patient day in June

Cost per patient day is typically used to describe incremental costs of care associated with a particular unit or point of service and helps middle-level managers make budgeting and financial projections. APN CMs can also use this calculation to report savings accrued when patients are redirected to alternative levels of care as a result of changes made in care delivery processes.

Cost per Discharge

Calculation:

$$\times = \frac{\text{Sum of total costs accrued from admission to discharge}}{\text{Count of all patients discharged in the population of interest}}$$

Example:

- Total costs for patients discharged with DRG 127 (CHF) = $3,538,784
- Total number of patients discharged with DRG 127 = 914
  ✔ $3,538,784 ÷ 914 = $3,871.75 per case

Cost per discharge is often used to evaluate cost of care trends for a particular case type or population over time. It is reported as an average (mean). This measure is even more meaningful when the population of interest is risk or severity adjusted. In the case of a CHF population, a more meaningful indication of cost could be achieved if costs were calculated for each of the four levels of New York Heart Association (NYHA) classifications of CHF; however, obtaining the data necessary to risk adjust a population based on physiological variables requires a dedicated medical record review effort and is often not sustainable over time. For this reason, many heath care organizations invest in automated risk adjustment methodologies that use coded claims data, such as the 3M APR DRG grouper software, which uses ICD-9 diagnosis and procedure coding, along with other demographic information that is commonly available in electronic source data to risk adjust patients into varying levels of intensity and severity.

Mean Cost per Covered Life

Calculation:

$$\times = \frac{\text{Cost of all care provided over course of year to all enrollees}}{\text{Count of all enrollees in the health plan}}$$

Example:

- Total cost of care provided by health plan = $18,487,234
- Total number of enrollees during the year = 2,421
  ✔ $18,487,234 ÷ 2421 = $1488.38 per enrollee

The calculation of mean cost per covered life is a difficult measure to capture for most health-care organizations because it requires claims data from the payors to determine all costs associated with care across the continuum. Ideally, this would include claims data from inpatient, emergency, outpatient, skilled nursing, rehabilitation, hospice, physician office visits, home health care, and pharmaceuticals. Despite the difficulty in gathering the data necessary to produce this measure, it is of particular interest to administrators in capitated managed care environments because it illustrates cost shifting that results when patients are redirected to alternative levels of service. It is an important fiscal measure to APN CMs who are evaluating population health management models.

Readmission Rates

Calculation:

$$X = \frac{\text{Count of all nonelective inpatient encounters within 15 days of discharge}}{\text{Count of all inpatients discharged alive with DRG 127}}$$

Example:

- The denominator identifies the population of interest. In this example there were 914 patients who had an inpatient hospital encounter for heart failure as identified by DRG 127 and who were discharged alive. Patients who expired during their first (index) encounter were excluded from the population.
- The numerator identifies the readmission event within 15 days of discharge. In this example, there were 82 of 914 patients who had a return inpatient encounter with any diagnosis (not just limited to heart failure) within 15 days of discharge from their index encounter. Patients who were admitted for "elective" or outpatient procedures were excluded from the count.
  ✔ 82 ÷ 914 = .089
  ✔ 089 × 100 = 8.9% readmission rate

The readmission rate is one of the most commonly calculated indicators in case management; however, it remains one of the most controversial because of differing methodologies for computing the measure. Readmission rates are valuable because they are viewed as an indicator of the effectiveness of the treatment plan and the patient's readiness for discharge. Patients that are discharged too early or with insufficient supports in place tend to "bounce back in" and in theory are considered case management failures, although in some cases the natural disease trajectory and unforeseeable complications that are beyond medical or case manager's control contribute to the readmission.

When calculating readmission rates, most hospitals rely on their IS to identify these occurrences; however, the APN CM should be aware of several problems associated with the computation of readmission rates using electronic source data. First, most hospital IS cannot "look forward" from the date of discharge and track a true readmission rate that occurs in the future. In reality, the majority of hospital ISs actually "look backward" from the date of discharge and count patients that had any inpatient encounter *prior* to the specified date; what is essentially being measured is a "preadmission rate," which is often used as a proxy measure for readmission. As a result, many hospitals still devote time to reviewing charts and collecting readmission statistics manually. In addition, there appears to be some debate about whether to count only patients who were readmitted for the same diagnosis they had during their index admission, or whether to count readmissions regardless of the clinical reason for returning, as long as it was not due to an elective procedure or outpatient visit. Although there are some hospital and case management IS that can provide "true" readmission rates by looking forward in the database, the APN CM must know how the index encounters are being identified, and have a clear understanding for how readmissions are being qualified at their organization.

Once readmission rates are obtained, it may be quite informative for the APN CM to view readmission patterns sorted by elapsed days between discharge and readmission. Figure 18-6 illustrates a histogram of 30-day readmission patterns. Although the overall readmission rate is reported to be 13.2%, what is most significant is that 75 of 164 (46%)

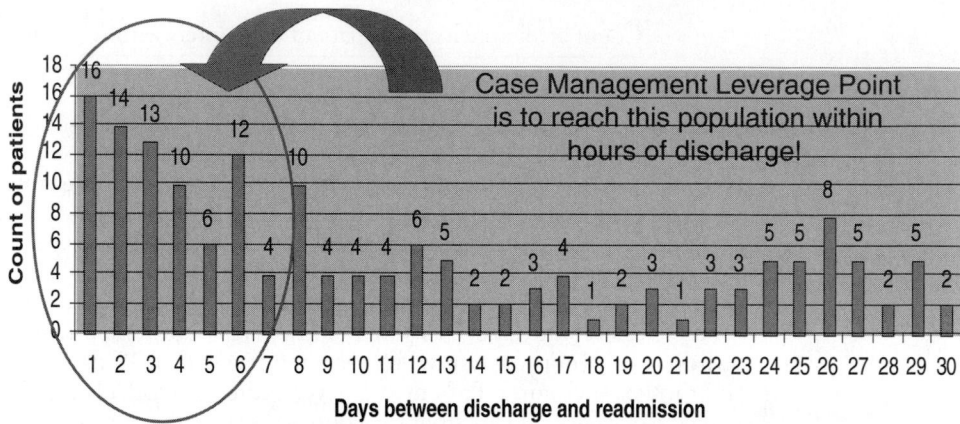

FIGURE 18-6 • Histogram of readmission rates reveals leverage points for case management. (Copyright 1998-2003 by ACS MIDAS+, Tucson, Arizona; reprinted with permission.)

of all readmissions occurred within the first 7 days following discharge. This information provides the APN CM with greater insight into where in the process to intervene. In this example, the home follow-up visit that took place for CHF patients at 1 to 2 weeks following discharge needed to be shifted to 1 to 2 days following discharge (Lamb, Mahn, & Dahl, 1996).

Productivity and Acuity

Productivity reports should capture direct patient care (e.g., hospital, home, or provider visits; telephone contacts) and indirect care (e.g., documentation, patient conferences, and travel time). All of these items should be recorded by the payor in order to calculate an average cost per case. Other time related to committee meetings or continuing education may or may not be averaged into the payor breakdown. Another method when measuring productivity is to include nurse case management intervention activities during visits. A study by Papenhausen (1996) demonstrated that community NCMs spent their visit time performing the following intervention activities: 30% assessing and monitoring, 17% teaching and informing, 7% in direct service, 23% supporting and sharing, and 11% exploring alternatives and goal setting. When APN CMs have this type of information, they can establish targets with NCMs, administrators, and contracted providers related to productivity and contract accountability. Productivity information and cost-benefit analyses enable the organization or private practice to negotiate better contracts for its services.

Acuity addresses the level and complexity of care for case-managed patients. This information must be captured in order to demonstrate the costs and benefits of APN CM interventions. For example, Ward and Rieve (1997) illustrated an acuity-based framework for CMs in a disease management/episodic-based case management model. In this model, patients who are at the lowest levels of complexity and risk and who require only 1 to 2 hours of CM intervention are assigned an acuity level of 1. Patients requiring extensive diagnostic testing, multiple complex treatments, and over 15 hours of CM intervention are assigned an acuity level of 5. Acuity tools that objectively quantify risk are necessary to establish valid selection criteria for triggering a case management referral. Without such criteria, other providers who initiate referrals for case management may make inappropriate referrals to case management services. As a result, undue workload on case management staff is created. Case management should not be viewed as a dumping ground for all discharge planning or continuum transition issues but rather as a distinct level of service provided to clients who demonstrate a specific need. Acuity measures are also needed to differentiate which patients need APN CM services, as opposed to NCM services.

Indirect Costs

Other business items the APN CM must consider relate to the general business elements of daily operations, such as office telephone, beeper, cellular phone, copying, faxing, invoicing/billing abilities, procedural coding (when appropriate), support staff, and rental space. These indirect expenses need to be tracked and calculated into reimbursement structures. For APN CMs who choose to practice independently, additional considerations must be given to obtaining and maintaining a business license, Federal Identification Number, worker's compensation insurance, liability insurance, business structuring (e.g., sole proprietor, partnership, or corporation), and attorney and certified public accountant services (see Chapter 20).

Reimbursements

Depending on the employment environment, the APN CM may receive reimbursements from a number of different sources. If the APN CM is working for a hospital or integrated delivery network (IDN), the APN CM will want to establish a mix of reimbursement vehicles. Conversely, the independent APN CM may negotiate directly with the MCO, employer, or insurance carrier for services. In this case, additional credentialing needs may be anticipated. The following business issues should be considered within the various reimbursement structures.

Fee-for-Service (Indemnity). A fee-for-service contract with insurance companies, third-party administrators, employers, and MCOs is just what it means: the APN CM is paid a fee for services delivered. The appropriate hospital/IDN departments involved in contracting (e.g., legal, contracts, finance) will assist in formulating a proper contract that includes scope of services to be provided, reporting needs, reimbursements, and billing requirements. In most cases, the APN CM will receive authorization for the initial visit and then must submit an authorization request for a certain number of additional anticipated visits needed along with a plan of care.

Capitated Contract. A capitated contract is established between an MCO and the hospital or provider based on a per member per month reimbursement. In this contract, the hospital negotiates a monthly capitation payment, and the APN case management cost center will be allocated a fixed payment. This type of arrangement must also be clearly defined in scope of services (e.g., hospital and home visits, service authorization capabilities) and reporting needs (e.g., outcomes of visits, service use). Another critical component in this type of arrangement is activity tracking. The APN CM must track time, broken down by payor, related to direct and indirect patient care. The APN CM can use this information to develop special services/programs such as group education for hospitalized CHF patients or a CHF clinic. Finally, through activity tracking, the APN CM can let administrators know if the capitated fee covers the cost of APN CM services being delivered.

Subcontracting ("Carve Outs"). Subcontracting or "carve outs" are another form of contract that occurs in specialized areas such as worker's compensation, behavioral health, or disease management. These contracts are set up by vendors who need an APN CM in a particular geographic area to deliver a specialized service. This type of arrangement is conducive to the APN CM in private practice. For example, the private practice APN CM will subcontract with a company to be its representative for worker's compensation cases. Depending on the needs of the patient, the private practice APN CM may need to establish special financial arrangements with local providers to deliver care on behalf of the worker's compensation company.

Billing Methods

Billing methods depend on the contractual arrangement between the contractor and the organization. The APN CM must collaborate with the finance department (if employed by an organization) or with a certified public accountant (if in private practice) regarding the preferred method for billing. Unfortunately, nurse case management is not recognized as a billable service under Medicare guidelines and therefore NCMs cannot bill independently as can some other APNs (CMS, 1998).

Marketing

Marketing APN CM services must take place both externally and internally across the organization and to the appropriate contracted providers. Zazworsky and Hospodar (1996) demonstrated a marketing plan approach that included target markets; competition analysis; strengths, weaknesses, opportunities, and threats (SWOT) analysis; and product development, pricing, and promotions applied to nurse case management. It is imperative that both internal and external markets be addressed, because success rests not only on desired outcomes but also on appropriate referrals. Internal and external marketing require assistance from the organization's public relations and/or marketing department for theme/message design, a communication plan, material development, and implementation assistance. Internally, the APN CM may communicate otherwise complex case management referral criteria in a simple, user-friendly format such as a referral form checklist or decision algorithm. Externally, the APN CM may offer the same referral form checklist to contracted providers (e.g., physicians, NPs, social workers, MCO authorization personnel). More comprehensive policies and procedures may then be developed to supplement such tools (see Chapter 21).

Certification and Credentialing Requirements

There is no certification credential specific to the APN CM role, and to our knowledge, there is no plan for one in the near future. As an evolving role (see Chapter 19), this is not surprising. Currently, APNs practicing in the APN CM role tend to pursue some type of certification in case management as well as advanced specialty certification when it is available. Since credentialing and regulation of APNs are a major health policy focus, readers are advised to consult their state boards on such matters. In this section, we outline the various credentialing "avenues" available to APN CMs (see Chapter 22).

The ANA offers special "modular" certification for NCM, which is available from the ANCC (American Nursing Credentialing Center). Modular certification is described as a way to "allow the nurse to continue lifelong learning and to be recognized in areas that involve new technologies, settings, advancements, procedures, techniques that cut across numerous specialties" (ANA, 2003b). The credential for this certification is the RN, C (Registered Nurse, Certified), which is not an APN credential. Since this credential is available to Associate and Diploma nurses who also are (or wish to become) certified in various clinical specialties, use of this credential alone by APN CMs may be confusing or misleading. This credential therefore seems incongruent with the fact that the core definition of NCM is a nurse with a baccalaureate degree.

ANCC offers a number of specialty certification examinations for CNSs. After passing the exam, the CNS uses the title of APRN, BC (Advanced Practice Registered Nurse, Board Certified). However, selected specialty organizations do support certification for advanced practice roles. For example, the American Association of Critical Care Nurses, the American Board of Occupational Health Nurses, and the Association for Rehabilitation Nurses now offer an advanced certification and their standards of practice incorporate role elements of the APN CM role. However, these advanced certifications are dependent on the need and marketability of the advanced practice role within their given settings. The advanced certification in Rehab (CRRN-A), for example, is being phased out in 2009 as a result of the small number of people requesting the certification and the limited success of states securing recognition of the advanced practice licensure. When there is no APN specialty exam, APN CMs may elect to sit for the "basic" specialty exam that RNs can take. With the adoption of second licensure as a requirement for APN practice, APN CMs, especially those in new specialties or in clinical areas for which no APN exam exists, APN CMs and policymakers will need to collaborate to define credentialing requirements that protect the public while ensuring the APN CM's scope of practice is not constrained.

Regardless of the availability of advanced certification within one's specialty, the APN CM should continue to meet the basic requirements for certification in their clinical specialty (e.g., gerontology, rehabilitation, oncology, adult medical-surgical, critical care) in addition to certification in case management. Depending on the job market and hiring organization, case management certification may or may not be a requirement.

A variety of certification bodies for case management are available, each with its own eligibility requirements and practice standards (Table 18-3). Some certifications, such as the Commission for Case Management Certification (CCMC) and the American Institute of Outcomes Care Management (AIOCM), offer an interdisciplinary case management certification. Others, such as the ANA, offer case management certification and standards of practice specific to nurse case management. Currently, not all case management certification bodies endorse the minimal requirement of a postsecondary degree in a health-care–related area; however, all require extensive experience and employment as a CM. In addition, all certifying bodies require the candidate to submit an extensive profile of her or his practice and pass a written examination.

One of the newest certifications available is the Administrative Case Management Certification offered by the Center for Case Management. This certification was developed

TABLE 18-3 CASE MANAGEMENT CERTIFICATIONS AND AGENCY OVERSIGHT		
CERTIFICATION CREDENTIAL	TARGET PROFESSIONALS AND ELIGIBILITY	ORGANIZATION CONTACT INFORMATION
CCM—Certified Case Manager	Multidisciplinary case managers who practice in multiple practice settings. Includes nurses, social workers, psychologists, rehab therapists, physicians, and other specialties	Commission for Case Manager Certification (847) 818-0292 www.ccmcertification.org
CDMS—Certified Disability Management Specialist (formerly Certified Insurance Rehabilitation Specialist)	Any discipline working with individuals with disabilities, including disability managers, insurance-based rehabilitation specialists, and vocational counselors	The Commission for Disability Management Specialists (847) 394-2106 www.cdms.org
CMAC—Case Management Administrator, Certified	Experienced Case Managers with bachelor's or master's degree preparation; active case management certifications from A-CCC, CRRN, CCM, or CDMS may substitute for academic eligibility criteria; not limited to nurses	The Center for Case Management (508) 651-2600 www.cfcm.com
CMC—Case Management Certified	Provides national Case Management certification to individuals involved in outcomes management; candidates may be from any discipline and are certified based upon national examination or a review of their professional portfolio in which educational background, work experience, and relevant training in outcomes management are taken into consideration	American Institute of Outcomes Care Management (562) 945-9990 www.aiocm.com
CRC—Certified Rehabilitation Counselor	Geared toward rehab counselors with a master's degree or higher in Rehabilitation Counseling or a related field with experience in Rehab Counseling and/or Case Management.	The Commission on Rehabilitation Counselor Certification (847) 394-2104 www.crccertification.com
CRRN-A—Certified Registered Rehabilitation Nurse-Advanced	Registered nurses with a practice specialty in rehabilitation; being phased out; last exam scheduled for June, 2004, with certification until June 30, 2009	Association of Rehabilitation Nurses (800) 229-7530 www.rehabnurse.org
COHN-S—Certified Occupational Health Nurse–Specialist	Registered nurses with a practice specialty in Occupational Health with a bachelor of science degree or higher and provides direct care, management, education, consulting, and case management	American Board for Occupational Health Nursing (888) 842-2646 www.abohn.org
RN, C—Registered Nurse, Certified	Registered nurses who complete a modular credentialing examination for Nursing Case Management regardless of education	American Nurses Credentialing Center (800) 284-2378 www.nursingworld.org/ancc

based on the belief that there is a distinct level of knowledge and experience required by those who are responsible for the development, implementation, and evaluation of case management programs. This certification advocates a master's degree in health-care–related areas but acknowledges the competencies of those individuals with baccalaureate preparation in conjunction with substantial case management experience by permitting nonmaster's-prepared individuals to become certified. This certification tests for competencies in management, human resources, employment issues, and budgetary issues. Although there is a small component focused on clinical competency in the management of chronic diseases such as asthma, cardiovascular disease, and diabetes, this certification is primarily geared toward those in administrative positions responsible for the oversight of the business and operational management aspects of case management. APN CMs who assume such responsibilities are excellent candidates for this certification, although it does not appear to be directly relevant to the APN CM role as described in this chapter (K. Bower, personal communication, June, 1999).

The AIOCM offers certification for health-care professionals who have attained expertise in managing data and information used to improve the performance of case management–related processes and outcomes. This credential recognizes those individuals who are proficient in outcomes management implementation projects, data management methodologies, health-care economics, statistics, quality improvement, and linking outcomes data to health-care decision making. The AIOCM certification is not limited to NCMs or social workers. Medical doctors, executives, respiratory therapists, pharmacists, or any allied health professional may become certified. Certification criteria include meeting standards of general education, 3 to 5 years of health-care experience, education in outcomes case management, and successful completion of the AIOCM certification examination.

CONCLUSION: LOOKING TOWARD THE FUTURE OF APN CM PRACTICE

The APN CM role as described in this chapter is one that requires clinical expertise and system stewardship. The combination of these skills and competencies are likely to be of increasing importance as chronic conditions increase and as the emphasis in health-care shifts to patient safety and cost-effective quality care. According to the Institute of Medicine (2001), the need for leadership has never been greater, and the emphasis in health care is on "creating an infrastructure to support evidence-based practice, facilitating the use of information technology, aligning payment incentives and preparing the workforce to better serve patients in a world of expanding knowledge and rapid change" (p. 5).

The APN CM's contribution in creating and sustaining a culture of organizational learning is a natural outcome of the role when realized to its fullest potential. APN CMs are in an ideal position to promote the diffusion of evidence-based best practices into a health-care organization, as well as to evaluate outcomes. Because of current economic incentives that reward adherence to best practice protocols and evidence-based care standards by individual providers and provider systems, APN CMs will find that their contributions will be highly valued. For example, the CMS is currently conducting a Medicare demonstration project to incorporate incentives for quality into its standards and payments. Based upon the JCAHO and CMS Core Quality Measures for Acute MI, Pneumonia and Heart Failure, participating community health plans and hospitals will receive payment (between 1% and 2% of their annual Medicare DRG reimbursement) for performance that meets and exceeds national standards for practice standards such as appropriate administration of aspirin and beta blockers to acute myocardial infarction (MI) patients, timely and appropriate administration of antibiotics to pneumonia patients, and assessment of left ventricular function and discharge teaching for heart failure patients (CMS, 2004). Because of their system focus, the APN CM will be in an excellent position to identify process barriers that prevent compliance to such evidence-based care practices, and because of their clinical credibility and collaborative skills, the APN CM will be highly instrumental in promoting adherence to such guidelines by individual medical providers.

The APN CM's strengths in data and information management will also be invaluable as computerized physician order entry and electronic medical record systems are implemented. Because of the increasing complexity in health-care systems and technologies, it is likely that some APN CMs will shift their expertise towards nonclinical specialty roles such as outcomes management and nursing or systems informatics, while others retain a more distinct clinical focus. Increasingly, graduate nursing programs are offering such specialized education, confirming the need for these skills in the marketplace.

Because the health-care environment is increasing in complexity, it may become increasingly difficult for APN CMs to remain equally expert at both clinical care and systems management. For this reason, it is possible that the APN CM role may evolve into two distinct roles: one to manage clinical care and the other to manage the system. Unless a greater emphasis on outcomes and system management is placed on the traditional APN roles (e.g., NPs and CNSs), the need to continue the preparation of clinical experts who are also system advocates will remain high.

REFERENCES

American Case Management Association. (2003). [2002-2003 National Case Management Survey]. Unpublished raw data.

American Nurses Association. (1988). *Nursing case management*. Kansas City, MO: Author.

American Nurses Association. (1997). Telehealth: A tool for nursing practice. In *Nursing Trends & Issues*, ANA policy series. Washington, DC: Author.

American Nurses Association (2003a). *American Nurses Credentialing Center Certification*. Retrieved January 10, 2004, from http://nursingworld.org/ancc/certification/catalogs/PnPCat.pdf

American Nurses Association (2003b). *Frequently asked questions—about ANCC certification*. Retrieved May 18, 2004, from http://www.nursingworld.org/ancc/certification/cert/certfaqs.html

Baird, S. (1995). The impact of changing health care delivery on oncology practice. *Oncology Nursing: Patient Treatment and Support, 2*, 1-13.

Becker, M. H. (1974). *The health belief model and personal health behavior*. Thorofare, NJ: Charles B Slack.

Bodenheimer T., Lorig, K., Holman, H., & Grumbach, K. (2002). Patient self-management of chronic disease in primary care. *Journal of the American Medical Association, 288*(19), 2469-2475.

Boult, C., Pacala, J. T., & Boult, L. B. (1995). Targeting elders for geriatric evaluation and management: Reliability, validity, and practicality of a questionnaire. *Aging: Clinical and Experimental Research, 7*, 159-164.

Brooten, D., Gennaro, S., Knapp, H., Jovene, N., Brown, L., & York, R. (1991). Functions of the CNS in early discharge and home follow-up of very low birthweight infants. *Clinical Nurse Specialist, 5*, 196-201.

Brooten, D., Naylor, M., York, R., Brown, L., Munro, B., Hollingsworth, A., et al. (2001). Lessons learned from testing the quality cost model of advanced practice nursing (APN) transitional care. *Journal of Nursing Scholarship, 34*, 359-375.

Brooten, D., Youngblut, J., Deatrick, J., Naylor, M., & York, R. (2003). Patient problems, advanced practice nurse (APN) interventions, time and contacts among five patient groups. *Journal of Nursing Scholarship, 35*, 73-79.

Brooten, D., Youngblut, J. M., Deatrick, J., Naylor, M., & York, R. (2002). *APN transitional care: patient problems and outcomes, APN interventions, time and number of APN contacts in 5 patient groups*. Paper presented at the Advancing Nursing Practice Excellence: State of the Science Conference, Washington, D.C. Retrieved September 6, 2003, from http://stti.confex.com/stti/sos13/techprogram/paper_12247.htm

Bryson, K., Naqvi, A., Callahan, P., & Fontenot, D. (1990). Brief admission program: An alliance of inpatient care and outpatient case management. *Journal of Psychosocial Nursing, 28,* 19-23.

Bushnell, F. K. (1992, October). Self-care teaching for congestive heart failure patients. *Journal of Gerontological Nursing, 18,* 27-32.

Calkin, J. (1984). A model for advanced nursing practice. *Journal of Nursing Administration, 14,* 24-30.

Case Management Society of America. (1995). *Standard of practice for case management.* Little Rock, AR: Author.

Case Management Society of America. (2002). *Standards of practice for case management.* Little Rock, AR: Author.

Centers for Medicare and Medicaid Services (1998, November 2). Rules and regulations. *Federal Register, 63,* 58871-58874.

Centers for Medicare and Medicaid Services. (2004, March). *Hospital quality initiative overview.* Retrieved May 18, 2004, from http://www.cms.hhs.gov/quality/hospital/overview.pdf

Cesta, T. (1993). The link between continuous quality improvement and case management. *Journal of Nursing Administration, 23,* 55-61.

Cesta, T., & Tahan, H. (2003): *The nurse's guide to managed care.* St. Louis: Mosby.

Chen, A., Brown, R., Archibald, N., Aliotta, S., & Fox, P. D. (2000). *Best practices in coordinated care* (Mathematica Policy Research, Inc., Reference No. 8534-004). Retrieved on September 7, 2003, from http: //www.mathematica-mpr.com/3rdLevel/bestprac.htm/.

Chin, P., & Papenausen, J. (2002). Integrating concepts of managed care and nursing case management into academic curricula. In Cesta, T., (Ed.), *Survival strategies for nurses in managed care* (pp. 196-217). St. Louis: Mosby.

Connors, H. (1993). Impact of care management modalities on curricula. In K. Kelly & M. Maas (Eds.), *Managing nursing care: Promise and pitfalls* (pp. 190-207). St. Louis: Mosby.

Cooper, D. M. (1990). Today—assessment and intuition: Tomorrow—projections. In D. M. Cooper, P. A. Minarik, & P. S. A. Sparacino (Eds.), *The clinical nurse specialist: Implementation and impact* (pp. 285-298). Norwalk, CT: Appleton & Lange.

Cronin, C., & Maklebust, J. (1989). Case-managed care: Capitalizing on the CNS. *Nursing Management, 20,* 38-47.

Daleiden, A. (1993). The CNS as trauma case manager. *Clinical Nurse Specialist, 7,* 295-298.

Doell Smith, L. (1994). Continuity of care through nursing case management of the chronically ill child. *Clinical Nurse Specialist, 8,* 65-68.

Donagrandi, M. A., & Eddy, M. (2000). Ethics of case management: Implications for advanced practice nursing. *Clinical Nurse Specialist, 14,* 241-246.

Eichert, J. H., & Patterson, R. B. (1997). Factors affecting the success of disease management. *Infusion, 3,* 31-38.

Eichert, J. H., Wong, H., & Smith, D. R. (1997). The disease management development process.

In W. E. Todd & D. Nash (Eds.), *Disease management: A system approach to improving patient outcomes* (pp. 27-60). Chicago: American Hospital Publishing.

Ethridge, P. (1991). A nursing HMO: Carondelet St. Mary's experience. *Nursing Management, 22,* 22-27.

Falter, E. J., Cesta, T. G., Concert, C., & Mason, D. J. (1999). Development of a graduate nursing program in case management. *Journal of Case Management, 5,* 50-56.

Flynn, A., & Kilgallen, M. (1993). Case management: A multidisciplinary approach to the evaluation of cost and quality standards. *Journal of Nursing Care Quality, 8,* 58-66.

Fralic, M. (1992). The nurse case manager: Focus, selection, preparation, and measurement. *Journal of Nursing Administration, 22,* 13-14, 46.

Friedman, N. M., Gleeson, J. M., Kent, M. J., Foris, M., & Rodriguez, D. J. (1998). Management of diabetes mellitus in the Lovelace Health Systems' Episodes of Care Program. *Effective Clinical Practice, 1,* 5-11.

Gaedeke-Norris, M., & Hill, C. (1991). The clinical nurse specialist: Developing the case manager role. *Dimensions of Critical Care Nursing, 10,* 346-352.

Gournic, J. (1989). Clinical leadership, management, and the CNS. In A. B. Hamric & J. A. Spross (Eds.), *The clinical nurse specialist in theory and practice* (2nd ed., pp. 227-250). Philadelphia: W. B. Saunders.

Hamric, A. B. (1989). History and overview of the CNS role. In A. B. Hamric & J. A. Spross (Eds.), *The clinical nurse specialist in theory and practice* (2nd ed., pp. 3-18). Philadelphia: W. B. Saunders.

Hamric, A. B. (1992). Creating our future: Challenges and opportunities for the clinical nurse specialist. *Oncology Nursing Forum, 19*(Suppl. 1), 11-15.

Hamric, A. B., & Taylor, J. W. (1989). Role development of the CNS. In A. B. Hamric & J. A. Spross (Eds.), *The clinical nurse specialist in theory and practice* (2nd ed., pp. 41-82). Philadelphia: W. B. Saunders.

Hartigan, M., Cesta, T. G., Mapes, D., Burrows-Hudson, S., Prathikanti, R., Lamb, G., et al. (2003). The anemia demonstration management demonstration project: Development, implementation and testing of a multidisciplinary action plan (MAP) for hemodialysis patients in the community. *Care Management, 9,* 19-28

Hopkins, S. C., Mundinger, M. O'Neil, Lenz, E. R., Lin, S. X., & Clark, J. (2002, September 27). *Patterns of NP practice: Results from a national survey.* Paper presented at the Advancing Nursing Practice Excellence: State of the Science Conference, Washington, D.C. Retrieved on September 6, 2003, at http://stti.confex.com/stti/sos13/techprogram/paper_11412.htm

Hospodar, J. A., & Zazworsky, D. (1997, September/October). Population health management development through a national Medicare demonstration project. *The Alliance for Healthcare Strategy and Marketing,* 9-11.

Hospodar, J. A., & Zazworsky, D. (1999, January). High-risk efforts. *The Alliance for Healthcare Strategy and Marketing, 6*-7.

Institute of Medicine (2001). *Crossing the quality chasm: A new health system for the 21st century.* Washington, DC: National Academies Press.

Jenkins, M., & Sullivan-Marx, E. (1994). Nurse practitioners and community health nurses: Clinical partnerships and future visions. *Nursing Clinics of North America, 29*, 459-471.

Kotler, P., & Zaltman, G. (1971). Social marketing: An approach to planned social change. *Journal of Marketing, 35*, 3-12.

Ladden, M. (1991). On-site perinatal case management: An HMO model. *Journal of Perinatal-Neonatal Nursing, 5*, 27-32.

Lamb, G., Mahn, V., & Dahl, R. (1996). Goals of an effective delivery system for the chronically ill. *Managed Care Quarterly, 4*, 46-53.

Lamb, G., & Stempel, J. (1994). Nurse case management from the client's view: Growing as insider-expert. *Nursing Outlook, 42*, 7-13.

Lamb, G., & Zazworsky, D. (1999, January). *Disease management* [slide presentation]. Presentation conducted at the Carondelet Health Network Executive Team Meeting, Tucson, Arizona.

Lamb, G., & Zazworsky, D. (2000). Improving outcomes fast: The FAST approach to disease management. *Advance for Providers of Post-Acute Care, 3*, 28-29.

Landesberg, P. (1999). In the beginning, there were Deming and Juran. *Journal for Quality & Participation,* November/December, 59-61.

Lynn-McHale, D., Fitzpatrick, E., & Shaller, R. (1993). Case management: Development of a model. *Clinical Nurse Specialist, 7*, 299-307.

Madden, M., & Reid Ponte, P. (1994). Advanced practice roles in the managed care environment. *Journal of Nursing Administration, 24*, 56-62.

Mahn, V. (1993). Clinical nurse case management: A service line approach. *Nursing Management, 24*, 48-50.

Mahn, V. (1999). Use of claims data to identify the right population to case manage: Pandora's box or the wave of the future. *MIDS Monitor,* July Supplement. MIDS, Inc. Tucson, AZ.

Mahn, V. A., & Spross, J. A. (1996). Nurse case management as an advanced practice role. In A. B. Hamric, J. A. Spross, & C. M. Hanson (Eds.), *Advanced nursing practice: An integrative approach* (pp. 445-465). Philadelphia: W. B. Saunders.

Mahn, V. A., & Zazworsky, D. (2000): The advanced practice nurse case manager. In A.B. Hamric, J.A. Spross, & C.M. Hanson (Eds.), *Advanced nursing practice: An integrative approach* (pp. 549-606). Philadelphia: W. B. Saunders.

Marash, S., Berman, P., & Flynn, M. (2003). Fusion management: Harnessing the power of Six Sigma, Lean, ISO 9001:2000, Malcolm Baldrige, TQM, and other quality breakthroughs of the past century. Fairfax, VA: QSU Publishing Company.

Martin, K. S., & Scheet, N. J. (1992). *The Omaha system: Applications for community health nursing.* Philadelphia: W. B. Saunders.

Milliman & Robertson, Inc. (1999). *Healthcare management guidelines.* San Diego: Author.

Newman, M. (1990). Toward an integrative model of professional practice. *Journal of Professional Nursing, 6*, 167-173.

Newman, M. (1994). *Health as expanding consciousness* (2nd ed.). New York: National League for Nursing Press.

Newman, M., Lamb, G., & Michaels, C. (1989). Nurse case management: The coming together of theory and practice. *Nursing & Health Care, 12*, 404-408.

Nugent, K. (1992). The clinical nurse specialist as case manager in a collaborative practice model: Bridging the gap between quality and cost of care. *Clinical Nurse Specialist, 6*, 106-111.

Office of Technology Assessment. (1986). *Nurse practitioners, physician assistants, and certified nurse midwives: A policy analysis* (Health Care Technology Study No. OTA-HCS-37). Washington, DC: Author.

Papenhausen, J. L. (1996). Discovering and achieving client outcomes. In E. L. Cohen (Ed.), *Nurse case management in the 21st century* (pp. 257-268). St Louis: Mosby.

Parker, M., Quinn, J., Viehl, M., McKinley, A., Polich, C., Detzner, D., et al. (1990). Case management in rural areas: Definition, clients, financing, staffing, and service delivery issues. *Nursing Economics, 8*, 103-109.

Peterson, K., & Kane, D. (1997). Beyond disease management: Population-based health management. In W. E. Todd & D. Nash (Eds.), *Disease management: A systems approach to improving patient outcomes* (pp. 235-259). Chicago: American Hospital Publishing.

Plocher, D. W. (1996). Disease management. In P. R. Kongstvedt (Ed.), *The managed health care services* (3rd ed.). Gaithersburg, MD: Aspen Publishers.

Porter-O'Grady, T. (1996). Nurses as advanced practitioners and primary care providers. In E.L. Cohen (Ed.), *Nurse case management in the 21st century* (pp. 10-20). St. Louis: Mosby.

Powell, S. K. (2000). *Advanced case management: Outcomes and beyond.* Philadelphia: Lippincott.

Prochaska, J. O., & DiClemente, C. C. (1999). *Transtheoretical models/stages of change.* Retrieved on September 14, 2003, from http://hsc.usf.edu/~kmbrown/Stages_of_Change_Overview.htm

Prochaska, J. O., DiClemente, C. C., & Norcross, J. C. (1992). In search of how people change: Applications to addictive behaviors. *American Psychologist, 49*, 1102-1114.

Rieve, J. A. (1999). Case identification and selection outcomes. *The Case Manager, 10*, 22-25.

Riley, T. (1992). HIV-infected client care: Case management and the HIV team. *Clinical Nurse Specialist, 6*, 136-140.

Rosenfeld, P. McEvoy, M. & Glassman, K. (2003). Measuring practice patterns among acute care nurse practitioners. *Journal of Nursing Administration, 33*(3), 159-165

Rotz, N., Yates, J., & Schare, B. (1994). Application of the case management model to a trauma patient. *Clinical Nurse Specialist, 8*, 180-186.

Schroer, K. (1991). Case management: Clinical nurse specialist and nurse practitioner, converging roles. *Clinical Nurse Specialist, 5*, 189-194.

Shelton, P., Sager, M.A., & Schraeder, C. (2000). The Community Assessment Risk Screen (CARS): Identifying elderly persons at risk for hospitalization or emergency department visit. *The American Journal of Managed Care, 6*, 925-933.

Sherman, J., & Johnson, P. (1994). CNS as unit-based case manager. *Clinical Nurse Specialist, 8*, 76-80.

Smith, M. (1993). Case management and nursing theory-based practice. *Nursing Science Quarterly, 6,* 8-9.

Stempel, J., Carlson, A., & Michaels, C. (1996). Working in partnership. In E. L. Cohen (Ed.), *Nurse case management in the 21st century* (pp. 124-132). St Louis: Mosby.

Strong, A. (1991). Case management of a patient with multi-system failure. *Critical Care Quarterly, 11,* 10-18.

Strong, A. (1992). Case management and the CNS. *Clinical Nurse Specialist, 6,* 64.

Tidwell, S. (1994). The critical care clinical nurse specialist as case manager. In A. Gawlinski & L. Kern (Eds.), *The clinical nurse specialist in critical care* (pp. 62-79). Philadelphia: W.B. Saunders.

Todd, W. E., & Nash, D. (Eds.). (1997). *Disease management: A systems approach to improving patient outcomes.* Chicago: American Hospital Publishing.

Trinidad, E. (1993). Case management: A model of case management. *Clinical Nurse Specialist, 7,* 221-223.

Tweed, V. (1998) The brave new reality of telemedicine. *Business & Health, 16,* 34-39.

Ulrich, C.M., Soeken, K.L., & Miller, N. (2003). Ethical conflict associated with managed care: Views of nurse practitioners. *Nursing Research, 52,* 168-175.

Utilization Review Accreditation Commission. (2002, August 6). URAC announces its first disease management accreditations: Program empowers patients to manage chronic care needs. Retrieved May 17, 2004, from http://www.urac.org/news_release.asp?navid=news&pagename=news_release&id=143

Wagner, J., & Menke, E. (1992). Case management of homeless families. *Clinical Nurse Specialist, 6,* 65-71.

Ward, M. D., & Rieve, J. A. (1997). The role of case management in disease management. In W. E. Todd & D. Nash (Eds.), *Disease management: A systems approach to improving patient outcomes* (pp. 235-259). Chicago: American Hospital Publishing.

Ware, J. E., Snow, K. K., Kosinski, M., & Gandek, B. (1993). *SF-36 Health Survey manual and interpretation guide.* Boston: The Health Institute, New England Medical Center.

Zalta, E., Eichner, H. L., Henry, M.E., et al. (1994). New trends in disease management. *Managing Employee Health Benefits, 2,* 1.

Zander, K. (1993). The impact of managing care on the role of a nurse. In K. Kelly & M. Maas (Eds.), *Managing nursing care: Promise and pitfalls* (pp. 65-82). St Louis: Mosby.

Zazworsky, D. (2002a). Disease management in managed care. In T. Cesta (Ed.), *Survival strategies for nurses in managed care* (pp. 376-397). St Louis: Mosby.

Zazworsky, D. (2002b). The nurse on a TV news team, in policy and politics. In D. J. Mason, J. K. Leavitt, and M. W. Chaffee (Eds.), *Nursing and health care* (4th ed.). St. Louis, W. B. Saunders.

Zazworsky, D., & Hospodar, J. A. (1996). Marketing nurse case management services. In E. L. Cohen (Ed.), *Nurse case management in the 21st century* (pp. 202-210). St. Louis: Mosby.

Zitter, M. (1994). *The Zitter Group special report: Disease management.* San Francisco: The Zitter Group.

CHAPTER 19

Evolving and Innovative Opportunities for Advanced Practice Nursing

JEANNE SALYER • ANN. B. HAMRIC

INTRODUCTION

Technological advances and economic and sociocultural conditions have sustained a climate of change in the health-care environment, and opportunities for advanced practice nursing have emerged in the wake of these changes. As specialties have emerged, many new roles have evolved from specialty nursing practice and have expanded to incorporate the core attributes of advanced practice nursing (see Chapters 1 and 3). Some of these roles have clearly evolved as advanced practice roles, while others are in various stages of evolution. Not all specialties, however, will evolve into advanced practice roles, for a variety of reasons. For example, some specialties evolve away from the core definition of advanced practice nursing, which encompasses direct clinical practice and clinical expertise as essential ingredients (Chapter 3). These specialties, such as informatics and nursing administration, arise as specialties and remain specialties because direct clinical practice is not a requisite role component.

The purpose of this chapter is to examine some currently evolving specialties and characterize stages in their continuing evolution from specialty nursing practice to advanced nursing practice. These specialties have not yet fully evolved to an advanced level. The focus of the discussion is on the various specialties—not on particular advanced practice nursing roles, such as clinical nurse specialist (CNS), nurse practitioner (NP), certified nurse midwife (CNM), or certified registered nurse anesthetist (CRNA). Specialties selected for inclusion in this discussion were chosen for one or more of the following reasons: (1) the specialty has the potential to evolve to advanced practice because of the complexity of care required by the patient population; (2) the specialty has arisen due to technological advances and the influence of these advances on the delivery of health care; (3) the specialty is growing because of the rising incidence of health problems in the population; and/or (4) the specialty's patient population needs sophisticated care across settings in the complex health care environment. Opportunities in these evolving specialties for advanced practice nurses (APNs) are discussed, and a framework for evaluating progress toward advanced practice status is illustrated. Exemplars provided by APNs in the specialty were deliberately chosen to illuminate the added value of advanced practice competencies to these evolving specialties.

PATTERNS IN THE EVOLUTION OF SPECIALTY TO ADVANCED PRACTICE NURSING

Before discussion of the evolution of specialty nursing practice into advanced practice, it is important to make a distinction between the two, as well as to clarify the use of the term "subspecialty" in this chapter. *Specialization* reflects a concentration in a selected clinical area in nursing. Specialties can be further characterized as "nursing practice that intersects with another body of knowledge, has a direct impact on nursing practice, and is supportive of the direct care rendered to patients by other registered nurses" (American Nurses Association [ANA], 2003). As the profession of nursing has responded to changes in health care, the need for specialty knowledge has increased. The classic specialties in nursing have been pediatric, psychiatric/mental health, obstetrics (now termed *women's health*), community/public health, and medical-surgical nursing. Newer specialties that have emerged include, for example, concentrations in critical care or geriatric nursing. As a given specialty coalesces out of practitioners' needs to share practice experiences and specialty knowledge, nurses often form specialty nursing organizations. Some examples include the American Association of Critical-Care Nurses (AACN), the Oncology

Nursing Society (ONS), and the Association of Women's Health, Obstetric, and Neonatal Nurses (AWHONN). Scope and standards of practice statements legitimize specialty designation and prompt efforts to provide opportunities for specialty education and certification.

Advanced practice nursing *includes* specialization but goes beyond it—involving *expansion*, which legitimizes role autonomy, and *advancement*, which is characterized by the integration of a broad range of theoretical, research-based, and practical knowledge (ANA, 2003; see Chapter 3). Thus, advanced practice nursing reflects concentrated knowledge in a specialty that offers the opportunity for expanded and autonomous practice based on a broader practical and theoretical knowledge base.

The term *specialty* suggests that the focus of practice is limited to *parts of the whole* (ANA, 1995). For example, family NPs, who classically see themselves as generalists, have in fact specialized in one of the many facets of health care, namely primary care. *Subspecialization* further defines the focus of practice. In subspecialty practice, there is *further expansion* of knowledge and skill in a delimited clinical area. With this expanded knowledge and skill, there is potentially further advancement of theoretical, evidence-based, and practical knowledge in caring for a specific patient population base. Examples of subspecialty practices within the specialty of medical-surgical nursing include diabetes, transplant nursing, and palliative care nursing. Examples of subspecialty practice within the specialty of psychiatric/mental health nursing include substance abuse/addictions and geriatric psychiatry. Notably, most of the practice opportunities chosen for discussion in this chapter are subspecialty practices. This distinction is important, particularly for certification and regulatory reasons. However, for the sake of brevity in the remainder of the chapter, we will refer to both specialty and subspecialty practices as *specialties*. The expansion of advanced practice nursing is increasingly occurring in subspecialty practice. Indeed, expanding the boundaries of specialty nursing practice into subspecialties places APNs on the cutting edge of clinical care delivery in a complex, ever-changing, health-care environment.

The evolution of specialty nursing practice to advanced nursing practice follows a trajectory that has been described by several authors (Beitz, 2000; Bigbee & Amidii-Nouri, 2000; Hamric, 2000; Lewis, 2000; see Chapter 1). Hanson and Hamric (2003) synthesized these observations and characterized this evolution as having three distinct stages (Table 19-1). Initially, the specialty develops in response to changing patient needs—needs that are usually a result of new technology, new medical specialties, and/or changes in the health care workforce. For example, a lack of pediatric residents created an opportunity for development of the neonatal NP role (De Nicola et al., 1994). A second phase of development is characterized by progress to the point that organized "training" in the specialty begins. This training is often institution-specific, on-the-job training that develops experts in the specialty. Some of these institution-specific programs develop into certificate programs; however, the content may not be standardized, and the quality of these programs may vary. In the third phase, the knowledge base required for specialty practice becomes more extensive, and the scope of practice of the nurse with specialty training expands. There is growing recognition of the additional knowledge and skill needed for increasingly complex practice in the specialty. It is not unusual at this stage to see APNs in other specialties migrate into an evolving specialty and further expand the specialty by infusing it with advanced practice core competencies, making the specialty resemble advanced practice and creating new calls for evolution to this higher level. Over time, pressure for standardization of education and skills involved in the specialty arise from clinicians, the profession, and regulators. Certificate-level training programs are moved into graduate schools that assume responsibility for preparing nurses for these evolving

TABLE 19-1	THREE STAGES IN THE EVOLUTION OF ADVANCED PRACTICE NURSING
STAGE	CHARACTERISTICS
Stage I	SPECIALTY BEGINS Specialty develops in practice settings • Development driven by increasing complexity in care demands, new technology, changing workforce opportunities • On-the-job training and expansion of practice • Not exclusively nursing
Stage II	SPECIALTY ORGANIZES Organized training for specialty practice begins • Institution-specific training develops • Initially uses apprenticeship model • Progresses to certificate training • Specialty organization forms • Certification exam develops but may not be nursing-specific • Writings appear on role of nurse in specialty
Stage III	PRESSURES MOUNT FOR STANDARDIZATION Knowledge base grows; pressures mount for standardization and graduate education • Knowledge base keeps growing, and scope of practice expands for practitioners in the specialty • Expanded practice leads to expanded regulatory oversight • Leaders call for transition to graduate education and differentiated practice to standardize practice in the specialty • APNs migrate to specialty, or specialty nurses return to school • Articles appear differentiating APN role in specialty

Adapted from Hanson, C.M., & Hamric, A.B. (2003). Reflections on the continuing evolution of advanced practice nursing, *Nursing Outlook, 51*, p. 204.

specialties – improving standardization, elevating the status of the specialty, and fostering its emergence as an advanced practice role. In this final stage of the trajectory, graduate education becomes an expected level of preparation (Hanson & Hamric, 2003).

It is important to note that these stages are dynamic and not mutually exclusive. It is not unusual for specialties to show characteristics of more than one stage simultaneously (e.g., graduate programs may begin to develop at the same time that most practitioners in the specialty are still prepared in certificate programs). In addition, the duration of each stage may significantly vary by specialty.

It is our contention that the evolution from specialty to advanced practice nursing can represent a natural maturation that should result from deliberate, logical planning to strengthen the education and broaden the scope of practice of specialty nurses. Some of these roles evolve to fulfill needs of specific patient populations or the needs of organizations. In some cases, changes in the legal recognition and regulation of practice also influence the movement toward advanced practice nursing. Complex and often controversial issues must be addressed both prior to and during this process (Box 19-1). In the following sections, the evolution of particular specialties to advanced practice nursing is described and these issues are discussed. Some specialties are struggling to evolve, and change is haphazard. Others are following a course of planned change and have emerged (or will soon do so) at the advanced practice level. Two challenges all evolving specialties share are the need to gain support both within and external to nursing for these roles and the need to clearly delineate their potential contributions in the health-care environment.

BOX 19-1 • ISSUES IN THE EVOLUTION OF SPECIALTY TO ADVANCED PRACTICE NURSING

1. Defining the attributes of advanced practice in the specialty
2. Delineating the core competencies of the specialty as encompassing the core competencies of advanced practice
3. Delineating a vision of advanced practice that may step outside of nursing's traditional vision of what constitutes an advanced practice role and gaining support within nursing and the health care community for the role
4. Standardizing curricula for achieving competency at the advanced practice level
5. Clarifying certification and credentialing requirements
6. Overcoming legal and regulatory issues that are barriers to patient and/or consumer access to advanced practice nurses
7. Promoting recognition of advanced practice nurses and nursing as a profession
8. Clarifying APN role titles to be consistent and decrease confusion

---

Adapted from Hanson, C.M., & Hamric, A.B. (2003). Reflections on the continuing evolution of advanced practice nursing, *Nursing Outlook*, 51, p. 205.

INNOVATIVE PRACTICE OPPORTUNITIES: STAGE I

The initial stage of the evolution from specialty practice to advanced practice is characterized by the development of a specialty focus. Numerous examples are apparent in the history of nursing, which is replete with accounts of nursing's response to unmet patient needs. As a consequence, definable specialties emerge as nurses expand their practice to include the knowledge and skills necessary to meet the needs of patients requiring specialty care. Examples include the specialty of enterostomal therapy (ET) nursing, now known as wound, ostomy, continence (WOC) nursing, and forensic nursing, which encompasses the care provision in correctional facilities, psychiatric settings, and emergency departments as nurse examiners care for sexual assault and child abuse victims (Doyle, 2001; Hutson, 2002; Maeve & Vaughn, 2001; McCrone & Shelton, 2001). As specialties begin to coalesce, the practice may not be viewed as a nursing role. However, as the specialty evolves, the valuable contributions of nurses begin to distinguish them from other care providers.

Several evolving roles in nursing are characterized as being "innovative." Some of these roles do not reflect the core competencies of advanced practice nursing, and the role components differ significantly, in some cases, from those of an APN. For example, if the focus of practice in forensic nursing is on the gathering of legal evidence, not sustained clinical practice using advanced practice core competency elements, the role will not evolve to an advanced practice level. Regardless, nurses functioning in these specialties, some of whom are APNs, make unique contributions to the health of specific populations of patients. One such role to be explored as a Stage I specialty is that of the parish nurse.

Parish Nursing

Recognized as a specialty by the ANA in 1998 when *The Scope and Standards of Parish Nursing Practice* was published (Health Ministries Association, 1998), parish nursing is an innovative practice model that promotes healthier communities and facilitates community partnerships (Brown et al., 1996). A parish nurse is a registered professional nurse who serves as a member of the ministry staff of a faith community to promote "health-as-wholeness" within the faith community, its family and individual members, and the community it serves. Parish nurses do this through the independent practice of nursing, as defined by the nurse practice act in their jurisdiction (Health Ministries Association, 1998). Direct nursing care is not the focus; rather, parish nurses function as liaisons between the medical and faith communities (Boland, 1998). Parish nurses expand home health and public health provider roles by providing health education, screening and health assessment, counseling, and referral (Brown et al., 1996). While these role functions encompass some of those characterizing advanced practice, the scope of practice as described is limited, and direct clinical practice is not a central competency.

There are two basic models of parish nursing: institution based and congregation based. In institution-based models, the congregation contracts with hospitals or multi-institutional health-care organizations (Coldewey, 1993; DeSchepper, 1999; Drummond, Buss, & Ladigo, 1992) or other institutions (Lough, 1999; Rydholm, 1997) to provide or organize parish nursing services for the congregation. In this model the parish nurse may be employed by the hospital or community agency that provides salary, benefits, resources, supervision, and support for the position. The second form is a congregation-based model in which a congregation develops a parish nurse program. In this model, the parish nurse may be employed by the congregation with salary, benefits, support, and supervision provided by the church itself. In both models, volunteer nurses work to supplement the services provided by the parish nurse, and in some cases all services may be provided by volunteers rather than paid staff (Lloyd & Solari-Twadell, 1994; Solari-Twadell & Westberg, 1991; Striepe, 1989).

Parish nurses, like nurses in every specialty, are prepared at a variety of educational levels—from diploma to doctoral degree—and in a variety of settings, including divinity schools. Because of the need to plan programs that target community needs, parish nursing consultation is often provided by nurses prepared at the master's and doctoral educational levels (Magilvey & Brown, 1997). This particular model predominates when university schools of nursing consult or form partnerships with faith communities to assist parish nurses with program development, implementation, and evaluation. Thus, different levels of parish nursing practice appear to be emerging. Because parish nurses may reach as much as 40% of the U.S. population in any given week (Ryan, 1995), APNs who function as parish nurses in faith communities need to carve out a niche for themselves and take the opportunity to advance the contributions of nursing to health care in this nontraditional setting.

Although there is limited support in the literature for this position, Magilvey and Brown (1997) believe that parish nursing should become an APN role requiring graduate education because of the independent nature of practice in the context of a community-based setting. Parish nursing is congruent with the movement toward building healthier communities, with its attention to primary health care of populations across the life span and to primary, secondary, and tertiary prevention. Health promotion and care management interventions are integral parts of an advanced practice nursing role in a community-based delivery system. Despite the fact that some advanced practice nursing role components are enacted by parish nurses, the evolution of this specialty into an advanced practice role may be limited by a focus on aggregate populations (the faith community) and an inability to delineate the core competencies of the specialty as encompassing the core competencies of advanced practice nursing. Furthermore, although parish nursing is a specialty, nurses in the specialty are only beginning to organize, suggesting that the specialty has not fully coalesced, despite the development of standards of practice. Thus, the potential for this role to evolve to an advanced practice role seems limited and uncertain at present.

As depicted in Exemplar 19-1, within the specialty of parish nursing, the opportunity is emerging to work with specific populations, similar to those of an APN within a more traditional health care setting. As will be seen in other specialty practices, the exemplar also illustrates that parish nursing is being influenced by APNs, such as NPs and CNSs, who

EXEMPLAR 19-1

THOUGHTS ON PARISH NURSING

As a neuroscience CNS, for many years I assisted my neighbors, friends and church members with health-care concerns and questions. Most of the assistance came in the form of answering questions about a new diagnosis or making suggestions for a specialty referral. Over the past few years, there have been dramatic increases in the number and complexity of requests from church members for assistance with health-care concerns. The requests have, in part, been driven by demographic changes and technical advances that have resulted in an increasingly elderly and chronically ill population. The increase in requests has also arisen out of the crisis that currently exists within the health-care system: people need information because of a lack time and resources on the part of health-care personnel and institutions to meet their needs. Additionally, there is increased consumer need for advocacy within the health-care environment.

Specifically within my own congregation, the needs for assistance are diverse. As a parish nurse, I serve an inner-city, culturally diverse, 900-member church. In part, the increased requests for help with health care have been due to the "graying" of the membership, with the church predominantly consisting of senior citizens and frail elderly people. Requests for assistance most often come in the form of asking for help in navigating the health-care system and to obtain information and services that can only be obtained from someone with "insider" knowledge of the system. Because of these needs within my church, a parish nursing program was developed and a paid parish nursing position was created.

The emphasis in many parish nursing education programs, including my own, has been to improve holistic health through health education and health promotion within the congregation. However, I have found my practice as a parish nurse to be an experience that extends well beyond those areas. Health education and health promotion have been a small part of my role in the church – including activities such as conducting an annual health fair, blood pressure screening, and health education classes. However, in serving the elderly and chronically ill members of the congregation, most of my practice has been aimed at helping individual church members and families successfully navigate their health-care experience.

My parish nursing colleagues have heard me comment frequently that the complexity of the issues that I have had to address in my role have, at times, been well beyond my area of clinical expertise. Success in meeting these role challenges has come from being guided by a spiritual model of caring coupled with my experience as an APN. As a parish nurse, I have used every skill that I developed as a nurse, particularly as an APN focusing on direct practice, education, collaboration, and consultation. My role as a paid parish nurse working with a health advisory committee also puts me in a leadership role. The health care issues I have faced with church members in 18 months of practice have ranged from assisting families to negotiate end-of-life care issues to assisting a brittle diabetic through an amputation and loss of independence and to dealing with church members with severe psychiatric disorders. Several of my parishioners have been terminally ill. I intervened by obtaining referrals, facilitating symptom management, attending doctor's visits with patients and families, educating patients and family members about medications, treatments, and the disease process—and, most important, how to become their own advocates. I have provided psychological and spiritual support—being present with the family when the patient wished to die at home. I have collaborated with nurses in hospital settings and home care and hospice agencies to obtain needed services for church members. I have also collaborated with physicians to advocate for patients to obtain needed services. My care did not end with the deaths of the church members but instead extended to grief support for their families. These and similar experiences prompted me to organize a grief support group for church members.

Continued

EXEMPLAR 19-1

THOUGHTS ON PARISH NURSING—cont'd

Because of the complexity of the needs in the congregation I serve, I often found it difficult to provide health education programs to meet the needs of church members. After a year of practice, I developed a health advisory committee to assist with the health programming for the church. The committee consists of other nurses in the congregation with varied clinical backgrounds, as well as a church member with training as an emergency medical technician. Other church members with social work, physical therapy, and medical backgrounds also provide assistance.

Although it has been suggested that parish nursing is a subspecialty of community health nursing, I would argue that this is not the case. While parish nursing is being incorporated into the curricula of schools of nursing, the majority of parish nurses are currently educated within a nonacademic spiritual model, such as through a seminary program or divinity school. The focus of these programs is the promotion of health based on a spiritual foundation. While the care of parish nurses is delivered within the faith community, the care delivered to the congregation by the nurse is *focused on individuals* as they exist within that faith community. Certainly a core focus in the care of members of a congregation is to provide health education and health promotion within a spiritual context. However, once a parish nurse enters the "real world" of the individuals who constitute a faith community and begins to address the special needs of members, parish nursing practice moves well beyond health education and health promotion as practiced in community health to something much more individualized and complex.

It is reasonable to suggest that parish nursing practice has elements that indicate the potential to evolve to an advanced practice role. The practice for many congregational parish nurses arises from the needs of that congregation. My parish nursing practice has become a practice that addresses the needs of the elderly and the chronically ill while others target the needs of children and adolescents within the faith community.

We gratefully acknowledge Sherry Fox, PhD, RN, Richmond, Va., for her assistance with this exemplar.

bring their competencies, skills, and specialty expertise to that practice. As these nurses continue to practice as parish nurses, their presence may well have an impact on parish nursing practice and create the momentum required to move it toward the advanced practice level.

Parish nursing, while not an advanced practice specialty, is a unique and innovative role. Because it is in its infancy, it is difficult to predict whether it will emerge at the advanced practice level. Despite this uncertainty, members of the faith community are benefiting from parish nursing and the added value that an APN brings to the specialty.

Commentary: Stage I

For the Stage I specialty to evolve to an advanced practice level, a number of issues must be addressed (see Box 19-1). Parish nursing provides a good example. Although some authors consider parish nursing to be an advanced practice role, others do not. The strong emphasis of parish nursing on the faith community is noted in Exemplar 19-1; however, there is also a component of direct clinical practice with individuals—an aspect of parish nursing that is not thoroughly described in the literature. Thus, the functions of the parish nurse seem to be determined by the aggregate congregation, the individual(s) in need of care or support, and the knowledge and skills of the individual parish nurse. With this variability, there is as yet no clarification of advanced practice attributes necessary for parish nursing practice, nor is there a unified vision of this specialty evolving in the APN direction. Training programs have recently been developed, but there is no standardization, nor is there certification for this practice. Many parish nurses are volunteer members of their congregations, so legal and regulatory issues are moot. In all of these ways, parish nursing exemplifies characteristics of the early coalescing seen in Stage I specialty development.

SPECIALTITES IN TRANSITION: STAGE II

Stage II roles are characterized by progress in the evolution of the specialty to the point that organized training in the specialty begins. This training is often institution-specific, on-the-job training that develops experts in the specialty. The two roles that are discussed as demonstrating predominantly Stage II characteristics are the clinical transplant coordinator (CTC) and the childbirth educator. One of these roles, that of the CTC, is clearly subspecialty practice, while the other, that of the childbirth educator, can best be characterized as a specialty component of women's health practice.

Clinical Transplant Coordinator

There is evidence that the role of the CTC is evolving to the level of advanced practice in response to patient care requirements in the referral and evaluation phase and in the pre- and post-transplant management phase of candidates and recipients. Organized training in the specialty in the form of an introductory course and continuing education is offered by the North American Transplant Coordinators Organization (NATCO), but institution-specific, on-the-job training is widely embraced. Continuing education opportunities are also offered by organizations such as the International Transplant Nurses Society (ITNS) and specialty scientific societies. Unlike the efforts to move specialty education into graduate nursing programs described by WOC nurses (Gray, Ratliff, & Mawyer, 2000), health-care providers in diabetes care (Melkus & Fain, 1995), and other established advanced practice roles (Bjorklund, 2003; Lynch et al., 2001; Murphy-Ende, 2002; Naegle & Krainovich-Miller, 2001), expertise in nephrology and renal transplantation nursing is gained in clinical practice and through continuing education (McNatt & Easom, 2000). Recently, ITNS began the development of a core curriculum for the specialty (International Transplant Nurses Society, 2003).

CTCs are essential for the continuity of care provided to transplant recipients. Most transplant centers employ coordinators; however, in many centers the role does not require that coordinators possess skills that reflect the core competencies of an advanced practice nurse (Reel, 1999). Specialty nurses with expertise in transplant nursing recognize the complex needs of their patients. Many obtain graduate education to better prepare them to deal with the realities of transplant nursing. To the benefit of their patients, these coordinators have expanded the specialty by incorporating advanced practice core competencies. It can be argued that the complex needs of patients with end-stage organ disease require higher levels of clinical reasoning and analytical skills, such as those possessed by advanced practice nurses; however, to advance the CTC role (not just individuals in the role) to this higher level, attention to several issues is necessary. First and foremost, leaders in the specialty must systematically determine whether advanced practice core competencies (see Chapter 3 and Part 2) are required to fully enact the role, or whether two levels of differentiated practice—general professional and APN—should be defined for the specialty. Second, the specialty's leadership must agree that the role is a *nursing* role. Making these decisions may disenfranchise many committed and experienced transplant professionals who are essential care providers. Similar to the levels of certification proposed for diabetes educators (Daly, Kulkarni, & Boucher, 2001; Hinnen Hentzen, 1994; see next section), some similar method of differentiation, which would recognize the added value that advanced practice knowledge and skill brings to the CTC role, might serve to acknowledge the contributions of both APNs and other transplant professionals.

Certification as a transplant coordinator is conferred by the American Board of Transplant Coordinators (ABTC) by written examination. Advanced education is not required for certification. Because this organization credentials all categories of transplant professionals, licensure as a registered nurse is also not a requirement. Recertification is achieved through continuing education. The issue of specialty versus subspecialty certification is an issue for all evolving advanced practice nursing specialties. We consider the case of transplantation in some detail to illustrate the complex issues surrounding the certification process for any evolving role.

A model proposed by McNatt and Easom (2000) addressed the credentialing and certification of APNs in nephrology nursing and renal transplantation. Currently, nephrology nurses are certified through the American Nephrology Nursing Association (ANNA), a subspecialty certification that does not require specific educational preparation. McNatt and Easom suggest that nephrology APNs should have a graduate nursing degree in a defined clinical specialty, national specialty certification in their area of advanced practice (e.g., as NPs or CNSs), and be board eligible for or certified in nephrology nursing. Transplant coordinator certification (CCTC) would be an additional certification for renal transplant APNs. They would be differentiated from other transplant professionals who hold the same certification by their expanded scope of practice as well as their credentials as CNSs or NPs. McNatt and Easom's model essentially depicts a modular certification configuration for nephrology and renal transplantation nurses that may have utility for other transplant specialties (e.g., cardiac, lung, liver).

This conceptualization is similar to an option proposed by Lyon (2002) regarding specialty versus subspecialty certification of CNSs, in which she described an examination process to test for core competencies (for legal recognition) and a subspecialty certification to test advanced clinical knowledge. Hanson and Hamric (2003) suggest expanding on this idea, with different modules being developed to evaluate advanced practice core competencies as well as knowledge required for functioning in various advanced practice roles (e.g., CNS, ACNP, CNM). Because some advanced practice is subspecialty practice (e.g., organ transplantation, oncology), a model that incorporates subspecialty certification (when available), in addition to a credentialing process that evaluates core competencies and knowledge required for a particular APN role, should be considered as long as the process is not unnecessarily restrictive. McNatt and Easom's model addresses this modular certification approach as well as the need for standardization of education and skills involved in the specialty. It can facilitate role and scope of practice differentiation among renal transplantation professionals and may have utility for other evolving subspecialties beyond the transplantation arena.

Educational institutions that prepare APNs must consider the certification options available and address methods of preparing students for certification beyond currently available credentialing requirements. They must also ensure that their graduates are eligible to sit for APN certification examinations approved for legal recognition of an APN role.

The transplant coordinator role in organ transplantation is evolving from a traditional model focusing on coordination of services to one incorporating the knowledge and skill of an advanced practice nurse (Martin, 1999; Morse, 2001; Reel, 1999). This evolution has been haphazard as a result of inattention to several issues. Most notably, the lack of recognition that the role requires advanced practice competencies and the lack of opportunities for subspecialty certification may impede expansion into an advanced practice nursing as an expectation of coordinator roles. There is also some disagreement about the preferred advanced practice role for the specialty, with some authors advocating the CNS and others the blended CNS/NP or acute care NP (Martin, Morse, & Reel). Clearly, a commitment to advanced practice nursing is needed, and given that commitment, more attention to these issues will be necessary in order for the CTC role to evolve.

Exemplar 19-2 demonstrates the complexity of care required for transplant candidates, recipients, and their families. In addition to expertise in advanced practice core competencies, the exemplar also highlights the skill of the CNS role in dealing with systems issues and staff education, both important components of providing care to this challenging patient population. It is our view that the knowledge and expertise of advanced practice nursing could fully enable the potential of the CTC position.

EXEMPLAR 19-2

HEART TRANSPLANT COORDINATOR

Given the complexity of care associated with solid organ transplant patients, most transplant programs have multidisciplinary teams that care for candidates and recipients (Donaldson, 2003). The clinical transplant coordinator's role is to facilitate the care of the patient, in collaboration with the multidisciplinary team, throughout the transplant process—a process that begins with the patient's initial referral to the transplant program and often continues for the rest of the patient's life.

As a CNS, my clinical transplant coordinator position affords me the opportunity to incorporate the core competencies of advanced practice nursing. My clinical practice role includes both direct and indirect care activities. For example, key direct care activities involve coordinating detailed discharge planning; seeing patients in transplant clinic, and triaging telephone calls from candidates, recipients, and family members. Indirect care activities include participating in interdisciplinary clinical rounds (for example, transfer conferences as patients transition from the intensive care unit to the intermediate care unit); developing protocols and patient education materials; participating in performance evaluation and improvement activities; initiating referrals to other health-care specialists, and facilitating staff support groups. One example of staff support involved a transplant candidate with biventricular mechanical support who remained hospitalized for over 12 months until a suitable donor organ became available. Over the course of this prolonged hospitalization, the nursing staff encountered several challenging problems. Many of the patient-staff conflicts revolved around the patient's desire for autonomy and the staff's need to provide care in a timely manner (e.g., dressing changes and physical therapy). Consultative sessions with the transplant team's neuropsychologist and social worker were held biweekly. The neuropsychologist enhanced the staff's understanding of the patient's cognitive status, and the social worker helped the staff articulate their frustrations. Over time, in concert with the patient, mutually acceptable strategies were devised and implemented. For example, staff members negotiated with the patient in developing a daily schedule that permitted him to "sleep in" on weekends when the census was typically low and the staff had more flexibility in providing care. In turn, the patient agreed to follow a more rigid schedule on weekdays.

My role affords many opportunities for staff and patient education. Staff education is both formal (e.g., teaching in the critical care nurse internship program) and informal (e.g., answering staff nurses' questions during rounds). Patient education involves extensive teaching sessions with prospective transplant candidates and their family members. The purpose of these sessions is to provide patients with information so they can make informed decisions about

Continued

EXEMPLAR 19-2

HEART TRANSPLANT COORDINATOR — cont'd

whether they wish to proceed with transplantation. Once a patient decides to proceed and is placed on the waiting list, additional education is provided during monthly support group meetings. Following the transplant procedure, recipients and family members attend comprehensive discharge education sessions. Postdischarge education is provided through newsletters, support group meetings, and individual counseling sessions during clinic visits.

One example of my role as collaborator is my participation with the interdisciplinary team that discusses, plans, implements, and evaluates the ongoing care of transplant candidates and recipients. One of our major responsibilities is to determine whether a particular patient meets the heart transplant program's physiological and psychosocial eligibility criteria for placement on the waiting list. A second example concerns technology transfer, more specifically, the transfer of scientific advances of mechanical assist device technology into clinical practice. When the heart transplant team was about to discharge our first patient with a left ventricular assist device (LVAD), I collaborated with the heart transplant research nurse, social worker, NP, physicians, hospital administrators, MedStar flight crew members, and community resource providers (e.g., the local power company) in facilitating this process. The purpose of this collaborative effort was to establish physiological and psychosocial criteria for discharge and to develop policies and procedures regarding emergent and routine follow-up care.

Lastly, I have had the opportunity to collaborate with an international, multidisciplinary task force in reviewing the literature pertaining to the biopsychosocial outcomes of cardiothoracic transplantation, evaluating the strength of the evidence, and developing specific recommendations for future research designed to improve psychosocial and clinical outcomes.

We gratefully acknowledge Sandra A. Cupples, DNSc, RN, Washington, D.C., for assistance with this exemplar.

Childbirth Educator

Childbirth education provides a different perspective on evolving specialties and is used here to illustrate a Stage II specialty practice that may become incorporated into existing advanced practice role in women's health, rather than evolve into a distinct advanced practice specialty. Childbirth educators play an important part in the preparation of expectant parents for childbirth. The practice of childbirth education is broad, extending from the preconception period through the early parenting period and may include other family members as well as the expectant parent(s). It takes a competent, well-informed, scientifically grounded, and articulate childbirth educator to teach consumer-oriented childbirth classes (Nichols, 2000). Childbirth educators may also serve as leaders, change agents, consumer advocates, consultants, entrepreneurs, and managers. Although some authors have argued that activities reflecting the role components of childbirth educators encompass the core competencies of advanced practice nursing (Nichols, 2000), this role has not emerged within maternal-child nursing as one requiring advanced practice competencies. One reason may be that it is overshadowed by emphasis on other advanced practice maternal-child nursing roles (e.g., NP and CNM). Another reason may be that some experts believe that the competencies are not unique to nursing practice, although some overlap between nursing and childbirth education is acknowledged (Lothian, 1996). The core issue is that the current practice of most childbirth educators is of limited scope and does not require advanced practice status. Moreover, tension exists between the medical community and the community of childbirth educators, whose values and perspectives reflect their view that birth is a normal, natural process instead of a medical event (Humenick, 1996, 1997; Lothian, 1997; Nichols, 1994; Zwelling, 1994). This tension may inhibit specialty nurses who are childbirth educators from seeking advanced practice education or may inhibit APNs in maternal-child health, such as CNSs, NPs and CNMs, from incorporating childbirth educator role functions into their practice. Regardless of the reasons that childbirth education has not evolved, commitment to advancing childbirth education to include an advanced practice level must involve expanding the contours of the practice. In addition, nursing leaders within the various organizations must address creating an advanced level of childbirth educator practice.

Currently, three organizations educate and certify childbirth educators, but none are nursing-specific: Lamaze International, the International Childbirth Education Association (ICEA), and the Childbirth and Postpartum Professional Association (CAPPA). These organizations embrace the participation of non–health-care professionals in various roles. Lamaze International Certification Program is the only one of these programs that is accredited by the National Commission for Certifying Agencies (NCCA), the accreditation body of the National Organization for Competency Assurance (NOCA) (Lamaze International Governing Body, 2001). Other organizations that are certified by NCCA include, for example, the ANCC Commission on Accreditation, Wound, Ostomy, and Continence Nursing (WOCN) Certification Board, International Board of Lactation Consultant Examiners, and the American Association of Critical-Care Nurses Certification Corporation.

Lamaze International educates (through university and chapter programs) and certifies childbirth educators and then credentials them (Lamaze Certified Childbirth Educator [LCCE]) for a 3-year period. Standards of practice were published by their governing body in 2001. The ICEA, which began as a federation of local consumer groups that convened as a result of published accounts of the cruelty of maternity practice (Ondeck, 2000), educates and certifies childbirth educators, doulas, postnatal educators, and perinatal fitness educators (ICEA, 1995). CAPPA, which was founded in 1998, offers education and certification for childbirth educators, lactation educators, labor doulas, antepartum doulas, and postpartum doulas. CAPPA's certification process varies from advanced practice certification; it more closely resembles specialty certification in that it requires experience but no formal education (CAPPA, 2003).

According to Sasmor and Grossman (1981), who surveyed childbirth educators in 1980 (n = 238), a majority of respondents agreed that there was a need for national guidelines for the preparation of childbirth educators. Despite this finding, many routes to preparation and certification have emerged, and these varied routes have created competition among the various organizations. At this point in time, there is little recognition in these organizations of the contributions APNs could make to these specialties. Because of the number of women in their childbearing years, advanced practice nurses who incorporate childbirth education have a tremendous opportunity to promote recognition of APNs and of nursing in general. The knowledge base for childbirth educators has become more extensive as a result of multidisciplinary research. Furthermore, there is a growing recognition of the additional knowledge and skill needed for increasingly complex practice in the specialty (Nichols, 2000). Thus, there is now an opportunity to better illuminate the potential value-added contributions that APNs can make to this role. Exemplar 19-3 illustrates how an APN who incorporated childbirth education into her practice was able to use her APN skills to achieve a positive outcome for both a patient and an institution.

EXEMPLAR 19-3

INCORPORATING CHILDBIRTH EDUCATION INTO ADVANCED PRACTICE NURSING

As a CNS at a large private medical center in the southern United States, I coordinated patient care, consulted on high-risk obstetric cases, implemented a staff education program, and directed and taught the childbirth education program. Patients were given my contact information when they registered for prenatal care. I often made rounds with the obstetricians, and on one particular day after rounds, one of the obstetricians requested a meeting with me to discuss a patient. She was a 39-year-old woman who was pregnant with her second child. During her last prenatal visit, she expressed concern about being *allowed* to take the Lamaze classes. He reported that she was adamant about having a "natural birth."

I called the woman to query her statement regarding being *allowed* to take classes. At first, she seemed taken aback that her physician had followed up with me. I described my role as CNS and childbirth educator for the Women's Health Department. I explained that health care providers often referred women to me who had special needs. During the conversation, she related that it had been 13 years since she had delivered a baby. During that pregnancy she had received no formal prenatal education. Her labor was long, and she received medication that "made me feel crazy." After we had established a rapport, I asked about enrollment in prenatal classes and her concern about being allowed to take the classes. At this point, her voice quivered, and she said, "I am all alone in this."

My initial thought was to tell her that other women have to come to classes without the father of the baby, but somehow I felt that this might terminate our contact. Instead, I asked if she would like to come for a tour of the birthing area; I felt like there was more going on than could be uncovered in a telephone conversation. We set up a time for her visit. On the day the visit was scheduled, she called and cancelled because her daughter had stayed home from school. During this brief conversation, her voice still told me that she was acutely stressed. I asked if I could drop off some information for at her home. She seemed shocked that I would be willing to make a home visit.

As we sat in her kitchen reviewing the various childbirth education classes and discussing her birth plan, she appeared to be very tense. I sat quietly while she looked at the material, then I noticed tears in her eyes, and she said, "I feel so alone, he left me." She explained her concern about going through labor alone. I reminded her of her inquiry about being allowed to take classes because "I won't have a husband to be with me." She explained that all the reading described the importance of a supportive partner during labor and birth. About that time, her daughter came in and volunteered to be her mother's coach, but her mother reminded her that the hospital rules would not allow her to be in the labor and delivery area as a support person. To help this woman maintain her privacy about her personal marital situation and regain some of her inner strength, I decided to teach private childbirth preparation classes in her home.

I reviewed the hospital and women's health unit policies to determine the hospital policy regarding a 13-year-old being allowed in the labor suite. Siblings were allowed to visit on the postpartum units, but not in the birthing area. I also called other area hospitals to determine their policies on this issue. I reviewed the research literature on the presence of siblings during labor and delivery and found that those siblings who were adequately prepared had a positive experience, overall, and felt more connected to the new baby. I followed up with the physician and inquired about how he felt regarding the daughter's presence during the labor and delivery. After our discussion, he called and asked the mother to bring her daughter to her next prenatal visit.

The next challenge was to get nursing administration to agree to the plan to have this 13-year-old serve as her mother's labor support. This meant meeting with both nursing administration and the staff of the labor unit and assuring them that this could be a positive experience for everyone involved. Initially, I did meet some resistance, but we were able to agree on a plan that would allow the daughter to support her mother during the labor and delivery. I agreed to be "on call" as a resource for the mother-daughter dyad and the staff during the labor event.

Mother and daughter both did well during the labor and delivery. Afterwards, the staff made the daughter a card with her handprints and those of her mother and baby brother, declaring the daughter a "world-class support person." As a result of this intervention, both practice and policy in the institution changed, and mother and daughter experienced an empowering event that was life-affirming for all.

We gratefully acknowledge Sheila A. Smith, PhD, RN, Charleston, SC, for assistance with this exemplar.

It is our view that childbirth education is a specialty within women's health. The exemplar illustrates the outcomes possible when the specialty is incorporated into an APN's practice. The educator and systems change components of the CNS role are demonstrated in this exemplar, as are the positive outcomes for the patient and the organization. However, a number of issues will need to be addressed in order for the role and functions of a childbirth educator to become an expectation of CNS practice in hospital-based women's health settings. One important question is whether the leaders of the organizations that educate and certify childbirth educators (CAPPA, ICEA, Lamaze International) support the specialty's evolution toward becoming a component of advanced practice roles. There is little evidence of this at present. If such support were to develop, the competencies and attributes of advanced practice nursing in the specialty must be defined. The exemplar describing the practice of one advanced practice nurse/childbirth educator demonstrates the problem-solving abilities of an advanced practice nurse, particularly in addressing a systems issue. Such examples can help differentiate the advanced nursing practice of childbirth education from that of other individuals who provide childbirth education. This differentiation is necessary for the certification and regulation of advanced practice, basic professional, and nonnurse childbirth educators.

Commentary: Stage II

In Stage II, the specialty becomes more organized and visible. Formal training programs develop, specialty organizations form, and certification moves beyond individual institution-based certificates for completion of training to national certification examinations. All of these developments lend strength and credibility to the specialty and its practitioners.

One of the major challenges in Stage II is demonstrating that the specialty is a *nursing* specialty. There are a number of evolving specialties, such as clinical research coordinators, childbirth educators, and clinical transplant coordinators, whose practitioners include nonnurses as well as nurses. Clearly, these roles cannot emerge as advanced practice nursing roles without clear distinctions being drawn between nonnursing practice and nursing practice in the specialty. Specialty organizations with members who are non-health-care providers, such as NATCO, must face this challenge. WOC nursing, which evolved from being a service offered by lay providers, moved from these early beginnings to nursing being recognized as the disciplinary basis for the specialty; WOC nurses now advocate for the role of APNs.

Although the practices among the emerging subspecialties discussed here are very different, they are similar with regard to some of the issues they have faced (or will face) in their evolution. One possibility is that the specialty will evolve as a component of an APN's practice. In the case of childbirth educators, whose role builds upon the core competencies of advanced practice nursing, a process of certifying them (e.g., CNSs, NPs, and CNMs) as childbirth educators (a type of modular certification package for these maternal-child APNs) might expand their sphere of influence in the settings in which they practice. In other cases, such as transplantation, recognition of an APN level of practice or a sanctioning of practice at the APN level for all specialty providers may evolve. For CTCs or other nurses working with transplant candidates or recipients, a mechanism for certifying basic professional and advanced practice transplant nurses (e.g., through ITNS) is necessary in order to recognize nursing's essential role in transplantation without diminishing the contributions of others who also provide essential care and services.

EMERGING APN ROLES: STAGE III

In the third stage of evolution to advanced practice, a specialty's knowledge base is growing and the scope of practice of nurses with specialty education is expanding. There is growing recognition of the additional knowledge and skills needed for increasingly complex practice in the specialty (Hamric, 2000). Pressures for standardization of education and skills required for specialty practice create incentives to move certificate-level training programs into graduate-level educational settings both as a means of increasing standardization and to raise the status of the specialty to an advanced practice level (Hanson & Hamric, 2003). According to Hanson and Hamric (2003), antecedents to legitimizing advanced practice roles must be addressed for a given specialty to evolve to advanced levels of practice (see Box 19-1, p. 681). Three organizations that have addressed (or are addressing) the issues necessary to legitimize advanced practice roles in their specialties include the Wound, Ostomy & Continence Nurses Society (WOCNS), the American Association of Diabetes Educators (AADE) (in collaboration with the American Diabetes Association, American Dietetics Association, and American Pharmaceutical Association), and the International Society of Nurses in Genetics (ISONG). Although these organizations have adopted differing approaches to advancing practice in their respective specialties, the process, in each case, was *unified* and *proactive* and depicts a framework that can guide other specialty organizations as they chart a course to advanced levels of practice.

Wound, Ostomy, and Continence Nursing

Wound, ostomy and continence (WOC) nursing, a specialty that developed in response to unmet patient needs following fecal or urinary diversion surgery, has evolved significantly since its inception in the 1960s. Historically, lay persons developed the specialty, dedicated exclusively to the care of ostomy patients (WOCNS, 1998). As health care changed and new patient needs arose, the original enterostomal therapist (ET) role evolved into a nursing specialty, whose scope of practice expanded to include wound, skin and continence care in addition to ostomy care. These WOC nurses became increasingly valued team members in acute care, outpatient settings, extended care facilities, and home care (Doughty, 2000).

The educational preparation for WOC nurses, which began as clinical training programs based heavily on experiential knowledge about ostomy management, has been provided within postbaccalaureate educational programs. Some of these programs have begun to offer graduate-level course work in the specialty. Thus, the content has been integrated into graduate curricula of some universities throughout the United States (Gray et al., 2000), and nurses can now become WOC specialists and obtain advanced practice credentials simultaneously (Beitz, 2000). Growing expectations for research (Bryant, 1995; Gray, 1998; Palmer, 2000) and evidence-based practice (Roe & Moore, 2001) require research skills best taught in graduate nursing programs. Thus, the WOCNS may soon be faced with the choice of recommending advanced practice education as minimal preparation for specialty certification as WOC APNs. Because WOC nursing practice already encompasses many core competencies of advanced practice nursing (e.g., direct clinical practice, expert guidance and coaching, consultation, and collaboration), this recommendation may offer several advantages. First, it will acknowledge the additional knowledge and skill required for increasingly complex practice (Beitz, 2000), which has been and remains "a strong motivating factor favoring development of graduate-level programs" (Hamric, 2000, p. 46). Second, nurses progressing to the advanced practice level will enjoy more autonomy, and their practice will be more visible as compared with that of basic professional-level specialty practice colleagues. Advanced practice status, however, is acknowledged by the state board of nursing or other credentialing body only when the specific qualifications of an advanced practice role are obtained (Bryant, 1993). For the WOC nurse, this requires advanced practice specialty education at the graduate level, credentialing as an APN by a national credentialing organization, and subspecialty certification as a WOC nurse. Despite differentiated levels of practice and education, certification (CWOCN) awarded by the Wound Ostomy Continence Nursing Certification Board (WOCNCB) remains at the basic professional level regardless of educational preparation. Thus, one issue facing the WOCNS is whether there should be both basic professional and advanced practice certifications (Beitz, 2000; Gray et al., 2000) or whether all practice should be at the advanced practice level.

This is a critical decision point for all specialties in Stage III. If WOC nursing is redefined as an advanced practice role, the unique characteristics that justify this redefinition must be identified (Gray, 1998) and must encompass advanced practice core competencies, appropriate credentialing, and regulatory recognition for these expanded activities. Attention to these issues is important for clinicians seeking to offer their services in a changing health care environment that includes nontraditional settings (Hamric, 2000). Although WOC nurses are considering whether their practice should be at the advanced level, no resolution has been reached. Alternative recognition for advanced practice competency for some nurses with graduate education in wound, ostomy, and/or continence nursing might be sought through certification as a wound management specialist (CWS) awarded to qualified clinicians by the American Academy of Wound Management, a multidisciplinary organization, or as a urological specialist, for CNSs or NPs, by the certification board of the Society of Urologic Nurses and Associates.

EXEMPLAR 19-4

ADVANCED PRACTICE IN WOUND, OSTOMY, AND CONTINENCE NURSING

I work as a blended role CNS/NP in the position of co-director of an outpatient wound center. Mr. L., a 60-year-old white male, was referred to me for management of a large nonhealing wound on his posterior left lower extremity. The patient was referred by a vascular surgeon who had already debrided the majority of the black necrotic tissue from the wound bed. The etiology of the wound was unclear. The patient's medical history included lymphoma, psoriasis, and obesity. He denied allergies and was not taking any medications. Employed as an accountant, the patient is married and lives with his wife in a condominium. He has one son, 30 years old, who is alive and well. After several weeks of therapy, the lateral half of the wound closed by reepithelialization. Over several months, there was an increase in the size, amount of exudate, and odor from the remaining wound bed. Based on wound culture results, I prescribed several courses of organism-specific oral antibiotics. In addition, every 2 to 3 weeks, I modified the protocol for topical wound therapy in order to modulate the wound environment and promote healing.

Approximately 6 months after the start of care in the wound center, the patient presented for his semiweekly visit in the wound center with a marked increase in the odor from his wound. After his dressings were removed, examination revealed that 50% of the wound bed was covered with new black necrotic tissue. In an institution where APNs cannot admit patients to the hospital, I consulted with the vascular surgeon about admitting the patient for surgical debridement, intravenous antibiotic therapy, and possible negative pressure wound therapy using the V.A.C. dressing. The vascular surgeon referred the patient to the admitting department for direct admission to the inpatient vascular unit.

During the next 8 days of hospitalization, the patient underwent two surgical debridements, consultation with dermatology, and wound biopsy. The wound biopsy eliminated neoplasm and autoimmune conditions as etiologies of the wound. A wound culture revealed moderate amounts of two types of *Eschrechia coli* and enterococcus, as well as a moderate amount of methcillin-sensitive *Staphylococcus aureus* and nonhemolytic streptococcus. He was started on two organism-specific oral antibiotics.

Continued

EXEMPLAR 19-4

ADVANCED PRACTICE IN WOUND, OSTOMY, AND CONTINENCE NURSING — cont'd

The V.A.C. therapy was initiated at a negative pressure of 125 mmHg. Within 4 days, the surface area of the wound bed decreased by almost 2 cm. The depth of the wound bed decreased by 2 mm—3 mm as a result of the formation of new granulation tissue. In addition, the edema in the wound edges had resolved, improving the likelihood of epithelial migration from the margins of the wound bed. The patient was discharged home with skilled nursing visits for V.A.C. dressing changes 3 times per week. I have continued to see this patient in the wound center postdischarge, and his wound has continued to heal without further incident.

We gratefully acknowledge Virginia Capasso, PhD, RN, Boston, MA, for assistance with this exemplar.

Advanced Diabetes Manager

The rising incidence of diabetes mellitus (DM) has created new opportunities for APNs. Advances in the technology of diabetes care and findings from two clinical research trials have redefined the roles of health care providers in diabetes care. Both the Diabetes Control and Complications Trial (DCCT) (DCCT Research Group, 1993) and the United Kingdom Prospective Diabetes Study (UKPDS) (UKPDS Group, 1998) demonstrated the value of multidisciplinary teams consisting of dieticians, nurses, and pharmacists in the clinical management of individuals with DM. Prior to the results of these clinical trials being released, however, the AADE (1992) published multidisciplinary scope and standards of practice guidelines. An advanced practice task force was established in 1993, and the dialogue among the three major disciplines constituting the membership of the association (nurses, dieticians, pharmacists) and their credentialing bodies was begun (Hinnen Hintzen, 1994; Tobin, 2000). These collaborative efforts resulted in a definition of advanced practice in diabetes as the highest of various levels of practice utilized along the full continuum of diabetes care (Hinnen Hintzen, 1994; Tobin, 2000). These levels are identified as the Generalist Diabetes Educator (GDE), Certified Diabetes Educator (CDE), and the Advanced Diabetes Manager (BC-ADM). The GDE is any health-care provider who interacts with individuals who have DM; the credential requires registration/licensure in a health-care profession. The generalist can provide basic assessment, survival knowledge, skill development, and referral for education and follow-up care (Hinnen Hentzen, 1994). The CDE is a health-care provider who meets educational and practice requirements, successfully completes the certification examination for diabetes educators, and is credentialed by the National Certification Board for Diabetes Educators (NCBDE). The CDE can provide case management; diabetes education program development, coordination, and implementation; and referral to advanced practitioners, other health care team members, or community resources (Hinnen Hentzen, 1994). The BC-ADM, credentialed by the American Nurses' Credentialing Corporation (ANCC), focuses on management of diabetes, including prescribing medications, rather than diabetes education. Thus, this credential distinguishes between two sets of skills (Daly et al., 2001). This level of credentialing is designed for licensed health care professionals, including registered dieticians, registered nurses, and registered pharmacists, who hold graduate degrees and have recent clinical diabetes management experiences after they have been licensed. Credentialing as a CDE is not required to take the advanced management examination.

Notably, the BC-ADM designation is unique. It is the first multidisciplinary approach to certifying nurses, dieticians, and pharmacists ever developed by the American Nurses' Credentialing Corporation (ANCC) (Daly et al., 2001). The fact that ANCC supported

AADE's request to support the advanced-level examination for disciplines other than nursing, to promote team collaboration and improve quality of care for individuals with diabetes, may represent the emergence of a new model of collaboration among practitioners who, in the past, may have competed for recognition by patient/consumer groups. The potential benefits of moving toward multidisciplinary certification include increased credibility (with colleagues, patients/consumers, employers, and other health-care professionals) as a result of a shared knowledge base, differentiation of these providers as having advanced-level expertise in diabetes management, greater autonomy in the delivery of care and services, and improved reimbursement (similarly, the CDE is now being recognized by third-party payors) (Daly et al., 2001). In this multidisciplinary model, APNs will fill a niche in the care of these patients.

Many nurses specializing in diabetes care obtain graduate education. Few graduate programs, however, offer subspecialty education in diabetes management. Because of the rising incidence of type 2 DM in the adult and adolescent populations, graduate nursing programs need to consider incorporating subspecialty course work into their curricula. This course work could either be *required* for preparation in a distinct advanced practice role or *elective* content. Melkus and Fain (1995) describe such a program and advocate for APNs taking lead roles in improving the quality of care delivered to individuals with this chronic health problem. Because nurses constitute the largest group of health care professionals who deliver care to individuals with DM across the life span and in a variety of settings, graduate-level preparation for APNs in diabetes management (consistent with American Diabetes Association standards) would fulfill the need for care providers in both acute and primary care settings.

Genetics Advanced Practice Nurses

Mapping of the human genome and the relevance of the Human Genome Project to health and disease are revolutionizing the provision of genetics services (specifically) and health care (generally). New genetic discoveries have made available an increasing number of genetic technologies for carrier, prenatal, diagnostic, and presymptomatic testing for genetic conditions. These discoveries are creating changes in the delivery of genetic services, the most immediate being the integration of genetics into primary health care delivery (Lea, 2000). Although brought to the forefront of public awareness by the mapping of the human genome, genetics services initially emerged out of a need for professionals who could provide genetic information, education, and support to patients and families with current and future genetic health concerns. Genetics specialists in academic medical, public health, and community-based settings have traditionally provided these services. In each setting, genetics professionals, including medical geneticists, genetics counselors, and genetics APNs, provide genetics services to patients and families. Working with other team members, genetics specialists obtain and interpret complex family history information, evaluate and diagnose genetic conditions, interpret and discuss complicated genetic test results, support patients throughout the genetics counseling process, and offer resources for additional individual and family support. Over time, through interaction with these specialists, patients and family members come to learn and understand relevant aspects of genetics, to make informed health decisions, and receive support in integrating personal and family genetics information into their daily lives (Lea et al., 1998).

According to ISONG, the scope of genetics nursing practice is both basic and advanced. At the basic level, genetics nurses are prepared to perform assessments to identify risk factors, plan care and provide interventions such as information, and evaluate for referral to genetic services. At the advanced level, nurses provide genetics counseling, case management, consultation, and evaluation of patients, families, resources or programs (ANA/ISONG, 1998). Nurses in genetics clinical practice are certified by the Genetic Nursing Credentialing Commission (GNCC), established in 2001 in cooperation with ISONG. Two levels of practice and certification, which correspond to the scope of genetics nursing practice, currently exist: the genetics clinical nurse (GCN) and the advanced practice nurse in genetics (APNG). The credentials conferred by GNCC mandate that specific educational, practice, and professional service requirements are met. The process is accomplished using a portfolio review. Eligibility for the APNG exam requires a minimum of 3 years experience as a clinical genetics nurse, completion of 300 hours of genetics practicum experiences (supervised by graduate nursing faculty with research or clinical emphasis in genetics, an APN in a genetics health care setting, board-certified health care professionals, or other clinicians who have a genetics research or clinical background in their specialty area), and extensive documentation of patient care experiences reflecting ISONG standards of clinical genetics nursing practice (ANA/ISONG, 1998). Noteworthy is the fact that GNCC is collaborating with ANCC on this process, with the intent that the portfolio review become a benchmark for the profession (GNCC, 2002).

The National Coalition for Health Professional Education in Genetics (NCHPEG), established in 1996 in cooperation with the ANA, the American Medical Association, and the National Human Genome Research Institute at the National Institutes of Health, has provided leadership in bringing advances in genetics to health-care providers. NCHPEG is a coalition of more than 100 professional organizations collaborating to promote professional education about advances in genetics. An interdisciplinary working group is developing recommendations for core competencies in genetics essential for all health-care professionals. Additionally, a core curriculum in genetics is being developed for all health professionals. There are, however, very few programs that offer graduate-level genetics programs for nurses. Educational preparation for APNs occurs in master's programs in nursing; genetics content is obtained later within postbaccalaureate educational programs or through continuing education courses. Course content must reflect information in human genetics; molecular and biochemical genetics; ethical, legal, and social issues in genetics; genetic variations in populations; and clinical application of genetics, including genetics counseling to meet requirements for certification. Growing expectations for evidence-based practice, which has the potential to transform health care due to integration of genetics knowledge (Jenkins, 2000), requires the knowledge and skill acquired in graduate nursing programs. In addition, the ethical decision-making skills of APNs are important to this specialty (see Chapter 11). Thus, ISONG may soon be faced with the choice of recommending advanced practice nursing education as minimal preparation for nurses practicing in this specialty. This seems a particularly pressing issue because graduate nursing educational preparation, required for the APNG credential, will place these nurses at the same level as other genetics services providers and has the potential to foster professional diversity and interdisciplinary collaboration.

The American Board of Genetics Counselors (ABGC) certifies some nurses; however, this avenue is not open to nurses unless they complete graduate education and clinical practice requirements in genetic medicine, human genetics, and/or genetic counseling. Those nurses who wish to pursue graduate education in nursing are not eligible for this certification. Because the scope of practice for the APNG is much broader than that of a genetics counselor, differentiation based on credentials is appropriate; however, collaboration among these professionals is necessary for appropriate genetics services delivery. Therefore it will be helpful for ISONG to collaborate and identify unique niches that nurses in these roles may fill. Failure to do so may undermine the relationship between professionals in these roles and affect the quality of genetics care and services.

Commentary: Stage III

The specialties discussed here that are in Stage III are characterized by a growing knowledge base and an expanding scope of practice that is differentiated from basic professional practice in the specialty. Changes in the law and regulation of practice, particularly those expanding the scope of practice for APNs, have also affected this stage. As shown in Exemplar 19-5, the commitment of leaders in the specialty organizations has been the driving force behind the evolution of these roles to the advanced practice level. In each instance, the advancement efforts have been unified and proactive. However, attention to several issues is still necessary for the roles to fully emerge at the advanced level (Box 19-2). For example, WOC nurses need to define levels of WOC nursing practice in order to differentiate advanced practice from basic professional practice—or decide that WOC nursing is advanced practice nursing and certify only those nurses with graduate nursing degrees. In contrast, ISONG and AADE have made tremendous progress in defining various roles for health care providers and differentiating levels of practice within multidisciplinary teams. These efforts provide an excellent example to other organizations that are considering advanced practice opportunities in their specialties. Although ISONG has differentiated basic from advanced genetics nursing practice, differentiating APNGs' contributions to genetics care and services from those of genetics counselors continues to require consideration to build practice models characterized by collaboration instead of competition.

BOX 19-2 • QUESTIONS FOR LEADERS TO ADDRESS IN CHARTING THE COURSE OF SPECIALTY EVOLUTION

1. Are advanced practice nursing competencies *required* to fully enact specialty practice, or are they an *added value?*
2. What are the distinct advanced practice nursing roles within the specialty?
3. How can the organization best recognize and value existing providers while moving to new expectations?
4. How should certification and educational expectations be structured, especially if differentiated practice between non-APNs and APNs continues within the specialty?
5. How should subspecialty certification within the context of advanced practice nursing regulation be addressed?
6. How can the centrality of direct clinical practice be maintained?

EXEMPLAR 19-5

INSIGHTS FROM LEADERS IN THE SPECIALTY

In 1976 the Genetic Diseases Act was passed by Congress, and the Genetic Diseases Services Branch of the Office of Maternal Child Health, Health Services Administration, Department of Health and Human Services, was established. At this time, a small and academically diverse group of nurses were working with genetics programs in tertiary health-care settings. They tended to come from practice backgrounds in pediatrics or obstetrics, which made sense, since genetic services at that time were centered primarily on the delivery of prenatal diagnostic procedures and evaluation of the dysmorphic child or the child with developmental delays. There also existed a relatively small number of masters-prepared genetics counselors working in settings similar to those of the nurses. In the 1980s, however, medical geneticists started to employ nurses rather than counselors for a variety of reasons, including the limited number of counselors available and the broader scope of practice of nurses.

Differing perspectives emerged regarding basic requirements for certification and the appropriate credentialing body for awarding certification. Genetics counselors required a

Continued

EXEMPLAR 19-5

INSIGHTS FROM LEADERS IN THE SPECIALTY—cont'd

degree from an approved master of science in genetics counseling program and were credentialed through the American Board of Medical Genetics (ABMG). In contrast, nurses advocated for a professional nursing organization as an appropriate credentialing body and graduate education in nursing as an acceptable educational route.

The number of genetics counselors increased faster than the number of genetics nurses in the 1980s. This led to the educational meetings of the National Society of Genetics Counselors (NSGC) becoming focused on the learning needs of genetics counselors—not consistently and sufficiently addressing the issues that confronted genetics nurses. After the initial NSGC educational meetings, a bond was formed among those nurses working in genetics and monies were found to form the Genetics Nurse Network. In 1987 there was significant discussion among the members of the network regarding the benefits of establishing a formal professional organization for genetics nurses. The lack of a professional "home" and the inability to obtain certification that would be recognized by the nursing profession led to the development of ISONG. Membership in the organization has continued to grow since 1987; however, the issue of certification remained unresolved. Nurses working in genetics had academic preparation ranging from diplomas to doctoral degrees. Some were already certified as genetics counselors, and others were certified as nurse practitioners in their specialty area. After significant discussion among the membership of ISONG, it was felt that the core knowledge required by genetics nurses was broader, but there was also the issue of recognition of a credential provided by a nonnursing organization being accepted by the nursing community. In addition, it was understood that at present there would not be a critical mass of nurses to sit for a written exam to provide for test item validation. Therefore, GNCC was established to investigate alternatives that would address these issues. After extensive work, the GNCC announced the establishment of the Advance Practice Genetics Nurse (APNG) credential and awarded the first credentials in 2001.

As genetics knowledge continues to develop, genetics will become an integral part of the clinical practice of all nurses. ISONG has worked with the National Coalition of Health Professionals Education in Genetics (NCHPEG) to develop competencies for health-care professionals at both the generalist and specialty levels and has collaborated with the ANA to publish competencies specific to nurses. ISONG continues to grow and develop to meet the needs of nurses who are anywhere on the novice-expert continuum and who focus on clinical practice, professional or consumer education, or research.

We gratefully acknowledge Shirley Jones, PhD, RN, Rockville, MD, and Judith Lewis, PhD, RN, Richmond, VA, for their assistance with this exemplar.

SUMMARY AND CONCLUSIONS

As can be seen from Chapter 1, the evolution of specialties in nursing has a long and rich history that continues in the present. Many nursing specialties are evolving towards advanced practice along a trajectory that for some has been haphazard, while others have evolved as a consequence of a cohesive vision communicated by leaders in the specialty. The progress made by members of specialty organizations that have evolved their specialties to advanced levels of practice (Stage III) can serve as examples for others that are struggling to evolve (Stage II) or are newly emerging (Stage I).

In this chapter we have examined each of these stages in the context of selected specialty groups and the evolving and innovative roles that characterize progression toward advanced nursing practice. Clearly, the ability to be deliberate in efforts to evolve the specialty toward advanced practice speeds progress, as demonstrated by organizations such as the WOCNS, AADE, and ISONG. Some specialties have haphazardly evolved. Others may not evolve into advanced practice nursing; without commitment from the nursing community and attention to the issues noted in Boxes 19-1 and 19-2, the move toward advanced practice may be an unrealistic goal. It is important to recognize that progression to advanced levels of practice is neither inevitable nor necessary. For example, staff development educators are a respected specialty group within the nursing profession, yet their competencies are not consistent with advanced practice nursing (Hanson & Hamric, 2003). As specialties move through the stages described here, one important question for the specialty's leadership is whether the specialty is best advanced by deliberate evolution to the advanced level of practice, development of differentiated levels of practice with distinct expectations and certifications, or continued development as a specialty (see Box 19-2). In these decisions, it is critically important to affirm the roles and value of ALL providers in the specialty, even as differentiation occurs for advancement and strengthening of specialty roles.

Concern over whether a role is a nursing role (versus *exclusively* a nursing role) is an issue that will need to be examined in particular specialties. In the history of nursing, there are examples of roles that were characterized as sharing attributes with other types of health-care providers. For example, some psychiatric CNSs attained the credentials to practice as licensed professional counselors. Other health-care providers (e.g., counselors, psychologists) also receive this same credential, despite educational differences. Failure to acknowledge the value of multidisciplinary teams, shared knowledge, and overlapping expertise may limit opportunities for APNs in the current health-care environment and impede advancement of specialties within the discipline. As a profession, nursing must embrace the notion that some roles are not *exclusively* nursing and endorse differentiated practice models.

At the same time, the profession must define the advanced level of practice within the interdisciplinary model. This is critical for regulatory purposes, for standardization of APN competencies in the practice, and for recognition by the public and insurers. In addition to the AADE, there are other multidisciplinary specialty organizations (Table 19-2) that certify health care providers who share a common knowledge base. These organizations are models of collaboration that communicate to consumers, other providers, third-party payors, and other stakeholders that there are national standards in the specialty that are upheld by these specialty care providers. These multidisciplinary collaborative models may represent a trend in health care that will give rise to a fourth stage in the evolution of advanced practice: a stage characterized by APNs who are mature, expert practitioners in a subspecialty, secure in understanding the unique contributions that they make in the direct care of patients, yet embracing the notion that some aspects of their practice are shared by experts from other disciplines essential to the care of their patients.

The proliferation of role titles seen in evolving specialties requires special attention as APNs begin practicing in the specialty. For example, within the transplant specialty, role titles such as "clinical transplant coordinator," "transplant coordinator," "transplant nurse," "transplant NP," and "transplant CNS" have been used in practice settings. The advanced practice role titles of CNS, NP, and CNM need to be consistently applied to APNs who are practicing in particular specialties to decrease role confusion. In addition, such consistency is important for promoting the recognition of advanced practice nursing within evolving specialties and the profession as a whole. For specialties that develop both nonadvanced and advanced levels of practice, consistent titles are necessary to avoid confusion among providers and patients.

This is an extraordinarily interesting time in the history of the nursing profession. Opportunities and challenges for advanced practice nursing abound. What will the history books say about this period in the evolution and expansion of the nursing profession? As the second author (Hamric, 2000) wrote in addressing the WOC specialty group, "[Our] hope is that they will say [we] clearly saw patients' needs and developed [our] skills to meet those needs; that [we] grasped the role opportunities that were possible and created new ones; and, most importantly, that [we] moved forward together" (p. 47).

TABLE 19-2 SPECIALTY ORGANIZATIONS OFFERING ADVANCED-LEVEL CERTIFICATION

SPECIALTY ORGANIZATION	CREDENTIALING ORGANIZATION/CREDENTIAL AWARDED	GRADUATE NURSING EDUCATION REQUIRED?
American Academy of HIV Medicine*	American Academy of HIV Medicine/HIV Specialist	Implied—must be licensed as an NP
American Academy of Wound Management*	American Academy of Wound Management/CWS	Yes (for diplomate or fellow status)
American Association of Critical-Care Nurses	AACN Certification Corporation/CCNS	Yes
American Association of Diabetes Educators*	American Nurses Credentialing Commission/BC-ADM	No (master's in nursing or related field)
Association of Nurses in AIDS Care	HIV/AIDS Nursing Certification Board/AACRN	Yes
Hospice and Palliative Care Nurses Association	National Board for Certification of Hospice & Palliative Care Nurses/APRN, BC-PCM	Yes
International Society of Nurses in Genetics	Genetic Nursing Credentialing Commission/APNG	Yes
International Nurses Society on Addictions	Addictions Nursing Certification Board/CARN-AP	No (master's in nursing or related field)
Oncology Nursing Society	Oncology Nursing Certification Corporation/AOCN	Yes
Society of Urologic Nurses & Associates*	Certification Board of Urologic Nurses & Associates/CUNP or CUCNS	Yes (must already be nurse practitioners or clinical nurse specialists)

*Multidisciplinary membership.

REFERENCES

American Association of Diabetes Educators. (1992). The scope of practice for diabetes educators and the standards of practice for diabetes educators. *The Diabetes Educator, 18,* 52-56.

American Nurses Association. (1995). *Nursing's social policy statement.* Washington, DC: Author.

American Nurses Association. (2003). *Nursing: Scope and standards of practice,* Washington, DC: Author.

American Nurses Association/International Society of Nurses in Genetics. (1998). *Statement on the scope and standards of genetics clinical nursing practice.* Washington, DC: American Nurses Association. Retrieved September 5, 2003, from http://www.genrticnurse.com

Beitz, J. M. (2000). Specialty practice, advanced practice, and WOC nursing: Current professional issues and future opportunities. *Journal of Wound, Ostomy, Continence Nursing, 27,* 55-64.

Bigbee, J. L., & Amidii-Nouri, A. (2000). History and evolution of advanced nursing practice. In A. B. Hamric, J. A. Spross, & C. M. Hanson, (Eds), *Advanced nursing practice: An integrated approach* (2nd ed.). Philadelphia: W. B. Saunders, p. 3-32.

Bjorklund, P. (2003). The certified psychiatric nurse practitioner: Advanced practice psychiatric nursing reclaimed. *Archives of Psychiatric Nursing, 17,* 77-87.

Boland, C. S. (1998). Parish nursing: Addressing the significance of social support and spirituality for sustained health-promoting behaviors in the elderly. *Journal of Holistic Nursing, 16,* 355-368.

Brown, N. J., Congdon, J. G., & Magilvy, J. K. (1996). An approach to care management for rural older adults: Parish nursing. *New Horizons, 5,* 7.

Bryant, R. (1993). ET nursing: Advanced practice, specialty practice, or both? *Journal of Enterostomal Therapy Nursing, 20,* 229-231.

Bryant, R. (1995). Establishing a WOCN research program. *Journal of Wound Ostomy Continence Nursing, 22,* 1-3.

Childbirth and Postpartum Professional Association. (2003). *General information.* Retrieved September 5, 2003 from http://www.cappa.net/CAPPAbout.asp

Coldewey, L. J. (1993). Parish nursing: A system approach. *Health Progress, 74,* 54-57, 66.

Daly, A., Kulkarni, K., Boucher, J. (2001). The new credential: Advanced diabetes management. *Journal of the American Dietetic Association, 101,* 940-943.

DeNicola, L., Klied, D., & Brink, L. (1994). Use of pediatric physician extenders in pediatric and neonatal intensive care units. *Critical Care Medicine, 22,* 105-106.

DeSchepper, C. (1999). Healthier communities through parish nursing. *Health Progress, 80,* 56-58.

Diabetes Control and Complications Trial (DCCT) Research Group. (1993). The effect of intensive treatment of diabetes on the development and progression of long-term complications in insulin-dependent diabetes mellitus. *New England Journal of Medicine, 329,* 977-988.

Donaldson, T. A. (2003). The role of the transplant coordinator. In S. A. Cupples & L. Ohler (Eds.), *Transplantation nursing secrets* (pp. 17-26), Philadelphia: Hanley & Belfus.

Doughty, D. (2000). Integrating advanced practice and WOC nursing education. *Journal of Wound, Ostomy, Continence Nursing, 27,* 65-68.

Doyle, J. (2001). Forensic nursing: A review of the literature. *Australian Journal of Advanced Nursing, 18,* 32-39.

Drummond, M., Buss, T. F., Ladigo, M. A. (1992). Volunteers for community health. *Health Progress, 73,* 20-24.

Genetic Nursing Credentialing Commission, Inc. (2002). *Home page.* Retrieved September 5, 2003, from http://www.geneticnurse.org/index main.htm

Gray, M. (1998). Continence research in the JWOCN: A report card. *Journal of Wound Ostomy, Continence Nursing, 25,* 61-62.

Gray, M., Ratliff, C., & Mawyer, R. (2000). A brief history of advanced practice nursing and its implications for WOC advanced nursing practice. *Journal of Wound, Ostomy, Continence Nursing, 27,* 48-54.

Hamric, A.B. (2000). WOC nursing and the evolution to advanced practice nursing. *Journal of Wound Ostomy Continence Nursing, 27,* 46-47.

Hanson, C. M., & Hamric, A. B. (2003). Reflections on the continuing evolution of advanced practice nursing. *Nursing Outlook, 51,* 203-211.

Health Ministries Association. (1998). *The scope and standards of parish nursing practice,* Washington, DC: American Nurses Association.

Hinnen Hentzen, D. (1994). AADE moves to advanced practice model for diabetes education and care. *The Diabetes Educator, 20,* 190.

Humenick, S. (1996). Lamaze body-wise preparation. *The Journal of Perinatal Education, 5,* v-vii.

Humenick, S. (1997). The normalcy of birth. *The Journal of Perinatal Education, 6,* v-vi.

Hutson, L.A. (2002). Development of sexual assault nurse examiner programs. *Nursing Clinics of North America, 37,* 79-88.

International Childbirth Education Association. (1995). *Welcome to ICEA.* Retrieved September 5, 2003 from http://www.icea.org/info.htm

International Transplant Nurses Society. (2003). *Transplant curriculum.* Retrieved December 8, 2003 from http://www.itns.org/education/curriculum.html

Jenkins, J. F. (2000, September 30). An historical perspective on genetic care. *Online Journal of Issues in Nursing, 5*(3), manuscript 2. Retrieved December 8, 2003, from http://nursingworld.org/ojin/topic13/tpc13_2.htm

Lamaze International Governing Body. (2001). *Standards of practice: Lamaze childbirth educators and Lamaze education series.* Retrieved September 5, 2003, from http://www.lamaze.org

Lea, D. H. (2000). A new world view of genetics service models. *Online Journal of Issues in Nursing, 5.*

Retrieved September 5, 2003 from http://nursing-world.org/ojin/topic13/tpc13_6.htm

Lea, D. H., Jenkins, J., & Francomano, C. A. (1998). *Genetics in clinical practice: New directions for nursing and health care*. Sudbury, MA: Jones & Bartlett Publishers.

Lewis, J. A. (2000). Advanced practice in maternal/child nursing: History, current status, and thoughts about the future. *Maternal Child Nursing, 25*, 327-330.

Lloyd, R. C., & Solari-Twadell, P. (1994). Organizational framework, functions and educational preparation of parish nurses: A comparison of national survey results. In *Proceedings of the Eighth Annual Westberg Symposium on Ethics and Values: A framework for parish nursing practice* (pp. 105-115). Northbrook, IL: National Parish Nurse Resource Center.

Lough, M. A. (1999). An academic-community partnership: A model of service and education. *Journal of Community Health Nursing, 16*, 137-149.

Lothian, J. (1996). Childbirth education: Why become certified? *The Journal of Perinatal Education, 5*, ix-xi.

Lothian, J. (1997). Are you really teaching Lamaze? *The Journal of Perinatal Education, 6*, vii-ix.

Lynch, M. P., Cope, D. G., & Murphy-Ende, K. (2001). Advanced practice issues: Results from the ONS Advanced Practice Nursing Survey. *Oncology Nursing Forum, 28*, 1521-1530.

Lyon, B. L. (2002). The regulation of clinical nurse specialist practice: Issues and current developments. *Clinical Nurse Specialist, 16*, 239-241.

Maeve, M. K. & Vaughn, M. S. (2001). Nursing with prisoners: The practice of caring, forensic nursing or penal harm? *Advances in Nursing Science, 24*, 47-64.

Magilvey, J. K. & Brown, N. J. (1997). Parish nursing: Advanced practice nursing model for healthier communities. *Advanced Practice Nursing Quarterly, 2*, 67-72.

Martin, R. K. (1999). The role of the transplant advanced practice nurse: A professional and personal evolution. *Critical Care Nursing Quarterly, 21*, 69-76.

McCrone, S., & Shelton, D. (2001). An overview of forensic psychiatric care of the adolescent. *Issues in Mental Health Nursing, 22*, 125-135.

McNatt, G. E., & Easom, A. (2000). The role of the advanced practice nurse in the care of organ transplant recipients. *Advances in Renal Replacement Therapy, 7*, 172-176.

Melkus, G. D., & Fain, J. A. (1995). Diabetes care concentration: A program of study for advanced practice nurses. *Clinical Nurse Specialist, 9*, 313-316.

Morse, C. J. (2001). Advance practice nursing in heart transplantation. *Progress in Cardiovascular Nursing, 16*, 21-24, 38.

Murphy-Ende, K. (2002). Advanced practice nursing: Reflections on the past, issues for the future. *Oncology Nursing Forum, 29*, 106-112.

Naegle, M. A., & Krainovich-Miller, B. (2001). Shaping the advanced practice psychiatric-mental health nursing role: A futuristic model. *Issues in Mental Health Nursing, 22*, 461-482.

Nichols, F. (1994). Mastering the winds of change. *The Journal of Perinatal Education, 3*, ii.

Nichols, F. H. (2000). Philosophy and roles. In F. H. Nichols & S. S. Humenick (Eds.). *Childbirth education: Practice, research and theory* (pp. 3-17). Philadelphia: W. B. Saunders Company.

Ondeck, M. (2000). Historical development. In F. H. Nichols & S. S. Humenick (Eds.), *Childbirth education: Practice, research and theory* (pp. 18-31). Philadelphia: W. B. Saunders Company.

Palmer, M. H. (2000). The RU-3 project: Research utilization and practice. *Journal of Wound Ostomy Continence Nursing, 27*, 98-99.

Reel, V. K. (1999). Utilization of the acute care nurse practitioner in lung transplantation. *Clinical Excellence for Nurse Practitioners, 3*, 80-83.

Roe, B., & Moore, K. N. (2001). Utilization of continence clinical practice guidelines. *Journal of Wound Ostomy Continence Nursing, 28*, 297-304.

Ryan, J. (1995). *A parish nurse preparation institute: Wisconsin model* [brochure]. Milwaukee, WI: Marquette University College of Nursing.

Rydholm, L. (1997). Patient-focused care in parish nursing. *Holistic Nursing Practice, 11*, 47-60.

Sasmor, J. L., & Grossman, E. (1981). Childbirth education in 1980. *Journal of Obstetrics and Gynecological Nursing, 10*, 155-160.

Solari-Twadell, A., & Westberg, G. (1991). Body, mind, and soul. *Health Progress, 72*, 24-28.

Striepe, J. M. (1989). *Nurses in churches: A manual for developing parish nurse services and networks* (2nd ed.). Park Ridge, IL: The National Parish Nurse Resource Center.

Tobin, C.T. (2000). A rainbow of opportunities: Advanced practice. *Diabetes Educator, 26*, 216, 326-327.

United Kingdom Prospective Diabetes Study (UKPDS) Group. (1998). Intensive blood glucose control with sulfonylurea or insulin compared with conventional treatment and risk of complications in patients with type 2 diabetes. *Lancet, 352*, 837-853.

Wound, Ostomy, and Continence Nurses Society. (1998). Commemorative program for opening session: 30th Anniversary Conference. Laguna Beach, CA: The Society.

Zwelling, E. (1994). Women: first, last, always. *The Journal of Perinatal Education, 3*, 1-6.

PART IV

Critical Elements in Managing Advanced Nursing Practice Environments

CHAPTER 20

Business Planning and Reimbursement Mechanisms

CHARLENE M. HANSON • CHRISTINA C. KING

INTRODUCTION

Today's patients need and demand health services beyond those that have been traditionally available. From the patient's perspective, services must be accessible and affordable. From the payor's perspective, they must be cost-effective. Both groups desire and demand high-quality services. The work of the health-care system and, subsequently, the advanced practice nurses (APNs) practicing within it, is to fulfill the health-related needs of the patient within an increasingly demanding and complex environment. There are many different processes that contribute to this system, most of which may be classified either as those related to direct patient care (with a clinical focus) or as those that support the patient care process indirectly (with an administrative focus). Successful APNs develop, implement, and continuously analyze the direct and indirect processes of care used to meet patient outcomes, while being cognizant of the other critical environmental elements that affect advanced nursing practice. The success of the resulting health-care system is measured by the ability of the APN provider using these existing processes to attain desired patient outcomes within the constraints of available resources and reimbursement. The price of system failure is measured in terms of human suffering.

Innovation in health care often stems from the professional and ethical commitment of nurses and other health-care providers to improve patient care, either directly or indirectly. Innovations in both direct patient care and the supporting indirect care infrastructure receive increasing attention from health-care providers, insurers, and regulating bodies as resources decrease and need increases. One particular innovation that has been successful in patient care settings, such as hospitals and larger group practices, is the conceptualization and organization of the direct and indirect processes of patient care within the context of systems thinking (HCA Quality Resource Group, 1992a, 1992b).

The current health-care environment provides significant tension for change. Through the political leadership of national organizations and the active participation of nurses in the political process, nursing has the ability to influence the direction of that change (see Chapter 9). The APN is uniquely poised as the viable alternative to the traditional physician provider and, as such, demonstrates the expertise, knowledge, and skills to do things differently. Factors providing support for new behaviors include the acceptance of the need for change by health-care organizations, the commitment of APNs to nursing's professional ethics, and the covenant nurses hold with society.

Simply put, any system represents the flow of resources through a process that results in the desired outcomes (Figure 20-1). The size and complexity of the developed system is dependent upon the number and complexity of processes being used to attain the desired outcome. Evaluation of the system includes assessment and evaluation of the resources used, the processes utilized, and the outcomes attained. This chapter focuses on the process of APN business planning from a systems approach. Although the emphasis is on an APN-managed practice, all APNs need to be aware that patient care delivery is conceptualized as comprising the direct and indirect patient care processes that ensure that available resources are allocated in such a manner as to meet desired patient outcomes. Business planning is itself a process that focuses primarily upon the development, implementation, and evaluation of those indirect processes that support patient care. It stands in contrast to a business plan, which is a document used by legal and financial advisors to evaluate the success potential of a particular business venture, such as an individual APN

We wish to thank Colleen M. Prophet, M.A., R.N., and Barbara Head, Ph.D, R.N., of the Center for Nursing Classification for their guidance and input related to the potential use of nursing classifications by APNs.

practice. The business plan may be conceptualized as an outcome product of the business planning process. Reimbursement, as part of overall business planning, is another indirect process supporting patient care and is one of the critical elements affecting the success of advanced nursing practice. Examples are provided to illustrate these important concepts. It is important to note that much of the information discussed throughout this chapter changes from year to year. Federal, state, and professional websites contain the most current information and should be consulted for latest changes.

BUSINESS PLANNING

Success in and satisfaction with one's APN role revolve around the right match between APNs and the work they do and the ability to be flexible and innovative within the scope of that role. As noted, APNs participate in two different groups of processes within the advanced practice role: direct and indirect care processes. Examples of indirect processes are the steps taken to register a patient and collect demographics, the process of third-party billing, and the identification of a medical and office supplies vendor (Table 20-1). Both direct and indirect processes are essential to the successful management of any health-care system, whether it be a small, self-contained APN practice or a large, multi-hospital network.

Over an APN's career, the balance between direct and indirect process involvement, and the size of the system in which these processes occur, may vary. One way of characterizing the shift in this balance and size of the system is to consider that the APN adopts an entrepreneurial approach, an intrapreneurial approach, or a mixture of both at any given time. Both entrepreneurs and intrapreneurs are individuals who continually search for and who are receptive to opportunities and innovation. Innovation comes through the creation of a new process (whether direct, indirect, or both) or through radical changes to an existing process so that it seems "like new." An entrepreneur plans, organizes, finances, operates, and participates in a new health-care delivery organization. Entrepreneurs have control over and responsibility for an increased proportion of indirect processes of care in their roles as compared with intrapreneurs. An intrapreneur is generally an employee of an existing health-care system, in which many of the indirect processes of the care delivery system may be controlled and managed by other employees or departments. The intrapreneur improves, redesigns, or augments an employer's current direct care processes, with a lesser role in day-to-day business administrative functions. Entrepreneurs function within the context of the larger, societal health-care system. Intrapreneurs function within an institutional health-care system, a microcosm of the larger arena. When

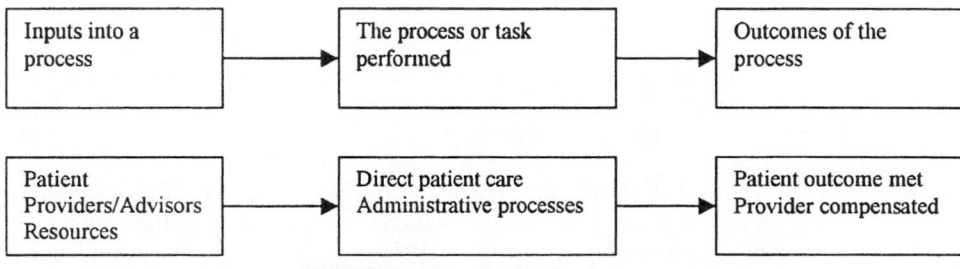

FIGURE 20-1 • Flowcharts of processes.

TABLE 20-1 EXAMPLES OF DIRECT AND INDIRECT PROCESSES AND SKILLS	
CLINICAL/DIRECT PROCESSES AND SKILLS	ADMINISTRATIVE/INDIRECT PROCESSES AND SKILLS
Wound management	Support staff supervision
Childbirth education	Presentation/teaching/precepting experience
Lactation consultation	Grant-writing capabilities
Suturing	Computer literacy
Intrauterine contraceptive device insertion	Budget development
Pain management	Medical billing
Intubation	Word processing/desktop publishing

embarking on program or practice oversight, the APN needs to understand the balance between direct and indirect processes as well as the size the business will have over time. The decision about the proportion of one's role to devote to direct care versus indirect processes is based upon the professional and personal values and goals of the APN. Determining one's professional values may be a complex process because these values may have been internalized and therefore may be difficult to articulate. Professional values include those tenets of nursing practice that provide significance and meaning to the APN's practice of nursing. Some sources of professional values include the various publications of the nursing profession, such as the *Code of Ethics for Nurses* (American Nurses Association, 2001), writings of nursing theorists to which the APN has been exposed, and artwork depicting care and compassion (Donahue, 1985). The mission and goal statements of the APN national organizations clearly portray these values as well.

Married to one's professional values are one's personal values, especially one's comfort with risk-taking and one's preference as to the arena in which care is delivered. Risk-taking is a key characteristic of the APN who is considering involvement in an entrepreneurial practice. A desire to function within an organizational setting is a key characteristic of an intrapreneurial approach. Some questions that may assist the APN in clarifying professional and personal values include the following (these sample questions are intended to be illustrative only, and are not assumed to be exhaustive):

- *To clarify one's internalized theoretical basis for practice:* What model of nursing practice, or approach to care delivery, best describes how I perceive my own nursing practice? Do the options before me favor this model or some other approach? If they favor another approach, how compatible is it with my own beliefs? (See Chapter 2.)
- *To determine one's tolerance for being entrepreneurial (requires increased risk-taking):* Do I thrive on risk-taking, like some risk, or prefer situations with a conservative level of risk involved? How is a "loss" or being "unsuccessful" defined? If I like taking risks, how much of a loss can I afford to take—both professionally and personally—should my venture prove unsuccessful?
- *To determine one's preference for an intrapreneurial approach:* Do I prefer being a part of a team or being on my own? If I like being on a team, what other team members would I like to be included on this team? How big a team am I most comfortable with? If I prefer working on my own, how will I interact with my colleagues? (See Chapters 6, 7, and 10.)

An ideal skills inventory serves as the springboard for the clarification of the APN's professional goals. The extent to which the APN balances the clinical role with administrative demands depends on the APN's skills and preferences and begins with an inventory of those clinical skills and administrative talents that the APN would like to bring, or acquire, in an ideal advanced practice role. Table 20-1 lists examples of clinical versus administrative skills. Some questions that may refine one's ideal inventory include the following:

- *To clearly articulate one's existing area of clinical expertise:* Do I have well-developed advanced clinical skills? If so, what are they?
- *To better articulate one's ideal role:* What tasks do I particularly enjoy, feel neutral about, and particularly dislike? Of those that I dislike but that need to be performed, do mechanisms exist for those tasks to be performed by someone else?
- *To identify one's areas for growth:* What processes would I like to do more of or learn more about? Does the current situation provide opportunities for me to do them?

The ability to actualize one's ideal APN role provides a strong incentive toward managing one's program or practice. However, APNs must realize that they will be the "boss" and may need to manage not only their own work but the work of a support staff as well (Stewart, 1989). Being in charge may include attention to the rules and regulations of many different entities governing APN clinical practice, grant execution and reporting, and general business practice. Because business and managerial skills are not taught in basic nursing programs, these skills will need to be learned. Graduate nursing programs are responding to this need and to the demands of dynamic and changing practice environments by incorporating business and practice management concepts into APN education. Many APNs have sought dual degrees in nursing and business administration. Some questions related to one's ability to assume an increased managerial role in indirect processes include the following:

- *To determine internal and external loci of support:* Do I have the unflagging support of those closest to me, both personally (significant other, children, friends, etc.) and professionally (physician collaborators, APN colleagues, financial and legal advisors, etc.)?
- *To determine basic management skills:* Do I have well-honed organizational skills? Do I enjoy paying attention to details? Am I comfortable in a leadership position? (See Chapter 9.)
- *To determine basic financial management skills:* Am I familiar with, or willing to learn, the budgeting cycle and processes of my employer? Have I participated in budget preparation and resource allocation in the past? Am I comfortable developing a budget for my own practice?
- *To determine external regulatory guidelines affecting practice:* Do I know where to locate copies of the applicable regulations affecting this program? Do I understand, or do I have access to advisors who understand, the specific ramifications of state and federal laws applicable to this program, such as those pertaining to the Clinical Laboratory Improvement Amendments (Centers for Medicare and Medicaid, 2004b). Are there any institutional rules and regulations that may limit my ability to practice within the full scope of my role? What are the procedures for obtaining approval of the various institutional committees that may be involved? (See Chapter 22.)
- *To determine financial resources:* Where will funding for the program (capital for start-up expenses) come from? Do I have the financial ability to live without a steady income or for at least 1 year while the practice is growing if the grant is not refunded?
- *To determine human resources skills and systems:* Am I willing to be responsible for the work of others? What does that entail? Are administrative systems in place for hiring, evaluating, and terminating staff for the duration of the program/practice?

These are among the many questions to be answered by APNs prior to deciding how extensive their role will be in the management of their program or practice. Fortunately, there are several resources to help clinicians better understand the indirect processes, or "business," of clinical practice. The reader is referred to Buppert (2004) for an in-depth discussion of nurse practitioner (NP) business and legal concerns. The American Medical Association (AMA) (1996, 1999, 2002a, 2002b, 2002c), in collaboration with the Coker Group, has published a series regarding independent practice management that is useful for any APN role. *Entrepreneur* and other business magazines provide useful information related to business management and administration. The Small Business Administration (www.sba.gov) provides general and specific information regarding business management and referral to local supports, including the local office of the Service Corps of Retired Executives (SCORE). There are many online resources related to business management. Some specific websites that may be useful to the development of small businesses include the following:

- *www.americanexpress.com* (American Express Company, 2003): go to "small business network" to find advice about business start-up and community networking.
- *www.smallbizsearch.com*: this website offers information about a wide variety of issues around financing, technology, and business opportunities.
- *www.dol.gov/osbp*: the Department of Labor, Office of Small Business Programs, offers good information about minority- and women-owned businesses.

An excellent resource that has in-depth coverage of all of the above concerns can be found at www.pftweb.org in the Building Your Practice Section of the Partnerships for Training website (Association of Academic Health Centers, 2002). This interactive, interdisciplinary Web resource offers a wealth of resources, information, and pearls of wisdom for clinicians who wish to develop a practice.

DIRECT PROCESSES OF CARE

The way to think about practice environments is that they represent small health-care systems based upon a patient population with an identified need. This patient population is identified through a variety of ways, including individual APN preference based upon the role and scope of practice of the individual APN. For certified nurse-midwives (CNMs) and certified registered nurse anesthetists (CRNAs), the patient population is essentially defined by their roles with childbearing women and their families and with patients undergoing surgical anesthesia, respectively. Nurse practitioners (NPs) and clinical nurse specialists (CNSs) have a broader population base, although their clinical subspecialty describes their patient population (e.g., family NP, psychiatric CNS; see Part III). Sometimes APNs identify patient populations through other modifiers, such as age, health promotion specialty, or disease state specialty, for example, CNMs who care for adolescent mothers-to-be, CNSs who have expertise in cardiac risk factor modification and rehabilitation, and adult NPs or CNSs who specialize in management of asthma or diabetes. In other instances, it is the geographical location or organizational setting that differentiates one's patient population of interest. Examples of these populations are the rural underserved populations cared for by National Health Service Corps providers, veterans cared for by the Veterans Affairs Medical Centers, and participants in Kaiser Permanente's managed care program who are cared for by their own staff of providers. APNs must be able to clearly and succinctly define the patient population being served by their clinical practice (marketing to this population is discussed in Chapter 21).

Mission, Vision, and Values

After the patient population has been identified and the patient care processes have been outlined, the APN may choose to formalize this information in a mission and vision statement. The mission and vision statement describes to patients and prospective funding agencies the APN practice's reason for existence and future direction; at times, the statement serves to remind the APN entrepreneur about where the program or practice's priorities should lie. The written summary of program or practice values may be combined with the mission and vision statements into one document, such as a brochure or program information sheet. This summary is available for review by any interested party and should be given to every patient at the time of the first program or practice encounter.

The mission states the goal of the direct processes of care in one sentence. The vision describes the "ideal" 5-year goal; that is, what the APN envisions the direct processes of care to be 5 years from inception. The mission and vision statements enhance interdisciplinary collaboration as APNs clearly articulate their goals and vision of patient care to existing and potential colleagues, consultants, and third-party payors. If the APN is functioning through an intrapreneurial approach, the program's mission and vision should be examined with knowledge of the organization's mission and vision to ensure that the program fits into the overall goals of the organization. If the program's mission conflicts with that of the organization, problems may take the form of delays in funding, changes to the program's direct or indirect processes of care, barriers to program implementation, and outright denial of program development. If other providers, individuals, or groups have a stake in the program, the mission and vision statement should be determined through consensus of the group.

The values of a practice or program describe those ethical precepts that govern relationships between the provider, the practice, the patients, and external groups. They may be related to direct or indirect care processes. Professional ethics are discussed in Chapters 11 and 21. Ethical precepts pertaining to patient-focused values are described briefly here.

INFORMED CONSENT

Informed consent is both an ethical and legal mandate requiring that any provider obtain a competent patient's fully informed and voluntary consent prior to any medical or nursing treatment. The APN must describe the general nature of the treatment and any consequences involved, the normal risks and hazards inherent to the treatment, any known side effects or complications that may occur, and any alternative treatments available to the patient. The patient's informed consent comprises the patient's understanding of this information and the agreement to proceed with treatment. Both the APN's information and the patient's agreement within the informed consent discussion must be documented as part of the patient's medical record.

PRIVACY AND CONFIDENTIALITY

Privacy and confidentiality are important ethical issues that require careful consideration. The balance between the patient's right to privacy and society's need to be protected is important. State laws clearly explicate those patient issues, such as sexually transmitted diseases, abuse, or tuberculosis that are reportable by law. Patient confidentiality is critical to the provider-patient relationship. Other than legal reporting obligations, it is the patient's right to decide what information the APN and all other members of the health-care team may share with others. Protecting confidentiality extends to any communication between the APN and the patient, all personal data, information contained in the medical record, and any billing information related to the patient's care. The federal Health Insurance Portability and Accountability Act (HIPAA) became law in 1996, but mandatory compliance with federal regulations was not required until 2003. HIPAA mandates the proper use and disclosure of personal health information. Providers must have policies and trained personnel in place to implement privacy standards (see Chapter 22 and Buppert, 2003).

HIPAA guidelines are detailed on the website www.cms.hhs.gov/hipaa. This site provides a good overview of the Privacy Rule as well as answers to frequently asked questions about implementation.

In addition to the right to confidentiality regarding their health information, patients are entitled to a degree of personal privacy within the clinical encounter. Courtesy commands that the patient's dignity be maintained, including providing the patient with well-fitting patient gowns and cover sheets during the physical examination. Attention should be paid to the physical layout of the patient encounter area, ensuring that conversations cannot be overheard and that the room is secure from line of gaze through open doors and/or windows. Unless the patient agrees or is a minor (*not* seeking certain types of reproductive health, substance abuse, or mental health care, as determined by individual states' laws), family members should not be invited into the patient encounter.

SECURITY

Both the patient and the APN should feel as if the patient care area is a safe and secure place for the encounter. Policies should clearly articulate how to maintain patient, provider, and staff safety, including provisions for securing a patient's valuables during procedures and for managing hostile persons in the area (including a policy for managing violent and armed persons). The level of security needed is dependent upon the APN's practice environment and available resources within the facility.

RESOLUTION OF COMPLAINTS

It is essential to monitor patient satisfaction with the clinical experience from the time the patient enters the waiting room through the time the final bill is paid for services. There are many patient satisfaction tools available to health-care providers to measure patients' responses to the way care is delivered (Kleinpell, 2001; see also Chapter 25). Despite one's best efforts, however, patients may be dissatisfied with some aspect of their experience at some point during an APN's career. It is important that any patient complaint or sign of dissatisfaction be addressed immediately, preferably at the time of the complaint (Buppert, 2002). A formal policy related to the management of patient complaints includes how patient complaints are recorded, who investigates and responds to the patient's concerns, and how quickly the complaint is addressed. Specific guidelines for managing patient complaints may be supplemented by risk management information provided by the APN's malpractice carrier.

COMMUNICATION

Ethical clinical practice demands honesty and integrity in all patient interactions. Under the best circumstances, communication lines will be open and both the APN and the patient will understand each other and feel as if they have been understood. When misunderstandings occur, it behooves the APN to manage the issue as if it were a patient complaint—seeking to address the concerns in an objective and timely manner. Communications of a vital nature to patient care, such as the reporting of a critical diagnostic test result or the termination of the provider-patient relationship, demand that additional steps be taken to ensure the patient is notified and that he or she understands the implications of the communication. In the instance of an abnormal test result, all telephone conversations should be documented with the date and time of the patient contact, along with any specific plans for treatment or follow-up testing resulting from the initial test result. Termination of the provider-patient relationship may be accomplished in a three-step process. First, a policy describing those scenarios under which the APN will terminate the relationship is clearly articulated and made available to the patient if requested. Second, the APN speaks directly with the patient, detailing the behaviors that meet the criteria for termination. Third, a summary of the discussion is promptly sent to the patient in a certified, return-receipt letter. A copy of the letter sent to the patient is kept in the patient's medical record with the signed postal receipts. Some states have regulations regarding the termination of the provider-patient relationship, and APNs should refer to individual state-specific guidelines from the board of nursing and/or boards of medicine and osteopathy for further information.

Clinical Relationships

Although the APN is assumed to be the primary care provider in this discussion, attention must be paid to the development of clinical relationships with APN, physician, pharmacist, and other allied health colleagues. (In-depth discussions related to clinical mentorship, consultation, and collaboration are found in Part II.) To be successful, the APN must maintain a collegial relationship with other health-care providers (Almost & Laschinger, 2002; Hanson, 1993). An important legal consideration is defining the parameters of the association with a collaborating physician through the development of a collaborative practice agreement (see Chapter 21 and 22). Most state statutes for APNs require some form of medical collaboration. A strong relationship with a collaborating physician or group of physicians is essential to the success of APN practice.

Consultants and Referrals

APNs need to find consultants and referral sources for patients whose medical problems require additional expertise from a specialist. Locating referrals for indigent or uninsured patients who need medical care or hospitalization may be difficult because of the lack of services for these populations. A list of consultants and referral sources, one that outlines the services offered and their willingness to accept referrals, should be generated. Their participation in third-party payor plans, such as health maintenance organization (HMO) networks or preferred provider organizations (PPOs), also should be noted and clearly understood by the APN entrepreneur. Consultants are identified through word-of-mouth recommendations from clinical mentors and colleagues, through the recommendation of lay public support groups who have worked with certain specialty groups, and through direct provider interviews. For example, a local chapter of the American Heart Association may be aware of the providers offering heart-healthy nutrition classes. Over time, the APN develops a referral and consultation base and develops strong relationships with those providers who are able to assist the APN in meeting patients' needs. Once the relationship is established, acknowledging the consultant's assistance and support is equally important. This acknowledgment may be as simple as learning from the consulting registration staff what demographic information they need in order to schedule the patient, providing the most recent office notes to the consultant in time for the patient's appointment, and sending seasonal cards thanking them for their support.

INDIRECT PROCESSES OF CARE

Indirect processes support patient care and center on administrative and operational structures and functions. Although they require a different set of advisors, staff, and equipment, indirect processes are equally important to the successful APN practice. Business relationships and business structures are necessary to define the context and framework under which clinical practice is performed. Knowledge of the external regulatory bodies that have an impact on APN practice is essential in today's complex and rapidly changing health-care arena. The subsequent discussion presents an overview of these issues but in no way is intended to be comprehensive. The APN is referred to business consultants for up-to-date information reflective of the laws and guidelines within a particular state and practice setting.

Business Relationships

Separate from, but as important as, the clinical advisors and resources described earlier are the administrative advisors and resources required to develop and maintain smooth indirect processes to support patient care. An independent practice will need to contract or consult with an accountant, attorney, banker, and insurance agent for specific services (Stewart, 1989). In addition, the services of a practice management consultant with medical billing expertise should be enlisted (Association of Academic Health Centers, 2002). The accountant should assist the APN in setting up an accounting system, establishing internal controls, and preparing an operating budget (AMA, 1996d). The accountant should set up the practice to ensure that the best tax advantages and flexibility are obtained (AMA, 1996d; Buppert, 2004). Attorneys with expertise in health-care law should establish the legal structure of the practice and provide advice on an as-needed basis for special purposes (AMA, 1996d). The attorney and accountant should have a working relationship so that the legal structure selected provides the best legal, financial, and tax advantages for the providers involved. The banking relationship serves to establish a line of credit or business loan (if needed) and to establish business banking needs (AMA, 1996d; Association of Academic Health Centers, 2002). A business insurance agent provides expertise in the areas of health, liability, and worker's compensation insurance programs. The practice management consultant serves to develop policies and procedure manuals, billing procedures and fee schedules, and job descriptions for an entrepreneurial enterprise (AMA, 1996d; Letz, 2002). A medical billing expert provides guidance in both the efficient completion and processing of billing forms in order to receive third-party reimbursement or capitation payment for the provider's services and the thorough and accurate completion of any third-party payor's contracting paperwork required for the APN's participation in selected contracts. The APN needs to carefully decide which of these functions can be done independently and which need to be purchased as externally contracted services. It is important for the APN entrepreneur to ask the following: Is this an area of strength and interest, or is this an area that I do not want to attend to? Is this an indirect process of care to which I want to devote time and energy?

The selection of day-to-day administrative support staff services (separate from the services of business advisors) revolves around the processes of care being delivered and the environment in which services are delivered. Once the APN knows what the direct patient care process will include and has identified those indirect processes that will support the patient encounter, additional ancillary personnel may be identified to meet process needs. In the community-based primary care setting, a practice requires someone to assist in patient registration and scheduling (the first process box in Figure 20-1), someone to assist the clinician in certain elements of patient care (the second box), and someone to collect or process patient fees (the third box). Any additional administrative roles support these primary roles and may include someone to manage patient medical records, someone to triage acutely ill patients by telephone, and someone to perform office cleaning functions. The actual individuals who fill these roles, along with their skills and qualifications, need to be matched with APN and practice goals for patient care. In hospital-based settings, CRNAs, CNSs, and CNMs often collaborate with the nurse managers of the area in which they practice to obtain the assistance of the unit's support staff and ancillary personnel. An organizational chart and job descriptions of the roles required should be developed, placed in a common personnel manual, and shared among staff members so that everyone is aware of his or her role within the successful functioning of the system. An example of an organizational chart is presented in Figure 20-2. Some payors require a copy of the organizational chart prior to enrolling the provider, as Medicaid does for APNs providing children's services. The experience, education, and other qualifications of the APN, other professionals providing services, and support staff should be described briefly and made available to interested parties.

Program and Business Structure

The structure that a particular intrapreneurial program takes is dependent upon the organization's overall guidelines for program development. An entrepreneurial program structure is often dictated by the requirements of whichever funding agency has provided the start-up and operating capital. The APN developing a program dependent upon the guidelines of other organizations is referred to the particular organization participating in program sponsorship. Many grant-funding agencies have criteria for funding and program guidelines available on the World Wide Web.

APN practice may assume one of several business structures depending upon the organizational context in which the practice is set. Practices may be hospital based or community based. Hospital-based practices may be inpatient or ambulatory in nature. Community-based practices are usually primary care settings or freestanding health centers or birthing centers, but may also be a part of a PPO, HMO, or other payor-based primary care site. Practices may be established on a for-profit or not-for-profit basis. APNs should consult with business advisors to determine the best business structure to match their values and goals. It is not the intent of this chapter to provide professional legal, business, or accounting advice, only to provide basic information for the establishment of those applicable business relationships. The APN is referred to professional advisors for the clarification of specific questions or issues.

There are three basic ways to structure the practice: a sole proprietorship, a partnership, or a corporation (Vogel & Doleysh, 1994). The primary differences between these structures lie in differing tax restrictions and liability. The simplest form of business

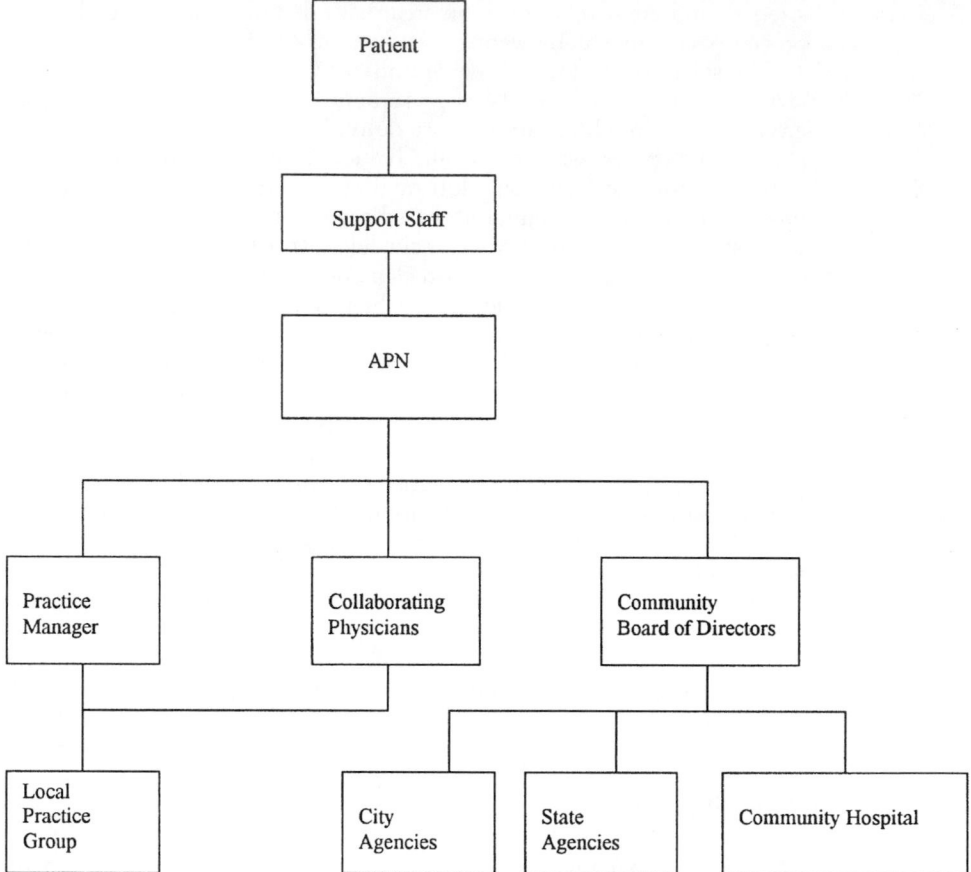

FIGURE 20-2 • Example of an organizational chart. (Based on data from Mercy Maritime Family Practice, Peaks Island, ME.)

organization is a sole proprietorship, which involves one owner. It is relatively straightforward and inexpensive to establish, and control remains with the sole owner. For tax purposes, the business income is taxed at the personal tax rate. The major disadvantage of the sole proprietorship is the unlimited liability that accompanies the structure. The owner assumes all liability, including that for any negligent acts of employees.

Most medical practices are for-profit partnerships. A general partnership may be advantageous for the APN because partnering with another professional may attract venture capital. The unlimited liability for each individual partner remains, as does the personal tax rate on business income. A disadvantage of this structure is the possibility of personality conflicts and disagreements arising between the partners over control and decision making. As mentioned previously, the legality of relationships between different professionals is often dictated by state law. CRNAs can join business arrangements as consultants to hospitals and anesthesia groups. Freestanding birthing centers are a respected alternative to tertiary hospitals for uncomplicated deliveries.

A corporation is a separate legal entity for both tax and liability purposes. Incorporation protects the owners from some, though not all, liability because a corporation's liability is limited. Consequently, because the medical professional owners retain a portion of any liability incurred, it is strongly advised that APNs and other providers have an individual liability policy. A professional corporation can elect a small business (Subchapter S) status, which allows owners to retain the benefit of taxation at the personal rate or, as is sometimes said, to avoid double taxation—first on corporate income and second on shareholder dividends. Other advantages of a corporation include the ability to start pension and profit-sharing plans and the possibility of attracting venture capital investors. The main disadvantage for a corporation not electing small business status is the higher tax rate incurred by corporations. A corporation may also be more expensive to establish and operate.

Selecting a name for the practice may be an option worth considering in certain situations. Rather than using an individual's name, a specific practice name may assist in describing the services offered and reflect the business focus, for example, Women's Health Services, Access to Continence Care and Treatment (Newman, 1996), and The Family Health and Birth Center (see Chapter 16). Many professionals use their own name to connote a more personalized service, as well as to promote themselves. Most individual states regulate the selection and registration of business names as part of the registration of the business structure process. The process entails registering the business name, conducting a formal state agency search to ensure that the name is not being used by another business, paying a registration fee, and awaiting the receipt of a formal document confirming assignment of the business name to the APN (Letz, 2002).

External Regulatory Bodies

An interwoven fabric of regulations and guidelines serves as the basis upon which APN professional practice is built and developed (see Chapter 22 and the individual APN chapters in Part III for an in-depth discussion of APN credentialing and regulation). Federal and state regulations, policies of private insurance companies, and, in some instances, local politics determine which business structures and practice environments an APN may work within and obtain reimbursement and whether this practice is independent, collaborative, or supervised. Although APN students routinely learn about the importance of the rules and regulations established by many different stakeholders to health-care systems, the impact upon daily practice may not be appreciated until the student becomes a practicing clinician. The major external regulatory vehicles affecting APN practice include the following:

- Those state and federal statutes pertaining to the regulation and credentialing requirements for advanced practice nursing
- Guidelines for health-care organizations regarding multiple facets of the management, environment, and delivery of health care established by the Joint Commission on Accreditation of Health-Care Organizations (JCAHO) (www.jcaho.org)
- Occupational Safety and Health Administration (OSHA) regulations related to safe working conditions for employees (www.osha.gov)
- CLIA regulations pertaining to laboratory services (www.cms.hhs.gov/clia)
- Additional Centers for Medicare and Medicaid regulations pertaining to Medicare reimbursement processes (www.cms.hhs.gov/medicare)
- Those additional regulations and guidelines determined by certain funding agencies, such as grant providers (reimbursement regulations specific to major health-care insurers)
- The JCAHO (1995) evaluates a health-care organization's system performance in both patient-focused (direct care) and organizational (indirect care) areas in order

to improve the quality of care provided to the public. Patient-focused functions include patient rights and organization ethics, assessment of patients, care of patients, education, and continuum of care. Organizational functions include improving organization performance, leadership, management of the environment of care, management of human resources, management of information, and surveillance, prevention, and control of infection. Additionally, the JCAHO examines an organization's governance, management, and functions related to medical and nursing staff. Each year, the JCAHO publishes detailed information about the performance-focused standards upon which a health-care organization is evaluated. These standards are described in the first volume of the accreditation manual for the particular health-care organization of interest (e.g., manual for hospitals, for ambulatory care clinics, etc.). The second volume of the manual contains the scoring guidelines used for accreditation purposes during JCAHO site surveys. Surveys are performed every 3 years by JCAHO-employed provider and nonprovider survey teams. The teams spend several days evaluating the organization using the scoring guidelines found in volume II of that year's manual. An overall score is determined along with any recommendations for improving scoring deficiencies. Accreditation is based upon the organization's compliance with JCAHO guidelines and implementation of any recommendations to resolve deficiencies (JCAHO, 2004 and www.jcaho.org).

As a result of being expert clinicians, APNs are often involved in patient-focused processes of interest to the JCAHO. Their level of involvement in organizational processes depends on the degree of individual APN responsibility for indirect care processes. Regardless of how many standards may directly relate to an individual APN's practice, all APNs should be aware of the guidelines upon which their organization is being evaluated. On an individual level, many of the APN competencies discussed in Part II are touched upon by some or many of the JCAHO standards. The JCAHO standards may also assist APNs in the development of their own standards of patient care and professional performance. In this manner, the JCAHO serves as a valuable resource to augment professional nursing standards and guidelines related to the delivery of clinically excellent patient care in caring, compassionate, high-quality health-care organizations.

Health-care safety management and hazard control are proven processes that produce results by preventing accidents, reducing injury rates, and increasing organizational efficiency (Tweedy, 1997). Areas include emergency planning and fire safety, general and physical plant safety, managing hazardous materials, managing biological waste, safety in patient care areas, and health-care support area safety (Tweedy, 1997). In terms of external regulators, safety management is carefully scrutinized by both the JCAHO and OSHA (Occupational Safety and Health Administration). APNs functioning as entrepreneurs or employers must be well versed in the rules, regulations, and implementation of safety programs governing these areas of safety management and hazard control. All APNs should be aware of their individual responsibilities regarding workplace safety, especially with respect to the management of biological waste and OSHA guidelines regarding blood-borne pathogens.

Created as part of the Department of Labor, OSHA was charged by the Occupational Safety and Health Act of 1970 to ensure safe and healthful working conditions for American workers. The general duty clause required every employer to furnish "a place of employment which is free from recognized hazards that cause or are likely to cause death or serious physical harm to employees." In 1991 the act was amended to include blood-borne pathogens as a specific occupational exposure to be managed. Under this amendment, occupational exposure is defined as the reasonably anticipated skin, eye, mucous membrane, or parenteral contact with blood or other potentially infectious materials that may result from the performance of an employee's duties. In order to prevent the employee's exposure, the employer is required to develop an exposure control plan.

Diagnostic Services

Any provider or laboratory service planning to collect, prepare, and analyze patient specimens is bound by CLIA rules and regulations (CMS, 2004b). Congress adopted the CLIA in response to published findings about the quality of laboratory testing (Hurst, Nickel, & Hilborne, 1998). Enacted to safeguard the public, the CLIA establish minimum acceptable criteria standards for all categories of laboratory testing in the United States. Providers offering laboratory services meet the criteria and apply for the appropriate level of CLIA certification. Certification is based on the complexity of testing being performed. Fees for the certificates are based upon the test complexity, the number of specimens being processed, and the cost of surveyor inspection (Schwartz, 1996). There are four categories of laboratory testing defined by the CLIA: waived tests, provider-performed microscopy (PPM), moderate-complexity procedures, and high-complexity procedures. If laboratory specimens are going to be performed by the APN, the first two categories of CLIA testing apply to the usual level of procedures performed. Moderate- and high-complexity procedures are generally performed by independent or hospital-based laboratories.

Waived tests are simple laboratory examinations and procedures cleared by the Food and Drug Administration for home use. They are simple and accurate (making the likelihood of error minimal) and pose no significant harm to the patient. Examples of CLIA-waived tests include fecal occult blood, nonautomated dipstick or tablet urinalysis, urine pregnancy visual color comparison tests, and all qualitative color comparison pH testing of body fluids. The laboratory would apply and pay for a CLIA Certificate of Waiver, allowing the laboratory to perform only waived tests. The certificate is valid for 2 years. PPM (Provider-Performed Microscopy Procedures) is a subcategory of the moderate-complexity level of testing. These examinations may be performed by physicians, dentists, or midlevel providers during the patient visit on a specimen obtained from the provider's patient or a patient of the group practice (American Academy of Family Practice, 2004). Other key criteria related to PPM stipulate that the primary instrument for the test be the microscope; that the specimen must be labile, or a delay in the testing could compromise test accuracy; and that limited specimen handling is required. Examples of PPM procedures include wet mounts, including preparation of vaginal, cervical, or skin specimens; all potassium hydroxide (KOH) preparations; pinworm examinations; and nasal smears for eosinophils. The certificate for this level of laboratory service, the Certificate for Provider-Performed Microscopy Procedures, allows the provider to perform waived tests as well.

Moderate- and high-complexity laboratories are allowed to perform procedures of increasing complexity, requiring additional pieces of instrumentation and necessitating increased amounts of specimen handling during processing. In addition to a specific listing of tests related to the appropriate level of complexity, moderate- and high-complexity laboratories are required to meet personnel and quality assurance/quality control proficiency testing and survey requirements in order to obtain a Certificate of Registration. These laboratories are also required to obtain Certificates of Compliance and Accreditation verifying compliance with all the applicable CLIA and Centers for

Medicare and Medicaid Services (CMS) requirements. With the new structure at CMS, quality and personnel rules for clinical laboratories have been streamlined and simplified. CLIA information may be obtained at the following sites: www.cms.hhs.gov/clia and www.aafp.org/pt.

If the APN does not intend to perform laboratory testing within the practice setting, the APN will need to identify providers of diagnostic testing services who will accept requisitions for diagnostic tests. In the absence of an in-house laboratory, external laboratory services basically include specimen collection, specimen processing, and reporting of results. Some APN practices choose to collect specimens themselves, then have them transported to the laboratory for processing and reporting. These practices require a separate refrigerator and/or freezer for specimen storage pending transfer to the processing area, along with the containers and media for proper specimen collection. For those practices choosing to collect and process their own specimens, additional equipment and supplies will be needed depending on the nature of the tests being performed. Local laboratories may be identified by asking for assistance from a local hospital or by speaking with a laboratory service representative directly. The APN should inquire about issues such as how the lab's specific requisition forms should be completed; specimen collection, pickup, and drop box availability; how results are reported (by telephone, fax, dedicated computer printer, or mail); what patients should expect; and how they are billed. In addition to laboratory services, imaging services need to be identified. Often local hospitals will allow providers to refer patients for radiological services through the outpatient referral process. As with the laboratory services, issues related to the requisition of testing, the testing process (including any patient preparation requirements), the reporting of results, and patient billing should be discussed and recorded for future reference.

Recent revisions in Medicare regulations have resulted in the heightened enforcement of the policy of medical necessity with respect to diagnostic services. In an attempt to decrease costs related to inappropriate diagnostic testing, certain laboratory and radiological services have been identified as requiring proof of medical necessity in order for them to be covered by Medicare, Medicaid, and other carriers. In order to have these services covered, the provider must ensure that they are medically appropriate for the patient's diagnosis or symptoms. The determination of medical necessity is made by CMS and codified through a listing of those *International Classification of Diseases: Clinical Modification* (ICD-9-CM) (AMA, 2004) diagnoses and symptoms that will justify the diagnostic service requested. For example, in order to have thyroid-stimulating hormone (TSH) testing paid for by Medicare, the patient must have a certain ICD-9-CM diagnosis on the listing for TSH testing, such as goiter (ICD-9-CM codes 240.0–240.9), acquired hypothyroidism (ICD-9-CM codes 244.0–244.9), or malaise and fatigue (ICD-9-CM code 780.7). (N.B.: Other diagnoses and symptoms are allowed for TSH testing. These diagnoses and symptoms are for use as examples only.) Those diagnostic tests for which medical necessity has been determined in specific locales of the United States are listed in local Medicare medical policies found either through the laboratory service or directly from the local Medicare intermediary newsletter. Most other carriers follow the Medicare medically necessary requirements. It is important to note here that CMS uses private companies, termed "fiscal intermediaries," that contract with Medicare to pay Medicare Part A and some Part B bills. These fiscal intermediaries influence what procedures and tests are covered at the local level.

If the patient's diagnosis does not comply with CMS guidelines but testing is determined to be necessary by the provider, the patient must be notified, in advance, that the cost of this testing may become the responsibility of the patient. This notification is formalized in the completion of an Advanced Beneficiary Notice (ABN), detailing the test requested, the symptoms or disease state necessitating the testing, and that the patient has been advised that the testing may not meet the guidelines for Medicare reimbursement. The patient signs the ABN, and the signature is witnessed by another staff person. Although on the surface this process may seem to limit provider discretion, underlying this process is a deepening of the provider's knowledge of appropriate utilization of diagnostic testing and recognition that diagnostic testing is an expensive and limited resource with significant financial impact on the health-care system. This process would also hold true for certain procedures that may be considered cosmetic, such as some lesion removals. A new ABN for lesion removal was developed in 2002.

PROCESS RESOURCES: EQUIPMENT/SUPPLIES/CAPITAL FUNDING

To follow in the paradigm of systems thinking, the processes of care to be delivered and the setting in which these processes occur will determine the tools needed to deliver that care. Equipment and supplies to deliver home-based primary care to an elderly population will be different from those required to implement a hospital-based wound care clinic for children who have sustained burns. The most effective way to determine what is needed for a program or practice is to flowchart all the processes of care (both direct and indirect) with all the items needed for a particular step itemized below their respective boxes (Figure 20-3). A secondary gain is that this process allows the APN to clearly identify the costs linked with particular services delivered. Table 20-2 depicts the initial cost-based inventory of the steps illustrated in Figure 20-3. This approach is the basis for cost-based analysis. Cost-based analysis examines the actual costs of the supplies, equipment, and personnel needed to perform a particular process of care. Additional costs related to business operations overhead are calculated into the final cost, which is then used to determine the charge to the patient for that process of care. The actual charge for each service should be based on the Medicare relative value analysis times a conversion that is not only necessary for the practice but is consistent with other services in the area. By using this system APNs will be assured that they will not be overcharging or undercharging for clinical services. The charge profile should be reviewed on a yearly basis. (The reader is referred to Neumann and Boles [1998] for an in-depth discussion of cost-based analysis.)

Additional methods available for identifying needed equipment and supplies include the following:

- Relying on clinical expertise of the APN and her or his familiarity with the items needed to deliver the identified service
- Referring to a clinical procedures manual that lists the equipment needed
- Consulting with the collaborating physician
- Interviewing other providers who are performing the same or similar services
- Interviewing support staff to determine what they require to perform their roles
- Referring to standardized equipment listings

After determining the program/practice needs, lists or inventories are generated. These equipment and supply inventories serve to accomplish the following:

- Establish an initial budget and time line for business-planning purposes, and provide information related to budgetary requests required by lenders and grantors. (These inventories may be included in any business plan, grant application, or office procedure manual, thus eliminating the need to rewrite them for each application.)

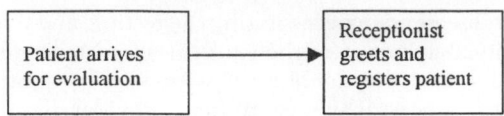

Who Performs:	Patient
	Receptionist
Related Processes:	Triage
	Scheduling
	Registration
	Patient confidentiality
	Medical records
Required Resources:	<u>Office space</u>: leased/purchased office

<u>Durable equipment</u>: desks, chairs, end tables, lamps/lights with bulbs, magazine rack, patient education brochure rack, bulletin board, decorative plants, pictures, curtains/draperies for the windows, rugs/carpet/floor covering, waste baskets, telephone, photocopying machine, locked cash box/drawer, calculator, credit card equipment and electronic transfer linkage, computer system, fax machine

<u>Reuseable items</u>: magazine subscriptions, patient education brochures, tacks/fasteners for bulletin board displays, actual bulletin board displays, telephone answering system/software, computer software

<u>Disposable items</u>: facial tissues, coloring books, crayons, pencils/pens, erasers, business cards, appointment book, demographic/registration forms, office encounter form (superbill), patient medical record folders/dividers, patient chart stickers (allergy, year, alphabetical), photocopy/fax paper

FIGURE 20-3 • Itemization of a patient care process.

- Create an initial ordering or shopping list.
- Record business assets.
- Establish minimum par levels for an inventory of disposable supplies.
- Identify the locations where items are kept in the office to facilitate inventory management.

The initial inventories for medical and office equipment and supplies follow the same template and could be set up as comparable spreadsheets within any commercial office

TABLE 20-2	COST-BASED INVENTORY OF PATIENT REGISTRATION PROCESS: DISPOSABLE ITEMS*			
ITEM	VENDOR	PAR LEVEL	UNIT COST ($)[†]	TOTAL COST ($)[†]
Facial tissues	ABC Office Supply	12 boxes	0.75	9.00
Coloring books	State Children Program	36	FREE	FREE
Crayons	State Children Program	36 packs	FREE	FREE
Pencils	ABC Office Supply	5 boxes of 12	2.00	10.00
Pens: black	ABC Office Supply	10 boxes of 12	3.00	30.00
Erasers	ABC Office Supply	5	0.50	2.50
Business cards	Printing Shop	2 boxes of 1,000	40.00	80.00
Appointment book	ABC Office Supply	1	15.00	15.00
Demographic forms	Printing Shop	2 pads of 100	10.00	20.00
Superbills	Printing Shop	1 box of 2,000	275.00	275.00
Medical record folders	XYZ Forms	1 box of 100	20.00	20.00
Medical record dividers	XYZ Forms	1 box of 100 sets	20.00	20.00
Chart stickers: allergy	XYZ Forms	1 roll of 100	5.00	5.00
Chart stickers: year	XYZ Forms	1 roll of 500	5.00	5.00
Chart stickers: alpha	XYZ Forms	1 set of 20 each	15.00	15.00
Photocopy paper	ABC Office Supply	1 box of 10 reams	75.00	75.00
Fax paper	ABC Office Supply	1 box of 6 rolls	45.00	45.00

*If the APN sees 2,000 patients in a 12-month period, and the above disposable items are depleted in the same amount of time, then the cost of the disposable items used during patient registration process per year is TOTAL COST/TOTAL NUMBER OF PATIENTS = COST PER PATIENT PER YEAR (approximate), or $626.50/2000 = $0.31 (approximate).
[†]Prices are approximate and are used for illustration only.

software package. The AMA (1996c) suggested creating three separate inventories: durable equipment, reusable equipment/supplies, and disposable supplies. One advantage to this separation is that it enables the program administrator/practice manager to quickly assess how much money is needed to set up the program/practice, as opposed to how much will be needed on an ongoing basis for replenishment of supplies. The first lists the furniture and equipment needed to set up the office and examination room(s). This list includes durable equipment (e.g., desks, chairs, file cabinets, examination tables, autoclave, electrocardiograph, computers). The second lists the reusable equipment needed, such as trash cans, staplers, tape dispensers, linen baskets, otoscope, stethoscope, and computer software (Rehm & Kraft, 1998). The third lists the disposable supplies needed. It is helpful to separate the disposable supplies into two lists, one for office supplies and one for medical supplies. The office supply list includes items such as pens, pencils, tape, staples, and photocopy/printer paper. The medical supply list includes items such as alcohol swabs, gauze pads, bandages, examination table paper, and syringes. For accounting and budgeting purposes, request professional advice to separate these items into capital and noncapital expenses. Each list includes the specific name of the equipment or supply needed and the number of units required. Quotes from potential vendors for the item should be sought on a yearly basis. Once a vendor is identified, the price per unit (unit cost) and a total price for that item (total cost) is added to the inventory template. It is possible to obtain some disposable supplies free of charge from other sources. For example, in primary care, often the laboratory analyzing the blood specimens drawn at the practice will provide alcohol swabs, small gauze pads, Band-Aids, and other supplies used during venipuncture or other specimen collection as part of its service to the practice. Many pharmaceutical representatives are often willing to provide pens, note pads, and clipboards for free, although these items will have the names of the pharmaceutical company's products on them as part of its marketing plan. Some larger facilities operate in-house supply "swaps" in which the excess supplies of one department are offered in trade for the excess supplies of another department. Although these sources of inexpensive disposable supplies are available, it is essential when planning an initial budget to calculate that the program/practice is responsible for purchasing these items from traditional vendors.

Decisions related to which processes will be performed in house, as opposed to being contracted externally, will affect the types of equipment and supplies needed. Examples of indirect processes of care include the following:

- *Creating a patient database.* There are several medical office computerized systems available, of varying complexity and cost, for the management of patient information. Some of the processes supported by these programs are appointment scheduling, generation of patient encounter forms (Superbills), and electronic claims filing. Electronic claims filing is essential to any practice as a way to keep the accounts receivable under control and should be HIPAA compliant (Buppert, 2003).
- *Transcription services.* For intrapreneurial APNs, transcription services may be available through the larger organization's facilities. For independent APNs, the decision to contract for transcription services should include a review of the available voice-to-text computer software programs that allow the APN to directly dictate the patient's progress note (or other printed material) into a commercially available word processing or desktop publishing program. There are several voice-to-text programs available with different degrees of complexity and adaptability and varying sizes of medical vocabulary lexicons. The prices for these programs range from $150 for a basic voice-to-text program to more than $4,000 for a complex system that may be used by several providers at once.
- *Ensuring staff safety.* Material safety data sheets (MSDSs) are required for all items that pose a potential occupational risk to the employees working with them, such as alcohol, povidone-iodine (Betadine), or cancer chemotherapeutic agents. The MSDS information is available from the manufacturer upon request at no cost. Other OSHA regulations, such as those pertaining to biomedical waste disposal and blood-borne pathogen exposure, must also be implemented into practice, and appropriate records kept for review. As with transcription services, personnel safety systems may be available within the larger institution or will need to be either developed or purchased for a freestanding practice.
- *Patient education materials.* Patient education materials are available in a variety of formats, including videotape, interactive computer software, and traditional written brochures or pamphlets. The APN should review the direct patient care processes for which educational materials can be anticipated. Part of the initial planning process includes reviewing available materials that can be incorporated into the APN's practice. Educational material should be evaluated for quality, readability/literacy level, availability in different languages, and cost. Oral presentations to individuals or groups are also an important component of patient education.

One process of care that requires particular attention is the use of pharmaceutical agents in direct patient care by APNs with prescriptive privileges. Some of the supporting processes involved in writing a patient prescription include the following:

- *Writing the physical prescription.* Because APNs have prescription privileges in the state in which they practice, the APN will need to have prescription pads available that comply with state regulation. The prescription pads will include the APN's name and credentials and the name of the APN's practice setting on the pad. In several states, the name of the collaborating physician must be on the prescription pad. Free prescription pads are available through Medi-Scripts, a prescription printing service funded by a collaboration of pharmaceutical companies. Box 20-1 provides further information. Prescription pads should never be left where they may become accessible to patients, family, or unauthorized staff.

- *Receiving drug samples.* A system to track lot numbers, expiration dates, and the patients to whom the drug was dispensed needs to be developed to address the issue of lot number recalls and to meet certain states' requirements for oversight.
- *Including controlled substances in the course of patient care.* In states where APNs can prescribe controlled substances, the APN must obtain an individual Drug Enforcement Agency (DEA) number. A completed DEA registration form will be required, with the registration fees paid, before the APN is able to prescribe controlled substances allowed by statute. The DEA registration is renewable every 3 years. Cost for NP registration in 2002 was $210 for the 3-year period. Forms may be requested on the Internet (see Box 20-1). In addition to a DEA number, a locked, secure location for storage needs to be established, and a procedure for access must be determined prior to acceptance of a supply, should the APN dispense controlled substances from the office.

The use of medications within a program or practice depends on the nature of the services to be delivered but is also constrained by the scope of practice granted by individual state nurse practice acts. When the decisions regarding the use of pharmaceutical agents have been made, a listing of anticipated pharmacy supplies, along with cost, vendor, and par level information, may be generated from the same software spreadsheet as the other inventories. When a pharmaceutical inventory is prepared, those practices that provide children's services will find enrollment in the state immunization program extremely

---

BOX 20-1 • USEFUL BUSINESS PLANNING RESOURCES FOR APNs

Centers for Medicare and Medicaid Services
7500 Security Blvd
Baltimore, MD 21244-1850
877-267-2323 (toll free)
410-786-3000

Medi-Scripts
500 Rt. 17 South, Suite 308
Hasbrouck Heights, NJ 07604
800-283-0140
201-727-1555
fax 201-727-9824
www.medipromotions.com

Pharmaceutical Research and Manufacturers of
   America (PhARMA)
1100 Fifteenth Street NW
Washington DC 20005-1707
202-835-3400
fax 202835-3414
www.phrma.org

Drug Enforcement Administration (DEA)
2401 Jefferson Davis Highway
Alexandria, VA 22301
1-800-882-9539
www.usdoj.gov/dea

Joint Commission on Accreditation of
   Healthcare Organizations (JCAHO)
One Renaissance Blvd.
Oakbrook Terrance, Il 60181
630-792-5000
www.jcaho.org

useful. States provide immunizations free to children who fall within certain eligibility guidelines (e.g., Medicaid recipients, uninsured patients, or participants in a federally funded health center). These programs involve practice enrollment, a monthly vaccine utilization report, and some record-keeping regarding recipient eligibility. Some state programs have established a web-based system, allowing practices to report monthly usage and to reorder vaccine online. The maximum benefit of the web-based system is that it allows confirmation of childhood vaccinations to other enrolled practices within a secure and confidential network environment. When choosing a pharmaceutical agent for their patients, APNs are also aware of the financial impact of the drug on the patient. With the advent of managed care came the start of insurer-based drug formularies that limit the medications covered by a patient's prescription plan. Most managed care organizations have copies of their formularies available to providers so that patient needs may be matched with the insurer's cost-containment guidelines. If a patient takes a medication that is not on the formulary, possible substitutions should be evaluated. If there is no suitable alternative, all formularies have a vehicle by which a provider may appeal the formulary decision for a particular patient need.

For patients who are indigent or who meet low-income guidelines, many pharmaceutical companies offer subsidized and free prescriptions. A listing of which drugs are covered by these programs is usually available from the local sales representatives of the parent company. The process for obtaining free medications for an indigent patient entails completion of a brief form by the provider and the patient, who attest that the patient meets the income criteria for the particular program of interest. A written prescription, usually for a specific period of time as designated by the pharmaceutical program (e.g., 1 month, 3 months), accompanies the completed form. The medications are sent directly to the provider's office on behalf of the patient, who then needs to be notified that they have arrived. (A compilation of prescription assistance programs is available from Pharmaceutical Research and Manufacturers of America [2004]. The address may be found in Box 20-1, and full eligibility requirements for patients are available on the website).

It is important to note that certain third-party payors, government agencies, and mail-order prescription drug companies will not accept prescriptions from APNs. The primary reason for this exclusion is that the state to which the prescription and enrollment form are sent does not permit APNs to write prescriptions. The secondary reason for this exclusion is that the parent company is unaware of revisions to the state practice act that allow APNs to write prescriptions in that particular state. The solution for the first scenario is through the development of a prescribing policy whereby the APN's collaborating physician writes the prescription for that patient's medications. The solution to the second scenario is continued efforts on the part of APNs to educate and collaborate with pharmaceutical companies to ensure that accurate, timely information is being used. Patients who mail away for their prescriptions through their insurance prescription plan may also suffer from the inconvenience of being told that the APN is unable to write their prescriptions. The solutions for this group of patients are the same.

THE BUSINESS PLAN SUMMARY

Once the process of business or program planning has been accomplished, the APN should summarize in one document the mission, vision, values, and processes of care and required resources to meet the patient's needs. Traditionally this summary has taken the form of a business plan, which was then distributed to potential sources of financial backing. Even if the program is not seeking external funding, a summary is needed to describe the available services to others. One way of writing this summary is to modify the traditional business plan so that it reflects a systems-thinking approach to patient care (Box 20-2 provides an outline of a business summary). The reader is referred to Buppert (1999, 2004), the AMA (2002c), Letz, (2002), the Small Business Administration, and local business advisors for additional information and advice.

BOX 20-2 • OUTLINE OF A PROGRAM/PRACTICE SUMMARY

I. Introductory Elements
  A. Cover page
  B. Overview/summary
    1. Mission and vision statements
    2. Overarching program/practice values
    3. Other required elements
  C. Table of contents
II. Description
  A. Background information
  B. Direct processes of care to be delivered
  C. Key factors in the delivery of patient care
III. Market
  A. Description of the patient population to be served
    1. Patient demographics
  B. Analysis of the market
  C. Marketing strategy
    1. Initial
    2. Ongoing
  D. Competition
  E. Advertising and promotion
IV. Program/Practice Structure
  A. Structure/ownership
  B. Management
  C. Clinical advisors and services offered (includes APN)
  D. Business advisors and services offered
  E. Support staff and services offered
V. Resources
  A. Budget
    1. Projected income
      a. Start-up capital: business loans, grants
      b. Ongoing capital: patient revenues, other funding
    2. Projected expenses
      a. Office space and overhead
      b. Durable equipment
      c. Reuseable equipment
      d. Disposable items
      e. Provider and staff compensation
VI. Compliance
  A. Federal and/or state regulations
    1. JCAHO
    2. OSHA
    3. CMS
  B. Other agency regulations
  C. Provider-specific licensing, credentialing, privileging
VII. Outcome Evaluation
  A. APN performance measures
  B. System performance measures
  C. Internal review parameters and timeline
  D. External review parameters and timeline

Consideration must be given to the audience for whom the summary is being prepared. As discussed earlier, grant-funding agencies have specific guidelines for the compilation of the program's operational documentation. If the summary is written for the community of patients being served, issues related to literacy, language, and emphasis need to be addressed. If the summary is written for potential investors or potential physician colleagues, issues related to capital expenditures, numbers of patients to be served, and services to be delivered need to be emphasized. Consequently, the first step in preparing the summary is to identify the anticipated audience.

The summary should start with a cover page that details the name, address, and contact telephone number of the program or practice; the name(s) and credentials of the involved APNs, collaborating physicians, and any other team members; and the date that the summary was prepared. The next page of the summary should include the brief mission and vision statements written during the planning process. Any organizational values (separate from those that are patient focused and described elsewhere) should be included in the summary. Some business plan formats request that mention be given to the numbers of patients to be served and the estimated amount of capital required for start up and maintenance. A table of contents should be included for quick reference to key areas of the summary. The second section of the summary describes the direct processes of patient care to be rendered and any background information that affected the determination of these services. The third section describes the patient population to be served and provides information about the particular marketing strategies to be employed to build the practice or program (see Chapter 21). The fourth section compiles the organizational chart and the description of the program structure and management and provides the reader with information regarding the advisors the APN has gathered to ensure the success of the program. The fifth section focuses specifically on the monetary aspects of the program or practice. Detailed budgetary information is summarized here in a spreadsheet or other accepted business accounting format. The sixth section focuses on how the program will comply with the applicable regulations and guidelines. The final section describes the performance measures against which the APN and the system will be evaluated. Parameters and time lines for internal and external review are defined.

A successful system is able to describe what it does, how it does it, and how it evaluates the outcome (Kleinpell, 2001). A successful APN develops, implements, and evaluates both patient care and indirect processes that support outcomes by organizing these tasks as a system. Today's health-care environment demands that patient care delivery be innovative and resource efficient. Today's health-care consumers demand that patient care delivery be individualized, compassionate, and effective. A sound knowledge of the system in which care is delivered enables APNs to meet the demands of today's complex environment and the patients they serve.

Choosing the type of practice to engage in as an APN is a difficult and challenging task, one that the APN will have to live with on a daily basis. Decisions around practice type require careful planning, research, and discussions with other APNs who have entered into various types of practice arrangements. The following exemplar describes one potential practice arrangement.

This exemplar is instructive in that it illustrates the extended time frame that may precede the ability to engage in private practice. First, Ann needed to fine-tune her clinical skills so that she was a truly competent provider; second, she needed to fully understand the market, the business aspects, and the reimbursement implications of independent practice; last and most important, Ann needed time and patience to build relationships with her physician colleagues and to demonstrate her clinical and interactive skills as a viable professional partner.

EXEMPLAR 20-1

Ann is a gerontologic nurse practitioner (GNP) who was in a salaried position as a staff GNP in a large nursing home for the first 2 years after APN graduation. During this time she was able to gain insight into many facets of GNP practice and to build her APN skills and confidence. Recently, Ann, her husband, and their two teenagers moved to a metropolitan area in the southwestern United States. This area is a haven for retired persons, and the need for geriatric care is high. As her children are preparing to enter college soon, this seemed like a good time for Ann to consider going into joint practice with a local geriatrician. Ann realized that this was a long-term goal and one that would be achieved through multiphased planning.

Ann engaged in a per diem contract practice in a nursing home for 6 months while she explored opportunities for independent practice in the area. At the same time she carefully researched APN licensure and credentialing, business licensure rules and regulations, and reimbursement provisions in her new state. She also explored the mix and distribution of physician and other APN practitioners who care for elderly patients. She attended community functions to get a feel for community-based needs and concerns. Ann made an appointment and visited the five nursing homes in the area to better understand the level of care and opportunities that existed in each one. She talked with as many geriatric health-care providers as possible and watched and listened to see who might be looking for a professional partner.

At a local geriatric care meeting, she heard that a new geriatrician was coming to town, and she made plans to meet and talk with her. This meeting led to exploratory discussions about various practice arrangements that might be advantageous and challenging for both of them. As a next step, Ann contracted her services with this physician and the nursing home while continuing with her exploration of joint practice opportunities. Her goal was to move toward an eventual full partnership arrangement.

Ann's carefully orchestrated plan was fruitful. She was asked to attend a local medical association meeting, and three internists who carried a heavy caseload of nursing home patients proposed that she follow their patients as part of a shared endeavor. This arrangement gave Ann an opportunity to care for patients and to better understand reimbursement and operational issues attending a geriatric practice.

Six months later, Ann noticed a call for proposals from a national philanthropic organization to develop a model practice environment for community-based elders. She and one of the geriatrician colleagues with whom she was working received funding to implement a model practice that would serve as the basis for a joint practice arrangement to serve the community. As part of this grant proposal, Ann approached a psychiatric CNS to become a part of the model team. The model community idea was funded for 5 years and became a successful practice site. At the close of the grant cycle, Ann and the geriatrician became partners in a successful private practice.

REIMBURSEMENT MECHANISMS

Reimbursement refers to the monetary compensation of the clinician for services provided to patients and their families. The process of reimbursement is perhaps the most important and complex indirect process supporting patient care. Figure 20-4 provides an overview of the process of reimbursement. As with other indirect care processes, the level of APN involvement in this process depends on the individual APN's role in indirect processes as a whole. All APNs are involved in the completion of the patient's clinical encounter, the documentation of the encounter in the patient's medical record, and, frequently, the completion of the patient's bill for services. Some APNs may be involved in the subsequent steps in the reimbursement process: the actual payment collection, either from the patient or from the third-party payor, and the posting of the payment to the patient's account in the provider's office. All APNs should be cognizant of the major concepts and issues related to third-party reimbursement and to APN compensation. As illustrated in Figure 20-4, reimbursement builds bridges between the clinical encounter, the patient's medical record, the patient's bill for services, the claim submitted to the appropriate third-party payor (if any), and the payment of the APN for services delivered. In this section, an overview of documentation

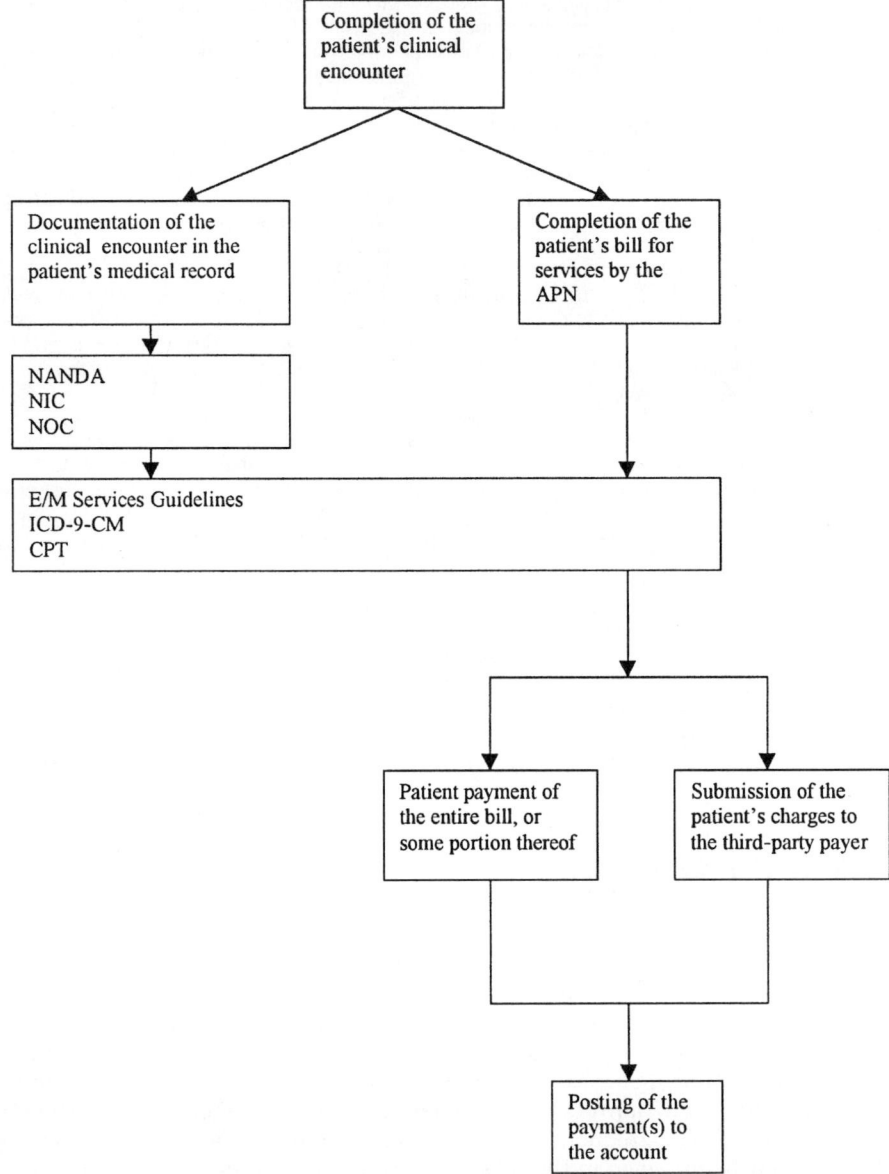

FIGURE 20-4 • An overview of reimbursement.

is presented, along with a description of the major third-party payment schemes. The patient's financial responsibility for self-pay is presented. Examples are used to illustrate steps in the reimbursement process.

Documentation

NURSING CLASSIFICATION SYSTEMS

Clinically excellent, holistic patient care delivered by APNs includes both nursing and medical diagnoses, interventions, and outcomes. Consequently, patient medical record documentation by an APN would reasonably include a combination of both nursing and medical diagnoses, interventions, and outcomes language. According to CMS, patient medical record documentation is required to chronologically record pertinent facts, reason for the visit, findings, and observations as to an individual's health history, including past and present illnesses, examinations, tests, treatments, and outcomes (CMS, 2004a). The undergraduate education of nurses emphasizes the nursing process and the use of standardized languages for nursing diagnoses, interventions, and outcomes in the record-keeping of nursing care. APNs, however, are not routinely prepared at the graduate level to continue the use of this nursing-sensitive language. One possible reason for this may be economically driven. In today's health-care arena, APNs are unable to bill third-party payors, or obtain reimbursement, for nursing diagnoses and/or interventions unless the diagnosis or intervention is recognized as a medical one. (The reader is referred to Henry, Holzemer, Randell, Hsieh, & Miller [1997] for a review of nursing interventions as compared with medical terminology.) The ramifications to nursing of this bias in monetary compensation are far reaching and beyond the scope of this discussion. However, the value of nursing care and the strides being made in standardizing and codifying what nurses do is being recognized and incorporated into various elements of reimbursement strategies, such as state nursing association recommendations for standardized language and automated billing software. (The reader is referred to www.alternativelink.com for information related to the integration of nursing interventions into the ABC Coding Systems for Third Party Billing.) In the future, direct financial compensation may be paid for nursing diagnoses and interventions that are independent of a medical model counterpart.

The nursing profession has organized nursing knowledge into three main areas: nursing diagnoses, nursing interventions, and nursing-sensitive patient outcomes (Bulechek & McCloskey, 1999). These areas correspond well to patient medical record documentation capturing the components of the patient's assessment, plan, and evaluation. The North American Nursing Diagnosis Association (NANDA) has worked toward the establishment and implementation of a classification system for nursing diagnoses since 1973 (Carpenito, 1999). In review, a nursing diagnosis is a clinical judgment about individual, family, or community responses to actual or potential health problems/life processes (Carpenito, 1999). The current strategic goals of NANDA include plans to incorporate NANDA diagnoses in standardized language systems and health-care databases and to promote the use of nursing diagnoses in nursing practice, education, and research. The Strategic Plan for NANDA International 2004-2010 can be found at www.nanda.org.

Nursing diagnoses provide the basis for the selection of nursing interventions that achieve the identified patient outcomes for which the nurse is accountable. An outcome is defined as a variable concept representing a patient or family caregiver state, behavior, or perception that is measurable along a continuum and responsive to nursing interventions. Ideally, outcomes should be chosen to optimize health as well as alleviate problems

(McCloskey & Bulechek, 1992). The Nursing Outcomes Classification (NOC) exists to codify a standardized language of nursing-sensitive patient outcomes (Iowa Intervention Project, 1997). The Iowa Intervention Project developed an evolving codified taxonomy of nursing interventions, the Nursing Intervention Classification (NIC), to list the treatments that nurses perform, to assist practitioners in documenting their care, and to facilitate the evaluation of nurse-sensitive patient outcomes (McCloskey & Bulechek, 1992). Familiarity with these standardized languages that capture the nursing care provided by APNs, as well as their consistent use in clinical practice and documentation, provides APNs with valuable tools in support of APN practice now and in the future.

MEDICAL CLASSIFICATION SYSTEMS

Familiarity with the medical-model guidelines and external regulations that govern reimbursement programs enables the APN to obtain health-care reimbursement through compliance with existing structures, and demonstrates to third-party payors that the APN is a knowledgeable participant in health care. This degree of professional accountability may reduce barriers to full APN participation as independent providers in their own right and expand the inclusion of nursing care within the realm of reimbursed elements of patient care. The foundation of the reimbursement process is proper patient medical record documentation of medical necessity. According to the AMA (2000), payors require the following information to determine medical necessity:

- Knowledge of the emergent nature or severity of the patient's concern or condition
- The signs, symptoms, complaints, or background facts describing the reasons for care

This information must be substantiated by the patient's medical record, and it must be available to payors upon request with a signed patient authorization (AMA, 2000). Failure to document services rendered translates into the nonperformance of the service, which may leave the APN open not only to questions regarding the medical necessity of the encounter but also to potential liability issues. Any and all services submitted for reimbursement must be supported by appropriate documentation in the patient's medical record. Notation of unusual services or extenuating circumstances should leave no room for misinterpretation or assumption. From a financial standpoint, insurance carriers will frequently limit or deny reimbursement for services because of insufficient documentation. In addition, they may request refunds from the provider if audited medical records do not substantiate the reported services.

To bill for services, many insurance carriers require the use of specific medical documentation guidelines, classifications, and reimbursement codes. Documentation guidelines provide standardization and structure for the clinical encounter record. The various classifications available provide a standard language, used by both insurance carriers and health-care providers, to provide a uniform interpretation of medical conditions and to identify the billable services of the provider. There are three main systems used to record and classify care delivered: the evaluation and management (E&M) services documentation guidelines (CMS, 2004a), the ICD-9-CM codes (Practice Management Information Corporation, 2003), and the *Current Procedural Terminology* (CPT) codes (AMA, 2003) at ama-assn.org/ama/pub.

The *E&M Services Guidelines* (CMS, 2004a) were developed to compensate providers for clinical and cognitive effort, rather than time expended. (They are available online at the CMS website [www.cms.hhs.gov] or through the local Medicare intermediary). There are seven components of E&M services, with the first four bearing the most weight:

1. *Nature of the presenting problem:* The reason or need for the client's office visit.
2. *History:* The client's chief concern, a brief history of the present issue or illness, and a related systems review. A family and/or social history is included.
3. *Physical examination:* Focused, addressing only the affected body area or organ system, or comprehensive, addressing a complete examination of a single system of concern, or a multiple system physical examination.
4. *Medical decision making:* The complexity in establishing a diagnosis and selecting a certain management strategy. It includes a list of all possible medical diagnoses (the differential diagnoses) and management options, an analysis of medical records, all diagnostic tests, and other information analyzed.
5. *Counseling:* Discussions or meetings with client, family, caregivers, and nursing staff (as in long-term care). Counseling can include discussions about disease process, results of diagnostic tests, prognosis, education and instructions on management, and treatment options.
6. *Coordination of care:* Time spent working with other health-care providers and agencies to direct care. This process must be well documented in the client's medical record if it is intended to denote the level of service, or care, delivered.
7. *Time:* In the case of encounters that predominantly consist of counseling or coordination of care, time is the key component used to determine the level of E&M services provided. Time is defined as "face-to-face" time in the office; time spent reviewing records and tests and arranging further services; or time spent with staff, such as in the nursing home. Time should be averaged in minutes and recorded in the client's medical record. Time is only relevant when coordination, chart review, and counseling services represent more than 50% of the visit.

As noted, the major elements used to determine the level of service provided under the E&M system are the patient history, the physical examination, and the complexity of medical decision making required to manage the patient. Elements of at least these three components must have been performed and consequently documented in the patient's medical record. The documentation guidelines provide minimum assessment data points within each component that will support a particular level of E&M service. Each level of service is assigned a separate five-digit CPT code. The codes vary for new patients and existing patients even if the same level of service has been provided (Box 20-3).

The ICD-9-CM codes are diagnostic codes that identify the diagnosis, symptom, or condition to be treated. Their purpose is to aid in standardizing coding practices across the United States (AMA, 2004) as directed by the CMS. The CMS has prepared guidelines for use of the ICD-9-CM codes in the area of medical billing. These guidelines are available online at the CMS website (www.cms.hhs.gov) and from Medicare's local fiscal intermediaries. The codes are published each year in two volumes that are combined into one spiral-bound text for ease of use. Volume 1 contains the Tabular List of Diseases, based upon the ICD-9-CM code attached to the diagnosis, symptom, or condition of concern. Volume 2 contains the Alphabetic Index to Diseases, published by Practice Management Information Corporation. To identify the appropriate code for a particular symptom, a clinician would begin the search in Volume 2 under the alphabetical listing. Once the code is obtained from Volume 2, the clinician then turns to the tabular listing of the code itself to determine any additional modifiers necessary to clarify the entity being coded. For example, if an NP diagnoses otitis media, Volume 2 indicates that "Otitis" is coded as

---

BOX 20-3 • EXAMPLE OF IMPLEMENTING DOCUMENTATION GUIDELINES:
SUBJECTIVE, OBJECTIVE, ASSESSMENT, PLAN, EVALUATION

S: R.M. is a 6-year-old boy brought to the office by his mother. He is an existing patient. She reports that R.M. has had a 24-hour history of severe sore throat, headache, and fever at home to 102°F. She states he is unable to swallow solids because of throat pain but is taking fluids well. R.M. reports that his best friend has also been ill with similar symptoms. Denies ear pain, nasal congestion, nausea, vomiting, or diarrhea. Mom has been treating his symptoms at home with over-the-counter medications for fever management, salt water gargles, rest, and increased amounts of fluids, with fair symptom relief.

R. M. has been a healthy child, with no prior episodes of acute illness, injury, or hospitalization. He has no known drug or environmental allergies. His only medication is a children's multivitamin. He takes no prescription medications or alternative modality supplements.

O: *GEN:* Alert, well-developed, well-nourished, flushed child in mild distress. *VS:* T, 101.9°F oral; HR, 115; RR, 20; Wt, 35 kg. *HEAD:* NC, AT. No frontal or maxillary tenderness with palpation or percussion. *ENT:* Bilateral external auditory canals clear. Bilateral tympanic membranes pink, translucent, neutral, and freely mobile. Bony landmarks clearly visible. Nasal mucosa pink, moist, mildly edematous. Nasal passages partially obstructed by swollen turbinates. Clear rhinorrhea in the vaults. Buccal mucosa pink and moist. Tonsillar pillars, tonsils, and posterior pharynx beefy, swollen, and covered with white purulent exudate. *NECK:* Supple with significant tonsillar and anterior cervical adenopathy. *QUICK STREP TEST:* positive (CPT 8788QW Rapid antigen strep testing).

A./P:
1. Strep pharyngitis (ICD-9-CM 041.00 Streptococcus, unspecified)
2. Fever (ICD-9-CM 780.6 Fever)
   - Throat swab for culture and sensitivity (CPT 99000 Laboratory specimen handling)
   - Antibiotic regimen based upon weight
   - Supportive measures including symptomatic management of fever and throat pain with over-the-counter medications (NIC 3900 Temperature regulation)
   - Anticipatory guidance provided to mother and child regarding streptococcal infection, anticipated course of illness, and treatment implementation (NIC 5602 Teaching: Disease process; NIC 5616 Teaching: Prescribed medication; NIC 7040 Caregiver support)
3. Risk for infection transmission
   - Anticipatory guidance provided to mother and child regarding meticulous handwashing and other activities that decrease the spread of infection (NIC 7040 Caregiver support; NIC 5618 Teaching: Procedure/treatment)

E: Mother to be notified of throat culture results and any need to alter antibiotic therapy based upon sensitivities. If child does not improve or worsens in next 48 hours, he is to return to clinic for reevaluation. R.M. due for next well-child check in 7 months.

E & M: 99213 Expanded services, existing patient.

382.9. Volume 2 also indicates that additional information is needed to determine which code best matches the type of otitis media the patient has: acute (382.9), with effusion (381.00), allergic (381.04), serous (381.01), with spontaneous rupture of ear drum (382.01), and so on. A listing of common ICD-9-CM codes used in family practice may be found on the American Academy of Family Practice website (www.aafp.org).

The primary function of the ICD-9-CM is to facilitate medical billing. Therefore it is sometimes used at the point of care to classify the patient's diagnosis (or diagnoses) on the patient's billing form, or superbill. The superbill is so named because all subsequent forms generated for that encounter are based upon this first bill completed at the time of service. The superbill may have a listing of frequently seen diagnoses or symptoms accompanied by the appropriate ICD-9-CM code for the provider to check off. This practice is discouraged by CMS because of a concern that diagnostic bias may be introduced by the presence of preprinted diagnoses. The CMS would prefer that the provider write the diagnosis or symptom independently, without the possible influence of the preprinted list. The billing coder for the medical practice then transcribes this code onto a uniform billing form (CMS-1500 claim form) that is submitted for reimbursement, preferably by electronic means. If the provider does not know the code assigned to her or his assessment findings, the coder assigns the code based on the diagnosis (or diagnoses), sign(s), or symptom(s) written on the patient's superbill. In addition, each service or procedure performed for a client must be represented by a diagnosis that would substantiate those particular services or procedures. In other words, the procedure performed must match the diagnosis coded. For example, if a urine dipstick was performed in the office, the superbill should show diagnoses related to urinary tract infection, polyuria, dysuria, and the like. This practice has received particular attention in the realm of diagnostic testing through the use of ABNs (see previous discussion in this chapter) for those services that may not fall within Medicare or any other insurer's guidelines for medical necessity. In addition to its role in reimbursement, the ICD-9-CM serves as a guide to the practicing clinician for the classifications of diseases and symptoms. It is a useful tool in the evaluation of morbidity data for indexing medical records, medical care review, ambulatory and other medical care programs, and basic health statistics (see example in Box 20-4). Supplemental coding information is located in the ICD-9-CM to capture those patient encounters with the health-care system that may not entail a disease or injury classified elsewhere in the manual. There are three main types of encounters that fall into this category and receive a "V code":

- When a well person encounters the health-care system for some specific purpose (e.g., organ or tissue donation [V42.0 for kidney recipient], prophylactic vaccination [V04.8 for influenza vaccination]).
- When a person with a known disease or illness encounters the system for a specific treatment related to that disease or illness (e.g., chemotherapy [V58.1]).
- When some circumstance exists that influences the person's health status but is not in itself a current illness or injury (e.g., inadequate housing [V60.1], no other household member able to render care [V60.4]).

Environmental events, circumstances, and conditions that are the cause of injury, poisoning, and/or other adverse effects are assigned "E codes." Examples of E codes include those pertaining to motor vehicle traffic accidents (E810 through E819); accidental poisoning by drugs, medicinal substances, and biologicals (E850 through E858); and accidents caused by fire and flames (E890 through E898). Both V and E codes may be found in volume I of the ICD-9-CM manual. The ICD-9-CM codes and user-friendly cross-indices are available in paper, disc, and CD-ROM formats from the AMA.

CPT codes are those listed in the *Current Procedural Terminology* manual published annually by the AMA (2004). This text is a listing of the descriptive terms and identifying codes for reporting medical services and procedures (AMA, 2003). As with the ICD-9-CM, the CPT manual serves to provide a uniform language that accurately describes medical, surgical, and diagnostic services. The CPT codes for reimbursement should accurately reflect the services or procedures performed for those ICD-9-CM codes assigned to the patient's diagnosis (or diagnoses) or symptom(s). All services or procedures are assigned a five-digit code and represent procedures consistent with contemporary medical practice and performance by many providers in multiple locations. The CPT manual is divided into several sections: Evaluation and Management (see previous discussion), Anesthesiology, Surgery, Radiology, Pathology and Laboratory, and Medicine.

BOX 20-4 • EXAMPLE OF THE DEMOGRAPHIC USE OF THE ICD-9-CM CODES

An adult NP wants to know which symptoms or diagnoses are most common in her practice. Collaborating with the medical billings administrator in her practice, the APN defines a sort of the administrative billing data base by ICD-9-CM code. The sort tallies the numbers of patient encounters associated with each code. The resulting list captures the most frequent diagnoses seen in her practice. Among the top five ICD-9-CM codes represented, hypertension, unspecified (401.9), and type 2 diabetes mellitus, uncontrolled (250.22), rank numbers 1 and 2. Based on this information, the NP commits to implementing the Seventh Report of the Joint National Committee on Prevention, Detection, Evaluation, and Treatment of High Blood Pressure guidelines (U.S. Department of Health and Human Services, 2003) for the management of hypertension, and the American Diabetes Association (2003) guidelines for the management of diabetes. Flow sheets for blood pressure readings, urinalysis results, glycosylated hemoglobin testing, and scheduled referrals to specialists and routine follow-ups are developed. The following year, the NP commits to evaluating what percentage of patients with hypertension are reaching the goal of systolic blood pressure less than 140 mm Hg and diastolic blood pressure less than 90 mm Hg, and what percentage of patients with diabetes are reaching the goal of a glycosylated hemoglobin below 7 gm/dl.

Medicare and state Medicaid carriers are required by law to use CPT codes for the payment of health insurance claims; all insurance carriers recognize and use CPT codes. Although there may be a CPT code that describes a current medical procedure, an insurance carrier is not obligated to reimburse the provider for that service.

Occasionally, modifiers are used to indicate that a service or procedure has been performed and not changed in its description or code but altered by some specific or extenuating circumstance. The use of modifiers attached to the end of CPT codes eliminates the need for separate procedure codes in these instances. Understanding the proper use of modifiers substantially affects insurance claim reimbursement. The reader is referred to the CPT manual for an in-depth explanation of the use of modifier codes. CPT codes are also available in paper, disc, and CD-ROM formats from the AMA.

Reimbursement for APNs

At the conclusion of the patient encounter, two parallel processes occur (see Figure 20-4). The APN documents the clinical encounter in the patient's record and completes the patient's superbill. Ideally, the medical record should provide data in support of the level of service selected, the ICD-9-CM diagnoses used, and the CPT codes utilized. As discussed previously, it is anticipated that the record will also document nursing diagnoses and interventions appropriate to the clinical scenario. Both medical and nursing outcomes and plans for evaluating the efficacy of the plan of care are expected to be included. Viewed through the lens of process improvement and innovation, the implementation of these external resources allows APNs to improve the existing processes of patient medical record documentation while establishing baseline information for reimbursement. Improvement may be obtained through the use of guidelines both to support the appropriate level of third-party reimbursement and to capture key elements of patient care. Guidelines can be adapted by individual APNs to create encounter forms incorporating the anticipated elements of the patient's history, physical examination, and diagnostic testing for any particular APN practice. Today's health-care economic landscape presents several obstacles to the inclusion of APNs in reimbursement strategies, from the barriers related to scope of practice (see Chapters 22 through 24) to the lack of recognition of nursing diagnoses and interventions through monetary compensation. From a systems-thinking approach, APNs must continue efforts to rectify these inequities through an understanding of, active participation in, and knowledge-based improvement of the current processes of reimbursement. An overview of the patient payor and third-party payor reimbursement strategies is presented here. The reader is referred to the individual programs described for the most recent legislation and information affecting APN participation or enrollment.

FOSTERING PATIENT RESPONSIBILITY

Clients need to assume some level of self-care and financial responsibility for their health care. Self-care measures include active participation in the development and implementation of the plan of care for wellness maintenance and/or illness management. Financial responsibility includes recognition of the valuable services provided by the APN and subsequent compensation of the APN for those services. Patients should be familiar with their insurance programs, particularly with regard to understanding that many programs do not provide the "blanket insurance" elements that were common in the past. Patients without insurance should expect to pay for the services rendered at the time of their delivery unless prior arrangements have been made with the APN. This policy obviously will not apply to patients being seen in free care clinics or enrolled in Medicaid or other subsidized programs.

Financial Responsibility Statement. The billing process includes the development of clear and concise written procedures and policies that will enhance the efficiency of the practice, allow review of individual patient bills to assure accuracy, and clearly communicate to clients where their responsibilities for payment lie (AMA, 2002b). A clearly written patient financial responsibility statement, specifically describing payment expectations, should be provided to and signed by each client upon entry into the APN's practice. These expectations not only include what is expected from the patient but also describe what the patient may expect from the APN's billing procedures and staff. It would be advantageous to include a signed statement allowing the assignment of insurance benefits directly to the APN as part of the financial responsibility statement. This release expedites the processing of insurance claims when the patient's signature is required and should be renewed annually. Annual renewal of financial responsibility not only complies with most insurance payors but also acts as a reminder to the patient of their responsibility. It is extremely important to check the patient's insurance card at every visit because one release form does not carry to another company.

Installment Plans. In the event that the uninsured, or self-pay client is unable to pay for services at the time they are rendered, offering alternative payment plans provides financial flexibility while supporting the patient's financial responsibility to pay for the care delivered. These alternatives should be negotiated and documented prior to the patient's appointment. The agreed-upon payment should then be collected at the time of service. Based upon systems developed by consumer lenders, installment payment plans enable patients to pay their bills in regularly scheduled partial payments. These plans are negotiated between the APN's practice and the patient on a case-by-case basis, according to predetermined policies established by the practice. Interest is not added to the install-ment payment because the payment is not considered a financial loan per se.

Sliding Fee Scales.

Sliding fee scale programs set up by the business using state and federal guidelines may be offered to eligible applicants who have been denied Medicaid because they exceed that program's income guidelines. Often, the income guidelines for a sliding fee program allow individuals and families to earn up to 150% of the federal poverty-level income, thus enabling access to health care by the working poor, the underinsured, and the uninsured. Practices offering sliding fee scales require that the patient apply for and be refused other forms of medical financial aid prior to applying for the practice's program. From a patient's perspective, the information needed to complete the application for sliding fee scale is often identical to that used for a state Medicaid application. Consequently, it is possible for the patient to have to compile the mandatory financial information only once, while applying to two different funding programs.

Charity Care and Bartering Arrangements. Other reimbursement strategies employed by providers are charity care and barter system arrangements. Charity care is usually offered by larger practice groups or hospital facilities because they are more financially able to absorb direct reimbursement losses incurred by caring for those unable to pay for services. Hospitals, in particular, may have designated charity care as part of their mission or may have access to foundation and trust funding designated to sponsor care for those unable to pay. Barter systems have recently been instituted in health-care facilities as an innovative option for patients having difficulty paying their bills (P. Tucker, personal communication, May 1999). Issues related to potential indi-vidual income taxation need to be addressed prior to the initiation of a bartering sys-tem. APNs interested in exploring this option are advised to seek legal and taxation advice from professional advisors before entering into this innovative financial arrangement.

Failure to Pay. Consequences for failure to meet the agreed-upon payments under prac-tice-based aid programs may result in collection services being initiated against the patient, and/or the decision by the provider to not offer services to the patient any longer. As discussed earlier, issues related to denial of care must be clearly documented prior to any action being taken by the provider and must include providing the patient with an opportunity to secure the services of another provider.

PAYMENT MECHANISMS

There are as many different payment mechanisms as there are different health insurance companies. Each company has its own process for becoming a recognized provider and obtaining reimbursement for care delivered to its beneficiaries. Because of the wide diver-sity of rapidly changing third-party plans and the increase in managed care entities and because the ability for APNs to obtain reimbursement in part depends on the individual state practice acts governing advanced practice, any discussion of specific third-party payor plans should be approached with caution. The information for each plan varies quickly from month to month and state to state. The need for uniformity is ever present as health-care reimbursement becomes more difficult and costly to obtain. The basic process involved in reimbursement, as an independent provider, is illustrated in Figure 20-5. As discussed previously, the individual APN may not be directly involved in the daily processes related to obtaining reimbursement. Nevertheless, APNs should be familiar

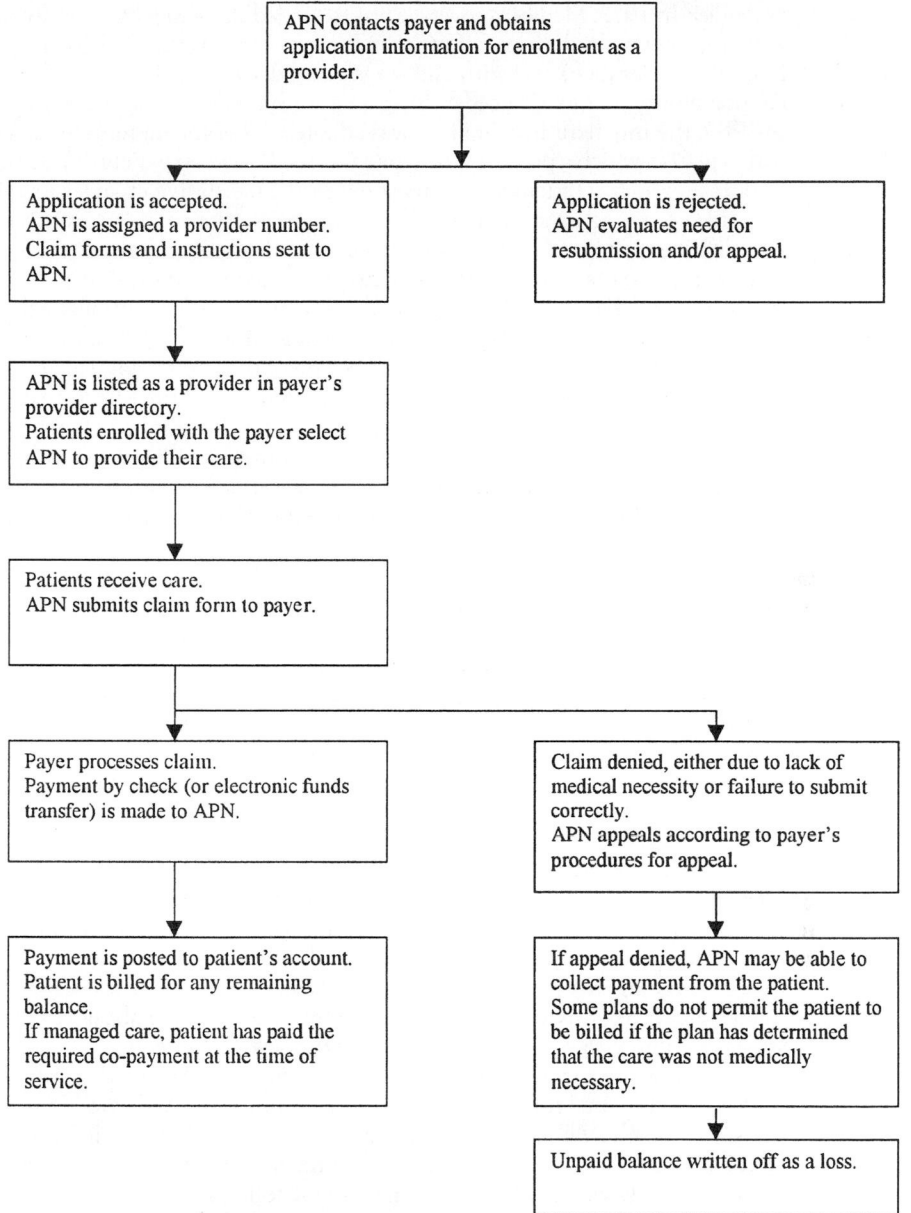

FIGURE 20-5 • The basic third-party payor reimbursement process.

with and participate in the major programs and concepts that provide the mainstay of American health care.

Medicare. Medicare provides health insurance benefits for 39 million beneficiaries in the United States (www.cms.hhs.gov/medicare). Since its authorization by Title XVIII of the Social Security Act in 1965, Medicare has provided access to care to individuals 65 years of age and older. In 1972, Medicare coverage was extended to include those individuals under age 65 with long-term disabilities (of at least 2 years' duration and eligible for Social Security Disability Insurance) and with end-stage renal disease. In 1982, the Tax Equity and Fiscal Responsibility Act introduced a risk-based option, facilitating the involvement of HMOs. In 1983, the inpatient hospital PPS was adopted. This system replaced cost-based payments with a plan in which a predetermined rate was paid based on patients' diagnoses. The Balanced Budget Act of 1997 included the most extensive legislative changes for Medicare since its inception. Among these changes are the expansion of covered preventive benefits and the establishment of Part C (Medicare + Choice), which creates new managed care and other health plan choices for beneficiaries (www.cms.hhs.gov/ medicare). In 1997, Medicare opened up to private company HMOs to provide beneficiaries with additional benefits at a proposed lower cost (Northeast Health Care Quality Foundation, 1999). Some of these private HMOs have already left the Medicare program because of the negative impact on their business and financial viability. (See Chapter 23 for further discussion of the Medicare program.)

Medicare coverage consists of two parts. Hospital insurance (Part A) covers inpatient hospital services, short-term care in skilled nursing facilities, postinstitutional home health care, and hospice care. Those individuals eligible for Social Security are automatically enrolled in Part A. Other qualified beneficiaries need to initiate the enrollment process. Supplementary Medical Insurance (Part B) covers physician services, outpatient hospital services, home health care not covered by Part A, and other medical services such as diagnostic testing, durable medical equipment, and ambulance costs. Enrollment in Part B is voluntary to beneficiaries receiving Part A. Medicare Part A is funded primarily through payroll taxes, although beneficiary cost sharing in the form of deductibles and co-insurance may apply. Beneficiaries participating in Part B pay into the system through monthly premiums that are established yearly based upon system expenses as well as through deductibles and co-insurance programs for various services. Medicare + Choice (Part C) benefits are available through participation in coordinated care or private fee-for-service plans and medical savings accounts (www.cms.hhs.gov/medicare).

Providers either can participate in Medicare or be nonparticipating providers. For participants, the Medicare fee schedule for physicians' professional services, services and supplies provided incident to physicians' professional services (e.g., certain medications and biological agents), and patient physical and occupational therapy services, diagnostic tests, and radiology services is 5% higher than for nonparticipants (National Heritage Insurance Company [NHIC], 1999). At present, NPs, CNSs, and CNMs are permitted to bill Medicare as individuals. Payments are set at 85% of the physician's fee schedule. Visit www.cms.hhs.gov/provider/ for the 2003 physician fee schedule.

APNs who are Medicare providers must be participating providers, which means they will accept "assignment," the allowable charge determined by Medicare. To become a participating provider, the APN must apply to Medicare for a Universal Provider Identification Number (UPIN). The qualifications for NPs requesting a Medicare UPIN were revised in the CMS 2000 Physician Fee Schedule regulation as follows.

As of January 1, 2001, the NP was to possess the following qualifications:

- A state license
- National certification in an advanced nursing specialty

As of January 1, 2003, the NP must possess the following qualifications:

- A state license
- National certification in an advanced nursing specialty
- A master's degree in nursing

The UPIN number is the APN's permanent identification number with the Medicare program, irrespective of the practice location. In other words, even if the APN moves to another state and establishes a practice there, the UPIN number will remain the same. A local provider number is also assigned that is to be used within the local Medicare fiscal intermediary's cachement area. Applications for the UPIN may be obtained from the local Medicare intermediary. A listing of local intermediaries may be obtained from the CMS by telephone at 1-800-MEDICARE.

Medicaid. Medicaid provides health insurance benefits as well as other assistance for eligible low-income individuals and families. Medicaid is a jointly funded state-federal insurance program. Coverage varies by state according to federal requirements that stipulate eligibility and basic services covered. Payment is usually lower than is available through other insurance groups. In 1989, Congress mandated that state Medicaid agencies provide direct reimbursement to family NPs, pediatric NPs, and CNMs. Some states cover the services of other APNs; however, the resulting inconsistencies have caused significant confusion. APNs receive Medicaid reimbursement in 49 states, 39 of which reimburse at 80% to 100% of a physician's rate (Pearson, 2003). As with Medicare, the APN must apply for a provider number and be knowledgeable of the local state Medicaid regulations. The Medicaid site at www.cms.hhs.gov/medicaid offers links to individual states and their Medicaid rules and regulations. Every state publishes a handbook of Medicaid rules complete with updates, and Medicaid publishes newsletters periodically. A recent change in Title XXI of the Social Security Act offers services for children through the State Children's Health Insurance Program (SCHIP) (see Chapter 23 and visit www.cms.hhs.gov/schip for detailed information about this payment mechanism for APN services).

A new service offered through the newly configured Centers for Medicare and Medicaid at the Department of Health and Human Services (DHHS) is especially helpful to APNs. Regularly scheduled "Open Door Forums" are accessible by phone, on the World Wide Web, or on site in which APN participants may discuss current issues and concerns about Medicare, Medicaid, and other federal reimbursement programs. To access this resource, go to www.cms.hhs.gov and click on "Open Door Forums," then proceed to the nursing and allied health section to schedule admission to the forum or to read current and recent minutes.

Federal Employee Health Benefit Program (FEHBP). The FEHBP is the health insurance plan for the approximately 10 million federal employees and their dependents. This is a voluntary, contributory program open to all employees of the federal government. Contracts are held with private health insurance carriers to offer health insurance plans to federal employees. Public Law 101-509, enacted in 1990, allows federal employees enrolled in the FEHBP direct access to NPs, CNSs, and CNMs, thus enabling direct reimbursement for APN services. Under this provision, insurance carriers for federal plans must make payment directly to these APNs if their services are covered under the plan. Collaboration with or supervision by a physician or any other health-care provider is not needed. The payment level is determined by the individual health insurance plan. Additional information is available at the Office of Personnel Management website under Federal Employee Insurance Programs (www.opm.gov/insure/).

Private Health Insurance—Fee-for-Service Plans. Private health insurance plans include carriers such as Blue Cross/Blue Shield, Aetna, Prudential, and Metropolitan. Many of these carriers are merging into larger entities as the move to managed care demands system-wide changes and efficiencies. These traditional fee-for-service plans reimburse providers for patient charges according to the usual and customary charges for that local area. An insurance policy does not explicitly need to include the coverage of nursing services for APNs to be reimbursed for their services. APNs' direct reimbursement by private insurance carriers varies from state to state (Pearson, 2003). When considering application for third-party reimbursement, the nurse needs to be familiar with the state's nurse practice act, state insurance laws and codes (including reimbursement amendments), judicial decisions, and opinions by the attorney general. State health insurance laws do not necessarily prohibit third-party reimbursement to nurses. In Florida and Maine, for instance, direct third-party reimbursement is essentially a 1:1 process. The individual nurse applies to the third-party insurer and requests provider status. If reimbursement is rejected, familiarity with the state's nursing practice act and the state's health insurance laws can assist the nurse in appealing the decision

Managed Care. Managed care denotes a spectrum of arrangements that entail some connection between financing and delivery of care, usually with cost containment (American Academy of Nursing, 1993). In managed care, the financial risk associated with health-care delivery is shared between the payors, the contracted providers, and the enrolled beneficiaries. Risk is lessened for payors by the exclusive enrollment of beneficiaries with a particular health status profile. Risk is lessened for any one provider by the addition of providers to the pool of providers sharing the care for a particular population of patients. Risk is lessened for the beneficiaries through the utilization of providers who are within the contracted pool, or "network," of providers. The distribution of financial risk has received increased media coverage recently as some managed care companies face financial difficulties. Such turmoil is evidenced by the alteration of key components of typical managed care contracts. Examples include changes in patient population (e.g., the disenrollment of Medicare beneficiaries), pharmaceutical coverage (e.g., the increased practice of allowing a decreased supply of chronic medications to be dispensed at one time to increase collection of co-payments), and departure of companies from a particular cachement location (e.g., the withdrawal of the Tufts Plan from Maine). Managed care companies base their reimbursement to providers on a combination of historical area charge data, relative value scales, and actuarial data. Managed care entities either will usually discount a physician's fee for services or require that a predetermined fee be charged. However, the majority of managed care companies pay providers a "capitated fee" (the provider cares for a client population for a pre-arranged fee per client). Capitation amounts typically vary by age, gender, and risk status and are negotiable. The capitated fee is paid to the provider monthly, based upon the number of plan enrollees who have selected that provider as their primary care provider. Key areas of managed care contracts include practice exclusivity, sign-on bonuses to the practice for new members recruited to the HMO, and profit sharing (Jenkins & Torrisi, 1995). Managed care programs are offered by commercial insurance carriers and include PPOs and HMOs, among others. HMOs encompass any variety of prepaid group practice arrangements. These programs usually offer health-care services to members enrolled in the plan for a predetermined, prepaid, or discounted fee. *Prepaid* means that the organization receives a fixed payment or premium to care for members of a certain population and that the organization bears the financial risk for the care that members receive. Participating providers are required to provide services for contracted reimbursement amounts. This reimbursement can range from a discounted fee for service to a lump sum for all services required. There are four main types of HMOs (Knight, 1998):

1. Staff-model HMOs employ salaried physicians who work in the HMOs' own clinics.
2. Group-model HMOs contract with a large multispecialty group practice.

3. Individual practice association (IPA) model HMOs contract with individual physicians or affiliations of independent physicians.
4. Network HMO models are similar to IPAs except that they contract with several larger physician groups. Some models are mixed combinations of group, staff, network, or IPA models.

A PPO is a network of providers, usually physicians and hospitals, that have discounted their fees for an increased volume of patients (Meazy & McGivern, 1993).

Some HMOs make extensive use of APNs in order to increase the cost-effectiveness of primary care. Jenkins and Torrisi (1995) stated that many private and public HMOs and other managed care organizations, however, have been slow to enroll primary care APNs as providers who receive direct capitation payments. California APNs have experienced "lock out" from some managed care contracts. As discussed earlier, APNs must provide the data needed by states to demonstrate cost efficiency and must work together at the policymaking level to eliminate these financial restraints to trade (Safriet, 1998; see also Chapter 23).

Reimbursement Summary

Reimbursement is an indirect process supporting patient care that provides a vehicle for APN compensation for the services rendered to patients. The process begins with the appointment for the patient's clinical encounter and ends with the posting of the patient's payment, either through individual accountability or through third-party reimbursement. The involvement of APNs in the reimbursement process depends on whether the APN is allowed by the applicable state and federal regulations to practice independently and is able to obtain direct reimbursement for those independently delivered services. The level to which the APN is involved in the administrative procedures depends on whether the APN has chosen to practice in an entrepreneurial or intrapreneurial manner. Most of the time, the process of reimbursement is, and should be, delegated to an individual familiar with medical billing, who is able to dedicate the time and effort required to become expert in this level of practice management. If the APN decides to become directly involved in reimbursement procedures, it is strongly urged that a professional billing advisor, similar to the attorney or accountant consulted during business planning, be contracted or hired. This advisor serves to provide the APN with the latest and most accurate information regarding this vital process in the APN's financial viability.

Some authors report that reimbursement should equal 90% of the patient's billable charges (Buppert, 1999). The reality of health-care economics is that this number varies considerably over time depending on the payor mix, specifically upon the percentage of Medicare, Medicaid, other payments to be received, and the amounts charged to patients. Medicaid usually pays a lower proportion of billed charges than Medicare, based on the local Medicare fee structure. Capitated contracts can result in financial losses if enrolled beneficiaries utilize the health-care system more frequently than the anticipated risk calculation had allocated. Patients who are unable to pay or who refuse to pay create a percentage of "bad debt" that is written off as a business loss. During the business planning phase, the APN should become intimately familiar with the reimbursement rates in the local area, the anticipated mix of the patient population to be served, and the available resources and personnel to design and implement a reimbursement process that meets the APN's financial expectations. APNs should never allow one payor to dominate their practice and should set goals based on the percent of each payor for their practice. As with any system, the reimbursement process should undergo periodic evaluation to determine where improvements in the process may be made, including electronic claim submission, tighter internal audit controls, and efficient cross-training of staff to ensure consistency during staff absences.

CONCLUSION

Through the development of innovative programs and practices grounded in a systems-thinking approach, APNs define, demonstrate, document, and thereby claim their contributions to patient care. Business planning establishes a clear picture of how the APN will function on a daily basis, as well as how midrange and long-term goals are to be met. Knowledge of the processes involved in care delivery increases the sharing of information between APNs and their patients, other health-care providers, and colleagues. Reimbursement is identified as the major indirect process of care that has a direct impact on the success of the APN's business planning efforts. Equally important to success is the APN's candid self-evaluation and determination of whether an entrepreneurial or intrapreneurial approach is the most appropriate model under which to deliver patient care. The recognition that others, such as other APNs, physicians, attorneys, and practice managers, in the greater health-care system have skills and expertise to offer provides the APN with a "safety net" of advisors who can play an active role in the actualization of advanced nursing practice. Above all, the success of the APN is grounded in the professional recognition of and active participation in the larger system to ensure that the needs of patients are met through the delivery of clinically excellent, holistic health care.

REFERENCES

Almost, J., & Laschinger, H. K. (2002). Workplace empowerment, collaborative work relationships, and job strain in nurse practitioners. *Journal of the American Academy of Nurse Practitioners, 14,* 408-420.

American Academy of Family Physicians. (2004). *CLIA and other regulatory information.* Retrieved March 14, 2004, from http://www.aafp.org

American Academy of Nursing. (1993). *Managed care and national health care reform: Nurses can make it work.* Washington, DC: Author.

American Diabetes Association. (2003). *American Diabetes Association: Clinical practice recommendations 2003.* Retrieved May 26, 2004, from http://www.diabetes.org

American Express Company. (2003). *Small business exchange: Creating an effective business plan.* Retrieved May 27, 2004, from http://www.americanexpress.com/smallbusiness/resources/starting/bizplan

American Medical Association. (1996). *Integration strategies for the medical practice: The physician's handbook to integration alternatives.* Norcross, GA: Coker Publishing Company.

American Medical Association. (1999). *Automating the medical record.* Norcross, GA: Coker Publishing Company.

American Medical Association. (2000). *Current procedural terminology.* Chicago: Author.

American Medical Association. (2002a). *Financial management of the medical practice: The physician's handbook for successful budgeting, forecasting and cost accounting* (2nd ed.). Norcross, GA: Coker Publishing Company.

American Medical Association. (2002b). *Managing the medical practice: The physician's handbook for successful practice administration* (2nd ed.). Norcross, GA: Coker Publishing Company.

American Medical Association. (2002c). *Starting a medical practice: The physician's handbook for successful practice start-up* (2nd ed.). Norcross, GA: Coker Publishing Company.

American Medical Association. (2004). *International classification of diseases. 9th revision: Clinical modification (ICD-9-CM 2004)* (vols. 1 and 2). Dover, DE: Author.

American Nurses Association. (2001). *Code of ethics for nurses with interpretive statements.* Washington, DC: Author.

Association of Academic Health Centers (2002). *Partnerships for training.* Retrieved March 15, 2004, from http://www.pftweb.org

Bulechek, G. M., & McCloskey, J. C. (1999). *Nursing intervention: Effective nursing treatments* (3rd ed.). Philadelphia: W. B. Saunders.

Buppert, C. (1999). *Nurse practitioner's business practice and legal guide*. Gaithersburg, MD: Aspen Publishers.

Buppert, C. (2002). *Avoiding malpractice. 10 rules, 5 systems, 20 cases*. Annapolis, MD: Law offices of Carolyn Buppert.

Buppert, C. (2003). HIPAA patient privacy. *The American Journal for Nurse Practitioners, 7*, 17-22.

Buppert C. (2004). *Nurse practitioner's business practice and legal guide* (2nd ed.). Boston: Jones & Bartlett.

Carpenito, L. J. (1999). *Handbook of nursing diagnosis* (8th ed.). Philadelphia: J. B. Lippincott.

Centers for Medicare and Medicaid Services. (2004a). *Evaluation and management documentation guidelines*. Retrieved March 15, 2004, from http://www.cms.hhs.gov

Centers for Medicare and Medicaid Services. (2004b). *CLIA: General program description*. Retrieved May 28, 2004, from http://www.cms.hhs.gov/clia

Donahue, M. P. (1985). *Nursing: The finest art*. St. Louis: Mosby.

Hanson, C. (1993). Our role in health care reform: Collegiality counts. *American Journal of Nursing, 93*, 16A-16E.

HCA Quality Resource Group. (1992a). *Organizing hospital care as a system: An annotated guide*. Nashville, TN: Author.

HCA Quality Resource Group. (1992b). *Organizing work as a system*. Nashville, TN: Author.

Henry, S. B., Holzemer, W. L., Randell, C., Hsieh, S. F., & Miller, T. J. (1997). Comparison of nursing interventions classification and current procedural terminology codes for categorizing nursing activities. *Image: The Journal of Nursing Scholarship, 29*, 133-138.

Hurst, J., Nickel, K., & Hilborne, L. H. (1998). Are physician's office laboratory results of comparable quality to those produced in other laboratory settings? *Journal of the American Medical Association, 279*, 468-471.

Iowa Intervention Project (Johnson, M., & Maas, M. [Eds.]). (1997). *Nursing outcomes classification*. St. Louis: Mosby.

Jenkins, M., & Torrisi, D. (1995). A nurse practitioner, community nursing centers, and contracting for managed care. *Journal of the American Academy of Nurse Practitioners, 7*, 119-124.

Joint Commission on Accreditation of Healthcare Organizations. (2004). *2004 Comprehensive accreditation manual form ambulatory care*. Oakbrook Terrace, IL: Author.

Kleinpell, R. M. (2001). *Outcome assessment in advanced practice nursing*. New York: Springer.

Knight, W. (1998). *Managed care: What it is and how it works*. Gaithersburg, MD: Aspen.

Letz, K. (2002). *Business essentials for nurse practitioners: Essential knowledge for building your practice*. Fort Wayne, IN: Previcare Inc. Publishing.

Meazy, M. D., & McGivern, D. O. (Eds.). (1993). *Nurses, nurse practitioners: Evolution to advanced practice*. New York: Springer-Verlag.

McCloskey, J. C., & Bulechek, G. M. (Eds.). (1992). *Nursing interventions classification* (2nd ed.). St. Louis: Mosby.

National Heritage Insurance Company. (2004). *Second update to Medicare physical fee schedule database*. Retrieved May 27, 2004, from http://www.medicarenhic.com

Neumann, B. R., & Boles, K. E. (1998). *Management accounting for health care organizations* (5th ed.). Chicago: Precept Press.

Newman, D. K. (1996). Program and practice management for the advanced practice nurse. In A. B. Hamric, J. A. Spross, & C. M. Hanson (Eds.), *Advanced nursing practice: An integrative approach* (pp. 545-568). Philadelphia: W. B. Saunders.

Northeast Health Care Quality Foundation. (1999). *Health matters for Medicare consumers* (vol. 3). Dover, NH: Author.

Pearson, L. (2003). The fifteenth annual legislative update. *The Nurse Practitioner: The American Journal of Primary Health Care, 28*, 26-58.

Pharmaceutical Research and Manufacturers of America. (1997). *Directory of prescription drug patient assistance programs*. Washington, DC: Author.

Practice Management Information Corporation. (2003). *ICD-9-CM*. Los Angeles: Author.

Rehm, S., & Kraft, S. (1998). *How to select a computer system for a family physician's office*. Retrieved April 11, 2003, from http://www.aafp.org/fpnet/guide/

Safriet, B. (1998). Still spending dollars, still searching for sense: Advanced practice nursing in an era of regulatory and economic turmoil. *Advanced Practive Nursing Quarterly, 4*(3), 24-33.

Schwartz, I. (1996). Private office laboratories: Coping with federal guidelines. *Infections in Urology, 9*(6), 175-183.

Stewart, P. (1989). The CNS in private practice. In A. B. Hamric & J. A. Spross (Eds.), *The clinical nurse specialist in theory and practice* (2nd ed., pp. 435-455). Philadelphia: W. B. Saunders.

Tweedy, J. T. (1997). *Healthcare hazard control and safety management*. Bethesda, MD: Board of Certified Healthcare Safety Management; and Delray Beach, FL: GR/St. Lucie Press.

U. S. Department of Health and Human Services. (2003, May). *The seventh report of the Joint National Committee on Prevention, Detection, Evaluation and Treatment of High Blood Pressure*. Washington, DC: Author.

Vogel, G., & Doleysh, N. (1994). *Entrepreneuring: A nurse's guide to starting a business*. New York: National League for Nursing.

Additional Readings

American College of Nurse-Midwives. (1994). *Joint statement of practice relations between obstetrician/gynecologists and certified nurse midwives (reaffirmed)*. Available at http://www. acnm.org/prof/jnstat.htm

American College of Nurse-Midwives. (1997). *Collaborative management in midwifery practice for* medical, gynecological and obstetrical conditions (rev.). Available at http://www.acnm.org/prof/collab.htm

American College of Nurse-Midwives. (1997). Definitions (rev.). Available at http://www.acnm.org/prof/defcnm.htm

American College of Nurse-Midwives. (1997). Guidelines for the incorporation of new procedures into nurse-midwifery practice. Available at http://www.acnm.org/prof/guide.htm

American College of Nurse-Midwives. (1997). Independent midwifery practice (rev.). Available at http://www.acnm.org/prof/independ.htm

American College of Nurse-Midwives. (1997). State and federal action on primary care and direct access to obstetrical and gynecological providers. Available at http://www.acnm.org/prof/diracces.htm

American College of Nurse-Midwives. (1998, January). States in which certified nurse-midwives have prescriptive authority. Available at http://www.acnm.org/prof/prescrip.htm

American College of Nurse-Midwives. (1998, February). Third party reimbursement for CNMs; State laws. Available at http://www.acnm.org/prof/mandate.htm

American Nurses Association. (n.d.). States recognizing advanced practice under independent acts, separate titles of advance practice acts, or regulations. Available at http://www.ana.org/gova/tiltrial.htm

American Nurses Association. (1996). Scope and standards of advanced practice registered nursing. Washington, DC: American Nurses Publishing.

American Nurses Association. (1997). States which recognize clinical nurse specialists in advanced practice. Available at http://www.ana.org/gova/cns.htm

Berwick, D. M. (1998, June). Managing for world-class improvement: Distinctive characteristics of the future outstanding health care organization. Paper presented at Quality Day, Dartmouth Medical School, Hanover, NH.

Blair, C. (1997). Advanced practice nurses as entrepreneurs. American Journal of Nursing, 97, 16AAA-16DDD.

Blondell, R. D., Norris, T. E., & Coombs, J. B. (1992). Rural health and family medicine. American Family Physician, 45, 2507-2510.

Bulechek, G. M., & McCloskey, J. C. (1999). Nursing intervention: Effective nursing treatments (3rd ed.). Philadelphia: W. B. Saunders.

Buppert, C. (1997). Employment agreements: Clauses that can change an NP's life. Nurse Practitioner, 22, 10-119.

Buppert, C. K. (1995). Justifying nurse practitioner existence: Hard facts to hard figures. Nurse Practitioner, 20, 43-48.

Carlson, E. (1998). What's happening: Emerging roles for the gerontological nurse practitioner. Journal of the American Academy of Nurse Practitioners, 10, 403-405.

Cavanah, C. (1998, November). Entrepreneur's complete guide to software. Entrepreneur, 129-139.

Centers for Disease Control and Prevention. (1998). New study shows lower mortality rates for infants delivered by certified nurse midwives. Available at http://www.cdc.gov/nchs/releases/98news/98news/midwife.htm

Covey, S. R. (1989). The seven habits of highly effective people: Restoring the character ethic. New York: Simon & Schuster.

Davies, A. R., Doyle, M. A. T., Lansky, D., Rutt, W., Stevic, M. O., & Doyle, J. B. (1993, March). Outcomes assessment: Implementation workbook. (Functional Outcomes Program; supported by Grant 92-005 by the Henry J. Kaiser Family Foundation). Boston: New England Medical Center, Inc.

DeBarth, K., & Kelly, K. (1996). Successfully sharing a private practice with MDs: Overlooked business opportunities for NPs and PAs. The Clinicians Reference Guide: A Supplement to Clinician Reviews, 6(Suppl), 108-112.

Freedman, E. (1999, March). Your so-called life. The overachieving entrepreneur's guide to making time for a real life. Entrepreneur, 146, 148-151.

Garr, D., Rhyne, R., & Kukulka, G. (1993). Incorporating a community-oriented approach in primary care. American Family Physician, 47, 1699-1702.

Henry, P. F. (1996). Analysis of the nurse practitioner's legal relationships. Nurse Practitioner Forum, 7, 5-6.

Internal Revenue Service. (1995). Understanding your EIN (Employer Identification Numbers) (Publication No. 1635–Revised [Rev. 6-95]; Catalog Number 14332X). Washington, DC: U. S. Department of the Treasury.

Jones, J. E., & Bearley, W. L. (1986). Participative management tree [Pocket reference card]. King of Prussia, PA: Organization Design and Development, Inc.

Jones, K. R., Jennings, B. M., Moritz, P., & Moss, M. T. (1997). Policy issues associated with analyzing outcomes of care. Image: The Journal of Nursing Scholarship, 29, 261-267.

Keepnews, D. (1994). The reimbursement manual: How to get paid for your advanced practice nursing services [Supplement]. Washington, DC: American Nurses Publishing.

Michalek, M. R. (1994, Spring/Summer). The advanced practice job search. Advanced Practice Nurse, 12-41.

Mohr, W. K. (1996). Dirty hands: The underside of marketplace health care. Advances in Nursing Science, 9, 28-37.

Nugent, K. E., & Lambert, V. A. (1997). Evaluating the performance of the APN. Nurse Practitioner, 22, 190-198.

Peters, S. (1998, October). States of the nation: Progress for NPs in South Carolina. Advance for Nurse Practitioners, 6, 14.

Reid, A. H. (1999, March). Grant writing. Presentation provided through Maine Bureau of Health, Division of Community and Family Health, York, ME.

Richards, R. N. (1998). How to select a practice site and practice type. *Medscape Orthopedics & Sports Medicine, 2*. Available at http://www.medscape.com/Medscape/OrthoSpo02.n04/mos4514.rich/pnt-mos4514.rich.html

Rodgers, S. (1998, October). Profession's leadership needs to address NP glut. *Advance for Nurse Practitioners, 6*, 93.

Rodkin, D. (1998, October). Full speed ahead: 15 shortcuts to business success. *Entrepreneur*, 132-138.

Ruberry, B. (1998, November). Danger zone: When bad things happen to good entrepreneurs: What every small business owner needs to know about crisis management. *Entrepreneur*, 153-157.

Shay, L. E., Goldstein, J. T., Matthews, D., Trait, L. L., & Edmunds, M. W. (1996). Guidelines for developing a nurse practitioner practice. *Nurse Practitioner, 21*, 72-81.

Simpson, L., & Lee, P. R. (1993). Primary care: An idea in search of a paradigm? *American Family Physician, 47*, 323-326.

Smith, A. (1998). The job market: What does the future hold for PAs and NPs? *Clinician News, 2*, 1, 8.

Smith, S. S. (1999, March). Future speak: Interview with Alvin and Heidi Toffler. *Entrepreneur*, 127-130.

Stodder, G. S. (1997, July). Independence days: Entrepreneurs offering a compassionate option to nursing homes are fueling the $12 billion assisted living industry. *Entrepreneur, 130*, 132-133.

Stodder, G. S. (1998, July). Goodwill hunting: Who cares about socially responsible business practices? Seventy percent of consumers, that's who. *Entrepreneur*, 118-125.

Taylor-Seehafer, M. (1998). Point of view: Nurse-physician collaboration. *Journal of the American Academy of Nurse Practitioners, 10*, 387-391.

CHAPTER 21

Marketing and Contracting Considerations

DONNA R. HODNICKI • SUSAN E. D. DOUGHTY

HEALTH CARE AS A BUSINESS: A CALL TO ACTION FOR ADVANCED PRACTICE NURSES

Despite the fact that advanced practice nurses (APNs) have been around for decades and that there are increased numbers of APNs providing health care today, there still remains a lack of knowledge among health-care colleagues and consumers about who APNs are and what they do. Many persons still are unaware that the term *advanced practice nurse* (APN) refers to four groups of nurses—certified nurse midwife (CNM), clinical nurse specialist (CNS), certified registered nurse anesthetist (CRNA), and nurse practitioner (NP)—or of when these groups came into being. In the 20th century, CNMs answered a call for safe birthing practices while CNSs responded to a need for expert practitioners at the nurse-patient interface. The practice realm of the CRNAs was established to provide anesthesia services long before the medical specialty of anesthesiology was developed (see Chapter 1). The establishment of NPs was the result of a nursing-medical cooperative effort to answer the health-care crisis of the 1960s, when increased numbers of health-care providers were needed to provide patient care services.

Currently, market forces drive health and illness care. In spite of the overall wealth and technological excellence in the United States as a whole, a serious problem still remains in that many Americans cannot obtain or afford even minimum health services. APNs have helped to alleviate some of this health-care disparity, but expanded use of APNs is needed to effect significant improvement in health-care outcomes. For the public to be informed about the services APNs can provide, it is necessary to market both the role and the services. In order to effectively market themselves, APNs must understand marketing concepts and utilize marketing strategies. APNs who cannot get beyond an aversion toward marketing themselves will be left behind, both as a group and as individuals. This chapter outlines key marketing concepts and strategies, delineates marketable properties of advanced practice nursing, itemizes essentials for effective external and internal marketing, and helps both the new graduate and the experienced APN to develop a personal marketing plan. Contracting considerations such as employment contracts, service contracts, and managed care contracts are addressed.

WHAT IS MARKETING?

Marketing is anything and everything APNs do to promote their role and practice. It is about meeting the needs of the consumer and positioning services and businesses in the marketplace. Nurses have the respect of the public. It is imperative that this respect not be eroded and that APNs work to enhance the public's trust through education and marketing strategies to communicate the role of the APN in the provision of health care and the services that are rendered. APNs provide quality care similar to that offered by physicians, and they are cost-effective providers (Office of Technology Assessment [OTA], 1986; Safriet, 1992). Government and national studies indicate that satisfaction with APN care has remained high over the years (Brown & Grimes, 1995; Druss, Marcus, Olfson, Tanielian, & Pincus, 2003; Mundinger et al., 2000; OTA, 1986; Rekevics, Harte, Meyer, Shively, & Ebersole-Kauffman, 1999). Therefore APNs need to continue to educate and inform consumers using common marketing strategies. The four categories of marketing that need to be addressed are product, price, place, and promotion (Chang, Pfoutz, & Price, 2001; Letz, 2002).

The authors would like to acknowledge Jennifer M. Keller, RN, MSN, for her contributions to this chapter in the second edition.

Product. A product is that entity which is offered to the market. An APN offers health-care services that may be specialized and serve a market niche. A growing number of individuals are seeking care from providers other than physicians. A study by Druss et al. (2003) reported that "between 1987 and 1997 the proportion of patients who saw a nonphysician clinician rose from 30.6 to 36.1 percent" (p. 130). With increasing numbers of individuals seeking care from alternative nonphysician sources, it is important that APNs make certain patients are cognizant that the care being provided is by an APN who is prepared to meet their holistic health-care needs. The office staff can also play a vital role in creating a positive perception of the care provided by an APN. If staff members have an accurate understanding of the APN's uniqueness and skills, they can have a positive impact on a patient's perception of APN care. One strategy that fosters this perception occurs when staff members offer the services of the APN if a patient's preferred provider is unavailable or a walk-in appointment is requested. It is important that the public understand the differences and complementary aspects of APNs in comparison with other providers.

Disseminating information about APNs to the public is essential. Master's-prepared APNs have built their knowledge and skills on a strong nursing foundation. This foundation is holistic in that APNs consider the physical, psychological, spiritual, and environmental aspects of the individual, aspects that emerge in assessment, interventions, and overall health care. Evidence of a holistic perspective is demonstrated by the APN when questions are asked about health promotion needs and other concerns beyond the primary reason for the visit. Thus, health and wellness are major components of the holistic perspective. Information about APN products and services should emphasize the uniqueness of advanced practice nursing – that is, using a holistic approach, promoting health, identifying health risks, and preventing illness in addition to diagnosing and treating disease. A consumer who is being seen by an APN not only receives a broader range of services relative to maintaining and restoring health but also begins to understand how APN practice differs from that of other providers.

Price. Price is the amount of money that the individual will be asked to pay for the product. Price will be strongly influenced by many factors. The expectations of the individual APN regarding financial rewards from the practice may vary due to locale and the differences in NP salaries across the United States. While good statistics on nationwide salaries are difficult to obtain, the APN needs to be familiar with regional and local salaries, compensation, and benefits in order to be competitive in the market (Hayes, Allen, Gruen, Wilson, & Kalmakis, 2001). The quality of care given by APNs has been shown to be cost-effective. If the cost of care by the APN is lower than that of competitors in the area, providing price information may be a useful marketing strategy. If lower costs are part of the marketing strategies, APNs can inform consumers that health promotion and early intervention services may prevent more costly care in the future.

Place. *Place* refers to accessibility and the various tasks that are necessary to make the product more available to the market (Chang et al., 2001). A needed product at a good price must be accessible to be successful. Historically, APNs have been in the forefront of providing care to vulnerable populations and remain willing to provide care to these groups. Positioning the APN clinic in an area of need, where care is lacking, is one strategy. Selecting a location that is safe, has parking, and is near public transportation will support the establishment of a practice site. Locating convenient office space and developing an aesthetic environment are important considerations (Letz, 2002).

Promotion. Promotion encompasses those activities that communicate the value of the product to the market (Chang et al., 2001). Promotion depends on making the consumer aware of the availability of APN services. A lack of recognition by consumers is a barrier to APN practice that can be removed (Lindeke, Bly, & Wilcon, 2001). Indeed, nurse practitioners identified the lack of public knowledge about NPs as the primary barrier to practice. Limitations of space and/or facilities were the second highest ranked barriers (Washington Consulting Group, 1994). APN promotional activities that address such barriers include the following:

- Changing a health-care company's promotional materials to ensure that APNs are explicitly mentioned
- Asking clients on their first visit how they found out about the APN's services
- Encouraging word-of-mouth referrals
- Sending a thank-you note to the individual who provided a referral

Another critically important endorsement for the nursing profession that also promotes APN practice is for APNs to be sure to use other APNs for personal care as well as for family care. Clearly, it is important for the public to understand the role of the APN in providing health care. Miller (2000) noted that successful promotion depends on APNs getting out into their target communities and being visible. In order to market one's practice, APNs will need to invest time, money, or both to have any chance of success.

Although advertising or promotion is a small but important part of marketing, advertising has a bad reputation for being focused on materialism. Almost no one believes advertising's claims, yet advertising thrives because it works! Health-care professionals may be uncomfortable with the notion of self-promotion, but consumer demands and constantly changing reimbursement mechanisms for health-care providers necessitate marketing to both clients and payors (Kendig, 2001). In today's health-care market, which is becoming more diversified and competitive, it is important that APNs understand and utilize multiple marketing strategies, including advertising.

KEY MARKETING CONCEPTS FOR APNs

Marketing is focused on satisfying the needs and desires of consumers. An important marketing concept is that of organizing information about client needs through a marketing survey using two components: service differentiation, that is, identifying aspects of a service valued by clients yet unmatched by competitors, and market segmentation, or dividing clients into groups according to factors that influence selection and use of services (Pakis, 1997). Determining service differentiation for an NP practice might include gathering data from a group of people about their preferences for a preferred location, hours of service, or availability of follow-up care. Market segmentation data in the survey might include individual and group characteristics such as age, gender, socioeconomic status, population density, and benefits sought.

Good marketing is designed to educate others about nursing and sell a service from a position of strength (Kendig, 2002). It is important for APNs to take a position regarding marketing as it relates to the provision of health care today. APNs cannot afford to be passive. Nursing values and information oriented toward the well-being and goals of the client can support ethical marketing. Marketing strategies to compete for finite health-care resources include health-care marketing seminars, hiring of health-care marketing consultants by agencies, and the development of marketing positions in most health-care organizations. Until recently, nursing's values have not embraced marketing. However, developing marketing skills and markets for advanced nursing practice could literally determine the survival of advanced practice nursing. Corporate marketing strategies can work for APNs (Shaw, 2002). The slogans "Because I'm worth it" and "We bring good things to life" positioned L'Oréal and General Electric for success. The slogan "Nurses care" has been incorporated by nursing organizations in a variety of ways to market nursing. The slogan has been placed on carry-all bags, pins, and bumper stickers to communicate the fact that the essence of nursing is caring and that the individual person matters to the nurse. Oncology nursing is using the slogan, "All heart, All mind, No limits," to promote its specialty (J. Spross, personal communication, May 24, 2004). APNs can use similar promotional strategies to position themselves as unique providers of certain service niches so that consumers automatically think of the APN when they seek that particular service. Examples of marketing service niches for APNs can be found in Box 21-1. While strategies to market APN services are integrated throughout the chapter, a few are summarized here and include the following: community public speaking, giving interviews to reporters, using office stationery, legislative lobbying, distributing fact sheets and business cards, and networking with colleagues to educate other professionals and the public about the role of the APN in providing quality health care. In all interactions with patients and consumers, it is essential to identify oneself as an APN and to answer questions as they arise about the advanced practice nursing role.

Based on the overview of marketing just presented, key marketing goals for APNs include the following:

- Educating consumers and colleagues about advanced nursing practice
- Generating income and obtaining funding
- Developing broad-based, interdisciplinary support for advanced nursing practice
- Meeting existing, but unmet, client needs
- Making health problems visible
- Creating new job opportunities and stable niches in changing delivery systems
- Understanding how to work with a variety of health-care practice configurations

Areas of growth in nursing are to be found at the edges of traditional practice. The continuing evolution of health-care provides APNs areas in which to expand. The acceptance of the APN as a core provider instead of a peripheral provider existing only on the edge of health-care delivery services provides opportunities for the development of specialized care by the APN and collaborative interdisciplinary partnerships, which create unique networks (Buchanan, 1997; see Chapter 10). APNs must broaden their knowledge base to include becoming familiar with economic, political, and marketing literature outside of nursing in order to learn about issues that affect care and to become familiar with strategies that would improve the context and care of the service provided. For example, the revolutionary business concept of cooperative competition, or "co-opetition" (Brandenburger & Nalebuff, 1996) offers a way for today's competitors to find new common ground for business collaboration tomorrow. Coile (1999) wrote, "When competitors reach a standoff in market advantage, they can switch to cooperation to increase their mutual strengths and benefits" (p. 5). Creating shared business alliances using "co-opetition" is one of many concepts APNs can borrow from the corporate world. Integrating business principles with caring practices enhances one's ability to market APN services.

MARKETABLE PROPERTIES OF APNs

Realistic self-appraisal of marketable skills is essential, not only for new graduates and APNs who lose jobs or move to a new area but for all APNs in the current health-care environment. The ability to market oneself is necessary whether one is (or wishes to be) an employee or an entrepreneur. Much of what we understand about marketing advanced nursing practice is based on the experiences and writings of nurse entrepreneurs.

BOX 21-1 • EXAMPLES OF ADVANCED NURSING PRACTICE MARKETING NICHES OR SERVICES

Adolescent gynecology specialist
Architectural consultant
Birthing center
Brokering services (e.g., elder care)
Chronic illness management
Correctional health care
Day care consultant
Diabetes management
Elder care
Employee programs for health-care cost-containment
Ethics counseling
Fitness/exercise consultant
Health policy consultant
Health/wellness promotion
HIV/AIDS care
Homeless shelters
Lactation consultant and equipment rental
Mammography, breast health counseling
Medical, nursing, health-care writing
Menopause center
Mobile health services (e.g., mammography van)
Multidisciplinary clinical practice
Nurse case manager
Nurse educator
Occupational health/worker's compensation consultant
Pacemaker center
Pain management
Product development (e.g., pharmaceutical, toys, personal care, therapeutic devices)
Psychiatric counseling
Radio/TV/media consultant
Retirement center
Risk management consultant
Same-day surgery center
School/college health
Special populations (e.g., lesbian/gay health, Latino health, immigrant health)
Stress management consultant
Women's health
YMCA/YWCA/Boys'/Girls' club

APNs cannot develop markets and sell themselves if they do not clearly recognize their unique skills and how these skills can meet client needs. Such an appraisal helps APNs to determine what areas of practice need to be developed in order to better position themselves for the marketplace. Many NPs are tempted to skip this step because they do not have the time or interest; they may think that the exercise is not valuable (Fitzgerald, 1999). APN entrepreneurs have invested tremendous energy and resources in their careers and owe it to themselves to perform a self-appraisal, a key step in determining one's marketability (Fitzgerald, 1999). Questions that can help APNs make an inventory of their skills and identify opportunities for applying these unique skills might include the following:

1. What motivates me in my practice?
2. What do I do best in my practice?
3. Where do I get the most satisfaction in my practice?

4. What am I most proud of about my practice?
5. Do I have a skill a consumer or organization would pay for?
6. How might I attract a consumer or organization to pay for my skills?

In his book *What Color Is Your Parachute?* Richard Bolles (2002) amply described how individuals can determine their best fit in a career and how they can market themselves to attain that goal. Readers are instructed to formulate a picture of their ideal job by identifying the specific wants and needs that allow them to flourish. By applying these strategies APNs can identify strengths, such as favorite transferable skills, favorite tasks, favorite people with whom to work, and favorite kinds of information with which to work, the APN can identify the unique services that she or he has to offer. Many APNs have successfully developed unique practices that fit a vital need. Exemplars 21-1 and 21-2 describe APNs' self-appraisals of marketable knowledge and skills.

 EXEMPLAR 21-1

The second author (SDD) was prepared as a CNS in critical care nursing with a master's degree in medical-surgical nursing in 1975 and found a great deal of satisfaction establishing a nurse-managed center for patients with pacemakers. After marketing the concept to the hospital administrators, the center became an excellent revenue source as well as a marketing tool for the hospital (Doughty, 1989). Because work with pacemaker patients demanded more primary care skills than she had learned in her graduate program, she completed an additional year in the adult and aging NP track. When she discovered, upon moving to Maine in 1983, that positions for CNSs were scarce, she accepted a position as the director of critical care nursing at a tertiary center. While SDD employed a new repertoire of management skills in this position, the aspect of direct patient care was missing. Missing the creativity and satisfaction of working directly with patients, she stated an intention to return to the clinical area. She realized that what she loved to do was listen to her pacemaker patients' stories and help them solve problems and create a healthy lifestyle. Within 1 month SDD received three job offers. One was as an NP in a holistic obstetrics-gynecology (OB-GYN) practice with another NP and three gynecologists. The prospect of listening to women's stories and helping them create health appealed to SDD, to the extent that she volunteered in a family planning clinic to refresh her gynecology skills. She left the executive position and built a practice at the holistic center. Most of the practice involved working with perimenopausal and menopausal women, which SDD found greatly satisfying. She marketed herself through community lectures and groups for menopausal women as well as in newsletter articles and radio interviews, emphasizing her unique contributions to the public as alternative ways to create health through menopause. Today she has her own interdisciplinary, holistic women's health center. (The development of this new center, which is the culmination of many dreams, is discussed later in this chapter in the section entitled "Marketing Strategies: Marketing a Service.")

 EXEMPLAR 21-2

This second exemplar describes two family nurse practitioners, KB and SB, who are graduates of the first author's (DRH) Master of Science in Nursing Family Nurse Practitioner (FNP) program. KB began the graduate program with the goal to establish a health-care clinic in her hometown, because the closest physician practice for the rural community was 30 miles away. The only other provider in the town was her dentist-husband. Together they purchased a building and refurbished it into a combined clinic, with his dentist office on one side and her primary care

Continued

EXEMPLAR 21-2—cont'd

clinic office on the other side. The entrance foyer, waiting room, receptionist area, and kitchen are shared in common. To open the clinic, KB negotiated with the regional hospital to set up and fund the clinic. She established a collaborative practice agreement with one of the area physicians as required by the Georgia Board of Nursing state practice act for APNs. In addition, she successfully led the effort to have her small town of 1200 persons redesignated as a health professional shortage area (HPSA). Almost 10 years later, the clinic is thriving, and KB has purchased the clinic from the hospital. She became an FNP because she saw a need. She developed a plan, marketed her clinic, and established a very successful health-care center.

SB was employed by a physician for several years. When the physician decided to make changes in his life, she purchased the primary care practice from him and is now the owner/employer, and hired several physicians to provide care to the underserved population of coastal Georgia. SB advertises her practice as offering health care and wellness throughout the life span. Working in multiple roles, she is the business administrator and a clinician in this nurse-owned primary care practice (Hanson, 2002). Over time, these two FNP entrepreneurs have worked and supported each other professionally in their practices. Their example shows how APNs can be successful entrepreneurs and demonstrates that a sound marketing plan helps to produce positive outcomes.*

*We gratefully acknowledge Kim Baird, MSN, ARNP, BC, Woodbine, GA, and Sally Bennett, MSN, ARNP, BC, Kingsland, GA, for their contribution to this exemplar.

ADVANCED PRACTICE NURSING, PUBLIC RELATIONS, AND THE MEDIA

Public relations and promotion are closely linked in that promotion incorporates a variety of public relations strategies. Certain public relations barriers need to be addressed in order for the marketing of APN services to be successful. These barriers are as follows:

- *Invisibility of nursing* and a general lack of knowledge about advanced nursing practice
- *Effects of negative publicity*, which includes inaccurate portrayals of APNs by other entities, or adverse publicity, as when a nurse is arrested for deliberately harming a patient or making a medication error
- *Traditional images of nurses* in the media that portray them as tyrants, sex symbols, ditsy females, or physicians' handmaidens

Invisibility of Nursing

Although the American Nurses Association (ANA) and other APN role-specific groups speak for APNs at the national level, APNs have the responsibility to market themselves at the state and local levels by educating legislators, physicians, and consumers about what services APNs are educationally prepared to provide. The lack of knowledge about advanced nursing practice in medical schools was boldly illustrated in the January 1999 issue of the *Reporter*, a monthly publication of the Association of American Medical Colleges. The article was positive about what it referred to as "physician extenders," including physician assistants (PAs) and CNMs. However, any mention of NPs, CRNAs, and CNSs was glaringly absent. The reality is that advanced nursing practice invisibility is a pervasive problem not only among consumers but among health-care professionals as well. In an interview, Robert J. Blendon, director of the Harvard Opinion Research

Program, stated that national polls regularly do not include questions on nursing, and as a result, more is known about the public's opinion of physicians than nurses (Buerhaus, 2000). In spite of the negative perspective on advanced practice nursing of organized medicine and the lack of public opinion information on nursing, the health-care community is becoming more aware of APNs, particularly NPs, in part because of new federal guidelines that include their services (Diamond, 2000). Language can be a powerful influence on the visibility or invisibility of particular APN providers. When one says the word "doctor," everyone knows who is being identified. The terms "nurse-midwife" and "nurse anesthetist" are also clear. However, when one says "advanced practice nurse" or "nurse practitioner" or "clinical nurse specialist," some consumers are not only unfamiliar with these terms but are often uncomfortable using them. For example, a young administrator (Marie) was describing her child's health-care provider to a nurse researcher who had previously practiced as an APN. During the conversation, Marie said "the doctor" did this and that. At the end of Marie's description of her child's visit to the provider, the nurse researcher said, "Marie, the person you are describing sounds a lot like a nurse practitioner." Marie said with some embarrassment, "Well . . . she is a nurse practitioner." When asked, Marie said that her only reason for using the term "doctor" was that it was easier to say. A teachable moment had arisen, and the nurse researcher had a collegial discussion with Marie about the power of language and its role in concealing nursing's contributions to health care. As a result of the conversation, Marie realized the negative impact (invisibility, unintentional invalidation) that is perpetuated when the appropriate identity of the APN is not utilized in conversations with others.

The lack of consistent terminology in nursing for APNs contributes to the invisibility of nursing and confusion within the profession as well as the public. For instance, the titling for nurse practitioner in the 50 states includes Certified Registered Nurse Practitioner (CRNP), Advanced Practice Registered Nurse (APRN), Advanced Practice Nurse (APN), and Certified Nurse Practitioner (CNP) (Miller, 2001). When NPs (and other APNs) have such varied legal titles, how can the public be expected to know what to call APNs? This conundrum may worsen as new roles evolve and as the nursing profession deals with advanced practice credentialing and licensing (see Chapter 22).

Effects of Negative Publicity

Physician dominance in the health-care market and its link to adverse publicity about advanced nursing practice has also proven to be an obstacle to effective marketing for APNs. Fear of encroachment and a lack of understanding about the services APNs are educationally prepared to provide to patients have caused some physicians and organized physician groups to attempt to block legislation that would allow for the full scope of APN practice activities. As health-care reform has evolved, some state laws that established barriers to APN practice have been challenged and changed to affect a broader APN practice base. These legislative victories, occurring within the context of a complex health-care market, have led to rising tensions between nursing and medicine. The medical profession has become more vocal and has initiated specific activities aimed at limiting APN scope of practice. As a result of these actions, the American public has been exposed to "negative marketing" campaigns directed against APNs.

In 1994, the American Medical Association (AMA) conducted an expensive campaign to convince the public that the quality of health care would be compromised if APNs were "allowed" to practice primary care. The nursing profession had a choice as to how to respond and might have ignored the smear campaign, as it had ignored other such efforts in the past, because it could only reflect poorly on the AMA. However, recognizing that the media are powerful in presenting a position, Virginia Trotter Betts, RN, JD (ANA president at the time) used this opportunity to market APNs' safety records. She responded to the AMA board by pointing out how their accusations against their nurse colleagues were inaccurate and ill-advised in the face of the desperate need for primary health care for all Americans. She did not confine her rebuttal to correspondence with the AMA but also took her message to the popular press, including *The Wall Street Journal* and *USA Today*.

In 1995, the AMA House of Delegates voted to adopt a resolution that would place tighter restrictions on NP practice (AMA Board of Trustees, 1995). The resolution called for "supervision" of the NP and listed guidelines. These guidelines were restrictive and did not take into consideration that the NP is licensed separately from the MD and is responsible and accountable for his or her own practice (Romaine-Davis, 1997).

From a public relations standpoint, it is crucial that APNs support their medical colleagues who do value and understand the role of APNs and who refuse to participate in the AMA's attempts to discredit APNs. It is important to delineate major differences in the practice scope and the range of services that nurses and physicians are prepared to provide (Moody, Smith, & Glenn, 1999). It is imperative that those who write health-care policy are clear about how APNs can help to meet the health-care needs of the country. APNs must also be proactive in contacting state and federal representatives to help them understand the role of APNs as health-care providers.

Traditional Images of Nurses

Traditional images of nurses in the media indicate that improved, widespread strategic promotion is a particularly important marketing concept for APNs to grasp. Over 20 years ago, Kalisch and Kalisch's (1981) classic work on nurses and the media recommended that nursing specialties work with the media to improve their image, that the public be informed that the primary role of the nurse is to promote health and not serve as handmaiden to the physician, and that nurses are knowledgeable and accountable, as well as sympathetic, caregivers. This advice, given over 20 years ago, is still accurate today. The media continue to present the traditional nurse-physician relationship in a stereotypical fashion as noted by nonphysician and nonnurse researchers from other disciplines (Corser, 2000). In spite of efforts to correct these portrayals, inaccurate perceptions of nursing still exists in many arenas. The media are not solely to blame for their traditional, negative, or stereotypical images of nursing or the current paucity of nursing coverage in the media. Nurses must bear some responsibility for these misperceptions. In order to be successful in the evolving health-care industry, nurses must be active in promoting positive images of nursing in the mass media. "Without counterbalancing examples of nursing reality in the serious and influential media, the power of trivialized or negative images is enhanced" (Buresh, 1998, p. 72).

Newer research suggests that Americans use the media as their primary source of information about health. "This finding is enormously important to nursing. It means that nursing cannot ignore or underestimate the power of the media to influence nursing's public credibility and prestige both now and well into the 21st century" (Buresh, 1998, p. 69). The public needs to be constantly oriented toward several functions that nurses serve in many settings: Nurses promote health, teach disease prevention strategies, and diagnose and treat common illnesses. In addition, some APNs are specially educated to deliver anesthesia and pain management; to provide safe prenatal, intrapartum, and postpartum care; and to broker services for the elderly or chronically ill. In order to change the public's perceptions of nursing, APNs must make themselves available to consult with entities such as health policy writers, health-care journalists, and health planning boards in order to help establish more pro-APN health policies and to increase the number of APN-led health-care centers.

In April 1998, the CBS network's *60 Minutes* aired a segment entitled "The Nurse Will See You Now." The feature was about CAPNA, the Columbia Advanced Practice Nurses primary care practice in Manhattan. Throughout the segment, the featured APNs answered all of Morley Safer's questions positively, a fine example of avoiding negative marketing techniques. For example, when asked, "Why aren't you a doctor?" Edwidge Thomas, NP, replied, "I chose to be a nurse. As medicine has progressed, nursing has progressed." APNs were often referred to as "prevention specialists" in the segment. The focus was on the nurses' abilities to engage people; to know their patients well; and as a result, to know when things are not normal. Using Columbia University affiliations and fund-raising, Mary Mundinger, dean of the College of Nursing, raised money from various foundations to pay for a $1 million advertising campaign to get the word out about CAPNA, an acronym for Comprehensive Accessible Personalized Now Available (see www.capna.com). The television commercial featured a voice-over with the slogan "Gotta go to CAPNA: Columbia Advanced Practice Nurses . . . Primary Care Specialists." The video footage featured a montage of images including fit, healthy bodies interspersed with NPs at work. Superimposed words that kept repeating over the images included "Choices," "Experienced," and "Responsible." Morley Safer concluded the segment by citing the results of a 1993 Gallup poll suggesting that 86% of Americans would be willing to have an NP for primary care. The CAPNA website provides information on APNs and the services that are provided. A study on the care provided by the NPs from 1995 to 1997 indicated, among other findings, that there were no differences in satisfaction ratings following the initial appointment ($P = .88$) for overall satisfaction between the care provided by the NPs and that provided by the physicians (Mundinger et al., 2000). These findings are consistent with observations from those outside the profession. In a *Harvard Business Review* article, the authors suggested that NPs could take on more complex roles than they are currently doing. Nurse practitioners are capable of treating many ailments that in the past were within the realm of physician's care (Christianson, Bohmer, & Kenagy, 2000). Widespread reporting of outcomes of APN care, including the public's level of satisfaction with the care provided by NPs, can influence the development of a more positive image of advanced nursing practice. Box 21-2 summarizes other public relations strategies.

The public's lack of understanding about nurses contributes to an inaccurate image of nursing and a lack of persons interested in the profession. In 2002, Johnson and Johnson began a national multiyear, multilevel media effort, The Campaign for Nursing's Future, to promote interest in nursing careers and a positive image of nursing. A phone survey conducted by Penn, Shoen, and Berland Associates in December 2001 of 1005 adults over 18 years of age in the United States found that only 53% knew that a registered nurse (RN) must have a bachelor's degree or an associate's degree. Fewer than one in five respondents (13%) knew that an RN must be licensed. Fewer than half knew that an NP must have a master's degree, and over two thirds did not know that NPs could prescribe medications (Johnson & Johnson, 2002). The data suggest that the lack of information about nurses is associated with the public's lack of understanding regarding the role that nurses and APNs have in health-care decision making. (For more information on The Campaign for Nursing's Future, see the website at www.jnj.com/news/jnj_news.)

The nursing community has undertaken a national effort to improve the image of nursing. *Nursing's Agenda for the Future* (ANA, 2001), a national plan developed by a steering committee comprising 19 national nursing organizations, is designed to provide guidance for improving nursing's future and the public's right to high-quality health care. The plan is designed around 10 domains. One of the domains is communication, and a primary objective is improving communication with the public about the role nurses play in health care (ANA, 2001). Both of these national efforts are, in part, aimed at improving nursing's image. As the public's understanding of APN practice, quality of care, and outcomes increases, existing barriers to practice can eventually be removed. However, as health care evolves and comes under continued intense scrutiny, more barriers to effective marketing for APNs can also arise. To counteract current and future barriers, APNs must be willing to go beyond conventional thinking and to perceive barriers as opportunities.

One strategy to improve the public image of nursing is to disseminate the positive, and, cost-effective outcomes of care provided by APNs to the lay literature as well as professional journals. The findings of a study by Brooten et al. (2002) in which seven clinical studies of care provided by APNs were reviewed over 22 years indicated that APN interventions consistently resulted in improved patient outcomes and reduced health-care costs across the groups studied. Stressing the economic outcomes of care provided by APNs is a marketing strategy that could be used to more advantage. For example, a comparative study looking at the cost-effectiveness of neonatal nurse practitioners (NNPs) with medical house staff was conducted (Bissinger, Allred, Arford, & Bellig, 1997). This retrospective chart review in a 36-bed neonatal intensive care unit investigated length of stay, days on ventilator, days on oxygen, mortality, morbidity, and cost of care with infants between 500 and 1250 grams. The infants cared for by the NNP had a 14-day shorter stay and a mean of 11 days fewer on oxygen. While the quality of care provided by both groups of providers was determined comparable in the study, economic findings favored the NNP. The cost of care by the NNP was significantly lower at $88,932, whereas the cost of medical staff care was $105,070. Economic outcomes such as these and other studies related to APN practice (Mundinger et al., 2000) can be used effectively to market the APN as a cost-effective, quality health-care provider. In light of rapidly escalating health-care costs, these types of information must be shared with the public in a way that is readily understood.

Nurses need to distribute press releases on innovative and effective clinical programs as well as important research findings to the popular press. This strategy can interest journalists in nursing and generate interviews and other media activities that will generate public interest in and commitment to advanced nursing practice. These actions need to be ongoing, as all efforts do not result in information being picked up by the popular press. Numerous opportunities exist for APNs to meet client needs and to improve the public's perception of the image of nursing, the role of nursing, and the variety of ways that nurses improve health-care services. Box 21-2 provides additional media and public relations strategies for marketing APN services.

MARKETING STRATEGIES FOR NOVICE AND EXPERIENCED APNs

Considerations for New Graduates

Marketing oneself as a new graduate is one of the most challenging tasks for APNs. The transition period from student to APN provides many exciting new opportunities, but it can also be the source of much anxiety. Helping students to develop skills to make the transition to new graduate APNs is essential to the success of future marketing strategies.

Brown and Olshansky's (1998) research-based model identifies the "Limbo to Legitimacy" transition stages that take into account the experiences of the new NP during the first year in primary care practice. Stage 1 of this developmental, nonlinear model is

---

BOX 21-2 • MEDIA AND PUBLIC RELATIONS STRATEGIES

Network with health journalists
Gain television news show exposure
Write magazine and journal articles
Send out press releases
Produce public service announcements
Publish research reports
Write for daily newspapers and news magazines
Give radio news interviews
Establish a site on the Internet/World Wide Web
Volunteer to give community presentations
Volunteer to work in a free clinic and/or provide free services (e.g., homeless shelter)
Join community organizations
Get involved with politics (e.g., run for public office)

---

relevant to all APNs in the first year of practice and raises important marketing considerations. This stage is characterized by a period of recovering from school, seeking employment, negotiating bureaucracies, and worrying about meeting role expectations. Maintaining positive self-esteem is key to a successful completion of this transition (see Chapter 4 for further discussion of APN role development).

Bolles (2002) suggested teaching students five approaches to sustaining a positive outlook during transition periods:

- Keep physically fit by developing an action plan that makes time for positive self-care.
- Deal with emotions by building an effective support network.
- Monitor mental stamina and focus on positive views.
- Utilize spirituality for support in difficult times.
- Keep active by using time and talents within the community.

According to Payne (1997), the role of executives, recruiters, and faculty is to help new graduates stay open to alternative options in health care. Key elements include helping them to remain enthusiastic, to market their unique skills, and to understand the need for flexibility. Strategies would include encouraging new graduates to view a part-time position as a potential bridge to full-time employment, to perceive cross-training as a challenge, and to consider new or unusual job opportunities as pathways to a rewarding professional nursing career.

Seeking Employment as a Novice APN

As previously noted, seeking employment is a primary task for new graduates. During the course of graduate education, students should learn strategies for seeking an APN position. Specific elements to cover included résumé preparation, the differences between a résumé and a curriculum vita, preparation of query letters, preparing for an interview, and accepting/negotiating for a position. These issues are briefly covered here.

Résumés and curricula vitae. Most graduates will work on preparing résumés to use as they seek employment. Résumés are generally one or two pages long and cover relevant experience and responsibilities appropriate to the position sought as well as educational background (give expected graduation date if one is still in school). Résumés may begin with a brief profile of the applicant and a goal statement. Relevant experience is usually organized chronologically with most recent experience first. It is not sufficient to list places and dates of employment; bulleted phrases under each position describing key responsibilities and accomplishments are necessary (e.g., "was responsible for developing and implementing an oncology certification review course; 20% of staff RNs (N = 10) became certified in oncology nursing within 18 months of program initiation," or "supervised 20 RNs and 10 CNAs"). Do not include salary requirements or other expectations about benefits. Because of concerns about identify theft, the résumé should not have your social security number or RN license number. It is sufficient to say that you are licensed (or have applied for a license) in a particular state or states. The résumé is your introduction to a prospective employer and should be visually interesting, brief but substantive. To maximize the possibility that a résumé will be considered, it is advisable to tailor the résumé to highlight the relevance of the applicant's experience to the position.

Curricula vitae (CVs) are more comprehensive—they are usually representative of one's entire career, and APN graduates who seek a joint appointment as a clinician and a faculty member may need to have both a résumé and a CV. While most APN graduates are unlikely to need a CV immediately upon graduation, those APNs who envision teaching at some point in the future may want to create one and update it annually. It is difficult to recreate a comprehensive CV 10 years after graduation if one has not developed some system for keeping track of the professional experiences and activities that are included in a CV.

For both résumés and CVs, accurate contact information must be included (address, telephone and fax numbers, and e-mail addresses). Readers can consult such resources as www.resume.com or job search resources such as www.Monster.com for additional information on résumé preparation. Many job sites have advice on résumé and CV preparation for those seeking positions in health care. Résumés and CVs should be carefully proofread. New graduates are advised to have a colleague or faculty member look at the résumé (and the position advertisement or description, if available) prior to sending it out to prospective employers.

Query and cover letters. APNs who are seeking employment can expand the opportunities for obtaining desirable positions by crafting a well-thought-out letter. Query letters are used to determine whether possibilities for employment exist, especially when no positions have been advertised and/or to request an informational interview. The first sentence or two must engage the reader—for example, you might indicate your familiarity with the setting and/or the staff, its vision, or mission; identify the person who referred you to the organization; or state why you want to work there. A query letter should conclude positively and assertively—"I look forward to speaking with you"—and include accurate contact information. If you receive no response within a week of sending a query letter, it is acceptable to follow up with a telephone call or e-mail message.

Cover letters are usually written in response to an advertisement or job board posting about a specific position. Prior to preparing a cover letter, it is advisable to consult the organization's website and/or marketing material to help you tailor the letter. The cover letter should be brief and, as with the query letter, should engage the reader in the first sentence or two. As with a query letter, you indicate why you are interested in the position; you also highlight the specific strengths you bring to the position. The letter is an opportunity to add additional, relevant information that a prospective employee would find useful. For example, your résumé may indicate that you have experience in medical surgical nursing. If you are applying for a job at a comprehensive cancer center, you can indicate in the letter additional knowledge and skills that may be specific to an oncology setting—those acquired in the med-surg setting as well as any additional skills acquired during graduate education. One variation on the cover letter that some human resources staff have recommended is a "T-letter," in which the applicant, after the first two, "engaging" sentences, creates a brief table (N. Solomons, personal communication, May 21, 2004). In the left-hand column, list, in bulleted phrases, the job requirements; in the right-hand column, list bulleted substantive phrases of your related experience. Such a letter highlights your relevant knowledge and skills as they relate to the specific requirements of the position.

Interviews. Prior to an interview, you must do some homework. As with the cover letter, it is advisable to be familiar with an organization's public "face"—website, brochures, and other marketing materials—as well as the position description. Using this information, you can prepare questions that will help you better understand the setting and the position expectations. Determine whether you are meeting with more than one person. Sometimes human resources staff does an initial interview by phone or in person to verify that a candidate should proceed with an interview with other providers. Other points to attend to are the following: dress appropriately, scout the location (if the interview is being held in an unfamiliar location, do a dry run to estimate time), and arrive a few minutes early. If you have an interview and you are not selected for the position, you may ask for some feedback that will help you improve your interviewing style/skills.

Accepting/negotiating for a position. Although it is not appropriate to discuss salary in résumés or initial interviews, it is wise to be aware of salary ranges for the type of position you are seeking in your local area. When an offer is made, this knowledge can help you negotiate a mutually acceptable salary and benefit package. Other elements to consider when negotiating once an offer has been made are reporting relationships, productivity expectations, administrative and staff support, on-call responsibilities, and orientation plan. Many of the issues discussed under contract considerations and listed in Boxes 21-5 and 21-6 may be relevant for APNs, such as CNSs, who will be employees of institutions.

Developing a Personal Marketing Plan and Creating a Personal Portfolio

An accurate self-assessment of individual strengths and a clear conceptualization of one's desired practice arena are essential first steps in developing a personal marketing plan for new graduates and experienced APNs. Developing a professional marketing portfolio is a useful strategy to aid in this process (Burgess & Misener, 1997). A professional portfolio is defined as a representative sample of documents about who you are professionally and what you have to offer (Letz, 2002). A portfolio differs from a résumé or curriculum vitae in that, in addition to containing a list of all previous positions and educational background, the portfolio contains examples of one's work. Professional portfolios contain a description of skills and provide a profile of the applicant's major accomplishments and contributions (Box 21-3). When a specific employment opportunity arises that an APN desires, the APN chooses from the portfolio those materials that best relate to the desired position, such as a résumé listing previous positions and responsibilities, a curriculum vitae listing academic experience and achievements, publications authored by the APN, project results, letters of recommendation from former employers, client and colleague recommendations, honors, and awards. Restifo (1999) recommends using the portfolio for communicating personal strengths in situations such as performance appraisals, job and return-to-school interviews, presentations, job fairs, and networking sessions. In addition, an APN who precepts or mentors students or graduate APNs can use her or his personal

---

BOX 21-3 • COMPONENTS OF A PROFESSIONAL PORTFOLIO FOR APNS

- Business documents such as your résumé or curriculum vitae (CV), letters of recommendation, list of references
- Nursing documents such as license, professional certificates, malpractice insurance information, NCLEX-RN results, diplomas and grade transcripts, contact-hour certificates, and continuing-education course information (course descriptions, outlines)
- Identification such as a driver's license, birth certificate, Social Security card, passport, and work visa
- Health information such as PPD or chest x-ray results, immunization record and titers

- Items showing special recognition you've received, such as honors and awards, newspaper clippings, and photos
- Evidence of your teaching, including programs, presentations evaluations, lesson plans, and handouts
- Items from your on-the-job work, such as performance appraisals, thank-you letters, reports papers, research findings
- Professional activities, including articles or a list of publications and photos (e.g., of posters, exhibits)

From Restifo V. (1999, February 8). Your professional portfolio. *Nursing Spectrum,* p. 17; reprinted with permission.
NCLEX-RN, National Council Licensure Examination for Registered Nurses.

---

professional portfolio as an exemplar about how a career develops over time, presenting activities and choices made and providing anticipatory guidance to the novice.

Scanland (1990) described an excellent example of marketing oneself by using a portfolio. She sought a new work environment that provided more flexibility, learning, and growth opportunities and a setting in which she could use both her expertise in geriatrics and her NP skills. She targeted a family practice residency program in the area and gathered data about the gap between the needs of the elderly in that area and the supply of physician services. She contacted the program director and convinced him to hire her to conduct both a clinical practice and a resident geriatric education program by matching information from her survey with that from her portfolio.

An APN might also find it useful to include information in the portfolio that helps differentiate what physicians do from the services that APNs can provide. Also helpful are studies that describe the role differentiation between physicians and APNs and how primary care, for example, differs when provided by an APN (Kassirer, 1994; Mundinger et al., 2000; Safreit, 1992). Fact sheets and brochures from professional organizations that describe the advantages of working with particular APNs might also be included in one's portfolio (Box 21-4 contains suggested websites that provide fact sheets). Thus, the

---

BOX 21-4 • NATIONAL NURSING ASSOCIATION WEBSITES

American Nurses Association (ANA)	www.ana.org
American Academy of Nurse Practitioners (AANP)	www.aanp.org
American Association of Colleges of Nursing	www.aacn.nche.edu
American College of Nurse Practitioners (ACNP)	www.acnpweb.org
American Holistic Nurse's Association	www.ahna.org
Association of Pediatric Nurse Practitioners (NAPNAP)	www.napnap.org
Oncology Nursing Society (ONS)	www.ons.org
American College of Nurse-Midwives (ACNM)	www.midwife.org
American Association of Nurse Anesthetists (AANA)	www.aana.com
National Association of Clinical Nurse Specialists	www.nacns.org

portfolio serves as a data bank from which the APN can construct a position-specific marketing tool.

External and Internal Marketing

Two facets of marketing that are useful to clarify the role(s) of APNs in every setting include external and internal marketing. *External marketing* refers to all the techniques that APNs can use to promote themselves or their practices to their consumers or the public at large. Suggestions include speaking at community meetings, circulating business cards, writing a column in the newspaper, advertising in the yellow pages, and sending out fliers or brochures about the practice. In addition, utilizing the positive opinions of respected resources to support practice outcomes and the use of APNs is beneficial. *Internal marketing* involves differentiating the unique capabilities of APNs in their practice environment and showing how what they have to offer is different from the care provided by anyone else, whether it is of higher quality, more complex, more accessible, or less expensive (Brunk, 1992). Hallums (1994) considered internal marketing an important, holistic management process that is important work undertaken by an organization to motivate and train its "internal customers" (employees) to work as a unified group to deliver customer service and satisfaction. Grasping the importance of internal marketing is crucial for APNs. Internal marketing strategies are often central to establishing credibility and developing collaborative, interdisciplinary relationships.

Capitalizing on creativity is the hallmark of both external and internal marketing for APNs. Tapping into one's creativity often gets overlooked when performing routine care and management of patient problems. In Exemplar 21-3, Keller (Doughty & Keller, 2000) used a unique, creative internal marketing strategy that was very successful.

EXEMPLAR 21-3

While working in a multispecialty group practice in the Southwest several years ago, NP/PA colleagues met regularly to discuss practice issues. The group decided that it was necessary to educate physicians, administrators, and clinical and clerical support staff about the role of NPs and PAs in the organization. A presentation was developed titled "A Day in the Life of an NP and a PA." With a total of 85 physicians and 13 NPs/PAs in the practice, the group felt that it was very important for the entire medical staff and top administrators to be in attendance. It was determined that the best forum for the presentation was during the health center's monthly medical and administrative staff meeting. Since this presentation would be a first within the organization, two things were certain: This might be the only chance to capture the attention of physician and administrative colleagues, and the presentation had to be extremely well-prepared in order to enhance the credibility of the NP/PA group.

After much brainstorming, a creative, humorous, and informative presentation was developed. A listing of the most memorable questions that had been asked of the group was developed. Examples of the questions included, "What do all those letters after your name mean?" "When are you going to become a doctor?" "Do I have to pay the full $5.00 co-pay to see you instead of a doctor?" "I am so confused . . . what is the difference between an NP and a PA?" "As an NP, are you the one who stands in the room with the doctor when he does a Pap smear?"

The group then enlisted the help of collaborative physicians to serve as "plants" in the audience. Each collaborating physician was provided with the question that was to be addressed

Continued

EXEMPLAR 21-3—cont'd

by the NP or PA in her or his dyad. "Dyad" was the term that had been mutually agreed upon with the medical director to define the relationship between each NP or PA provider and her or his collaborating physician in the practice. It was felt that the dyad recognition in the presentation was important because some of the physicians had historically been uncomfortable referring patients to NPs and PAs if they were not aware of the dyad arrangement. The overall mood during the presentations was humorous and informal. On cue during the program, each physician "plant" stood up and asked the question assigned to her/him. The corresponding NP or PA then answered the question with factual information illustrating the role of the NP or PA. For example, in response to the question "When are you going to become a doctor?" an NP replied with enthusiasm about positive reasons for choosing to be an APN instead of a physician. In response to the question "As an NP, are you the one who stands in the room with the doctor when he does a Pap smear?" an NP addressed the need for consumer education and widespread external and internal marketing of APNs. Other issues that were addressed in the question-and-answer format were the educational requirements for NPs and PAs, quality-of-service issues, and the role of NPs and PAs as primary care providers.

Before the start of the program, the NPs and PAs were seated in front of the audience with large nametags and were given the opportunity to introduce themselves individually in a brief biographical format (e.g., name, department, site, collaborating physician name, education, related work/volunteer background, and special interests clinically and personally). Many of the staff members had never met each other, so this provided the opportunity for recognition and networking. The feedback the group received was tremendous. Many physicians, administrators, and human resources representatives made a special point to thank the group for a most informative and interesting program. The outcome of the presentation was an overall increase in the numbers of internal referrals to NPs and PAs. As a result of this success, further marketing projects were launched. A presentation for receptionists and medical assistants about the role of NPs and PAs in health care was provided.

The result of this effort was more appropriately scheduled appointments and no more receptionists being overheard to say, "You can't see the doctor today, just the NP or PA. Sorry!" One of the most important outcomes of this overall marketing effort by the NP/PA group was the appointment of the first NP on the medical center's new board of directors. In this setting, it was determined that an aggressive internal marketing strategy was necessary before branching out to external strategies. In this exemplar, thoughtful assessment of the practice situation, group discussions, and strategic planning for the best possible implementation resulted in positive outcomes. One caveat to remember is that it is important never to assume that all of the administrators or physician colleagues have a clear understanding of the role an APN in a practice setting. Internal and external marketing strategies can help improve the practice milieu and thus have a positive impact on APN job satisfaction.

CONTRACTING CONSIDERATIONS

Obtaining a working knowledge of negotiation skills is the foundation for handling contract considerations. Negotiating and advocating for patients is much easier than negotiating a new contract, salary, and/or benefits package. Historically, nurses have been inexperienced with establishing contractual and legal relationships, which are common in the business world. However, a political and economic reality of the current health-care environment is that there is resistance to recognizing APNs as legitimate providers of care. As members of a largely female profession, nurses may be less comfortable when it comes to self-promotion. Keller advised nurses to avoid the "burnt toast" syndrome—a term she coined to describe the self-effacing behavior demonstrated by mothers who make toast for breakfast and keep the burnt piece for themselves while giving the nicely toasted pieces to family members. Nurses can no longer afford to eat "burnt toast." (Doughty &

Keller, 2000). Despite nurses' inexperience and possible discomfort with self-promotion, gender differences can play a significant role in negotiating contracts that help APNs achieve their goals (Wyatt, 1999).

Robbins' (1998) Negotiation Framework outlines five steps that can help APNs become more comfortable with negotiating

- Step 1: Prepare and plan
- Step 2: Define the ground rules
- Step 3: Clarify and justify
- Step 4: Bargain and problem-solve
- Step 5: Close and implement

By learning to be a strong negotiator, the APN can increase the probability of achieving desired outcomes. Negotiating a contract is an important marketing skill. As APNs share the market place with other health-care providers, they have to acquire new skills, especially in the area of business and leadership (Munden, 2001). The most common contracts or agreements that APNs are likely to encounter are employment contracts, managed care contracts, collaborative practice agreements, and service contracts.

Employment Contracts

An employment contract helps the APN to clarify all parameters of a new position, including a section that outlines the requirements for ending the professional relationship. The value of an employment contract is still being debated, but, at the very least, some type of written agreement should be obtained. APNs should avoid agreeing to unreasonable restrictive covenants (Buppert, 1999). Noncompete and gag clauses are restrictive covenants that may be included in a contract. A noncompete clause provides a barrier to future practice in the employer's service area for a period of time after the professional relationship has been terminated between the employer and the APN. Noncompete clauses refer to areas such as geographic location, patient referrals, and employment opportunities (Zaumeyer, 2003). Depending on applicable state laws, a noncompete clause may be governed by a state statute and is still considered by some to be a restraint of trade (Herman & Zeil, 1999). Box 21-5 lists elements of an employment contract, and a sample employment agreement can be found in Appendix A.

APNs must also be alert to gag clauses that constrain clinical practice or interactions with patients during employment and after severance of the professional relationship with the employer. Gag clauses can limit the ability of the provider to provide information to a patient as to why, for example, tests are not covered under a carrier or about other providers outside of the health-care organization. The AMA came out in strong opposition to gag clauses in health maintenance organization (HMO) contracts, which limited the physician's ability to provide needed information to patients. On January 17, 1996, the AMA's Council on Judicial and Ethical Affairs, the division of the AMA that maintains its Code of Ethics, stated that certain confidentiality or gag clauses found in some managed care contracts were unethical and could subject physicians to sanctions if enacted by the health plans (AMA, 1996). The federal government has passed regulations to ban gag clauses in certain contracts. The regulation, which covers the 350 health insurance companies offering coverage to federal employees and retirees, prohibits companies from including so-called "gag clauses" in contracts with doctors, hospitals, and other health-care providers (Fiel, 1998). In light of the current environment, APNs must read

---

BOX 21-5 • ELEMENTS OF AN EMPLOYMENT CONTRACT

Your contract should include:

1. Official relationship with physician partnership, medical group, or corporation
2. Terms of employment
   Start date
   Probation period
   Criteria for probationary review
   Duration of contract
   Annual review
   Salary increases
3. Clinical responsibilities and supervision
   Supervising/consulting MD responsibilities
   Job description or expected duties
   Work hours
   Call hours and responsibilities
   PA/NP cross-coverage
   Work sites
4. Compensation
   Salary and method of calculation
   Bonuses and/or incentives, profit sharing
5. Benefits
   Insurance
   —Medical
   —Dental
   —Vision
   —Disability (short and long term)
   —Life
   —Automobile
   Medical malpractice coverage
   Retirement plan
6. Business expenses
   State licensure and supervisory fees
   Certification fees
   Hospital medical staff fees
   Automobile costs and insurance
   Association dues
   Books and professional journals
   Equipment
7. Vacation and sick time
   Vacation conditions
   Holiday time
   Sick leave and limits
   Maternity leave
8. Continuing education
   Conditions and amounts
   Listed separately from vacation
9. Contract renewals and terminations
   Paid leave
   Option to review
   Clinician evaluation criteria
   Termination "for cause" specifics
   Termination "without cause"
      —Notice period
      —Compensation/benefit buyout
10. Other standard clauses
    Contract is total agreement (no verbal agreements accepted—neither contract negotiations nor contract changes)
    Contract modifications must be signed by both parties
    Conduct differing from the contract does not waive the right to uphold all contract clauses
11. Proper signatures with names and title typed below
12. Date of signing

Adapted from Woomer, S. (1994). Negotiating an employment contract. *The Clinician's Reference Guide 1994* (a supplement to *Clinician Reviews*), pp. 21-28; reprinted with permission.

the contract carefully to ascertain that all essential areas are covered and that unreasonable restrictions are not included. All areas of a contract are negotiable, including restrictive clauses. Consider the clause carefully before signing the contract (Buppert, 2001). In addition, it would be prudent to have a lawyer review any contract before signing it.

When negotiating an employment contract/agreement, the APN should know what is desired and needed ahead of time. Although this might seem obvious, nurses often do not anticipate or negotiate for important personal and professional benefits. In addition to salary, other negotiable contract items, which APNs should consider in advance, are noted in Box 21-5.

The essence of a contract will vary according to the nature of individual APN practices, but the goal of negotiating a contract is always to protect the APN by including expectations, objectives, and the nature of the relationships with those with whom the contract is being formed. In addition, APNs must always attend to the certification, licensing, and authorization requirements in states where they will practice (see Chapter 22).

In terms of vacation, APNs should aim for the physician standard in the setting/practice. For continuing education time, they should aim for at least 4 to 5 paid days per year and a minimum of $1000 for continuing education expenses (Fitzgerald, 1999). Buppert (1999) notes additional items that may be desirable to address in an employment contract:

- Extent of support service to be provided to APN
- Expectation as to the number of patients to be seen daily
- Administrative work to be expected
- Listing of APN's name on outside clinic sign, doors, directories, and advertisements
- Use of APN's name when phone is answered
- Release to the APN of the APN's quality performance as measured by health plan auditors
- Release to the APN of the amount of profit brought into the practice by the APN

Managed Care Contracts

Contracts are required by insurers and fall into two categories, managed care and indemnity insurers (Buppert, 1999). Box 21-6 lists the key components of a managed care contract. The goal of managed care is to decrease overall health-care costs and to provide more services for less reimbursement through a contract on a capitated or fee-for-service basis. A contract is essential to clarify the responsibilities of a position when participating in managed care; it should provide the details of the services that will be provided and a description of the arrangement between the APN and the MCO (Buppert, 1999). A practice must be recognized in the MCO provider panels in order to participate. Managed care contracts with providers include an agreement for the APN to provide certain kinds of services for a company, such as pre-employment histories and physical examinations. Provision of health education to employees of a company may or may not include the employee's family members, and this should be clarified by the contract. It is important to make sure that contracts with the MCO specify the APN as a legitimate provider of care in order to protect APNs from being eliminated as providers of care.

While indemnity insurers pay provider fees, unlike an MCO, they have no relationship with the provider other than to pay the bill for the care received by the covered patient (Buppert, 1999). Not all insurers cover care provided by APNs, and a contract with the insurer may need to be negotiated for coverage of services. Newer legislation is continuing to open doors for APNs to ensure that they are included in the primary care medical provider panels and will be reimbursed.

Collaborative Practice Agreements

Depending on the regulatory requirements of particular states (see Chapter 22), APNs may need to make formal arrangements with physicians to ensure that medical backup is available for patients' health-care issues that are out of the APN's scope of practice. Typically, such agreements address the nature of the collaborative relationship, parame-

---

BOX 21-6 • KEY COMPONENTS OF A MANAGED CARE CONTRACT

Negotiating a contract with a managed care organization (MCO) will demand the assistance of an attorney experienced in negotiating these contracts, because the contract will cover much more than just compensation.

- What is included? What is excluded?
- Requirements for:
  - Utilization management
  - Quality assurance
  - Credentialing
  - Member grievance
  - Record-keeping
  - Claims submission
  - Hours of operation
  - Appointment response times
  - On-call coverage
  - Employing other providers
  - Arranging backup with other groups
  - Maximum/minimum number of patients
  - Antidisparagement
  - Business confidentiality
- Fee (capitation) schedule
- Special needs programs (carve outs): criteria, process for transfer of care for those eligible
- Stop-loss provisions
- Referral pools
- Withholds
- Level of distribution from withhold/referral pools over prior five years
- Bonus system
- Provisions for closing the practice to additional practice from the MCO
- Claims processing: in-house or contracted out?
- Who does lab work?
- Renewal of contract: based upon? Renewal rate with provider
- MCO's review of office practices
- Directory listing: How will it read?
- Any prohibition on joining other MCOs?
- Definitions of "experimental emergency" and "preexisting condition"
- Who bears the brunt of a mistake in eligibility or coverage determination?
- Can preadmission or referral approval be rescinded retroactively?
- Formulary contents
- System for verifying member eligibility
- Routine for notification of members selecting practice
- Provisions for dispute resolution
- Marketing provided
- Who owns the records/data?

Adapted from Buppert, C. (1999). *Nurse practitioner's practice and legal guide* (pp. 259-261, 341-344). Boston: Jones and Bartlett.

ters for consultation, and physician availability for consultation and emergency care. Such agreements may refer to interdisciplinary guidelines, medical references, and particular standards of care that are to be followed. The agreement should meet the state regulatory requirements and be signed by all involved parties. A sample collaborative practice agreement is found in Appendix B.

Service Agreements

Service agreements that outline services to be provided over a specified period of time are often negotiated between APNs and other parties. For example, an oncology clinical nurse specialist employed in a comprehensive cancer center may negotiate with a consortium of rural hospitals in his or her state to provide two chemotherapy certification workshops annually. The service agreement would outline the responsibilities of each party, contingencies for insufficient registration, a budget or specified dollar amount to cover honoraria and expenses (overhead expenses would be included if the contract were negotiated with the CNS's agency as opposed to the CNS as an independent contractor), and other relevant details. In this example, the CNS would meet with his or her department head and the financial officer for the CNS's agency to discuss the contract and identify the appropriate agency person to sign the contract. The CNS would estimate the number of days it would take to prepare and deliver the programs, the human and material resources needed, and travel expenses; the CNS would anticipate factors that might require cancellation/rescheduling (e.g., weather, insufficient registration); and the CNS would indicate the dates (agreed to by the CNS and the consortium representatives) on which the program is to be delivered and identify "in-kind" resources that would not require financial support (e.g., the consortium would be responsible for copying and collating the training manuals). Together, the CNS and a financial officer would determine the appropriate activities and budget to discuss with the consortium prior to signing an agreement. Another example of a service agreement would be when a nurse researcher contracts with an NP to provide certain services for research subjects. Similar details would need to be considered for this type of service agreement.

Professional Development Plan

A final and important aspect of professional development includes making an informal contract with oneself to reevaluate short-term and long-term goals. It is to the APN's advantage to review objectives at least quarterly to be able to determine if progress is being made along the anticipated career path and to recommit to the most important employment components in order to attain personal satisfaction in a position. A critical part of this personal contract includes balancing the physical, intellectual, emotional, and spiritual dimensions of the individual. Reviewing the position to determine whether it is consuming an unbalanced amount of energy is essential in order to ensure that the interests of the APN, patients, and the organization are being served.

MARKETING STRATEGIES: MARKETING A SERVICE

To be successful, a business must be well-planned, and the owners must be prepared to offer and market a service that others need and value. Before one can market a service, it is important to prepare a business plan. This section describes preparing a business plan for making advanced practice nursing services available and strategies for marketing these services (Box 21-7).

Writing a Successful Business Plan

According to Haag (1997), approximately 1 million new businesses are started each year in the United States alone. Of those 1 million new businesses, only about one in five will survive to see their fifth anniversary. "A business owner who fails to plan, plans to fail"

BOX 21-7 • INTERNET RESOURCES RELATED TO BUSINESS PLANNING AND MARKETING

APN Business and Law Resource Center www.medscape.com	Latest on business and legal topics for both new and experienced APNs
www.legalnurses.net/opportunity/homestudy	Homey site about working from home as an NP. Helpful for working mothers
www.buppert.com/trainingmodules	Site describes training modules for purchase to start a business in the health-care field
www.sba.gov	Help from the government to start your business
www.startupjournal.com	Information from the *Wall Street Journal* on how to start a business
www.business.com	Leading business search engine and business directory designed to help users find the information needed to make business decisions
www.businessknowhow.com	Lots of pithy advice on real problems faced in starting and early stages of a business

---

(Covello & Hazelgren, 1995). Although writing a successful business plan is not usually a component of traditional advanced nursing practice curricula, it is a vital aspect of the entrepreneurial movement in advanced nursing practice. The process of writing a business plan includes the following steps (Haag, 1997, p. 26):

- Define the business concept.
- Gather data on the feasibility and specifics of the concept.
- Focus and refine the concept.
- Outline the specifics of the business.
- Put the plan in a compelling form.

The survival of a small business can also depend on other critical factors such as identification of consumer needs, financial resources, timing of entry into the marketplace, and planning for growth to meet future demands (Gardner & Weinrauch, 1998). An important resource for a new business is the Service Corps of Retired Executives (SCORE) (www.score.com), which provides multiple formats of support through consultation, Web links and, useful resources and the Small Business Survival Committee (www.sbsc.org). Many "how-to" guides exist on what critical elements to include in a business plan (see Box 21-8 for more information) (Buppert, 1999; Letz, 2002; Robert Wood Johnson Foundation, 2003; Zaumeyer, 2003).

Approaches to Marketing A Service

It is helpful for the APN to remember that people usually will not appreciate what a professional does unless they are educated to the facts (Abraham, 1994). People want to know more about unique services, yet potential customers (employers, patients, physicians, and other providers) may have no concept of the expertise APNs could bring to their businesses or practices and, therefore, would never advertise for one (Weill et al., 1989). In fact, those who have worked with APNs or contracted for APN services, often wonder how they ever got along without them. APNs have many strengths that increase their marketability and these strengths are rooted in basic nursing practice.

BOX 21-8 • BUSINESS PLAN COMPONENTS

Cover/Title Page
Executive Summary
Table of Contents
Business Description and History
Business Structure
Product/Service Description
Market Analysis and Strategy (Plan)
Operations
Management Team
Financial Data/Projections
Appendix

From Haag, A. B. (1997). Writing a successful business plan. *AAOHN Journal, 45*(1), 27; reprinted with permission.

Marketing is a social and managerial process by which individuals and groups obtain what they need and want through creating, offering, and exchanging products of value with others (Chang, Price, & Pfoutz, 2001). According to Stern (1997) using multiple marketing techniques is not an outdated practice because people seek information from traditional sources, not just the Internet. The keys to marketing a service are variety and reinforcement. The basics of marketing are keeping focused by not varying the presentation of the image widely (e.g., using one logo on all marketing materials), selecting the media format carefully to reach the intended population, tracking marketing results, and remaining flexible in order to change to more effective strategies when necessary.

Differentiation, that is, how a proposed service differs from that provided by others, is important. These services may include such things as higher quality, more accessibility, or different hours of service. Services targeted toward specific market segmentation data, such as retirement centers, hospital staff, individuals living with chronic pain, or new mothers needing breastfeeding counseling, help the APN to tailor marketing plans for success based on client needs.

Establishing, growing, and improving a business takes a sophisticated mix of entrepreneurial vision, business management know-how, and specialized knowledge. Through free, small business counseling and support services, the Service Corps of Retired Executives (SCORE) volunteers provide marketing advice and financial and business plan development assistance that could benefit the APN just forming a business or implementing the marketing of a service (see www.score.org). Exemplar 21-4 provides an example of how one APN developed and marketed a unique service to a defined population with health care needs.

EXEMPLAR 21-4

As an NP in a holistic OB-GYN practice, the second author (SDD) recognized a need in the community for women in midlife to have access to information about whether to take hormones or herbs, how to improve quality of life, and how to prevent problems of aging that start in midlife. Certain obstacles prevented universal access in that practice, and SDD dreamed of an interdisciplinary holistic center on a bus line, a center with handicapped accessibility and a fund for indigent women. Intrinsic to her dream was the concept of circle leadership among the disciplines without a medical hierarchy, consistent with the work of Christina Baldwin (1998). According to Baldwin, "The circle is an organizational structure that locates leadership

Continued

EXEMPLAR 21-4—cont'd

along the rim and provides an inclusive means for consultation. Circling is a useful structure for learning, governance, creating community, providing services, envisioning in starting long-range goals and observing ritual" (p. 38).

After a year of planning with a nurse massage therapist and a highly skilled medical receptionist, SDD completed the business plan and went to the bank. She hoped to get partial funding as a business loan and to secure a personal loan for the remainder of the start-up costs. The bank officials were so impressed with the marketing projections and data in the business plan that they funded the entire start-up cost.

Critical to the success of the women's center was the agreement of a close friend and colleague, another experienced women's health NP with a background in business and a master's degree in business administration, to buy in as a partner. Many of the business decisions that had to be made in the infancy of the practice were tempered with expertise and practical orientation. The new partner believed in the vision, and both practitioners remained connected to the constant question, "How will this decision affect the women who want our services?"

Initially, the other disciplines included massage, mental health, movement, and nutrition. A physical therapist and a gynecologist were recruited. The team sat in "circle" weekly to discuss how the center was doing and how they were doing with the center. They held retreats quarterly to bond as a team. A naturopath also joined the group. Their marketing efforts are detailed in Box 21-9.

Obstacles to third-party reimbursement for APN autonomous practice in Maine precipitated legislation to ensure reimbursement. The state NP group hired a lobbyist who helped them forge this legislation. SDD's business partner was extremely active in this effort, gathering data and testimonials. Prior data that had been generated on cost and efficacy influenced the banking and insurance committee, who first heard the bills. Patient testimonials were what convinced all involved that APNs made a difference and needed to have separate identification numbers and reimbursement. A unanimous vote supporting eligibility for reimbursement for certified NPs and CNMs went from the committee to both houses, where it passed without debate.

This exemplar emphasizes how marketing a service effectively depends on making others aware of its unique features. It is helpful to gather data on how clients discovered a service so that future energy and resources can be channeled into what is known to be successful. Brochures, articles in the newspaper, newsletters, letterhead stationery, business cards, flyers, personal interviews with the media, and group community classes all help promote a unique service. Yellow Pages advertising is expensive, so it is wise to routinely audit how often clients use the publication to initiate contact. Groups such as Rotary, American Association of Retired Persons, American Association of University Women, Junior League, and Kiwanis often invite speakers to address health topics. These opportunities allow the APN not only to promote a service but also to dispel misinformation about APNs and clarify their role. Joining professional and civic organizations is an important part of marketing a service as well, and the opportunity to sit on a board of directors or a health-related committee does much to enhance one's professional reputation (Box 21-10). To help APN students think about marketing their services, some faculty have students develop a personal website that can be used for creative marketing, employment searching, and patient education purposes (C. Hanson, personal communication, September, 2003). Lastly, with whatever marketing is done the APN must make sure that it is HIPAA compliant. For example, if mothers who have given birth are sent invitations to attend a patent education session on caring for the toddler, the APN must make sure that only those mothers who have given consent are contacted. If a patient gave birth and was keeping it secret, an invitation opened by a family member would violate both her privacy and HIPAA rules (Advisory Publications, 2002).

BOX 21-9 • MARKETING EFFORTS FOR HOLISTIC OB-GYN PRACTICE

Marketing the concept to the bank for start-up costs
The business plan included detailed data based on experience as well as income projections.
Marketing to the community
1. Other providers
   - Contracts with three gynecologists to provide backup care on an urgent basis
   - Community letters and meetings with internists and gynecologists about the niche our service provided to help women with complex midlife needs or hormone therapy that was not working
   - Meetings with a community breast surgeon, oncologist, and nurse practitioners about complex menopausal symptom relief for women who could not take estrogen
2. Potential women clients
   - Open houses highlighting the services of the center
   - Day-long workshops presented by the team about midlife issues. Topics included
     —Osteoporosis: Reframing Your Frame
     —Heart Disease: Finding Your Heart's Desire
     —Mental Clarity: Mysteries of the Menopausal Mind
     —The Joy of Soy: Cooking with Soy Made Easy
   - Free monthly menopause support group supported by the American Menopause Foundation, which helped market to area media
   - Multiple community education workshops and lectures to YWCA, women in business, insurance executives
   - Lunch meetings and tours through center
   - Newspaper stories featuring third-party reimbursement hassles for an APN practice
   - Newspaper columns about women's health
   - Newspaper advertisement
   - Promotional fact sheet about center
3. Other APNs who wanted to start similar practices
   - Reprints about the practice
   - Panel discussions with slide show at state APN meetings
   - Meetings, tours, and opportunities for shadowing in the practice (professional fee charged for time spent with us)
   - Lectures to the university NP programs in the city
   - Preceptor to one APN graduate student each semester

BOX 21-10 • STRATEGIES FOR MARKETING APN SERVICES

Advertise in local phone book
Direct mail to specific groups (teens, housing complex for the elderly)
Distribute flyers with services provided, philosophy and credentials
Mail patient birthday cards
Mail reminder cards for heath promotion examinations or call ahead
Distribute useful materials with your name or practice's name and contact numbers
Provide free Pap smears on occasion for an underserved population
Offer to teach sex education classes for community or local schools
Ask your patients to refer family and friends
Establish collaborative relationships with other health-care providers in the area
Establish hours that meet patient needs, such as evening and weekends
Distribute business cards and practice brochures generously in the community (grocery store, fitness club, alternative health-care businesses)
Donate a day for specialty consultation in areas that are hard to manage in primary care
Send a generalized brochure about your practice by bulk mail to a targeted zip code
Network with local businesses and banks; join the local chamber of commerce

Marketing to Physicians, Consumers, and Others

Presenting oneself to the medical community is an important marketing strategy in promoting a service. During the process of business plan development, an APN has opportunities to meet with physician colleagues and begin building relationships that can lead to referrals. Having self-confidence about one's skills, knowing one's particular areas of expertise and limitations, and having a collaborative approach are important. Establishing credibility with regard to one's competency and abilities is essential. Successful APN-physician collaboration, including those interactions that lead to positive patient outcomes, helps alleviate such fears (see Chapter 10). When one is outlining possible benefits to physicians for including an APN in their referral network, it is important to stress the APN's unique areas of expertise: prevention, counseling, education, and the ability to see patients with special, time-consuming needs.

The office staff has a role in helping APNs in this process by having a thorough understanding of the APN's uniqueness and skills and sharing that knowledge with the public. APNs and staff should be able to describe the aspects of APN care that are different from and complementary to other providers' services.

When APNs deal with pharmaceutical representatives, it is important to educate them about the differences between what an APN does and what a physician does. Representatives should be asked to have APNs included as providers in their patient-oriented product brochures. To constantly see the word "doctor," such as "see your doctor with any questions," sends a distinct message to potential clients, health policy decision makers, and legislators (Smithing & Wiley, 1990). Finally, a critically important endorsement for the nursing profession is for the APN to be sure to use an APN for personal as well as for family care.

Avoiding Common Marketing Mistakes

In 1989, Weill and colleagues projected that the biggest obstacle to future viability of the APN's role was lack of consumer awareness and minimal demand for preventive services as a result of inadequate marketing by APNs. Today, we are experiencing a greater demand for preventive services, and yet a lack of consumer awareness about the APN role remains. An understanding of this notion, a strong belief in oneself and in the APN role, and a strong understanding of one's own APN philosophy are critical to reversing this trend and enhancing the return on the time and energy invested in marketing. When marketing a service, APNs should strive to avoid the common marketing mistakes noted by Abraham (1994) by doing the following on a regular basis:

1. Audit clients and others to find which particular strategies provide the best return (Calmelat, 1993).
2. Continuously ascertain needs for unique services and develop them.
3. Differentiate APN practice from that offered by the competition.
4. Always give clients a reason to return for repeat services.
5. Address clients' needs as a priority.
6. Educate and inform clients about any changes made in the practice, such as an increase in prices.
7. Maintain enjoyment in providing the service in order to avoid burnout.

APNs can learn from other professionals' experiences with marketing mistakes. A casebook of scenarios of marketing mistakes, successes, analyses, and practical tips are presented by Hartely (2000).

CONCLUSION

Buppert (1999) summarized some general principles of marketing a practice that APNs need to consider. To educate consumers about APNs and engage their interest in APN services, APNs must do the following:

- Repeat the marketing message over and over in order to be heard.
- Create in clients a sense of affiliation with the practice.
- Create an image of the practice and a marketing message.
- Strive to exceed the expectations of clients (they not only will stay with the practice but will share their perceptions with others and encourage them to seek APN services) and
- Remember that a new patient is worth the price of the visit, whereas a patient who values and stays with the practice is likely to generate more revenue.

Marketing oneself and one's services is critical to the survival of APNs and might well influence the future of the nursing profession itself. As the health-care environment changes, clients are becoming sophisticated about what they want as well as about what they need. APNs must become familiar enough with marketing concepts and be flexible enough so that they can position themselves to meet client needs. As a result of successful marketing strategies, clients will specifically request APNs, and they will demand their services, recognizing the value they provide in the ever-expanding and complex world of health care.

In his book *Not What the Doctor Ordered: How to End the Medical Monopoly in Pursuit of Managed Care*, Dr. Jeffery Bauer (1998) underscored the reason APNs need to market their services effectively and successfully. He wrote, "I do not argue that nurses should replace primary care physicians, merely that advanced practice nurses provide a desirable competitive alternative and a different approach to basic healthcare. This point is important to the future of our nation's health" (p. 103).

REFERENCES

Abraham, J. (1994). *The Abraham experience*. Rolling Hills Estates, CA: Citation Publishing Group, Inc.

Advisory Publications. (2002). Make sure your marketing is HIPAA compliant. *Financial Management Strategies, 1,* 5-6. Retrieved May 29, 2003, from http://www.medscape.com/viewarticle/446400

American Medical Association Board of Trustees. (1995). *Model guidelines for physician and nurse practitioner integrated practice* (Report 6-A-95). Chicago: AMA.

American Medical Association. (1996, January 17). *Statement on ethical concerns regarding managed care physician gag* [AMA press release]. Retrieved May 28, 2003 from http://www.ebglaw.com/article_330.html

American Nurses Association (2001). *Nursing's agenda for the future*. Retrieved May 26, 2004, from http://nursingworld.org/naf/

Baldwin, C. (1998). *Calling the circle*. New York: Bantam Books.

Bauer, J. (1998). *Not what the doctor ordered: How to end the medical monopoly in pursuit of managed care* (2nd ed.). New York: McGraw-Hill.

Bissinger, R. L., Allred, C. A., Arford, P. H., & Bellig, L. L. (1997). A cost-effectiveness analysis of neonatal nurse practitioners. *Nursing Economics, 15,* 92-99.

Bolles, R. N. (2002). *What color is your parachute?* Walnut Creek, CA: Ten Speed Press.

Brandenburger, A. M., & Nalebuff, B. J. (1996). *Co-Opetition*. New York: Doubleday.

Brooten, D., Naylor, M. D., York, R., Brown, L. P., Munro, B. H., Hollingsworth, A. O., et al. (2002). Lessons learned from testing the Quality Cost Model of Advanced Practice Nursing (APN) Transitional Care. *Journal of Nursing Scholarship, 34,* 369-375.

Brown, M., & Olshansky, E. (1998). Becoming a primary care nurse practitioner: Challenges of the initial year of practice. *Nurse Practitioner, 23,* 46, 52-66.

Brown, S. A., & Grimes, D. E. (1995). A meta analysis of nurse practitioners and nurse midwives in primary care. *Nursing Research, 44,* 332-339.

Brunk, Q. (1992). The clinical nurse specialist as an external consultant: A framework for practice. *Clinical Nurse Specialist, 6,* 2-4.

Buchanan, L. (1997). The acute care nurse practitioner in collaborative practice. *Journal of the American Academy of Nurse Practitioners, 8,* 13-20.

Buerhaus, P. I. (2000). A conversation with Robert Blendon about public opinion and health care, nursing and the 2000 presidential election. *Nursing Outlook, 48,* 203-210.

Buppert, C. (1999). *Nurse practitioner's business practice & legal guide*. Gaithersburg, MD: Aspen Publishers.

Buppert, C. (2001). *Agreeing not to compete. The green sheet, 3*(7). Retrieved May 29, 2003, from http://www.medscape.com/viewarticle/407075

Buresh B. (1998, Spring). Healthcare forms new media partnership—nursing must participate. *Revolution— The Journal of Nurse Empowerment, 8,* 68-75.

Burgess, S. E., & Misener, T. R. (1997). The professional portfolio: An advanced practice nurse job search marketing tool. *Clinical Excellence for Nurse Practitioners, 1,* 468-471.

Calmelat, A. (1993). Tips for starting your own nurse practitioner practice. *Nurse Practitioner, 18,* 58, 61, 64, 67-68.

Chang, C. F., Pfoutz, S. K., & Price, S. A. (2001). *Economics and nursing: Critical Professional Issues*. Philadelphia: F.A. Davis.

Christianson, C. M., Bohmer, R., & Kenagy, J. (2000, Sept-Oct). Will disruptive innovations cure health care? *Harvard Business Review, 78,* 103-111.

Coile, R. C. (1999). The three C's: Consumerism, cyberhealth, and co-opetition. In R. Gilkey (Ed.), *The 21st century health care leader* (pp. 3-21). San Francisco: Jossey-Bass.

Corser, W. D. (2000). The contemporary nurse-physician relationship: Insights from scholars outside the two professions. *Nursing Outlook, 48,* 263-268.

Covello, J., & Hazelgren, B. (1995). *Your first business plan*. Naperville, IL: Sourcebooks, Inc.

Diamond, F. (2000, August). Nurse practitioners inch onto the field. *Managed Care, 9,* 24-30.

Doughty, S. (1989). The CNS in a nurse managed center. In A. Hamric & J. Spross (Eds.), *The clinical nurse specialist in theory and practice* (pp. 415-434). Philadelphia: W. B. Saunders.

Doughty, S., & Keller, J. M. (2000). Marketing and contracting considerations. In A. B. Hamric, J. A. Spross, & C. M. Hanson (Eds), *Advanced nursing practice*: An integrative approach (2nd ed., pp. 655-677). Philadelphia: W. B. Saunders.

Druss, B. G., Marcus, S. C., Olfson, M., Tanielian, T., & Pincus, H. A. (2003). Trends in care by non-physician clinicians in the United States. *New England Journal of Medicine, 348,* 130-137.

Fiel, B. (1998). *'Gag clauses' banned in federal health plans*. Retrieved May 28, 2003 from http://www.govexec.com/dailyfed/0898/081198b3.htm

Fitzgerald, M. A. (1999). Negotiating your future: Employment, contract and practice issues for the nurse practitioner. *Clinical Letter for Nurse Practitioners, 3,* 1-11.

Gardner, K., & Weinrauch, D. (1988). Marketing strategies for nurse entrepreneurs. *Nurse Practitioner, 13,* 46, 48-49.

Haag, A. B. (1997). Writing a successful business plan. *AAOHN Journal, 45,* 25-32.

Hallums, A. (1994). Internal marketing within a health care organization: Developing an implementation plan. *Journal of Nursing Management, 2,* 135-142.

Hanson, C. M. (2002). Nurse practitioner entrepreneurs bring care to coastal Georgia. *Nurse Practitioner World News, 7,* 1, 3, 10-11.

Hartely, R. F. (2000). *Marketing mistakes and successes*. Indianapolis, IN: Wiley Publishing.

Hayes, E., Allen, J., Gruen, S., Wilson, J., & Kalmakis, K. (2001). Nurse practitioner practice patterns, compensation, and professional participation: Western Massachusetts. *Clinical Excellence for Nurse Practitioners, 5,* 52-60.

Herman, R., & Zeil, S. (1999). Collaborative practice agreements for advanced practice nurses: What you should know. *AACN Clinical Issues: Advanced Practice in Acute and Critical Care, 10,* 337-342.

Johnson and Johnson. (2002). *Knowledge gap about opportunities for nurses contributing to escalating nursing shortage*. Retrieved May 18, 2003, from http://www.jnj.com/news/jnj_news/20020506_0949.htm

Kalisch, P. A., & Kalisch, B. J. (1981). Communicating clinical nursing issues through the newspaper. *Nursing Research, 30,* 132-138.

Kassirer, J. P. (1994). What role for nurse practitioners in primary care? *New England Journal of Medicine, 330,* 204-205.

Kendig, S. M. (2001). Every woman deserves an NP: Getting your message across. *Women's Health Care, 1,* 29-32.

Letz, K. K. (2002). *Business essentials for nurse practitioners*. Fort Wayne, IN: PreviCare, Inc.

Lindeke, L. L., Bly, T. R., & Wilcon, R. A. (2001). Perceived barriers to rural nurse practitioner practice. *Clinical Excellence for Nurse Practitioners, 5,* 218-221.

Miller, S. K. (2000). Marketing your practice. *Patient Care for Nurse Practitioners, 3,* 52-53.

Miller, S. K. (2001). What's in a name? *Patient Care for Nurse Practitioners, 4,* 44.

Moody, N. B., Smith, P. L., & Glenn, L. L. (1999). Client characteristics and practice patterns of nurse practitioners and physicians. *Nurse Practitioner, 24,* 94-103.

Munden, J. (Ed). (2001). *Nurse practitioner's legal reference*. Springhouse, PA: Springhouse.

Mundinger, M., Kane, R. L., Lenz, E. R., Totten, A., Tsai, W., Cleary, P. D., et al. (2000). Primary care outcomes in patients treated by nurse practitioners or physicians. *Journal of the American Medical Association, 283,* 59-69.

Office of Technology Assessment. (1986). *Health technology case study 37: Nurse practitioners, physician assistants, and certified nurse midwives: A policy analysis* (Publication OTA-HCS-37). Washington, DC: Government Printing Office.

Pakis, S. (1997). Managing the marketing function for advanced nurse practitioners in a managed care environment. *Seminars for Nurse Managers, 5,* 149-153.

Payne, M. E. (1997, July/August). Counselling new graduates to find jobs. *Recruitment, Retention & Restructuring Report, 10*, 4-7.

Rekevics, C., Harte, S., Meyer, K., Shively, M., & Ebersole-Kauffman, D. (1999). Patient satisfaction with nurse practitioners. *1998/99 APN Sourcebook*, 14-16.

Restifo, V. (1999, February 8). Your professional portfolio. *Nursing Spectrum, 3*, 17.

Robbins, S. (1998). *Organizational behavior* (8th ed.). Englewood Cliffs, NJ: Prentice-Hall.

Robert Wood Johnson Foundation. (2003). *Partnerships for training*. Washington, DC: American Association of Academic Health Centers. Retrieved May 3, 2004, from http:// www.pftweb.org

Romaine-Davis, A. (1997). *Advanced practice nursing. Education, roles, trends*. Sudbury, MA: Jones and Bartlett.

Safriet, B. J. (1992). Health care dollars and regulatory sense: The role of advanced practice nursing. *Yale Journal on Regulation, 9*, 417-487.

Scanland, S. (1990). What's happening: The nurse teaches the doc. *Journal of the American Academy of Nurse Practitioners, 2*, 174-177.

Shaw, C. (2002). What can you learn from Coca-Cola? *Nursing Spectrum, 11*, 12.

Smithing, R. T., & Wiley, M. D. (1990). Marketing and management. See your physician. *Journal of the American Academy of Nurse Practitioners, 2*, 38.

Stern, M. (1997). *Marketing for small business*. Retrieved May 26, 2004, from http:/www.digitalstore.com/ marketing/mstern/ trad_mktg.html

Washington Consulting Group. (1994). *Survey of certified nurse practitioners and clinical nurse specialists: December 1992*. Rockville, MD: Division of Nursing, Health Resources and Services Administration.

Weill, J. A., Love, M. G., Pron, A. L., Tesoro, T. A., Grey, M., Hickel, M., et al. (1989). Future potential, phase I: Nurse practitioners look at themselves. *Journal of Pediatric Health Care, 3*, 76-82.

Wyatt, D. (1999, January). Negotiation strategies for men and women. *Nursing Management, 30*, 22-25.

Zaumeyer, C. R. (2003). How to start an independent practice. Philadelphia: F. A. Davis.

Additional Readings

Ball, G. B. (1990). Perspectives on developing, marketing, and implementing a new clinical specialist position. *Clinical Nurse Specialist, 4*, 33-36.

Boccuzzi, N. K. (1998). CAPNA: A new development to increase quality in primary care. *Nursing Administration Quarterly, 22*, 11-19.

Buppert, C. (1999, February 8). Malpractice insurance: To have or to have not? *Nursing Spectrum (New England Edition), 3*, 13-14.

Cawley, J. F. (1998). Whither independence? *Clinician News, 2*, 40.

Crow, G. (1998). The entrepreneurial personality: Building a sustainable future for self and the profession. *Nursing Administration Quarterly, 22*, 30-35.

Curtin, L. (1993). Barbarians at the gate. *Nursing Management, 24*, 9-10.

Gelman, E. (1999, January 5). Be prepared—with a master's degree [editorial]. *Patient Care for the Nurse Practitioner, 2*, 5.

Giordano, B. P. (1994). Watch out for "friendly fire" from our medical allies! *AORN Journal, 59*, 360, 362.

Hau, M. L. (1997). Ten common mistakes to avoid as an independent consultant. *AAOHN Journal, 45*, 17-22.

Henry, P. F. (1996). Analysis of the nurse practitioner's legal relationships. *Nurse Practitioner Forum, 7*, 5-6.

Hodges, L. C., Satkowski, T. C., & Ganchorre, C. (1998). Career opportunities for doctoral-prepared nurses. *MEDSURG Nursing, 7*, 114-120.

Kowal, N. (1998). Specialty practice entrepreneur: The advanced practice nurse. *Nursing Economics, 16*, 277-278.

Leccese, C. (1998, January). Who's making what—and where? *Advance for Nurse Practitioners, 6*, 30-35.

Levin, T. E. (1993). The solo nurse practitioner: A private practice model. *Nurse Practitioner Forum, 4*, 158-164.

MacDonahue, D. (1997). Interviewing hints. *Massachusetts Nurse, 67, 9*, 14.

Manthey, M., & Avery, M. D. (1996). Remembering the nurse in the business of advanced practice. *Advanced Practice Nursing Quarterly, 2*, 49-54.

Monahan, B. B. (1996). The nurses' media handbook: A reference for nurses planning to meet the media . . . first in a two part series. *Massachusetts Nurse, 66, 2, 6*, 12.

Niederlitz, P. (1997). Laid off? What's next? The job search process. *AORN Journal, 66*, 502-503.

Pearson, L. J. (1999). Stands on legislative issues affecting advanced nursing practice. *Nurse Practitioner, 24*, 18–24.

Porter-O'Grady, T. (1998). The private practice of nursing: The gift of entrepreneurialism. *Nursing Administration Quarterly, 22*, 23-29.

Price, J. L. (1998). A reflective approach to career trajectory in advanced practice nursing. *Advanced Practice Nursing Quarterly, 3*, 35-39.

Price, S. A., & Frank-Lightfoot, L. (2001). Evolving roles and professional practice models for nursing. In C. F. Chang, S. A. Price, & S. K. Pfoutz (Eds), *Economics and nursing. Critical professional issues* (pp. 243-273). Philadelphia: F.A. Davis.

Scarano, R. M. (1998). PA/NP practice and contract law: Avoiding pitfalls of managed care. *Clinician Reviews, 2*, 33.

Schaffner, R. J., & Bohomey, J. (1998). Demonstrating APN value in a capitated market. *Nursing Economics, 16*, 69-74.

Schneider, B. (1997). Have you thought of entering business as an entrepreneur or intrapreneur, a satisfying alternative career in nursing? *Washington Nurse, 27*, 45.

Sebas, M. B. (1994). Developing a collaborative practice agreement for the primary care setting. *Nurse Practitioner, 19*, 49-51.

Selph, A. K. (1998). Negotiating an acute care nurse practitioner position. *AACN Clinical Issues, 9,* 269-276.

Shepard, P. M. (1997). Medicine and the Internet. *Clinician News, 1,* 12, 14-15.

Sherrod, D. R. (1997). Advising nursing students in a tightened job market. *Journal of Nursing Education, 36,* 344-346.

Simpson, R. L. (1998). From nursing to nursing informatics consultant: A lesson in entrepreneurship. *Nursing Administration Quarterly, 22,* 87-90.

Sloan, A. J. (1995). Employment contracts—who needs them? (Parts I and II). *Virginia Nurses Today, 3*(4), 28, 30; *3*(5), 20-21.

Smithing, R. T., & Wiley, M. D. (1990). Marketing and management. Marketing techniques in person. *Journal of the American Academy of Nurse Practitioners, 2,* 88–89.

Steiger, N., Hagenstad, R., & Anderson, A. (1996). Budget development and implementation for the APN in independent practice. *Advanced Practice Nursing Quarterly, 2,* 41-48.

Straka, D. A. (1996). Are you your resume? *Advanced Practice Nursing Quarterly, 2,* 75–77.

Thomas, B. (1997). A successful job search begins with a realistic resume and a positive approach to the market. *AORN Journal, 66,* 702-703.

Waldrop, J. B. (1999, April). Getting the word out. *The Clinical Advisor, 2,* 84.

Ward, R. (1998). Public relations for advanced practice nurses. *AWHONN Lifelines, 2,* 47-48.

Waxman, K. T. (1998, August). Marketing your skills outside the hospital walls. *Nursing Management, 29,* 48-51.

White, K. R., & Begun, J. W. (1998). Nursing entrepreneurship in an era of chaos and complexity. *Nursing Administration Quarterly, 22,* 40-47.

Woomer, S. (1994). Negotiating an employment contract. *The Clinician's Reference Guide 1994* (a supplement to *Clinician Reviews*), *4*(Suppl), 21-28.

CHAPTER 22

Understanding Regulatory, Legal, and Credentialing Requirements

CHARLENE M. HANSON

INTRODUCTION

Impressive strides have been made over time in the areas of credentialing and regulation of advanced practice nurses (APNs). The health care provided by APNs has had far-reaching effects on members of society, and thus the evolution of advanced practice nursing in the United States is a source of pride to nurses. However, with success comes ever higher accountability and the need for more standardized ways to credential, certify, regulate, and sanction competent practice for a growing number of APNs. At both federal and state levels, this is a time of shifting priorities and changing models for nursing practice in all settings. Advanced practice nurses are meeting regularly in national forums to discuss evolving roles and to conceptualize new dimensions for practice (see Chapters 2 and 19). It is an environment in which any discussion of regulatory issues is, by definition, fluid, dynamic, and subject to rapid change. APNs must influence health policy at both national and grass-roots levels to ensure regulatory configurations that allow for successful advanced nursing practice and reimbursement. This activity may be as simple as interpreting health policy decisions to patients and co-workers locally, or as complex as negotiating equitable regulatory decisions about reimbursement with the Centers for Medicare and Medicaid Services (CMS) in Washington, DC.

Mary Wakefield, a noted nurse policymaker, stated:

We don't have Florence Nightingale to share with us a vision of exactly what the solutions might be to unburden us and the people for whom we care. Nevertheless, we know that in very difficult times, she exerted influence at both the bedside and in the halls of statesmen to craft solutions to the problems of her day. Her footprints are there. Will our organizations, through the work of each of us, follow them and in the process, leave new footprints behind? (Wakefield, 2002, p. 16)

The challenge to provide standards of quality upon which advanced practice nursing can be framed, defended, and regulated is a serious one that requires constant attention. Issues involving education, scope of practice, specialty practice, reimbursement, and prescriptive authority are all embedded in regulatory language. Regulatory issues are governed by multiple federal, state, educational, and professional entities whose work occurs in different venues, and these differences complicate efforts to collaborate (Hanson, 1998). The complexity of regulatory issues and the multiplicity of stakeholders are the bases for the 1998 recommendations by the Pew Health Professions Commission that national policy initiatives are urgently needed to research, develop, and publish national scopes of practice and continuing competency standards for state legislatures to implement (O'Neil & the Pew Health Professions Commission, 1998). This work continues to be vitally important and requires regular and careful input from APNs.

This chapter describes basic national and state credentialing and regulatory realities and provides a discussion of the critical elements of health policy and regulation that currently affect APNs. (Chapter 23 deals with major health policy issues confronting healthcare providers and consumers nationally.) For specific questions about up-to-the-minute, current APN rules and regulations—especially those that pertain to specific state statutes regarding licensing of APNs, prescriptive authority, and reimbursement—the reader should refer to individual local and state regulatory bodies for practice requirements.

The skills required for successful policy activism and advocacy, which are crucial to negotiating regulatory mechanisms, are part of the advanced practice nursing core competency of clinical and professional leadership. The concepts and skills outlined in Chapters 9 and 10 are crucial to the role APNs play in setting credentialing and regulation policy mechanisms and should be considered as this chapter is read.

CURRENT PRACTICE CLIMATE FOR APNs

During an era of global turbulence, recession, and unsettled health-care change, stakeholders must give serious and thoughtful consideration to the appropriate preparation and employment of APNs. The differences in education, certification, and individual scope of practice regulations from one advanced nursing specialty to another complicate issues for policymakers and regulators (Hanson & Hamric, 2003). The climate within nursing practice is greatly affected by what is happening in other health-care disciplines. For example, the move toward group practice and away from solo medical practice has implications for APNs (Rentmeester & Kindig, 1994; Deighton, 2003).The continued preference of physicians for speciality practice and away from primary care practice is important for APNs to consider. Within the nursing profession, serious shortages in bedside nurses and nursing faculty have profound implications for advanced practice nursing education and practice (American Nurses Association [ANA], 2002). Currently, the combined health-care needs of an aging population and a period of economic retrenchment in health care have fostered mixed trends for advanced nursing practice. Community-based health-care systems that rely on interdisciplinary health-care team approaches have positively benefited from APN specialties but in some instances have heightened tensions between the disciplines of medicine and nursing. In addition, recent issues around physician malpractice and tort reform directly affect APNs and require constant vigilance (Deighton, 2003). Health policy issues surrounding practice parameters, reimbursement, and choice of provider require careful exploration. All of these environmental phenomena have an impact, either directly or indirectly, on the credentialing and regulatory policies that govern advanced nursing practice. Nursing's earliest efforts to establish professional identity for APNs focused on advancing APN education as well as gaining independent authority for nursing practice and autonomy from the medical community. These efforts were critical to the evolution of advanced practice in nursing, and great strides have been made over the years (see Chapter 19). At the same time, complex health-care systems and patient population needs that require a multifaceted approach to multiple problems demand effective interdisciplinary team-building. "Parallel play," or working side by side, is not enough; a true blending of nursing and medical models to offer a comprehensive health-care approach is needed. Larger teams of health-care providers must collaborate fully to provide comprehensive care to families and whole communities. To be able to move forward as full-fledged team members in cooperation with other interdisciplinary health-care providers, APNs need to shift their practice ideal from one of complete autonomy to a truly collegial interdisciplinary paradigm. This change in practice stance is necessary and long overdue. Does any health-care professional, including the most renowned vascular surgeon, practice with full independence? Or does this surgeon call upon the internist, the clinical nurse specialist (CNS), and the physical therapist to assist with providing competent and expert care? Will APNs do themselves a disservice if they maintain an isolationist stance based on barriers and professional turf issues? Have APNs reached a point in their evolution at which they can feel comfortable as peers and colleagues with providers in other disciplines? These are all questions that APNs struggle to answer.

It is important to understand that when APNs seek to change statutes and regulations, it is not because they see themselves as needing to practice in a vacuum of independence apart from the rest of the health-care team. It is a hard fact that APNs must have authority over their own practices and the decisions they make about patient care. They must be able to defend their actions within the legal system based on nursing-driven standards and regulation. Only in this way can an APN move out of the darkness of being a "shadow provider" (Wilcox, 1995). Issues related to being a "shadow provider" are best exemplified by "incident to" billing by nurse practitioners (NPs) using the physician's Medicare number. Advanced practice nursing care is invisible to regulators and reimbursers with this type of billing procedure. This is an example of the challenges for APNs across the nation who are working to clarify statutory policies within state boards of nursing. It may be that APNs will feel comfortable only when their position within the health-care community is fully secure in all states, and this will require focused and coordinated political and legislative work related to credentialing and regulatory issues.

SCOPE OF PRACTICE FOR APNs

By definition, scope of practice describes practice limits and sets the parameters within which nurses in the various advanced practice nursing specialties may practice. Scope statements define what APNs can do for and with patients, what they can delegate, and when collaboration with others is required. Scope-of-practice statements tell APNs de facto what is beyond the limits of their nursing practice (Cady, 2003). The scope of practice for each advanced practice nursing specialty group is explicated in Chapters 12 through 18. Scope-of-practice statements are key to the debate about how the U.S. health-care system employs APNs as health-care providers; scope is inextricably linked with barriers to advanced practice nursing. The ability to diagnose disease and treat patients that is inherent to the role of the APN is fluid and evolving and is, in many instances, tied to the collaborative relationships that APNs have with physician colleagues. Certified registered nurse anesthetists (CRNAs), who administer general anesthesia, have a markedly different scope of practice from that of the primary care NP, for example, although both have their roots in basic nursing. In addition, it is important to understand that scope of practice differs from state to state and is based on state statutes promulgated by the various state nurse practice acts and the rules and regulations for APNs (Pearson, 2003). On the Internet, scope-of-practice statements can be found by searching state government Web pages in the areas of licensing boards, nursing, and advanced practice nursing rules and regulations or by visiting the National Council of State Boards of Nursing (NCSBN) site at www.NCSBN.org.

Accountability becomes a crucial factor as APNs move toward increasing authority over their own practices. First, it is important that scope-of-practice statements identify the scope of each advanced practice nursing role. Furthermore, it is crucial that scope-of-practice statements presented by national certifying entities are carried through in scope-of-practice language in state statutes. APNs must recognize that, because they live in a highly mobile society, their scope of practice will vary from state to state; and in a worst-case scenario, one can be an APN in one state but not meet the criteria in another state. This factor is discussed more fully later in this chapter in the section on telehealth and telepractice.

APNs owe Barbara Safriet, Associate Dean at Yale Law School, a debt of gratitude for her vision and clarity in helping APNs understand and think strategically about scope-of-practice and regulatory issues. In her landmark 1992 monograph, Safriet noted that APNs are unique in that there is a multiprofessional approach to their regulation based on ignorance and the fallacy that medicine is all-knowing, particularly about advanced nursing practice. Safriet (1992) reports that

States have used a variety of approaches to extend the scope of practice of nursing. Some have revised their Nurse Practice Acts (NPAs) to delete the absolute prohibition on diagnosis and treatment, or to add "nursing diagnosis." Some have added an "additional acts" clause to the NPA, authorizing some specially trained nurses to "perform acts of medical diagnosis and treatment" as specified by rules of the state nursing and/or medical boards or as "agreed upon by the professions of nursing and medicine." Some have added a generic category, or specific categories, of advanced practice nurses and have either defined their scope of practice or have authorized state nursing and/or medical boards to promulgate rules that do so. Some have revised their Medical Practice Acts (MPAs) to authorize physicians to "delegate" diagnosis and treatment tasks to nurses who have the necessary additional training." (pp. 445-446)

As her quote implies, restraints on advanced nursing practice result from ignorance about APNs' abilities, rigid notions about professional roles, and turf protection.

In a recent monograph, Safriet (2002), cites new reforms in scope of practice in Colorado and in Ontario, Canada, that are encouraging solutions to long time tensions over control of practice between organized medicine and nursing. In Colorado, the new provision defines practice authority in terms of ability and thus redirects the regulatory focus from providers' status to the APN's training and skills. The Regulated Heath Professions Act of Ontario, Canada, establishes a new regulatory framework for the health-care professions, making the professions accountable to the public. This shifts the regulatory focus from profession-centered regulation to public interest regulation. These examples offer hope that, in the future, policies can be formulated that will close the gap between what APNs can do and what they are allowed to do by scope-of-practice statutes.

LEGAL CONCERNS SURROUNDING APN TITLING

The ANA's definition of an APN requires that the role be clinically focused and that the APN give direct clinical care to patients (ANA, 1996). The definition developed in this text goes beyond this definition and is further explicated in Chapter 3. Currently, four established advanced practice nursing roles are generally recognized: NPs in primary and acute care, certified nurse-midwives (CNMs), CRNAs, and CNSs. In addition, emerging advanced practice nursing roles can be included in these groups (see Chapters 15, 18, and 19). From a legal and regulatory perspective, inclusion in the designation of what constitutes an APN is primarily driven by two factors: the ability of APNs to be directly reimbursed and the degree to which nurses desire prescriptive and admitting privileges. While this may seem restrictive to some, there must be a well-defined and efficacious way for state boards, insurers, prescribing entities, and the like to monitor the scope of practice, prescribing, and reimbursement patterns of APNs. There must be clear criteria that can be validated in order to ensure patient safety and to monitor proper certification and credentialing. Credentialing of APNs to ensure that they meet competency and safety standards that will protect the public has developed rather haphazardly. To try to impose some uniformity on credentialing and licensure of APNs, professional nursing organizations and the NCSBN have moved toward second licensure. Second licensure means that an APN must meet certain criteria established by a state board of nursing in order to receive an additional license or recognition and be authorized to practice at an advanced level of nursing. The notion of second licensure is unprecedented among the health professions but, given the various routes of entry into the nursing profession, seems the only way to ensure a minimum set of competencies or requirements. The issue of titling and second licensure is a "bread and butter" issue for all APNs, and they must pay attention to these issues to protect their ability to practice.

The issues surrounding the titling and credentialing of APNs have been difficult since the inception of the role. There is an ongoing dialogue between national certifying bodies and state regulators, as well as among agencies that accredit educational programs, to bring standardization to the multiple APN specialties. CRNA and CNM certification and credentialing are the most clearly uniform and standardized based on their longevity, singleness of purpose, and specialty. However, the issue of CNM education is at variance with advanced practice nursing standards (see Chapter 16). The credentialing and oversight of NPs and CNSs is less clear because of the multiplicity of programs and specialties and the continuing need to develop certification examinations in some areas (see Chapter 12). As new APN roles evolve the problems around credentialing become increasingly acute.

There are several reasons that the multiplicity of titles and roles for APNs is a problem from a policy viewpoint. The foremost reason is that it is confusing to policymakers and regulators, especially at agencies such as the CMS, where major designations for Medicare and Medicaid reimbursement set the standard for all reimbursement of APNs across the country. In addition, discrepancies in advanced practice nursing definition and licensing criteria among states make mobility difficult for APNs in terms of prescriptive authority and reimbursement. APNs are primarily responsible to and are disciplined by individual state boards of nursing. One of the licensing and credentialing difficulties faced by APNs is the variance in board regulations from state to state. In some states advanced nursing practice is governed only by the board of nursing; in others, it is jointly administered by the boards of nursing and medicine; and in still others, it is governed by the boards of nursing and pharmacy. In many states CNMs are answerable to nurse-midwifery boards that are attached to boards of medicine. CNSs who are not in prescribing roles may be regulated by the board of nursing with no additional sanctions. Although written prescriptive statements delegating medical acts to the APN that are approved by the board of medicine and must be co-signed by a physician preceptor are not as prevalent as they were in the 1980s, they are still the norm in some states, predominantly in the South. Currently, states that have delegated medical authority for APNs often require collaborative agreements for APNs who diagnose diseases, manage treatment, and prescribe medications for patients. As implied, collaborative agreements provide a written description of the professional relationship between an APN and a collaborating physician that defines the parameters by which the APN can perform delegated medical acts. (See further discussion later in this chapter and in Chapter 21 for a sample collaborative agreement).

STANDARDS OF PRACTICE AND STANDARDS OF CARE FOR APNs

Standards of practice for nursing are defined by the profession nationally and help to further explicate and delineate scope of practice. Standards are overarching, authoritative statements that the nursing profession uses to describe the responsibilities for which its members are accountable (ANA, 1996; ANA, 2003). APNs are held to both the standards of practice promulgated by the nursing profession and to standards of the various advanced practice nursing specialties. At both levels, standards of practice describe the basic competency levels for safe and competent practice (e.g., see Chapters 16 and 17 for the standards of practice for CNMs and CRNAs, respectively). Professional standards of practice match closely with the core competencies for APNs, outlined in Chapter 3, which undergird advanced practice nursing.

Standards of care differ from the standards of practice set forth by the nursing profession described previously. These standards are often termed *practice guidelines*. Practice guidelines provide a foundation by which health-care providers administer care to patients. These guidelines crosscut the health professions disciplines and are the frameworks or standards by which basic safety and competent care are measured. For APNs this means that the standard used to evaluate advanced practice is often the same as the standard used to review medical practice. Standards of care are derived from evidence-based practice and are continuously evolving. The Agency for Healthcare Research and Quality (formerly the Agency for Health Care Policy and Research), at the federal policy level, has responsibility for conducting the research needed to evaluate clinical practice guidelines that define a standard of appropriate care in some specific areas (Buppert, 1999; Agency for Healthcare Research and Quality, 2004). The Centers for Disease Control and Prevention and many professional medical and nursing specialty organizations promulgate guidelines for practice. It is very important that APNs be part of interdisciplinary teams that develop and test practice guidelines for care. The ability of APNs to download cutting-edge practice guidelines onto handheld personal digital assistants for use in clinical settings is a major step toward competent and safe practice.

COMPONENTS OF APN CREDENTIALING AND REGULATION

Several definitions and concepts are central to the discussion of credentialing and regulation of APNs in the United States. As APNs become more mobile across state and international boundaries and as communications allow for increased interaction, it is important that credentialing and regulatory parameters be well understood.

Credentialing is an umbrella term that refers to the regulatory mechanisms that can be applied to individuals, programs, or organizations (Styles, 1998). Credentialing can be defined as "getting your ducks in a row" for the purpose of meeting standards, protecting the public, and improving quality. For the purposes of this text, credentialing (as it relates to APNs) is defined as follows: *Credentialing is furnishing the documentation that one is authorized by a regulatory body to engage in certain activities and to use a certain title. Credentialing in health care is used to assure the public that the individual meets proposed standards and is prepared to perform the duties implied by the credential.* As an example, for the individual APN, credentialing may include, but is not limited to, the following:

- Graduation from an approved graduate nursing program
- Attainment of national certification
- State licensure/recognition as a registered nurse (RN) and APN
- Collaborative practice agreement with a physician
- Approval as a nurse prescriber
- Medicare/Medicaid provider numbers
- Approval of hospital privileges

For a graduate nursing program preparing APNs, credentialing may include accreditation by the Commission on Collegiate Nursing Education (CCNE) or the National League for Nursing Accreditation Center (NLNAC); regional and state university boards and commissions; or groups such as the American College of Nurse-Midwives or the American Association of Nurse Anesthetists (Faut-Callahan & Caulk, 1998). For an institution, credentialing may include adhering to Joint Commission on Accreditation of Healthcare Organizations (JCAHO) or Occupational Safety and Health Administration (OSHA) guidelines.

Credentialing may be mandatory, as in state licensure, or voluntary, as with some national certification processes. In some instances, bodies that regulate APNs to ensure public safety may recognize voluntary credentialing bodies, such as national nursing certification organizations, as a part of the mandatory state credentialing mechanism.

APN program accreditation and approval, scope of practice, standards of practice, practice guidelines, and collaborative practice agreements all have important implications for APNs in terms of proper credentialing and interactions with the court system. These documents create the standard by which advanced practice nursing is monitored and regulated and deemed safe or unsafe and by which APNs are disciplined from state to state. The components of advanced practice nursing education and practice are described in the following sections.

Master's Education

The first criterion that the new APN must meet is successful graduation from an approved APN program. Over time, most educational programs have moved their curricula to the graduate nursing level. For example, the year 2007 is the projected time by which all NPs who use the title *APN* are to be prepared in master's of nursing programs (Buppert, 1999). In many states, both eligibility to sit for national certification and the ability to obtain advanced practice nursing licensure or recognition by the state require a transcript showing successful completion of a master's degree from an approved university in the designated nursing specialty. This is rapidly becoming the norm for APN licensure or recognition in all states, with the exception of credentialing for midwifery.

APN PROGRAM ACCREDITATION

Graduate programs in nursing and related fields that prepare APNs must be accredited as educationally sound, with appropriate content for the specialty and adequate clinical hours of supervised experience. As noted, the National League for Nursing Accreditation Center and the Commission on Collegiate Nursing Education accredit graduate programs in the nursing major (Commission on Collegiate Nursing Education, 1998). The accreditation process provides an overall evaluation of the graduate program for the most part but currently does not deal with the specifics of approval of specialty advanced practice nursing content. Oversight of specialty education for APNs occurs with the use of several different models. The clearest models are those administered by The American College of Nurse-Midwives and the American Association of Nurse Anesthetists, which oversee and review CNM and CRNA educational programs, most but not all of which are graduate programs. These bodies provide a process to review and regulate CRNA and CNM programs across the country that is separate from but feeds into the overall graduate nursing accreditation process.

The review and monitoring of NP education at the specialty level is much more complex because of the multiplicity of specialties. The National Organization of Nurse Practitioner Faculties (NONPF), the National Certification Board of Pediatric Nurse Practitioners and Nurses (NCBPNP/N), and other like bodies provide curriculum guidelines, program standards, and competencies to assist NP programs with curriculum planning and monitoring of programs of study. The most clearly established review processes for NP programs are those administered by the NCBPNP/N, which approves pediatric NP programs, and the National Association of Women's Health, which accredits women's health programs (Association of Women's Health, Obstetric, Neonatal Nurses & the National Association of Nurse Practitioners in Reproductive Health, 1996). In 1997, the National Task Force on Quality Nurse Practitioner Education established national criteria by which to monitor and evaluate NP programs according to broad-based criteria in six overarching areas (Box 22-1). In 2002, The National Task Force Guidelines for Quality NP education were updated and revised. They are available on the NONPF website at www.NONPF.com.

BOX 22-1 • NATIONAL TASK FORCE CRITERIA FOR NURSE PRACTITIONER PROGRAM EVALUATION

Criterion I—Organization and administration nurse practitioner programs
　Institutional support
Criterion II—Students
　Student admission and progression
Criterion III—Curriculum
　Content areas, competencies, basic course work
Criterion IV—Resources, facilities, and services
　Physical resources, clinical site and preceptorship resources
Criterion V—Faculty and faculty organization
　Faculty preparation, credentialing, and clinical practice
Criterion VI—Evaluation
　Program, students, faculty, clinical sites

Data from the National Task Force on Quality Nurse Practitioner Education (2002).

The National Task Force Criteria for Evaluation of Nurse Practitioner Programs (1997, 2002) were developed and endorsed by a consortium of NP education and practice associations, NP regulators, and NP national certifiers and accreditors. These criteria, in conjunction with the American Association of Colleges of Nursing's (AACN's) *Essentials of Master's Education for Advanced Practice Nursing* (1995), which define graduate nursing core and advanced practice nursing core (pathophysiology, physical assessment, and pharmacology) curriculum requirements provide the needed structure and guidance for NP nursing education. From the late 1990s to the present, good progress has been made by NP educators to bring the multiplicity of NP educational programs into a standardized approval process for NP education (CCNE, 2004; National Association of Neonatal Nurses, 1995; NONPF, 1995, 2002).

CNS education is fully embedded within the nursing paradigm. The CNS community is working toward clear structure and progression of CNS specialty education to ensure compliance with credentialing and regulation as advanced practice nursing providers (NACNS, 2003a, 2003b). Currently, there is strong momentum among nursing accreditors, advanced practice nursing certifiers, and advanced practice nursing specialty organizations such as the NONPF and NACNS to better align the overarching accreditation process (NACNS, 2004). Furthermore, certifying agencies review programs, to some degree, to sanction eligibility for advanced practice nursing graduates to sit for national advanced practice nursing certification exams, but many educators feel that this process comes too late. There is a need to be proactive and oversee program appropriateness and strength before students graduate and are ready for credentialing. Given the increased numbers of advanced practice nursing programs in a variety of nursing specialties, the work being done to standardize education for APNs is of major importance. The proposed standardization of the approval process for NP educational programs provides one example that would greatly assist state boards of nursing in their role of recognizing and regulating APNs for practice (Hanson & Hamric, 2003). The use of grandfathering mechanisms to protect APNs during transition periods of standardization provides leeway for positive change to occur.

POSTGRADUATE EDUCATION

The number of postgraduate advanced practice nursing programs targeted to students who have already attained a graduate degree in nursing but who wish to become APNs or want to work in a different advanced practice nursing role markedly increased in the late 1990s but has leveled off more recently (AACN & NONPF, 1999; Berlin, Stennett, & Bednash, 2003b; NONPF, 1996). Post-master's advanced practice nursing education is often tailored to meet the individual needs of post-master's students. Standardization of post-master's APN programs is needed because many of these programs, depending on the specialty, currently do not fall within the purview of formal graduate nursing accreditation. Additional education to meet requirements of a new specialty needs to be met from both a didactic and a clinical standpoint regardless of educational programs. It is important that master's-prepared nurses who aspire to do post-master's work to acquire a new or additional advanced practice nursing credential identify programs that offer curricula that meet the standards of eligibility for national certification and state licensure for the particular APN role they seek to attain.

DUAL AND BLENDED ROLE EDUCATION

New configurations of programs and tracks for specialty APNs that are dual or blended (see Chapters 3 and 15 for clarification of these roles) are widespread (Berlin, Stennett, & Bednash, 2003a). These programs require careful consideration of content and clinical experiences to ensure mastery of basic advanced practice nursing competencies and clinical experiences in both specialty areas. Dual and blended advanced practice nursing programs are by necessity longer and require more clinical experiences. New certification examinations and program review processes are being developed to meet the quality assurance and regulatory needs of these new specialties. Many APNs are dually prepared and thus should sit for more than one national certification. Today's complex health-care system makes this a viable option for many APNs who are functioning in diverse settings.

National task forces at the NONPF and the AACN are exploring whether a clinical or practice doctorate should be a new level of APN nursing (Mundinger et al., 2000; NONPF Task Force, 2004). At this point it is premature to say what the outcome will be, but this issue bears careful watching.

State Licensure/Recognition

Individual state nurse practice acts define the practice of nursing for RNs throughout the 50 states. State laws overseeing advanced nursing practice are divided into two forms: statutes as defined by the nurse practice act enacted by the state legislature and rules and regulations explicated by state agencies under the jurisdiction of the executive branch of state government. There are three types of regulation: registration (title protection), certification, and licensure (Crawford, 2001). Licensure is the authority delegated to the individual states by the federal Constitution, which provides standards to ensure basic levels of public safety. In most states, the board of nursing has sole authority over advanced nursing practice; however, in 11 states, there is joint authority with the board of medicine (Buppert, 2003). The states require that all APNs carry current licensure as RNs. Advanced nursing practice status is achieved through rules and regulations developed from individual state nurse practice acts. Authority to practice is tied to scope of practice and varies from state to state, depending on the degree of practice autonomy the APN is granted. Most states require national certification and proof of completion of an approved advanced practice nursing program. In addition, many states require evidence of collaboration and/or consultation expectations with physicians. Current status of advanced practice nursing licensure and scope of practice and application information can be easily obtained by accessing the NCSBN website, which has a link to each individual state board of nursing.

Most states require a temporary permit for a new APN graduate to practice as an APN while awaiting national certification results. New graduates should contact the board of nursing and submit the required application for a temporary advanced practice nursing permit if the state allows such practice.

PRESCRIPTIVE AUTHORITY

Credentialing and licensure for prescriptive authority also occur at the state level. Pharmacology requirements vary from state to state, although currently, most states require a graduate core pharmacotherapeutics course during the advanced practice nursing educational program and yearly continuing education (CE) credits thereafter to maintain prescriptive privileges. Prescriptive authority may be regulated solely by the board of nursing, as it is in several states; jointly by the board of nursing and the board of pharmacy, as it is in several others; or by a triad of boards of nursing, medicine, and pharmacy. It is incumbent upon the APN to clearly understand the mechanism of prescriptive authority regulation in his or her state.

As prescriptive authority has evolved over the past several years, certain basic requirements have become fairly standard (although not entirely) for APN prescribers (Box 22-2). These requirements vary from state to state but provide a core regulatory process for prescriptive authority (Buppert, 1999; Hanson, 1996). A good resource for understanding differences in prescriptive practice from state to state is the yearly journal update provided by Pearson each January, which provides a chart that lists prescribing regulations in all 50 states (Pearson, 2003).

State boards of nursing need to clearly document the numbers of hours of pharmacology required for an APN to receive and maintain prescriptive privileges in terms of both educational program and year-to-year CE. APN programs that previously integrated pharmacological content within clinical management courses have moved toward offering separate pharmacology courses in order to comply with recent state requirements for a designated amount of pharmacology content in advanced nursing education. Pharmacology content should be taught by faculty pharmacists or a nurse-pharmacist faculty team who have an in-depth knowledge of therapeutic prescribing. Some states are currently requiring that APN nursing programs verify specific course and content hours in order to be used in an application for prescriptive authority. Furthermore, several states require documentation of the number of hours of CE for pharmacology per year or per cycle. The direction is clearly to require APNs to attend ongoing CE in pharmacology in order to maintain prescriptive privileges. Therefore states need to move toward contracting with universities or other

---

BOX 22-2 • REQUIREMENTS FOR APN PRESCRIBERS

- Graduation from an approved master's-level APN program
- Licensure/recognition in good standing as an APN
- National certification in an APN specialty
- Recent pharmacotherapeutics course of at least 3 credit hours (45 contact hours)
- Evidence of a collaborative practice arrangement (in some states)
- Ongoing CE hours in pharmacotherapeutics to maintain prescribing status
- State prescribing and national Drug Enforcement Administration numbers in some instances

educational providers to offer timely CE offerings and distance learning modalities (e.g., interactive television or Web-based offerings) in order to meet the needs of isolated rural clinicians. Over time, the states will most likely move in the direction of interdisciplinary pharmacology education for both nurses and physicians. New innovations, including hand-held personal digital assistants that offer clinicians on-site information about prescribing modalities and state-of-the-art drug information, are a positive response to the increasing evidence of medication prescribing errors (Huffstutler, Wyatt, & Wright, 2002).

REGULATION FOR REIMBURSEMENT PURPOSES

There are several areas in which reimbursement schemes directly affect the regulation of advanced nursing practice. Managed care organizations (health maintenance organizations and preferred provider organizations) build networks of providers by hiring, purchasing services from, or contracting with physicians and APNs, hospitals, and others to provide health-care services to patient members. Generally, these systems are capitated; that is, providers are prepaid a fixed amount to care for a population of patients. When APNs join a managed care provider network, they must meet all of the requirements, regulations, and standards of care established by the plan (Knight, 1999). For example, a primary care NP applying for a position in managed care would need to meet all of the criteria, listed in Box 22-2, and obtain appropriate Medicare and Medicaid provider status, malpractice history and coverage. Some managed care groups choose to hire credential verification organizations that are distant from the practice or conduct searches of national databases to verify credentials (Knight, 1999). It is incumbent upon the APN to have all credentials and regulatory documentation in good and accessible order when preparing to practice in a managed care environment that may be governed by managed care administrators in a distant state.

National Certification

Over time, national certification for APNs has served several purposes, including regulation and licensure, entry into practice, validation of competence, and recognition of expert practice (Lewis, Camp, & Rothrock, 1996). Advanced practice nursing certification is national in scope and is a mandatory requirement for APNs to obtain and maintain credentialing in most but not all states (Pearson, 2004). Multiple stakeholders for certification such as the ANA, faculty groups (e.g., NONPF), specialty organizations (AANP, American Association of Nurse Anesthetists, the Oncology Nursing Society), and many others have worked to accomplish the multifaceted tasks needed for successful advanced practice nursing certification. These efforts have resulted in a broad range of certification and credentialing requirements. Typically, certification mechanisms develop when a role delineation study is undertaken to define the competencies that provide evidence for appropriate testing within the APN specialty. More and more state regulatory bodies are currently using national certification examinations as a component of their advanced practice nursing credentialing mechanism. CRNAs are credited with the first national certification in 1945, with other advanced practice nursing specialties following suit, although there were few standards for certification in place early on (Hodnicki, 1998). A perceived weakness of advanced practice nursing certification is the multiplicity of certification configurations for advanced nursing practice. See Table 22-1 for a comparison of certification requirements for APNs.

Although there is consensus within the advanced practice nursing community that regulation for practice is needed for public safety and protection and that the public has a right to rely on the credentials of health-care providers in making choices and decisions

TABLE 22-1 COMPARISON OF CERTIFICATION REQUIREMENTS FOR APNs

CRITERIA	ANCC (NP)	ANCC (CNS)	PNCB	AANP	NCC (WHNP OR NNP)	ACC (CNM)	DOA (CRNA)
Education	Master's	Master's	Master's in nursing or post-master's certification	Master's in nursing or post-master's certification	Master's	Certificate, master's, doctoral	Master's
RN licensure in United States or its territories	Yes	Yes	Yes	Yes	Yes	Yes	Yes
Program length	Master's or 12 months with ⅓ didactic, ⅔ clinical	Master's	Master's or 12 months with ⅓ didactic and ⅔ clinical	Master's or 12 months with ⅓ didactic and ⅔ clinical	9 months minimum with 200 hrs didactic and 600 hrs clinical	Master's or 12 months	24 months minimum
Practice requirements	No	Per specialty	No	No	No	No	No
Curriculum outline	Yes	Yes*	Yes	Yes	Yes	Yes	Yes
Clinical hours mandated	500 hrs	500 hrs*	500 hrs plus national competencies met prior to exam	500 hrs	600 hrs	Not stated	450 cases and 800 clinical hrs
Program accreditation or preaccreditation required	Yes CCNE, NLNAC, or regional	Yes CCNE, NLNAC, or regional	Yes, curriculum review required per national competency standards.	Yes	No	Yes	Yes

Adapted from Hodnicki, D. R. (1998). Advanced practice nursing certification: Where do we go from here? *Advanced Practice Nursing Quarterly, 4*, 34-43, © Aspen Publishers, Inc. reprinted with permission.

ANCC = American Nurses Credentialing Center; NP = nurse practitioner; CNS = clinical nurse specialist; PNCB = Pediatric Nurse Certification Board; AANP = American Academy of Nurse Practitioners; NCC = National Certification Corporation; WHNP = women's health nurse practitioner; NNP = neonatal nurse practitioner; ACC = American College of Nurse-Midwives Certification Council Inc.; CNM = certified nurse-midwife; DOA = Division of Accreditation; CRNA = certified registered nurse anesthetist; CCNE = Commission on Collegiate Nursing Education; NLNAC = National League for Nursing Accreditation Center.

*The 2004 Statement on Clinical Nurse Specialist Practice and Education outlines a general CNS curriculum and recommends 500 clinical hours. Some APN specialties have no certification exams because there are too few applicants for valid testing (NACNS, 2004).

regarding health care (NCSBN, 2002), there is tension among stakeholders about how the process plays out for specific advanced practice nursing roles. The NCSBN and many others believe that advanced practice nursing licensure should be designated in relatively broad categories of practice and not at the subspecialty level in order to ensure baseline competency and experience with common health-care problems (NCSBN, 2002). This requirement puts CNSs in a difficult position because many, if not most, CNSs are prepared in subspecialties such as oncology, critical care, and orthopedics. Some subspecialties have certifications at the advanced practice level and others do not. While it would make sense, as Hamric & Spross (1989) proposed, to have CNSs sit for the highest-level specialty exam available, this would make it difficult to regulate this group of APNs. When an advanced practice nursing exam has not been created, there is concern that the proliferation of subspecialties and the slow pace with which CNS certifications in subspecialties have been developed make for an unwieldy regulatory process that, at least in theory, could compromise patient care. On the other hand, the pattern of specialty development (Hanson & Hamric, 2003; see Chapter 1) suggests that, over time, specialties do conduct the role delineation studies needed to document advanced practice, establish standards aimed at protecting the public, and create appropriate certification examinations.

Prior to the promulgation of the latest requirements for Uniform Advanced Practice Registered Nurse Licensure/Authority to Practice (NCSBN, 2002), CNSs could meet the requirements for licensure by an "alternative mechanism" (such as a portfolio) if no exam existed. The latest requirements delete this option (NACNS, 2003). CNSs argue that they practice almost exclusively within the domain of nursing, that other methods of ensuring competence are needed to meet the needs of patients requiring CNS skills, and that they are different from other APNs who move into the broader domain of medical practice (NACNS, 2003). At the same time, state boards of nursing are striving for a way to regulate all APNs who diagnose, prescribe, and are reimbursed for services. Medicare and Medicaid issues also come into play. The reality is that more and more CNSs are falling into this broader category of practice as the regulatory arena softens. These observations, in part, explain some of the tensions that CNSs will encounter as they make decisions about certification and pursue second licensure. The situation also creates challenges for graduate programs as they develop and revise curricula to prepare students to be eligible for particular advanced practice nursing credentials. With the variability of master's education and the multiplicity of certification exams, there is no easy solution to this dilemma; open and respectful dialogue among stakeholders is required to bring this issue to closure.

RECERTIFICATION

Overall, APNs must fulfill CE and practice requirements to successfully maintain their national certification, although differences in requirements exist from specialty to specialty. Each advanced practice nursing certification entity clearly lays out the requirements and time frame for recertification. Generally, national certification for most specialties lasts from 5 to 8 years and requires that the candidate retest unless the established parameters are met. Table 22-2 provides a comparison of recertification requirements for advanced practice nursing specialty groups.

MANDATORY CONTINUING EDUCATION REQUIREMENTS

CE requirements differ from specialty to specialty as to the type and amount of CE needed to maintain current national certification. Individual advanced practice nursing specialties determine the number of hours required for successful recertification. Instruction should be

TABLE 22-2   COMPARISON OF RECERTIFICATION REQUIREMENTS FOR APNs

CRITERIA	ANCC (NP)	ANCC (CNS)	PNCB	AANP	NCC (WHNP OR NNP)	ACC (CNM)	DOA (CRNA)
Due date	5 years	5 years	7 years, certification maintenance program required	5 years	3 years	8 years	2 years
RN licensure	Yes	Yes	Yes	Yes	Yes	Yes	Yes
Retest option	Yes	Yes	Yes	Yes	Yes— must take prior to recertification expiration date	Yes or complete 3 certification maintenance modules	Yes but provisional recertification available
Practice hours	1000 hrs	1000 hrs	None, certification maintenance program required	1000 hrs	None	None	850 hrs over 2 years recommended
Continuing education from accredited provider	75-150 contact hrs plus other categories	75 contact hrs plus other categories	70 contact hrs	75 contact hrs	45 contact hrs	20 contact hrs	40 contact hrs
Random audit performed	20%	20%	20%	20%	20%-30%	10%	All applications reviewed
Lapsed recertification option	Reactivation up to 2 years; >2 years retest	Reactivation up to 2 years; >2 years retest	Retest	Retest	Retest only	Retest and appeal process	May be granted late start on recertification

Adapted from Hodnicki, D. R. (1998). Advanced practice nursing certification: Where do we go from here? *Advanced Practice Nursing Quarterly, 4,* 34-43, © Aspen Publishers, Inc., reprinted with permission.
ANCC = American Nurses Credentialing Center; NP = nurse practitioner; CNS = clinical nurse specialist; PNCB = Pediatric Nurse Certification Board; AANP = American Academy of Nurse Practitioners; NCC = National Certification Corporation; WHNP = women's health nurse practitioner; NNP = neonatal nurse practitioner; ACC = American College of Nurse-Midwives Certification Council Inc.; CNM = certified nurse-midwife; DOA = Division of Accreditation; CRNA = certified registered nurse anesthetist.

in the area of advanced practice nursing specialty, although it may be interdisciplinary. For example, CRNAs may choose to attend a conference with collaborating anesthesiologists, or family NPs may attend a conference with family practice physicians. It is encouraging to note that more and more conferences are offering interdisciplinary speakers and panels at discipline-specific conferences. APN expert clinicians are serving as conference faculty for medical CE and vice versa. Ongoing CE hours can be met by attending CE courses and workshops; working toward degree requirements; completing journal CE offerings; writing for publication; and completing online offerings, simulations, audiotape and CD-ROM materials, and the like. Many nursing and medical journals offer CE credit to subscribers. The move to interdisciplinary offerings has broadened the scope of information available.

MANDATORY PRACTICE REQUIREMENTS

Most, but not all, advanced practice nursing specialties have built in specific requirements for an adequate number of clinical practice hours between the years of recertification to ensure that APNs are remaining clinically current and competent through regular practice. Each certification process clearly spells out the clinical hour practice requirement for the specialty. Some advanced practice nursing specialties accept clinical teaching and other modalities as part of the practice requirement. APNs who do not meet stipulated CE and practice requirements must retake the national certifying exam to continue to practice.

The goal of national certification is to ensure national consistency of professional standards and to help the public to understand scope of practice (AACN, 1995). One concern is that standardization of quality will be lost in the face of multiple advanced practice nursing specialties and specialty certifications. Certification is one way to make sure that competent APNs provide needed health care to patients and families. Therefore standardization of advanced practice nursing certification and recertification processes is critical in order to ensure the credibility of advanced practice nursing specialties (Hodnicki, 1998). Box 22-3 presents Internet website addresses for major advanced practice nursing accreditation, regulatory, and certification organizations.

"Certification is a form of credentialing and credentialing is a form of regulation" (Styles, 1998, p. 1). At no time has it been more important that APNs understand and

---

BOX 22-3 • INTERNET ADDRESSES TO NATIONAL ADVANCED PRACTICE NURSING ACCREDITATION, REGULATION, AND CERTIFICATION WEBSITES

American Academy of Nurse Practitioners (AANP)	www.aanp.org
American Association of Colleges of Nurses & Commission on Collegiate Nursing Education (AACN and CCNE)	www.aacn.nche.edu (links to CCNE)
American Association of Nurse Anesthetists (AANA)	www.nursecredentialing.org
American College of Nurse-Midwives (ACNM)	www.acnm.org
American Nurses Credentialing Center (ANCC)	www.nursecredential.org
Pediatric Nursing Certification Board	www.pncb.org
National Certification Corporation for Obstetrical, Gynecological and Neonatal Nursing Specialties (NCC)	www.nccnet.org
National Council of State Boards of Nursing (NCSBN)	www.ncsbn.org
National League for Nursing and National League for Nursing Accreditation Corporation (NLNAC)	www.nln.org/nlnac
National Association of Nurse Practitioner in Women's Health (NPWH)	www.npwh.org

value the important relationships that underpin the complex processes and systems that regulate practice. New models of health care and varying configurations of how APNs practice in interdisciplinary teams escalate the importance of regulatory considerations to new levels. The growth of telehealth and telepractice modalities makes the picture even more complex. APNs will need to provide leadership and clear direction to policymakers to ensure the development of broad-based practice standards that will satisfy state statutes and "fit" all of the advanced practice nursing specialties.

Collaborative Practice Arrangements

The general term *practice guidelines* can be confusing to the APN in that it is used in several different contexts. First, as defined earlier, it is an evidence-based standard of care. Practice guidelines are used by health-care providers and provide interdisciplinary support for state-of-the-art practice. However, the term may sometimes be used to refer to a collegial agreement between the APN and the physician to define parameters of practice for the APN. A collaborative agreement or arrangement may take many forms, from a one-page written agreement defining consultation and referral patterns to a more specific prescribed "protocol" for specific functions based on state statutes for advanced nursing practice. Collaborative agreements need to be written as broadly as possible to allow for practice variables and new innovations.

The term *protocol* in relation to advanced nursing practice was common several years ago as a physician-directed, specified guideline for the medical aspects of practice that defined each patient problem and the care directive. Some states used this "cookbook" approach to NP practice as a way to oversee prescriptive and other treatment modalities. For the most part, specific protocols for care are no longer used in most settings because it is difficult to update them and tailor them to the individual needs of patients and practices. More importantly, advanced nursing practice has evolved. As APNs have proven their ability to provide competent care with positive outcomes, protocols have been replaced by evidenced-based practice guidelines and collaborative practice agreements. However, it is important to note that the specificity of the collaborative arrangement is most often based on trust and respect between the collaborating APN and physician colleague. For example, a newly graduated APN might have a more tightly drawn collaborative agreement than a more experienced one in a new practice arrangement. APNs must often "earn their stripes" as competent health-care providers in the medical world before they are granted more autonomous practice. Although it should not be this way, physicians are, de facto, assumed to be competent in the workplace while APNs need to prove their worth.

The norm today in advanced practice nursing regulation is shifting toward loosely configured collaborative relationships that offer support to all parties and protect the safety of patients. In any case, to achieve compliance with state regulations for practice, the collaborative agreement, if required in a given state, must have a current signature and provide relevant and up-to-date information. Collaborative relationships vary widely from advanced practice nursing specialty to specialty. The chapters in Part III of this text help to explain the differences in collaborative structures for APNs. Chapter 21 offers an example of a collaborative practice agreement.

Institutional Credentialing

The need for hospital privileges for APNs varies according to the nurse's practice. For example, CNMs and many rural NPs cannot properly care for patients without the ability to admit to the hospital should the need arise. Conversely, many CNSs are employed by hospitals and have no need for admitting privileges. CRNAs and some NPs have not needed to admit patients to the hospital independently in order to give comprehensive care, but they may need to see patients in the emergency room.

The rules for practice as part of the hospital staff are even more specific and variable than those for prescriptive authority and are bound to the local hospital or medical facility and the medical staff of the granting institution. Unfortunately, most of the criteria and guidelines are written exclusively for medical practitioners and therefore are not compatible with the APN's education and supporting credentials. In many hospitals, professional privileges are granted by a committee made up of physicians and administrators. The first step for APNs seeking hospital privileges is to seek out the nurse administrator and find out how the credentials committee is organized, who makes up the membership, and what support there is for nonphysician applicants. Is there a process for nurses or others to petition for privileges? Nursing administrators are often members of these committees, and the APN should meet with nurse colleagues for advice and support prior to the application process.

A second step is to obtain the application package and begin to collect the necessary documents, which include licenses and certifications, transcripts, letters of support, provider numbers, and so on. Support from collaborating physicians is key; in some committee structures, a collaborating physician may serve as the petitioner for a nurse colleague. Dialogue between the hospital administration, physician staff, and other stakeholders such as APN colleagues and other team members is necessary if admitting privileges are required for the desired practice role. Alliances with consumers often add support to the application. Some hospitals have specific guides and protocols for all nonphysician providers; others do not.

The determination of the specific privileges desired is critical to the process. For example, is it necessary to be able to admit or discharge patients; write orders; perform particular procedures; visit in-hospital patients; or take an emergency room call? Many hospitals have different levels of hospital privileges, ranging from "full" to modified privileges for specific functions. Asking for full privileges may not be prudent or useful in a particular setting. A good rule is to ask for what is needed, establish a solid track record, and expand privileges later as the need arises. It is important to remember that the attainment of hospital privileges is often a professional turf issue and fraught with political overtones. The task of overcoming this barrier to practice requires astute planning, negotiating, and careful attention to the stakeholders and set policies of the institution.

ISSUES THAT AFFECT APN CREDENTIALING AND REGULATION

Reimbursement

On a par with the need to be able to prescribe medications for patients is the need to be appropriately reimbursed for care. Clearly, APNs must be paid for services rendered for health care whether they work independently, share a joint practice with a physician colleague, or are employed within a managed care system or provider network. Although the insurance industry is regulated by the individual states, many of the private-pay insurance standards that are used to set payment mechanisms are modeled after federal Medicaid and Medicare policy (see www.cms.gov). Federal mandates that encourage direct payment of nonphysician health-care providers are often blocked at the state level by discriminating rules and regulations. The terms *nonphysician provider* and *mid-level provider* both

EXEMPLAR 22-1

MEETING THE REQUIREMENTS FOR CREDENTIALING AND REGULATION

Jeni is in the final semester of her master's family nurse practitioner (FNP) program at a state university. She is in the process of negotiating a contract with a provider network of physicians and advanced practice nurses (APNs) in a satellite health maintenance organization (HMO) practice. Jeni knows that she must begin the process of acquiring the necessary credentials in order to be able to practice in her state. When she applied to her FNP program, she made sure that the university and graduate program were accredited in good standing. Now that she is ready to leave, she must prepare for a new and challenging professional life.

In her seminar class, Jeni received the application to sit for national certification the month after she graduates and has sent the application forward to ensure her seat at the examination. Her next step is to access the Internet and download the advanced practice nursing rules and regulations for her state as well as the application for a temporary permit to practice as an APN for the interim between graduation and the time that she gets the results from her national certifying exam. Jeni reviews both of these documents carefully so that she fully understands the application process and the materials and fee that she will need to submit.

Jeni carefully notes in the advanced practice nursing rules and regulations that, to be able to prescribe in her state, she must show proof that she has completed a 45-contact-hour approved course in pharmacotherapeutics and that she must complete 6 hours of CE in pharmacotherapeutics each year to maintain her status as a prescriber. She makes a note to request the transcript for her pharmacotherapeutics course to attach to her application for her advanced practice nursing license.

The HMO where Jeni plans to practice has sent her several documents that she must complete in order to be able to practice. First, upon signing her contract, she will need to negotiate a written collaborative arrangement with the precepting physician colleague, who will see the patients who are beyond her scope of practice. Second, she needs a Medicaid provider number in order to see children in the Medicaid program and a Medicare number in order to see elders. In addition, this managed care system requires that Jeni apply to the local hospital and nursing home privileging committees so that she can see patients on rounds, do admitting and discharge planning, and follow nursing home patients on a regular basis.

As part of her "package," Jeni has negotiated for the employer to pay the premium on her malpractice insurance as an APN. She needs to call her insurance carrier to discuss the transfer of her student policy to a full policy to cover her as a certified APN with the appropriate scope of practice that she will need in her new position. Jeni uses the support of her colleagues and mentors as she works though this important process of preparing her credentials to practice as an APN.

denote caregivers who are not prepared as medical doctors. This category includes NPs, CNSs, CNMs, CRNAs, physician assistants, psychologists, and other reimbursable providers of care. Many third-party reimbursers, including some major insurance companies, are now reimbursing APNs and other nonphysician providers directly; others are not. As states move more directly into reimbursement models for APNs, in both the private and public sectors, and into large purchasing groups in which APNs are providing care as part of interdisciplinary teams, reimbursement is becoming more readily available. However, tensions persist with regard to provider status and membership on patient panels. From a credentialing standpoint, attention to CMS rules, Medicare and Medicaid provider numbers, Clinical Laboratories Improvement Act (CLIA) (www.cms.hhs.gov/clia/) regulations, and provider requirements is extremely important to ensure that APNs are reimbursed. How APNs fit into reimbursement systems is a critical issue for nurses. It is important for APNs to know how to contract for their services at the individual level as they negotiate employment packages, but, even more importantly, they need to be present at the negotiating table as members of management teams who are setting the policies for provider services where the rules for payment are made.

Payment for advanced practice nursing services has long been controversial. Issues surrounding substitutive care offered by nonphysician providers versus care by APNs that enhances medical care is a complex issue that profoundly affects direct and indirect reimbursement. It is important that APNs differentiate and be able to clearly articulate the differences between their practices and those of physician extenders. The argument continues about whether nurses should be paid the same fee for service as a physician or be paid only a percentage of the physician payment. Should APNs demand equal pay for equal service or should they cast themselves as more cost-effective providers to patients? This is always a negotiable issue, and there is disagreement within medicine and nursing alike. Payment by private insurers is contract specific and varies with each state's insurance commission. The current climate of large-scale mergers between major private insurance companies to accommodate complex managed care structures has important relevance for reimbursement for APNs. It is critical that APNs position themselves to sit on policymaking boards for private enterprise. To accomplish this, APNs must have visibility with local, state, and national entities that make the important decisions for health care. A prime example comes from the 1980s, a time when NPs lost their liability coverage nationally. NPs worked with the National Alliance of Nurse Practitioners and, through negotiation and education, gained access to the executive board at the major liability carrier as part of an advisement group. This activity cemented a long-term relationship that has resulted in a clear understanding about the practice of NPs and a newsletter for risk management with this carrier (Hanson, 1985).

There is another key issue with regard to reimbursement for APNs. In managed care contracts, the level of reimbursement is immaterial. APNs and all other providers must deliver care at a fixed, preset price; this can be an advantage if APNs are less costly to employ. Thus it becomes critical for APNs to fully understand how much it costs them to provide care for patients with a variety of preventive, episodic, and chronic health problems and to be able to articulate to contractors that they are competitive in the marketplace.

Policy issues surrounding the reimbursement of APNs require careful reflection before strategies to remove constraints to payment are undertaken. For all health-care providers, outcomes of care will take precedence in reimbursement over all other issues, so attention to quality of care is a paramount consideration. Several other important questions should be considered when policy is being shaped. For example, what services do APNs want to be paid for? Are they different from physician services or the same? Are there specific nursing services that need to be reimbursed? Is direct payment the issue, or does it matter who gets the payment? Will the payment level be the same as or lower than what physicians receive for equivalent service? These are important questions because, in most states, APNs historically have been reimbursed indirectly, "incident to" physicians and at a considerably lower rate. As mentioned earlier, "incident to" billing is a difficult issue. An APN can charge the full physician rate if billing is incident to, but only 80% to 85% if billing is done directly by the APN, an unfortunate disincentive for doctors to let APNs bill independently. Most physicians desire to bill under their own Medicare number in order to receive the highest rate of reimbursement. On the other hand, APNs want and need to bill independently in order to be viewed as the caregivers of record. There are many rules associated with incident to billing, including the need for the physician to be on the premises. The CMS is currently studying incident to billing to better understand the prevalence of advanced practice nursing provider care and the cost to the system for billing APN services through the physician for a higher fee for service. It is advantageous for APNs who are planning to practice clinically, no matter what the setting or physician relationship, to seek counsel about the reimbursement realities in their state and in their particular practice setting(s) before beginning to care for patients. In particular, it is important to identify the third-party payors of the majority of patients the APN will be caring for and to learn their requirements for reimbursement of APNs. Only then are APNs in an appropriate position to seek status as reimbursable providers with Medicare, Medicaid, and the many private payors.

Risk Management, Malpractice, and Negligence

Although malpractice suits involving APNs are rare, malpractice issues are ever present for all providers of health care, regardless of credential or setting. In an unstable health-care environment, patients look to the tort system to ease their apprehension and anxiety about the care they receive. Patients are more likely to seek redress if they mistrust their provider or believe they have been harmed by the system. First and foremost, APNs need to clearly understand what constitutes negligent practice and grounds for malpractice and to put safeguards in place so that they do not have to confront the legal system.

By definition, negligence is the failure to act in a reasonable way as a health-care clinician. Negligence may lead to malpractice and legal action. The following four factors must exist in order for a malpractice suit to be valid:

1. A duty of care must be owed to the injured party, either through direct office or hospital care OR through phone or e-mail advice, and a patient-nurse relationship must be established.
2. The accepted standard of care must be breached.
3. The patient must have sustained an injury.
4. There must be causation demonstrated, that is, the patient suffered an injury that was caused by the APN clinician. (Often there are multiple causation implications based on care by several caregivers over time.)

Within the court system, care is evaluated by preset criteria in the form of medical and advanced practice nursing standards. National professional organizations set the standards for appropriate care. APNs are often held to the medical standard of care as advanced practice nursing standards continue to be developed. There is much blurring between medical and nursing standards, leading toward a need for truly interdisciplinary standards of care that will hold care providers to the same standards as their peers (Buppert, 2002; Letz, 2002). There are several ways that legal standards of care are established in a particular case. By far the most common is through expert testimony offered by a person who is qualified by education, experience, knowledge, and skill level to judge the actions of the providers in the case. Other mechanisms include review of professional literature, manufacturers' package inserts, and documented professional standards of care. Letz (2002) suggested four ways to prevent malpractice events: establish a good rapport with patients over time; follow an established standard of care to ensure competence; document accurately and completely; and take a course in risk management.

Many risk management resources to assist APNs are available through professional advanced practice nursing organizations and though public and private entities. Visit the professional websites suggested throughout this text to find comprehensive risk management tools and a current discussion of legal questions confronting APNs. Box 22-4 provides a list of 10 rules compiled by Buppert (2002) to help APNs avoid malpractice.

BOX 22-4 • RULES TO AVOID MALPRACTICE

1. Know the "red flag" complaints and conditions for your specialty.
2. Rule out the worst thing first.
3. Know the risk factors that call for screening tests.
4. For diagnostic tests or referrals ordered, be able to answer "yes" to these three questions:
   Was it done?
   Are results on record?
   If abnormal, was the condition, symptoms, or finding followed up to a definitive diagnosis or rule-out?
5. Revisit an unresolved problem until it is resolved.
6. With every prescription, go through a script analysis: Side effects; Contraindications; *R*ight patient, right drug, right dose, frequency, duration, and route; *I*nteractions; *P*recautions; *T*ransmittal legible.
7. Have office systems and policies in place for ensuring follow-up.
8. Audit charts for mistakes or omissions.
9. Treat every medical opinion you give as if it were rendered during an office visit.
10. If the patient doesn't really need something, don't order it.

Adapted with permission from Buppert, C. (2002). *Avoiding malpractice: 10 rules, 5 systems, 20 cases.* Annapolis, MD: Law Offices of Carolyn Buppert. www.bupport.com

LIABILITY INSURANCE

APNs need a thorough understanding of liability insurance coverage, types of policies, and extent of coverage required. It is important to understand the difference between the two most common types of professional liability insurance plans—"Claims-Made" and "Occurrence." A "Claims-Made" insurance policy covers claims made against the APN only while the policy is in effect. Coverage must be continued indefinitely to ensure coverage for claims filed in the future for actions that occurred in the past. On the other hand, with an "Occurrence" policy, the APN is covered for alleged acts of negligence that occurred during the time when the policy was in effect. The benefit of occurrence coverage is that even if the policy is cancelled at some future date, coverage for events that occurred while the policy was in effect will be honored. For more information about advanced practice nursing liability insurance, see the Cotterell, Mitchell, and Fifer Group website at (www.cmfgroup.com). It is also important to understand the extent of coverage per incident and how personal legal costs are covered.

As APNs move in and out of what is considered the domain of medicine, serious thought must be given to the standard by which APNs will be judged if they are deemed to have made an error. Although there are not many documented cases citing APNs who have injured patients by wrongful actions, the question about whether APNs should be tried by the courts according to medical or nursing standards is important and needs to be clarified. It is incumbent upon APNs to set clear standards for practice that are based on clinical competency.

Privacy Issues

HEALTH INSURANCE PORTABILITY AND ACCOUNTABILITY ACT

The federal Health Insurance Portability and Accountability Act (HIPAA) became law in 1996. Legal requirements were finalized by the U.S. Department of Health and Human Services in 2002, and mandatory compliance with federal regulations was required by

April 14, 2003. Visit www.hhs.gov to view the ruling and its latest amendments and documentation.

HIPAA establishes a mandatory requirement for implementing uniform minimum patient privacy standards within the states. The main goal of HIPAA is to protect the privacy of a patient's identifiable health information that is maintained or transmitted by health-care providers and insurers. This information includes any information that would identify the patient, the patient's problem, the plan of care, or the way that care is paid for. The regulations for privacy established by HIPAA place a new level of legal responsibility on health providers including APNs. If APNs accept third-party reimbursement or transmit any health information in any form, they are required to comply with HIPAA regulations.

Providers and facilities need to adhere to several operating standards in order to be in compliance with HIPAA regulation. Standard 1 lays out the proper use and disclosure of personal health information in any form (oral, written, TV and Web-based, etc.). Standard 2 allows patients to request access to their information, request amendments to it, and receive an annual report of all the uses and disclosure of personal information that they did not authorize in writing. Patients must also receive notice of the privacy practices of their health-care provider. The third set of standards requires facilities to complete several administrative tasks, including the appointment of a privacy officer. The rules state that providers are required to train all of their staff members regarding HIPAA rules and on-site procedures. Facilities and providers can design their own policies and procedures to meet the needs and scope of their practice, but the policies must adhere to all of the standards that are included in the operating standards of HIPAA. Penalties are severe and include civil monetary fines and, in some cases, felony criminal penalties. There are several templates and kits available online to assist in the development of appropriate compliance procedures; these may be obtained at www.hhs.gov/ocr/hipaa/privacy.html or www.buppert.com and others (Buppert, 2003; Ziel, 2002). APNs need to be familiar with their institution's implementation procedures, as these vary.

Telehealth and Telepractice

Regulatory issues surrounding the changes in the way health-care providers practice based on electronic capabilities will continue to challenge policymakers and APNs well into the new millennium. A model described as "mutual recognition" refers to the use of a system much like that used for driver's licenses, whereby states share the jurisdiction, discipline, and information needed to regulate practice based on an interstate compact (NCSBN, 1998; Williamson & Hutcherson, 1998). An APN is licensed in a home state, but other states recognize the licensure. The mutual recognition model would hold the APN accountable for the laws and regulations in the state where the APN provides the health care but would rely on the licensure from the home state (Williamson & Hutcherson, 1998). In August of 2002, the NCSBN Delegate Assembly approved the adoption of model language for a licensure compact for advanced practice registered nurses (APRNs). Only those states who have adopted the RN and LPN/VN Nurse Licensure Compact may implement a compact for APRNs. Implementation issues for the APRN Compact are addressed by the advanced practice task force at NCSBN, which meets four times a year. The reader can follow this discussion at www.NCSBN.org. Exemplar 22-2 illustrates an interstate practice.

EXEMPLAR 22-2

INTERSTATE PRACTICE

As a pediatric NP in a health maintenance organization practice, Alice has been co-managing, with Dr. Pete Johnson, the health care of 4-year-old David since he was born in North Carolina. David has insulin-dependent diabetes mellitus. The child and his mother have grown to trust and depend on Alice's care for David over time. While at Disneyland in Florida, David develops diarrhea and vomiting. His mom chooses to e-mail Alice for advice rather than take David to an unfamiliar emergency room and provider. Alice responds back to the mother with directions about management of the gastroenteritis and potential changes in David's insulin dosage if needed. In providing this guidance, Alice has cared for David in a state other than the one in which she is licensed and recognized as an APN. However, a system of mutual regulatory recognition between Florida and North Carolina would allow for Alice to care for David using her North Carolina advanced practice nursing credentials.

Interestingly, new technologies and a system of "virtual practice," as described in the previous example, focus attention on pervasive barriers that have plagued APNs for many years (Safriet, 1998). Although implementation of a mutual recognition system is well underway for RNs, the same type of recognition is lagging behind for APNs because of the lack of stability and standardization of regulatory schemes from state to state with regard to scope of practice, prescriptive authority, and reimbursement. Although the dysfunctional aspects of this current regulatory climate for APN providers are problematic, they may provide a basis for positive change. Based on the Comprehensive Telehealth Act of 1997 (Senate Bill 385), physicians and other health-care providers, including nurses, fall within the boundaries of electronic practice and all require regulation. Therefore the potential for policymakers to focus on "what is being done" rather than on "who is doing it" is positive for APNs (Safriet, 1998). Telehealth legislation could provide the catalyst needed to ensure that all states recognize and authorize key elements of scopes of practice for APNs (e.g., prescriptive authority). Since some states are lagging behind, a national strategy such as this legislation could bring these states into alignment with the rest of the country. In addition to identifying issues that arise in their own practices, it will be important for APNs to carefully monitor the development of practice across state boundaries and work closely with advanced practice nursing associations to effect regulatory change that removes barriers and augments practice.

From a legal and regulatory standpoint, clear statutes are needed that offer broad practice standards to allow for mobility across state lines. This change will require national standards of practice as well as certification and credentialing requirements that can satisfy many different jurisdictions and advanced practice nursing specialty groups—not an easy task! These standards will require diligent collaboration between educators, state boards of nursing, the specialty professional associations, and all practicing APNs (Hanson, 1998). Part of the professional agenda that APNs must address is the need for accountability and responsibility for competence in practice. As a professional group, APNs must build strong national standards of practice, scope, and skills. Experienced practitioners need to help novices gain greater competence and new skills. It is important that APNs not lose sight of the need to support each other and to mentor colleagues as the practice arena broadens.

Cost Containment Initiatives

The national health-care reform debate that began with the Clinton administration has served as a catalyst for change at all levels of government throughout the past decade. A myriad of configurations of systems of care have evolved that require nurses to understand, more than ever before, how much it costs to treat patients as well as how to interface with new systems as providers. A decade ago, Buerhaus (1994) suggested four overarching issues that nurses facing competition in practice needed to address. These four concerns are still of critical importance to APNs who are moving into practice settings. First, APNs must realize the range of opportunities for APNs in fee-for-service, prepaid, and privatized markets and proceed appropriately into these markets. Second, as part of that effort, APNs must ensure that the minimum package of patient benefits includes advanced practice nursing services. Third, any care system must meet both the clinical and economic interests of APNs. Fourth, nurses must make sure that the turmoil does not detract from the value of nursing services. When these four issues are studied in conjunction with the direct care chapters and Chapter 20, they form the context within which APNs practice today.

Research has shown that APNs are viable and cost-effective alternatives to physician-based health care (see Chapter 25). This increased visibility makes it imperative that APNs monitor the competencies of their own practices and clearly understand the costs of providing care to patients. Recent acts of Congress that have cut federal programs for the poor will augment the need for APNs even while funds to pay for this care are reduced, which increases the stress placed on underserved populations with health problems. The ANA's *Nursing's Agenda for the Future* (2002) provides needed leadership in these unsettled times for health care and is an important reference for APNs who want to better understand how to improve access and reduce cost. It addresses several imperatives: access to health care, leadership by nurses, political savvy, emphasis on primary and preventive care, shared consumer and provider accountability for health-care decision making, and holistic health-care services that emphasize quality.

INFLUENCING THE REGULATORY PROCESS

APNs can directly influence the regulatory process in several ways in addition to using political strategies. At all levels, regulators are keen to find practicing APNs and advanced practice nursing educators who will take an active role in assisting them to develop and implement sound regulatory policies and procedures. Chapter 9 provides an in-depth discussion of skills needed for leadership and political advocacy. Following are some additional ways that APNs can actively engage in any regulatory process that affects their practice.

- Seek out a gubernatorial appointment to the board of nursing or to the advanced practice committee that advises the board of nursing in your state.
- Seek membership as the APN member of the advisory council for either the state medical board or the state board of pharmacy.
- Seek appointment to the board of accreditation or the test-writing committees for national certification examinations.
- Seek appointment to CMS panels where Medicare and Medicaid provider issues are decided.
- Seek appointment to hospital privileging committees and ensure that privileging materials are appropriate for APNs.
- Seek appointment on advisory committees and task forces that are advising the NCSBN.
- Offer testimony at state and national hearings where proposed regulatory changes in advanced practice nursing regulation, prescriptive authority, and reimbursement schemes will be aired.
- Respond to offers to review/edit/provide feedback on circulated draft regulatory polices that directly affect advanced practice nursing education and practice.

In order to accomplish these activities, APNs need to use research data, a powerful tool for shaping health policy (Hamric, 1998). By actively participating in the regulatory process, APNs assure themselves of a strong voice in regulatory and credentialing processes. At the very least, it is incumbent upon the practicing APN to carefully monitor the process through websites and newsletters to stay informed.

FUTURE REGULATORY CHALLENGES FACING APNs

Two health professions reports disseminated by the Pew Health Professions Commission documented the need for generic benchmarks and standards for health-care education and practice (Gelmon, O'Neil, Kimmey, & the Task Force on Accreditation of Health Professions, 1999; O'Neil & the Pew Health Professions Commission, 1998). Furthermore, the Pew Commission recommended interdisciplinary competence for all health-care professionals. More specifically, advanced nursing practice leaders were charged to "develop standard guidelines for advanced nursing practice and reinforce them with curriculum guidelines, examination requirements, and accreditation regulations" (O'Neil & the Pew Health Professions Commission, 1998).

The future requires that APNs promulgate clear, competency-based standards for both education and practice that will allow for growth and movement across state lines. It is important that APNs accomplish this work in preparation for the next phase—interdisciplinary credentialing and regulation based on defined patient outcomes—because this phenomenon will become a reality in the not too distant future (see Chapter 19). The wave of the future is to move to interdisciplinary regulation—whereby, for example, family practice physicians, family NPs, and CNMs caring for menopausal women would all be held to a like standard of education and practice. Porter-O'Grady (1998) suggested that regulation for the health professions will require a new approach that dispels notions of exclusivity, exclusion, or independence from other disciplines. This move toward overarching regulation for the health professions, when and if it comes to pass, will require much higher levels of collaboration among the disciplines and specialties than now exist and, most importantly, broad-based standards and regulations for advanced nursing practice.

Dr. Loretta Ford, founder of the modern NP movement, offered sound advice to APNs: "The problems and issues of the day—in seeking independence and control of practice, reimbursement, nitpicking skirmishes on the scope of practice, and relationships with medicine— are but a bump in the road along the way to solving the world's problems" (Tumulo, 2003, p. 1). What really matters are the patients and the benefits patients will realize through care provided by APNs.

REFERENCES

Agency for Healthcare Research and Quality. (2004). *Clinical guidelines index.* Retrieved March 20, 2004, from http://www.ahrq.gov

American Association of Colleges of Nursing. (1995). *Essentials of master's education for advanced practice nursing.* Washington, DC: Author.

American Association of Colleges of Nursing & National Organization of Nurse Practitioner Faculties. (1999). *1998–1999 Enrollment and graduations in baccalaureate and graduate programs in nursing* (Publication No. 98-99-1). Washington, DC: American Association of Colleges of Nursing.

American Nurses Association. (1996). *Scope of practice and standards of advanced nursing practice.* Washington, DC: Author.

American Nurses Association. (2002). *Nursing's agenda for the future.* Washington, DC: Author.

American Nurses Association, (2003). *Nursing's social policy statement 2003* (2nd ed.). Washington DC: Author.

Association of Women's Health, Obstetric and Neonatal Nurses & the National Association of Nurse Practitioners in Reproductive Health. (1996). *The women's health nurse practitioner: Guidelines for practice and education*. Washington, DC: Authors.

Berlin, L. E., Stennett, J., & Bednash, G. D. (2003a). *Enrollment and graduations in baccalaureate and graduate programs in nursing*. Washington, DC: American Association of Colleges of Nursing.

Berlin, L. E., Stennett, J., & Bednash, G. D. (2003b). *2002-2003 Enrollment and graduation in baccalaureate and graduate programs in nursing*. Washington, DC: American Association of Colleges of Nursing.

Buerhaus, P. I. (1994). Managed competition and critical issues facing nurses. *Nursing and Health Care, 15*, 22-26.

Buppert, C. (1999). *Nurse practitioner's business practice and legal guide*. Gaithersburg, MD: Aspen.

Buppert, C. (2002). *Avoiding malpractice. 10 rules, 5 systems, 20 cases*. Annapolis, MD: Law Offices of Carolyn Buppert.

Buppert, C. (2003). HIPAA patient privacy. *The American Journal for Nurse Practitioners, 7*, 17-22.

Cady, R. F. (2003). *The advanced practice nurse's legal handbook*. Baltimore: Lippincott–Williams & Wilkins.

Commission on Collegiate Nursing Education. (1998). *Procedures for accreditation of baccalaureate and graduate nursing education programs*. Washington, DC: Author.

Commission on Collegiate Nursing Education (2004). *Commission on collegiate nursing education amends accreditation standards* [Press release]. Retrieved May 19, 2004, from http://www.aacn. nche.edu/ Accreditation

Comprehensive Telehealth Act of (1997), S. 385, 105th Congress (1997).

Deighton, B. (2003, February 28). *The effect of the medical liability insurance crisis on physician supply and access to medical care*. Presented at the Georgia Health Strategies Council Meeting. Atlanta: Georgia Board for Physician Workforce.

Faut-Callahan, M. F., & Caulk, S. S. (1998). Credentialing of certified registered nurse anesthetists. *Advanced Practice Nursing Quarterly, 4*, 54-62.

Gelmon, S. B., O'Neil, E. H., Kimmey, J. R., & the Task Force on Accreditation of Health Professions Education. (1999). *Strategies for change and improvement: The report of the Task Force on Accreditation of Health Professions Education*. San Francisco: Center for the Health Professions, University of California at San Francisco.

Hamric, A. B. (1998). Using research to influence the regulatory process. *Advanced Practice Nursing Quarterly, 4*, 44-50.

Hamric, A. B., & Spross, J. A. (1989). *The clinical nurse specialist in theory and practice* (2nd ed.). Philadelphia: W. B. Saunders.

Hanson, C. M. (1985). *Personal archives*. Statesboro, GA: National Alliance of Nurse Practitioners.

Hanson, C. M. (1996). Health policy issues: Dealing with the realities and constraints of advanced practice nursing. In A. B. Hamric, J. A. Spross, & C. M. Hanson (Eds.), *Advanced nursing practice: an integrative approach* (pp. 496-515). Philadelphia: W. B. Saunders.

Hanson, C. M. (1998). Regulatory issues will lead advanced practice nursing challenges into the new millennium. *Advanced Practice Nursing Quarterly, 4*, v-vi.

Hanson, C. M., & Hamric, A. B. (2002). Reflections on the continuing evolution of advanced practiced nursing. *Nursing Outlook, 51*(5), 203-211.

Hodnicki, D. R. (1998). Advanced practice nursing certification: Where do we go from here? *Advanced Practice Nursing Quarterly, 4*, 34-43.

Huffstutler, S., Wyatt, T., & Wright, C. P. (2002). The use of handheld technology in nursing education. *Nurse Educator, 27*, 271-275.

Knight, W. (1999). *Managed care: What it is and how it works*. Gaithersburg, MD: Aspen.

Letz, K. (2002). *Business essentials for nurse practitioners: Essential knowledge for building your practice*. Fort Wayne (IN): Previcare Inc.

Lewis, C. K., Camp, J., & Rothrock, J. (1996). *The trilateral initiative for North American nursing: Nursing specialty certification in the United States. An assessment of North American nursing*. Philadelphia: Commission on Graduates of Foreign Nursing Schools.

Mindinger, M. O., Kane, R. L., Lenz, E. R., Totten, A. Tsoco W., Cleary P. D., et al. (2000). Primary care outcomes in patients treated by nurse practitioners or physicians: A randomized trial. *Journal of the American Medical Association, 283*, 59-68.

National Association of Clinical Nurse Specialists. (2003a). Regulatory credentialing of clinical nurse specialists. *Clinical Nurse Specialist, 17*, 163-169.

National Association of Clinical Nurse Specialists. (2003b). NACNS responds to the national council of state boards of nursing uniform advanced practice registered nurse licensure/authority to practice requirements. *Clinical Nurse Specialist, 17*, 58-65.

National Association of Clinical Nurse Specialists. (2004). *Statement on clinical nurse specialist practice and education*. Harrisburg, PA: Author.

National Association of Neonatal Nurses. (1995). *Report of NANN neonatal nurse practitioner program accreditation*. Washington, DC: Author.

National Council of State Boards of Nursing, Inc. (1998). *APRN licensure: Draft uniform requirements*. Chicago: Author.

National Council of State Boards of Nursing, Inc. (2002). *Regulation of advanced practice nursing: 2002 national council of state boards of nursing position paper* (pp. 1-8). Chicago: Author.

National Organization of Nurse Practitioner Faculties. (1995). *Advanced nursing practice:*

Curriculum guidelines and program standards for nurse practitioner education. Washington, DC: Author.

National Organization of Nurse Practitioner Faculties. (1996). *Workforce policy project technical report for nurse practitioner educational programs 1988-1995* (pp. 7-41). Washington, DC: Author.

National Organization of Nurse Practitioner Faculty Practice Doctorate Task Force (2003). The practice doctorate in nursing: Future or fringe. *Topics in Advanced Practice Nursing eJournal, 3*(2) 2003 Medscape, Posted May 19, 2003. Retrieved May 19, 2004.

National Task Force on Quality Nurse Practitioner Education. (1997). *Criteria for evaluation of nurse practitioner programs.* Washington, DC: Author.

National Task Force on Quality Nurse Practitioner Education. (2002). *Criteria for evaluation of nurse practitioner programs.* Washington, DC: Author.

O'Neil, E. H., & the Pew Health Professions Commission. (1998). *Recreating health professional practice for a new century.* San Francisco: Pew Health Professions Commission.

Pearson, L. (2004). The sixteenth annual legislative update: How each state stands on legislative issues affecting advanced nursing practices. *The Nurse Practitioner: The American Journal of Primary Health Care, 29*(1), 26-31.

Porter-O'Grady, T. (1998). A new age for regulation. *Advanced Practice Nursing Quarterly, 4,* 94-95.

Rentmeester, K., & Kindig, D. A. (1994). *Physician supply by specialty in managed care organizations.* Madison: School of Medicine, University of Wisconsin.

Safriet, B. (1992). Health care dollars and regulatory sense: The role of advanced practice nursing. *Yale Journal of Regulation, 9,* 417-487.

Safriet, B. (1998). Still spending dollars, still searching for sense: Advanced practice nursing in an era of regulatory and economic turmoil. *Advanced Practice Nursing Quarterly, 4,* 24-33.

Safriet, B. (2002). Closing the gap between can and may in health care providers scopes of practice: A primer for policymakers. *Yale Journal of Regulation, 19,* 301-334.

Styles, M. M. (1998). An international perspective: APN credentialing. *Advanced Practice Nursing Quarterly, 4,* 1-5.

Tumulo, J. (2003). *NP spotlight: Miles to go. An interview with Loretta Ford.* Retrieved March 7, 2003, from http://www.advancefornp/NPcover.htm

Wakefield, M. (2002). What would Florence do? *Reflections on Nursing Leadership, 28,* 12-16.

Wilcox, P. (1995, April). *Advanced practice model response to needs of women at risk for female malignancies.* Abstract presented at the Oncology Nurses Society national conference, Anaheim, CA.

Williamson, S. H., & Hutcherson, C. (1998). Mutual recognition: Response to the regulatory implications of a changing health care environment. *Advanced Practice Nursing Quarterly, 4,* 86-93.

Additional Readings

Antrobus, S., & Brown, S. (1997). The impact of the commissioning agenda upon nursing practice: A pro-active approach to influencing health policy. *Journal of Advanced Nursing, 25,* 309-315.

Brent, N. J. (1997). *Nurses and the law: A guide to principles and applications.* Philadelphia: W. B. Saunders.

Gorenberg, B. D., Alderman, M. C., & Cruise, M. J. (1991). Social policy statements: Guidelines for decision making. *International Nursing Review, 38,* 11-13.

Hebda, T., Czar, P., & Mascara, C. (1998). *Handbook of informatics for nurses and health care professionals.* New York: Addison-Wesley.

Koerner, J. (1998). Tapping into uncommon wisdom through mentorship. In C. Vance & R. K. Olson (Eds.), *The mentor connection in nursing* (pp. 7-233) New York: Springer-Verlag.

Mason, D. J., & Leavitt, J. K. (1998). *Policy and politics in nursing and health care* (3rd ed.). Philadelphia: W. B. Saunders.

Milstead, J. A. (1997). A social mandate: APN leadership for the whole policy process. *Advanced Practice Nursing Quarterly, 3,* 1-8.

Milstead, J. A. (1998). *Health policy and politics: A nurse's guide.* Gaithersburg, MD: Aspen.

Mundt, M. H. (1997). Books on health policy and health reform: How is nursing represented? *Journal of Professional Nursing, 13,* 19-27.

Penney, N. E., Campbell-Heider, N., Miller, B. K., Carter, E., & Bidwell-Cerone, S. (1996). Influencing health care policy: Nursing research and the ANA social policy statement. *Journal of the New York State Nurses Association, 27,* 15-19.

Pew Health Professions Commission. (1995). *Critical challenges: Revitalizing the health professions for the twenty-first century, third report.* San Francisco: Center for the Health Professions, University of California at San Francisco.

Starfield, B. (1997). Primary care and health policy. The future of primary care in a managed care era. *International Journal of Health Services, 27,* 687-696.

Sullivan, T. J. (1998). *Collaboration: A health care imperative. Part III, intraorganizational collaboration.* New York: McGraw-Hill.

Whitman, M. (1998). Nurses can influence public health policy. *Advanced Practice Nursing Quarterly, 3,* 67-71.

CHAPTER 23

Health Policy Issues in Changing Environments

JEAN JOHNSON • L. GREGORY PAWLSON

INTRODUCTION

Although clinical practice is the hallmark of advanced practice nurses (APNs), health policy issues influence virtually all aspects of clinical practice. Policies established at the federal, state, and corporate levels influence, for example, which patients are seen by APNs, what services are reimbursed, what and how APNs are paid, how quality of APN care is measured and the scope of APN practice. Health policy also defines issues of concern to APNs beyond direct clinical practice, including the financing of health care in general and the overall tax burden resulting from health-care expenditures. This chapter discusses health policy in a broad perspective, including (1) the definition of health policy, (2) financing and cost of health care, (3) access to health care, and (4) quality. Specific issues related to APN practice are integrated into these general topics.

While recognizing that there are areas of conflict between nursing and medicine, this chapter is written by an APN and a physician in the hope that we can convey the possibility and desirability of collaboration. Given the extraordinary pressures on health-care providers from purchasers, government, corporations, and others, it is important to try to find the common concerns among health professionals, particularly medicine and nursing, rather than automatically taking adversarial positions based on discipline. When the well-being of individual patients and the health of our nation are at stake, we firmly believe in the importance of working together. However, we also have not omitted or underestimated those areas in which conflict is present or likely.

This chapter also complements several other chapters in the book, specifically Chapters 9, 20, and 22. No single chapter can cover all the topics relevant to practice issues, and many issues can be more fully understood when viewed from a different perspective. For these reasons, the reader is strongly encouraged to refer to the other chapters noted.

WHAT IS HEALTH POLICY AND WHY IS IT IMPORTANT?

Health policy in its broadest sense can be taken to mean any decision that affects health care at a group or macro level, including access, finance, reimbursement, delivery, quality, and cost. Longest (2002) stated that policy decisions are intended to direct or influence the actions, behaviors, or decisions of others. In a more limited sense, health policy is often used to mean public policy related to health-care delivery, specifically decisions regarding health care that are made in a public forum, mostly through local, state, or federal government actions by their legislative, judicial, or executive branches. However, this latter definition leaves out the increasing number of decisions about health care that are made by insurers, providers, purchasers, or others outside of government who nonetheless form and shape health-care systems.

The importance of health policy stems from a number of factors. The most obvious factor is that health care has become a major economic activity in the United States. The health-care industry is one of the top three employers in this country, and health-care expenditures represented 14.1% of our gross domestic product (GDP) in 2001. GDP is the value of all goods and services produced in the United States (Heffler et al., 2003). Health-care spending is expected to reach 17.7% of GDP by 2012. In order to understand the magnitude of public interest in health-care spending, it is important to know the amount of public funds used (Table 23-1). In 2001, total health-care expenditures amounted to $1.4 trillion (Levit et al., 2003). Federal and state public funds accounted for

TABLE 23-1	HEALTH-CARE EXPENDITURES (IN BILLIONS)	
Public		647 (45%)
Federal		455
Medicare		242
Medicaid		129
Other		83
State and Local		191
Private		777 (55%)
Employer sponsored insurance		496
Self-pay		205
Other		76
Total		1.4 trillion

just over 45% ($647 billion) of this spending. Federal funds paid for 37% ($242 billion) of Medicare costs, 20% ($129 billion) of Medicaid costs, and 18% in other costs. State and local government spending constitutes 30% ($191 billion) of public spending. Private funding accounted for the other 55% ($778 billion) of health spending. The majority of private funding was from employer-sponsored insurance at 64% ($496 billion), self-pay at 26% ($205 billion), and other private funding at 10% ($76 billion) (Levit et al., 2003).

The portion of total health-care spending in the United States financed directly by government is the lowest among developed countries; however, state, federal, and local tax dollars still account for 46% of all health-care expenditures (Levit et al., 2003). Although the United States spends more on health care, measured either per capita or as a percentage of GDP, than any other developed country in the world, the United States has the highest proportion of its citizens with no insurance and ranks near the bottom of this group of developed nations in a number of key health indicators, such as perinatal and maternal mortality, and life expectancy (World Health Organization [WHO], 2003). The weakening economy and increasing cost to consumers for health insurance are expected to increase the number of uninsured individuals.

The Basis of Health Policy in the United States: Health Care as a Right Versus the Free Market

Although there is no legal or statutory "right" to health care in the United States, most of the public sees health care as a "right" (Curran, 1989). One of the main arguments for health care being a "right" is that, like other basic rights, health care and health are a prerequisite to allow citizens some equitable chance at "life, liberty, and the pursuit of happiness" (Daniels, 1985). If health care is a basic human right, like freedom of religion or speech, it can be argued that the public (government) should have a primary role in ensuring that everyone has some measure of equitable access to health care. In this formulation, a key role of government would be to ensure that health care is equitably distributed among its citizens.

Much of the history of health policy in the United States can be seen as a struggle between those who see health care as a right and government as the guarantor of that right, and those who hold that health care is best handled in the "free market" and therefore see most government intervention as either undesirable or actually harmful.

Both traditions have a strong place in U.S. history. Those who hold to the idea of the free market believe that the best means to distribute goods and services (except perhaps defense, fire, and police services) is by an open and direct transaction between those who desire a good or service and those who wish to sell a good or service. Inherent in this belief is that goods and services should be distributed on the basis of willingness and ability to pay a negotiated price. In a market-based economy, government interventions are usually seen as distorting the free market. The most prominent example of the failure to come to a resolution of these opposing forces is the patchwork health-care systems created for different groups in the United States. There are systems fully financed and delivered by the federal government (veterans, active-duty military, and Indian Health Service), a system that is federally financed and privately delivered (Medicare), a system financed by federal and state revenues and privately delivered (Medicaid), systems in which care is largely financed and provided by local government (public and county hospitals and clinics), and, finally, our largest sector, with private financing and delivery (private insurance purchased individually or through an employer) (Table 23-2).

The origins of this patchwork can be traced to public support for legislation covering specific groups who were felt at the time to be especially needy or deserving or for whom the free market did not seem to work well. These groups include the aged, blind, or disabled (Medicare); veterans (Veterans Affairs [VA] health care); active-duty military (Department of Defense); children living in low-income, single-parent families (Medicaid); and Native Americans (Indian Health Service). Although there have been repeated attempts in virtually every decade of this century (most recently in 1994-1995) to enact some level of government-sponsored or mandated health insurance for all citizens, in the end, the fear of federal government control and the tax burden of the very large dollar amounts created by pooling current health expenditures into one program have resulted in a failure to enact universal coverage (Heclo, 1995). It is likely that another effort to enact legislation to address the growing numbers of uninsured will be mounted. The future effort is likely to have broader support than in the past as more middle income families struggle with the cost of health-care premiums.

Public distrust of government, especially at the federal level, has a long history. Indeed, the Constitution includes the phrase "all powers not herein specified are reserved to the states." This distrust has recently led to a shift of some health policy decisions and other public services to the state level. This is known as the "New Federalism movement." A number of states (Hawaii, Minnesota, Washington, and Vermont, among others) have tried to set up state-based programs that would provide insurance coverage to most people who are uninsured. However, these attempts have not been fully successful (Holahan, Weiner, & Wallin, 1998). Thus the United States remains the only economically developed nation that does not have government-financed or mandated health insurance available to all, or nearly all, its citizens (Anderson & Poullier, 1999).

TABLE 23-2	PROGRAMS, FINANCING, AND DELIVERY BASED ON PUBLIC AND PRIVATE BASES		
PROGRAM		**FINANCING**	**SERVICE DELIVERY**
Veterans Administration, military health care, county hospitals		Public	Public
Medicare, Medicaid		Public	Private
Employer or individually purchased insurance		Private	Private

Organizations and Institutions Shaping Health Policy

Formulation of most health policy through law and regulation lies with the executive, legislative, and judicial branches of government at the federal, state, and local levels. Typically the initial formulation of health-care law has resided within the legislative branch, while the role of the executive branch has been to implement those laws through regulation and program development. The judicial branch ensures that laws enacted by the legislative branch are consistent with state or federal constitutions, and that the executive branch follows the wishes of the legislature. Given that the executive and legislative branches can be, and often are, controlled by different parties, health policy reform has often been a major point of conflict between the executive and legislative branches. At the federal level, jurisdiction over health care in Congress is highly fragmented among different committees that oversee the various systems of publicly financed health care. For example, health-related committees in the U.S. Senate include Veterans Affairs (VA program), Armed Services (military), Labor and Human Resources (Public Health Service), and Finance (Medicare and Medicaid).

There are also a large number of nongovernmental groups that attempt to influence health policy. These can be classified as follows (examples in parentheses): provider groups (American Nurses Association), suppliers (Pharmaceutical Research and Manufacturers Association), insurers (Health Insurance Association of America), disease-related interest groups (American Cancer Society), purchasers (National Association of Manufacturers), "the public" (AARP), and groups purporting to represent payors (American Taxpayers Union). Most major health policy issues call forth a remarkable effort on the part of these special interest groups—they engage in direct advertising and mobilize their memberships to do "grassroots" lobbying. The influence they have is determined by many factors, including the size of campaign contributions, their ability to influence elections by "getting out the vote" and mobilizing public opinion, and their capacity to provide critical information to legislators or regulators.

For policies promulgated through laws, the focus of intervention by such groups may come at any point in the process. The intervention may be exerted during the legislative process when the Senate or House writes a bill, as a bill is amended in committee, on the floor, or in House-Senate conference committee meetings. In addition, lobbying groups have an opportunity to influence how legislation is operationalized during the writing of regulations. The regulatory system establishes the rules and guidelines for the implementation of policies. Finally, the judicial system offers another road for influence through a court challenge to some aspect of the law or regulation (Feldstein, 1988).

Examples of APN Involvement in Health Policy

APN influence during the legislative phase of policy development is exemplified in the success of achieving Medicare payment to APNs in 1997. A coalition of nursing organizations influenced key senators and representatives to insert language into the Medicare bill that allowed for direct reimbursement for APN services without requiring physician supervision or restricting the types of visit for which they could be paid. An extensive grassroots effort, during which nursing organizations reached out to members to call and write their Congressional representatives, was highly effective. APNs tracked the legislation throughout the regulatory process to ensure that the intent of Congress was upheld in the regulations. Without careful monitoring of the regulatory phase, gains that were achieved in the legislation phase could have been greatly reduced.

APNs have become politically sophisticated over the past several decades and have exerted considerable influence over health legislation. Although APN organizations have limited funds to invest in lobbying as compared with some other organizations such as the American Medical Association (AMA) and the American Hospital Association (AHA), APN groups have developed the ability to form coalitions to work together targeting specific issues that have a high benefit for practice and patients, rather than having limited input on a broad set of issues. Results of this strategy were seen when certified nurse-midwives (CNMs) obtained Medicaid reimbursement in the 1970s and when nurse practitioners (NPs), clinical nurse specialists (CNSs), and CNMs expanded Medicare reimbursement in 1997.

Nursing has often been accused of not speaking with a unified voice. As APN groups have become more politically adept, the level of comfort and trust has increased in working as a coalition of groups for a common interest and remaining silent, when necessary, if there is not a common interest. During the Clinton Health Reform era, nursing groups of all types came together and developed a strategy to make nursing's health-care agenda integral to the reform plan. Even though the reform act was eventually defeated, the nursing profession proved it could be an influential and unified force in the policy arena.

Professional Practice and Health Policy

Laws and regulations governing who can provide health care have their origins in the early 1900s, with the rise of "professionalism." A profession is usually defined by a set of knowledge and skills acquired through training and education, coupled with a self-generated set of standards and values. The public has been willing to allow individuals from most professions to have a strong influence in promulgating laws that define the level of education required as well as the scope of activities provided within the profession. These laws usually restrict others not educated in a similar manner from practicing that profession.

There is clearly a large degree of trust required between professionals and society to allow this model to flourish. It is helpful to remember that, prior to these laws being established, there were virtually no barriers to anyone practicing in health care. For example, anyone could designate herself or himself a physician or nurse. Over time, each state passed laws that defined and regulated what constitutes the practice of medicine and nursing as well as other professions and who can engage in the practice of these professions. In many states the oversight of these laws, including administrative enforcement, is given over to publicly appointed bodies (such as state nursing or medical boards) whose members are drawn largely from the profession.

Even though barriers to entry into a profession and restrictions as to who may engage in some set of services may protect the public from harm, they also clearly restrict competition and the free market. Although professionalism is still flourishing, there is growing evidence of greater distrust of professionals as self-defining entities, particularly when self-regulation leads to economic advantages at the expense of the public. As time has passed, the courts have created limits on the ability of professionals to use restricted entry into practice, or other means, to restrict competition in health care. Some notable decisions include several preventing fee-setting by professional societies, a decision enjoining the AMA from attacks on chiropractic doctors, and a number of antitrust restrictions on monopolistic practices of hospitals or large physician groups.

Over the opposition of some medical groups, APNs have taken on responsibilities that had previously been the sole prerogative of medicine. By contrast, APNs and physicians have worked together effectively in the clinical area for decades, and some of the strongest supporters of APNs have been physician colleagues. However, economic pressures in the health system together with expanding numbers of physicians and APNs have created tensions, particularly at the level of national organizations. These economic tensions will likely intensify as physician salary and employment choices decrease. The AMA has taken a strong stand and established guidelines for members that facilitate physician con-trol of patient care (AMA, 1995). As recently as 2003, the American Academy of Pediatrics (AAP) has taken a position that APNs must be supervised by pediatricians (AAP, 2003). The paradox about the current context of interprofessional politics is that economic territorialism is occurring simultaneously with the need to develop efficient and effective health-care teams. The renewed impetus to develop health-care teams has been spurred by population-based health care as well as an increased chronic illness burden, each requiring varied expertise in order to deliver effective and efficient care.

THE HEALTH-CARE MARKET AND FINANCE ISSUES

Fundamentally, the health-care market is, like all markets, the interaction among those who use and purchase health care and those who provide health-care services. However, it is a very "distorted" market because of the complexity of financing and the presence of "third parties" in the form of insurers, purchasers, and payors other than the patient. Economists describe a "free" or perfect competitive market by four major characteristics: (1) the presence of a large number of buyers and sellers, (2) the unrestricted mobility of resources that allows easy exit and entry of both suppliers and buyers to the market, (3) a homogeneous (standard) product, and (4) possession of all relevant information by both supplier and buyers. The further a market is from these characteristics, the more imperfect the market, which for some may indicate a greater need for governmental intervention. In considering the health-care market, none of the four characteristics noted is even close to optimal. Although there would seem to be a large number of buyers and suppliers, health care is now purchased by an ever-shrinking number of insurance companies and govern-ment agencies from ever-larger, consolidated hospital systems and larger medical groups. Furthermore, in many emergent situations, or in rural settings, the patient may be able to exercise little or no choice of provider. Professionalism and training, the life-or-death needs for health care in some situations, and the high cost of hospital technology all miti-gate against easy entry and exit. Finally, health care is far from a "standard" product. Large variation is seen throughout the United States in basic procedures such as the rate of cesarean sections, the rate of bypass surgeries, and so on. Most would argue that consumers are not particularly well informed about health-care services. A noted economist, Paul Feldstein, observed years ago that the health-care market is far from perfect, thus produc-ing a need for government intervention (Feldstein, 1988). The question of the type and extent of government intervention has been debated for decades without resolution.

Health-Care Financing

Health-care finance can be best understood as the flow of money from the source of funds to those providing services. In health care, the proximate source of the funds for the provider is often an insurer, or other entity, that collects the dollars and pools the risk for health-care costs. The ultimate source of financing is individuals who earn money, who purchase health care or private insurance directly, who pay taxes that are earmarked for health care, or who forgo some of their earnings/wages in the form of fringe benefits that allow employers to purchase health care on their behalf. An important point is that neither government nor employers are really the source of the funds. Rather, the funding comes from employees who forgo wages to get insurance as a fringe benefit, taxpayers who pay Medicare, and various other state and federal taxes.

In most developed countries there is a dominant system of financing using tax funds with the government acting as insurer and purchaser. In a few instances, such as in Great Britain, the government serves as provider as well. A few other countries, including Germany and the Netherlands, rely primarily on employer-based insurance, but these countries mandate coverage by all employers and provide government-financed insurance for nearly all those not employed. As noted, the financing of health care in the United States is more complex than that in most other countries and uses a combination of direct payment (out-of-pocket expenses) and insurance purchased through fringe benefits by employers or via multiple forms of public (government) insurance.

The most direct means of health-care financing is purchasing and payment by private citizens, as occurs with cosmetic plastic surgery. This type of payment is the norm with non–health-care goods and services. However, as health-care technology evolved, it became obvious that some health-care services were beyond the means of most people to pay directly out of pocket.

TRADITIONAL PRIVATE HEALTH INSURANCE

One of the first examples of private health-care insurance was developed in the 1930s with the creation of Blue Cross. The first Blue Cross plan was started to enable a group of teachers in Texas to pool contributions to an insurance plan to pay for hospital care. Private health insurance expanded rapidly during and after World War II. During World War II there was both a shortage of workers and a government freeze on wages. To retain or attract employees, companies began to offer health insurance as a fringe benefit. Health-care benefits were not only exempt from the wage freeze but, through legislation passed by Congress, were exempt from federal taxes as well. Economic studies show that most workers, except those at very low pay levels, are often willing to trade off some portion of wages for fringe benefits. Their tendency to do so is greatly enhanced by the favorable tax treatment of health insurance. This tax exemption accounts for billions of dollars per year in forgone taxes (Reinhardt, 1993). As with most income tax exemptions, this benefit is realized most by those with higher incomes and, along with employer "payment" of health care, greatly reduces the apparent cost of health care for most employed people.

The concept of insurance as a means to protect against catastrophic events has become distorted in health care by the inclusion of insurance coverage for expenses that are neither rare nor particularly expensive. Insurance coverage for common and relatively inexpensive events such as office visits to a physician or APN do not fit the definition of insurance (rare and costly events) but instead are a form of prepayment of expenses that are likely to be incurred (such as paying one's electric bill in even payments rather than as it varies with seasonal use). The distortion of the health-care market created by insurance, and even more by prepayment, is termed "the moral hazard" of health insurance. This is simply the tendency to overuse (or undervalue) services for which the person consuming the service does not have to pay the full cost. It is helpful in understanding the phrase "moral hazard" to consider how consumers might behave if they "insured" themselves or, more accurately, prepaid and pooled funds for groceries. If groceries were paid for by insurance, most people would probably choose to shop at a high-quality, expensive gourmet grocery store since the cost of the groceries would be paid by "insurance" regardless of the cost. Both insurance and tax subsidies (discussed later) introduce moral hazard by lowering (sometimes to zero) the direct cost of health-care services to the consumer.

Until the mid-1980s, the most common form of health insurance in the United States was "indemnity" insurance. The concept of indemnity is that the insurer agrees to "indemnify" (protect) those who are insured from losses sustained up to some set amount. In classic indemnity insurance (which is nearly nonexistent in health care at present), a person would go to a health-care provider of his or her choice, would pay the provider for the service, and would then file a claim with the insurance company for reimbursement at some preset level. An early modification to indemnity insurance that was quickly adopted by most insurers was the positioning of the insurer as the direct payor of the service provider. This protected the insured individual from having to come up with funds to pay the provider first and allowed the insurance company to negotiate with providers for lower rates based on volume purchasing or other issues negotiated between payor and providers. Note that this introduced a fundamental change in the health-care market. While the consumer of health-care services (the patient) remains the same, the entity that negotiates the price and pays for the service is now an insurance company. This shift, accelerated by the growing consolidation of insurers and the rise of large, often for-profit provider entities (hospitals, physician groups, home care providers, nursing home chains) has been termed by Starr (1982) the "corporatization" of American health care.

Many small to moderate-sized employers offer employees one or more insurance plans that can be purchased as an employment-related fringe benefit, usually along with some additional direct payment by the employee. In this case, the insurance company becomes the "at risk" entity, which means that the insurance company agrees to pay the cost of all covered health-care benefits for enrolled employees. The "risk" is that the premiums paid by the employee and employer may not be sufficient to cover the costs. A growing number of larger employers are "self-insured." This means the company accepts the risk for paying the costs of health-care services covered by the health-care benefits provided by the company. Most self-insured companies use insurance companies to perform such tasks as estimating the probable cost of health benefits (actuarial or risk analysis), overseeing eligibility and enrollment, and management of claims made by providers.

HEALTH MAINTENANCE ORGANIZATIONS

With their roots in traditional indemnity insurance, most health insurance companies saw themselves primarily as actuaries (i.e., predicting how much they would have to pay out) and did not see themselves as directly trying to control costs or utilization or as providing health-care services themselves. A few industries, such as railroads and timber, provided health care directly for their workers as long ago as the late 19th century. These companies hired and paid for their own health-care providers and in some cases built their own hospitals. During World War II, the Kaiser Aluminum Corporation created a company-sponsored health-care plan for its employees. After the war, Kaiser began to offer membership in their plan to other employers and individuals for a set yearly payment. In a similar way, and prior to the war, consumer groups in Washington, DC, and Seattle, Washington, had started "group health cooperatives." Like the Kaiser plan, these consumer-"owned" entities acted as risk pool manager (insurer) but also hired health-care providers, including physicians, to care for people who joined the cooperative. Membership was defined by a yearly "membership" payment. Kaiser and the two consumer cooperative health plans were termed "prepaid health plans". When the Nixon administration and Congress created a government incentive program to encourage the creation of similar organizations elsewhere in the country as a potential cost-controlling approach, the new organizations were termed "health maintenance organizations (HMOs)." The basic concept was that, for some predetermined "prepaid" premium, the health plan itself would provide all needed care directly by an employed health-care staff (thus the designation *staff-model HMO*). Later forms of HMOs moved away from the staff model to insurers that contracted with one or a small number of organized medical groups and, later, large open networks of providers via contractual relationships (network or independent practice association "IPA" models). The critical difference, when compared with more traditional health insurance, is that HMOs worked actively to influence the cost, utilization, and quality of health care provided to their members, in addition to their actuarial and risk pool management functions as insurers. HMOs were much more aggressive than traditional insurers in competitive contracting with a limited group of providers, reducing prices paid for services, and intervening in the process of health care to try to reduce utilization or improve quality. As HMOs evolved from staff and group models to individual practice associations and point of service plans (plans in which a person can choose any provider but pays more to do so), and traditional insurers began to implement fee schedules and utilization management and create "preferred provider organizations" (PPOs), the distinction between HMOs and other insurers blurred under the term "managed care." In many regards, all care is now "managed care" since only classic indemnity insurance does not try to affect provider utilization or payment.

PUBLIC FINANCING

A final form of health-care financing that is dominant in all other developed countries is publicly financed health care through taxation by government. Unlike private insurance, public funding for health care nearly always involves coverage for some people who cannot afford to purchase private health-care insurance on their own. For public (government-financed) programs, the source of funds is taxpayers, with the government serving as funds collector, manager, and payor (as in the traditional Medicare and Medicaid programs). The government may also serve as purchaser (as with the Medicare+ Choice program) or as funds collector, manager, and provider, as for active-duty military through the Department of Defense, for military veterans through the VA, or for Native Americans through the Indian Health Service. The advantages of public financing include lower administrative costs, creation of the largest possible risk pool, and maximal equity in the quality and accessibility of health care. Finally, as noted earlier, one of the largest and often least noted sectors of public financing of health care is the tax subsidy provided by the tax-exempt status of private health-care insurance that is purchased directly or provided as a fringe benefit of employment.

Reimbursement

Reimbursement is simply the way those who purchase health-care services pay those who provide services. Payment in health care is complicated by the fact that, presently, the payor is most often not the person who receives the services but rather an insurance company. Historically, indemnity insurers reimbursed the insured individual a set amount for any service that was covered by the insurance plan. The patient could go to any provider who was defined in the insurance contract as qualified to deliver the service. *Qualification* was usually defined as anyone licensed as a specific type of provider. The patient, not the insurance company, paid the provider the amount charged, and then would file a claim with the insurer and receive the amount defined in the insurance contract. The amount received by the patient could be more, the same, or less than the amount charged by the provider.

With the emergence of the insurer as active purchaser rather than as passive payor, insurers began to restrict reimbursement to those providers who signed an agreement or contract with the insurer. These contracts defined the terms and often the level of reimbursement provided by the insurer. This trend was greatly accelerated by the emergence of HMOs and "managed care." In addition to limits on whom they would pay, insurers moved to directly pay providers based on one of the following: the amount charged by the provider (fee for service [FFS]), a set level of reimbursement set by the insurer (fee schedule), or a capitation payment (per-member-per-month payment, regardless of the services provided). It is vital for APNs to understand and monitor reimbursement, particularly because of their ability to be directly reimbursed by Medicare and Medicaid (for some APNs). As APNs become recognized providers and contract directly with managed care organizations, it is critical that they understand payment mechanisms.

CHARGE OR COST-BASED FEE FOR SERVICE

In the simplest form of FFS reimbursement, the provider sets a price (charge) for a defined service provided to a patient, and the patient pays that amount. This is the way that we pay for most goods and services. As insurers attempted to control costs and to pay providers directly, more complex variations of FFS arrangements were developed. The most common of these arrangements bases the amount that the insurer reimburses either the patient or the provider for a given service on the lesser of the "actual, customary, prevailing, or reasonable" charge (Table 23-3). The actual charge is the amount on the bill from the provider; the customary charge is the average charge that the same provider charged for the same service in the past (usually over a 1-year period); the prevailing charge is some percentage of the average charge for all providers in a given area for the specific service; and reasonable charge is the amount determined by the insurer to be "reasonable" for the service.

The proportion of reimbursement based on FFS has been steadily declining, especially with the enactment of the Medicare fee schedule for physicians. Some large insurers and, by definition, preferred provider organizations (PPO) negotiate a discount on what the provider usually charges. This is termed "discounted FFS" and can take the form of a fixed percentage reduction of the charges. An example of the discounted FFS is a PPO group in

TABLE 23-3	TRADITIONAL PAYMENT METHODS		
ACTUAL	CUSTOMARY	PREVAILING	REASONABLE
Amount on the bill from the provider	Average charge of provider for the same service in the past (usually averaged over a year)	A percentage of the average charge for all providers in a given area for a specific service	Amount determined by insurer to be "reasonable" for the service

which an insurer negotiates a special discounted rate with a specific provider group who is willing to accept the discounted payment.

APNs have had limited success in gaining access to FFS reimbursement. Much of the reason for this was timing. Just as APNs gained enough influence and political strength to be recognized by insurers, there was a shift away from the traditional FFS reimbursement.

A variation of charge-based reimbursement is cost-based reimbursement, which has been used for payment to hospitals. In cost-based reimbursement, the provider and insurer negotiate a contract in which the provider is reimbursed the "allowable costs" of producing a service. The contract defines what costs are "allowable" or considered to be legitimate costs of producing the service. Until recently, cost-based reimbursement was used extensively by Medicare and some private insurers to pay hospitals, nursing homes, and home care providers. Very few insurers now pay on the basis of cost-based reimbursement.

FEE SCHEDULES

A fee schedule is when the price paid for a single service or group of services ("bundled services") is determined in advance by the insurer. This is often done in negotiation with providers. However, the critical difference between this and FFS reimbursement is that the insurer, not the provider, has the final say in setting the reimbursement. The fee schedule may be developed based on some percentage of historical charges or costs or on an analysis of the work and expenses that go into producing a given service, as with the Medicare resource-based relative value scale. In the case of Medicare and most other insurers at this time, providers must sign an agreement to accept the fee schedule, in most cases as full payment, if they want to be reimbursed by Medicare for seeing the patient. Patients who obtain services from providers who are not under contact with the patient's insurer will usually have to pay for those services themselves. Most health plans, most notably Medicare, either limit or altogether forbid (through contract or, in Medicare, through statutory law) the provider from charging the patient the difference between what the provider "charges" to patients paying FFS and the fee schedule amount. Payments under Medicare's various "prospective payment" programs (hospitals, skilled nursing facilities, and most recently home care services) are basically variants of a fee schedule developed using a fraction of historical costs as the basis of paying for the service. A per diem payment—that is, a set amount per day of services—is also, in effect, a type of fee schedule.

Unlike FFS, APNs have made considerable inroads into reimbursement under fee schedules. As with reimbursement for physicians, APN reimbursement under Medicare and Medicaid is through a fee schedule. APNs are paid a set percentage of the fee that a physician receives. For instance, CNSs and NPs eligible for Medicare reimbursement receive 85% of the physician rate if billing independently or 100% if the billing is "incident to" a physician visit. The policy dilemma for APNs is whether to politically position themselves as "cost-effective" providers and continue to accept 85% of an already-low reimbursement rate, or push to get 100% of the physician rate based on the premise that the same or a very comparable service is provided.

CAPITATION

Just as a fee schedule changes the control of reimbursement from the provider to the insurer, capitation changes the locus of financial risk from the insurance company to the provider entity that accepts capitation. With capitation, providers are paid a negotiated amount per member per month or per year. For that fixed amount, the provider agrees to provide all necessary health-care services that are covered by the insurance benefit and specified in the provider's capitation contract. Capitation can cover total or limited services (as for primary care, specialty care, or hospital care only). Because of the risk of adverse selection (i.e., getting patients who require more services than average), providers cannot afford to accept full risk capitation unless they are part of a large group.

The fundamental challenge to APNs under the capitation reimbursement mechanism is to be a recognized provider who can contract with a managed care entity or be accepted as part of a group practice. In either situation, APNs need to fully assess the financial risk associated with capitation. For primary-care-only capitation, there is a lower risk of financial losses from adverse selection, and it may be possible for individual or groups of APNs to negotiate capitation contracts with HMOs.

SALARY

In addition to these three mechanisms of reimbursement, providers may be salaried. Although this is a relatively new phenomenon for physicians, it has been the standard form of payment for most APNs. Thus, while a provider or provider group may be reimbursed via a mix of capitation, FFS, and fee schedule, the individual providers may pay themselves or be paid a salary or a salary plus incentive based on charges or resource-based relative value units (RBRVUs) generated. RBRVU was implemented by Medicare in 1992 to replace the customary, prevailing, and reasonable charges. It is a payment calculation derived from the "relative value" of services provided and the resources those services consume. The components of the relative value are as follows: amount of health-care provider work that goes into a service, the practice expense associated with the service, and the professional liability expense associated with the service. The relative value of each service is adjusted by a Geographic Practice Cost Index (GPCI) for each Medicare locality.

ETHICAL ISSUES RELATED TO REIMBURSEMENT

Each form of reimbursement introduces certain economic and ethical issues. In FFS or charge-based reimbursement, providers can set prices at whatever level they choose, which is the way most businesses operate. Although this is the way most non-health-care markets operate, FFS tends to result in overuse of health-care services and high costs. Like FFS, cost-based reimbursement results in high costs because there is no incentive for the provider to keep costs down. In these modes of reimbursement, the economic interest of the provider is to maximize the price, or allowed cost, and the number of services provided.

With a fee schedule, salary with incentives, billings, RBRVUs, or net revenues, there are economic incentives for providers to minimize the costs of producing the service while still providing as many services as possible. This method of payment has been shown to encourage providers to supply services that are of small or, in some cases, of no benefit to the patient. With capitation, or a salary plus incentives based on controlling utilization of services, providers have an incentive to minimize both the cost of producing a given service and the number of services. This creates the pressure for providers to withhold services that may be of substantial benefit to the patient. An example of this situation is failure of a physician to order a diagnostic test that may be expensive. Finally, when providers are paid a salary, there is no direct incentive related to the number or price of services provided to a given patient. However, salary also removes any incentive to increase productivity or provide services quickly and efficiently. In many group practices, whether dependent on fee schedules or capitation, providers are often paid by salary, plus or minus some incentives or risk pools. Even where pure salary is used, the provider's salary is ultimately affected by the balance of practice revenues and practice expenses.

From the patient's perspective, it would be most desirable to get the maximum number of useful services at the lowest cost. If the patient's insurance fully pays, with no out-of-pocket payments, there is a strong incentive for the patient to use services that may be of very small benefit. For the taxpayer in public programs or the insurer and employees who pay for private insurance, the goal is to try to pay for only those services that are essential and at the lowest possible overall cost. The ethical dilemmas raised by different types of reimbursement arise where the interests of the provider, the patient, the insurer, and those who pay for insurance are in conflict. Thus each mode of reimbursement presents the patient, provider, and insurer-financier with ethical dilemmas. In FFS the challenge is for the provider and patient not to oversupply and overuse services; in capitation, it is for the provider not to withhold needed services.

Cost and Cost Containment

The total expenditures on health care as a percentage of all goods and services (the GDP) have been growing in the United States throughout the 20th century. Since the 1950s, with the widespread introduction of insurance for most Americans and the acceleration of health-care technology development, health-care cost increases have pushed the proportion of GDP devoted to health care to nearly 15%.

Most studies of health-care cost increases have found that there are three major factors driving the rise in health-care costs relative to GDP or general inflation (Newhouse, 1993). While these factors were identified a decade ago, they are even more relevant today. These factors are technology, demographics (growth and aging of the population), and health-care price inflation. The most powerful factor, accounting for well over half of the cost increase, is the ever-growing use of health-care technology. In U.S. society, there is a very high value on individual autonomy, which adds to the imperative in health care to do "everything possible." In addition, the use of insurance and tax exemptions means that the person receiving the services does not see the total cost of the service, further driving the use of technology.

In addition, with more effective treatments that create little risk for the patient, problems such as hypertension, hypercholesterolemia, impotence, and infertility are constantly redefined to include everyone with a low level of risk or with slight functional declines, rather than a more narrowly defined group with an identified disease or markedly impaired function. Artificial joints, laser eye surgery, laparoscopic surgery, and virtually risk-free diagnostic procedures, such as magnetic resonance imaging, constantly lower the risk-benefit barriers of diagnostic and therapeutic interventions. This removal of patient risk as a barrier to using technology, along with insurance and tax exemptions, gives rise to increased use of technology, including procedures that are very expensive and provide limited benefit in prolonging life or enhancing the quality of life. An example is the total body scan offered in many cities. This diagnostic technology is being promoted as the means to early detection of a variety of diseases, including colon cancer and heart disease, yet is largely unproven in terms of cost/benefit. Moreover, most technologies do not totally replace existing ones but are simply added to existing procedures, thus increasing total cost.

Those interventions that do prolong life exacerbate another major factor leading to higher health-care costs, namely population growth and the aging of the population. Between 1900 and 1960, average life expectancy rose from 45 years to nearly 70 years, and between 1960 and the present, life expectancy has risen from 70 to 78 years. The most rapidly growing portion of the population is people over 85 years. In addition to longer survival rates, people are also living longer with major disease and disability, which further adds to cost.

Another major factor driving escalating health-care costs is that price increases for health care have in most years exceeded price increases in other sectors of the economy. Prices charged for a defined service, such as an office visit, rose faster than GDP or general inflation, especially in the period from 1950 to 1975. The spread of insurance and the enactment of Medicare, with their use of FFS and cost-based reimbursement, contributed to the rise in inflation. Again, however, technology played a role because what was being delivered as part of a unit of service (e.g., an emergency room visit for a person with a myocardial infarction) was modified by new technologies. Many of these new technologies, such as the use of tissue plasminogen activators, not only add costs directly but may require the use of more highly trained, and often more costly, personnel to deliver the technology. Thus the cost of producing and the price charged for a "standard" unit of service, such as the emergency room visit, are increased.

There have been numerous attempts to try to reduce the rate of increase of health-care costs, most of which have totally failed. Even those that appear to have had some impact have only provided a brief, usually one-time reduction. The reasons that health-care costs are so difficult to control include the moral hazard of insurance, with its disconnect between the benefits received by the patient and the perceived cost; our society's drive to prolong life regardless of the cost (the rescue mentality); ample public financing of basic research and technology development (most notably through the National Institutes of Health); our fascination with technology; a strong history of focus on the individual; and, until recently, a relative undersupply of providers in the face of failure of market forces to control prices.

Some of the mechanisms by which government and private insurers attempt to control costs have included payment and market reforms, utilization management strategies, and shifting costs to reduce demand (Box 23-1). All of these interventions have been present in the health-care market for the past decade or more, many of them under the general title of "managed care." Although medical sector cost inflation has been affected at times, especially by some of the payment and market reforms, health-care costs have, in most years, continued to rise 1% to 3% faster annually than either general inflation or the GDP. The various pronouncements that health-care inflation has been tamed have proved to be untrue. While in 1996-1997, health-care costs actually rose less rapidly than other costs or GDP (Health Care Financing Administration [HCFA], 1998), in the past 3 years there has been rapid growth in health-care costs at a time of low inflation and slow growth in the GDP (Heffler et al., 2003). Taming the increase in health-care technology has been thus far unsuccessful. The double-digit rise in the cost of pharmaceuticals in the past 4 years, and of hospital costs in the last two years, is just one manifestation of this seemingly uncontrollable sector. Short of a major economic depression or adoption of national health insurance with a set budget, health-care costs appear to be destined to continue to rise faster than inflation or GDP for the foreseeable future.

ACCESS

Access to care has been a major policy issue for many years. It is of growing concern and, along with concern about rising costs, was a key factor that drove the health-care reform initiative during the early years of the Clinton administration. Concern about access has

---

BOX 23-1 • SUMMARY OF COST CONTROL STRATEGIES

Payment Reforms
- Imposition of fee schedules instead of cost-based reimbursement (Medicare's Prospective Payment System [PPS] for hospitals and Resource Based Relative Value System (RBRVS) fee schedule for doctors)
- Limiting total increases in PPS and RBRVS to some index of inflation or GDP and reducing the fee schedule rates if volume increases occur
- Use of capitation payments to give providers incentive to reduce both costs and volume of services as well as to cap total expenditures

Market Reforms
- Mergers that increase the relative economic power of insurers to set price
- Contracting only with selected providers who agree to lower fees
- Competitive contracting (bidding out services to the lowest bidder)
- Profiling providers on the basis of utilization and price (total cost) and eliminating the high-cost provider from the plan
- Use of a specific group rating instead of community rating (charging an enrolled group a premium based on the specific group's risks and utilization, rather than on the average risk and utilization in the community as a whole)

Utilization Management
- Requiring second opinions for expensive services such as surgery
- Concurrent and retrospective reviews resulting in denial or payments
- Guidelines, case management, disease management, and other attempts to change the way medicine is practiced

Reducing Demand by Shifting Costs to Consumers
- Higher co-pays
- Higher deductibles
- Higher self-pay premiums
- Excluding services (contraception, transplants, infertility services)

---

been significant during times of economic prosperity and has become of even greater concern with the current downturn in the economy and rising health-care costs. Access to health care is a complicated issue. Barriers to access are related to a number of factors, including inability to pay for health care, as well as lack of availability of specific types of health-care providers or institutions, and potentially in some cases because of provider bias toward special populations, such as minorities (IOM, 2002). It can be argued that health care is inaccessible if it is not available within a geographically convenient area for a specific type of provider, such as a CNM or NP, or if patient and provider do not share a common cultural background, values, and language. There is an increasing body of empiric evidence that links reduced access to care to a lack of insurance. The number of uninsured in 2002 is estimated to be 41.2 million people (14.6% of the population), representing an increase of 1.4 million since 2001. Among the 41.2 million uninsured, there are 8.5 million children (U.S. Census Bureau, 2002). Of the total number of uninsured, nearly 20 million are non-Hispanic white, 12.4 million are Hispanic, 6.8 million are black, and 2.3 million are Asian and Pacific Islander (U.S. Census Bureau, 2002).

Lack of access has been operationally defined by several measures. The most traditional measure is the number of uninsured individuals. Individuals are considered uninsured if they have no insurance coverage, through either employer-sponsored insurance or public safety net programs such as Medicare or Medicaid. It is important to note that some uninsured may be eligible for coverage through a safety net program but, for many reasons, do not apply. Additional measures include the number of individuals unable to obtain care, the number of emergency room visits for nonemergent care, and reports of fair or poor health with no physician visits in the past year (Berk & Schur, 1998). The Institute of Medicine (2002) identified a number of health consequences of being uninsured:

- Uninsured with chronic illness are less likely to receive appropriate care
- Uninsured with diabetes are less likely to receive recommended services
- Uninsured with HIV are less likely to receive highly effective medications
- Uninsured with end-stage renal disease begin dialysis with more severe disease
- Uninsured are less likely to receive preventive and screening services
- Uninsured cancer patients are in poorer health and more likely to die prematurely because of a delay in diagnosis

APNs have been a forceful voice to ensure access to comprehensive care. Access concerns by APNs are linked to the roots of advanced practice nursing. APN roles largely developed as a policy response to access problems for those in rural and other underserved areas. Much of the focus of the Department of Health and Human Services' (DHHS') Division of Nursing, which implements the funds appropriated by Congress to support nursing education and special projects through Title VIII of the Nurse Practice Act, has been to support programs that increase the number of APNs in order to enhance access.

AFFORDABILITY

The rise in health-care costs, coupled with a stagnating economy, has created significant problems in the affordability of health care for many people in the United States. Although the public perception has been that the uninsured are individuals who did not want to work, most studies show that the majority of uninsured individuals work either full- or part-time, and often in multiple jobs. Eight out of ten uninsured are from working families. Two thirds of uninsured families earn less than 200% of the Federal poverty level, about $35,000 for a family of four (DHHS, 2003). The estimated cost of caring for the uninsured is between $34 and $38 billion dollars per year (IOM, 2002).

Several reasons (in addition to the state of the economy) have been advanced for the increased numbers of uninsured people, including a change in immigration patterns, a shift in employment to small firms or self-employment, and, most important, the growing cost of health care. Kronick and Gilmore (1999) proposed that the rise in the uninsured is related more to rising health-care expenditures making insurance unaffordable for increasing numbers of workers, even when it is offered by their employers, and the shift to group rating from community rating by insurance companies. The group rating may narrow the pool of people on which insurance premiums are calculated, and if one person in a small group has high health-care costs, the premiums in that firm may be double or triple the rates of other similar companies. Thorpe and Florence (1999) found that a growing number of workers cite as their reason for refusing coverage the high cost of their employee contribution for insurance. As a result of this and reductions in Medicaid and other safety net programs, the number of people uninsured and underinsured will likely grow during hard economic times.

It is important to understand the profile of individuals who are uninsured. Because Medicare covers nearly all Americans 65 years and older, most uninsured are under 65. The likelihood of being uninsured increases if one works for a small business (fewer than 100 employees), is self-employed or a temporary worker, or is an employee in a low-wage firm (Gabel, Hurst, Whitmore, & Hoffman, 1999). Collins, Schoen, Colasonto, and Downey (2003) noted that low-wage workers are less likely to work in companies that offer health insurance; if they do work in companies offering coverage, they are less likely to be eligible for health insurance benefits, and if they are eligible, the cost is prohibitive. However, the major reason that low-wage workers do not have health insurance is that small employers do not offer it.

Lack of insurance is a major factor limiting access to and use of health services. However, there is substantial reason to be concerned also about the population who are "underinsured." Although there is no clear definition of what "underinsured" is, being underinsured relates to the degree of financial exposure for the care of illness. One measure of underinsured is out-of-pocket expenses exceeding 10% of family income for a serious illness. Using this measure, Short and Banthin (1995) estimated that 18.5% of the population, or nearly 40 million people, were underinsured.

State and federal government-sponsored programs have been the backbone of providing access to care for those who otherwise could not financially afford insurance. The federal programs include Medicare and the VA; federal-state programs include Medicaid and the Child Health Initiative Program.

Medicare

PROGRAM DESCRIPTION

Medicare was enacted in 1965 to provide health coverage to individuals over 65 years of age and to those who are blind or disabled. Many at the time considered Medicare as the first step to providing universal health insurance coverage, starting with a specific group (the elderly, blind, and disabled) of whom many were poor (nearly 20% under the poverty level at the time) and who had relatively high health-care costs. Although the expansion to other groups (with the exception of those with kidney failure) has not occurred, Medicare now covers approximately 41 million Americans with a total expenditure in 2002 of $266 billion (Centers for Medicare and Medicaid [CMS], 2003a). Medicare Part A, primarily funded from a payroll tax as a special part of the Social Security Tax, covers hospital stays, skilled nursing facilities, home health care, hospice care, and certain products. Part B, funded from general tax revenues (75%) and premiums paid by enrollees (25%), which had been $54/month in 2002, covers most costs of physician and APN visits; outpatient medical and surgical services; supplies; physical, occupational, and speech therapies; diagnostic tests; and durable medical equipment. Part B also covers outpatient clinical laboratory services, home health care (if the individual is not covered by Part A), and outpatient hospital services and blood products (as an outpatient) (Table 23-4). Medicare expenditures represented 2.6% of GDP in 2002, a figure that is expected to rise as a percent of GDP over the next several decades. An increasing portion of payment for Medicare will likely come from beneficiary premiums and general revenues and less from payroll taxes (Board of Trustees of the Federal Hospital Insurance and Supplemental Insurance Trust Funds, 2003).

Even though Medicare provides coverage for a broad array of services, individuals with Medicare coverage can experience considerable out-of-pocket expenses as a result of co-payment and deductible costs and the costs of noncovered services, such as long-term care and pharmaceuticals. Other products and services not included are eyeglasses, most dental care, hearing aids, and routine eye exams.

Although nearly 80% of Medicare recipients have additional coverage through private Medicare supplemental insurance or Medicaid, few of the private insurers cover

TABLE 23-4 MEDICARE-COVERED SERVICES	
PART A	PART B
Hospitalization, including semiprivate room, meals, and general nursing	Medical expenses, including physician and APN services; inpatient and outpatient medical and surgical services; occupational, physical, and speech therapy; diagnostic tests, and durable medical equipment
Skilled nursing facility, including semiprivate room, meals, skilled nursing and rehabilitative services	Clinical laboratory services, including blood tests, VA, and others
Home health care, including intermittent skilled nursing, physical therapy, speech-language services, home health aide services, and durable medical equipment	Home health care (if patient does not have Part A)
Hospice (including pain) and support relief, home care, inpatient care	Outpatient hospital services for diagnosis or treatment of an illness or injury
Blood during a hospital or skilled transfusion facility stay	Blood transfusion as an outpatient

long-term care or pharmaceuticals. Thus a substantial number of Medicare enrollees are underinsured relative to their personal financial risk. These uncovered costs can be catastrophic for elderly individuals and couples. The cost of a hospital stay followed by a period of rehabilitation, along with home care costs and drug costs, can be financially devastating. For instance, the out-of-pocket expenses related to stroke may easily exceed $10,000 in the first year. These costs include the hospital co-pay, the co-pay on the first 100 days of skilled nursing care and the full costs (often more than $300 per day) for each skilled nursing home day thereafter, the full costs of drugs outside the hospital, and the 20% co-pay for all outpatient physician or APN care and durable medical equipment, such as a wheelchair, that may be needed. Individuals experiencing prolonged stays in skilled nursing facilities with recurrent hospitalizations can also exhaust their Medicare hospital benefits, resulting in expenses that can overwhelm all but the very wealthy.

As noted previously, many older persons purchase supplemental private insurance known as Medigap Supplemental Insurance. These policies are designed to pay primarily for the deductibles, co-pays, and long hospital stays not covered by Medicare. Medigap policies are regulated by federal and state governments and grouped into 10 "standard" policies, each offering a slightly different combination of benefits (CMS, 2003b). Most of these policies cost $3500 or more a year, and individuals must purchase them from personal funds. Elderly and disabled individuals with severe illness and low incomes cannot afford this expense, and, as noted, few of these policies cover long-term care or pharmaceuticals. The CMS offers a Medigap Compare tool to help beneficiaries find insurance companies in their locale that offer Medigap policies. The website to visit for further information is www.cms.hhs.gov/MGCompare/home.asp.

Medicare coverage for pharmaceuticals has been frequently considered and debated since the program's inception in 1965. A Medicare drug benefit was actually enacted as part of the "Catastrophic Coverage Act of 1987" but was repealed the following year largely because of fears of its impact on higher taxes and of government control of pharmaceuticals. While legislators are anxious to meet the needs of a group of citizens with a powerful lobby machine and who comprise a formidable voting block, concern about cost implications has kept a bill from passing. The cost of the most recent drug benefit proposal is $200 billion over 10 years. Critics of Medicare's failure to provide a drug benefit cite numerous anecdotes of individuals who experience an acute illness because they were not able to pay for the prescriptions that would prevent or treat the illness. The politics surrounding this issue are complex and involve potential conflict with the pharmaceutical companies.

MEDICARE FINANCING

Much of the current policy debate about Medicare centers on the viability of Medicare Part A, which is funded through the Medicare Trust Fund. The Trust Fund receives revenues from the Medicare part of the Social Security Tax, which are then used to pay expenses of Medicare Part A. Projections of the viability of Part A of Medicare are based on the balance between the rate of future expenditures and anticipated revenues. The projections are very dependent on both the anticipated rate of growth of health-care expenditures and on employment, which determines payments into the Medicare Trust Fund as well as general tax revenues. Prior to changes made in the program in 1997, even the most optimistic projections predicted that the Trust Fund would be depleted in the early years of the 21st century. Expenditures in Part B of Medicare, which is funded largely from general federal tax funds (mostly income tax revenues), have become one of the largest single federal expenditures. Concerns about the viability of the Part A Trust Fund and the drain on general revenues by Part B have led Congress to enact a steady stream of mostly ineffective cost-control measures.

The political pressures surrounding changes in the Medicare program are considerable, with the more than 41 million persons who benefit from the program pushing for benefit expansion and with those who pay Social Security and income taxes in favor of holding costs down. Given these political pressures and the lack of effective ways of controlling costs, policy makers have focused most of the changes on trying to control expenditures by changing reimbursement procedures from cost or FFS to fees that can be controlled by Medicare. The evolution of hospital payments from cost-based reimbursement to prospective payment using diagnosis-related groups (DRGs) and of physician payments from FFS to a fee schedule based on RBRVUs are two changes that were enacted in the 1980s and early 1990s that illustrate this trend. The 1997 Balanced Budget Act (BBA) removed the remaining cost-based reimbursements and extended prospective payment to skilled nursing facilities, hospital outpatient settings, home care, and rehabilitation hospitals, as well as reducing the rate of increase of prospective payment and RBRVU-based payments to physicians and hospitals. The current Medicare fee schedule payment to APNs represents an example of how pressure to allow APNs to bill directly was combined with a cost-control measure.

Attempts to control expenditures through limiting Medicare benefits, requiring higher-income elderly to pay higher premiums for Part B, or any other measure directed at recipients have met strong opposition from politically active elders. President Bush floated an option to offer a drug benefit to those enrolling in managed care plans. After much criticism from groups representing the elder constituency, he backed away from that proposal. Efforts to link the Part B premium paid by recipients to 25% of total program costs and to limit skilled nursing and home care benefits with restrictions on prior hospital stays are just two types of measures that have been enacted to control costs on the recipient side.

The decision to cut provider rates has had significant consequences. Many hospitals, particularly academic health centers and hospitals providing care to uninsured populations, are experiencing severe financial difficulty. Health plans are choosing to scale back or eliminate their Medicare + choice options. Actual and proposed Medicare cuts to primary care physicians have created significant financial hardship, leading many physicians to refuse any new Medicare patients and to lobby CMS and Congress to roll back the cuts. CMS recognized that there was an error in their calculations, resulting in bigger cuts than should have been instituted. The error was acknowledged, and a cut to be instituted in January 2003 was rescinded. APNs need to be knowledgeable about changes in Medicare in order to know how efforts to control costs may affect the financial viability of practice. Updates on changes in Medicare can be obtained at www.cms.hhs.gov/medicare. In addition, the administrator of CMS has instituted an Open Door Forum for providers and one specifically for nursing and allied health. Times to meet and give comment about CMS policies and procedures have been established (CMS, 2003c). APNs can also e-mail questions directly to CMS. To access information go to www.cms.hhs.gov/opendoor/physicians-nurses-alliedhealth.asp.

Medicaid

The Medicaid program was enacted in 1965 as Title XIX (along with Medicare, which is Title XVIII) of the Social Security Act. In 2002, 47 million low-income or needy individuals were covered by Medicaid, including children; the aged, blind, and/or disabled; and those eligible to receive federally assisted income maintenance programs (CMS, 2003d). Medicaid provides health insurance coverage for certain groups of individuals and families with specified levels of low income and assets. It is a program funded jointly by the states and the federal government. The formula used to determine the state contribution is based on the average per capita income of the state. Thus, states with low per capita income contribute less than the 50% maximal match required of wealthier states.

Although the federal government through intermediaries, carriers, and other contractors administers Medicare, Medicaid is administered by individual states, with substantial latitude in terms of eligibility standards, scope of service, payment rates, and the administering entities. States have some discretion in determining eligibility requirements, but there are some groups that states must offer coverage to in order to get federal matching dollars. These mandated groups include U.S. citizens who are

- In families who meet requirements that previously applied to the Aid to Families with Dependent Children (AFDC) program
- Recipients of Supplemental Security Income (SSI)
- Infants born to Medicaid-eligible mothers
- Children below the age of 6 and pregnant women who meet the state's earlier AFDC financial requirements or whose family income is at or below 133% of the federal poverty level
- All children up to age 19 born after September 30, 1983, in families with incomes at or below the federal poverty level
- Medicare beneficiaries who meet Medicaid income and asset restrictions

Note that people eligible for Medicaid must both meet the income/asset tests *and* be a member of one of the defined groups. In addition, with the loss of automatic enrollment linked to cash assistance programs such as ADFC, many low-income people do not apply for Medicaid coverage until they are hospitalized or have some other major health need.

Within the broad national guidelines noted above, states can establish their own eligibility standards; determine types, amount, duration, and scope of services; set payment rates for services; and administer its own program. States have the option of providing Medicaid coverage to other "categorically needy" groups. Eligibility criteria applicable to all states for these groups are more flexible than the mandatory groups—for example, infants up to 1 year and pregnant women whose family income is up to 185% of the poverty level are eligible. In addition, states have the option to have a "medically needy" program to extend coverage to individuals who have too much income to qualify under the mandatory or optional categorically needy groups but who have high medical care costs. This medically needy option allows individuals to "spend down" to Medicaid eligibility by incurring medical care expenses to offset their excess income. An example is an individual entering a nursing facility with income and assets in excess of Medicaid limits but who, after paying for nursing home care for a period of time, depletes his or her assets and has an income that is less than the cost of the nursing home plus the Medicaid income limit. If the state offers a "medically needy" program under Medicaid (and 38 states do so), the remainder of the nursing home stay may be covered under Medicaid. (Table 23-5 provides a summary of Medicaid services.)

The Medicaid program is often thought to cover poor children. In fact, attempts to cut Medicaid costs have often been based on reducing "abuse" in the system by welfare

TABLE 23-5 MEDICAID SERVICES		
REQUIRED FOR CATEGORICALLY NEEDY	REQUIRED FOR MEDICALLY NEEDY	FEDERALLY FUNDED COMMON OPTIONAL SERVICES
Inpatient hospital	Prenatal care and delivery services	Clinic services
Outpatient hospital	Ambulatory services to individuals under age 18	Nursing facility services for individuals under age 21
Physician services	Home health services to individuals entitled to nursing facility services	Intermediate care facility/ mental retardation services
Medical and surgical dental services		Optometrist services and eyeglasses
Nursing facility for individuals age 21 and over		Prescribed drugs
Home health care for those eligible for nursing facility		Tuberculosis (TB)-related services for TB-infected individuals
Family planning services and supplies		Prosthetic devices
Rural health clinic services		
Laboratory and x-ray		Dental services
Pediatric and family NP services		
Federally qualified health center services		
Nurse-midwifery services		
Early and periodic screening, diagnosis, and treatment for individuals under age 21		

mothers. However, approximately 70% of enrollees are children and nondisabled adults, but two thirds of spending goes to the elderly and disabled (Weil, 2003). A 1996 comparison of Medicaid payment by age of recipients show that those 85+ years received $12,169 per year while those 0 to 5 years received services valued at $1406 per year (HCFA, 1998).

Policymakers have pursued a variety of strategies to contain the cost of Medicaid, mostly focused on the nonelderly portion of the program. States have looked to managed care to help control some costs. In 1991, 9.5% of Medicaid enrollees were in a managed care plan. In 2002, more than 58% of (nonelderly) Medicaid beneficiaries were enrolled in managed care arrangements (Hurley & Somers, 2003). In a number of states, movement of Medicaid enrollees to managed care has been beset by problems of disenrollment, loss of Medicaid eligibility, and failure of those enrolled to understand HMO restrictions on use of non-HMO resources, such as the continued use of emergency rooms in public hospitals. In this situation, the HMO receives the payment for providing care, but the public hospital provides the care with no HMO reimbursement.

Because of the federal match, many states have tried to expand Medicaid programs, which can substitute for programs that are fully state funded. This tendency has been a factor that has increased the cost of Medicaid at the federal level.

However, the federal government has also created ways to limit expense. An example is the enactment of the Welfare Reform Act in 1996. Prior to enactment of this bill, enrollment in Medicaid was automatic for persons receiving cash assistance under a number of federal low-income assistance programs, most notably AFDC, which was abolished by the Welfare Reform Act. The de-linking of Medicaid enrollment from cash assistance programs such as AFDC has resulted in substantial decreases in the number of low-income nonelderly enrolled in Medicaid. In addition, the Welfare Reform Act prohibited states from enrolling noncitizens in Medicaid other than in very limited situations.

The weakened economy and resultant high unemployment has increased the number of unemployed workers, thus increasing the potential number of Medicaid recipients. As states continue to struggle to balance their budgets, efforts to control costs will likely be focused on increasing eligibility requirements to limit the number of enrollees or decrease the benefits, or both.

Currently, only specific groups of APNs are eligible for Medicaid reimbursement. These groups include pediatric NPs, family NPs, and CNMs. A major policy agenda of NPs is to extend Medicaid reimbursement to all APNs.

Children's Health Insurance Program

The Children's Health Insurance Program (CHIP) was passed as a part of the BBA as Title XXI of the Social Security Act. Congress set aside $24 billion from general tax revenues over a 5-year period to create this program to expand health-care insurance coverage for low-income children. CHIP is intended to extend insurance to children in low-income families who are not eligible for Medicaid but who do not have or cannot afford private health-care insurance. Like Medicaid, CHIP is a program in which federal funds must be matched by a set proportion of state funds.

CHIP represents the largest investment in children's health since the enactment of Medicaid in 1965. The impetus for CHIP was the recognition of the growing number of uninsured children in low-income families. Over 11 million children in 1996 were uninsured, a number that had grown by nearly 800,000 in just 1 year (Congressional Budget Office, 1999). Projections when the program was enacted indicated that 3.8 million uninsured children would be eligible for CHIP, or about 1 in 4 uninsured children in this country (Selden, Banthin, & Cohen, 1999). Even with CHIP, it is estimated that 8 million children remain uninsured.

To date, all states and territories have approved CHIP plans. However, some states were slow to implement CHIP because of the requirement for matching funds and the provisions requiring active enrollment efforts for both CHIP- and Medicaid-eligible children. It is now ironic that Congress anticipated that federal funding for the CHIP program would come from the federal tobacco settlement. As events unfolded, the federal settlement was scuttled, but most states participated in an agreement with the tobacco companies. However, the income from the settlement was not earmarked for CHIP or any other health program. Even with significant opportunity for states to improve health through the use of the tobacco money, many states are using the funds to close budget gaps to avoid deficits. States such as Wisconsin have sold their rights to future funds (the payout is over many years) because of the need for cash now. As states struggle to balance budgets, there is concern over the viability of the CHIP program when it comes up for reauthorization.

There were three alternative forms for implementation of the CHIP program. Nineteen states and territories have implemented CHIP as part of the Medicaid program; 16 have developed a separate child health insurance plan; and 21 have a combination plan (CMS, 2003e) (Table 23-6). States also have several benefits plan options. One benchmark plan is the standard Blue Cross/Blue Shield preferred provider option offered under the Federal Employees Health Benefits Program. Another is a benefit plan generally available to state employees, and the third uses the benefit plan of the HMO with the largest commercial enrollment in the state (HCFA, 1997).

Policymakers are concerned that parents or employers might see CHIP as a substitute for offering private insurance coverage to employees. In a survey of low-wage employers,

TABLE 23-6 CHIP MANAGEMENT PLAN		
SEPARATE STATE CHILD HEALTH PLAN (16)	MEDICAID EXPANSION (19)	COMBINED PLANS (21)
Alabama	Arkansas	California
Arizona	Alaska	Connecticut
Colorado	American Sumoa	Delaware
Georgia	Commonwealth of the	Florida
Kansas	Northern Mariana Islands	Iowa
Mississippi	District of Columbia	Illinois
Montana	Guam	Indiana
North Carolina	Hawaii	Kentucky
Nevada	Idaho	Massachusetts
Oregon	Louisiana	Maryland
Pennsylvania	Missouri	Maine
Utah	Nebraska	Michigan
Vermont	New Mexico	Minnesota
Washington	Ohio	New Hampshire
West Virginia	Oklahoma	New Jersey
Wyoming	Puerto Rico	New York
	South Carolina	North Dakota
	South Dakota	Rhode Island
	Tennessee	Texas
	Virgin Islands	Virginia
		Wisconsin

nearly one fifth said they would stop paying premiums if CHIP was available (Aston, 1999). However, most employers stated they would not drop their contributions if there was a waiting period for eligibility; thus numerous states have established waiting periods as a disincentive for employers to opt out of offering health insurance.

A greater concern related to the program is enrollment of uninsured children (Rosenbaum, Johnson, Sonosky, Markus, & DeGraw, 1998). Significant efforts have been made to reach out to families and communities through schools, churches, and day care centers to let parents know about the availability of coverage. Over 5.3 million children have been enrolled in CHIP since its inception (CMS, 2003f). APNs need to be part of the effort to identify children who are eligible for CHIP.

CHIP payment to APNs has presented some challenges. Although states recognize payment to family NPs, pediatric NPs, and CNMs through Medicaid, it has been difficult in some states, such as New York, for eligible APNs to get payment if the program was implemented under a separate state health plan and not through Medicaid. State and national organizations representing APNs have been active in working with these states to ensure access to APN care. Information about outreach for CHIP can be obtained at www.cms.hhs.gov/schip/stateplans/statepln.asp.

AVAILABILITY

In addition to affordability, availability is an important dimension of access. Availability can be viewed as convenient geographic access; access to providers with specific expertise, such as midwifery or cardiology; and access to providers who understand or share their patients' cultural values. It is estimated that 53 million people currently live in communities without access to primary care (National Health Service Corps, 2002).

APNs have their policy roots in enhancing geographic access. CNMs have a long history of providing services to traditionally underserved populations. They secured Medicaid reimbursement in the 1970s, enabling them to deliver services to poor women living in areas with no accessible providers. Governmental concern in the 1960s about substantially unmet health-care needs of society, particularly among individuals in rural and poor urban areas, strengthened the growth of NP roles. The Rural Health Clinics Act of 1979 implemented Medicaid and Medicare reimbursement to APNs to address availability issues.

In the 1990s there were projections of too many health-care providers of all types; now significant shortages are projected, particularly of nurses, including APNs. As of June 2003, there were 3000 federally designated health professional shortage areas (HPSAs). Reducing the number of HPSAs has proved to be an intractable problem. Federal attempts to address geographic accessibility have had limited success. The policies have focused on two main strategies: recruitment of individuals from underserved areas, in the hope that they will come to educational programs and then return to their home communities, and transplantation of graduates into underserved areas, in the hope that they will remain in these communities. A new strategy is being employed using distance learning to take educational programs to qualified individuals already living in underserved areas (Johnson & Posey, 2003).

The National Health Service Corps (NHSC), a federal agency within the Department of Health and Human Services charged with addressing the problem of geographic access, has used the first two strategies. It offers a scholarship and loan repayment program for health professionals who agree to work in underserved areas for a specific period of time. The NHSC has proposed to use funds to support the type of health professional that communities want. APNs are not usually requested first, mainly because communities do not fully understand the benefits of having an APN. This could jeopardize the funding available to APNs. However, the NHSC is taking the idea of a partnership approach with APN organizations to work with communities to enable them to better understand the advantages of having services provided by APNs. To check whether a site is a designated HPSA, go to www.bphc.hrsa.gov/database/newhpsa/newhpsa/cfm.

Availability of specific services is a problem. An example of limited availability is that of mental health services. Physical health needs have always taken priority in the eyes of most policymakers. Chronic mental illness, like chronic physical illness, often has multiple biopsychosocial and financial effects; however, mental health needs have not had equal parity with physical health needs. The Mental Health Parity Act (MHPA) of 1996 (P.L. 104–204) requires insurers to offer the same benefits for mental health care as for other health benefits. All employers with more than 50 employees must offer mental health insurance benefits, but, because of the Employee Retirement Income Security Act, employers that self-insure are exempt. In effect, access to mental health services continues to be problematic, mainly because of limited reimbursement through the many exclusions and limits on the MHPA, which in turn has reduced the number of health providers willing to work specifically in mental health.

Fourteen states have passed more stringent mental health laws than the federal law. Even with this legislation addressing mental health issues, Mark and Coffey (2003) found that employer-based health insurance spending on mental health benefits decreased from 7.2% in 1992 to 5.1% in 1999. Although insurance plans offer mental health and substance abuse coverage, mental health benefits usually carry substantial limits for inpatient stays and substance abuse counseling and may require higher co-pays and deductibles than physical health coverage (Buck, Teich, Umland, & Stein, 1999). Attempts to expand mental health services have fallen short mainly because of concerns about the costs of mental health parity, yet there is little evidence to support this fear. Psychiatric/mental health APNs have a significant challenge. Even though their services can be reimbursed, significant problems continue to exist with regard to access because of the constraints noted here.

QUALITY

Quality of care as a policy issue is rather new to health care. In the past, quality of care was seen largely as the exclusive domain of the health professions. There was an implicit assumption by the public that quality was uniformly high and was ensured by the presence of the norms of professionalism that placed the interests of the patient before those of the professional. Many of the early approaches to policy were either efforts from within the profession, like accreditation of educational programs, or certifying of health professionals or regulatory efforts, which were dominated by professional input, like licensing. One of the first direct incursions of public policy into quality was a result of the enactment in 1965 of the Medicare and Medicaid programs. The Health Care Financing Administration (HCFA), and now CMS, was charged with ensuring the effective and efficient use of public funds, including assessment and assurance of the quality of care. This quality-related function of HCFA/CMS has grown slowly over the years.

In addition, changes in the health system, such as heightened competition and ongoing pressure to reduce costs, created federal and state interest because of constituent concerns about the possible harmful effects of cost reduction, or imposition of "managed care" on quality. In a similar fashion, purchasers other than the federal government, such as business groups, have pushed to hold managed care organizations and, in a few instances, hospitals or physicians more accountable for quality. Finally, there has been a small but growing body of research on quality that has demonstrated wide variation in health-care quality and in patterns of utilization of services and a lack of congruence, in many instances, between cost and quality. These research findings have been brought to the attention of the public largely by a series of reports from the Institute of Medicine. The first report, *To Err is Human* (IOM, 2000), which reviewed studies of medical errors, received widespread media attention with its estimation that between 50,000 and 100,000 Americans die each year from medical errors in the hospital (IOM, 2001). The report also suggested that research in health care and other areas, such aviation safety, demonstrate that most errors are the result of poorly designed systems rather than the fault of a single individual. A second report, *Crossing the Quality Chasm* (IOM, 2001), summarized the extensive studies, most notably of Robert Brook and Jack Wennberg, demonstrating the high degree of variation in quality and utilization and major defects in quality of care for persons with chronic illness. This report noted that improving systems by creating valid and reliable measures of quality, providing feedback and benchmarking, and making other systems changes, rather than blaming individuals, is the key to improving quality (IOM, 2001). Subsequent reports have looked at the infrastructure and quality of public health, access to care, and, most recently, defining priority areas for quality improvement action (IOM, 2002, 2003a, 2003b).

Nursing has been invested in quality for decades. Seminal work on nursing outcomes has been supported by the National Institute of Nursing Research. Recently, nursing staff levels have been related to patient mortality and morbity in hospitals (Aiken, Clarke, Sloane, Sochalski, & Silber, 2002; Needleman, Buerhaus, Mattke, Stewart, & Selvinsky, 2002). However, the efforts within nursing to measure and promote quality from a national perspective have been severely limited compared with the activities focused on medical care. For example, there are no standardized nursing performance measures that are identified, collected, and reported for all hospitals in this country. As a result, there are no national and regional benchmarks by which the public or payors can compare the quality of nursing care, and nursing care in hospitals remains nearly invisible.

Many different types of organizations and agencies are currently influencing quality of care, thereby creating a complex landscape. There are accrediting bodies such as the Joint Commission on Health Care Organizations that accredit hospitals. State agencies certify nursing homes for reimbursement through Medicaid and Medicare. The National Committee on Quality Assurance accredits managed care organizations. The primary driving organization for accreditation of health-care institutions is the CMS, to ensure that they are paying for at least a baseline level of care. In addition to CMS and the accrediting bodies, a number of organizations are dedicated to institutionalizing already-existing measures or developing new quality measures, such as the federal Agency for Healthcare Research and Quality (AHRQ), and privately run organizations, such as National Forum for Quality (NQF) and National Committee on Quality Assurance (NCQA). Professional associations are also involved in helping members improve care.

What Is Quality of Care?

Quality of care has been defined by the Institute of Medicine (1990) as "the degree to which health services for individuals and populations increase the likelihood of desired health outcomes and are consistent with current professional knowledge" (p. 4).

Quality of care issues have been conceptualized as problems related to underuse (providing too little of care that is effective), overuse (providing care that is not effective or efficient), and misuse (providing care that is unsafe or inappropriate). Again, health services research has demonstrated major gaps in all three areas. For example, in regard to underuse, recent studies have shown that only half of the patients with hypertension, diabetes, or asthma are receiving appropriate screening and/or medication (NCQA, 2002). Pain management has also been identified as a significant problem related to underuse of treatment. Overuse is characterized by providing excessive and unnecessary services that do not contribute to improving health. Use of antibiotics to treat colds and acute bronchitis is an example of overuse. Gonzales, Steiner, and Sande (1997) found that nearly half of all patients diagnosed with acute bronchitis received antibiotics. Misuse of services can result in injury to patients, high costs, and sometimes death or major disability. Use of more expensive antibiotics to treat ear infections was associated with more adverse effects and worse outcomes than use of less expensive antibiotics (Brennan et al., 1991). Medication errors also constitute misuse of services and can frequently be prevented (IOM, 2001).

The IOM provided a framework for quality and defined six critical domains: (1) patient safety (providing services and an environment that is safe), (2) effectiveness (interventions that have a good likelihood of improving health or function), (3) patient centeredness (putting the needs of the patient at the center of the health system), (4) efficiency (services provided in the most cost-effective manner), (5) timeliness (services provided when they are really needed), and (6) equity (a just distribution of services based on health need rather than ability to pay) (IOM, 2001). The report also noted that quality is affected by actions at all levels of the health-care system: those of the patient, clinician, the "micro-environment (such as the outpatient office or hospital unit), the organization (hospital, medical group, etc.), and environment (financing and reimbursement, public policy, etc.). For an examination of overuse, underuse, and misuse and improvement of health-care quality, a systems approach in all six domains of quality will be required; that is, initiatives must be undertaken at all levels of the system, from patients to the environment, including policies related to access, financing, and reimbursement.

PATIENT SAFETY

While all six domains of quality are important, patient safety is seen by the public, and by most experts in quality, to be the foundation for a high-quality system. Patients should be able to enter the health-care system knowing that everything reasonable is being done to keep them safe from harm by the health-care system itself. Public policy in safety is still, for the most part, mired in the belief that most harm to patients is the result of errors by "bad" health-care providers and that malpractice is a major deterrent to such errors. There is strong evidence not only of the large number of adverse patient events but also of the fact that most adverse events are the result of systems failures rather than individual human error (IOM, 2000). The IOM report points out that all humans are subject to making errors and that the systems of care in which we work are the most important factors in determining which errors will occur. For example, there were a number of patient deaths caused by a gas other than oxygen being administered as ventilation during surgery. Blaming, firing, or educating the anesthesiologist, nurse, or technician who connected the wrong tubing did little to change the error rate. These deaths were virtually eliminated when the connectors for oxygen to ventilators were made so that it is essentially impossible to connect any other gas to the machine.

It should be noted that most errors (providing care in a manner that does not conform to acceptable practice) do not result in adverse events (harm to patients), and conversely, most adverse events are not the result of errors. Since it is sometimes difficult to determine whether an error has occurred, some experts in the field feel that we should focus our attention on adverse events regardless of whether it is the result of an apparent error. The IOM report and subsequent research and educational programs have begun to shift how patient safety issues are analyzed and how improvement is pursued. Use of techniques such as root cause analysis and factor analysis is becoming more common.

While consumers are not yet fully aware of the shift, the business community has supported change in patient safety practices through the "Leapfrog" group (www.leapfrog group.org). This coalition of large corporations has encouraged hospitals, through public reporting and selective contracting, to increase their adherence to three evidence-based safety "leaps," including computerized order entry, the use of intensivists in intensive care units, and referral of highly complex surgery to high-volume hospitals. AHRQ has funded multiple patient safety research projects and a center for evidence-based research in safety, as well as providing leadership for a group that is coordinating pubic sector efforts in patient safety. With the Division of Nursing in the Department of Health and Human Services, AHRQ co-funded the study noted previously by Needleman et al. (2002) to examine the link between nurse staffing and patient outcomes. The National Quality Forum (NQF), a congressionally mandated, public-private membership organization of providers, consumers, purchasers, and researchers, has identified and developed consensus on a set of "safe practices" and "never" events (adverse events, such as wrong site surgery, wherein even one occurrence is a major defect). The American Nurses Association is creating a report card for nursing care in hospitals. Over 200 hospitals participate in the program.

Quality-of-Care Monitoring Activities

A necessary first step in assessing and improving quality is to have accurate and reliable ways of measuring it. The basic approaches to measuring quality, as defined by Donebedian (1980), the grandfather of health-care quality, include measure of structure (how many registered nurses are present), process (are wrist bands checked when medications are given?) and outcomes (how many patients are injured or die from medication errors?). There are a very limited number of ways to measure quality, including direct observation, the use of administrative data (data collected for billing or other nonclinical purposes), surveying participants (either patients or clinicians), and extraction of data from clinical records (paper or electronic medical records). Major challenges exist that have retarded the development and deployment of accurate and reliable measurement. A few of these challenges include the resistance of some providers to being measured, the cost of measurement, the lack of rewards for providing high-quality care, and unreliable and inconsistent data recorded in administrative and clinical records.

While small scale experiments and research have measured quality for several decades, one of the first widespread efforts to measure and publicly report on the quality of care was in the HMO sector, with the creation of the Healthplan Employer Data and Information Set (HEDIS) by the National Committee on Quality Assurance (NCQA). HEDIS includes more than 50 standardized measures of health plan performance, many of which are measures of clinical care. HEDIS is consistently updated by the NCQA and includes measures such as immunization rates, mammography screening, and cholesterol management.

Reporting of HEDIS measures is now required for NCQA-accredited health plans, and some of the measures are used as part of the accreditation itself (accreditation of hospitals and most other health-care entities is driven by adherence to written standards rather than by performance). This data is now released to the public in the form of "report cards" on individual HMOs (see NCQA website, www.healthchoices.org). NCQA releases an annual report on health-care quality. The most recent report suggested that there has been a continuing improvement in care for many millions of Americans (NCQA, 2002). It also reported that more than 6000 deaths and 22 million sick days could have been prevented with "best practices." New NCQA programs include Bridges to Excellence, which involves large corporations such as UPS, Verizon, and Ford Motor Company; health plans; and consumers in paying providers for quality. The NCQA also has a diabetes recognition program that identifies practices that provide high quality in diabetes care. There is also a Health Plan Report Card that employers and others can use in reviewing health plan quality to make decisions about offering those plans to employees.

Recently CMS has developed a set of measures and a public reporting system on nursing homes. At this point, any patient or consumer can go to the CMS website and look up a few meaures of quality on specific nursing homes (CMS, 2003g). CMS is also in the process of developing a Hospital Consumer Assessment of Health Plan Survey that will collect and report standardized patient information from all hospitals. This instrument includes numerous questions related to patient assessment of the quality of nursing care (CMS, 2003h). In addition, the CMS Hospital Quality Initiative will make information about hospital performance available to consumers. CMS has also initiated a home health quality project that has begun reporting 11 home health measures from the Outcome and Assessment Information Set (OASIS) in eight states and will expand it to all states.

The Agency for Healthcare Research and Quality (AHRQ) (formerly the Agency for Health Care Policy and Research) was established in 1988 by congressional mandate to foster health-care research that contributes to high quality, cost-effective services; accountability to consumers and purchasers; and improvement of the health status and quality of life of all citizens. In 1989 AHRQ established the Center for Outcome and Effectiveness Research to support studies on outcome and effective diagnostic, therapeutic, preventive health services and procedures (AHRQ, 2003a). In 1997, AHRQ funded 10 evidence-based centers to promote evidence-based clinical decisions in everyday practice. The agency expanded this number to 13 in 2002 (AHRQ, 2003b).

Businesses, because of their role in purchasing health care on behalf of employees, have also gotten involved in quality activities. For instance, the Pacific Business Group on Health (PBGH) has been a leader in establishing performance measures for more than a dozen of the largest health plans in California. The PBGH negotiated on behalf of health purchasers who put $8 million at risk if the plans did not meet their performance measures (Schauffler, Brown, & Milstein, 1999). The purpose of building a financial incentive for meeting specific targets based on information (including consumer satisfaction as well as a number of specific clinical measures, such as immunization rates) is to provide a monetary reason for plans to provide quality care.

Finally, NQF has been charged with creating a national strategy for health-care quality measurement and reporting. NQF has reported a framework for quality and has developed a process for creating a consensus around quality measures that can be applied to a variety of institutional settings, including hospitals, nursing homes, and other health-care entities. NQF is currently working to identify measures that reflect quality of nursing care in hospitals.

The efforts to improve quality of care are occurring piecemeal and in a highly charged political climate. Numerous organizations have a stake in how quality is defined and measured. Providers are concerned about being measured accurately, particularly if reimbursement may be tied to performance at some time in the future. Performance measures are being developed when there is a special interest, but without an overall strategic plan for assessing the areas that can be measured in a valid and reliable process, there will likely be heightened competition among professional associations, accrediting agencies, payors, and purchasers.

While APNs have been involved in quality of care issues, the central focus of activity at the national and state level has been on the physician community. APNs need to be involved in quality improvement activities at all levels. Nurses, and specifically APNs, are a critical part of the systems changes that are essential to improving the quality of care. Moreover, APNs are frequently asked to be on the quality staff of both provider organizations and organizations such as JCAHO and NCQA, which address quality issues. There is a major opportunity for well-informed APNs to be leaders in the growing effort to enhance quality of care, both within provider organizations and at the level of public policy, both within their own profession and in health care in general.

Fraud and Abuse

To ensure the efficient use of taxpayer dollars, the government is committed to detecting fraud and abuse in billing. Fraud and abuse detection initiated by the CMS is one method being used to ensure appropriate use of Medicare and Medicaid dollars. Fraud is defined by the CMS as "the intentional representation that an individual knows to be false or does not believe to be true and makes, knowing that the representation could result in some unauthorized benefit to himself/herself or some other person" (CMS, 2003i, p. 1). Abuse is defined as "actions that are inconsistent with accepted, sound, medical, business, or fiscal practices. Abuse directly or indirectly results in unnecessary costs to the program through improper payments" (CMS, 2003i, p. 1). Each Medicare contractor, whether an intermediary or carrier, has a Medicare Fraud Unit in place. Once an investigation takes place and there is sufficient evidence to warrant potential prosecution, the case goes to the U.S. Department of Health and Human Services Office of the Inspector General (OIG). The OIG's office then prepares the case for referral to the Department of Justice for criminal and/or civil prosecution. If a provider or institution is found guilty of committing fraud or abuse, penalties can range from a civil penalty of $5000 to $10,000 per false claim and treble damages under the False Claims Act to imprisonment up to 10 years. The penalties associated with fraud or abuse can clearly be substantial.

Every APN needs to be familiar with the laws regarding fraud and abuse. There are a number of potential billing errors that could be construed as fraud or abuse. Examples of billing fraud and abuse that APNs need to be careful about are "incident to" billing as well as kickback issues. The Medicare legislation enabling APN billing under Medicare creates opportunities as well as responsibilities. Ignorance of billing requirements will not be a justification for billing practices that could be construed as fraud or abuse. Confusion about "incident to" billing has arisen because of the limited guidelines from CMS about the requirements for this billing procedure. Johnson and Torras (1999) have provided a number of criteria that must be met for "incident to" billing for supplies or services; they must be

- An integral, although incidental, part of the physician's services
- Commonly rendered without charge or included in the physician's bill
- Of the type that is commonly furnished in an office or clinic
- Furnished under the physician's direct supervision
- Furnished by an individual who qualifies as an employee of the physician or clinic

All of these criteria must be met in order to comply with the requirements for "incident to" billing. It is important for APNs to note that services "incident to" APN services can be billed. That stipulation as part of the BBA provides an avenue for billing that has previously not been open to APNs.

The anti-kickback statute could also be inadvertently abused by APNs if there are grounds for the APN to get a financial benefit from a particular arrangement—for instance, if an APN orders a specific drug and gets payment from the drug company as a result. APNs must be careful about what can be construed as an arrangement for financial enhancement for the clinician. It is difficult to identify specific examples of problems related to "incident to" billing or kickback schemes because there have been no reported incidents involving APNs as of this writing.

APNs and Physicians

At the beginning of the chapter, the importance of nursing and medicine working together for the welfare of patients and the health of the nation was recognized. The policy arena, although a potential avenue for important collaboration, often serves as a forum where both disciplines are adversaries in economic competition. Because the basis for nearly all policy decisions rests on economics, many national organizations have staked out policy positions that maintain or enhance the economic positions of their respective disciplines, rather than substantive health policy issues such as access, quality, and safety. The cost-containment emphasis of health-care financing has led to reductions in inflation-adjusted physician income. In addition, under managed care, physicians feel they have experienced significant loss of control over how they practice medicine. These actual and perceived losses make it difficult for physicians to embrace expanded practice for APNs, who may be seen as competitors for jobs and income.

An understanding of this economic and policy landscape allows physicians and APNs to recognize the factors that may create an adversarial relationship in order to look for common ground in the pursuit of better patient care. Over the past few years, each discipline has tried to strengthen its own position. However, the major opportunities for improving the effectiveness, safety, and efficiency of health care and addressing the increasing problem of assuring a decent level of access to basic health care for all with fair payment for services delivered are imperatives for cooperative action.

Despite the competitive, sometimes adversarial policy stances of nursing and medicine, physicians and APNs have collaborated and created new practice models that deliver care efficiently and effectively to elderly, underinsured, and disabled populations. These models demonstrated that APNs and physicians can invent policy approaches and craft interdisciplinary models of care that recognize the strengths of each discipline. There are many geriatrics practices in which NPs and physicians work together and care for this very challenging population. Neither nursing nor medicine alone can care for individual patients with multiple, interacting health and social problems, high needs for prevention, care, and case and/or disease management. For instance, the Program of All Inclusive Care of the Elderly (PACE) has a core team of providers, including an APN, physician, social worker, home health aide, and others, who provide care to keep elderly disabled individuals out of nursing homes. The PACE team meets regularly for case conferences and shares accountability and responsibility for frequent and effective communication. This collaboration demonstrates and uses overlapping as well as distinctive areas of expertise among team members and has had remarkable outcomes in terms of decreasing hospitalizations and keeping elderly persons in their homes for as long as possible (Wieland et al., 2000).

BOX 23-2 • URL ADDRESSES TO NATIONAL APN ACCREDITION REGULATION AND CERTIFICATION WEB SITES

American Association of Nurse Practitioners (AANP)	www.aanp.org
American Association of Colleges of Nurses and Commission on Collegiate Nursing Education (AACN and CCNE)	www.aacn.nche.edu (links to CCNE)
American Association of Nurse Anesthetists (AANA)	www.aana.com/index.htm
American College of Nurse-Midwives (ACNM)	www.acnm.org
American Nurses Credential Center (ANCC)	www.nursingworld.org/ancc
National Certification Corporation for Obstetrical, Gynecologic and Neonatal Nursing Specialists (NCC)	www.nccnet.org
National Council State Boards of Nursing (NCSBN)	www.ncsbn.org
National League for Nursing Accreditation Corporation (NLNAC)	www.nln.org/nlnac
Pediatric Nursing Certification Board	www.pncb.org

Another example of a policy problem for which physicians and APNs have a shared concern is the growing number of uninsured individuals. National attention could effectively be focused on this issue and solutions identified with medicine and nursing working together. A model of interdisciplinary collaboration was demonstrated by an initiative entitled Primary Care Action (more information can be found at www.futurehealth. ucsf.edu/primarycareaction.html). Numerous nursing and medical professionals representing major organizations have joined together to identify a common set of policy goals and to develop a plan for attaining those goals that includes enhancing the quality of primary care and providing universal coverage.

CONCLUSION

Policy advocacy needs to be a part of every APN's professional role. Membership in professional organizations that advance issues critical to APN practice and the health of the nation is vital to the continued viability of APNs. The first step to being involved in policy formulation is to be knowledgeable about the policy process and issues. In order to be involved, APNs need to understand the details related to funding issues, measures of quality and how they reflect APN practice, and specific programs designed to improve access. Box 23-2 lists websites that can provide APNs with current and comprehensive information about important policy issues. The important lesson in policy is that a single person, after understanding an issue, can make a difference. An individual backed by organizational strength, particularly by coalitions of organizations, can make an even more significant difference.

REFERENCES

Agency for Healthcare Research and Quality. (2003a). *Overview: Center for outcomes and effectiveness research.* Retrieved July 14, 2003, from http://www.AHRQ.gov/about/COER/overview.htm

Agency for Healthcare Research and Quality. (2003b). *Evidence-based practice centers: Overview.* Retrieved July 14, 2003, from http://www.ahrq.gov/clinic/epc/

Aiken, L., Clarke, S. P., Sloane, D.M., Sochalski, J., & Silber, J.H. (2002). Hospital nurse staffing and patient mortality, nurse burnout, and job dissatisfaction. *Journal of the American Medical Association*, *288*, 1987.

American Academy of Pediatrics. (2003). Scope of practice issues in the delivery of pediatric health care. *Pediatrics*, *111*, 426.

American Medical Association. (1995). *Physicians' assistants and nurse practitioners*. Chicago: American Medical Association.

Anderson, G. F., & Poullier, J. P. (1999). Health spending, access and outcomes: Trends in industrialized countries. *Health Affairs*, *18*, 178.

Aston, G. (1999). States act to reserve CHIP funds to cover uninsured children. *American Medical News*, *42*, 1.

Berk, M. L., & Schur, C. L. (1998). Measuring access to care: Improving information for policymakers. *Health Affairs*, *19*, 180.

Board of Trustees of the Federal Hospital Insurance and Supplementary Medical Insurance Trust Funds. (2003). *2003 Annual report of the Board of Trustees of the Hospital Insurance and Supplementary Medical Insurance Trust Funds*. Retrieved July 20, 2003, from http://www.cms.hhs.gov/publications/trusteesreport/2003

Brennan, T. A., Leape, L.L., Laird, N. M., Hebert, L., Localio, A. R., Lawthers, A. G., et al. (1991). Incidence of adverse events and negligence in hospitalized patients: Results of the Harvard Medical Practice Study I. *New England Journal of Medicine*, *324*, 370-376.

Buck, J. A., Teich, J. L., Umland, B., & Stein, M. (1999). Behavioral health benefits in employer-sponsored health plans, 1997. *Health Affairs*, *18*, 67-78.

Centers for Medicare and Medicaid. (2003a). *Highlights—National Health Care Expenditures*. Retrieved May 2, 2004, from http://www.cms.hhs.gov/statistics/nhe/historic/highlights.asp

Centers for Medicare and Medicaid. (2003b). *Medigap insurance*. Retrieved May 20, 2003, from http://www.medicare.gov/MGCompare/Home.asp

Centers for Medicare and Medicaid. (2003c). *Open door forum: Nurses and allied health professions*. Retrieved May 20, 2003, from http://www.cms.hhs.gov/opendoor/nurses-alliedhealth.asp

Centers for Medicare and Medicaid. (2003d). *State Medicaid toll-free lines*. Retrieved May 20, 2003, at http://cms.hhs.gov/medicaid/mcontact.asp

Centers for Medicare and Medicaid. (2003e). *State Child Health Insurance Program plan activity*. Retrieved May 20, 2003, from http://cms.hhs.gov/schip/chip-map.asp

Centers for Medicare and Medicaid. (2003f). *Fiscal year 2002 number of children enrolled in SCHIP—Preliminary data*. Retrieved May 20, 2003, from http://cms.hhs.gov/schip/schip02.pdf

Centers for Medicare and Medicaid. (2003g). *Nursing Home Compare*. Retrieved May 20, 2003, from http://www.medicare.gov/NHCompare/Home.asp

Centers for Medicare and Medicaid. (2003h). *Overview of hospital CAHPS (HCAHPS)*. Retrieved May 20, 2003, from http://cms.hhs.gov/quality/hospital/HCAHPSqanda3.pdf

Centers for Medicare and Medicaid. (2003i). *Fighting fraud and abuse*. Retrieved May 20, 2003, from http://www.cms.hhs.gov/providers/fraud/

Collins, R. R., Schoen, C., Colasonto, D., & Downey, D. A. (2003). *On the edge: Low wage workers and their health insurance coverage* (Issue Brief). New York: The Commonwealth Fund.

Congressional Budget Office. (1999). *Expanding health insurance coverage for children under Title XXI of the Social Security Act 1998*. Retrieved May 24, 2003, from www.cbo.gov/byclasscat.cfm?class-0&cat-9

Curran, W. J. (1989). The constitutional right to health care: Denial in the court. *New England Journal of Medicine*, *320*, 788-789.

Daniels, N. (1985). *Just health care*. Cambridge, England: Cambridge University Press.

Department of Health and Human Services. (2003). 2003 HHS Poverty Guidelines. *Federal Register*, *66*(33): 6456. Retrieved May 24, 2003, from http://aspe.hhs.gov/poverty/01poverty.htm

Donebedian, A. (1980). *Exploration in quality assessment and monitoring* (Vol. 1). Chicago: Health Administration Press.

Feldstein, P. (1988). *The politics of health legislation*. Ann Arbor, MI: Health Administration Press.

Gabel, J., Hurst, K., Whitmore, H., & Hoffman, C. (1999). Class and benefits at the workplace. *Health Affairs*, *18*, 144-150.

Gonzales, R., Steiner, J., & Sande, M. (1997). Antibiotic prescribing for adults with colds, upper respiratory tract infections, and bronchitis by ambulatory care physicians. *Journal of the American Medical Association*, *278*, 901-904.

Heclo, H. (1995). The Clinton Health Care Plan: Historical perspective. *Health Affairs*, *14*, 86.

Health Care Financing Administration. (1997). *Children's Health Insurance Program Answers to frequently asked questions—released September 11, 1997 (first set)*. Washington, DC: Author.

Health Care Financing Administration. (1998). *Medicare and Medicaid statistical supplement: Health Care Financing Review OHHS*. Washington, DC: Author.

Heffler, S., Smith, S., Keehan S., Clemens, M. K., Won, G., & Zezza, M. (2003) Health spending projections for 2002-2012. *Health Affairs*, *22*, 12.

Holahan, J., Weiner, J., & Wallin, S. (1998). *Health policy for the low income population: Major findings from Accessing the New Federalism* (Occasional Paper #18). Washington, DC: Urban Institute.

Hurley, R. E., & Somers, S. A. (2003). Medicaid and managed care: A lasting relationship? *Health Affairs*, *22*, 77.

Institute of Medicine. (1990). *Medicare: A strategy for quality assurance*. (K. N. Lohr, Ed.). Washington, D.C., National Academy of Science Press.

Institute of Medicine. (2000). *To err is human: Building a safer health system*. Washington, DC: National Academy of Science Press.

Institute of Medicine. (2001). *Crossing the quality chasm: A new health system for the 21st century*. Washington, DC: National Academy of Science Press.

Institute of Medicine. (2002). *Care without coverage*. Washington, DC: National Academy of Science Press.

Institute of Medicine. (2003a). *Priority areas for national action: Transforming health care quality*. Washington, DC: National Academy of Science Press.

Institute of Medicine. (2003b). *A shared destiny: Community effects of uninsured*. Washington, DC: National Academy of Science Press.

Johnson, D., & Torras, H. (1999). *NP billing and coding tips*. Washington, DC: American College of Nurse Practitioners.

Johnson J., & Posey, L. (2003). *Partnerships for training grantees*. Retrieved May 1, 2003, from www.pftweb.org

Kronick, R., & Gilmore, T. (1999). Exploring the decline in health insurance coverage, 1979-1995. *Health Affairs, 18*, 30.

Levit, K., Smith, C., Cowan, C., Lazenby, H., Sensenig, A., & Catlin, A. (2003). Trends in US health care spending, 2001. *Health Affairs, 22*, 154.

Longest, B. B. (2002). *Health policy in the United States* (3rd ed.). Chicago: Health Administration Press.

Mark, T. L., & Coffey R. M. (2003). What drove private health insurance spending on mental health and substance abuse care, 1992-1999. *Health Affairs, 22*, 165.

National Committee on Quality Assurance. (2002). *State of health care quality report*. Retrieved June 4, 2003, from www.ncqa.org /communications/news/sohc2002.htm

National Health Service Corps. (2002). Welcome to the National Health Service Corps. Retrieved June 4, 2003, from http://nhsc.bphc.hrsa.gov

Needleman, J., Buerhaus P., Mattke, S., Stewart, M., & Selevinsky, K. (2002). Nurse-staffing levels and the quality of care in hospitals. *New England Journal of Medicine, 346*, 1715.

Newhouse, J. P. (1993). An iconoclastic view of health care cost containment. *Health Affairs, 12*(Suppl), 152-171.

Reinhardt, U. E. (1993). Recognizing the financial flaws in American healthcare. *Health Affairs, 12*(Suppl), 172-193.

Rosenbaum, S., Johnson, K., Sonosky, C., Markus, A., & DeGraw, S. (1998). The children's hour: The State Children's Health Insurance Program. *Health Affairs, 17*, 75-89.

Schauffler, H. H., Brown, C., & Milstein, A. (1999). Raising the bar: The use of performance guarantees by the Pacific Business Group on Health. *Health Affairs, 18*, 134.

Selden, T. M., Banthin, J. S., & Cohen, J. W. (1999). Waiting in the wings: Eligibility and enrollment in the State Children's Health Insurance Program. *Health Affairs, 18*, 126.

Short, P., & Banthin, J. (1995) Caring for the uninsured and underinsured. *Journal of the American Medical Association, 274*, 1302.

Starr, P. (1982). *The social transformation of American medicine*. New York: Basic Books.

Thorpe, K. E., & Florence, C. S., (1999). Why are workers uninsured? Employer-sponsored health insurance in 1997. *Health Affairs, 18*, 213-218.

U.S. Census Bureau (2002). *Health Insurance coverage*. Retrieved May 14, 2003, from http://www.census.gov/hhes/hlthin02.html

Weil, A. (2003). There's something about Medicaid. *Health Affairs, 22*, 13.

Wieland, D., Lamb, V., Sutton, S., Boland, R., Clark, M., Friedman, S., et al. (2000). Hospitalization in the Program of All-Inclusive Care for the Elderly (PACE): Rates, comcomitants and predictors. *Journal of the American Geriatrics Society, 48*, 1373.

World Health Organization. (2003). Basic health indicators: 2002. Retrieved May 14, 2003, from http://www3.who.int/whosis/reported/reproted.cfm?path=whosis,basic,reproted

Strengthening Advanced Nursing Practice in Organizational Structures and Cultures

BRENDA M. NEVIDJON • MARY D. KNUDTSON

Continued

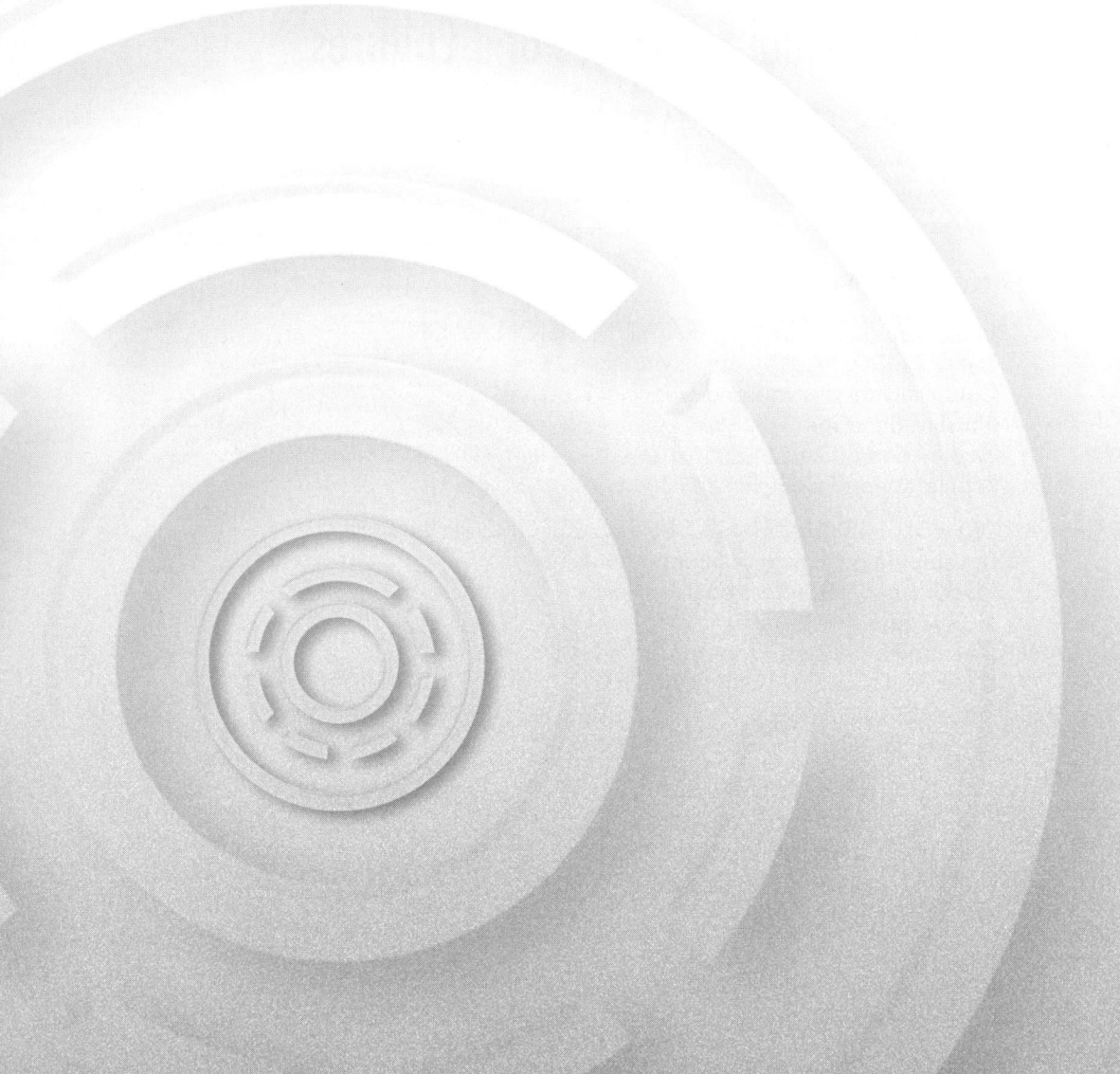

INTRODUCTION

Advanced practice nursing has had a recent history that can be compared to a sine wave (see Chapter 1). Both clinical nurse specialists (CNSs) and nurse practitioners (NPs) have been in and out of demand as the economic health of the health-care system waxed and waned. In the 1980s, administrators increased the number of CNS positions. In the turbulent 1990s, those positions rapidly diminished as employers felt the impact of managed care and other payor changes. The number of NPs grew when managed care organizations (MCOs) indicated they would need more primary care practitioners for their enrollees. The continuation of the CNS role, especially in acute care settings, was uncertain, given the financial challenges faced by hospital administrators. Many CNSs quickly returned to school to prepare as NPs because administrators, often on the advice of consultants, eliminated hospital-based CNS positions in the early cycles of budget reductions. In response to these changes, schools of nursing eliminated CNS programs and ramped up programs to prepare more NPs. However, managed care did not penetrate the health-care environment as originally expected, and nurse executives who eliminated CNS positions reintroduced them because they saw the negative impact on basic nursing care that resulted from the lack of CNSs. Schools of nursing are increasingly reintroducing programs to prepare CNSs. During this time, physician organizations publicly challenged the competencies of advanced practice nurses (APNs), and conflict between nursing and medical organizations intensified.

Other trends of the 1990s included the interest in acute care NPs (ACNPs) to compensate for the decreasing numbers of medical residents in teaching hospitals. A change in the graduate medical education (GME) requirements limited the residents' work week to 80 hours, causing academic medical centers and teaching hospitals to seek new models of providing care to patients. Certified registered nurse anesthetists (CRNAs) found their job security challenged by an abundance of anesthesiologists. Birthing centers gained a foothold as certified nurse-midwives (CNMs) offered women a choice in birthing experience. Primary care NPs continue to flourish, while the blended role of CNS and NP has gained popularity; and the evolving nurse case manager role is being discussed in the literature as a potential advanced practice role. Other job titles, such as *practice-based educators* and *clinical consultants*, are appearing in the literature as potential advanced practice roles, continuing the confusion for health-care administrators and other audiences that interact with nurses about nomenclature and what advanced practice nursing means (see Chapter 19).

Administrators who consider employing APNs in their health-care organizations must deal with internal issues, such as how to define the value an APN will bring and how to identify what groups APNs might threaten within the organization. Numerous internal and external factors in all health-care settings, whether community- or institutional-based, influence how advanced practice nursing is embraced and how care is delivered. For organizations that support APN roles, the fiscal well-being of the organization and politics among the various clinicians can shape how APNs are included in the model of care. Lack of consensus about the definition of roles, need for second licensure, reimbursement, prescriptive privileges, and scope of authority are some of the external, national environment issues that compound the internal issues about how organizations employ APNs. As changes regarding where and how health care is delivered continue, traditional and often inflexible organizational boundaries are disappearing. Thus administrators have opportunities to be creative and to build strong alliances among the health-care professions to meet society's needs for accessible and affordable health care.

The purpose of this chapter is to outline the factors that contribute to the justification and employment of APNs now and in the future. It provides information to help administrators champion the employment of APNs in their organizations, whether they are introducing a new position or promoting a current one. The chapter should also help APNs understand the needs of administrators within complex health-care systems and how to assist them in advocating for advanced practice roles in the organization. Factors such as organizational culture, policy, and finance are discussed. As our experience has shown, without an appreciation for and documentation of the contributions of APNs, administrators will eliminate financial support for them.

Administrators have a responsibility to remain knowledgeable about APN roles and what these roles can accomplish for patient care and for organizations. In hospitals, the nurse administrator is a critical ally and key voice of support for APNs. A clearly articulated vision of advanced nursing practice by the nursing leadership of an organization will sustain commitment to the roles through difficult times. In other settings, physicians, physician executives, or business managers decide on the structure and function of APN roles. In any setting, collaboration between APNs and administrators is essential to define the expected contributions of APNs, including innovative practices, improved patient outcomes, cost savings, and revenue generation.

TRENDS DRIVING ADMINISTRATIVE DECISION MAKING

Administrators must make decisions about pressing matters that can affect the organization's future on a daily basis. Some of the following trends are both challenges and opportunities in which administrators and APNs can partner to find creative solutions.

The Changing Health-Care Environment

The health-care system is an industry searching for definition. An increasingly diverse and demanding population now complicates the age-old dynamic tension inherent in a discussion of access, quality, and cost. Economics has been the driving force behind changes in the health-care environment since the 1980s. Both private and governmental payors led initiatives aimed at reducing the cost of health care. Their key issues include cost containment, new forms of payment, consumer preferences, health reform efforts, and technological developments (Levit et al., 2003; Shortell, Gillies, & Devers, 1995). Managed care was embraced in the 1990s as the way to contain costs. However, health care as a percentage of the U.S. gross national product has continued to rise. The uninsured now number more than 43 million, and that number is expected to increase as a result of the economic climate of the early 2000s (U.S. Census Bureau, 2002).

As shown in Table 24-1, there are many internal and external factors that create opportunities for or impediments to the practice of nursing and the delivery of patient care. The external factors drive many of the internal factors. For example, the external payor environment has frequently led to reactive decisions about services and the future of specific disciplines in hospitals. However, the predicted restructuring of care delivery has not occurred as deliberatively, uniformly, or quickly throughout the country as one might think from media coverage of this issue (Burns & Pauly, 2002; Urden & Walston, 2001). Nonetheless, administrators have been challenged by decreasing reimbursement, increasing regulatory controls, increasing cost of technology, and increasing acuity of care. In hospitals, nurse administrators have responded by changing the skill mix of staff, developing cross-training programs, eliminating certain types of positions, and expanding the scope of middle managers. Commitment to CNSs and blended role APNs has varied throughout this time, particularly when the positions are fixed costs in a nursing department's budget. On the other hand, in ambulatory care settings, physician groups have increased service availability (access) by employing NPs. Other examples of how access has been increased are employment of geriatric NPs who coordinate care of patients in skilled nursing facilities and employment of acute care NPs who coordinate care for a practice's hospitalized patients.

Population demographics are also affecting the health-care environment, and administrators are strategically planning services to meet a variety of populations. The large generation of baby boomers is aging into the decades in which chronic diseases such as heart disease, cancer, and diabetes are more common. This has raised questions about hospital capacity, skilled nursing facilities, community care, and alternative care systems. It is likely that the traditional way of delivering care will not meet the increased demand brought by aging baby boomers. Immigration, particularly of Hispanics, will continue to challenge administrators. The 2000 U.S. Census showed the shift occurring in the population, and Hispanics are expected to exceed African Americans as the largest minority in the near future (Miller, 2003). This has increased the need for providers with a multicultural philosophy and bilingual skills. Migrant health-care clinics offer an opportunity for APNs and administrators to resolve the problem of overcrowded emergency rooms. The number and needs of veterans are changing and the Veterans Administration system has redesigned its structure to create more options for care delivery.

Any and all of these changes in the health-care environment can result in challenges for administrators, which can become opportunities for APNs. The wide variability of organizational structures and cultures provides a rich setting in which APNs can practice.

Care Delivery Systems and Financial Pressures

The changing health-care environment has led to changes in the structure of the care delivery system. Loose alliances of formerly competing organizations or formal contractual

TABLE 24-1	PRESSURES ON HEALTH-CARE ADMINISTRATORS
EXTERNAL FACTORS	INTERNAL FACTORS
Managed care	Diminishing resources
Competition—market shifts	Restructuring work processes
Global pricing	Changes in skill mix
Emphasis on costs	Creation of new types of workers
Demand for outcomes data	Reduction in acute care beds
Interest in patient satisfaction	Increased acuity in all settings
Insurers as driving forces regarding clinical decisions	Need for standard outcomes data
Emphasis on primary care	Enhanced training needs
Technological advances	Fewer workers through retirement, buy-out, terminations
Increased Internet use	Application of technology/automation
Changing demographics	Emphasis on interdisciplinary efforts
Shift to less acute/ambulatory/home care	Changing organizational structures
Regulatory requirements	Expanded scope of nurse executives
Licensing/credentialing requirements	Job/career insecurity
Changes in the medical profession	New reporting relationships
Better informed consumers	Pressure to constrain wages
Federal and state health-care initiatives	Multisite practices, affiliations, networks
Labor shortages, especially nursing shortages	Administration-physician relationships
Increased union activity	Nurse-physician relationships

arrangements, such as integrated delivery networks (IDNs), have increased throughout the country. IDNs can be developed horizontally or vertically and be for profit or not for profit. In a horizontally integrated delivery network, several like organizations form a legal entity. One example is an IDN of several hospitals, with one hospital usually being the tertiary or quaternary site. A vertically integrated delivery network, in contrast, brings together organizations from along the continuum of care. This network would include primary care, an acute care hospital, home health, a skilled nursing home, and perhaps even an insurance product. IDNs can cover a wide geographic area or consolidate care options in one city. It is more common to see one or two IDNs in a community as opposed to the several hospitals that once existed. Ownership of the system may also be distant as regional consolidation occurs. In the case of national for-profit systems, such as Columbia HCA or Tenet, centralized administration exerts significant control over local operations. For-profit niche players, such as heart hospitals and cancer treatment facilities, have competed effectively against full-service institutions in many communities. Their strategy of having a joint venture with specialty physicians provides what physicians want: control and enhanced income. APNs are entering this market as major cost-effective members of the team.

Although the reorganization that is occurring should provide opportunities for APNs, support for their employment varies widely among MCOs and IDNs. Some of the reasons for this are that physicians do not want the competition, executives who set policy do not appreciate the benefits of APNs, and the managers who do know the benefits are usually not in positions of influence within the organization (Sinclair, 1997). Mason, Cohen, O' Donnell, Baxter, and Chase (1997) researched the ways in which 67 MCOs employed NPs as primary care providers in New York and Connecticut. They found that the MCO executives who employed NPs were highly satisfied with them. Their data indicate the need for intensive efforts to educate MCO leaders as well as the public about the role, scope, and strengths of NPs. The most effective way to employ APNs in IDNs is undetermined, but some characteristics of IDNs would indicate possibilities for APNs, particularly those in the blended CNS/NP role (see Chapter 15). These APNs are able to cross settings to follow specialty patients and are able to work with nurses in those multiple settings to meet the complex needs of these patients. Systematic planning and coordination of care across settings are necessary to ensure desired outcomes, patient satisfaction, and financial performance. APNs can fill gaps in services and cross boundaries. They can facilitate the integration of nursing into the overall mission of the organization and devise cost-effective and quality clinical program innovations. System-wide chief administrators, in particular, should find APNs to be excellent candidates for ensuring the standard of nursing practice across all sites, as demonstrated in Exemplar 24-1.

Barger (1997) outlined some of the ways in which an APN can be better prepared to be effective in managed care delivery systems. She cited an example of time management in which a director of a primary care network found NPs to be less efficient in using their time than physician assistants (PAs). NPs spent an average of 45 minutes with patients, more than the practice could afford. She attributed this difference to the educational preparation of NPs, which encourages spending more time with the patient than does traditional medical training. However, she sees APNs as being in the best position to bridge managed care and community partnerships because of their skills in networking, coordinating, and integrating tasks.

As the organizational structures for care delivery have been reshaped, the work and structures inside have been reshaped too. Some organizations have introduced a product line structure in which nursing is often decentralized. In a product line structure, services are integrated and coordinated by a defined focus. This focus could be age, as with chil-

EXEMPLAR 24-1

In a large integrated delivery network (IDN), the chief nurse executive proposed that the cancer services unit employ a blended role advanced practice nurse (APN) to join oncologists in conducting consultative clinics in rural communities that were part of the IDN. Historically, the rural sites had designated a staff nurse to work with visiting oncologists, but there was not consistency in the assignments and the oncologists had expressed frustration. At first, the oncologists were uncertain about how the APN would function in the clinic. However, using skills in collaboration and negotiating entry to new organizations, the APN built credibility not only with the oncologists but also with the nurses and physicians at the rural sites. Originally, the APN accompanied the oncologist, but over time, her practice became increasingly independent. Typically, the oncologists evaluated patients with new diagnoses of cancer. The APN managed the care of patients receiving chemotherapy or those being followed up after completion of treatments. She also provided education for nurses in the rural sites and assisted in their development of chemotherapy administration skills. Because of her relationship with the comprehensive cancer center, she was also a source of information on clinical trials for the physicians in these communities. As the value of having a blended role APN available to patients with cancer in rural areas was recognized and the network of rural sites increased, the IDN cancer services hired an additional APN.

dren's services; gender, as with women's health services; or disease, as with cancer services. The structure may result in a marginalized nursing leadership that cannot advocate for appropriate patient care delivery models. However, a product line or decentralized structure does not necessarily indicate a lack of senior nursing voices. In fact, many product line administrators are nurses who have backgrounds in both advanced practice and administration. Product line structures can result in internal variability in advanced practice roles, with each product line defining positions differently, unless the organization develops linkages across product lines.

Changes to reduce cost have resulted in fewer resources for patient care units, reductions in the overall number of hospital employees, changes in the skill mix of employees, and the introduction of new kinds of workers to provide direct and indirect patient care. An APN role that suffered through these changes is that of the CNS. Because the CNS was too often "all things to all people," the actual contributions made by the CNS to patient care have been underestimated. One of the more frequent administrative responses was to eliminate the position as a cost-containment initiative. However, the literature reveals that new and reconfigured roles for the CNS and other APNs emerged from the chaotic inpatient environment (Fitzpatrick, 1998; Genet et al., 1995; McNatt & Eason, 2000; Naegle & Krainovich-Miller, 2001; Payne & Baumgartner, 1996; Tobin, 2000; see Chapter 19). The prediction that hospitals in the future will be purely intensive care facilities may create a justification for nurse administrators who are considering reintroduction of the CNS role. Having a CNS available to consult with staff about complex patient care situations will be increasingly necessary to support the staff at the bedside. Early in the development of case management, many CNSs were asked to take the lead in role definition. These positions built on the CNS's expertise in patient care and corporate financial management. The evolution of the role of APN case manager in hospitals is one example of how organizations are responding to the need to ensure effective and efficient care across traditional institutional boundaries in order to remain competitive (see Chapter 18).

Another role that is emerging in hospital settings is that of the ACNP (see Chapter 14). Although, historically, neonatal NPs were present in pediatric acute care settings,

NPs have not been widely employed with other inpatient populations. Today, in contrast, ACNPs have roles with trauma services, long-term medical services, and perioperative services.

The prediction that hospitals in the future will be purely intensive care facilities may create a justification for nurse administrators who are considering reintroduction of the CNS role. Having a CNS available to consult with staff about complex patient care situations will be increasingly necessary to support the staff at the bedside. Subacute, transitional, or skilled nursing and hospice units exist today as freestanding organizations or within hospital systems. The goal of these units is to provide care in the most appropriate setting to meet patients' needs. In the process, it is expected that the cost of care will be reduced by enhancing efficiency, eliminating unnecessary activities, and reducing overhead costs. Nurse administrators face daily pressure to have models of care that will achieve those goals and help the organization be attractive to managed care businesses. They need clinical leaders who understand the continuum of the patient's needs and who can develop appropriate services. APNs will fulfill that need. Regardless of the care environment, APNs and administrators must work together to be successful in designing new nursing roles and to preserve and enrich nursing values and heritage within current and emerging systems.

APNs are eligible to receive direct reimbursement in the majority of states. However, obtaining reimbursement privileges from managed care and insurance organizations has been difficult. With the increase in IDNs, APNs may find that they are not recognized as primary care providers and thus are ineligible for reimbursement because they are not included on the provider list. However, state laws and private insurance companies tend to follow federal legislation, so gains at the national level are having a broader influence.

As a result of turbulent health-care reimbursement changes, the momentum of moving care to the outpatient arena accelerated and the role of "gatekeeper" emerged. MCOs are focused on reducing the cost of care by controlling utilization of services through exerting greater control over approval of services. Physicians have experienced increased workloads with flat or decreased income. The Health Care Advisory Board (1999) found that, across the United States, relationships between physicians and hospital administrators were seriously strained. Academic organizations have not been immune to the changes. Johnson (1994) suggested that, if the medical profession did not increase the supply of primary care physicians, the government should redirect GME funds to schools of nursing for NP education. However, this has not happened. The Balanced Budget Act (BBA) (1997) decreased funding for GME, which is creating pressures on the competing missions of academic medical centers (Dickler & Shaw, 2000; Iglehart, 1999). Faculty are faced with the competing demands of seeing more patients while maintaining the teaching and research activities required for academic advancement. The decline in the number of residents and the restrictions on the number of hours they can work have prompted teaching hospitals to consider APNs and other alternative providers such as house physicians. The dilemma for administrators is that an APN's or house physician's salary is more expensive than that of a resident physician and there is no GME reimbursement. However, if the cost of educating and supervising the resident is factored in, the difference in cost may be slight. The dilemma for an APN is whether the role is purely substitution for the physician or is structured to allow the full benefit that an APN can provide. For instance, in critical care units, the ACNP can bring a distinct benefit to care delivery through advanced nursing skills of guidance and coaching, provision of continuity of care, and creative management of patient symptoms. Pioro et al. (2000) found that care delivered by an NP in an inpatient hospital setting is associated with resource use and clinical and functional outcomes similar to care provided by attending and house staff physicians. While such comparisons of APNs and physicians have been helpful in demonstrating the safety of APNs, the value-added component of advanced nursing needs to be emphasized in marketing these roles to administrators (see Chapter 25 for supporting research).

States have experimented with modifications to their Medicaid plans to improve access for their citizens. Historically, Medicaid enrollees have been predominantly women and children; currently, an increasing share of the funds covers services for people with chronic diseases and disabilities (Licking & Sampson, 1995). The State Children's Health Insurance Program (SCHIP) was expected to reach an additional 5 million children without health-care coverage (Lowe & Havens, 1998). Under Medicaid, family and pediatric NPs are recognized and reimbursed as primary care providers and could be hired into health-care systems to meet the needs of these additional 5 million children. However, many of the SCHIP initiatives are underfunded or unfunded or have been subject to severe budget cuts because of state budget crises, and the predicted outcomes have not materialized (see www.cms.hhs.gov/schip and Chapter 23). Nurse administrators can and should advocate for APNs as programs and services are designed for vulnerable populations.

Nursing Shortage

At the beginning of the 21st century, while most attention was focused on Y2K concerns, a beginning recognition of a new and different nursing shortage surfaced (Buerhaus, Staiger, & Auerbach, 2000). While little about the shortage was published in the health-care literature at that time, newspaper articles from around the country showed the breadth of the issue and some of the strategies being implemented to counter the effect of declining nursing school enrollments (Nevidjon & Erickson, 2001). A number of national organizations have released reports on the shortage as projected by the Bureau of Health Professions (Human Resources and Services Administration, 2002). These reports outline many strategies for recruiting new nurses and retaining current nurses. While the focus is on the registered nurse (RN) workforce in total and not advanced practice specifically, APNs will face opportunities and challenges if the shortages worsen as predicted. Administrators face escalating contract labor costs to maintain services and again are making difficult decisions related to roles that are not direct care related. However, they are also faced with issues of patient safety and quality of care. APNs can be a key resource in managing this complex scenario and improving the work environment (Disch, Walton, & Barnsteiner, 2001).

Quality and Safety

The Institute of Medicine's report, *To Err is Human: Building a Safer Health System* (2000), attracted national attention to the issues of safety in the health-care system. The second report, *Crossing the Quality Chasm: A New Health System for the 21st Century* (Institute of Medicine, 2001), focuses broadly on how to design the health-care system to improve quality of care and ensure safety. Other studies have addressed questions about the outcomes of the 1990s' restructuring of hospitals and IDNs (Burns & Pauly, 2002; Knox & Gharrity, 2002; Urden & Walston, 2002). Aiken and her team at the University of Pennsylvania have a long record of research on the outcomes of health care, the health-care workforce, and health-care workforce policy, with the aim of improving the quality of health care (see the website at www.nursing.upenn.edu/research/centers/detail.asp?rcid=3). One challenge for administrators is achieving a balance between strengthening quality and containing costs. Data-driven care management through the use of evidence-based standards and technology enhance both safety and quality improvements but also has a high cost. The public has been greatly sensitized to this issue through several patient situations that gained national attention; therefore organizations must have safety and quality at the top of the priority list.

Regulatory and Compliance Issues

Radical health-care reform did not occur under the Clinton administration, but two key pieces of federal legislation left their mark on the health-care industry. The 1996 Health Insurance Portability and Accountability Act (HIPAA) increased flexibility in coverage, and the BBA affected reimbursement (http://www.cms.gov). The BBA also created SCHIP. The nursing community heralded the BBA as a victory for their lobbying efforts because it contains a provision to extend Medicare reimbursement for APNs to all geographic areas and clinical settings (Haber, 1997; Minarik, 1997). Prior to this legislation, reimbursement was limited to APNs in rural areas and only to NPs in nursing homes. Interestingly, Wilken (1995) found that more rural states had fewer primary care NPs available than the need would require. She also noted that increased numbers of NPs in urban areas occurring simultaneously with declining numbers in rural areas was important to health-care policy. Her research showed that the availability of NPs is influenced by state-level initiatives such as support of educational programs, recruitment and retention efforts, and the presence of direct third-party reimbursement.

Regulatory agencies, such as the Joint Commission on Accreditation of Healthcare Organizations (JCAHO), recognize the changing health-care environment. The JCAHO has revised its standards to reflect the dynamic nature of health care and reflect the shift in the locus of care. The JCAHO requires consistent standards of care across an organization's care delivery sites (i.e., inpatient units, ambulatory clinics, and hospital-affiliated physicians' practices or offices). In community-based settings, the Health Plan Employer Data and Information Set (HEDIS) captures key indicators and is also modified as the changing health-care environment requires. These indicators become especially important as regional and national networks of health-care providers are formed.

COMMON PROBLEMS AND STRATEGIES FOR SOLVING THEM

There are compelling reasons for administrators to consider advanced practice nursing roles as the answers to many of the important challenges of today's health-care environment. Box 24-1 lists some of the characteristics that provide justifications for advanced practice nursing roles. Descriptions of the core competencies of APNs and other attributes that make them invaluable to administrators can be found in Chapter 3 and in the role chapters in Part III. Many of the variables that contribute to the success of APN roles are within the control of the administrator, so the needs and concerns of the administrator are important. Likewise, many of the variables that are within the control of the APN can contribute to the administrator's success. The next sections are relevant for both administrators and APNs.

BOX 24-1 • JUSTIFICATION FOR APN ROLES

- Use of theory-based and evidence-based clinical care
- Knowledge of clinical practice, including both medical and nursing perspectives
- Knowledge of health-care systems
- Ability to develop and integrate practice within organizations, communities, and systems
- Ability to make independent judgments and ethical decisions
- Ability to practice in multiple care settings, such as tertiary, hospice, and home care
- Flexibility
- Ability to identify the nature and costs of nursing interventions and their effects on patient outcomes
- Expertise in specific areas of advanced nursing practice within the domain of nursing, such as pain management and women's health
- Ability to translate research into practice
- Ability to analyze care for a population, not only an individual
- Skill in educating staff

Developing a Climate of Support for APNs

Abdellah (1997) described APNs worldwide and noted that their frustrations included balancing components of blended roles, defending their roles, lack of involvement in decision making, and lack of authority to make change. The last two are an alert, particularly to nurse administrators. They indicate that nurse administrators may be missing an opportunity to position APNs effectively within the nursing organization. However, they may also indicate that APNs have not been assertive in taking a leadership role. Given today's health-care climate, clinical leadership is essential for redesigning care delivery (see Chapter 9). APNs should be the administrator's designees to lead redesign efforts because they are the experts in direct patient care and they interact with patients along the continuum of care. They are also ideal candidates to lead a multidisciplinary team in performance improvement initiatives.

Administrators want APNs who are able to build partnerships and work comfortably in interdisciplinary teams. Support from physician and nurse colleagues tops the list of factors that help or hinder an APN. Acceptance by colleagues creates a successful environment in which to develop a practice. The opposite holds if support and acceptance are absent. Resistance to the role may be due to beliefs about APN roles (whether they are part of nursing or not) or to concerns about reimbursement. Sometimes a simple lack of understanding of a particular role by colleagues raises a barrier to successful implementation. Woods (1999) presented preliminary findings of a longitudinal study of factors facilitating or inhibiting implementation of advanced practitioner roles in the United Kingdom. In addition to the support of colleagues, Woods found that other key factors for success were the APN's own confidence in her or his ability, having increased autonomy, being valued as a resource by staff, and good staffing levels. Inhibiting factors included lack of resources, lack of understanding/unrealistic expectations of the role, poor staffing levels, nurse colleagues feeling threatened, and inadequate compensation for the role.

Modulating Interprofessional Tensions

Whatever the specific practice role, APNs have experienced tensions with other professions and within nursing. A study by Martin and Hutchinson (1999) documented the social problem of discounting behaviors and found that physicians, nurses, and administrators all contributed. Those tensions can influence the commitment of administrators to advanced practice nursing roles if mediating a situation puts the administrator at risk of alienating physicians. At the same time that organizations need to be creative and take risks in developing new ways of delivering care, increasing financial constraints may be creating a conservative, risk-averse atmosphere.

Tensions occur between administrators who want to employ APNs and insurers who do not want to reimburse for their services. This is a key issue for health-care administrators and can also be an issue for employer benefits managers. Employees may want the choice of NPs on a plan's health-care provider panel, and the lack of this choice can make them dissatisfied with a plan. Tensions occur between APNs and other health-care professionals, such as PAs, who compete for the same jobs if both credentials are accepted. They may also vie for the same patients.

When there is conflict and lack of clarity about a role, administrators may shy away from introducing the role into an organization, even if there is a good business case. The administrator should be the voice to influence decisions but may also be someone who does not understand the value of the various APN roles. Thus APNs must build meaningful working relationships with key administrators. This includes assessing the administrator's understanding of the APN's potential contributions and undertaking sustained efforts to educate and inform the administrator about advanced practice if necessary. If the administrator is knowledgeable and committed to advanced practice, the partnership between administrator and APN can lead to innovative solutions to the stresses experienced in health-care organizations.

Confusion among physicians about the specific nature of advanced practice nursing roles may stop them from giving support. Administrators and APNs can alleviate this confusion in a number of ways. These include providing information and research data regarding the attributes of APN roles and the benefits of collaboration for clinical practice, research activities, and teaching responsibilities. The administrator needs to demonstrate the positive value APNs add to patient care. Information and relevant articles can be distributed at clinical and administrative meetings or when a budget request for a position is presented. The importance of using appropriate data to support one's point of view cannot be overemphasized. The demonstration of successful role implementation is the most powerful means by which administrators and APNs can garner organizational support. Building institutional success stories, the folklore about the roles, can be most helpful to administrators.

Regardless of the organization and its structure, the administrator is influential in preparing the organization for the successful implementation of the role. The administrator can broker relationships, making sure the APN is introduced effectively in the organization by using formal communication tools such as newsletters and by setting up meetings with key individuals during the APN's orientation. The administrator can align resources that help an APN achieve the expected outcomes, such as arranging for access to current technology versus providing a "hand-me-down" computer from another employee in the organization. Such actions demonstrate how the organization values the APN's contribution.

In hospitals, administrators need to ensure that there is a voice for nursing in the credentialing and privileging process. In some community practices, physicians and APNs

are credentialed through the practice organization. The chief nurse administrator or another senior nurse should be a member of the organization's credentialing committee. In some organizations, credentialing is delegated to a nursing review committee, with the organization's credentialing committee simply accepting the nursing committee's approval. In an organization with well-established acceptance of APN roles, this works. Where there is ambivalence or unfamiliarity with the roles, the administrator needs to be in a position to clarify a particular role and advocate for privileges for APNs. APNs share the responsibility with administrators in ensuring that they have the proper credentialing to support their practices. They can assist the administrator by having timely and well-prepared application portfolios that meet the criteria established by the institution's credentialing committee.

A collaborative effort between the administrative team and APNs ensures integration of both administrative and clinical perspectives. This greatly enhances the potential for successful implementation of advanced nursing practice and reduces interprofessional tensions.

Maximizing Reimbursement

Events of the past few years illustrate the pressure administrators and clinicians feel to maximize reimbursement and, at the same time, maintain fiscal integrity. Besides being expert clinicians, APNs must understand the different reimbursement mechanisms and their role in ensuring that their fiscal practices are legal and ethical. While Medicare allows direct reimbursement to all APNs, there is variability with Medicaid, MCOs, and private payors. Medicaid allows direct reimbursement to family and pediatric NPs, but some states have extended this to all NP specialties. Some private insurance companies recognize and credential NPs as participating providers in their health plans. By having an individual provider number for each plan, APNs can bill for their services and generate revenue for themselves or their organization. (See specific roles chapters for further explanation of reimbursement by advanced practice nursing specialty.)

APNs must learn about the operations and finances of their practice group or institution. Although most providers do not like to think of health care as a business venture (Bodenheimer & Grumbach, 2002), it is important to know whether the business is conducted through a nonprofit community clinic or a for-profit private practice. Obviously, if the institution or practice does not remain financially solvent, it will be unable to remain open and to continue to provide patient care services. All health-care providers must adjust to practicing in an era of finite resources, and APNs are integral to development of cost-containment strategies. They can demonstrate how to integrate quality care and fiscal restraint.

An increasing number of authors are emphasizing the need for health-care providers to broaden their view to encompass the health of the general population, as well as their focus on providing the best possible care for each patient. Eliminating ineffective and inappropriate care and administrative waste can be a painless cost control method that does not adversely affect the quality of care provided to individual patients in the practice. Professional ethics in health care must incorporate social accountability for resource use and population health, as well as clinical responsibility for the care of individual patients. APNs can be leaders in this effort and ensure that the chosen cost control strategies do not adversely affect the quality of the care that is provided to patients. APNs are in a unique position to contribute to changing practices in health care to reduce waste, increase efficiency, and enhance the quality of care that is provided to patients. In inpatient settings in particular, APNs may have a greater understanding of the system as a whole and recognize areas where improvements can be made that lead to cost savings without compromising quality patient care.

APNs must pay special attention to the patient base in their institution and their practice. Is the mode of payment for most of the patients Medicaid, Medicare, managed care, point of service (POS), preferred provider organization (PPO), health maintenance organization (HMO), or fee for service? In a practice in which most of the patients are in managed care plans, health promotion and disease prevention are usually covered as part of the plan. Developing a system to track glucose control for all patients with diabetes in the practice or emergency room visits made by patients with asthma or offering group appointments for patients with hyperlipidemia may be cost-effective strategies in this scenario. In some fee-for-service plans, preventive medicine services are not covered benefits. In order to develop appropriate types of programs for the practice or institution, APNs must know the most common payment methods and how they affect the care of patients (Bodenheimer & Grumbach, 2002).

Coding all patient encounters accurately requires familiarity with the *International Classification of Diseases, 9th Revision* (ICD-9) diagnostic codes and *Current Procedural Terminology* (CPT) billing codes (Buppert, 2000; Chapter 20). Coding has not been routinely taught in many advanced practice nursing programs but is now becoming the norm. In general, most APNs undercode, which loses revenue for the practice. Asking the person who does the office billing to informally audit the APN's chart to determine whether the appropriate billing code is routinely selected can be a good way to ensure accuracy (Henley, 2003).

A primary goal of community-based APNs is to build a practice. In establishing a patient base, the APN becomes a valuable asset to the practice or institution. Marketing the unique skills of the APN or his or her expertise as a clinician can help build the practice. A common method many new providers use to build a practice is to allow the APN to interact with many new patients. One way this can be accomplished is by developing a schedule template that allows the APN to be more available for urgent care or same-day patient appointments. Patients who have positive experiences are much more likely to return to the APN for subsequent appointments. Once a patient base has been established, the practice is much more likely to be willing to make concessions to the APN in order to retain the patients in the APN's practice.

Developing Policies, Procedures, and Protocols

Whatever the practice setting, administrators value and require policies, procedures, and protocols to guide practice. The health-care environment has become increasingly litigious, and policies, procedures, and protocols are the infrastructure for safety and quality. APNs can bring their expert knowledge to the development of general institution-wide policies and procedures, as well as those that specifically address advanced practice. In a hospital setting, an APN may be the best choice to lead the clinical practice council or the product selection committee. Administrators can also recruit APNs to translate health policy regulations into the practice setting. An example would be designating APNs as leaders in some of the HIPAA policy and procedure definitions.

Compliance with Regulatory Agencies

The health-care environment has many regulatory influences that affect everything from reimbursement to worker safety (Table 24-2). Whether the APN is an employee or an

TABLE 24-2 KEY REGULATORY AGENCIES	
ACUTE CARE OR INPATIENT SETTINGS	OUTPATIENT OR COMMUNITY-BASED SETTINGS
Joint Commission on Accreditation of Healthcare Organizations (JCAHO): JCAHO is an independent, not-for-profit organization that evaluates the quality and safety of care of health-care organizations. JCAHO has specific regulations that must be adhered to in order for the institution to be accredited. Website: www.jcaho.org	**Health Plan Employer Data and Information Set (HEDIS):** HEDIS is a tool used by more than 90% of America's health plans to measure performance on important dimensions of care and service. It is a set of standardized measures that specifies how health plans collect, audit, and report on their performance in important areas ranging from breast cancer screening, to helping patients control their cholesterol, to customer satisfaction. Website: www.ncqa.org/Programs/HEDIS/
	National Committee for Quality Assurance (NCQA): NCQA is a consumer-driven, nonprofit organization that accredits health plans. Plans are being made to accredit group practices in future. Website: www.ncqa.org
Health Insurance Portability and Accountability Act (HIPAA): Title I of HIPAA protects health insurance coverage for workers and their families when they change or lose their jobs. Title II of HIPAA requires the Department of Health and Human Services to establish national standards for electronic health-care transactions and national identifiers for providers, health plans, and employers. It also addresses the security and privacy of health data. Website: www.cms.hhs.gov/hipaa/	HIPAA rules apply to outpatient settings as well as inpatient settings.
Center for Medicare and Medicaid Services (CMS): CMS is the federal agency that administers the Medicare and Medicaid Programs. Both programs have regulations that affect the care of patients covered under these plans. Website: www.cms.hhs.gov	CMS rules apply to outpatient settings as well as inpatient settings.

employer, awareness of regulations that direct clinical practice and business operations is critical. Regulations specific to advanced practice may not be known by administrators, and the APN can educate administrators and physicians about the rules governing advanced practice and reimbursement of APNs. Many hospitals do not take advantage of the potential scope of advanced nursing practice because there is not a champion who understands the regulatory arena for APNs. For example, under Medicare, APNs can be reimbursed "incident to" the services of a physician at 100% of the physician fee schedule if all of the incident to rules are followed, or they may apply for their own Medicare provider identification number and be reimbursed directly at 85% of the physician fee schedules (Gosfield, 2001; see Chapter 20).

Many managed care plans monitor health-care providers' performance in providing care. Individual providers track performance-related information. A provider profile presents summarized statistics to reflect provider performance in the form of rates and averages pertaining to the care rendered to a specific population. Pharmacy claims are an important source of profiling information. They allow the health plan to measure preventive care and long-term management of chronic disease (such as prescription of inhaled steroids for patients with asthma). Measures of resource utilization are another common indicator used. Common indicators measuring resource utilization include the numbers of emergency room visits or the numbers of days of hospitalization for the patients in the provider's panel. Measures that directly address quality of care have gained a more prominent place in provider profiling in the last several years. Many of these measures are required for external reporting of total plan performance. A common measurement tool is HEDIS. Among the key areas of HEDIS reporting are immunization rates, mammography rates, cervical screening rates, and treatment of patients with a chronic disease such as asthma or diabetes. APNs need to be aware of the measures used to evaluate their effectiveness as providers in a practice (see Chapter 25).

The National Practitioner Databank was established under the Healthcare Quality Improvement Act of 1986. The intent is to improve the quality of health care by encouraging hospitals and other health-care agencies to restrict the ability of incompetent health-care providers to move from state to state without disclosure or discovery of previous malpractice. It is primarily a flagging system intended to facilitate a comprehensive review of health-care practitioners' professional credentials. Hospitals must query practitioners when they apply for privileges and every 2 years for practitioners who are on the medical staff or hold privileges. State licensing boards may query at any time. Health-care practitioners may self-query at any time (see www.npdb-hipdb.com).

Hospitals and other health-care agencies can also verify the state license status of an APN through their individual state board of nursing or the National Council of State Boards of Nursing (NCSBN). The NCSBN Nursys (Nurse System) is a computer system containing nurse license and license discipline information compiled by boards of nursing in the United States and its territories.

Ensuring Patient Safety

The Institute of Medicine's attention to safety and quality has progressed to a study and recommendations about health professions education. In the Institute's 2003 report, *Health Professions Education: A Bridge to Quality*, the five core competencies that all health clinicians should have are outlined. The five competencies are providing patient-centered care, working in interdisciplinary teams, employing evidence-based practice, applying quality improvement, and utilizing informatics.

APNs can be the champions for safety and quality initiatives in organizations. Because of the admission of more patients with acute and complex illnesses and the issues related to nursing staffing, APNs in hospitals can provide the expertise needed to identify performance improvement initiatives and to lead those initiatives. By virtue of education and experience, APNs should be role models of the five competencies, and administrators can turn to them as internal consultants rather than hiring external ones. While the national attention to safety and quality has focused primarily on the hospital environment, community practices also need to have ongoing performance improvement as part of their agenda.

Technology and Informatics

Technology and advances in the understanding of disease, especially through genetics, have affected the cost of care and led to changes in the care environment. The rate of discovery in the last two decades has been incredible and has translated new knowledge into clinical treatment. Advances in electronic communication, in particular access to the Internet, have meant immediate worldwide information distribution. Patients and their families can obtain in-depth details about their diseases in a matter of minutes and come to their providers with more information than the providers may have. With a more informed public, providers encounter patients who expect more time to discuss their disease and treatment options. At the same time, payors may be restricting access to certain technologies and pressuring providers to see more patients.

Organizations diligently deliberate choices of clinical and information technology because the demands are endless and the financial resources are not. Administrators often face difficult decisions related to capital expenditures. APNs can advocate for both clinical and informatics technology and are excellent members of committees that evaluate requests. Because they have a broad view of the organization and the patients being cared for, APNs can relate technology to work flow and identify cost/benefit factors. For example, handheld devices or personal digital assistants can store reference books, calculate complex medical results, keep track of patients and procedures, and serve as daily planners. There are even programs that create prescriptions to be automatically sent to a pharmacy or calculate CPT codes for billing.

STRATEGIES TO STRENGTHEN APN ROLES

Unless an APN establishes an independent practice, administrators decide whether to create a new APN role, whether to eliminate one, whether to transform the role, or whether to keep it as it is. They also can influence how an advanced practice nursing position is compensated and what resources will be made available for the APN. Thus, by understanding the needs of administrators, APNs can cultivate champions within the organization for their roles. Likewise, by understanding the contributions APNs can make, administrators can most effectively position APNs as leaders and achieve success in fulfilling the organization's mission.

An administrator can assess the organization's need for an APN and determine which advanced practice role will fulfill the need. Involving stakeholders in planning for the new position ensures commitment to the person who is hired. A well-developed position description and agreed-upon reporting relationships establish the foundation for the APN and facilitate entry to the organization. The process of recruiting the best APN includes a comprehensive interview process to ensure that all stakeholders have an opportunity for input about their expectations. Finally, an orientation to the organization, including communication about the expectations of the APN, is necessary to foster success.

Considerations When Applying for a Position

There are many factors for the APN to consider when applying for a position in an organization or practice (Box 24-2). Although it may seem that many of these factors relate to larger organizations, they can be equally important when an APN is considering entering a primary care practice or physician group. Being knowledgeable about the regulatory conditions in a particular state is important if the APN is considering relocation. Some states are more supportive of advanced nursing practice than others. Once there is an understanding about the state's regulatory environment, conditions specific to a position are critical.

Administrators provide the vision and shape the culture for nursing practice within hospitals, community-based practices, and many other health-care organizations. They derive their vision from the organization's visions, mission, and goals and their beliefs and values about nursing. For APN roles to be firmly established, administrators must promote a nursing philosophy that recognizes advanced nursing practice as central to the quality of care, access to care, and advancement of the profession. However, administrators are also faced with pressures of balancing cost and quality and a workforce shortage. APNs provide the clinical surveillance within an organization. They are able to see patterns of care, as well as assess and meet the individual needs of patients. Because APNs are able to move throughout the care continuum, they can collaborate with administration to identify ways to manage resources effectively. Also, they are able to address development needs among the nursing staff. When administrators understand this, it is easy to maintain a commitment to advanced practice even in difficult times. For example, one author refused to eliminate the CNS role in her organization, even though consultants were suggesting to administration that this was an easy budget cut.

The organization's mission and vision can orient an APN candidate to the potential support for the role. Organizations with a strong community focus may be seeking to develop APN-run clinics. Academic organizations—with their triple mission of patient care, teaching, and research—may seek doctorally prepared CNSs to influence the advancement of all nursing practice. IDNs may create a blended APN role that crosses boundaries of the discrete entities within the network to ensure a consistent standard of care for patients.

An important consideration for an APN applying for a position with a corporate MCO is that the chief operating structure and high-level administrators that control policy and budget may be several states away and virtually inaccessible. APNs need to assess for dissonance between midlevel management at the local level and the centralized hierarchy. In such structures, final decisions usually come from the central administration, and there may not be a nursing administrator to serve as a champion.

A candidate should assess how members of the organization understand the mission and vision and how an APN contributes to achieving them. Likewise, the nurse administrator will evaluate the APN candidate as to her or his interpretation and understanding of the organization and its goals. The nurse administrator will look for the fit between the mission and vision of the organization and the APN's personal abilities and reasons for seeking the position. In the interview process, the selection committee and hiring administrator will also evaluate the candidate's ability to negotiate the political environment of the organization, particularly if the position is new.

BOX 24-2 • ORGANIZATIONAL CONSIDERATIONS FOR APNs WHEN APPLYING FOR A POSITION

- Organization's mission, structure, strategic priorities, culture
- Nursing philosophy, share of organizational power, definition of APN roles
- Commitment to interdisciplinary care and continuous improvement principles
- Expected outcomes, financial objectives
- Reporting relationship, credentialing requirements, reimbursement potential
- Resources, other APNs
- Models of care delivery, clinical programs, patient populations
- State regulations for APNs

When an APN considers a position, he or she must evaluate the collaborative atmosphere of the organization, regardless of whether it is a large and complex system or a small group practice. The advertising of a position does not necessarily mean that all the people within the organization embrace an advanced practice nursing role. Learning about the partnerships that exist and seeking examples of past successes can be helpful in understanding who may be champions of the role. A champion is not just found in the physician or nursing arenas. Strategic alliances can be formed with any of the organization's formal and informal leaders. They are more likely to be supporters if they understand the purpose of the position and, as appropriate, participate in the interviewing process.

In an organizational culture with open and honest communication, the administrator and APN can identify key leaders and anticipate their needs for specific information. All organizations may not have that culture, and the administrator can help the APN understand the politics. Other APNs in the organization can also help a new APN by introducing the new APN to key leaders. Partnering with supporters builds a strong network that can prevent an APN from being seen as an intruder.

Entry in to the Organization

How an APN is introduced in the organization sets the stage for the APN's success. Being educated about organizational culture and politics, as well as being given the usual basic information of orientation, prepares the APN for the work environment. Larger organizations usually have well-developed orientation plans in place that introduce new employees to the organizational culture. However, even a small primary care practice needs to develop an orientation plan for a new APN. Having clear expectations on entry into an organization lays a foundation for success. The APN and administrator should collaborate in establishing goals and means of performance measurement to define success. Success may be defined as shorter waiting times for a new patient appointment, higher patient satisfaction scores, or decreased lengths of stay in the inpatient units. It can mean developing a new home care service for seniors who cannot travel to office practices. It can mean designing a clinical advancement program for staff nurses.

Whether the new position is in a private practice or in a hospital, establishing credibility as a clinician begins as soon as the APN joins the organization. Once physicians, administrators, nurses, and other staff have confidence in the APN's abilities and judgment as a clinician, they will begin to offer support for the APN's efforts. As a new employee in an institution, the most important priority for the APN is to establish a clinical practice and gain the respect of colleagues. One of the ways an administrator can expedite an APN's transition into the organization is to set up a peer review system for the first 30 to 90 days of employment. For example, a senior provider in a clinic practice can review the charts of patients who have been seen by the new APN. This is usually an expeditious way for the new APN to gain the confidence and trust of the other providers in the practice. Once the other providers have confidence in and respect for the APN, they will be more apt to support changes that remove barriers to the APN's practice. Another method is reporting and tracking satisfaction scores of patients who have been cared for by the APN. Recent randomized clinical trials in which NPs were compared with primary care physicians revealed no major differences in selected patient outcomes and higher patient satisfaction with NP care (Phillips, Harper, Wakefield, Green, & Fryer, 2002). The APN can also become a resource for the practice by training other staff or providers in the practice. As the APN gains credibility with administrators, the potential for the APN to become an influential leader in the organization is enhanced.

In most institutions and larger practices, committees make decisions about practice management. APNs should apply to be members on the different committees in the practice and the institution. Common committees are customer satisfaction, performance improvement, product/technology evaluation, practice management, utilization review, credentialing, and the executive committee. As a committee member, it is the responsibility of the APN to have an understanding of the economics of providing health care in the institution and a willingness and desire to participate in finding solutions to provide care cost-effectively. Institutions and practices cannot remain open unless they remain solvent. It is critical that APNs remain cognizant of the dual responsibility and goal of providing quality care in the most cost-effective manner possible.

Most primary care practice sites have a designated medical director whose role is to be the administrator of the practice at each clinic. In many institutions one of the requirements for becoming a medical director is being a physician. However, this requirement can be changed, and the second author has had the opportunity to serve as the co-medical director of a practice site. If the requirements are restrictive, APNs can lobby to have them changed to be more inclusive. If the bylaws are successfully changed, APNs can apply for the position. One approach is to make the changes in stages. The APN can begin as an associate medical director or co-medical director. APNs have the skills and knowledge to be leaders in primary care practices.

The "Fit" of the APN within the Organization

The requirements of the position will determine the educational preparation and previous work experiences needed by the APN. For example, an organization seeking ways to maximize its reimbursement potential may develop NP and CNM positions to achieve this goal. An academic organization faced with declining availability of residents may increase opportunities for APNs to ensure a standard of quality care. Neonatal NPs have managed care in intensive care nurseries for many years, and ACNPs are establishing themselves in critical care units and trauma programs.

The goals and objectives of the position determine the APN's responsibilities, such as primary care delivery, consultation, program planning, staff development, clinical research, and expansion of patient services. The nature of the clinical program will determine the selection of the appropriate APN role. The number and type of other disciplines and professionals within the practice setting are other considerations. A CNS position may be selected to enhance staff nurses' clinical and communication skills within a clinical program that includes physicians, PAs, and ACNPs. A blended role CNS/NP may be desired if the purpose is to manage the care of a group of patients across multiple settings in an IDN. A CRNA may be hired to cost-effectively enhance the day surgery program. The purpose of a position will also determine the licensure and credentialing requirements (see Chapter 22).

Nuccio and colleagues (1993) suggested that role expectations solicited from staff nurses could be useful in developing supportive relationships. Paul (cited in Paladichuk, 1998) also spoke to the importance of the APN–staff nurse partnership. Delineation of roles and clear communication and reporting structures strengthen these relationships. The emerging focus on advanced nursing practice within the context of work redesign affects other care providers in different ways. In some organizations, APNs are assuming functions previously performed by other professionals, including physicians, social workers, and clinical dietitians. Because APNs potentially affect the practice of other care providers, having well-defined expectations modulates what can become "territorial disputes." The broadest communication of the APN's responsibilities and goals helps ensure the APN's success. The administrator can minimize the potential for these disputes by maintaining the focus of decision making on patient care requirements and how to address them in the most cost-effective and efficient manner with the best possible outcomes. Sincerely expressed respect for the work of other professionals, coupled with sensitivity and diplomacy, modulates the potentially negative effects of these negotiations.

APNs may align with medicine's organizational structure and discount their nursing connection. APNs need to seek collaborative relationships within the nursing organizational structure because the nursing leaders can be essential advocates for APNs. For example, although CRNAs have worked for many years with their physician colleagues, there have been many occasions of conflict, and for this reason, organizations and practices may have concerns about hiring these APNs. Anesthesia is a recognized specialty in both medicine and nursing. Approximately 80% of CRNAs work as partners in care with anesthesiologists, while the remaining 20% function as sole anesthesia providers working and collaborating with surgeons and other licensed physicians. When anesthesia is administered by a CRNA, it is recognized as the practice of nursing; when it is administered by an anesthesiologist, it is recognized as the practice of medicine. In a hospital that employs CRNAs, the nurse administrator can be an effective voice in collaboration with them if interprofessional tensions arise.

Reporting Relationships

There is no singular reporting structure for APNs, regardless of the organization. APNs may report to another APN in organizations with many APNs, to a nursing director responsible for an acute care area, to a physician, or to a practice manager in a community-based agency. Specific roles, legal requirements, and other variables in the organization will shape the reporting relationship. For instance, NPs, CNMs, and CRNAs who practice in hospital settings must obtain privileges through the credentialing committee, which may require a designated physician supervisor/collaborator. The recent improvements in direct reimbursement for APNs may change the requirement for a physician supervisor/collaborator, but the authors' experience is that most hospital risk managers still expect this supervision/collaboration if APNs seek hospital privileges. Some APNs may also be accountable to a nurse administrator. While acute care CNSs are unlikely to need formal credentialing or require a collaborating physician, blended role CNS/NPs or CNSs in a physician practice may require both. The individual to whom the APN reports can indicate the importance of the position, but this should not be overvalued. Depending on the organization, where an APN is listed on an organizational chart may be much less important than what access the APN has to key leaders.

As noted, all APNs should carefully examine a potential practice setting before accepting a job offer. Consideration should be given to how the job is positioned in the organization and to the position or individual to whom the APN is accountable. Parrinello (1995) described three models of APN practice: the physician practice model, the nursing model, and the joint practice model. In the physician practice model, the APN typically joins a group practice and reports to a physician. In the nursing model, usually seen in hospitals, the APN typically reports to a nurse administrator and works with a specific group of patients, physicians, or units. This is the traditional CNS structure, but it is also how APN case managers may be assigned and it is often used with ACNPs, such as those in intensive care units. The joint practice model is a cohesive physician and nurse care delivery model in which the funding for the APN is a private enterprise between stakeholders or a combination of nursing/hospital and professional revenue funds. An additional model is the independent contractor model. In the independent contractor model, the APN establishes a private business and serves as both administrator and clinical provider to patients (see Chapter 20). The business may also be consultative in which the APN provides educational and project consultation to an organization. Table 24-3 outlines some of the advantages and disadvantages of each model.

In the physician practice model, three organizational structures exist: single clinics, multiple practice sites, and integrated delivery systems.

SINGLE CLINICS

The traditional model in United States medical care has been that of independent private physicians working as solo practitioners in single or small group practices dispersed throughout a region. In this model private physicians delivered most medical care under a fee-for-service arrangement. In the past, most hospitals were private nonprofit institutions, often run by a board of trustees composed of prominent individuals in the community. Most physicians in the traditional fee-for-service system were not employees of any hospital. They joined the medical staff of one or several hospitals to gain the privilege of admitting patients. Along with medical staff privileges came the responsibility and opportunity to serve on hospital committees that set the hospital's policies and standards. For many years, physicians were the dominant power in hospitals because they are permitted to admit patients to the hospital and hospitals require patients to receive income. Now the norm is larger physician group practices with shared risk and cost. With the changes in reimbursement mechanisms and the consolidation of practices and institutions, new opportunities exist for physicians, and subsequently, for APNs.

MULTIPLE PRACTICE SITES

Multispecialty group practice started with the Mayo Clinic in the 1890s (Boenheimer & Grumbach, 2002). In this early model, physicians worked in a group setting that preserved

TABLE 24-3	MODELS OF PRACTICE IN ORGANIZATIONS	
MODEL	ADVANTAGES	DISADVANTAGES
Physician Practice Model	Funding linked to the success of the group practice, not nursing budget; clinical work closely linked with physicians and clearly defined	Potential conflict in definition of collaboration versus supervision; isolation from nursing colleagues
Nursing Model	Clear identification with nursing, credibility with staff, focus on broader APN skills	Potential for decreased collaboration with physicians; risk for losing continued funding within the large nursing budget
Joint Practice Model	Captures the best of physician- and nursing-based models; interdependency is recognized	Complexity of a matrix structure and potential to be caught between two supervisors
Independent Contractor Model	Autonomy, minimal bureaucracy	Isolation, financial risk, professional liability

the private practice's traditional independence. The financing and delivery of health care remained separate. The practice billed patients and third-party plans under a fee-for-service structure. The clinics were owned and administered by physicians working in various specialty areas. They brought large numbers of physicians together in one practice structure. By formally integrating specialists in a single clinic structure, group practice attempted to promote a more collaborative style of care. Enhanced quality of care was expected as a result of the greater opportunity for peer review when colleagues worked together and shared responsibility for the care of patients.

INTEGRATED DELIVERY SYSTEMS

As noted, vertical integration refers to consolidating all levels of care under one organizational chart and ownership. It includes all levels of care, from primary to tertiary, and all the staff and facilities necessary to provide this full-spectrum level of care. The Kaiser-Permanente organizational model is typical of vertical integration. The Kaiser-Permanente Medical Care Program is the largest United States prepaid group practice model. It consists of three interlocking administrative units. The Kaiser Foundation Health Plan performs the functions of health insurer. The Kaiser Foundation Hospitals Corporation owns and administers Kaiser Hospitals. The Permanente Medical Group is the physician organization that administers the group practice and provides medical care services to Kaiser Plan members under a capitated contract plan (Bodenheimer & Grumbach, 2002).

In 1973 President Nixon enacted the Health Maintenance Organization Act into law. Independent Practice Association (IPA) model HMOs were included as legitimate HMOs along with prepaid group practice models. The HMO law required medium-sized and large businesses that provided health insurance to their employees to offer at least one federally qualified HMO as an alternative to traditional fee-for-service insurance. Under this model, physicians and other health-care providers remain in their own private practice offices but join together into physician groups called *independent practice associations*. There are different types of models under the umbrella term of *IPA*. In general, the IPA contracts with insurance companies to provide care to patients in their plan under a discounted fee-for-service or capitated contract arrangement.

In any of these models, APNs may also practice under a leased employee agreement. This allows a business to contract for the services of an employee of another business. The APN may be an employee of the hospital or of the physician group. One group may lease the employee from the other group.

In any of these physician models, the clinical experience of the APN is similar. Where APNs will find differentiation is in their ability to influence organization policy. In large complex organizations, such as large multidisciplinary/multisite groups or integrated delivery systems, decisions may be made remote from the APN's practice. In a smaller group practice, the APN may be integral to practice decisions. Additionally, the procedure for specialist referral may vary by the type of organization. In a small practice the APN may have more freedom to select specialists for consultation compared with large multidisciplinary groups where providers are expected to refer internally.

In deciding in which model to practice, an APN will want to assess a variety of variables including, but not limited to, the specific functions of the position, funding for the position, size and characteristics of the organization, outcomes expected, and scope of influence. No one model is preferable for APNs; rather, the APN must be aware of personal preferences and availability of positions.

Resources

To succeed, APNs need resources. Some are as simple as adequate space for direct and indirect patient care activities. Common practice-related expenses are telephone lines, computer, malpractice insurance, and a beeper for answering pages. In primary care practices, employment of a medical assistant or RN to admit patients to examination rooms, a medical billing person, and a receptionist are also needed resources. The organization needs to assure the APN of appropriate salary support and opportunities for raises or sufficient opportunities to generate income through professional fees. Assistive staff, such as clinical assistants, secretarial support, and data entry personnel, may be required. Access to automated systems is essential in today's environment. Financial and administrative support for continuing education opportunities in both academic and nonacademic programs is essential for maintaining skills. Asking to see a budget for the APN position is an easy way to evaluate whether the organization has planned for the needed resources. Finally, routine and regular contact with the administrator ensures that ongoing and new resources are provided (see Chapter 20).

Measuring the Impact of APNs

During the turmoil of the changing health-care payor environment, much has been written about the value of NPs to provide primary care. The lay media as well as the professional literature have viewed the use of this APN role as a way to increase access to care and to control costs. However, the literature also reinforces the necessity of measuring the impact of all advanced practice roles on the cost and quality of care (Byers & Brunell, 1998; Carroll & Fay, 1997; Fitzpatrick, 1998; Jackson et al., 2003; Mundinger, 1999; Schaffner & Bohomey, 1998). By demonstrating their ability to deliver high-quality, cost-effective care, APNs show their value and secure a position in the health-care marketplace. Box 24-3 lists Web-based resources APNs and administrators can use to develop measurement and monitoring strategies (see also Chapters 20 and 25).

Carroll and Fay (1997) reviewed the challenges APNs and administrators face in measuring the impact of advanced nursing practice. They discussed several considerations: defining the scope of practice of the APN; building consensus about the definition and the relationship of structure, process, and outcomes variables; designating the settings and systems of practice; influencing stakeholders; and ensuring the scientific rigor of a study. In making informed decisions about the employment of APNs in an organization, an administrator will often search the literature for studies that document cost and quality outcomes of employing APNs. Administrators are inundated with a tremendous amount of information, so it is helpful to the administrator when APNs forward articles to them, particularly reports about outcomes and cost savings attributed to APNs.

Evaluation strategies have typically focused on specific components of an APN's role. Chapter 25 details comprehensive models for evaluating the impact of APNs and examines the growing research literature supporting the varied outcomes of advanced practice nursing. Administrators need to consider allocation of resources to support APNs in practice evaluation beyond the basics required by regulatory agencies or performance management systems. Byers and Brunell (1998) advocated the development of a statewide or national database of APN-dependent measures, such as rate of complications following an APN-provided procedure, which would provide critical information for APNs.

BOX 24-3 • RESOURCES FOR SAFETY AND QUALITY MEASUREMENT

Agency for Healthcare Research and Quality	www.ahrq.gov
American Nurses Association	www.nursingworld.org
American Society for Quality	www.asq.org
Institute for Healthcare Improvement	www.ihi.og
Institute of Medicine	www.iom.edu
International Council on Nursing	www.icn.ch
Joint Commission on Accreditation of Healthcare Organizations	www.jcaho.org
Leap Frog Group	www.leapfroggroup.org
Medical Group Management Association	www.mgma.com
National Association for Healthcare Quality	www.nahq.org
National Guideline Clearinghouse	www.guideline.gov/index.asp
Medical Outcomes Trust	www.outcomes-trust.org
Health Outcomes Institute	www.health-outcomes-institute.com
Foundation for Accountability	www.facct.org
National Healthcare Practitioner Databank	www.npdb-hipdb.com,

---

In any organization, a clear definition of the APN roles, the roles' objectives, and the time frame for achieving them are required to measure and monitor APN contributions. The APN and the person or persons to whom the APN is accountable must understand these factors. Consensus about the scope of practice, definitions of outcomes, and practice setting are a few of the variables to consider. Ongoing communication about performance and achievement of objectives is one step in measuring the value of the role. Formal goal setting and review of performance according to the organization's performance management system should be done annually.

In a primary care practice, deciding the appropriate number of patients for whom the APN is responsible is based on the context and nature of the clinical practice and forms the basis for one measure: productivity. In Frampton and Wall's study (1994), NPs and PAs believed that 81% to 91% of the patients they saw were appropriately cared for and did not require the services of a physician (Grumbach, Hart, Mertz, Coffman, & Palazzo, 2003). Other factors that influence this number include the organization's standards of practice and the number and diversity of other staff members within the clinical practice. For example, Dang and Haller (1995) found a range of 7 to 16 patients per case manager in the academic hospitals surveyed. MCOs often have established targets for the numbers of patients seen by NPs or CNMs. Hummel and Pirzada (1994) noted that teams of "non-physician providers" (NPs or PAs) and physicians were extremely cost-effective when the number of patients cared for expanded.

As health-care administrators know, listening to patients' concerns regarding the operation of a practice is instructive. Besides receiving quality patient care and having confidence in the providers in the practice, patients choose to remain with a practice for many other reasons. Patient satisfaction surveys are a valuable means of obtaining feedback about how patients perceive the practice and what areas need improvement. Many standard surveys are available. An example used by many large clinics and hospitals is the Press Ganey Survey (www.pressganey.com). This survey, like others, measures a variety of factors that patients are concerned about including ability to schedule an appointment quickly and conveniently when needed, ability to obtain refills in a timely manner, adequate parking facilities, waiting time in the office and exam room before being seen, waiting time on hold trying to get an appointment, being able to speak with a real person, friendliness and efficiency of the front and back office, clinic location, office hours, and environment. Common provider factors that patients identify in this survey include being listened to, having their questions answered, and having confidence in the provider. APNs tend to score well on patient satisfaction surveys. In practices that use patient satisfaction surveys, positive scores increase the value of the APN to the practice. However, it is most helpful if the generic surveys can be modified to contain specific items that are more reflective of advanced practice nursing strengths and areas of emphasis. Data do not indicate that generic patient satisfaction instruments demonstrate significant differences between APNs and physicians (Girouard, 2000). Smaller practices can develop their own survey instrument if necessary.

CONSIDERATIONS FOR THE FUTURE

The turmoil of the current health-care environment is expected to continue for the next two decades. This holds both opportunities and threats for APNs. The passage of the BBA in 1997 offered opportunities for expanding practice options for NPs and CNSs (Keepnews, 1998), since direct billing by these APNs identifies the types of patients they see. The BBA also defined CNS practice for the first time in Medicare law, which gives CNSs the opportunity to serve Medicare beneficiaries. However, the BBA is also affecting physicians, and in a few years, APNs may find increased competition with physicians who are struggling to maintain their practices and their income. In addition, the rising cost of malpractice insurance is part of the turmoil in the health-care environment for both physicians and APNs.

A theme throughout this chapter has been reimbursement. Given the increasing pressure on institutions and practices to sustain financial viability, APNs and administrators must work together to maximize reimbursement for APN services.

In 1990 the National Practitioner Data Bank began collecting information about health-care practitioners who have had judgments in malpractice suits or disciplinary action taken against them. Between 1990 and December 31, 2001, general and advanced practice RNs have had 3615 malpractice payments against them (Croke, 2003). General RNs had the most malpractice payments, 2311 or 63%, followed by CRNAs with 820 or 22.7% and CNMs with 296 or 8.2%. NPs made the fewest malpractice payments (188 or 5.2%) (Croke, 2003).

It is essential that APNs define the value-added services they provide that complement both physician and nursing practices. According to Flanagan (1998), analyses of NP-physician collaborative practice show that patients benefit from the combination of complementary skill sets. Several studies of NP-physician teams have demonstrated cost and quality-of-care improvements in nursing homes, as well as in emergency, obstetrical, and surgical inpatient settings (Burl, Bonner, Rao, & Khan, 1998; Horrocks, Anderson, & Salisbury, 2002; Jackson et al., 2003; Naylor et al., 1999). Disease prevention and management of chronic conditions also benefit from NP-physician teams (Phillips, 2002). Studies have shown that physicians who work with NPs report improved job satisfaction, reduced workloads, and increased ability to offer a higher standard of care (Koperski, Rogers, & Drennan, 1997).

Berger and colleagues (1996) defined several future roles to promote the optimal use of knowledge, skills, and abilities of APNs. They do not all fit the advanced practice nursing definition in this book but do represent the reality of the marketplace in which new titles and role definitions continue to arise. Although these authors acknowledge the confusion that has existed in defining advanced practice roles and functions, they propose the following roles: case manager, clinical educator, clinical researcher, clinical consultant, NP, corporate/community NP, and patient care manager. These roles take into account the need to serve patients with increasingly complex health-care concerns while being cost conscious, and some of them incorporate the unique skills of APNs. Debate continues about whether nursing needs more advanced practice titles, but during a state of major change, more roles and titles are likely to develop (see Chapters 3 and 19). Nurse administrators in particular, but all executives, can assist in reducing the confusion about advanced practice nursing roles by not introducing more nomenclature into the job lexicon. Increasing clarity about the advanced practice nursing roles described in this text is an important responsibility of administrators as well as other nursing leaders.

Achieving such clarity will require that educational programs, whether formal education or continuing education, prepare nursing administrators to understand advanced practice nursing. As APN roles become more prevalent, administrators need program content on APN roles and outcomes. Further, managing a differentiated workforce requires attention to organizational positioning of APNs in order to maximize their contributions. Faculty in both nursing administration programs and health-care administration programs need to educate their students so that administrators are in a better position to promote and preserve advanced nursing practice.

Hester and White (1996) examined CNSs' perceptions of their future. They found that CNSs perceived that their roles were changing to meet the challenges of the changing delivery system. An area in which APNs can take a lead is in the research of patient outcomes, particularly related to quality and cost (see Chapters 8 and 25). This chapter has emphasized that APNs must become more knowledgeable about the "business" of health care and learn to speak the language of administrators. As early as 1989, Brown described the need for CNSs to serve as "shuttle diplomats" who interpret economic realities and administrative decisions to nursing staff and clinical realities to administrative staff. Brown (1989) described the CNS as able to be "the person in the middle, a person expected and required to speak the language of both subcultures, understand the issues and dilemmas of each, and participate in the problem-solving of both arenas" (p. 285). The need for shuttle diplomacy by all APNs, particularly those working in large, complex organizations, has never been more critical, especially in relating clinical activities to institutional costs. Administrators must help APNs with this development. The era of APNs being able to self-define their positions and be vaguely accountable within an organization is over. Additionally, changes in the organizational structures that support care delivery can present advantages for advanced practice nursing. APNs need to view the development of IDNs or community-based programs as realms in which they can advance their services and create new opportunities.

The APN's direct clinical practice is the foundation for advanced practice nursing success in the 21st century. As noted throughout this book, clinical care is increasingly complex; the aging population is living longer with multisystem chronic illnesses; increases in technology continue; and burgeoning research findings, particularly in genetics research, need to be incorporated into clinical care. Having a strong expert clinical practice base is critical for APNs to enact the clinical leadership and critical thinking skills so valued by administrators. The characteristics of APN direct clinical practice noted in Chapter 5 (use of a holistic perspective, formation of partnerships with patients, expert clinical thinking and skillful performance, use of research evidence, and diverse health and illness management approaches) are the sources of the APN's value-added contributions to patient care. Core competencies (see Chapter 3) emanate from this practice expertise. Administrators must be careful not to overload APNs with committee and project work to the extent that they lose these skills or become less visible in key practice arenas. Although this is tempting in the short term, weakening an APN's practice strength compromises the reason the positions were established and can diminish the APN's effectiveness in the long term. APNs must also be vigilant in communicating with their administrators when nonclinical activities require them to compromise their practice expertise.

According to Milstead (1997), the role of political activist is one that APNs should embrace. Certainly, APNs need to follow national and state legislation closely and make their views known. They can also be valuable educators of politicians and their staffs about the issues faced by patients and by nurses in advanced practice. Many of the APN's clinical skills, such as communication, conflict resolution, and critical thinking, transfer well into the political arena (see Chapters 9 and 23). Administrators can be allies to APNs in the political arena and present a strong voice for nursing.

SUMMARY

APNs and organizational leaders—whether nurse executives, administrators, or physicians—should think in terms of the skills that APNs bring to an organization, especially as changes continue in the provision and the location of care delivery within an organization and within the community. APNs should promote their skills as new opportunities and new relationships emerge, and administrators should assist them in doing so. Furthermore, the community's and the organization's needs and strategic imperatives are the context for current and future job-related opportunities for APNs. By committing to the mission and objectives of the organization and consistently developing and expanding their skills, APNs ensure their place in the future of health-care delivery.

REFERENCES

Abdellah, F. G. (1997). Managing the challenges of role diversification in an interdisciplinary environment. *Military Medicine, 162,* 453-458.

Barger, S. E. (1997). Building healthier communities in a managed care environment: Opportunities for advanced practice nurses. *Advanced Practice Nursing Quarterly, 2,* 9-14.

Berger, A. M., Eilers, J. G., Pattrin, L., Rolf-Fixley, M., Pfeifer, B. A., Rogge, J. A., et al. (1996). Advanced practice roles for nurses in tomorrow's healthcare systems. *Clinical Nurse Specialist, 10,* 250-255.

Bodenheimer, T., & Grumbach, K. (2002). *Understanding health policy: A clinical approach* (3rd ed.). New York: Appleton and Lange.

Brown, S. J. (1989). Supportive supervision of the CNS. In A. B. Hamric & J. A. Spross (Eds.), *The clinical nurse specialist in theory and practice* (2nd ed., pp. 285-298). Philadelphia: W. B. Saunders.

Buerhaus, P. I., Staiger, D.O., & Auerbach, D. I. (2000). Implications of an aging registered nurse workforce. *JAMA: The Journal of the American Medical Association, 283,* 2948-2954.

Buppert, C. (2000). *The primary care provider's guide to compensation and quality.* Boston: Jones & Bartlett.

Burl, J. B., Bonner, A., Rao, M., & Khan, A. M. (1998). Geriatric nurse practitioners in long-term care: Demonstration of effectiveness in managed care. *Journal of the American Geriatrics Society, 46,* 506-510.

Burns, L. R., & Pauly, M. V. (2002). Integrated delivery networks: A detour on the road to integrated health care? *Health Affairs, 21*(4), 128-143.

Byers, J. F., & Brunell, M. L. (1998). Demonstrating the value of the advanced practice nurse: An evaluation model. *AACN Clinical Nurses, 9,* 296-305.

Carroll, T. L., & Fay, V. P. (1997). Measuring the impact of advanced practice nursing on achieving cost-quality outcomes: Issues and challenges. *Nursing Administration Quarterly, 21,* 32-40.

Croke, E. (2003). Nurses, negligence and malpractice. *American Journal of Nursing, 103,* 54-64.

Dang, D., & Haller, K. (1995). *Analysis of non-physician provider roles.* Unpublished manuscript, The Johns Hopkins Hospital, Baltimore.

Dickler, R., & Shaw, G. (2000). The Balanced Budget Act of 1997: Its impact on U.S. teaching hospitals. *Annals of Internal Medicine, 132,* 820-824.

Disch, J., Walton, M., & Barnsteiner, J. (2001). The role of the clinical nurse specialist in creating a healthy work environment. *AACN Clinical Issues, 12,* 345-355.

Fitzpatrick, E. R. (1998). Analysis and synthesis of the role of the advanced practice nurse. *Clinical Nurse Specialist, 12,* 106-107.

Flanagan, L. (1998). Nurse practitioners: Growing competition for family physicians? *Family Practice Management, 5,* 34-43.

Frampton, J., & Wall, S. (1994). Exploring the use of NPs and PAs in primary care. *HMO Practice, 4,* 165-170.

Genet, C. A., Brennan, P. F., Ibbotson-Wolff, S., Phelps, C., Rosenthal, G., Landefeld, C. S., et al. (1995). Nurse practitioners in a teaching hospital. *Nurse Practitioner, 20,* 47-54.

Girouard, S. A. (2000). New directions for the advanced practice nurse in health care quality: Performance and outcome improvement. In A. B. Hamric, J. A. Spross, & C. M. Hanson (Eds.), *Advanced nursing practice: An integrative approach* (2nd ed., pp. 755-794). Philadelphia: W. B. Saunders.

Gosfield, A. (2001). The in's and out's of incident to reimbursement. *Family Practice Management, 8,* 23-27.

Grumbach, L., Hart, G., Mertz, E., Coffman, J. & Palazzo, L. (2003). Who is caring for the underserved? A comparison of primary care physicians and non-physician clinicians in California and Washington. *Annals of Family Medicine, 1,* 97-104.

Haber, J. (1997). Medicare reimbursement: A victory for APRNs. *American Journal of Nursing, 97,* 84.

Health Care Advisory Board. (1999). *The physician perspective: Key drivers of physician loyalty.* Washington, DC: The Advisory Board Company.

Henley, D. (2003). Coding better for better reimbursement. *Family Practice Management, 10,* 29-35.

Hester, L. E., & White, M. J. (1996). Perceptions of practicing CNSs about their future role. *Clinical Nurse Specialist, 10,* 190-193.

Horrocks, S., Anderson, E., & Salisbury, C. (2002). Systematic review of whether nurse practitioners working in primary care can provide care equivalent to doctors. *British Medical Journal, 324,* 819-823.

Human Resources and Services Administration. (2002, July). *Projected supply, demand, and shortages of registered nurses: 2000-2020.* Retrieved July 15, 2002, from http://bhpr.hrsa.gov/healthworkforce/rnproject/

Hummel, J., & Pirzada, S. (1994). Estimating the cost-effectiveness of nurse practitioner/physician team in long-term care facilities. *HMO Practice, 8,* 162-164.

Iglehart, J. K. (1999). Support for academic centers—revisiting the 1997 Balanced Budget Act. *The New England Journal of Medicine, 341*(4), 299-304.

Institute of Medicine. (2000). *To err is human: Building a safer health system.* Washington, DC: National Academy Press.

Institute of Medicine. (2001). *Crossing the quality chasm: A new health system for the 21st century.* Washington, DC: National Academy Press.

Institute of Medicine. (2003). *Health professions education: A bridge to quality.* Washington, DC: National Academy Press.

Jackson, D. J., Lang, J. M., Swartz, W. H., Ganiats, T. G., Fullerton, J., Ecker, J., et al. (2003). Outcomes, safety, and resource utilization in a collaborative care birth center program compared with traditional physician-based perinatal care. *American Journal of Public Health, 93,* 999-1006.

Johnson, S. J. (1994). GME financing: A well-kept secret. *Nursing Management, 25,* 43-46.

Keepnews, D. (1998). New opportunities and challenges for APRNS. *American Journal of Nursing, 98,* 62-64.

Knox, S., & Gharrity, J. (2002). Transitions in American hospitals: The necessary reshaping is taking place: "Turnaround" processes in organizations. *JONA's Healthcare Law, Ethics, and Regulation, 4,* 13-17.

Koperski, S., Rogers, S., & Drennan, V. (1997). Nurse practitioners in general practice—an inevitable progression? *British Journal of General Practice, 47,* 696-698.

Levit, K., Smith, C., Cowan, C., Lazenby, H., Sensenig, A., & Catlin, A. (2003). Trends in U.S. health care spending, 2001. *Health Affairs, 22,* 154-164.

Licking, M., & Sampson, D. (1995). HCFA regulations and financing. *Nurse Practitioner, 20*(12), 6-9.

Lowe, M., & Havens, D. H. (1998). Hot issues for NPs in 1998. *Journal of Pediatric Health Care, 12,* 161-163.

Martin, P., & Hutchinson, S. (1999). Nurse practitioners and the problem of discounting. *Journal of Advanced Nursing, 29*(1), 9-17.

Mason, D. J., Cohen, S. S., O'Donnell, J. P., Baxter, K., & Chase, A. B. (1997). Managed care organizations' arrangements with nurse practitioners. *Nursing Economics, 15,* 306-314.

McNatt, G. E., & Eason, A. (2000). The role of the advanced practice nurse in the care of organ transplant recipients. *Advances in Renal Replacement Therapy, 7,* 172-176.

Miller, S. (2003). *Hispanics replace African Americans as largest U.S. minority group.* US Department of State. Office of International Information Program on Diversity. Retrieved December 22, 2003, from http://www.usinfo.state.gov/usa/diversity/a012303.htm

Milstead, J. (1997). Using advanced practice to shape public policy: Agenda setting. *Nursing Administration Quarterly, 21,* 12-18.

Minarik, P. (1997). Medicare reimbursement for nurse practitioners and clinical nurse specialists passes; states' legislative and regulatory forum II. *Clinical Nurse Specialist, 11,* 274-275.

Naegle, M. A., & Krainovich-Miller, B. (2001). Shaping the advanced practice psychiatric-mental health nursing role: A futuristic model. *Issues in Mental Health Nursing, 22,* 461-482.

Naylor, M. D., Brooten, D., Campbell, R., Jacobsen, B. S., Mezey, M. D., Pauly, N. V., et al. (1999). Comprehensive discharge planning and home follow-up of hospitalized elders: A randomized clinical trial. *JAMA: The Journal of the American Medical Association, 281*, 613-620.

Nevidjon, B., & Erickson, J. (2001). The nursing shortage: Solutions for the short and long term. *Online Journal of Issues in Nursing, 6* (1). Retrieved from http://www.nursingworld.org/ojin

Nuccio, S., Costa-Lieberthal, K. M., Gunta, K. E., Mackus, M. L., Riesch, S. K., Schmanski, K. M., et al. (1993). A survey of 636 staff nurses' perceptions and factors influencing the CNS role. *Clinical Nurse Specialist, 7*, 122-128.

Paladichuk, A. (1998). Interview. Sara Paul, RN, MSN, FNPC. The advanced practice/staff nurse partnership: Building a winning team. *Critical Care Nurse, 18*, 92-97.

Payne, J. L., & Baumgartner, R. G. (1996). CNS role evolution. *Clinical Nurse Specialist, 10*, 46-48.

Parrinello, K. M. (1995). Advanced practice nursing: An administrative perspective. *Critical Care Nursing Clinics of North America, 7*, 9-16.

Phillips, R., Harper, D., Wakefield, M., Green, L., & Fryer G. (2002). Can nurse practitioners and physicians beat parochialism into plowshares? *Health Affairs, 21*, 133-142.

Pioro, M., Landefeld, C., Brennan, P., Fortinsky, R., Kim, U., & Rosenthal, G. (2000). Outcome based trial of an inpatient nurse practitioner service for general medical patients. *Journal of Evaluation in Clinical Practice, 7*, 21-33.

Sinclair, B. P. (1997). Advanced practice nurses in integrated health-care systems. *Journal of Obstetric, Gynecologic, and Neonatal Nursing, 26*, 217-223.

Shortell, S. M., Gillies, R. R., & Devers, K. J. (1995). Reinventing the American hospital. *Millbank Quarterly, 73*, 131-158.

Tobin, C. T. (2000). A rainbow of opportunities: Advanced practice. *Diabetes Educator, 26*, 216, 326-327.

Urden, L., & Walston, S. (2001). Outcomes of hospital restructuring and reengineering: How is success or failure being measured? *Journal of Nursing Administration, 31*, 203-209.

U. S. Census Bureau. *Health insurance coverage in the United States: 2002.* Retrieved December 22, 2003, from http://www.census.gov/prod/2003pubs/p60-223.pdf

Wilken, M. (1995). State regulatory board structure, regulations, and nurse practitioner availability. *Nurse Practitioner, 20*, 68-74.

Woods, L. P. (1998). Implementing advanced practice: Identifying the factors that facilitate and inhibit the process. *Journal of Clinical Nursing, 7*, 265-273.

Woods, L. P. (1999). The contingent nature of advanced nursing practice. *Journal of Advanced Nursing, 30*, 121.

CHAPTER 25

Outcome Evaluation and Performance Improvement

GAIL L. INGERSOLL • VICKY A. MAHN-DiNICOLA

INTRODUCTION

Increased demand for health-care system accountability and the changes occurring in the organization, delivery, and financing of health care have prompted the need for an accurate assessment of advanced practice nurse (APN) performance. Employers, consumers, insurers, competing providers, and others are calling for APNs to justify their contribution to health care and to demonstrate the value they add to the system. Verification of APNs' contributions to improved health requires an assessment of the structures, processes, and outcomes associated with APN performance and the care delivery systems in which APNs practice.

Assessment of individual APN impact occurs at multiple levels; supporting evidence is collected during annual performance reviews, outcomes measurement activities, process improvement analyses, and program evaluations, as well as from small- and large-scale clinical, health systems, and outcomes research. The extent of APN involvement in each of these activities is driven by individual interest, local and national reimbursement and accreditation expectations, availability of resources, and support of others. At the very least, individual performance review and outcomes measurement are required of all APNs, regardless of location of service, size of practice, or previous experience with impact assessment.

Outcomes evaluation and performance improvement are complex areas, but understanding them is critical to the success and survival of advanced practice nursing. This chapter focuses on measuring, monitoring, and managing the quality-of-care processes and outcomes achieved through APN performance at two levels: the aggregate level, focusing on evidence of overall APN impact, and the individual level, focusing on the outcomes of one APN's practice. The chapter first defines key terms and describes frameworks for quality and outcomes assessment. Advanced practicing nursing outcomes research is reviewed extensively, and recommendations are made for further study. The reader will find many ideas in these studies for APN–sensitive outcome indicators and strategies for evaluating and improving their own practices. Finally, the chapter discusses steps APNs can take to design and implement an outcome evaluation plan for their own practices. Resources available for APNs to use in outcomes assessment are also included.

REVIEW OF TERMS

Several new and interrelated terms are used to describe and define the components of performance improvement and outcomes assessment activities. The principal terms used in this chapter are defined as follows.

Disease management: An organized process focusing on the patient's disease as the target of interest, with improvements in outcomes seen as a result of attention to the attributes or characteristics of the disease. The intent is the same as outcomes management—to take some action or perform an intervention to achieve a desired effect. The principal difference is the focus, with disease management directed at the patient's underlying condition and outcomes management focused on the observed effect. Assessments of disease management effectiveness should indicate clearly what changes in care delivery approach affected the disease process or the symptoms seen.

Effectiveness: The extent to which interventions or actions performed in clinical settings have the desired results for defined populations (Armenian & Shapiro, 1998). Indicators of program or intervention effectiveness are commonly included in assessments of cost outcomes (e.g., cost-effectiveness analysis). In cost-effectiveness analysis, outcomes are measured both in terms of dollars expended and beneficial effects achieved (often for which no dollar amount can be readily assigned) (Hargreaves Shumway, Hu, & Cuffel, 1998). This measurement approach is different from cost-benefit analysis, in which dollars are used to compare money spent with money saved. In clinical practice, cost-benefit analyses are rarely possible or useful for determining which program or intervention is most desirable for achieving outcomes.

Efficacy: The extent to which interventions or actions performed in tightly controlled settings (e.g., laboratories) or situations (e.g., randomized controlled trials [RCTs]) have the desired results for defined populations (Hargreaves et al., 1998). Studies of an intervention's efficacy are often not immediately relevant to individual practice and must be considered in light of a full body of evidence that clarifies their usefulness for clinical decision making.

Efficiency: The effects achieved by some intervention in relation to the effort expended in terms of money, resources, and time. In outcomes assessment, efficiency measures are used to compare two equally effective interventions (Hargreaves et al., 1998), and for care providers, often include productivity considerations. In such cases, treatment patterns, service volumes, and costs of care are usually compared (Armenian & Shapiro, 1998).

Evidence-Based Practice: The integration of research findings (evidence) into clinical decision-making and care delivery processes. Best evidence for clinical practice is derived from methodologically sound research that is theory derived, consistent with patient needs and preferences (Ingersoll, 2000), and clinically relevant to the population of interest. The findings of these investigations support and enhance the clinician's clinical expertise; they do not replace it. This is particularly true for decisions concerning individual patients, when personal characteristics and circumstances may differ from those of the populations studied.

Impact Analysis: An assessment of the magnitude of some intervention or change (e.g., APN care delivery) on recipients, programs, policies, and stakeholders. An impact analysis may also be performed prior to the introduction of an intervention to determine whether a proposed action, theoretically, should produce better results than an alternative or the current standard of care. Some evaluators differentiate impact analysis from outcomes analysis by the length of time required to achieve an effect, with impact analysis denoting longer-term changes (Krueger, n.d.). In most cases, however, the term *impact analysis* is a more global statement for assessment of some intervention effect.

Outcome: A change or result in the recipient of some intervention or action. Recipients may be patients, families, students, other care providers, communities—and in some cases—organizations, if the organization as a whole is the recipient of the intervention. Outcomes may be intended or unintended, and both should be assessed in a comprehensive outcomes assessment.

Outcome(s) Assessment: An evaluation of the observed results of some action or intervention for recipients of services. Outcome assessments provide the data needed to support or refute the perceived beneficial effect of some clinical decision, care delivery process, or targeted action.

Outcome Indicators or Measures: Observable, measurable evidence of the effect of some intervention or action on a person, group, organization, or community. Although some authors distinguish between indicators and measures, most often the terms are used interchangeably, as they are in this chapter. Outcome indicators denote changes in the recipient of the service or action, not the provider. Acceptable measures should vary sufficiently to allow for the assessment of intraindividual and interindividual differences across providers, employers, insurers, and circumstances. They focus on changes over time and measure some aspect of behavior, cognitive process, or physiological response. An essential attribute of outcome indicators is their implied or explicit causal link to an intervention or action. One of the challenges for APNs in outcomes evaluation is determining which of several measures is the most reliable, valid, and sensitive to individual or program effect.

The most desirable indicators of care delivery outcome are suitable to the population or target of interest, are not overly costly to collect, and are sensitive to changes within and across individuals or departments. They can be global (applicable to any population or care delivery environment) or population specific. The more global the indicator, the more difficult is the determination of its relationship to advanced practice nursing intervention or action. The more specific the indicator, the less generalizable it is to other groups or circumstances. For example, "patient satisfaction" is a global indicator that is relevant to all patients but is influenced by a number of factors and a variety of care providers. As a result, distinguishing the APN's impact from everyone else's is difficult. On the other hand, the outcome indicator "birth complications" is specific to newborns, making it relevant only to APNs serving that particular patient population.

Intermediate Outcome Indicators: Observable evidence of some movement toward the achievement of a desired outcome. These indicators assist in determining whether any progress is being made in response to some intervention. They are most useful when the desired outcome is long-range or multidimensional and preliminary actions or changes are required before the final outcome is achieved.

Because APNs often influence patient outcomes through indirect means, the use of intermediate outcome indicators may be a desirable way to measure progress toward an overall goal of improving patient care. For instance, many APN role responsibilities include the mentoring of other nursing staff or the management of interdisciplinary teams. As a result, changes in team member behavior or staff nurse performance may be an indication of APN effect. When possible, the proposed relationships between these intermediate outcomes and subsequent patient outcomes should be clearly described.

Outcome(s) Management: Deliberate care delivery actions designed to achieve desired outcomes through the application of outcomes research to practice (adapted from Powell, 2000). Outcomes management is directed toward the refinement of care delivery processes for the purposes of maximizing care delivery outcome. According to Ellwood (1988), a comprehensive outcomes management program (1) emphasizes the use of standards to select appropriate interventions; (2) measures both disease-specific and generic, behavior-focused or perception-focused outcomes; (3) pools clinical and outcomes data for groups of patients; and (4) analyzes and disseminates information to decision makers. Decision-making action for individual patients is not necessarily the goal of outcomes management programs. Rather, the intent is directed toward the improvement of care to aggregate populations.

Outcome(s) Measurement: The collection and reporting of information about an observed effect. Outcomes measurement involves the identification of reliable and valid outcome measures; the selection of appropriate measurement methods; and attention to the timing of data collection, analysis, and reporting. Outcome findings may be influenced by the amount of time elapsed since an intervention and what has transpired during that period. They may also be affected by the circumstances evident at the time of data collection.

Outcome(s) Research: The use of rigorous scientific methods to measure the effect of some intervention on some outcome or outcomes (Ingersoll, 1998). It is directed toward populations of patients and is designed to establish care delivery standards or policy statements about best practices. The term *outcomes research* is a fairly new one; previous studies were focused on cause (intervention) and effect (outcome) relationships. In many respects, the intent of the research (interventional versus outcomes) is the same—to demonstrate a causal connection between some change in practice or process and improvement in some outcome observed. Because of its focus on formal research investigations, usually involving RCTs, the term should not be used synonymously with the terms *outcome evaluation* and *outcome management.*

Performance Benchmark: Most commonly defined in health care as an ideal target that has been achieved by some group or organization known for its quality of services. This benchmark serves as the gold standard against which others are compared. Some evaluators also use this term to denote intermediate steps, or milestones, that indicate progress toward the attainment of some desired outcome (LaCava, 2001). In this case, the long-range or desired outcome is broken down into smaller parts that can be achieved in a shorter period and tracked for evidence of progress.

Performance (Process) Improvement: Activities designed to increase the quality of services provided. The focus of attention shifts to the processes involved in care delivery rather than the outcomes that result from the actions taken. Although outcomes are monitored to determine whether the change in process has produced a desired effect, primary attention is focused on the interventions (care delivery processes) provided. In reality, outcome evaluation and performance improvement are two components of an iterative (back-and-forth) process in which the two activities simultaneously inform and appraise the service delivered and the actions taken to achieve it. The ultimate goal of each action is tied to quality care, with performance improvement activities directed toward excellence in care provider and organizational processes. Clearly linked with these actions is outcomes evaluation, which focuses on the impact of care delivery processes and areas in which additional improvements are needed.

Subsumed within performance improvement activities are those associated with quality improvement initiatives, also described by some as *continuous quality improvement* (*CQI*) or *total quality management* (*TQM*). Although subtle distinctions are assigned to each of these terms, the focus and the intent is the same—to ensure the delivery of care that is appropriate, safe, competent, and timely and to maximize the potential for favorable patient outcomes (Palmer et al., 1995). In most instances, the measurement of performance is guided by the use of established indicators of best practice, such as national guidelines for care. These performance indicators may be internally derived or externally developed by expert panels that use existing evidence to specify which indicators are most reasonable and which targets are most desirable for achievement.

Performance Evaluation (Assessment): Assessment of individual achievement and the attainment of personal, professional, and organizational goals. Performance assessment activities for APNs include those associated with evaluating and improving day-to-day interactions with individual patients and health-care colleagues, as well as those involving the measurement of APN impact on populations, organizations, and communities. During these self-assessment and peer- or supervisor-initiated reviews, areas for improvement are identified. These performance improvement activities may be directed toward technical skill enhancement, interpersonal style, productivity specifications, professional development, or other individual APN actions linked to improved processes of care or care delivery outcome. In this case, the focus is on the individual behaviors of the APN, with specific goals for improved performance in the upcoming quarter or year.

Process Indicator/Measure: A measure of visible behavior or action that a care provider undertakes to deliver care. Process indicators measure what care providers do during their interactions with patients and are necessary for demonstrating a cause-and-effect relationship between intervention and outcome. Process indicators are currently the focus of regulatory agencies such as the Joint Commission on Accreditation for Healthcare Organizations (JCAHO) (2000; 2001) and the Center for Medicare and Medicaid Services (CMS) (2003). Within the CMS, a national initiative has been undertaken to evaluate hospital compliance with evidence-based best practice standards (processes) of care for patients with AMI, heart failure, community-acquired pneumonia, pregnancy-related conditions, and surgical procedures (CMS, 2003). Process indicators such as the administration of aspirin to qualifying patients with AMI, the timely administration of antibiotics to patients with pneumonia, or the delivery of appropriate discharge instructions to patients with heart failure are currently being collected by acute care hospitals across the country. While these indicators may not directly reflect independent advanced nursing practice, APNs are in a unique position to influence the performance of interdisciplinary teams and care delivery systems.

Process-As-Outcome Indicators: The incorrect use of process-of-care indicators as evidence of improved patient or organizational outcome. A common example of a process-as-outcome indicator is nursing documentation, which is often identified in research reports and program evaluations as a desired outcome for some targeted intervention. The assumption is that improved documentation provides evidence of the delivery of better-quality care, which should result in improved patient outcome. The problem is that process-as-outcome indicators focus on the care providers and actions taken, not the recipients of services. There is no guarantee that the processes of care observed (or the documentation of their occurrence) will result in the desired outcome. Although process actions should be described fully and included in any discussion of how some program or action is expected to result in some outcome, they should not be identified as outcome indicators. At best, they are indications of intermediate effect, or process improvement; they are not acceptable outcomes by themselves. For example, any changes in documentation frequency, accuracy, or consistency must be tied to the changes in outcomes expected at the patient or organizational level.

For some APNs, particularly clinical nurse specialists (CNSs), whose role responsibilities include mentoring and teaching others, the recipient of the APN's intervention may be a staff member or group of staff. In this case, assessment of the CNS's impact may include an evaluation of change in staff nurse performance or level of understanding. This is a legitimate and acceptable indicator of APN effect. Ideally, the assessment should follow the performance changes by staff nurses with an evaluation of the impact of the staff's improved performance on organizational or patient outcomes. The overall impact of the change in staff nurse performance or level of understanding may be increased patient satisfaction with care, reduced incidence of adverse events, reduced length of stay, or reduced cost of care.

Structural Indicators: Measures of human, technical, and other resources that are used in the process of delivering care. These indicators are focused on characteristics of the setting, system, or care providers and include such elements as numbers and types of providers, provider qualifications, agency policies and procedures, characteristics of patients served, and payment sources. Examples of structural indicators are ratio of registered nurses or APNs to total nursing staff, nurse-to-patient ratio, nursing care hours per patient, nursing injury rates, and attrition rates. The assumption underlying these measures is that the provision of adequate structures will result in adequate outcomes. While structural indicators can provide important information for evaluating the impact of advanced practice, they cannot stand alone.

Program Evaluation: An assessment of a program's overall worth or benefit. In most cases, program evaluations are designed to provide decision makers with information about the costs and benefits of some program or service. They provide an indication of indirect APN impact when the APN designs or assists in the implementation and maintenance of some educational or health services program. Program evaluations may also determine the direct effect of APN performance when the APN's care delivery actions are the principal component of the program. Because programs generally involve multiple components, however, isolating the APN's impact is often difficult.

Proxy Indicators: An indirect measure of some anticipated outcome that is used when a direct measure cannot be obtained or when an accurate indicator has not been identified. An example of a proxy indicator is the collection of self-report data from parents or spouses when patients are unable to respond to questions about perceptions of care or previous health. Proxy indicators are less reliable than directly linked outcome indicators but sometimes provide the only route available for collecting outcome data. When used, they should be supported by direct measures if at all possible.

In the acute care hospital setting, case mix index, patient age, and co-morbidity are often used as proxy indicators of risk adjustment for given clinical populations. Risk adjustment is a process used to standardize groups according to some characteristic that might unduly influence an outcome. For example, the number and severity of co-morbid conditions might make one person less likely to achieve a favorable outcome simply because of physiological state, even when the best possible care is delivered. If patients with similarly high levels of co-morbid conditions are not standardized against other patients without those same conditions, an incorrect impression of intervention effect might occur. Those persons with fewer co-morbid conditions, who happen to be treated by one provider, might have better outcomes than patients with more co-morbid conditions, who happen to be treated by another. Comparing the outcomes of the two providers would erroneously suggest that one provider gives better quality care, when in fact the difference is the result of the patients' underlying conditions and the influence of those underlying conditions on the individual's ability to achieve an outcome.

Quality of Care: The degree to which health-care services for individuals and populations increase the likelihood of desired health outcomes and are consistent with professional knowledge (IOM, 1990; IOM, 2001). Quality of care is a dimension of the process of care; it is not an outcome. Outcomes are assessed to provide an indication of the level of quality achieved during the care delivery process. Some authors recommend focusing on the value of services, which they believe may be a more helpful framework for understanding the nature and relationship of quality in health care. The concept of value incorporates the patient's assessment of a particular diagnostic or treatment approach's importance or acceptability (Wing & Gay, 1990).

CONCEPTUAL MODELS OF CARE DELIVERY IMPACT

Because APNs usually work with other health-care professionals, their influence on care delivery outcome is difficult to assess. They may have a direct effect through their interactions with patients and families and/or they may have an indirect effect through their enhancement of the performance of others. Moreover, a number of factors influence advanced practice nursing irrespective of the direct or indirect efforts of APNs. Among these are state-defined and organizationally mandated scopes of practice, location of services, and care delivery structures (Carroll & Fay, 1997).

Measurement of the full range of APN effect may also be hampered by the organization's or clinician's philosophy underlying the care delivery process. For example, Murphy and Fullerton (2001) noted that a hallmark of midwifery practice is the "advocacy of nonintervention in the absence of complications" (p. 274). Measuring this advocacy process is difficult, and relating it to observed care delivery outcomes may be even harder. Linking noninterventions to outcomes, likewise, is a challenge. A further example is evident with APN case managers who advocate for the needs of their patients, while also striving to achieve the economic goals of their sponsoring organizations. In these cases, APN performance measures may reflect the biases of different stakeholders (Mahn & Zazworsky, 2000).

Quality of Care Models

Much of the difficulty associated with measuring APN impact can be minimized through the use of a conceptual model to guide assessment and monitoring activities. A number of outcomes measurement and role impact models have been proposed, with several of these evolving from an original quality-of-care framework proposed by Donabedian (1966; 1982). In this model, structural variables relate to the components of an intervention or system of care as defined earlier. Process variables pertain to the behavior or actions of the APN or the activities of an APN-directed educational or care delivery program. The result of the interactions among structure and process variables is an outcome. Structure, process, and outcome variables can be studied independently or as a model for overall advanced nursing practice. The more complete the model (e.g., inclusion of all or at least two of the components), the more likely is the successful isolation of the APN's impact on care delivery outcome.

Byers and Brunell (1998) used Donabedian's model (1966, 1982) to describe what they defined as the APN's value to the health delivery system. In their approach, value is equivalent to quality divided by cost. According to Byers and Brunell, the structural factors in this model refer to the characteristics of the APN and the practice setting. The stronger the structural elements of the setting or the provider, the greater is the likelihood that an APN can provide quality care and achieve desired outcomes. In this model, process elements include not only what the APN does but also whether the actions are appropriate and indicated for the circumstance. Ideally, process activities are guided by research evidence. Outcomes in this model are defined by evidence-based standards and are compared with benchmarks for determining APN impact. Byers and Brunell's model categorizes APN–sensitive outcomes as short-term clinical outcomes, long-term clinical outcomes, perceived outcomes, patient/family satisfaction with care versus need, functional status, and resource utilization. The patient/family satisfaction with care versus need outcome represents a fairly new approach to measuring patient and family satisfaction. It incorporates a comparison between an individual's perception of the value of (or need for) an intervention or structural characteristic and the individual's level of satisfaction with it. For example, if an item is not perceived as valuable or needed by patients, its satisfaction rating may not be particularly useful for assessing whether an individual's needs were met. On the other hand, if a patient or family member rates an item as highly valued or needed, the satisfaction rating provides a better indication of how well the service provided met the patient's or family's expectations.

A second Donabedian-guided model was designed by Holzemer (1994) and adapted by others (Cohen, Saylor, Holzemer, & Gorenberg, 2000; Wong, Stewart, & Gilliss, 2000). The value of this model is its program planning structure, which helps identify essential components of any outcomes evaluation plan. In Holzemer's model, essential outcomes measurement components are defined in a table consisting of inputs/context (structure), processes, and outcomes, which are identified along the horizontal axis. The vertical axis specifies three factors (client, provider, and setting) that contribute to outcomes and that should be assessed prior to any measurement activity (Holzemer, 1994). This breakdown of Donabedian's structure component into inputs and contexts helps clarify which dimensions are considered in the model and alleviates some of the previous awkwardness of including people (clients, providers) in the structure component.

For the APN, the client is any recipient of APN services (e.g., a patient, family, staff nurse, or physician). The provider is the person (APN) or the interdisciplinary group providing the service; a provider also could be a trained layperson who assists with the provision of services. The setting is the local environment in which the services are delivered and includes the resources available to provide the care. Table 25-1 contains an application of Holzemer's (1994) model to APN outcomes assessment planning. Included in the table are potential variables that may facilitate assessment of APN impact. Additional variables would be selected on the basis of specialty service; population specifics; and additional characteristics of the provider, client, or environment.

Dynamic Quality Health Outcomes Model

Mitchell, Ferketich, Jennings, and the American Academy of Nursing Expert Panel on Quality Care (1998) challenged Donabedian's one-way (linear) approach to measuring the effect of structure and process on care delivery outcome. They proposed a more dynamic model that moves away from a simple cause-and-effect relationship between processes and outcomes. They also extended Holzemer's (1994) refinement of Donabedian's model by replacing Holzemer's inputs/context terminology with the terms *system* and *client*. In the revised model, two-way relationships are proposed for all components of the model, with interventions (their equivalent of processes) always acting on outcomes through the characteristics of the system (individual, organizational, and group) and the client (individual, family, and community). Outcomes, likewise, influence both the system and the client, which subsequently affect decisions about which intervention to use.

Mitchell et al. (1998) also identified specific outcome indicators that support their model's dimensions and proposed interactions among components. These indicators address the functional, social, psychological, physical, and physiological aspects of an individual's experience in health and illness and are defined as achievement of appropriate self-care, demonstration of health-promoting behaviors, health-related quality of life, perception of being well cared for, and symptom management.

Radwin (2002) subsequently proposed a refinement of this model in light of the need to distinguish between client characteristics that are amenable to change (e.g., behavior,

TABLE 25-1 APN OUTCOMES PLANNING GRID*

	INPUTS/CONTEXT (STRUCTURE)	PROCESSES	OUTCOMES

Client (Patient)	Age
	Gender
	Ethnicity
	Marital status/social supports
	Educational background
	Health status (current & past)
	Previous experience with health system
	Special needs (e.g., visual, literacy, hearing)
	Expectations of provider & health system
	Access to care
	Insurance coverage
		Performance of self-care behaviors
		  Ability
		  Willingness
		Family involvement in care delivery process
		Use of alternative or complementary therapies
			Generic
			  Physical health
			  Mental health
			  Symptom control
			  Functional status
			  Perceived well-being
			  Satisfaction with care
			  Adherence to treatment regimen
			  Knowledge of condition, treatment program, & expected outcomes
			Specific (dependent on patient condition & need; representative examples)
			  Serum glucose level
			  Birth weight
			  Re-infarction rate
			  Transplant rejection rate
			  Smoking cessation rate
			  Length of stay
			  Ventilator days
			  Wound closure/healing

APN Provider	Educational preparation Specialty focus Years of experience Level of self-esteem Resourcefulness	Expert practice Collaboration Communication patterns Interactions with other care providers & staff	Productivity

Assertiveness

Expert coaching
Consultation
Clinical & professional leadership
Ethical decision making
Evidence-based practice
Case management
Care delivery according to practice standards
Documentation

Care provider credentialing process
Quality improvement process
Communication patterns
Governance process
Care provider documentation process
Annual performance review process
Provider credentialing process

Length of stay
Staff turnover rate
Cost of services
New program development
Revenue generated
Community satisfaction
Provider satisfaction
Staff satisfaction

Setting

Geographic location (rural, urban, mixed)
Type of facility (academic health center, acute care, clinic, industry)
Diagnostic equipment
Organizational culture & philosophy
Administrative structure
Standards of care
State regulations on advanced practice
Policies & procedures
Patient mix
Nursing practice care delivery model
Availability of other services in vicinity
Credentialing agency requirements
State health department regulations
Annual goals
Annual budget

Adapted from Holzemer, W. L. (1994). The impact of nursing care in Latin America and the Caribbean: A focus on outcomes. *Journal of Advanced Nursing, 20,* 5-12.
APN, Advanced practice nurse.
*Components are not exhaustive of advanced practice nursing–related outcomes planning, but serve as a guide for planning, activities.

perception) and those that are not (e.g., age, race, gender). In Radwin's revision, change-able client characteristics are defined as *state characteristics* and are included in the two-way pathway proposed by Mitchell et al. (1998). The client characteristics that cannot be changed are defined as *trait characteristics* and are distinguished from the others by their unidirectional relationship to the system, intervention, and outcome components of the model. According to Radwin, these distinctions help clarify the potential impact of each of the model's components on the client's ability to change.

An important aspect of each of these models is the limited testing done in clinical set-tings. The Holzemer (1994) model has been used in a few studies, and findings provide support for the model's components. Neither the modification by Mitchell et al. (1998) nor the one by Radwin (2002) has been tested, although the components of each are derived from prior research and are therefore reasonable models for exploration.

THE EVIDENCE THUS FAR

A review of the literature suggests that increasing attention is being given to assessment of APN performance. Much of the evidence, however, consists of short-term impact evalua-tions and descriptions of process activities that are not clearly linked to any observable outcome. Although useful for understanding the demands of the APN role, these process-focused studies require additional follow-up concerning how APN role behaviors con-tribute to outcomes achieved.

Prior to the 1990s, most reports of APN performance were descriptive in nature, with limited use of the experimental or quasi-experimental designs that allow for comparisons across studies. In a meta-analysis of nurse practitioner (NP) and certified nurse midwife (CNM) performance in primary care, Brown and Grimes (1995) identified 210 studies pertaining to NPs and CNMs. Of this number, only 53 met study inclusion criteria, which required evidence of NP or CNM intervention, data from patients in the United States or Canada, presence of a control group, outcome measures pertaining to process of care or clinical impact, use of an experimental or quasi-experimental design, and data availability to support the calculation of effect size or the determination of direct effect. Outcome indicators varied across studies, and no information was included to substantiate a cause-and-effect relationship between type of care provider (APN or physician) and outcomes observed (Brown & Grimes, 1995). Outcomes measured for NPs reflected more generic indicators of provider impact (e.g., patient compliance, patient satisfaction, functional status, and use of EDs), while CNM outcomes were more reflective of specialized practice and included number of cesarean deliveries, spontaneous vaginal deliveries, incidence of fetal distress, birth weight, and 2-minute Apgar scores. Findings suggested that NPs requested more laboratory testing than physicians and had more favorable outcomes pertaining to patient satisfaction, health promotion behaviors, time spent with patients, and number of hospitalizations. CNMs used less anesthesia, analgesia, intra-venous fluids, and fetal monitoring and performed fewer episiotomies, forceps deliver-ies, and amniotomies. Their patients were also more likely to have spontaneous vaginal deliveries, although these were accompanied by an increased number of per-ineal lacerations.

Since 1992, APN performance and impact have been investigated in a number of locales. For purposes of summarization, studies have been categorized according to whether they focused on role descriptions or practice characteristics, care delivery processes, process (or performance) improvement activities, program evaluation, disease management activities, outcomes management programs, or outcomes research.

Role Description Studies

Role description studies focus on defining and describing role components and job attributes of APNs. These foundational studies assist in identifying the direct and indirect APN actions that potentially influence care delivery outcomes; thus they provide information about the structure or process components of Donabedian's model (1966; 1982). Without information about the outcomes associated with the characteristics and role behaviors identified in these studies, however, little can be said about their impact on patient care. What these studies provide is evidence to guide the development of theories about which characteristics of advanced nursing practice or aspects of the APN role contribute to care delivery outcome. For example, do APNs, through expert coaching and collaboration processes, contribute to more favorable outcomes when compared with care providers whose use of these processes is less evident?

Role description studies have explored the role characteristics of psychiatric mental health APNs (Campbell, Musil, & Zauszniewski, 1998; Merwin, et al., 1997), ACNPs (Irvine et al., 2000; Kleinpell, 1998; Kleinpell-Nowell, 2001; Mezey, Dougherty, Wade, & Mersmann, 1994; Sidani et al., 2000); CNSs (Aiken, Taggart, & Tripoli, 1993; Hill, Ellsworth-Wolk, & DeBlase, 1993; Scott, 1999); neonatal nurse practitioners (NNPs) (Beal et al., 1999); pediatric nurse practitioners (Brady & Neal, 2000; Jackson et al., 2001); primary care NPs (Holcomb, 2000; Hooker & McCaig, 2001; Kane, Flood, Keckhafer, & Rockwood, 2001; Moody, Smith, & Glenn, 1999; Way, Jones, Baskerville, & Busing, 2001), CNMs (Mezey et al., 1994); certified registered nurse anesthetists (CRNAs) (McAuliffe & Henry, 1998; Mezey et al., 1994); APNs working in gastroenterology (Hillier, 2001) and with acute pain services (Musclow, Sawhney, & Watt-Watson, 2002); and NPs based in hospital outpatient clinics (Lin, Hooker, Lenz, & Hopkins, 2002), ambulatory services (Mills & McSweeney, 2002; Mills, McSweeney, & Lavin, 1998; Williams & Sidani, 2001), and local health departments (Hughes, 2000). Advanced practice nursing activities have been directed primarily toward the oversight and management of patients' needs, followed by administrative, teaching, research, program development, process improvement, and miscellaneous other demands. Some differences existed for locale and educational preparation (Hughes) and whether the APN is an NP or CNS (Aiken, Lake, Semaan, et al., 1993; Hillier, 2001; Kearnes, 1993; Lincoln, 2000; Mick & Ackerman, 2000). Studies in which NPs were compared with physician assistants (PAs) have also revealed differences between these two roles (Lin et al., 2002; Mills & McSweeney, 2002).

Role Perception/Acceptance Studies

Studies examining the acceptance of APNs have been conducted since the various roles were introduced and generally involve surveys of staff nurses, administrators, patients, and other care providers. The contribution of role perception studies to the assessment of APN impact lies with their potential for clarifying which contextual (structural) factors influence APNs' ability to perform maximally. If the environment in which an APN practices does not support the APN's delivery of services or the APN's colleagues view the APN's performance as unsatisfactory or unacceptable, outcomes may be affected. Using Mitchell et al.'s, (1998) framework, this organizational or group component of the system influences both the interventions provided and the outcomes observed. These studies serve to identify potential confounding factors that may need to be controlled when APN effect is measured.

Overall perception of APN performance has been favorable, with most care providers and clients giving the performance and contribution of APNs high ratings (Baldwin et al., 1998; Bergeron, Cash, Boulger, & Bergeron, 1997; Mitchell, Dixon, Freeman, & Grindrod, 2001; Murphy & Ericson, 1995; Riportella-Muller, Libby, & Kindig, 1995; Trotter & Danaher, 1994). Concerns expressed have focused on the proficiency of APNs covering in EDs on off-shifts and weekends and conducting hospital rounds. Increased workload, liability, and job competition were also concerns in a study of rural family physicians (Bergeron et al., 1997). In one study, perceptions differed according to respondent role. Attending physicians and medical residents reported the greatest levels of support, with administrators and nurses reporting moderate levels. Medical students were the least supportive (DeNicola et al., 1994). Physician perceptions about the role have also differed according to previous experience working with NPs and location of practice (Aquilino, Damiano, Willard, Momany, & Levy, 1999). In a study of emergency medicine residents' willingness to be treated by an APN for acute illness or injury, most residents were unwilling. Some reported they would do so if the illness or injury was minor and the APN could treat their condition sooner than an attending physician. An additional finding in this study was residents' concern over threat to practice, with one third of respondents perceiving APNs in the ED as a professional threat (Larkin Kantor, & Zielinski, 2001).

APN role receptivity studies have also explored physicians' acceptance of performance of specialized diagnostic screening and invasive interventions by APNs. In a study of skin cancer screening, between 60% and 70% of family physicians and internists were supportive of screening by NPs (Oliveria, Altman, Christos, & Halpern, 2002). Similar findings were noted for the acceptance of NP and CNM involvement in medical abortions (Beckman, Harvey, & Satre, 2002).

The acceptance of NNPs as expert practitioners was assessed in a study of NNP and physician involvement in a community hospital resuscitation team (Britton, 1997). In this descriptive report of a resuscitation team's performance in a community hospital, a medical record review of pre- and post-NNP resuscitation events showed a clear pattern of increased participation by NNPs. It also demonstrated the reduced involvement of newborn care physicians after the NNPs were hired. Because the physicians had the option of requesting that NNPs replace or assist them in resuscitations, the decline in physician involvement was considered evidence of a high level of comfort with the NNPs' assumption of resuscitation oversight.

In a more recent study, a phenomenological design was used to assess families' perceptions of the "essence" of NNP care (Beal & Quinn, 2002). Themes identified included being positive and reassuring, being present, caring, translating information, and making parents feel at ease. In this same study, expert practitioner ability was identified as an expectation families had of all care providers, regardless of background (medical or nursing) or level of practice (staff nurse or APN). Expectations for the NNP focused on interpersonal style and effectiveness of interactions with families.

An important pragmatic implication of this study's findings is the potential difficulty in placing a dollar amount on APN behavior. Because much of advanced nursing practice is reimbursement driven, intangible provider attributes such as interpersonal competence often go unrecognized or are disregarded in provider payment decisions. This is a serious concern because patient and family perceptions of intangible processes often influence overall impressions of care delivery experience and may contribute to more tangible outcomes. Additional research is needed to clarify the magnitude and the importance of this link.

A caution with each of these studies is the potential for respondent bias, with persons unfamiliar with the role being less likely to respond. In addition, many of the investigations are site specific, making them more useful for performance improvement activities rather than global indication of acceptance of APNs.

Care Delivery Process Studies

Studies in which care delivery processes are evaluated are often done in combination with role definition research. The distinction between these studies and role definition explorations is in their attention to what APNs do as part of their roles. Examples include the delivery of preventive services (Carroll, Robinson, Buselli, Berry, & Rankin, 2001; Courtney & Rice, 1997; Jessup & Harrell, 1996; Johnson, 2000; Lemley, O'Grady, Raukhorst, Russell, & Small, 1994; Sheahan, 2000; Windorski & Kalb, 2002; Zapka et al., 2000), the inclusion of alternative health-care treatments in care delivery processes (Sohn & Cook, 2002), the treatment of patients in the ED (Mabrook & Dale, 1998), the consultation services of the CNS role (Gurka, 1991), the ordering of diagnostic tests, and the performance of invasive and noninvasive procedures (Cole & Ramirez, 2000; Sole, Hunkar-Huie, Schiller, & Cheatham, 2001; Venning, Durie, Roland, Roberts, & Leese, 2000). In these descriptive studies, information is provided about the direct and indirect actions APNs take during the delivery of care. However, no statements can be made about the relationships between any of these processes and care delivery outcomes, although some hypotheses can be proposed based on study findings. As a result, these studies are useful for that preliminary step in outcomes assessment.

In some studies, APN care delivery processes were compared with those of physicians and other care providers. These studies indicated that NPs were more likely than physicians and other community health providers to spend more time with patients (Venning et al., 2000) and to discuss and encourage smoking cessation (Sheahan, 2000; Zapka et al., 2000), although this prevention-focused activity may not extend to other health risk needs (Sheahan, 2000).

Rudy et al. (1998) compared ACNP and PA care delivery activities with those of resident physicians. Activities were monitored prospectively through the use of activity logs, with outcomes data collected from medical records of patients overseen by ACNPs, PAs, and medical residents. A review of activity logs determined that ACNPs and PAs spent significantly fewer hours caring for patients. Residents were more likely to discuss patients during clinical rounds and to serve as preceptors or instructors for others. Residents also spent more time than ACNPs and PAs writing orders, consulting, completing procedures, and speaking with patients; while ACNPs and PAs spent more time in research and administrative activities. In addition, ACNPs and PAs were more likely to discuss patients with nursing staff and to formally present patients during rounds.

Other process-focused studies have identified differences between CNMs and physicians, with midwives spending more time in practice and less time in teaching and research (Yankou, Petersen, Oakley, & Mayes, 1993). CNMs also reported spending significantly more time during first and subsequent prenatal visits and providing significantly more teaching, which physicians delegated to others. In a separate study of differences in communication styles between CNMs and physicians, both groups used informational styles during interactions with patients (Lawson, 2002). However, intraindividual differences were noted for the CNM providers, suggesting they changed to a more controlling communication style with certain patients. Contrary to Lawson's expectations, communication style was not related to patient-perceived support for autonomy or patient satisfaction.

Process-focused studies have also been done to explore NP prescriptive writing patterns (Campbell et al., 1998; Hamric, Lindebak, Worley, & Jaubert, 1998; Mahoney, 1994; Shell, 2001). These studies provide clear evidence to counter early concerns about the potential for NPs to overprescribe. In a study of prescriptive decision making by primary care NPs and primary care physicians, NPs prescribed significantly fewer medications in response to hypothetical case vignettes. They also demonstrated significantly better decision making regarding which drugs to use and recommended significantly more nondrug therapeutic interventions (Mahoney, 1994). In one study of mental health NPs, however, analysis of prescribing patterns for managing depression suggested that they overuse drugs that are considered less desirable, discontinue medications prematurely, and minimize important patient characteristics such as age (Shell, 2001).

A few studies have been done to explore whether the availability of clinical guidelines improves primary care provider documentation of preventive and screening services (Gray, 1998; Windorski & Kalb, 2002) and care delivery outcome (Lund et al., 2001). In the study by Lund et al., the introduction of evidence-based practice guidelines and a consistent measure of skin condition resulted in improved skin condition in newborns admitted to 51 neonatal intensive care units (NICUs). In the documentation and screening studies, clinical guidelines improved NP documentation of preventive and screening services. When clinical guidelines were not used, however, the frequency of screening behaviors was less than desired. In one study, NPs reported rarely ordering cholesterol screening in children unless some evidence of family history for premature heart disease, stroke, or hypercholesterolemia was present (Windorski & Kalb, 2002)—a practice that clearly conflicted with recommended standards.

These process-focused investigations highlight some of the APN activities that are expected to contribute to care delivery outcome. However, because most of the studies have not assessed the relationship between process of care and any specific outcome, little is known about the actual impact of these actions on recipients of care. Some information about this potential relationship was provided in two reports of a process analysis conducted as part of an RCT of APN impact on early discharge of very low birth weight infants (Brooten, Gennaro, et al., 2002); women who had unplanned cesarean deliveries, high-risk pregnancies, and hysterectomies; and elders with heart disease (Brooten, Youngblut, Deatrick, Naylor, & York, 2003). (In most of these studies, CNSs were mentioned, although later reports by these authors used the generic term *APN*.) During each of these investigations, protocols guided APN care delivery; APNs also recorded what was done during their interventions, the number of patient contacts made, the time spent during contacts, patient outcomes, and health-care costs. In the study of mothers and infants, the majority of the APNs' time was spent on assessment activities (69%), with the remaining time devoted to interventions (Brooten, Gennaro, et al., 2002). Assessments of infants were focused on physical status, while assessments of mothers were directed at coping, health care, availability of support systems, and home environment. Assessments of mothers also addressed caretaking skills, understanding of procedures and medications, knowledge of infant growth and development, and recognition and prevention of infection. Intervention activities were devoted primarily to teaching, followed by liaison or consultation, and encouragement of self-care or infant care.

In the combined analysis, surveillance was identified as the most common intervention, with APNs spending the greatest amount of time on monitoring signs and symptoms of physical problems (Brooten et al., 2003). An important finding of this second analysis was the relationship between magnitude of APN interaction and improvement in patient and cost outcomes. The greater the amount of time spent by the APN, the better the outcomes. A second important finding was the difference in outcomes seen and the amount of APN involvement required across patient populations. This finding reinforces the importance of carefully describing the makeup of the patient population, the care delivery setting (both of which are contextual or structural components of the quality-of-care framework), and the processes of care when an APN impact is measured. Without this information, Brooten et al. (2003) might have erroneously concluded that some APNs performed better than others, when in fact, the differences were the result of patient condition and need.

Although no statement can be made as to which of the APNs' activities contributed specifically to the favorable outcomes seen (described later), the inclusion of a process assessment component provides preliminary indication of a cause-and-effect relationship between APN and patient outcome. Additional research is needed to determine whether selected aspects of the process are more important or whether favorable outcomes are achieved only through a combination of APN actions.

Process Improvement Activities

Few reports of process improvement activities specifically mention the involvement of APNs or their probable impact on care delivery outcome. In one approach, an individual APN served as the process improvement intervention (Counsell & Gilbert, 1999). The difficulty with this report is the limited information provided concerning how the outcome data were collected and analyzed and how any variables unrelated to APN intervention were considered in the data interpretation process. A report by Hylka and Beschle (1995) provides one example of an NP process improvement approach that resulted in cost savings and improved services to patients undergoing outpatient or short-stay (overnight admission) surgical procedures. Although not described as a process improvement activity by the authors, the back-and-forth actions the NPs used to assess care delivery impact suggests this approach. Data were used to understand the magnitude of costs associated with care delivery processes, and then several revisions were made to existing practice, including shifting the ordering of preoperative laboratory tests to a time when NPs were conducting preoperative visits, eliminating standing orders for physical therapy consults, reducing the use of sequential compression devices for short-stay patients, and redesigning the patient discharge teaching process. Each of these process changes resulted in considerable cost savings for the hospital. No information is provided about the impact of these process-related changes on other patient or organizational outcomes.

The use of interdisciplinary rounds as a process improvement approach was described by Halm et al. (2003). In this case, a CNS oversaw the shift of unit-based patient rounds to an interdisciplinary approach that involved all disciplines in the review and discussion of care delivery decisions. No information was provided about the impact of this change at the hospital involved. Instead, the authors reported the findings of an internet survey of APNs who summarized the processes they used to measure the impact of interdisciplinary rounds on patient outcomes and the outcomes APNs recommended for measurement of effect. However, several of the outcome indicators suggested are measures of process rather than outcome (e.g., case finding, consults/referrals, accomplishment of plan for patient, continuity of care, ethical issues addressed, quality initiatives for population, evidence-based protocols). Although these may indeed be useful indicators of improved processes of care and of the potential for better care delivery outcomes, they should not be labeled as patient/family outcome indicators.

Process-as-Outcome Studies

Evident in the literature is ongoing confusion about the use of process indicators to denote outcomes achieved. Among those proposed or examined by authors are resolution of nursing problems (Kleinpell-Nowell & Weiner, 1999), correct nursing diagnosis, correct medical diagnosis (Smith & Waltman, 1994), completeness of admission note (Rudy et al., 1998), collaboration among care providers, providers' recommendations for care based on need, frequency and type of procedures ordered (Ingersoll, McIntosh, & Williams, 2000), and prevention of readmission (Smith & Waltman, 1994). This last process indicator can easily be converted to a true outcome indicator by removing the word *prevention*. Readmission rate is a reasonable and acceptable outcome indicator. Whether it is influenced by advanced practice nursing, however, is an entirely different matter.

Rarely seen are studies that focus exclusively on processes as indicators of outcome. More commonly, investigators mistakenly report some process as an indication of intervention effect. For example, Rudy et al. (1998) identified completeness of admission note as one of seven clinical outcome indicators for their comparison of ACNP, PA, and medical resident practice. In this case, the completeness of an admission note measures care provider performance; it is not a measure of the care received by patients, and there are no data to support the proposed causal link with a true clinical outcome, such as pain intensity or complication rate. A second example is evident in a report by Kinnersley et al. (2000), who described secondary outcomes of a comparison between NP and general practitioner consultations as length of consultation, information provided, resources used (prescriptions, investigations, referrals), and follow-up consultations—all of which are structure (e.g., resources used) and process indicators (e.g., information given, referrals made). However, they did collect information about patient satisfaction, resolution of symptoms and concerns, and patients' intentions to deal with future similar illnesses, which constitute reasonable clinical outcome indicators. The ability to accurately measure patient intention to deal with future similar illnesses is questionable, however, and the authors provided no information about how they did this.

Disease Management Activities

Formal reports of the APN's role in disease management are few. The failure to identify disease management analyses may be due in part to their close linkages with other intervention and assessment activities. One example describes an ACNP disease management program for patients admitted to the hospital for treatment of uncomplicated heart failure (Dahle, Smith, Ingersoll, & Wilson, 1998). In this case, the ACNP used disease-specific protocols to manage and monitor the care of hospitalized patients. Prior to the ACNP's arrival, disease management processes were managed by hospital residents, who rotated through the cardiac service on a monthly basis. The ACNP's impact on organizational and patient outcomes was assessed by comparing administrative databases for the year prior to and following the ACNP's assumption of care. Overall costs, ancillary service costs, and use of electrocardiogram and respiratory care services declined significantly after the ACNP arrived. Mortality rates and lengths of stay were comparable prior to and following the initiation of disease management activities by the ACNP. While there was no difference in patient outcomes, the ACNP did have an impact on the resources used, which would be considered an organizational outcome.

The report of an outpatient NP case manager for patients with cardiovascular disease also constitutes a disease management approach (Dougherty, Spertus, Dewhurst, & Nichol, 2000), although it is not described as such in the article. The authors focused their attention on the case management aspects of the NP role instead, which they described as assessing the patient's needs for specific services and facilitating access to each of these. In this situation, case management was used to provide the services required to manage the disease of the targeted group. A concern with this report is the authors' contention that they evaluated the impact of case management on patient outcomes, when in fact, they evaluated the effect of different medication administration approaches. The case management process, per se, was not the intervention of interest. Consequently, the outcome findings reported by the authors provide no indication of whether that approach to disease management is better than any other.

A description of an APN-directed work-site disease management program is also available (Carioti, Lavigne, Stone, Tortoretti, & Chiverton, 2001). In this case, 54 employees were surveyed about their perceptions of disease control, behavioral change, and understanding of disease condition following program completion. A majority of respondents (who were primarily educated white men being treated for hypertension, dyslipidemia, and diabetes) reported behavioral changes as a result of the program. Those who were treated for dyslipidemia and for hypertension also reported greater understanding of their disorders. Participants with asthma reported no change in level of understanding or initiation of behavioral change. Overall, participants were highly satisfied with the program. Because the outcome indicators were self-reports of perceived changes that were measured after intervention only, however, caution is required when the impact of this intervention is considered. Additional indicators, including those that could validate self-reports, are desirable. Moreover, the collection of data prior to the intervention and at additional periods following program completion would help ensure that behavioral and perceptual changes did in fact occur and that the impact was sustained long enough to achieve a true outcome effect. Blood pressure, lipid level, pulmonary function, medication intake, blood glucose level, and other quantifiable measures collected longitudinally would assist with validation of self-reports.

Outcomes Management Activities

Reports of APN-directed outcomes management programs are few. Several descriptions of program development activities are available, with each of these highlighting the steps necessary for successfully designing and implementing such programs (Cook & Nolan, 1996; Davidson, 1999; Peters, Cowley, & Standiford, 1999; Wojner, 1996; Wojner, Rauch, & Mokracek, 1997). Three of these reports provided some information about the site-specific impact of the outcomes management approach on targeted patient outcomes. In the first, an outcomes management program for hospitalized patients who had experienced a stroke resulted in reduced lengths of hospital and intensive care unit (ICU) stay, time to wean from mechanical ventilation, need for tube feeding, and number of fevers of unknown origin (Wojner, 1996). In the second report, cesarean delivery rates in an obstetrical department were reduced by 6% over a 3-year period (Peters et al., 1999); in the third, preliminary cost estimations showed a reduction in costs for NP-directed care (Cook & Nolan, 1996). Patient satisfaction levels were high.

The results of an outcomes management approach at an academic health science center have also been described (Russell, VorderBruegge, & Burns, 2002). In this outcomes managed model, two ACNPs served as outcomes managers for a population of neuroscience patients. The impact of the model was assessed through a retrospective medical record review of outcomes directly linked to daily management by and interventions of the APNs. A significant reduction in length of hospital stay was seen for patients at risk. Reductions in ICU length of stay and incidence of urinary tract infection and skin breakdown were also evident, with overall cost savings approaching $2.5 million for a 1-year period.

Outcomes Research

Outcomes research has been carried out to investigate care delivery outcomes across providers and between different APN types. In most cases, physician groups (including medical residents) have been used for comparison. This process is a concern because it implies that physician practice is the gold standard for APNs and that it encompasses the full range of advanced practice nursing activity. In actuality, physician practice overlaps in some respects and diverges in others. In the process studies reviewed earlier, APNs routinely used strategies that were either not considered by physicians or were not incorporated to the extent evident in advanced nursing practice. Ideally, attention should be directed to indicators that accurately measure all care providers' impact and those that can serve as benchmarks for advanced practice nursing alone.

In this section of the review of the literature, outcomes studies are clustered together according to whether their focus was preliminary and attempted to identify outcome indicators used by APNs to measure impact or whether the studies measured the actual effect of advanced nursing practice on outcomes observed. The APN intervention studies are further divided into those that compare outcomes achieved by APNs with those achieved by other provider groups (e.g., physicians), those that compare APN outcomes with those achieved when usual care is provided, and those without comparison groups that measure outcomes prior to and following the introduction of an APN. This section includes representative reports highlighting the indicators measured in outcomes studies, the limitations evident in some of the research, and the findings described.

OUTCOMES IDENTIFICATION STUDIES

Ingersoll et al. (2000) investigated which outcome indicators APNs routinely use or would recommend using for measurement of APN impact. A modified Delphi survey was used to identify the top 10 outcome indicators APNs in Tennessee would recommend for assessment of performance regardless of specialty practice or location of service. The initial list of potential indicators was generated by APNs, who identified a combination of process and outcome indicators during multiple focus group sessions. These 27 indicators were then compiled into a survey and sent to practicing APNs throughout the state. APN respondents (N = 177) rated each indicator on the cost of using the indicator, the feasibility and burden of collecting indicator data, the relevance of the indicator to practice, and the indicator's overall usefulness for assessing advanced nursing practice. In the second survey, respondents were given the mean acceptance scores identified in the first round and the initial ranking of indicators. APNs were then asked to indicate whether they agreed with the ranking and how likely they would be to use the top 10 indicators to assess their practice. The top 10 indicators selected (in descending order) were satisfaction with care, symptom reduction or resolution, perception of being well cared for, compliance/adherence, knowledge level of patients and families, trust of care provider, collaboration among care providers, care provider recommendation according to need, frequency and type of procedures ordered, and quality of life. Of note in this listing is the inclusion of three process indicators (collaboration, care provider recommendation, and procedures ordered), which would not reflect the APN's impact on outcomes.

Findings from this investigation differed somewhat from those of an earlier study by Smith and Waltman (1994), who surveyed oncology CNSs about their perceived influence on care delivery processes and outcomes. In that study, CNSs rated 63 outcome- and barrier-related items identified through a review of literature, interviews with two oncology CNSs, and a small pilot study. Respondents rated each of the items on a scale ranging from 1 (seldom or 0-6 times/year) to 4 (constantly or at least once per week). What is not clear from the article is whether these response options pertained to how often the CNSs perceived they influenced the outcomes themselves or believed that CNSs did so overall.

With a mean rating of 3.0 or higher, the following were rated as frequently to constantly influenced by APNs: improved patient/family knowledge, comfort level, improved coping for patient/family, patient/family anxiety level, patient/family satisfaction, control of treatment side effects, self-care ability, correct nursing diagnosis, staff knowledge, staff skill, staff use of effective interventions, program development, consultation with caregiver, multidisciplinary cooperation, improved interdisciplinary communication, advocacy for patient/family, referrals to resources, and consultation with physician (Smith & Waltman, 1994). A serious concern with this report is its stated focus on patient outcomes but its inclusion of organizational, interdisciplinary/consultative, and research processes as indicators of such. This mixing of indicators, without a discussion of which pertain to processes (and therefore not patient outcomes), serves to confuse the outcomes measurement picture.

STUDIES COMPARING APN AND PHYSICIAN OUTCOMES

Studies in which APNs are compared with medical practitioners have been published in the United States, Canada, the British Isles, Europe, Australia, the Middle East, and elsewhere. Caution is needed when these studies are compared, however, because educational requirements for advanced practice differ by country. Graduate education is now the standard in the United States and is moving in that direction throughout Canada. In the British Isles and in other countries, certificate programs are often the norm. In addition, some reports label nurses as specialists or advanced practitioners solely because of their number of years of experience in the clinical setting (Chang et al., 1999; Sakr et al., 1999) or because their role behaviors are "typical" of APNs (Oddi & Cassidy, 1998).

NP Outcomes. Most studies of APN versus physician practice have compared NPs with primary care physicians. In a recent systematic review of this literature, RCTs and studies with prospective experimental designs conducted between 1966 and 2001 were reviewed if they included patient satisfaction, health status, health service costs, or process of care measures (Horrocks, Anderson, & Salisbury, 2002). In addition to searching electronic databases for studies from developed countries, investigators contacted schools of nursing offering NP training programs and authors of identified studies. When the study reports did not specify whether the nurse providing the care was an NP, the investigators used specific criteria to determine whether the study should be included. This process is a limitation and may have resulted in the inclusion of studies that should not have been considered. Thirty-five of 119 potential studies met review inclusion criteria. Overall, the research demonstrated that patient satisfaction with care provider was significantly greater for NPs. No differences were seen for health status or quality of life. Process indicators suggested NPs spent more time with patients, identified physical abnormalities more often, communicated more effectively, and recorded observations in the medical record more completely than physicians. The ordering and interpreting of x-ray films was comparable across groups (Horrocks et al., 2002). Evident from this review is the need for additional rigorous research concerning APN impact. Only 29.4% of studies in which NP outcomes were compared with primary care physician outcomes were sufficiently well designed to meet the review's inclusion criteria. Without this level of comparison, few recommendations can be made about which indicators are most reflective of and sensitive to advanced nursing practice.

Two recent RCTs of NP and primary care physician practice include one from the United States (Mundinger et al., 2000) and one from Wales and England (Kinnersley et al., 2000). In both studies more than 1000 patients were randomly assigned to either

NP or primary care physician practice. In the study by Mundinger et al., health status, patient satisfaction, service utilization, and physiological test results were comparable for NP and physician groups. Similar results were seen in the study by Kinnersley et al. (2000), although patients in that sample were significantly more satisfied with the care provided by NPs and reported receiving more information about their illnesses.

ACNP Outcomes. Rudy et al. (1998) used a longitudinal, matched group design to compare ACNPs' outcomes with resident physicians' outcomes at two medical centers. Outcomes data were collected from the medical records of patients overseen by ACNPs, PAs, and medical residents. During the 14-month period of the study, patient outcomes (lengths of stay, mortality rates, number of adverse drug reactions, and readmissions to the hospital within 2 weeks) were comparable across care providers. A shortcoming of this study is the mixing of ACNP and PA providers, which suggests that these two groups have comparable educational preparation and skill. Because of the distinctions between ACNPs and PAs, outcomes assessment initiatives should measure their impact separately.

CNS Outcomes. Favorable outcomes have been seen for patients with cancer treated by CNSs in outpatient settings (Moore et al., 2002). CNSs in this study managed patient care in nurse-led clinics and then contacted patients by phone for follow-up assessment. Patients treated by CNSs had significantly better levels of emotional functioning and less peripheral neuropathy than patients treated by physicians. Patients treated by CNSs were also significantly more likely to die at home than were patients treated by physicians. Costs of care were comparable for both groups.

CNM Outcomes. The outcomes of CNM-directed care are compared with those of physician-directed care in several reports of birth delivery outcomes. These studies demonstrated that the incidence of cesarean delivery for CNM providers was low (Greulich et al., 1994) and was significantly lower than that for physicians (Butler, Adams, Parker, Roberts, & Laros, 1993; Davis, Riedmann, Sapiro, Minoque, & Kazer, 1994). CNMs in one study also used significantly less epidural anesthesia during delivery and had significantly fewer labor abnormalities or episodes of fetal distress than physicians (Butler et al., 1993). In each of these studies, the incidence of cesarean delivery and the use of epidural anesthesia are considered patient outcomes because of their impact on patients and their potential for longer patient recovery and response to care. They also are indications of care provider process and reflect decision making and the selection of alternative practices by providers. When used as outcomes, they should be clearly linked to the patient responses that occur as a result of these interventions.

CRNA Outcomes. Two studies of CRNA outcomes are available in the literature; one pertains to a cost estimation model derived from case studies of four anesthesia services at four different hospitals—a large academic medical center, a large community hospital, a medium-sized community hospital, and a small community hospital (Cromwell & Snyder, 2000). Labor cost projections for 10,000 anesthetics delivered per year demonstrated that an all-CRNA care delivery model would require less than half the cost of an all-anesthesiologist model. The cost savings for a mixed model composed of anesthesiologists and CRNAs in ratios of 1:1 to 1:4 ranged from 33% to 41% of the total costs for an all-anesthesiologist model. In the second CRNA outcomes study, risk-adjusted mortality rates of patients undergoing carotid endarterectomy, cholecystectomy, herniorrhaphy, hysterectomy, knee replacement, laminectomy, mastectomy, or prostatectomy were compared for CRNAs and anesthesiologists (Pine, Holt, & Lou, 2003).

Medicare data were analyzed for a 3-year period, and no differences were seen for type of anesthesia provider.

NNP Outcomes. NNP resuscitation effectiveness was compared with that of junior medical staff in one institution in which a resuscitation team was introduced into the NICU (Aubrey & Yoxall, 2001). In this study, NNPs' and medical residents' intubation rates were similar, although NNPs intubated infants more quickly and administered surfactant earlier. Survival rates and adverse events for infants were comparable for both groups. The earlier intubation timing and the administration of surfactant suggested that the NNPs were more familiar with the institution's best-practice protocols, which stressed early intubation and early administration of surfactant for at-risk neonates.

An interesting and noteworthy finding of this study is the failure of the NNPs' improved care delivery processes (earlier intubation and administration of surfactant) to achieve better patient outcomes. This finding highlights the difficulty in identifying which factor or combination of factors contributes to the achievement of improved care delivery outcome. Clearly, factors other than timing of intervention and administration of surfactant were influencing the outcomes achieved. A strength of this study is its comparison of resuscitation process (reflected by frequency of intubation, timing of intubation, and administration of surfactant) with resuscitation outcome (infant survival rate and frequency of adverse events). Any time information about the comparability of or differences in actions taken during the delivery of care is included, the degree of comfort with probable cause-and-effect relationships is increased.

In several other studies, NNP outcomes were compared with those of other care providers, including PAs and resident physicians. Chart reviews assessing care delivery outcomes revealed comparable morbidity and mortality rates, costs of care, and lengths of stay in the NICU and the hospital as a whole (Bissinger, Allred, Arford, & Bellig, 1997; Carzoli, Martinez-Cruz, Cuevas, Murphy, & Chiu, 1994; Karlowicz & McMurray, 2000; Schultz, Liptak, Fioravanti, 1994). When prematurity was considered in the study by Schultz et al., however, significant reductions in length of stay and cost of care were seen for the NNPs' patients. These retrospective findings were supported in an RCT in which NNPs' and medical residents' outcomes related to morbidity, mortality, length of stay, parent satisfaction, and cost were comparable (Mitchell-DiCenso et al., 1996)

STUDIES COMPARING APN AND PHYSICIAN PRODUCTIVITY

One of the most difficult and contentious elements of APN outcomes measurement is the assessment of APN productivity, which is an organizational rather than patient outcome. Productivity is an indication of care provider efficiency rather than skill or capability, and as such, does not provide any guarantee of quality patient care. The issue with productivity is that reimbursement practices and the income generated by care providers are directly tied to productivity levels. Because APNs spend more time with patients, their overall productivity levels may result in the loss of potential income for the organization or practice. Until reimbursement decisions are shifted to a care delivery outcomes approach, this will continue to be a problem for APNs.

Relative Work Value of APNs. Payment for services provided to Medicare patients is determined through the use of a resource-based relative work value scale methodology (RBRV), which incorporates an estimate for the amount of work, practice expense, and professional liability insurance associated with various procedures. The total relative value of each procedure is multiplied by a standard dollar conversion factor to determine the allowable service charge care providers may request for reimbursement of services

(Sullivan-Marx & Maislin, 2000). Until 1994, all RBRVs were calculated solely from physician data. Since that time, NP data have been used to adjust the RBRVS for some payment codes, although considerable work is needed to clarify how NPs' work values differ from physicians' (Sullivan-Marx & Maislin, 2000).

Sullivan-Marx and Maislin (2000) and Sullivan-Marx, Happ, Bradley, and Maislin, (2000) have begun to explore this issue. In a survey mailed to expert practitioners, NPs quantified both the time and complexity of the work required to provide care during three office encounter vignettes. In quantifying the time required, NPs estimated preservice, intraservice, and postservice time in minutes. Complexity was measured by assessing mental effort, technical skill, and physical effort, and the psychological stress associated with an iatrogenic event related to the *Current Procedural Terminology* (CPT) code associated with the vignette. In all cases, NPs estimated relative work values comparable to those established for physician practice, suggesting that their practice patterns were similar for the scenarios described. Because the CPT codes and descriptors were designed with physicians in mind, however, other activities by APNs may not have been included in the estimation process. Until these are well defined and marketed by APNs, this process will continue to potentially underrepresent APNs' actual relative value in the delivery of care.

STUDIES COMPARING ADVANCED PRACTICE NURSING AND USUAL PRACTICE OUTCOMES

Some of the strongest APN outcomes research has focused on the impact of early hospital discharge by using a CNS-directed discharge planning and home follow-up intervention (Brooten, Naylor, et al., 2002). This care delivery model has been tested with women with high-risk pregnancies (York et al., 1997), women undergoing cesarean delivery (Brooten et al., 1994), older patients with cancer who have undergone surgery (McCorkle et al., 2000), and the elderly (Naylor et al., 1994; Naylor et al., 1999 [in this recent report the term *APN* was used, so NPs may have been interveners as well as CNSs]). In each of these investigations, a randomized controlled research design was used to compare CNS outcomes with those seen with usual care. In all cases, outcomes were superior for the CNS intervention groups. Cost of care for CNS-directed services was 29% (Brooten et al., 1994) to 44% (York et al., 1997) less than that of standard care. Most of the cost savings for the elderly group were the result of a significant reduction in the number of readmissions for patients treated by APNs (Naylor et al., 1999).

Other studies in which APN outcomes were compared with standard care have been conducted in long-term care facilities (Ryden et al., 2000), with women with recent diagnoses of cancer (Ritz et al., 2000), with rehabilitation patients discharged from an acute care facility (Rawl, Easton, Kwiatkowski, Zemen, & Burczyk, 1998), and with critically ill patients at risk for pulmonary complications (Hanneman, Bines, & Sajtar, 1993). In the long-term care facility, gerontological CNSs used evidence-based protocols to manage the care of newly admitted patients at risk for incontinence, pressure ulcers, depression, and aggressive behavior (Ryden et al., 2000). Care delivery outcomes were compared with those at a comparison site where residents received usual care. Findings suggested that CNSs influenced care delivery outcomes through direct and indirect means; reductions were seen in the number of episodes of urinary incontinence, the incidence of pressure ulcers, and the frequency of aggressive behavior. An overall 6-month composite change score was also significantly higher for patients treated by the CNSs. Missing from this report is an indication of how the direct versus indirect activities of the CNS influenced outcomes are seen. This component of impact assessment studies is difficult to determine, although steps in this direction are needed to clarify how APNs improve care delivery through direct intervention, as well as through the improved performance of others.

In one study of APN (type of provider not specified) impact on early adjustment to diagnosis of breast cancer, inclusion of an APN in delivery of services resulted in improved quality of life, less uncertainty, and fewer mood disturbances (Ritz et al., 2000). Overall costs of care were comparable for usual services and for those that were enhanced by advanced practice nursing, suggesting that this approach is cost-effective for improving care delivery outcomes in women with recent diagnoses of breast cancer. Findings with rehabilitation patients were less conclusive; anxiety and number of postdischarge phone calls declined significantly in experimental, but not control, groups. However, other measured outcomes demonstrated no difference between groups (Rawl et al., 1998).

In a study by Hanneman et al. (1993), both the direct and indirect effects of a unit-based CNS were considered. Preventable pulmonary outcomes were assessed for patients treated in an ICU in which a CNS rounded daily with nurses, conducted formal workshops related to care of patients with artificial airways, and provided one-on-one clinical training to nursing staff. Significant reductions were seen in the frequency of malpositioned endotracheal tubes and inadvertent extubation following the introduction of the CNS. These improvements occurred despite significantly higher acuity rates in the study unit. No changes were seen in the frequency of adverse outcomes or patient acuity in the comparison ICU. The addition of a unit-based CNS at another institution also resulted in favorable outcomes, with significant reductions seen in length of stay (Wheeler, 1999). A trend was seen for a reduction in complication rate, although the total number of complications was too small to detect significant differences.

STUDIES WITH NONCOMPARISON GROUPS

A number of studies have compared care delivery outcomes prior to and following the APN's introduction into clinical practice. In many of these studies, a preintervention/postintervention approach was used to test for differences. A weakness of these studies is the frequent reliance on retrospective reviews of medical records for evidence of outcomes prior to the APN's arrival. The absence of a comparison group also makes confirmation of the relationship between APN and outcome difficult. Nevertheless, they do provide useful information for further exploration in more controlled trials and should be viewed as preliminary indications of possible effect. In one such study, length of stay, patient satisfaction, use of laboratory tests (a process-as-outcome indicator), and overall costs for the year prior to the ACNP's arrival were compared with those during the 16 months afterward (Sarkissian & Wennberg, 1999). Length of stay, use of laboratory tests, and overall costs of services declined significantly following the arrival of the ACNP. Satisfaction, which was measured only after the ACNP's arrival by an investigator-developed scale, was high. Similarly high ratings were seen in a prospective, noncomparison study of psychiatric CNSs (Baradell & Bordeaux, 2001). Patients in this study also reported significant reductions in clinical symptoms and improvements in quality of life.

Several other studies have focused solely on patient or staff satisfaction with APN practice as an indicator of care provider effect (Benkert et al., 2002; Bryant & Graham, 2002; Knudtson, 2000; Larrabee, Ferri, & Hartig, 1997; Ramsey, Edwards, Lenz, Odom, & Brown, 1993; Stutts, 2001). In many cases, these studies used questionnaires with limited reliability and validity estimates and included single-site samples of patients. In most instances, no comparison groups were available. Because of the methodological issues associated with the measurement of satisfaction, reliance on this outcome indicator alone is generally not sufficient for assessing APN impact. Patient satisfaction data are often skewed, with only the most satisfied or dissatisfied patients responding. In addition, general satisfaction measures may not be sufficiently sensitive to detect differences across APN providers. Their use should not be avoided altogether, however, because they do offer one indication of care provider impact. When serious problems with delivery of services occur, satisfaction levels drop. In stable environments, the variation may not be sufficient to assist with effective outcomes monitoring activities.

Program Evaluation

Differentiating program evaluation initiatives from outcomes research is difficult, especially if an APN has been actively involved in developing and implementing the program. In most cases, outcome measures are used to assess program impact, contributing further to the confusion. For purposes of this review, program evaluation reports are those in which the authors describe the activity as an evaluation, those in which the advanced practice nursing activity is one component of several initiatives designed to provide some service or influence some outcome, and those in which the purpose of the assessment was to determine the worth or value of the intervention for purposes of decision making.

Evaluations of APN-involved programs have included initiatives designed to reduce smoking frequency in pregnant women (Gebaur, Kwo, Haynes, & Wewers, 1998), improve service delivery to and reduce the costs associated with patients admitted to the hospital for treatment of heart failure (Dahl & Penque, 2001) or for inpatient surgery (Hylka & Beschle, 1995), cover vacancies resulting from the loss of resident staff (McMullen, Alexander, Bourgeois, & Goodman, 2001), oversee the home nutritional support needs of discharged patients (Schaffner & Bohomey, 1998), provide counseling for high-risk drinkers (Ockene, Adams, Hurley, Wheeler, & Hebert, 1999), reduce maternal depression after cesarean section (Small, Lumley, Donohue, Potter, & Waldenstrom, 2000), improve the quality of diabetes care to primary care patients (Brown, Wolff, Elasy, & Graber, 2001), prevent disability in frail older adults (Leveille et al., 1998), and deliver school-based health care to children and their siblings (Jones & Clark, 1997).

In several of these evaluations, APN oversight of or involvement in program planning and implementation resulted in improved care delivery outcome (Brown et al., 2001; Gebaur et al., 1998; Gruelich et al., 1994; Hylka & Beschle, 1995; Jones & Clark, 1997; Schaffner & Bohomey, 1998), although in one study the improvements occurred in some but not all outcomes assessed (Leveille et al., 1998). Attending physician/NP collaborative services produced favorable patient perceptions of care delivery, physical health of patients, physician and nursing staff satisfaction (McMullen et al., 2001), and reduction in alcohol intake (Ockene et al., 1999). In addition, the costs of managing acute illnesses in children and siblings were reduced in one setting to one quarter of the comparison group's (Jones & Clark, 1997).

An evaluation of an NP care coordinator role, in combination with standing orders and a clinical pathway, demonstrated significantly improved care delivery outcomes following the introduction of a multidimensional program (Dahl & Penque, 2001). Length of hospital stay, mortality rate, and readmission rates at 30 and 90 days all decreased significantly in the year after program implementation. Highlighted in this study is an important outcome measurement issue relevant to advanced nursing practice. Although the overall length of stay for program patients was significantly less than for those prior to program implementation, patients seen by the NP had significantly longer lengths of stay. The authors suggested that this finding was the result of the complex needs of patients and the likelihood that the NP became more directly involved the longer the patient remained in the hospital. Had the investigators used this indicator alone as the sole measure of program effect, the outcome might have been perceived as unsupportive of the APN role. Because the investigators used several measures, however, and because they attempted to analyze which components of the program contributed to which results, the findings are more useful for practitioners interested in developing comparable programs.

Two other reports of APN impact are included here as examples of rarely performed, but highly desirable, first steps in advanced practice nursing program implementation and outcome evaluation activities: feasibility/pilot studies and instrument sensitivity testing. In each of these, a pilot study was conducted with a small sample of the population targeted for APN-directed care (Beeber & Charlie, 1998; Brown & Hanis, 1995). Feasibility/pilot studies are useful for preventing the implementation of interventions that will not be received favorably by targeted recipients or stakeholders (e.g., other care providers, community leaders). They also help identify unforeseen barriers that might interfere with the introduction of new programs and the assessment of their impact. In addition, they clarify the direct and indirect costs of program implementation and maintenance and uncover the strategies required to implement a new process and evaluate its results. Brown and Hanis's pilot project, for example, was conducted to determine whether a community-based diabetes education and group-support intervention provided by a bilingual Mexican American CNS, registered dietician, and community layperson could be implemented and evaluated successfully in the area targeted. The pilot intervention was shorter than the proposed full-scale program, and the number of subjects who completed the study (N = 5) was small. Nonetheless, the pilot study detected a trend in participant outcomes that supported the potential effectiveness of the intervention. It also identified several course content changes that would better address participants' needs and provided information about the most appropriate site for the intervention, the number of sessions desired for achieving learning objectives, and the acceptability of the intervention by targeted recipients.

Instrument sensitivity testing is also a common component of pilot studies and was undertaken in the feasibility/pilot studies by Brown and Hanis (1995) and Beeber and Charlie (1998). Instrument sensitivity testing provides information about the usefulness and appropriateness of the data collection tools proposed for measuring outcomes in the population targeted. In the study by Brown and Hanis, English and Spanish versions of investigator-developed instruments were evaluated for use with representatives of the targeted population. Beeber and Charlie, on the other hand, tested instruments used previously in a variety of studies to confirm their sensitivity to changes in the outcomes proposed for the targeted intervention group. Data from the pilot study supported reliability and validity estimates from other research.

COST ANALYSES

Comprehensive cost analyses of program performance are few, with most discussions reflecting charges associated with services rather than true cost of care. Two comprehensive cost analyses of APN-managed care facilities were identified in the literature. One focused on the delivery of primary care services in an underserved area (Saywell, Lassiter, & Flynn, 1995), and the other targeted women with low-risk pregnancies (Stone, Zwanziger, Walker, & Buenting, 2000). In the first analysis, the costs of NP-managed primary care were compared with the costs of primary care physician services in surrounding communities (Saywell et al., 1995). Investigators conducted general cost accounting, operational cost analysis, and scenario or sensitivity analysis procedures to identify actual costs and projected costs if productivity rates increased. The NP clinic costs were comparable to physician costs when volunteer time and donated resources were not included in the estimation. When actual costs were computed, however, NP service costs were higher. These higher costs were attributed to a productivity index (1.2) that fell below the minimum 2.25 clinic visits per hour that was required to keep the costs comparable to physician costs. This finding highlights a serious concern for APNs, especially when their productivity and cost outcomes are compared with those of physicians. The additional time APNs spend with patients may exceed efficiency requirements for maximum revenue generation. At issue is whether the reduced income per visit can be offset by the need for fewer visits overall because of the extra attention paid to patients by the APNs. Unfortunately, no research is available to answer this question.

In the second analysis, CNM provider costs for care delivered in a freestanding birth center were compared with physician costs for care delivered in a hospital setting (Stone et al., 2000). In both cases, costs were estimated according to maternity episode, with direct prenatal and childbirth costs calculated from institutional reports, census reports, office profit and loss statements, and billing records. A sensitivity analysis was performed to determine the effect of patient volume on cost of care. The costs of the CNMs' prenatal services were significantly higher than the physicians'; childbirth costs were significantly less. When combined over the episode of care, costs were comparable for both provider types.

A more comprehensive summary of APN outcome studies published since 1990, organized by outcome indicators, is provided in Table 25-2. Only studies that contained sufficient information about how the outcomes were measured and when they were measured in relation to APN intervention are included in Table 25-2.

Summary of the Research Thus Far

The evidence concerning APN impact on individual, organizational, and community outcomes suggests that the quality of care APNs deliver is comparable to or superior to that of other care providers in the specialty. A variety of studies have explored the direct and indirect processes APNs use to manage patient care and the outcomes achieved through practice. All have determined that advanced nursing practice overlaps with the practice of other care providers in some respects, while differing in others. These distinctions and their potential to confound comparisons with other care providers contribute to the complexity inherent in measuring APN effect. Moreover, the limited research linking specific APN processes to care delivery outcomes makes determining which role components achieve the effect difficult. Difficult or not, a clear distinction is needed if APNs are ever to receive the recognition they deserve or the financial reimbursement they are due.

This review of APN outcomes research suggests that intensive work is needed in several areas. The first and most preliminary of these areas involves the consistent use of a set of core outcome indicators relevant to and sensitive to differences in APN practice. To achieve this goal, networks of APN groups and institutions where APNs practice need to facilitate the collection of comparable data and the sharing of results for comparisons across groups, specialties, and locales. This approach is particularly important for those APNs whose practices are too small to generate the data needed to influence policymakers and make decisions about which performance measures to reward. A recommendation is to begin small, selecting evidence-based indicators that appear to be the most reliable, valid, and sensitive to differences in APN practice. Other indicators can be added as further investigations demonstrate evidence of cause and effect between APN and care delivery outcome. Ideally, these data should be relatively inexpensive to collect and the reporting methods should be comparable across sites. Table 25-2 lists the numerous APN-sensitive outcome indicators that have been used in previous studies.

National leadership groups should assume responsibility for coordinated efforts to evaluate APN outcomes, with recommendations for which indicators to choose and the allocation of funds to support the central collection of and dissemination of research findings. Collaborations between APNs and nurse researchers and the development of outcomes consortia will also facilitate this process. Bringing together clinical practice and research design and measurement experts from multiple locations and specialties is the best approach for identifying the most reliable and valid indicators of APN effect.

Second, there is an urgent need to reexamine reimbursement practices that reinforce productivity levels according to physician performance. Process-focused and cost-effectiveness studies demonstrate that APNs take more time with patients and therefore are at risk for failing to meet organizational or group practice productivity standards based on the medical model. Because researchers have not compared different types of productivity estimations, the true magnitude and impact of APN efficiency is unknown. A shift in focus from time spent during individual patient interaction to one that considers total time spent during an episode of care (as was done by Stone et al., 2000) might be more realistic for measuring and comparing APN practices. In the episode-of-care approach, total time and resources used per episode indicate level of productivity. In this case, the extra time spent by APNs and the number of interactions with patients at the outset of service may eliminate the need for longer-term, sustained interactions that occur when patients and families are not sufficiently prepared to manage their health-care needs. The additional time spent in education and counseling in the initial phase may eliminate the need for more costly care over the course of the episode. At this time, the evidence is insufficient to determine whether this or alternative approaches to measuring productivity can more accurately assess the efficiency and benefits of advanced practice nursing.

Closely linked with this issue is the third need to determine whether the increased patient and family satisfaction evident when APNs spend extra time also contributes to improvements in longer-term care delivery outcomes. Because APNs spend more time with patients and provide additional teaching and healthy behaviors counseling, their impact may be most evident in the long-term prevention of diseases and adverse outcomes commonly associated with poor health behaviors. In studies thus far, patient outcomes have been monitored for relatively short periods, usually 6 months to 1 year after APN intervention. Additional longitudinal studies are needed to determine the true long-term impact of these early outcomes on overall lifestyle, quality of life, and health.

Fourth, additional research is needed to compare APNs with other APN providers. To date, the focus has been consistently directed at comparisons of APNs with physicians, medical residents, or PAs. Although these studies are useful, evidence is unavailable concerning which outcome indicators are most sensitive to differences in APN practice. Benchmarking for the future should be based on the recognition and use of best practices for and by APNs in various roles and the extent to which individuals or groups of APNs practice according to these standards.

Fifth, this review makes evident the need to explore the value-added impact of APNs in collaborative practice with physicians and other care providers. Some preliminary work has begun in this regard, but additional work is necessary. Because APNs and physicians have different perspectives about care and demonstrate distinct but complementary behaviors, studies concerning how these combined practices reinforce and maximize the beneficial effects of one another are needed. This value-added approach may generate the data needed to alter reimbursement procedures and document the increased potential for favorable outcome when a collaborative APN-physician approach is used.

Text continued on p.913

TABLE 25-2 APN-SENSITIVE OUTCOME INDICATORS TESTED IN PRACTICE*

OUTCOME INDICATOR	AUTHORS (YR)	STUDY DESIGN	FOCUS OF INDICATOR (POPULATION-GENERIC, POPULATION-SPECIFIC, OR ORGANIZATIONAL)	FINDINGS
Activities of daily living (ADLs)	Leveille et al. (1998)	RCT	Population-generic	Significantly improved over control group
Adverse events/unplanned incidents, including drug reactions	Rudy et al. (1998)	Comparative analysis	Population-generic, organizational	Comparable to residents
Affect	Ryden et al. (2000)	Quasi-experimental comparison	Population-generic	Significantly improved over control group
Aggressive behavior	Ryden et al. (2000)	Quasi-experimental comparison	Population-generic	Significantly improved over control group
Alcohol consumption	Ockene et al. (1999)	Program evaluation	Population-specific	Significantly improved over control group
Amniotomy†	Brown & Grimes (1995)	Meta-analysis	Population-specific	Significantly fewer than physicians
Anxiety/depression; mental health status; emotional state	Brooten et al. (1994)	RCT	Population-generic	Comparable to control group
	Hill et al. (1994)	Single-blind, parallel-group comparison	Population-generic	Significantly better than physicians
	Leveille et al. (1998)	RCT	Population-generic	Comparable to control group
	McMullen et al. (2001)	Program evaluation	Population-generic	Comparable to physician service
	Moore et al. (2002)	RCT	Population-generic	Significantly better than physicians
	Naylor et al. (1994)	RCT	Population-generic	Comparable to control group
	Naylor et al. (1999)	RCT	Population-generic	Comparable to control group
	Rawl et al. (1998)	RCT	Population-generic	Significantly better than control group
	Ritz et al. (2000)	RCT	Population-generic	Significantly better than control group
	Ryden et al. (2000)	Quasi-experimental comparison	Population-generic	Comparable to control group
APGAR score	Davis et al. (1994)	Administrative record review	Population-specific	Comparable to physicians
	Greulich et al. (1994)	Medical record review	Population-specific	Low incidence of low score
	Murphy & Fullerton (1998)	Survey	Population-specific	Low incidence of low score
Autonomous decision making (patient perceived)	Lawson (2002)	Survey	Population-generic	Comparable to physicians

Outcome	Source	Method	Type	Finding
Birth weight	Brown & Grimes (1995)	Meta-analysis	Population-specific	Comparable to physicians
	Gravely & Littlefield (1992)	Cost-effectiveness analysis	Population-specific	Comparable to physicians
	Greulich et al. (1994)	Medical record review	Population-specific	Low incidence
	York et al. (1997)	RCT	Population-specific	Comparable to control group
Blood pressure	Cook & Nolan (1996)	Outcomes management program	Population-generic	Comparable to comparison group
	Mundinger et al. (2000)	RCT	Population-generic	Comparable to physicians
Caregiver psychosocial status	Jepson et al. (1999)	RCT	Population-generic	Comparable to control group
Cesarean section†	Brown & Grimes (1995)	Meta-analysis	Population-specific	Significantly fewer than physicians
	Butler et al. (1993)	Medical record review	Population-specific	Significantly fewer than physicians
	Davis et al. (1994)	Administrative database review	Population-specific	Significantly fewer than physicians
	Greulich et al. (1994)	Medical record review	Population-specific	Low incidence
Complication rate	Carzoli et al. (1994)	Medical record review	Population-generic	Comparable to physicians
	Mitchell-DiCenso et al. (1996)	RCT	Population-generic	Comparable to residents
	Rawl et al. (1998)	RCT	Population-generic	Comparable to control group
	Wheeler (1999)	Medical record review		Trend for fewer with APN present on patient unit
Cost of care	Bissinger et al. (1997)	Medical record review	Population-generic	Significantly less than residents
	Brooten et al. (1994)	RCT	Population-generic	Significantly less than control group
	Burl et al. (1998)	Administrative database review	Population-generic	GNP/MD team significantly less than physician alone
	Carr (2000)	Administrative database review	Population-generic	Significantly less than physicians
	Carzoli et al. (1994)	Medical record review	Population-generic	Comparable to physicians
	Cook & Nolan (1996)	Outcomes management program	Population-generic	Less than comparison group
	Cromwell & Snyder (2000)	Case study cost comparison	Population-generic	Significantly less with CRNA team model
	Dahle et al. (1998)	Pre/post comparison	Population-generic	Significantly less than physicians
	Gravely & Littlefield (1992)	Cost-effectiveness analysis	Population-generic	Significantly less per clinic visit than physician-directed care
	Jones & Clark (1997)	Program evaluation	Population-generic	Reduced to ¼ of comparison group
	Karlowicz & McMurray (2000)	Medical record review	Population-generic	Comparable to residents
	Mitchell-DiCenso et al. (1996)	RCT	Population-generic	Comparable to physicians
	Naylor et al. (1994)	RCT	Population-generic	Significantly less than control group
	Naylor et al. (1999)	RCT	Population-generic	Significantly less than control group

Continued

TABLE 25-2 APN-SENSITIVE OUTCOME INDICATORS TESTED IN PRACTICE* —cont'd

OUTCOME INDICATOR	AUTHORS (YR)	STUDY DESIGN	FOCUS OF INDICATOR (POPULATION-GENERIC, POPULATION-SPECIFIC, OR ORGANIZATIONAL)	FINDINGS
Cost of care—cont'd	Ritz et al. (2000)	RCT	Population-generic	Comparable to control group
	Russell et al. (2002)	Outcomes management program	Population-generic	Significantly reduced
	Sarkissian & Wennberg (1999)	Pre/post comparison	Population-generic	Significantly reduced
	Saywell et al. (1995)	Cost estimation	Population-generic	Comparable to physicians when adjusted for productivity
	Schultz et al. (1994)	Medical record review	Population-generic	Significantly less than residents
	Stone et al. (2000)	Cost estimation	Population-generic	Less than physicians, when adjusted for productivity
	Topp et al. (1998)	Administrative database review	Population-generic	Significantly lower than comparison group
	Venning et al. (2000)	RCT	Population-generic	Comparable to residents
	York et al. (1997)	RCT	Population-generic	Significantly less than control group
Disability (bed) days	Leveille et al. (1998)	RCT	Population-specific	Significantly fewer than control group
Disease activity	Tijhuis et al. (2003)	RCT	Population-generic	Comparable to multidisciplinary teams
Emergency department use	Aiken, Lake et al. (1993)	Survey	Population-generic	Comparable to physicians
	Brown & Grimes (1995)	Meta-analysis	Population-generic	Comparable to physicians
	Jones & Clark (1997)	Program evaluation	Population-generic	Significantly less than comparison group
	Leveille et al. (1998)	RCT	Population-generic	Comparable to control group
	Mundinger et al. (2000)	RCT	Population-generic	Comparable to physicians
	Naylor et al. (1994)	RCT	Population-generic	Comparable to control group
Episiotomy, with & without laceration†	Brown & Grimes (1995)	Meta-analysis	Population-specific	Significantly less than physicians
	Greulich et al. (1994)	Medical record review	Population-specific	Low incidence
	Lydon-Rochelle et al. (1995)	Observational cohort study	Population-specific	Incidence associated with client factors
	Murphy & Feinland (1998)	Observational cohort study	Population-specific	Low incidence
Fetal distress	Brown & Grimes (1995)	Meta-analysis	Population-specific	Significantly less than physicians
	Butler et al. (1993)	Medical record review	Population-specific	Significantly less than physicians
Five-minute APGAR score	Brown & Grimes (1995)	Meta-analysis	Population-specific	Significantly higher than physicians
	Davis et al. (1994)	Administrative database review	Population-specific	Comparable to physicians

Forceps/vacuum extraction delivery[†]	Davis et al. (1994)	Administrative database review	Population-specific	Significantly less than physicians
	Greulich et al. (1994)	Medical record review	Population-specific	Low incidence
Functional status/ability	Aiken, Lake et al. (1993)	Survey	Population-generic	Comparable to physicians
	Brooten et al. (1994)	RCT	Population-generic	Comparable to control group
	Brown & Grimes (1995)	Meta-analysis		Comparable to physicians
	Bula et al. (1999)	Secondary analysis		Significantly better than control group
	Leveille et al. (1998)	RCT	Population-generic	Comparable to control group
	Mundinger et al. (2000)	RCT	Population-generic	Comparable to physicians
	Tijhuis et al. (2003)	RCT	Population-generic	Comparable to multidisciplinary teams
	Naylor & McCauley (1999)	Secondary data analysis	Population-generic	Comparable to control group
	Naylor et al. (1994)	RCT	Population-generic	Comparable to control group
	Naylor et al. (1999)	RCT	Population-generic	Comparable to control group
	Rawl et al. (1998)	RCT	Population-generic	Comparable to control group
	York et al. (1997)	FCT	Population-generic	Comparable to control group
Gestational age	Gravely & Littlefield (1992)	Cost-effectiveness analysis	Population-specific	Comparable to physicians
	York et al. (1997)	RCT	Population-specific	Comparable to control group
Glucose level, serum	Brown et al. (2001)	Program evaluation	Population-specific	Significantly improved over time
	York et al. (1997)	RCT	Population-specific	Comparable to control group
Health state	Tijhuis et al. (2003)	RCT	Population-generic	Comparable to multidisciplinary teams
Hospitalizations, including readmissions[†]	Aiken, Lake et al. (1993)	Survey	Population-generic	Comparable to physicians
	Brooten et al. (1994)	RCT	Population-generic	Comparable to control group
	Brown & Grimes (1995)	Meta-analysis	Population-generic	Significantly less than physicians
	Dahl & Penque (2001)	Program evaluation	Population-generic	Significantly less than before program
	Jones & Clark (1997)	Program evaluation	Population-generic	Comparable to comparison group
	Leveille et al. (1998)	RCT	Population-generic	Comparable to control group
	McCorkle et al. (2000)	RCT	Population-generic	Comparable to control group
	Mundinger et al. (2000)	RCT	Population-generic	Comparable to physicians
	Naylor & McCauley (1999)	Secondary data analysis	Population-generic	Comparable to control group
	Naylor et al. (1994)	RCT	Population-generic	Significantly less than control group
	Naylor et al. (1999)	RCT	Population-generic	Significantly less than control group
	Rawl et al. (1998)	RCT	Population-generic	Comparable to control group
	Rudy et al. (1998)	Comparative study	Population-generic	Comparable to residents
	Schultz et al. (1994)	Medical record review	Population-generic	Comparable to residents
	York et al. (1997)	RCT	Population-generic	Comparable to control group
Incontinence, control of	Ryden et al. (2000)	Quasi-experimental comparison	Population-specific	Significantly greater than control group

Continued

TABLE 25-2 APN-SENSITIVE OUTCOME INDICATORS TESTED IN PRACTICE* —cont'd

OUTCOME INDICATOR	AUTHORS (YR)	STUDY DESIGN	FOCUS OF INDICATOR (POPULATION-GENERIC, POPULATION-SPECIFIC, OR ORGANIZATIONAL)	FINDINGS
Length of stay	Bissinger et al. (1997)	Medical record review	Population-generic, organizational	Comparable to residents
	Brooten et al. (1994)	RCT	Population-generic, organizational	Significantly less than control group
	Carr (2000)	Administrative database review	Population-generic, organizational	Significantly less than physicians
	Dahl & Penque (2001)	Program evaluation	Population-generic, organizational	Significantly less than prior to program (overall)
	Dahle et al. (1998)	Pre/post comparison	Population-generic, organizational	Comparable to physicians
	Karlowicz & McMurray (2000)	Medical record review	Population-generic, organizational	Comparable to residents
	Kearnes (1994)	Medical record review	Population-generic, organizational	Reduced with NP/MD collaboration
	Leveille et al. (1998)	RCT	Population-generic, organizational	Comparable to control group
	Lombness (1994)	Medical record review	Population-generic, organizational	CNS significantly less than PA
	Naylor & McCauley (1999)	Secondary data analysis	Population-generic, organizational	Comparable to control group
	Naylor et al. (1994)	RCT	Population-generic, organizational	Comparable to control group
	Naylor et al. (1999)	RCT	Population-generic, organizational	Significantly less than control group
	Rudy et al. (1998)	Comparative study	Population-generic, organizational	Comparable to residents
	Russell et al. (2002)	Outcomes management program	Population-generic, organizational	Significantly reduced
	Sarkissian & Wennberg (1999)	Pre/post comparison	Population-generic, organizational	Significantly reduced
	Schultz et al. (1994)	Medical record review	Population-generic, organizational	Comparable to residents
	Topp et al. (1998)	Administrative database review	Population-generic, organizational	Significantly less for units with APN
	Wheeler (1999)	Medical record review	Population-generic, organizational	Significantly less than comparison group
	York et al. (1997)	RCT	Population-generic, organizational	Comparable to control group
Length of survival/ survival rate	Bula et al. (1999)	Secondary data analysis	Population-generic	Comparable to control group
	Karlowicz et al. (2000)	Medical record review	Population-generic	Comparable to residents
	McCorkle et al. (2000)	RCT	Population-generic	Significantly greater for APN-directed home care

Outcome	Author (year)	Study design	Type	Findings
Maternal weight gain	Gravely & Littlefield (1992)	Cost-effectiveness analysis	Population-specific	Comparable to physicians
Morbidity	Bissinger et al. (1997)	Medical record review	Population-generic, organizational	Comparable to residents
	Brooten et al. (1994)	RCT	Population-generic, organizational	Significantly less than control group
	Lombness (1994)	Medical record review	Population-generic, organizational	CNS comparable to PA
	Murphy & Fullerton (1998)	Survey	Population-generic, organizational	Low incidence
Mortality	Aubrey & Yoxall (2001)	Medical record review	Population-generic, organizational	Comparable to residents
	Bissinger et al. (1997)	Medical record review	Population-generic, organizational	Comparable to physicians
	Brown & Grimes (1995)	Meta-analysis	Population-generic, organizational	Comparable to physicians
	Carzoli et al. (1994)	Medical record review	Population-generic, organizational	Comparable to physicians
	Dahl & Penque (2001)	Program evaluation	Population-generic, organizational	Significantly less than prior to program
	Dahle et al. (1998)	Pre/post comparison	Population-generic, organizational	Comparable to physicians
	Karlowicz & McMurray (2000)	Medical record review	Population-generic, organizational	Comparable to residents
	Mitchell-DiCenso et al. (1996)	RCT	Population-generic, organizational	Comparable to residents
	Murphy & Fullerton (1998)	Survey	Population-generic, organizational	Low incidence
	Pine et al. (2003)	Medicare database review	Population-generic, organizational	Comparable to anesthesiologists
	Rudy et al. (1998)	Comparative study	Population-generic, organizational	Comparable to physicians
Nurse satisfaction	Martin (1999)	Survey	Organizational	Highly satisfied
	McMullen et al. (2001)	Program evaluation	Organizational	Highly satisfied
One minute APGAR	Brown & Grimes (1995)	Meta-analysis	Population-specific	Comparable to physicians
Patient compliance/ adherence	Brown & Grimes (1995)	Meta-analysis	Population-generic	Significantly greater than physicians
Patient/family knowledge	Brown & Grimes (1995)	Meta-analysis	Population-generic	Comparable to physicians
	Hill et al. (1994)	Single-blind, parallel-group	Population-generic	Significantly greater than physicians
Patient/family perception of health	Naylor et al. (1994)	RCT	Population-generic	Comparable to control group
Patient/family satisfaction	Aiken, Lake et al. (1993)	Survey	Population-generic	Comparable to physicians
	Benkert et al. (2002)	Survey	Population-generic	Scores influenced by number of visits, type of contact, & respondent characteristics

Continued

TABLE 25-2 APN-SENSITIVE OUTCOME INDICATORS TESTED IN PRACTICE* —cont'd

OUTCOME INDICATOR	AUTHORS (YR)	STUDY DESIGN	FOCUS OF INDICATOR (POPULATION-GENERIC, POPULATION-SPECIFIC, OR ORGANIZATIONAL)	FINDINGS
Patient/family satisfaction—cont'd	Brooten et al. (1994)	RCT	Population-generic	Significantly greater than control group
	Brown et al. (2001)	Program evaluation	Population-generic	Highly satisfied
	Brown & Grimes (1995)	Meta-analysis	Population-generic	Significantly greater than physicians
	Bryant & Graham (2002)	Survey	Population-generic	Highly satisfied
	Chang et al. (1999)	RCT	Population-generic	Comparable to physicians
	Cook & Nolan (1996)	Outcomes management program	Population-generic	Satisfied with services
	Gravely & Littlefield (1992)	Cost-effectiveness analysis	Population-generic	Significantly greater than physicians
	Hamric et al. (1998)	Demonstration project evaluation	Population-generic	Highly satisfied
	Hill et al. (1994)	Single-blind, parallel-group	Population-generic	Significantly greater than physicians
	Kinnersley et al. (2000)	RCT	Population-generic	Significantly greater than general practitioners
	Knudtson (2000)	Survey	Population-generic	Highly satisfied
	Larrabee et al. (1997)	Survey	Population-generic	Highly satisfied
	Martin (1999)	Survey	Population-generic	Highly satisfied
	McMullen et al. (2001)	Program evaluation	Population-generic	Significantly greater for communication rate than physician services
	Mitchell-DiCenso et al. (1996)	RCT	Population-generic	Comparable to residents
	Moore et al. (2002)	RCT	Population-generic	Significantly greater than physicians
	Mundinger et al. (2000)	RCT	Population-generic	Comparable to control group
	Naylor et al. (1994)	RCT	Population-generic	Comparable to physicians
	Sarkissian & Wennberg (1999)	Postintervention, noncomparison survey	Population-generic	Highly satisfied
	Stutts (2001)	Program evaluation	Population-generic	Improved with program
	Venning et al. (2000)	RCT	Population-generic	Significantly greater than general practitioners
Perceived self-esteem	Naylor et al. (1994)	RCT	Population-generic	Comparable to control group
Perineal lacerations	Brown & Grimes (1995)	Meta-analysis	Population-specific	Significantly greater than physicians
	Murphy & Feinland (1998)	Observational cohort study	Population-specific	Low incidence

Outcome	Author(s)	Method	Level	Finding
Physician satisfaction/perception of APN performance	Brown et al. (2001)	Program evaluation	Organizational	Highly satisfied
	Hamric et al. (1998)	Demonstration project evaluation	Organizational	Highly satisfied
Postdischarge phone contact (for questions)	McMullen et al. (2001) / Stutts (2001)	Program evaluation / Program evaluation	Organizational / Organizational	Highly satisfied / Mixed response
	Rawl et al. (1998)	RCT	Population-specific	Significantly fewer than control group
Pressure ulcers; skin breakdown	Russell et al. (2002)	Outcomes management program	Population-specific	Significantly reduced
	Ryden et al. (2000)	Quasi-experimental comparison	Population-specific	Significantly less than control group
Preventable pulmonary complications	Hanneman et al. (1993)	Quasi-experimental comparison	Population-specific	Significantly less than control group
Productivity	Cromwell & Rosenbach (1990)	Survey	Organizational	Significantly greater with CRNA team model
	Gravely & Littlefield (1992)	Cost-effectiveness analysis	Organizational	Significantly greater than physicians
Provider contacts, appropriate use	Jones & Clark (1997)	Program evaluation	Organizational	Significantly more than comparison group
Quality of life	Moore et al. (2002) / Ritz et al. (2000)	RCT / RCT	Population-generic / Population-generic	Comparable to physicians / Significantly better than control group
	Tijhuis et al. (2003)	RCT	Population-generic	Comparable to multidisciplinary teams
Readmission to critical care unit	Schultz et al. (1994)	Medical record review trial	Population-specific, organizational	Comparable to residents
Smoking cessation	Gebaur et al. (1998)	Program evaluation	Population-generic	Significantly greater than control group
Spontaneous vaginal delivery	Brown & Grimes (1995)	Meta-analysis	Population-specific	Significantly greater than physicians
Status of presenting condition	Hamric et al. (1998)	Demonstration project evaluation	Population-generic	Improved following initiation of APN prescription writing
Symptom control	Hill et al. (1994)	Single-blind, parallel-group	Population-generic	Significantly greater than physicians
	Moore et al. (2002)	RCT	Population-generic	Comparable to physicians; neuropathy significantly less
Transfer to acute setting†	Greulich et al. (1994)	Medical record review	Population-generic, organizational	Low incidence

Continued

TABLE 25-2 APN-SENSITIVE OUTCOME INDICATORS TESTED IN PRACTICE* —cont'd

OUTCOME INDICATOR	AUTHORS (YR)	STUDY DESIGN	FOCUS OF INDICATOR (POPULATION-GENERIC, POPULATION-SPECIFIC, OR ORGANIZATIONAL)	FINDINGS
Transfer to acute setting—cont'd	Murphy & Fullerton (1998)	Survey	Population-generic, organizational	Low incidence
Urinary tract infection	Russell et al. (2002)	Outcomes management program	Population-generic	Significantly reduced
Ventilator days	Bissinger et al. (1997)	Medical record review	Population-specific, organizational	Comparable to residents
Visits to care provider	Brown & Grimes (1995)	Meta-analysis	Population-generic	Comparable to physicians
	Gravely & Littlefield (1992)	Cost-effectiveness analysis	Population-generic	Comparable to physicians
	Leveille et al. (1998)	RCT	Population-generic	Comparable to control group
	Mundinger et al. (2000)	RCT	Population-generic	Comparable to physicians

*Published studies since 1990.
†Constitute both a process (action by provider) and an outcome (condition or response in patient).
Definition of Terms for the Focus of the Indicator: population-generic—indicators that could be used with any patient population; population-specific—indicators that are relevant to specific populations only; organizational—indicators that focus on the outcomes of the setting rather than the patient.
Note: Some indicators that were used with specific populations in studies have been labeled as generic because they can be applied to multiple patient groups.

The literature also highlights the difficulties evident in generating widespread interest in measuring care delivery outcomes. Many APNs view the ongoing assessment of care delivery impact as an additional burden to an already full agenda. This mixed perspective was highlighted recently in a survey of oncology APNs who identified critical issues that warranted planning for future nursing society projects (Lynch, Cope, & Murphy-Ende, 2001). Only 2% of respondents included outcomes management as important content for advanced practice nursing programs. At the same time, outcomes documentation was identified as one of the top five priority issues for oncology APNs. Clearly, the foundational work pertaining to outcomes assessment needs to begin during graduate education. Because APN outcome measurement activities begin immediately once the APN is hired, preparation for identifying target outcomes, collecting data, and managing and reporting findings is the minimum information required. Mahn and Zazworsky (2000) have further recommended the inclusion of content on health-care financing, billing codes, health-care information systems, database query, and statistics. Without these skills at the outset, APNs are likely to be ill prepared to succeed in today's outcomes-driven environment.

The research to date suggests that APNs can contribute to the field of outcomes assessment in several ways. One of the simplest and most common mechanisms for monitoring advanced nursing practice is the routine documentation of what an APN does. This includes patient-specific documentation in medical records; process improvement reporting for groups of patients; descriptions of new program initiatives; annual performance self-assessment summaries; and published reports of projects, programs, evaluations, or research studies. As Boyle (1995) noted, the documentation of advanced practice nursing work should be considered an inherent job responsibility that contributes to the quantification of role impact, effectiveness, and value. It is the basic starting point for measuring care delivery outcome. Other APN impact assessments range from individual performance review to large-scale, multisite studies. In each of these situations, however, the common denominator is the consistency and quality of the process and outcome measures used.

Because standardized approaches to reporting advanced practice nursing work and care delivery impact are unavailable at this time, health-care organizations with more than one APN should ensure that comparable reporting mechanisms are used and that both generic (organization-wide) and specific (population-focused) indicators are included to evaluate overall effect. Ideally, decisions about which outcomes to measure and determinations about how to monitor the care delivery process are driven by existing evidence and expert panel standards or recommendations.

APNs can also take advantage of the quality initiatives underway in health-care organizations today. These data collection, performance monitoring, and outcome assessment activities provide excellent opportunities for documenting and understanding processes and outcomes of care. Several strategies for facilitating APNs' efforts to evaluate their care are described in the next section, with representative data collection planning and reporting formats provided. In addition, Box 25-1 lists some of the Web resources available to APNs and organizations interested in initiating outcomes measurement programs.

STRATEGIES TO FACILITATE PROGRAM DESIGN, QUALITY IMPROVEMENT, AND OUTCOME EVALUATION FOR ADVANCED PRACTICE NURSING

Much of health-care practice in today's economic market is data driven, with APNs assuming greater responsibility for collecting and using clinical, economic, and quality outcomes data. Moreover, their ability to recognize patterns in resource utilization and

BOX 25-1 • WEBSITE OUTCOME ASSESSMENT RESOURCES

RESOURCE	WEB ADDRESS
Agency for Healthcare Research & Quality (AHRQ)	www.arhq.gov

Information available:
- Reports from evidence-based practice centers; outcomes & effectiveness trials
- Outcome measures: www.qualitymeasures.ahrq.org
  - Consumer Assessment of Health Plans (CAHPS);
  - National Clearinghouse Quality Indicators
- Funding opportunities

American Health Information Management Association (AHIMA)   www.ahima.org

Information available:
- Documentation guidelines.
- Search engine for quality management topics; professional measurement tools; research

Center for Medicare & Medicaid Services (CMS)   www.cms.hhs.gov

Information available:
- Laws & regulations
- Quality initiatives
- Data collection instruments (Outcome & Assessment Information Set [OASIS]; Minimum Data Set [MDS 3.0])

Center for Evaluative Clinical Sciences, Dartmouth College   www.dartmouth.edu/~cecs/

Information available:
- Atlas of health care
- Centers for Medicare & Medicaid Services database

Centers for Disease Control and Prevention (CDC)   www.cdc.gov

Information available:
- Search engine for health topics
- Databases: health statistics
- Funding opportunities

Cochrane Library of Clinical Trials   www.cochrane.org

Information available:
- Systematic reviews of evidence
- Search engine for evidence-based reviews

Foundation for Accountability (FACCT)   www.facct.org

Information available:
- Quality measures
- Clearinghouse for health-care information

Health Resources & Services Administration (HRSA)   www.hrsa.org

Information available:
- Health interest area information: HIV/AIDS; primary health care; maternal child health; health professions; rural health
- Center for Quality: quality activities; providers' guide to quality   www.hrsa.org/quality

Institute for Healthcare Improvement (IHI)   www.ihi.org

Information available:
- Continuous improvement newsletter
- Search engine for quality; patient safety
- Quality improvement methods, measures, tools, & resources   www.qualityhealthcare.org

Institute for Safe Medication Practices (ISMP)   www.ismp.org

Information available:
- Bibliography
- Medication safety pathways
- Organizational self-assessment for medication safety practices

Institute of Medicine (IOM)   www.iom.edu

Information available:
- Reports: health related; reviews of evidence
- Best practices & quality improvement projects underway
- Topic-related information

BOX 25-1 • WEBSITE OUTCOME ASSESSMENT RESOURCES — cont'd

Joint Commission on Accreditation of Healthcare Organizations (JCAHO)   www.jcaho.org
Information available:
- Search engine for quality of health-care organizations
- Glossary of terms
- Performance measurement standards
- Core measures for evidence-based assessment of performance

Medical Outcomes Trust   www.outcomes-trust.org
Information available:
- Outcomes assessment instruments, including the SF-36 & SF-12 Health Surveys

Medscape   www.medscape.com/nurseshome
Information available:
- Updates on health issues information
- Search engine of selected health-care journals
- Resources for APNs: prescribing law; billing for services

MedWeb, Emory University Health Sciences Center Library   www.medweb.emory.edu/medweb
Information available:
- Search engine for evidence-based medicine; practice guidelines; databases

National Center for Nursing Quality, University of Kansas   www.nursingquality.org
Information available:
- ANA national database for nursing quality indicators (NDNQI)
- Bibliography of nursing quality articles
- Abstracts of research

National Committee for Quality Assurance (NCQA)   www.ncqa.org
Information available:
- Quality performance databases: Health Plan Employer Data & Information Set (HEDIS); Quality Compass
- Publications related to measurement of quality (for purchase)

National Guideline Clearinghouse (NGC)   www.guideline.gov
Information available:
- Evidence-based practice guidelines

National Institutes of Health (NIH)   www.nih.gov
Information available:
- Specialty-focused institutes' reports
- Search engine for health topics; clinical trials
- Funding opportunities

National Library of Medicine (NLM)   www.nlm.nih.gov
Information available:
- Reference databases: PubMed/ MEDLINE; MeSH
- Funding opportunities

National Patient Safety Foundation (NPSF)   www.npsf.org
Information available:
- Bibliography of safety-related articles
- Fact sheets

ZYNX Health Incorporated   www.zynx.com
Information available:
- Bibliography of evidence-based medicine (not nursing) articles
- Clinical pathway constructor (for purchase)

These resources can be located by using most search engines, and Google (www.google.com) is particularly helpful for identifying additional sites.
AIDS, Acquired immunodeficiency syndrome; *ANA,* American Nurses Association; *APNs,* advanced practices nurses; *HIV,* human immunodeficiency virus; *SF-36,* short form 36; *SF-12,* short form 12.

care delivery processes makes APNs ideal facilitators of quality improvement activities, in which data direct and support decisions about how to achieve best practices. This pattern recognition also facilitates the identification of system inefficiencies, barriers to continuity of care, and other ineffective ways of delivering health-care services. These in turn become opportunities for APNs to positively influence processes and outcomes—at both individual patient and system levels.

One vehicle for achieving quality patient outcomes is the use of interdisciplinary quality improvement teams, which are charged with improving care delivery outcomes or redesigning work flow processes for greater effectiveness or efficiency. Because APNs routinely attend to the ways in which care delivery systems work, they are in an ideal position to plan quality improvement initiatives by leading or actively participating in interdisciplinary quality improvement teams. As clinical experts, they are also well-suited to influence practice patterns and to develop meaningful standards, practice protocols, clinical guidelines, health-care programs, and health-care policies that promote teamwork, improve clinical outcomes, and reduce costs. These role expectations require a careful review of relevant literature and an understanding of the potential for application of research findings to individual practice (see Chapter 8). In the remainder of this chapter, a stepwise approach is proposed for developing and implementing an outcome evaluation plan that demonstrates an APN's value and contribution to the health-care setting. Although the term *outcome evaluation* is used throughout this section, these steps can be applied to impact analysis, outcomes measurement, performance evaluation, process improvement, program evaluation, and clinical research.

Three phases of inquiry are used as an organizing framework for the development of an effective outcome evaluation plan. The first of these involves defining the core questions that need to be answered. The second focuses on determining the data required to answer the questions, and the third is directed at deriving meaning from the data and acting on the results. Several steps within each of these phases are described to promote successful completion of the phase. Box 25-2 lists the phases and related steps in developing and conducting an outcomes evaluation.

Define the Core Questions

The demand for data-based information to objectively quantify the value of the APN role has increased significantly over the past 10 years. Before any useful data can be gathered, however, the questions foremost in key stakeholders' minds must be understood and described. These questions serve as the foundation for the development of an effective outcome evaluation plan. In formulating the core questions, the APN must ensure that the questions clarify the purpose of the APN's role within the organization, define the population targeted, identify the relevant stakeholders, and articulate the program goals and interventions to be evaluated. Once these foundational aspects have been established, the APN can formulate an approach to the outcome evaluation plan and determine whether and to what degree the APN's contributions are independent or value added.

CLARIFY THE PURPOSE OF THE APN'S ROLE

In developing an outcome evaluation plan, APNs are often required to revisit the purposes of their employment, their organization's mission, and the goals for their position. If

BOX 25-2 • SUMMARY OF OUTCOME EVALUATION PLANNING PROCESS

PHASE I: DEFINE THE CORE QUESTIONS

I-1. Clarify the purpose of the APN's role.
- Review organization's mission, vision, and goals.
- Clarify role expectations.
- Confirm clinical and reporting accountability.

I-2. Define the target population.
- Identify differences in patient characteristics within target population.
- Clarify relationships between APN role behaviors and population needs and outcomes.
- Compare target group with other groups monitored through performance improvement activities.
- Assess level of risk, complexity, and resource use of subpopulations within target group.

I-3. Identify the stakeholders.
- Facilitate participation by and input from key stakeholders.
- Isolate APN interventions and actions from those of other care providers.
- Secure early buy-in from stakeholders.

I-4. Articulate program goals and interventions.
- Review literature for supportive evidence.
- Consider resources needed to implement and maintain the intervention.
- Identify key strategies for managing target population.
- Formulate specific questions.

PHASE II: DEFINE THE DATA ELEMENTS

II-1. Identify the population of interest.
- Clarify inclusion and exclusion criteria.
- Identify electronic data sources for information about the target population.

II-2. Establish performance and outcome indicators.
- Identify measures to determine evidence of APN impact.
- Ensure alignment between program goals, proposed interventions, and outcome indicators.
- Consider the use of national databases for comparison and benchmarking purposes.

II-3. Identify and evaluate data elements.
- Evaluate ease of collecting data and compare with need.
- Identify data resources available.
- Link use of intermediate outcome indicators to target goals and outcome achievement.
- Formulate outcome evaluation plan and implement.

PHASE III: DERIVE MEANING FROM DATA AND ACT ON RESULTS

III-1. Analyze data and interpret results.
- Seek assistance from others as needed.
- Select data analysis and reporting procedures.

III-2. Present and disseminate findings.
- Prepare reports according to audience and stakeholder needs and interests.
- Select software programs and other resources to support presentation approach.

II-3. Identify improvement opportunities.
- Work with stakeholders to identify most appropriate opportunity for improvement.
- Select most effective tools to facilitate performance improvement planning process.
- Conduct pilot studies to assess new program feasibility, cost, and resource needs.

III-4. Formulate a plan for implementation and reevaluation.
- Summarize goals of performance improvement plan.
- Identify proposed interventions, responsible persons, and target dates for completion.
- Select indicators and measures based on goals and interventions identified.
- Provide educational programs to support intervention, as needed.

the purposes of their roles are unclear, APNs may need to engage in a discussion with administrators and collaborators about what role expectations are reasonable and appropriate. Before deciding on what outcomes to measure, APNs must be certain about the clinical populations they serve and their accountability for the structures and processes of care. Because the APN's role usually changes over time in response to new technology, changes in patient population, length of stay, and other care management mandates or organizational change, the desired outcomes for the APN role may also shift. Therefore APNs must have an accurate understanding of their employer's expectations at the time the outcome evaluation process is begun. In some cases, employers may not recognize the APN's full range of services or potential benefit to the organization. If that occurs, the APN may need to identify specific processes and areas of focus within the setting and set appropriate goals and performance objectives to meet these.

The APN's role may also change as a direct result of performance improvement and outcome evaluation studies. Findings may indicate that APN interventions are better suited to other points of care across the continuum of services or may be delivered more effectively or efficiently by other providers. As an example, Lamb, Mahn, and Dahl (1996) evaluated the effectiveness of hospital-based APN case management for patients with heart failure and found that readmission rates were higher than expected. In light of these findings, the APN case management intervention was shifted to the patient's home and provided within 24 to 48 hours of discharge. Subsequent assessment of this change in APN intervention on care delivery outcome determined that readmission rates declined significantly and that patient compliance with therapeutic regimens improved. Eventually, non-APN case managers assumed responsibility for the case management intervention and similar results were seen. This confirmation of comparable impact allowed the APNs to shift their attention to other high-risk populations. Conversely, findings may support the effectiveness and efficiency of the APN intervention, which could lead to program growth and expansion to other populations or points of care. In all cases, outcome evaluation and APN role definition and scope of practice go hand in hand.

DEFINE THE TARGET POPULATION FOR STUDY

Once the APN's role and purpose within the care delivery setting have been clarified, the APN defines the population targeted for evaluation. Because most APNs use a wide range of activities to manage heterogeneous clinical populations, it is necessary to focus on specific aspects of their practice with a particular patient group when an outcome evaluation plan is designed. This focus helps create a more manageable outcome evaluation plan and limits the impact of extraneous variables that could interfere with the interpretation of findings. Aspects of advanced practice nursing activities that are used with the target population should be identified so that they can be included in the design. Whenever possible, the target population should be comparable to other groups monitored through quality improvement initiatives at either the organizational or department level. For example, an adult NP may provide primary care for a variety of patients in an ambulatory care setting, yet the outcome evaluation plan may focus on outcomes specific to subpopulations of patients with human immunodeficiency virus (HIV) infection or patients with diabetes. The decision to target subpopulations of patients may be based on a desire to evaluate patients who are at high risk for complications, have complex care needs, or tend to use more services than others. Likewise, CNSs in a hospital setting may specialize in adult cardiovascular nursing and practice in critical care and telemetry step-down settings but limit their evaluation to patients undergoing heart transplantation because of their organization's expansion as a regional transplant center and the CNS's resulting emphasis on this patient group.

Other factors to consider when a target population is defined include patient satisfaction and financial performance. For example, when a large pediatric medical group hires a pediatric NP to perform routine physical examinations and give vaccinations, parent satisfaction is likely to be an important component of the outcome evaluation plan. An analysis of expenses and revenues versus profit margin is also an important dimension for this business decision. Additional factors to consider include patient volume, level of risk or complexity, and potential for development of adverse events. Patient factors such as insurance provider, age, ethnicity, and co-morbid condition may also be used to define the target population at risk for an adverse outcome. As an example, CNMs may examine outcomes of care associated with adolescent pregnancy or low birth weight rates in rural American Indian women. They may target this population because of multiple factors that increase the risk for adverse outcomes in these groups.

Finally, some populations are targeted because of the need for organizations to determine their level of compliance with national care delivery guidelines, best-practice standards, or regulatory requirements. Frequently, APNs are involved in the care of several populations of interest and therefore must prioritize which populations warrant first review and evaluation. In doing so, APNs must be sensitive to the resource requirements of any outcome study, working closely with information systems, quality improvement, and medical records staff for the support required to conduct the review. A tool developed by Mahn and Heller (1998) at Carondelet Healthcare Systems in Tucson, Arizona, provides one example of an approach to prioritizing performance improvement initiatives within larger health-care systems (Figure 25-1). The weighted scoring method used in this tool provides an objective method for obtaining input from other departments and stakeholders and for identifying and prioritizing target populations for outcome evaluation.

IDENTIFY THE STAKEHOLDERS

In addition to identifying the target population for study, APNs must identify the structures and processes of care for which they share accountability. Most often APNs are not the only or even the major stakeholders in the provision of care to the populations they serve. Often, however, they are "the glue" that holds the team together. As a result, they often find themselves moving the team, the health-care agency, and/or the system toward a shared vision of desired outcome. Creating this vision is not an isolated APN activity. APNs must also facilitate the contributions, ideas, and creativity of professionals who participate in the care of the target population. Among the stakeholders most commonly involved are medical providers, other nurses, pharmacists, administrators, and other members of the health-care team. In some cases, APNs will need to include stakeholders from outside their immediate practice settings. For example, a community-based APN serving fragile elderly patients with chronic diseases may need to include stakeholders from managed care agencies, primary care clinics, physicians' offices, skilled nursing facilities, home health-care agencies, and hospitals. While including all stakeholders in the development of an outcome evaluation plan may not be feasible or desirable, including primary stakeholders and considering their potential impact on care delivery outcomes will assist in understanding and measuring those processes and outcomes that are interdependent with advanced nursing practice. Because APNs are typically only one component of a greater whole, they usually cannot be granted exclusive credit for the results achieved. Therefore

Prioritization Tool for Performance Improvement Initiatives
Proposed Population or Process: _____

	Low 1 Point	Medium 2 Points	High 3 Points
Cost	<$5,000 ❑	$5,000 - $10,000 ❑	>$10,000 ❑
Annual Volume	<50 cases ❑	50-150 cases ❑	>150 cases ❑
Risk	<1/1000 deaths ❑	<1/100 deaths ❑	>1/100 deaths ❑
Problem Prone	Minor problems infrequently reported ❑	Minor to moderate problems reported occasionally ❑	Steady stream of minor to major problems reported ❑
Regional Variation	Process of care delivery generally consistent ❑	Normal or expected variation exists ❑	Process of care delivery highly variable ❑
Improvement Opportunity	Few if any opportunities to improve exist ❑	Minor to moderate opportunities to improve exist ❑	Significant opportunities to improve exist ❑
National Guidelines	No guidelines exist and rarely discussed in the literaure ❑	Topic widely discussed in the literature ❑	Guidelines exist and are recognized nationally ❑
Controversial Therapy	Process or procedure is widely accepted nationwide ❑	The literature suggests alternative approaches may be of value ❑	Process or procedure has widely accepted alternatives ❑
Market Interest	Little if any focus exists in the community ❑	Process or procedure is of general concern in the community ❑	Process of major concern to the community ❑
Physician/Staff Interest	Very few professional staff would agree this area is important ❑	Selected professional staff would agree this area is important ❑	There are many staff who would agree this area is important ❑
Total Number of Points			
	___ x 1 = [ ]	___ x 2 = [ ]	___ x 3 = [ ]
Note: *Lowest possible score is 10. Highest possible score is 30.* **TOTAL SCORE**			

FIGURE 25-1 • Prioritization tool for performance improvement initiatives. (From Mahn & Heller [1998]. Copyright ACS MIDAS+, 2003. Reprinted with permission.)

APNs must articulate advanced nursing practice–specific inputs and interventions that contribute to the team effect, so they can document and demonstrate their role's value to the organization. The need to carve out additional measures of role effectiveness results in a more complex outcomes plan, which typically requires multiple measurement methods, instruments, and analysis techniques. For instance, part of an outcome evaluation plan may incorporate quantitative methods to capture specific outcomes of treatment (e.g., average number of clinic visits per year, total costs, and number of diabetic patients with a normal hemoglobin A_{1c} level within 2 months of diagnosis), while another may employ a qualitative approach, using oral or written feedback from physician and dietician colleagues about APN effectiveness in facilitating the development of new patient care guidelines for managing the diabetic population.

Once the plan for an evaluation study is disclosed to stakeholders, buy-in to any proposed change must be ensured to improve care. Not only will APNs be change recipients as a result of the outcome evaluation, they will also serve as change implementers and change strategists for others and their organization. Identifying and including stakeholders early in the process of designing an outcome evaluation plan helps facilitate this process.

ARTICULATE PROGRAM GOALS AND INTERVENTIONS

Perhaps the easiest way to demonstrate positives outcomes of care is to do the right things, at the right times, for the right patients, in the right ways. After that, the task of measurement becomes an artful assembly of data and information necessary to reflect the outcomes and processes associated with the intervention. The determination of which interventions to implement for a given population and which to include in an outcome evaluation plan may be based in part on the resources required to accomplish the interventions and maintain them in practice. To begin, APNs should engage in a comprehensive review of the relevant literature to examine all standards of care, regulatory requirements, national guidelines, and established or emerging evidence-based best practices that are relevant to their clinical population. In searching the literature, APNs may wish to subscribe to one of the online services that provide systematic reviews of the medical and nursing literature, such as the Cerner ZYNXTM Critical Pathway Constructor (www.zynx.com), the Cochrane Collaboration (www.cochrane.org), or Medscape from WebMD (www.medscape.com/nurseshome), which also reviews some nursing literature applicable to advanced nursing practice. Box 25-1 identifies other relevant sites.

Using information from the literature and their clinical experience, APNs identify appropriate interventions for managing populations. Interventions may include attention to early detection and diagnostic modalities, timeliness of interventions, drug appropriateness, or patient education. In addition, the needs of the organization and any political agendas should be considered, although the number of interventions evaluated should be limited to keep the project scope manageable. Committing to too many interventions or unrealistic data collection activities may result in "project scope creep." This unplanned expansion of project activities can overwhelm available resources and undermine or stall performance improvement and outcome evaluation initiatives.

Once the program goals and interventions are defined, the APN can begin to formulate specific questions of interest to stakeholders. Sketching out some basic questions serves as a useful exercise for establishing the outcome evaluation plan. Some sample questions are as follows:

- How cost-effective is this program?
- How satisfied are patients with the services they received?
- How closely does the health-care team adhere to best-practice standards?
- How many patients have complications of care?
- What patient safety issues associated with this population should we examine?
- What can be done to reduce resource utilization for this population?
- What do we need to do differently to become a center of excellence for this population?
- How has the APN contributed to the training and development of other staff?

Once the core questions are formulated, the APN can begin designing the data collection method that will be used to answer key questions.

Define the Data Elements

After APNs determine the core questions to be answered, they are ready to define the outcome indicators and the data elements they will use to measure the intervention's success. This is the phase in the outcome evaluation plan that often poses the greatest challenge for APNs, particularly for those who have had little or no exposure to quality improvement principles and management information systems—both of which support outcome evaluation. Three steps are required for this phase. In the first step, APNs decide how they will capture the targeted patients or care episodes that qualify for the outcome study. In the second, they identify which indicators they will use to answer the study's core questions, and in the third, they determine which data elements will be collected for each indicator chosen for the study. APNs with limited expertise in these areas may wish to seek assistance from other health-care professionals with experience in continuous quality improvement principles, Six Sigma Theory (Marash, Berman, & Flynn, 2003), health-care statistics, nursing informatics, program evaluation, or nursing research.

IDENTIFY THE POPULATION OF INTEREST

While this may seem like an obvious first step, it is important to consider how patients that qualify for inclusion in the study will be initially identified. Actually enrolling particular patients in a study is often more difficult than simply identifying the general qualifying criteria. Identifying electronic data sources that contain information about the target population is generally the most efficient way to begin. For example, NPs who practice in a physician's office or clinic may be able to retrieve a list of all patients seen within a given time frame. This is possible because the NP's provider number identifies his or her patients in the claims database, which generates the bill for services rendered. The NP could further reduce this list to patients seen for a specific diagnosis or complaint through the use of *International Classification of Diseases, Ninth Revision* (ICD-9) codes, *CPT-4* codes, and/or Ambulatory Payment Classifications (APC) codes. In behavioral health settings, *Diagnostic and Statistical Manual of Mental Disorders, Fourth Edition* (DSM-IV) codes are generally more useful.

In contrast, CNSs who practice in acute care environments may have a more difficult time obtaining a list of patients whose care they have managed or influenced, simply because CNSs do not typically bill directly for services. As a result, they do not have a provider identification (ID) number, which is required for billing database queries. In this situation, the population of interest may be captured by a nonelectronic data source, such as a log or referral list. If the CNS's influence extends to a general clinical population, such as patients undergoing liver transplantation, the best approach may be to obtain a list of patients by using specified diagnosis-related group (DRG) or ICD-9 diagnosis or procedure codes. This information is generally available from hospital information systems. Other APNs, such as CRNAs, may also have difficulty retrieving electronic data for patients they have treated. For these APNs, many institutions maintain specialized surgery or other specialty databases that track such information and can be used as a source of data. APNs should become familiar with the data sources available in their organizations to assist with outcome evaluation.

The importance of such specificity in identifying the target population resides in the fact that these inclusion criteria generally become the denominator for specific indicators (which typically involve a numeric count, rate, or sum) that are used to monitor the effectiveness of APN interventions. For example, if a measure of NP effectiveness in a hospital-based wellness clinic is average number of hospital ED visits per year, specific inclusion and exclusion criteria for the population of interest will need to be defined (e.g., patients with type II diabetes older than 17 years are included; those younger than 17 years are excluded). Additional criteria may be needed to define the population further to ensure that the targeted patients are as similar (homogeneous) as possible. APNs should consult with experts in medical records coding to determine the most reliable and valid ways of isolating a specific clinical population of patients for their outcomes evaluation.

ESTABLISH PERFORMANCE AND OUTCOME INDICATORS

Once the patient population is defined, the APN begins to identify specific measures of performance that will be used to draw conclusions about how well the population was managed or the degree to which favorable outcomes were achieved. In general, measures are classified into three types: proportion measures (e.g., mortality rates, readmission rates, complication rates), ratio measures (e.g., falls per 1000 patient days, central line infections per 1000 line days, restraint episodes per psychiatric patient days), and continuous variable measures (e.g., median time to initial antibiotic administration, average length of stay). Some measures are direct counts of a particular phenomenon within a given period, such as number of allergic reactions in patients receiving antibiotics. Others are sums, such as total costs of care for a given population or total patient days. The type of measure selected is less important than how well it answers the core questions of the study (although, ultimately, the type of measure will determine the approach required for data analysis and presentation to stakeholders). The best approach is to create a draft list of indicators and obtain feedback from stakeholders about how well the indicators address their core questions and concerns. Only after stakeholder buy-in is secured should the APN formally establish the indicators for the evaluation plan. Otherwise, the APN runs the risk of conducting an outcome evaluation study that fails to determine how well the population is being managed in the eyes of the stakeholders.

Alignment between program goals, interventions, and performance and outcome indicators is another important consideration in the design of the outcome evaluation plan. This process ensures that the findings of the outcome evaluation can be traced back to the interventions associated with APN practice. For example, if average length of stay is selected as one outcome indicator for a population of patients with AMI under the direction of a hospital-based CNS, this variable should be linked in theory and in practice to an intervention for which the CNS has or shares accountability, such as discharge planning or management of complications. Measures that reflect the subprocesses of other providers, such as time from first incision for patients undergoing angioplasty to the time the wire crosses the lesion in the coronary artery, may be of interest to invasive cardiologists and other stakeholders from the cardiac catheterization lab. They may have little to do with the APN's ability to directly influence care delivery outcome, however, and should not be considered in the APN's outcome evaluation plan. Often, APNs are lured into coordinating data collection for other providers as part of the performance monitoring process. APNs may agree to perform these data coordination or data collection activities, but they must be careful not to overburden themselves with data collection responsibilities that diminish their own clinical effectiveness or assessment of intervention effect. Should this happen, APNs should quickly examine other potential resources within the organization, to gather data, so they can continue to perform to their highest level and provide the best service to the institution. Staying focused on the interventions and specific program goals for which they are responsible will assist APNs in formulating a meaningful and manageable outcome evaluation plan.

As decisions about which sources to use for measurement of interventions and outcomes are made, APNs may wish to consider data available from national comparative database services. Subscription to such services generally provides access to definitions for measures, along with benchmark or comparison data that may be helpful in evaluating level of performance. Table 25-3 contains a list of benchmark or comparison data provided by national database services that are available for various practice settings and that may be useful in evaluating outcomes or establishing potential thresholds for performance. As noted earlier, use of such benchmarking indicators can assist with building a consistent set of core APN–sensitive indicators to strengthen assessment of APN effect across providers and settings.

IDENTIFY AND EVALUATE DATA ELEMENTS

This is the point in the outcome evaluation plan at which APNs address the details of the data collection instruments and the actual processes required for data collection. To ensure a smooth and efficient data collection process, APNs should evaluate the relative ease of collecting each individual data element and balance that against the overall usefulness of the indicator for determining advanced practicing nursing effect. Indicators that require extensive, resource-intense data collection efforts may need to be eliminated in favor of indicators that better reflect the core questions of the study. To determine which indicators are essential versus those that are interesting but not essential, APNs can list each indicator on a separate piece of paper and then write down all aspects of data collection for it. If, for example, a rate or proportion measure is selected, then the specific definitions for the numerator and the denominator of the measure should be provided. Inclusion and exclusion criteria should be stated, and the data elements required to construct the indicator numerator and denominator should be listed. Finally, the specific data source for each data element should be identified. See Chapter 18, Box 18-2 (p. 658) for a list of data elements commonly available in most hospital management information systems.

Other types of information—such as time when a specific medication was administered or length of time waiting in the ED—must be abstracted from a careful review of the medical record. Still other types of information may be found in specialized information systems. As an example, surgery information systems may collect details relating to anesthesia type, anesthesia risk, return to surgery, and total anesthesia time. Risk management systems may provide details pertaining to medication errors, transfusion reactions, or other adverse outcomes; while pharmacy systems may track total number of doses for

TABLE 25-3	NATIONAL COMPARATIVE PERFORMANCE AND BENCHMARKING DATA RESOURCES	
SETTING	**DESCRIPTION**	**WEBSITE**
Acute care hospitals	**MEDPAR UB-92 (Uniform Billing):** Billing information sent to state intermediaries and available through Medicare Provider Analysis and Review (MEDPAR). This information is free and available to download from the CMS website. A limitation of this information is that it is 18 to 24 months old by the time it is released.	www.cms.hhs.gov/researchers/ statsdata.asp
	CMS QualityNet Exchange: The national data warehouse for CMS Seventh Scope of Work initiatives for AMI, heart failure, pneumonia, and surgical infections and procedures. All hospitals have access through their state quality improvement organizations (QIOs).	www.qnetexchange.org or go to www.cms.hhs.gov/contacts/ to obtain contract information on your State QIO agency
	JCAHO ORYX: Receives data from hospitals related to AMI, heart failure, pneumonia, and pregnancy-related complications. National comparison data are available through performance measurement systems listed with JCAHO for ORYX. Additional topics of surgical procedures and infections, critical care and ventilator management, and pediatric asthma are anticipated in 2004 and 2005.	www.jcaho.org
	Proprietary Software Vendors: A wide variety of for-profit vendor services exist for the provision of comparison data. Comparative data pool may vary in size, and hospital participation may be limited to selected states or hospital specialties (e.g., academic teaching facilities, behavioral health hospitals). See JCAHO website for a full listing.	www.jcaho.org
	California Nursing Outcomes Coalition Report: Statewide database linking patient outcomes to hospital nursing care. Benchmark data currently available for patient falls.	www.nursingworld.org/ snas/ca/calnoc/intro.htm
Managed care and employer	**Milliman USA, Healthcare Management Guidelines:** A set of utilization criteria that provide benchmark data for hospital ALOS for various managed care markets.	www.mnr.com
	Health Plan Employer Data and Information Set (HEDIS): A set of standardized measures used by purchasers and consumers to compare performance of managed health-care plans. HEDIS is sponsored by the National Committee for Quality Assurance (NCQA).	www.ncqa.org/ Programs/HEDIS/
Long-term care	**Minimum Data Set (MDS):** Provides data for quality improvement, benchmarking, and shared best practices for Medicare certified long-term care facilities. The MDS Version 2.0 contains a core set of screening elements that can be used for a comprehensive assessment of residents at time of arrival and at various points in time during their stay. The CMS is responsible for oversight of this data set.	www.cms.hhs.gov/medicaid/ mds20/man-form.asp
Home health care	**Outcome and Assessment Information Set (OASIS)** Used by home health agencies for quality improvement and client assessment. The CMS is responsible for oversight of this data set.	www.cms.hhs.gov/ providers/hha/
Public health	**Minnesota and Washington Departments of Health:** This project uses the Omaha System (Monsen & Martin, 2002a, 2002b) to assist public health departments with organizing, documenting, analyzing and disseminating data to the public. Public data are available for population characteristics, nursing interventions, and client outcomes according to the KBS (Knowledge, Behavior and Status) scale.	www.co.washington.mn. us/info_for_residents/ public_health

ALOS, Average length of stay; *AMI,* acute myocardial infarction; *CMS,* Center for Medicare and Medicaid Services; *JCAHO,* Joint Commission on Accreditation for Healthcare Organizations.

specific medications, day of initial administration, or total costs for medication. The determination of whether specific laboratory or radiology tests were conducted may be found in cost accounting systems that have access to charge information. If specific laboratory or radiology test results are required (e.g., lipid level or confirmation of pneumonia on admission), however, access to medical records may be required. Clinical documentation systems, if available, may also house data elements common to the medical record, such as New York Heart Association (NYHA) classification for heart failure, diagnostic test results, and disease history. In addition, nursing departments may collect data on patient acuity, information on continuous quality improvement (CQI) team activities, and other unit-based quality monitoring reports. APNs can avoid duplication of effort and data collection redundancy by becoming familiar with the many sources of data and information available in their respective organizations (Box 25-3).

Finally, each data element should be evaluated in terms of the relative degree of difficulty in obtaining it. Table 25-4 illustrates an analysis of the data required for a single indicator that examines the percentage of patients with pneumonia who receive antibiotics within 8 hours of arrival at the acute care hospital. In this illustration, the indicator is dissected into its component parts so that each data element can be carefully reviewed for ease of data collection. Only after all indicators within the study are evaluated, will APNs have an appreciation of the scope of their outcome evaluation project and the resources required for successful completion.

As a general rule, data that are available through electronic sources are considered easier to obtain, even if the APN lacks the specialized knowledge necessary for running such reports. Training in running queries and reports may or may not become an essential part of the APN's role. In most cases, experts are available within health-care systems to assist APNs in retrieving the information. Data that are available only through specialized or resource-intensive instruments such as phone surveys, home follow-up visits, or comprehensive chart reviews are considered difficult to obtain and should be evaluated carefully before a final decision is made to include them in the outcome evaluation plan. In some cases, questions about the effective management of clinical populations can only be answered through longitudinal studies. For example, for a diabetic population, clinical outcomes such as reduced hospitalization, improved functioning, reduced evidence of

---

BOX 25-3 • HIPAA SIDEBAR

When collecting patient identifiable data, APNs should be cognizant of the restrictions on their use. The Health Insurance Portability and Accountability Act of 1996 (Public Law 104-191, 104th Congress), commonly referred to as *HIPAA*, is an act designed to improve the continuity of health insurance coverage and combat waste and fraudulent use of health-care resources (see Chapter 22). This act includes significant restrictions on the manner in which identifiable patient information may be used for research and quality improvement activities. In general, health-care agencies are required to establish policies and procedures that protect patient confidentiality and access to information, which is granted on a need-to-know basis. Typically, information used for quality improvement and outcome evaluations is considered to be protected health information. In most cases, APNs are covered under their agency's policies. In some circumstances, particularly if they are contracted in a fee-for-service arrangement with the health-care agency, APNs may be required to sign a business associate agreement with the health-care provider. For more information about HIPAA regulations and impact on evaluation activities, APNs should refer to their organization's policies and procedures.

TABLE 25-4	ANATOMY OF A SAMPLE PROCESS INDICATOR USED IN PERFORMANCE IMPROVEMENT

Indicator	Percentage of patients admitted to hospital with pneumonia who receive initial antibiotic within 8 hours of arrival
Numerator Definition	Patients who receive any antibiotic, regardless of route, type, or dose within 8 hours of arrival to the hospital
Denominator Definition	All patients admitted to the hospital with a working diagnosis of pneumonia

Inclusion criteria:
- Patients admitted as inpatients
- Patients with a working diagnosis of pneumonia on arrival
- Patients 18 years of age and older
- Patients with a principal ICD-9 diagnosis code of pneumonia

OR
- Patients with a principal ICD-9 diagnosis of respiratory failure AND a secondary ICD-9 diagnosis code of pneumonia

OR
- Patients with a principal ICD-9 diagnosis of sepsis AND a secondary ICD-9 diagnosis code of pneumonia

Exclusion criteria:
- Patients admitted from other acute care hospitals, including other EDs
- Patients admitted for comfort care only

REQUIRED DATA ELEMENTS	DATA SOURCE
Encounter type (inpatient, outpatient, ED, short stay)	Hospital admit-discharge-transfer (ADT) system
Age on day of discharge	Hospital ADT system
Working diagnosis on arrival	Chart Review (physician orders, progress notes)
Admission source	Hospital ADT system
Time of arrival to hospital	Chart Review (ED record, progress notes, physician orders)
Admission for provision of comfort care only	Chart Review (physician orders, progress notes)
Administration of any antibiotic	Pharmacy drug system or medication administration record
Initial time of initial antibiotic administration	Chart review: Allowable data sources include medication record, physician orders, ED record

ED, Emergency department; ICD-9, International Classification of Diseases, Ninth Revision.

retinopathy, and reduced limb amputations may be sound, but such data are typically too long-range to be useful for performance improvement or outcome evaluation activities. In addition, the link between advanced practice nursing and the outcomes may be difficult to assess over long periods, making the assessment of intermediate outcomes more desirable for a short-term evaluation.

The usefulness of measures for intermediate outcomes will be most evident if they clearly indicate progress toward some desired endpoint or outcome. The case management literature provides a framework for identifying intermediate outcomes of nursing care that may be applicable to advanced practice. The Second Council for Case Management Accountability and the State of the Science Papers from the Council's annual meeting identify intermediate outcomes as improved patient adherence to therapeutic regimens, increased patient and family involvement in treatment plan, education and empowerment that lead to higher levels of self-management, and improved access to services (Braden, Lambe, & Koithan, 2002).

Once the indicators and the individual data elements have been finalized and the sources of data have been secured, APNs should summarize the outcome evaluation plan in a concise document that describes the plan. Table 25-5 illustrates a high-level outcome evaluation plan for an APN case manager charged with evaluating the effectiveness of a case management program for patients with heart failure. Specific interventions and key process steps are listed for each program goal. For clarity, the indicators that reflect the relative success of the interventions are listed alongside the goals and the interventions. Finally, specific sources of data, timelines, and accountability for data collection and analysis are included to highlight the full scope of the outcome evaluation plan. Such a plan simplifies implementation, as it clarifies the responsibilities of all involved.

When the population of concern spans a larger continuum of care and involves many stakeholders and information sources, creating a visual model of the data plan is useful. This approach facilitates stakeholder visualization of the relationships among the various points of service affected by the project. It also highlights the measures used to evaluate each point of service and the data sources required. See Chapter 18, Figure 18-5 (p. 660) for a conceptual data plan for a population of patients with congestive heart failure.

Derive Meaning from Data and Act on Results

The final phase of the outcome evaluation process involves the evaluation and dissemination of findings and the identification of opportunities for improvement. In these final steps, results are transformed into meaningful information that can be used to improve quality, cost, and customer satisfaction and to evaluate the contributions of the APN. Four steps are required for this final phase. They include the analysis and interpretation of study findings, the presentation and dissemination of study results, the identification of improvement opportunities, and the formulation of a plan to implement and reevaluate changes that occur as a result of the study.

ANALYZE DATA AND INTERPRET FINDINGS

Data analysis is typically the responsibility of the APN, although the inclusion of other peer reviewers is useful, especially when the APN has a vested interest in the outcomes. The inclusion of others helps eliminate any perceived bias during the final data analysis and reporting phases. In some cases, the APN may wish to enlist the support and guidance of a statistician or a doctorally prepared nurse researcher to ensure that the end product is methodologically sound and contains the information necessary to convince others.

The comparison of preintervention with postintervention performance data is one effective way of evaluating the degree of change resulting from APN interventions. Preintervention performance is commonly collected retrospectively and then compared with data collected either during or following an APN intervention. Retrospective data are generally available for measures constructed from electronic data sources. Some examples of data possibly available through these sources are raw counts or volume of patients in the targeted population, average length of stay, number of APN visits per patient, average charges or cost, payor mix, complication rate, mortality rate, discharge disposition following release from treatment, readmission dates, return for service, and other measures derived from the national coding taxonomy, claims data, or patient registration information.

When electronic data are insufficient to provide adequate baseline information, APNs may elect to collect more detailed data from nonelectronic sources, such as flow charts, progress notes, patient teaching records, and diagnostic reports commonly found in non-computerized medical records. While this approach generally requires a greater degree of effort, time, and planning, it may be warranted when specific processes of care are altered as part of the APN's intervention. For example, a CRNA evaluating the frequency of

TABLE 25-5   SAMPLE INSTITUTIONAL OUTCOME EVALUATION PLANNING GRID

GOAL	INTERVENTIONS	KEY PROCESS STEPS	INDICATORS	SOURCE OF DATA	DATA COLLECTION	DATA ANALYSIS	TIME FRAME
Reduce number of admissions and acute care bed utilization by 5%-10%	1. Identify patients in capitated risk groups	—Review all patients admitted with CHF during past 12 months	—No. inpatient days/year —Mean No. acute care days/quarter —No. ED visits/year	QA/UR System	Director of UR	CHF CM QA Medical Director PI Director	Quarterly
		—Mail out SF-36 survey	—No. returned SF-36 surveys/total	SF-36 software Care management log	Case manager Clerk	APN CM	Quarterly
		—Phone interview to patients with physical score <50	—No. with scores <50/total received —Hours/case/month —No. patients declined CM service —No. high-risk patients currently taking ACE inhibitor	Care management log	APN CM	APN CM	Monthly
	2. Patient & family education and monitoring	—Schedule home visits for patients taking more than 8 medications —CHF video	—No. home visits/month —No. of patients/zip code —Pretest/posttest improvement scores on CHF video	Care management log	APN CM	APN CM	Monthly
			—Pretest/posttest improvement scores on CHF video	Care management log	APN CM	APN CM	Quarterly
		—Assess KBS scores on admission and at 6-month intervals	—Mean improvement of Omaha KBS scores	Care management log	APN CM	APN CM	Biannually

Continued

TABLE 25-5 SAMPLE INSTITUTIONAL OUTCOME EVALUATION PLANNING GRID—cont'd

GOAL	INTERVENTIONS	KEY PROCESS STEPS	INDICATORS	SOURCE OF DATA	DATA COLLECTION	DATA ANALYSIS	TIME FRAME
Decrease overall cost of care by 10%	1. Daily rounds in critical care to triage	—Establish triage criteria with critical care committee	—No. critical care bed days/total days —Mean critical care cost/patient —Mean telemetry care cost/patient	QA/UR System	Finance Department	Director, Critical Care	Quarterly
	2. Home health referrals for patients who meet criteria	—Meet with home health liaison daily to review referrals	—Mean home health cost/case —Readmit rate 31 days after discharge from home health	CMS 1500 QA/UR System	Finance Department	Director, Home Health	Quarterly
	3. Establish CQI team to review opportunities to reduce radiology and pharmacy costs	—Secure membership for CQI team —Identify team facilitator —Develop mission statement —Schedule monthly meeting	—Mean cost per admission —Mean pharmacy cost/admission —Mean radiology cost/admission —Total CQI team meeting expenses/year	Cost Accounting System CQI meeting minutes	Finance Department Team Facilitator	CQI Team Director, Pharmacy Director, Radiology	Biannually

ACE, Angiotensin-converting enzyme; *CHF*, congestive heart failure; *CM*, case manager; *CMS*, Centers for Medicine and Medicaid Services; *CQI*, Continuous Quality Improvement; *ED*, emergency department; *KBS*, knowledge, behavior & status; *PI*, performance improvement; *QA*, quality assurance; *SF-36*, short form 36; *UR*, utilization review.

intraoperative hypotensive episodes may have to review medical records because this phenomenon is not contained in common electronic source data. In some cases, a baseline study must be conducted prior to the APN intervention to ensure that appropriate baseline data are available for comparison. For example, an NP who is implementing changes in clinic protocols to reduce waiting times in pregnant women undergoing glucose tolerance testing may have to conduct a preintervention time and motion study to establish a baseline against which to compare postintervention results. This need reinforces the importance of considering how data will be collected and analyzed early in the outcome evaluation planning process.

While baseline information is useful for evaluating outcomes, not everything measured by APNs will have suitable baseline data available for comparison. When this occurs, performance can sometimes be evaluated against a known standard of care or benchmark. This is particularly true when an area of practice is supported by evidence-based practice. When no best-practice standard of performance is known, APNs may use comparative data provided by a national database if the measures used for comparison are the same as those used by the national database.

PRESENT AND DISSEMINATE FINDINGS

The effective communication of data-based findings, conclusions, and recommendations for future practice is an essential component of the outcome evaluation process. The manner in which the findings are presented will depend on the audience receiving the information. Nonclinical audiences with a business focus, such as boards of directors or operations teams, will require briefings that summarize pertinent findings, draw conclusions, and provide reasonable options or recommendations for consideration. Clinical audiences generally require additional detail about how the evaluation was conducted and a more extensive discussion of the clinical and statistical strengths of the evidence. Clinical audiences are becoming more sophisticated in their understanding of data analysis techniques and their assessment of the applicability of evidence to practice.

One of the most effective methods for demonstrating change over time is statistical process control analysis, which examines process variation and its source. Statistical process control analysis uses control charts, which visually display performance data against upper and lower control limits reflective of normal variation in a system. Performance data lying outside these upper and lower limits and clusters of data within limits indicate the existence of some special cause of variation requiring exploration and elimination (Melum, Bartleson, Panzer, & Ron, 1995). Control charts document processes over time, eliminating the need to rely on isolated "snapshots" of performance, which may or may not capture the true picture of process variation. Figure 25-2 contains an example of a control chart displaying the time until antibiotics were initially administered to patients treated for pneumonia in an ED. Data for the control chart were used to detect meaningful changes that occurred as a result of an APN's implementation of standard protocols for treatment of patients with pneumonia. The longitudinal display of data provides a more accurate and informative representation of APN impact than would be evident by a simple comparison of average time before and after the intervention.

Six Sigma analysis is a method used with increasing frequency to define, measure, analyze, improve, and control health-care processes and outcomes (Marash et al., 2003). The term *Six Sigma* refers to a performance level that defines the number of acceptable defects or errors per opportunity. It serves as a quality goal for organizations, with existing processes compared for conformance to minimum acceptable error standards (Erwin, 1998; Perez-Wilson, 1997). A detailed discussion of these data analysis techniques is

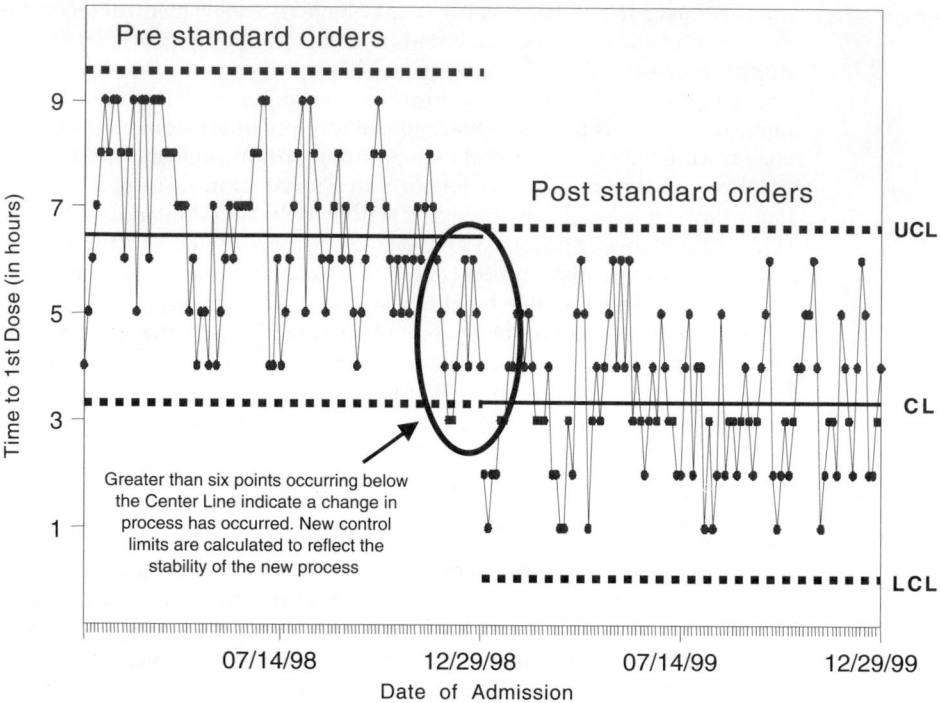

FIGURE 25-2 • Sample control chart for time to initial antibiotic administration for patients with pneumonia treated in an emergency department. UCL, Upper control limit; CL, center line; LCL, lower control limit. (Copyright 2004 by Vicky A. Mahn DiNicola, ACS MIDAS+, Tucson, AZ; reprinted with permission.)

beyond the scope of this chapter, although a basic knowledge of control charts is useful in most situations (Wheeler, 1993).

Packaging the study's findings for presentation to stakeholders may be the APN's responsibility. In some cases, assistance from the facility's media department may be required. Findings should be disseminated in the forms of graphs and summary documents to facilitate rapid review and comprehension of information. Microsoft PowerPoint and Excel programs are useful for this process. For APNs who wish to produce their own control charts, one low-cost and user-friendly tool that is used in conjunction with Microsoft Excel (QI Macros) is available for purchase at www.quantum-i.com. This software includes tutorials on how to produce a variety of quality improvement tools and control charts suitable for proportion, ratio, and continuous variable data. Findings are commonly presented in committee meetings and formal presentations, although the APN should also consider posters, newsletters, white papers, articles, and bulk e-mail communications as additional ways to disseminate information.

IDENTIFY IMPROVEMENT OPPORTUNITIES

Once the outcome evaluation findings have been interpreted and assembled for presentation, the APN begins working closely with stakeholders to identify potential opportunities for improvement and leverage points to better manage care. Leverage points are specific aspects of care delivery processes, technology resources, or points in time that can be altered to achieve greater efficiency or effectiveness within the health-care system. For example, an APN working in the acute care hospital may identify opportunities to improve performance in discharge teaching of patients with heart failure and approach this by leveraging the hospital's decision to participate in the American Heart Association's Get With The Guidelines Program, a national demonstration of best-practice performance for the treatment of AMI and heart failure. Participation in this program provides patient educational materials that can be downloaded from the Web and distributed to patients and family in order to improve discharge-teaching outcomes (www.outcomesciences.com/home/header.html). During this third step, the APN assists team members to develop a shared vision of which intervention(s) to adopt and why. Bringing stakeholders together to review existing processes of care and to isolate any process failures or barriers that have contributed to suboptimal performance is useful at this time. Useful tools for this purpose include flow charts, cause-and-effect (Ishikawa) diagrams, failure modes and effects analysis, SWOT (Strengths, Weaknesses, Opportunities and Threats) analysis, and formal brainstorming techniques. The reader is referred to Powell's book on advanced case management (2000) for additional information on these and other quality improvement tools.

The process for identifying opportunities for improvement is similar to any work redesign initiative. Champions and potential opponents of change should be identified. Careful specification of program components is also required, as is delegation of responsibility for project-related activities. During this process, change theory can serve as a useful foundation for APNs charged with informing stakeholders and overcoming resistance to new care delivery practices. Issues such as level of difficulty with implementing the intervention should be addressed, as should projected costs and the human and technology resources required to implement and sustain the plan (University of York, 1999). Consideration should be given as to how much time the APN will be engaged in the project and how this may affect other areas of practice. A staged pilot testing approach is useful for new or large-scale projects. As noted earlier, these smaller-scale versions help identify potential implementation problems and determine whether the intervention can achieve the desired effect. As an example, if one of the goals of a performance improvement plan is the timely initial administration of antibiotics to patients with pneumonia in an acute care setting, interventions might include using a risk appraisal tool or instituting fast tracking of admission orders to the pharmacy department. These interventions might be pilot tested on one shift in the ED for 2 to 3 weeks before the strategy is deployed across the hospital or used during all shifts.

FORMULATE A PLAN FOR IMPLEMENTATION AND REEVALUATION

Once the findings have been shared and the goals of the performance improvement initiative have been established, they should be summarized concisely in a document and distributed to all stakeholders. Each goal should specify the primary intervention or interventions that will be used to reach the goal, along with who is accountable for the actions required and the target dates for completion. When the interventions, accountabilities, and timelines are established, the APN can then use the identified indicators/measures to reevaluate the outcome. This in turn becomes the basis for future outcome evaluation plans. Once performance in a particular area is stabilized, the APN may elect to discontinue monitoring a given area of performance or periodically revisit performance through intermittent monitoring.

For interventions that focus on change in practice patterns or processes of care, the APN may be called upon to provide educational programs for other providers and disciplines affected by the new process or change. The educational content of these sessions should focus on the standards of practice expected for the population and the strategies, tools, and supports available (e.g., revised documentation systems, flow sheets, or computerized alerts) to assist in the adoption of the care delivery standard. Providers should also be informed about the measures that will be used to monitor performance. In some cases, this action will alter performance in and of itself simply because the providers know they are being observed and their performance is being monitored. This reaction, which is described as the *Hawthorne effect*, is troublesome for process measurement. As a result, the program should continue for a sufficient period to ensure that the novelty of the intervention has worn off and the changes in behaviors are a true reflection of intervention effect.

SUMMARY

The issues facing the profession in relation to justifying the use of APNs and measuring the effect of advanced practice nursing on patients and health-care systems are similar to but distinct from those faced by individual APNs needing to evaluate the outcomes of their particular practice. This chapter has examined both sets of issues. It is apparent that the need for well-designed, longitudinal assessments of APN impact has never been stronger. Because reimbursement decisions are driven by evidence of provider performance, APNs without reliable and valid data to substantiate their impact will struggle for equitable reimbursement for services. Moreover, reimbursement decisions made solely on the basis of physician-derived outcome indicators seriously limit the understanding of advanced nursing practice impact on patient care. Currently, the majority of managed care organizations that list APNs as primary care providers evaluate them according to physician standards (Mason, Cohen, O'Donnell, Baxter, & Chase, 1997). Furthermore, the magnitude of APNs' contributions to care is often lost because managed care organizations regularly attribute all outcomes to the collaborating physician (Mason et al., 1999). This invisibility in the health-care system further threatens the recognition of APNs as viable, important providers of health-care services.

Addressing the need for inclusion of APN-sensitive outcome indicators will require focused attention on the development of electronic information systems that support the identification and tracking of APN outcome data. A first step in this process is national agreement on a core set of outcome indicators relevant to APNs and the initiation of standards that support the collection of APN-sensitive data. Until health-care organizations and reimbursement agents begin demanding data to substantiate individual APN and APN group provider performance, no widespread action is likely.

This chapter highlights several frameworks for measuring and monitoring advanced nursing practice. Other approaches are also available, and the APN should begin the process of outcomes measurement and management by selecting one and refining it to meet individual and organizational needs. The best approach is to begin small and expand activities over time. In selecting indicators, APNs must consider the resources needed to collect the data, the time required to do so, and the fit between the data and the organization's mission. Networking with other APNs is useful for identifying beneficial outcomes and sharing personal experiences about what does and does not work in the integration of outcomes measurement into busy practices.

This discussion illustrates the interconnectedness of outcomes measurement with every other aspect of the APN role. Effective outcomes measurement and management require APNs to work collaboratively with others, to plan and organize processes of care and assessment of quality in highly complex health services environments, and to expose their individual practices to the scrutiny of others. Experience with organizational change behaviors and a willingness to seek information and assistance from others will assist with this process. In the end, the quality and value of care will improve, as will the community's recognition of the APN's impact on outcomes of care.

REFERENCES

Aiken, J. L., Taggart, J. R., & Tripoli, C. A. (1993). Evaluation and time documentation for the clinical nurse specialist. *Clinical Nurse Specialist, 7*, 33-38.

Aiken, L. H., Lake, E. T., Semaan, S., Lehman, H. P., O'Hare, P. A., Cole, C. S., et al, (1993). Nurse practitioner managed care for persons with HIV infection. *Image: The Journal of Nursing Scholarship, 25*, 172-177.

Aquilino, M. L., Damiano, P. C., Willard, J. C., Momany, E. T., & Levy, B. T. (1999). Primary care physician perceptions of the nurse practitioner in the 1990s. *Archives of Family Medicine, 8*, 224-227.

Armenian, H. K., & Shapiro, S. (1998). *Epidemiology and health services.* New York: Oxford University Press.

Aubrey, W. R., & Yoxall, C. W. (2001). Evaluation of the role of the neonatal nurse practitioner in resuscitation of preterm infants at birth. *Archives of Disease in Childhood, 85*, F96-F99.

Baldwin, K. A., Sisk, R. J., Watts, P., McCubbin, J., Brockschmidt, B., & Marion, L. N. (1998). Acceptance of nurse practitioners and physician assistants in meeting the perceived needs of rural communities. *Public Health Nursing, 15*, 389-397.

Baradell, J. G., & Bordeaux, B. R. (2001). Outcomes and satisfaction of patients of psychiatric clinical nurse specialists. *Journal of the American Psychiatric Nurses Association, 7*, 77-85.

Beal, J. A., & Quinn, M. (2002). The nurse practitioner role in the NICU as perceived by parents. *MCN, American Journal of Maternal Child Nursing, 27*, 183-188.

Beal, J. A., Richardson, D. K., Dembinski, S., Hipp, K. O., McCourt, M., Szlachetka, D., et al. (1999). Responsibilities, roles & staffing patterns of nurse practitioners in the neonatal intensive care unit. *MCN, American Journal of Maternal Child Nursing, 24*, 168-175.

Beckman, L. J., Harvey, S. M., & Satre, S. J. (2002). The delivery of medical abortion services: The views of experienced providers. *Women's Health Issues, 12*, 103-112.

Beeber, L. S., & Charlie, M. L. (1998). Depressive symptom reversal for women in a primary care setting: A pilot study. *Archives of Psychiatric Nursing, 12*, 247-254.

Benkert, R., Barkauskas, V., Pohl, J., Corser, W., Tanner, C., Wells, M., et al. (2002). Patient satis-faction outcomes in nurse-managed centers. *Outcomes Management, 6*, 174-181.

Bergeron, J., Cash, R., Boulger, J., & Bergeron, D. (1997). The attitudes of rural Minnesota family physicians toward nurse practitioners and physician assistants. *Journal of Rural Health, 13*, 196-205.

Bissinger, R. L., Allred, C. A., Arford, P. H., & Bellig, L. L. (1997). A cost-effectiveness analysis of neonatal nurse practitioners. *Nursing Economics, 15*, 92-99.

Boyle, D. M. (1995). Documentation and outcomes of advanced practice. *Oncology Nursing Forum, 22*(Suppl. 8), 11-17.

Braden, C. J., Lambe, G., & Koithan, M. (2002). State of the science: Involvement/participation, empowerment and knowledge outcome indicators of case management. Little Rock, AR: Case Management Society of America.

Brady, M. A., & Neal, J. A. (2000). Role delineation study of pediatric nurse practitioners: A national study of practice and responsibilities and trends in role functions. *Journal of Pediatric Health Care, 14*, 149-159.

Britton, J. R. (1997). Neonatal nurse practitioner and physician use on a newborn resuscitation team in a community hospital. *Journal of Pediatric Health Care, 11*, 61-65.

Brooten, D., Gennaro, S., Knapp, H., Jovene, N., Brown, L., & York, R. (2002). Functions of the CNS in early discharge and home followup of very low birthweight infants. *Clinical Nurse Specialist, 16*, 85-90.

Brooten, D., Naylor, M. D., York, R., Brown, L. P., Munro, B. H., Hollingsworth, A. O., et al. (2002). Lessons learned from testing the quality cost model of advanced practice nursing (APN) transitional care. *Journal of Nursing Scholarship, 34*, 369-375.

Brooten, D., Roncoli, M., Finkler, S., Arnold, L., Cohen, A., & Mennuti, M. (1994). A randomized trial of early hospital discharge and home follow-up of women having cesarean birth. *Obstetrics & Gynecology, 84*, 832-838.

Brooten, D., Youngblut, J. M., Deatrick, J., Naylor, M., & York, R. (2003). Patient problems, advanced practice nurse (APN) interventions, time and contacts among five patient groups. *Journal of Nursing Scholarship, 35*, 73-79.

Brown, A. W., Wolff, K. L., Elasy, T. A., & Graber, A. L. (2001). The role of advanced practice nurses in a shared care diabetes practice model. *Diabetes Educator, 27,* 492-500.

Brown, S. A., & Grimes, D. E. (1995). A meta-analysis of nurse practitioners and nurse midwives in primary care. *Nursing Research, 44,* 332-339.

Brown, S. A., & Hanis, C. L. (1995). A community-based, culturally sensitive education and group-support intervention for Mexican Americans with NIDDM: A pilot study of efficacy. *Diabetes Educator, 21,* 203-210.

Bryant, R., & Graham, M. C. (2002). Advanced practice nurses: A study of client satisfaction. *Journal of American Academy of Nurse Practitioners, 14,* 88-92.

Burl, J. B., Bonner, A., Rao, M., & Khan, A. M. (1998). Geriatric nurse practitioners in long-term care: Demonstration of effectiveness in managed care. *Journal of the American Geriatrics Society, 46,* 506-510.

Butler, J., Adams, B., Parker, J., Roberts, J. M., & Laros, R. K. (1993). Supportive nurse-midwife care is associated with a reduced incidence of cesarean section. *American Journal of Obstetrics & Gynecology, 168,* 1407-1413.

Byers, J. F., & Brunell, M. L. (1998). Demonstrating the value of the advanced practice nurse: An evaluation model. *AACN Clinical Issues, 9,* 296-305.

Campbell, C. D., Musil, C. M., & Zauszniewski, J. A. (1998). Practice patterns of advanced practice psychiatric nurses. *Journal of American Psychiatric Nurses Association, 4,* 111-120.

Carioti, C. A., Lavigne, J. E., Stone, P., Tortoretti, D. M., & Chiverton, P. (2001). Work site disease management outcomes: Expanding the role of the APN. *Outcomes Management for Nursing Practice, 5,* 179-184.

Carr, C. A. (2000). Charges for maternity services: Associations with provider type and payer source in a university teaching hospital. *Journal of Midwifery & Women's Health, 45,* 378-383.

Carroll, D. L., Robinson, E., Buselli, E., Berry, D., & Rankin, S. H. (2001). Activities of the APN to enhance unpartnered elders self-efficacy after myocardial infarction. *Clinical Nurse Specialist, 15,* 60-66.

Carroll, T. L., & Fay, V. P. (1997). Measuring the impact of advanced practice nursing in achieving cost-quality outcomes: Issues and challenges. *Nursing Administration Quarterly, 21,* 32-40.

Carzoli, R. P., Martinez-Cruz, M., Cuevas, L. L., Murphy, S., & Chiu, T. (1994). Comparison of neonatal nurse practitioners, physician assistants, and residents in the neonatal intensive care unit. *Archives in Pediatric & Adolescent Medicine, 148,* 1271-1276.

Center for Medicare and Medicaid Services (CMS). (2003). Quality efforts. Retrieved August 12, 2003, from http://www.cms.gov/quality

Chang, E., Daly, J., Hawkins, A., McGirr, J., Fielding, K., Hemmings, L., et al. (1999). An evaluation of the nurse practitioner role in a major rural emergency department. *Journal of Advanced Nursing, 30,* 260-268.

Cohen, J., Saylor, C., Holzemer, W. L., & Gorenberg, B. (2000). Linking nursing care interventions with client outcomes: A community-based application of an outcomes model. *Journal of Nursing Care Quality, 15,* 22-31.

Cole, F. L., & Ramirez, E. (2000). Activities and procedures performed by nurse practitioners in emergency care settings. *Journal of Emergency Nursing, 26,* 455-463.

Cook, T., & Nolan, W. (1996). A nurse practitioner-led, collaborative, outpatient practice: A case study in outcomes management. *Seminars for Nurse Managers, 4,* 154-162.

Counsell, C., & Gilbert, M. (1999). Implementation of a nurse practitioner role in an acute care setting. *Critical Care Nursing Clinics of North America, 11,* 277-282.

Courtney, R., & Rice, C. (1997). Investigation of nurse practitioner-patient interactions: Using the nurse practitioner rating form. *Nurse Practitioner, 22,* 46, 48, 54, 56-57, 60, 65.

Cromwell, J., & Rosenbach, M. (1990). The impact of nurse anesthetists on anesthesiology productivity. *Medical Care, 28,* 159-169.

Cromwell, J., & Snyder, K. (2000). Alternate cost-effective anesthesia care teams. *Nursing Economics, 18,* 185-193.

Dahl, J., & Penque, S. (2001). The effects of an advanced practice nurse-directed heart failure program. *Dimensions of Critical Care Nursing, 20,* 20-28.

Dahle, K. L., Smith, J. S., Ingersoll, G. L., & Wilson, J. R. (1998). Impact of a nurse practitioner on the cost of managing inpatients with heart failure. *American Journal of Cardiology, 82,* 686-688.

Davidson, J. U. (1999). Blending case management and quality outcomes management into the family nurse practitioner role. *Nursing Administration Quarterly, 24,* 66-74.

Davis, L. G., Riedmann, G. L., Sapiro, M., Minoque, J. P., & Kazer, R. R. (1994). Cesarean section rates in low-risk private patients managed by certified nurse-midwives and obstetricians. *Journal of Nurse Midwifery, 39,* 91-97.

DeNicola, L., Kleid, D., Brink, L., van Stralen, D., Scott, M., Gerbert, D., et al. (1994). Use of pediatric physician extenders in pediatric and neonatal intensive care units. *Critical Care Medicine, 22,* 1856-1862.

Donabedian, A. (1966). Evaluating the quality of medical care. *Milbank Quarterly, 44,* 166-206.

Donabedian, A. (1982). *Explorations in quality assessment and monitoring: The definition of quality and approaches to its assessment.* Ann Arbor, MI: Health Administration Press.

Dougherty, C. M., Spertus, J. A., Dewhurst, T. A., & Nichol, W. P. (2000). Outpatient nursing case management for cardiovascular disease. *Nursing Clinics of North America, 35,* 993-1003.

Ellwood, P. M. (1988). Outcomes management. A technology of patient experience. *New England Journal of Medicine, 318,* 1549-1556.

Erwin, J. (1998). Achieving total customer satisfaction through Six Sigma. *Quality Digest, 18,* 38-41.

Gebaur, C., Kwo, C. Y., Haynes, E. F., & Wewers, M. E. (1998). A nurse-managed smoking cessation intervention during pregnancy. *Journal of Gynecologic & Neonatal Nursing, 21,* 47-53.

Gravely, E. A., & Littlefield, J. H. (1992). Cost-effectiveness analysis of three staffing models for the delivery of low-risk prenatal care. *American Journal of Public Health, 82,* 180-184.

Gray, M. (1998). The impact of the "Put Prevention Into Practice" initiative on pediatric nurse practitioner practices. *Journal of Pediatric Health Care, 12,* 171-175.

Greulich, B., Paine, L. L., McClain, C., Barger, M. K., Edwards, N., & Paul, R. (1994). Twelve years and more than 30,000 nurse-midwife-attended births: The Los Angeles County + University of Southern California Women's Hospital Birth Center experience. *Journal of Nurse Midwifery, 39,* 185-196.

Gurka, A. M. (1991). Process and outcome components of clinical nurse specialist consultation. *Dimensions of Critical Care Nursing, 10,* 169-175.

Halm, M. A., Gagner, S., Goering, M., Sabo, J., Smith, M., & Zaccagnini, M. (2003). Interdisciplinary rounds. Impact on patients, families, and staff. *Clinical Nurse Specialist, 17,* 133-142.

Hamric, A. B., Lindebak, S., Worley, D., & Jaubert, S. (1998). Outcomes associated with advanced nursing practice prescriptive authority. *Journal of the American Academy of Nurse Practitioners, 10,* 113-118.

Hanneman, S. K. G., Bines, A. S., & Sajtar, W. S. (1993). The indirect patient care effect of a unit-based clinical nurse specialist on preventable pulmonary complications. *American Journal of Critical Care, 2,* 331-338.

Hargreaves, W. A., Shumway, M., Hu, T. W., & Cuffel, B. (1998). *Cost-outcome methods for mental health.* New York: Academic Press.

Hill, J., Bird, H. A., Harmer, R., Wright, V., & Lawton, C. (1994). An evaluation of the effectiveness, safety and acceptability of a nurse practitioner in a rheumatology outpatient clinic. *British Journal of Rheumatology, 33,* 283-288.

Hill, K. M., Ellsworth-Wolk, J., & DeBlase, R. (1993). Capturing the multiple contributions of the CNS role: A criterion-based evaluation tool. *Clinical Nurse Specialist, 7,* 267-273.

Hillier, A. (2001). The advanced practice nurse in gastroenterology: Identifying and comparing care interactions of nurse practitioners and clinical nurse specialists. *Gastroenterology Nursing, 24,* 239-245.

Holcomb, L. O. (2000). A Delphi survey to identify activities of nurse practitioners in primary care. *Clinical Excellence in Nursing Practice, 4,* 163-172.

Holzemer, W. L. (1994). The impact of nursing care in Latin America and the Caribbean: A focus on outcomes. *Journal of Advanced Nursing, 20,* 5-12.

Hooker, R. S., & McCaig, L. F. (2001). Use of physician assistants and nurse practitioners in primary care, 1995-1999. *Health Affairs, 20,* 231-238.

Horrocks, S., Anderson, E., & Salisbury, C. (2002). Systematic review of whether nurse practitioners working in primary care can provide equivalent care to doctors. *British Medical Journal, 324,* 819-823.

Hughes, W. J. (2000). Health department nurse practitioners as comprehensive primary care providers. *Family & Community Health, 23,* 50-65.

Hylka, S. C., & Beschle, J. C. (1995). Nurse practitioners, cost savings, and improved patient care in the department of surgery. *Nursing Economics, 13,* 349-354.

Ingersoll, G. L. (1998). Administrative issues in the measurement and management of outcomes. *Applied Nursing Research, 11,* 93-97.

Ingersoll, G. L. (2000). Evidence based nursing: What it is and what it isn't. *Nursing Outlook, 48,* 151-152.

Ingersoll, G. L., McIntosh, E., & Williams, M. (2000). Nurse-sensitive outcomes of advanced practice. *Journal of Advanced Practice, 32,* 1272-1281.

Institute of Medicine. (2001). *Crossing the quality chasm: A new health system for the 21st century.* Washington, DC: National Academy Press.

Institute of Medicine. (1990). *Medicare: A strategy for quality assurance, volume 1.* Washington, DC: National Academy Press.

Irvine, D., Sidani, S., Porter, H., O'Brien-Pallas, L., Simpson, B., Hall, L. M., et al. (2000). Organizational factors influencing nurse practitioners' role implementation in acute care settings. *Canadian Journal of Nursing Leadership, 13,* 28-35.

Jackson, P. L., Kennedy, C., Sadler, L. S., Kenney, K. M., Lindeke, L. L., Sperhac, A. M., et al. (2001). Professional practice of pediatric nurse practitioners: Implications for education and training of PNPs. *Journal of Pediatric Health Care, 15,* 291-298.

Jepson, C., McCorkle, R., Adler, D., Nuamah, I., & Lusk, E. (1999). Effects of home care on caregivers' psychosocial status. *Image: Journal of Nursing Scholarship, 31,* 115-120.

Jessup, A. N., & Harrell, J. S. (1996). Promotion of cardiovascular health in children by nurse practitioners and physicians in family practice. *Journal of the American Academy of Nurse Practitioners, 8,* 467-475.

Johnson, J. E. (2000). Assessment of older urban drivers by nurse practitioners. *Journal of Community Health Nursing, 17,* 107-114.

Joint Commission on Accreditation of Healthcare Organizations. (2000). *Mining ORYX data 2000: A guide for performance measurement systems.* Oakbrook Terrace, IL: Author.

Joint Commission on Accreditation of Healthcare Organizations. (2001). *Specifications manual for national implementation of hospital core measures.* Oakbrook Terrace, IL: Author.

Jones, M. E., & Clark, D. (1997). Increasing access to health care: A study of pediatric nurse practitioner outcomes in a school-based clinic. *Journal of Nursing Care Quality, 11*, 53-59.

Kane, R. L., Flood, S., Keckhafer, G., & Rockwood, T. (2001). How EverCare nurse practitioners spend their time. *Journal of American Geriatric Society, 49*, 1530-1534.

Karlowicz, M. G., & McMurray, J. L. (2000). Comparison of neonatal nurse practitioners' and pediatric residents' care of extremely low-birth-weight infants. *Archives of Pediatric & Adolescent Medicine, 154*, 1123-1126.

Kearnes, D. R. (1993). A productivity tool to evaluate NP practice: Monitoring clinical time spent in reimbursable, patient-related activities. *Nurse Practitioner, 17*, 50, 52, 55.

Kearnes, D. R. (1994). Impact of a nurse practitioner and physician collaborative practice on older adults admitted to a large urban hospital: Differences in treatment and outcome. *Nurse Practitioner, 19*, 32, 34-36.

Kinnersley, P., Anderson, E., Parry, K., Clement, J., Archard, L., Turton, P., et al. (2000). Randomised controlled trial of nurse practitioner versus general practitioner care for patients requesting "same day" consultations in primary care. *British Medical Journal, 320*, 1043-1048.

Kleinpell, R. M. (1998). Reports of role descriptions of acute care nurse practitioners. *AACN Clinical Issues, 9*, 290-295.

Kleinpell-Nowell, R. (2001). Longitudinal survey of acute care nurse practitioner practice: Year 2. *AACN Clinical Issues, 12*, 447-452.

Kleinpell-Nowell, R., & Weiner, T. M. (1999). Measuring advanced practice nursing outcomes. *AACN Clinical Issues, 10*, 356-368.

Knudtson, N. (2000). Patient satisfaction with nurse practitioner service in a rural setting. *Journal of American Academy of Nurse Practitioners, 12*, 405-412.

Krueger, R. A. (n.d.). *Outcome evaluation.* Retrieved July 29, 2003, from http://www.tc.umn.edu/~rkrueger/evaluation/oe.html

LaCava, L. A. (2001). *Identifying and measuring CYD outcomes.* Retrieved July 29, 2003, from http://www.cydjournal.org/Brandeis/lacava_1218.html

Lamb, G., Mahn, V., & Dahl, R. (1996). Goals of an effective delivery system for the chronically ill. *Managed Care Quarterly, 43*, 46-53.

Larkin, G. L., Kantor, W., & Zielinski, J. J. (2001). Doing unto others? Emergency medicine residents' willingness to be treated by moonlighting residents and nonphysician clinicians in the emergency department. *Academic Emergency Medicine, 8*, 886-892.

Larrabee, J. H., Ferri, J. A., & Hartig, M. T. (1997). Patient satisfaction with nurse practitioner care in primary care. *Journal of Nursing Care Quality, 11*, 9-14.

Lawson, M. T. (2002). Nurse practitioner and physician communication styles. *Applied Nursing Research, 15*, 60-66.

Lemley, K. B., O'Grady, E. T., Raukhorst, L., Russell, D. D., & Small, N. (1994). Baseline data on the delivery of clinical preventive services provided by nurse practitioners. *Nurse Practitioner, 19*, 57-63.

Leveille, S. G., Wagner, E. H., Davis, C., Grothaus, L., Wallace, J., LoGerfo, M., et al. (1998). Preventing disability and managing chronic illness in frail older adults: A randomized trial of a community-based partnership with primary care. *Journal of American Geriatrics Society, 46*, 1191-1198.

Lin, S. X., Hooker, R. S., Lenz, E. R., & Hopkins, S. C. (2002). Nurse practitioners and physician assistants in hospital outpatient departments, 1997-1999. *Nursing Economics, 20*, 174-179.

Lincoln, P. E. (2000). Comparing CNS and NP role activities: A replication. *Clinical Nurse Specialist, 14*, 269-277.

Lind, P. (2001). Disease management: Applying systems thinking to quality patient care delivery. In E. Cohen & T. Cesta (Eds.), *Nursing case management: From essentials to advanced practice applications* (3rd ed., pp. 37-48). St. Louis, MO: Mosby.

Lombness, P. M. (1994). Difference in length of stay with care managed by clinical nurse specialists or physicians assistants. *Clinical Nurse Specialist, 8*, 253-260.

Lund, C. H., Osborne, J. W., Kuller, J., Lane, A. T., Lott, J. W., & Raines, D. A. (2001). Neonatal skin care: Clinical outcomes of the AWHONN/NANN evidence-based clinical practice guideline. *Journal of Obstetric, Gynecologic, & Neonatal Nursing, 30*, 41-51.

Lydon-Rochelle, M. T., Albers, L., & Teaf, D. (1995). Perineal outcomes and nurse-midwifery management. *Journal of Nurse-Midwifery, 40*, 13-18.

Lynch, M. P., Cope, D. G., & Murphy-Ende, K. (2001). Advanced practice issues: Results of the ONS advanced practice nursing survey. *Oncology Nursing Forum, 28*, 1521-1530.

Mabrook, A. F., & Dale, B. (1998). Can nurse practitioners offer a quality service? An evaluation of a year's work of a nurse led minor injury unit. *Journal of Accident & Emergency Medicine, 15*, 266-268.

Mahn, V. A., & Heller, C. J. (1998). Prioritization of target populations for care management and process improvement activities. Tucson, AZ: ACS MIDAS+.

Mahn, V., & Zazworsky, D. (2000). The advanced practice nurse case manager. In A. B. Hamric, J. A. Spross, & C. M. Hanson (Eds.), *Advanced nursing practice: An integrative approach* (2nd ed., pp. 549-606). Philadelphia: W. B. Saunders Company.

Mahoney, D. F. (1994). Appropriateness of geriatric prescribing decisions made by nurse practitioners and physicians. *Image: Journal of Nursing Scholarship, 26*, 41-46.

Marash, S., Berman, P., & Flynn, M. (2003). *Fusion management: Harnessing the power of Six Sigma, Lean, ISO 9001:2000, Malcolm Baldrige, TQM, and other quality breakthroughs of the past century.* Fairfax, VA: QSU.

Martin, S. A. (1999). The pediatric critical care nurse practitioner: Evaluation and impact. *Pediatric Nursing, 25,* 505-510.

Mason, D. J., Alexander, J. M., Huffaker, J., Reilly, P. A., Sigmund, E. C., & Cohen, S. S. (1999). Nurse practitioners' experiences with managed care organizations in New York and Connecticut. *Nursing Outlook, 47,* 201-208.

Mason, D. J., Cohen, S. S., O'Donnell, J. P., Baxter, K., & Chase, A. B. (1997). Managed care organizations' arrangements with nurse practitioners. *Nursing Economics, 15,* 306-314.

McAuliffe, M. S., & Henry, B. (1998). Survey of nurse anesthesia practice, education, and regulation in 96 countries. *AANA Journal, 66,* 273-286.

McCorkle, R., Strumpf, N. E., Nuamah, I. F., Adler, D. C., Cooley, M. E., Jepson, C., et al. (2000). A specialized home care intervention improves survival among older post-surgical cancer patients. *Journal of the American Geriatric Society, 48,* 1707-1713.

McGlynn, E. A., Asch, S. M., Adams, J., Keesey, J., Hicks, J., DeCristofaro, A., et al. (2003). The quality of health care delivered to adults in the United States. *New England Journal of Medicine, 348,* 2635-2645.

McMullen, M., Alexander, M. K., Bourgeois, A., & Goodman, L. (2001). Evaluating a nurse practitioner service. *Dimensions of Critical Care Nursing, 20,* 30-34.

Melum, M. M., Bartleson, J. D., Panzer, R., & Ron, A. (1995). *Total quality outcomes management. A guide to interpreting outcomes measurement and TQM to improve health.* Methuen, MA: GOAL/QPC.

Merwin, E. I., Greiner, D., Barrell, L. M., Clement, J., Chisholm, M., Delaney, K. R., et al. (1997). Advanced practice psychiatric nursing: A national profile. *Archives of Psychiatric Nursing, 11,* 182-183.

Mezey, M., Dougherty, M., Wade, P., & Mersmann, C. (1994). Nurse practitioners, certified nurse midwives, and nurse anesthetists: Changing care in acute care hospitals in New York City. *Journal of the New York State Nurses Association, 25,* 13-16.

Mick, D. J., & Ackerman, M. H. (2000). Advanced practice nursing role delineation in acute and critical care: Application of the Strong Model of advanced practice. *Heart & Lung: Journal of Acute & Critical Care, 29,* 210-221.

Mills, A. C., & McSweeney, M. (2002). Nurse practitioners and physician assistants revisited: Do their practice patterns differ in ambulatory care? *Journal of Professional Nursing, 18,* 36-46.

Mills, A. C., McSweeney, M., & Lavin, M. A. (1998). Characteristics of patient visits to nurse practitioners and physician assistants in hospital outpatient departments. *Journal of Professional Nursing, 14,* 335-343.

Mitchell, J., Dixon, H. L., Freeman, T., & Grindrod, A. (2001). Public perceptions of and comfort level with nurse practitioners in family practice. *Canadian Nurse, 97,* 21-26.

Mitchell, P. H., Ferketich, S., Jennings, B. M., & American Academy of Nursing Expert Panel on Quality of Care. (1998). Quality health outcomes model. *Image: Journal of Nursing Scholarship, 30,* 43-46.

Mitchell-DiCenso, A., Guyatt, G., Marrin, M., Goeree, R., William, A., Southwell, D., et al. (1996). A controlled trial of nurse practitioners in neonatal intensive care. *Pediatrics, 98,* 1143-1148.

Monsen, K. A., & Martin, K. S. (2002a). Developing an outcomes management program in a public health department. *Outcomes Management, 6,* 62-66.

Monsen, K. A., & Martin, K. S. (2002b). Using an outcomes management program in a public health department. *Outcomes Management, 6,* 120-124.

Moody, N. B., Smith, P. L., & Glenn, L. L. (1999). Client characteristics and practice patterns of nurse practitioners and physicians. *Nurse Practitioner, 24,* 94-103.

Moore, S., Corner, J., Haviland, J., Wells, M., Salmon, E., Normand, C., et al. (2002). Nurse led follow up and conventional medical follow up in management of patients with lung cancer: Randomized trial. *British Medical Journal, 325,* 1145-1147.

Mundinger, M. O., Kane, R. L., Lenz, E. R., Totten, A. M., Tsai, W. U., Cleary, P. D., et al. (2000). Primary care outcomes in patients treated by nurse practitioners or physicians. *JAMA: The Journal of the American Medical Association, 283,* 59-68.

Murphy, J. E., & Ericson, J. R. (1995). Acceptance of nurse practitioner services by rural elderly. *Nurse Practitioner, 20,* 72-74.

Murphy, P. A., & Feinland, J. B. (1998). Perineal outcomes in a home birth setting. *Birth, 25,* 226-234.

Murphy, P. A., & Fullerton, J. T. (1998). Outcomes of intended home births in nurse-midwifery practice: A prospective descriptive study. *Obstetrics & Gynecology, 92,* 461-470.

Murphy, P. A., & Fullerton, J. T. (2001). Measuring outcomes of midwifery care: Development of an instrument to assess optimality. *Journal of Midwifery & Women's Health, 46,* 274-284.

Musclow, S. L., Sawhney, M., & Watt-Watson, J. (2002). The emerging role of advanced nursing practice in acute pain management throughout Canada. *Clinical Nurse Specialist, 16,* 63-67.

Naylor, M. D., & McCauley, K. M. (1999). The effects of a discharge planning and home follow-up intervention on elders hospitalized with common medical and surgical cardiac conditions. *Journal of Cardiovascular Nursing, 14,* 44-54.

Naylor, M. D., Brooten, D., Jones, R., Lavizzo-Mourey, R., Mezey, M., & Pauly, M. (1994).

Comprehensive discharge planning for hospitalized elderly: A randomized clinical trial. *Annals of Internal Medicine, 120,* 999-1006.

Naylor, M. D., Brooten, D., Campbell, R., Jacobsen, B. S., Mezey, M. D., Pauly, M. V., et al. (1999). Comprehensive discharge planning and home follow-up of hospitalized elders: A randomized clinical trial. *JAMA: The Journal of the American Medical Association, 281,* 613-620.

Ockene, J. K., Adams, A., Hurley, T. G., Wheeler, E. V., & Hebert, J. R. (1999). Brief physician- and nurse practitioner-delivered counseling for high-risk drinkers. *Archives of Internal Medicine, 159,* 2198-2205.

Oddi, L. F., & Cassidy, V. R. (1998). The message of SUPPORT: Change is long overdue. *Journal of Professional Nursing, 14,* 165-174.

Oliveria, S. A., Altman, J. F., Christos, P. J., & Halpern, A. C. (2002). Use of nonphysician health care providers for skin cancer screening in the primary care setting. *Preventive Medicine, 34,* 374-379.

Palmer, R. H., Duggar, B., DeLozier, J., Goldenberg, D., Lawthers, A. J., Banks, N. J., et al. (1995). Understanding and choosing clinical performance measures: Development of a typology (Publication No. 95-N001). Washington, DC: Agency for Health Care Policy and Research.

Perez-Wilson, M. (1997). Six Sigma strategies: Creating excellence in the workplace. *Quality Digest, 17,* 27-31.

Peters, C., Cowley, M., & Standiford, L. (1999). The process of outcomes management in an acute care facility. *Nursing Administration Quarterly, 24,* 75-89.

Pine, M., Holt, K. D., & Lou, Y. B. (2003). Surgical mortality and type of anesthesia provider. *AANA Journal, 71,* 109-116.

Powell, S. K. (2000). *Advanced case management: Outcomes and beyond.* Philadelphia: Lippincott.

Radwin, L. (2002). Refining the quality health outcomes model: Differentiating between client trait and state characteristics. *Nursing Outlook, 50,* 168-169.

Ramsey, P., Edwards, J., Lenz, C., Odom, J. E., & Brown, B. (1993). Types of health problems and satisfaction with services in a rural nurse-managed clinic. *Journal of Community Health Nursing, 10,* 161-170.

Rawl, S. M., Easton, K. L., Kwiatkowski, S., Zemen, D., & Burczyk, B. (1998). Effectiveness of a nurse-managed follow-up program for rehabilitation patients after discharge. *Rehabilitation Nursing, 23,* 204-209.

Riportella-Muller, R., Libby, D., & Kindig, D. (1995). The substitution of physician assistants and nurse practitioners for physician residents in teaching hospitals. *Health Affairs, 14,* 181-191.

Ritz, L. J., Nissen, M. J., Swensen, K. K., Farrell, J. B., Sperduto, P. W., Sladek, M. L., et al. (2000). Effects of advanced nursing care on quality of life and cost outcomes of women diagnosed with breast cancer. *Oncology Nursing Forum, 27,* 923-932.

Rudy, E. B., Davidson, L. J., Daly, B., Clochesy, J. M., Sereika, S., Balderissi, M., et al. (1998). Care activities and outcomes of patients cared for by acute care nurse practitioners, physician assistants, and resident physicians: A comparison. *American Journal of Critical Care, 7,* 267-281.

Russell, D., VorderBruegge, M., & Burns, S. M. (2002). Effect of an outcomes-managed approach to care of neuroscience patients by acute care nurse practitioners. *American Journal of Critical Care, 11,* 353-364.

Ryden, M. B., Snyder, M., Gross, C. R., Savik, K., Pearson, V., Krichbaum, K., et al. (2000). Value-added outcomes: The use of advanced practice nurses in long-term care facilities. *The Gerontologist, 40,* 654-662.

Sakr, M., Angus, J., Perrin, J., Nixon, C., Nicholl, J., & Wardrope, J. (1999). Care of minor injuries by emergency nurse practitioners or junior doctors: A randomized controlled trial. *The Lancet, 354,* 1321-1326.

Sarkissian, S., & Wennberg, R. (1999). Effects of the acute care nurse practitioner role on epilepsy monitoring outcomes. *Outcomes Management for Nursing Practice, 3,* 161-166.

Saywell, R. M., Lassiter, W. L. III, & Flynn, B. C. (1995). A cost analysis of a nurse-managed, voluntary community health clinic. *Journal of Nursing Administration, 25*(10), 17-27.

Schaffner, R. J., & Bohomey, J. (1998). Demonstrating APN value in a capitated market. *Nursing Economics, 16*(10), 69-74.

Schultz, J. M., Liptak, G. S., & Fioravanti, S. (1994). Nurse practitioners' effectiveness in NICU. *Nursing Management, 25,* 50-53.

Scott, R. A. (1999). A description of the roles, activities, and skills of clinical nurse specialists in the United States. *Clinical Nurse Specialist, 13,* 183-190.

Sheahan, S. L. (2000). Documentation of health risks and health promotion counseling by emergency department nurse practitioners and physicians. *Journal of Nursing Scholarship, 32,* 245-250.

Shell, R. C. (2001). Antidepressant prescribing practices of nurse practitioners. *Nurse Practitioner, 26,* 42-47.

Sidani, S., Irvine, D., Porter, H., O'Brien-Pallas, L., Simpson, B., McGillis-Hall, L., et al. (2000). Practice patterns of acute care nurse practitioners. *Canadian Journal of Nursing Leadership, 13,* 6-12.

Small, R., Lumley, J., Donohue, L., Potter, A., & Waldenstrom, U. (2000). Randomised controlled trial of midwife led debriefing to reduce maternal depression after operative childbirth. *British Medical Journal, 321,* 1043-1047.

Smith, J. E., & Waltman, N. L. (1994). Oncology clinical nurse specialists' perceptions of their influence on patient outcomes. *Oncology Nursing Forum, 21,* 887-893.

Sohn, P. M., & Cook, C. A. L. (2002). Nurse practitioner knowledge of complementary alternative health care: Foundation for practice. *Journal of Advanced Nursing, 39,* 9-16.

Sole, M. L., Hunkar-Huie, A. M., Schiller, J. S., & Cheatham, M. L. (2001). Comprehensive trauma patient care by nonphysician providers. *AACN Clinical Issues, 12,* 438-446.

Stone, P. W., Zwanziger, J., Walker, P. H., & Buenting, J. (2000). Economic analysis of two models of low-risk maternity care: A freestanding birth center compared to traditional care. *Research in Nursing & Health, 23,* 279-289.

Stutts, A. (2001). Developing innovative care models: The use of customer satisfaction scores. *Journal of Nursing Administration, 31,* 293-300.

Sullivan-Marx, E. M., & Maislin, G. (2000). Comparison of nurse practitioner and family physician relative work values. *Journal of Nursing Scholarship, 32,* 71-76.

Sullivan-Marx, E. M., Happ, M. B., Bradley, K. J., & Maislin, G. (2000). Nurse practitioner services: Content and relative work value. *Nursing Outlook, 48,* 269-275.

Tijhuis, G. J., Zwinderman, A. H., Hazes, J. M. W., Breedveld, F. C., & Vlieland, P. M. T. (2003). Two-year follow-up of a randomized controlled trial of a clinical nurse specialist intervention, inpatient, and day patient team care in rheumatoid arthritis. *Journal of Advanced Nursing, 41,* 34-43.

Topp, R., Tucker, D., & Weber, C. (1998). Effect of a clinical case manager/clinical nurse specialist on patients hospitalized with congestive heart failure. *Nursing Case Management, 3,* 140-147.

Trotter, C., & Danaher, R. (1994). Neonatal nurse practitioners: A descriptive evaluation of an advanced practice role. *Neonatal Network, 13,* 39-47.

University of York, The. (1999). Effective health care. Getting evidence into practice. Retrieved September 26, 2003, from http://www.york.ac.uk/inst/crd/ehc51.pdf

Venning, P., Durie, A., Roland, M., Roberts, C., & Leese, B. (2000). Randomised controlled trial comparing cost effectiveness of general practitioners and nurse practitioners in primary care. *British Medical Journal, 320,* 1048-1053.

Way, D., Jones, L., Baskerville, B., & Busing, N. (2001). Primary health care services by nurse practitioners and family physicians in shared practice. *Canadian Medical Association Journal, 165,* 1210-1214.

Wheeler, D. J. (1993). *Understanding variation: The key to managing chaos.* Knoxville, TN: SPC Press.

Wheeler, E. C. (1999). The effect of the clinical nurse specialist on patient outcomes. *Critical Care Nursing Clinics of North America, 11,* 269-275.

Williams, D., & Sidani, S. (2001). An analysis of the nurse practitioner role in palliative care. *Canadian Journal of Nursing Leadership, 14,* 13-19.

Windorski, S. K., & Kalb, K. A. (2002). Educating NPs to educate patients: Cholesterol screening in pediatric primary care. *Journal of Pediatric Health Care, 16,* 60-66.

Wing, D. M., & Gay, G. (1990). Determining alcoholism treatment outcomes: A cost-effectiveness perspective. *Nursing Economics, 8,* 248-255.

Wojner, A. W. (1996). Outcomes management: An interdisciplinary search for best practice. *AACN Clinical Issues, 7,* 133-135.

Wojner, A. W., Rauch, P., & Mokracek, M. (1997). Collaborative ventures in outcomes management: Roles and responsibilities in a service line model. *Critical Care Nursing Quarterly, 19,* 25-41.

Wong, S. T., Stewart, A. L., & Gilliss, C. L. (2000). Evaluating advanced practice nursing through use of a heuristic framework. *Journal of Nursing Care Quality, 14,* 21-32.

Yankou, D., Petersen, B. A., Oakley, D., & Mayes, F. (1993). A pilot study comparing certified nurse-midwives and physicians. *Journal of Nurse Midwifery, 38,* 159-164.

York, R., Brown, L. P., Samuels, P., Finkler, S. A., Jacobsen, B., Persely, C. A., et al. (1997). A randomized trial of elderly discharge and nurse specialist transitional follow-up care for high-risk childbearing women. *Nursing Research, 46,* 254-261.

Zapka, J. G., Pbert, L., Stoddard, A. M., Ockene, J. K., Goins, K. V., & Bonollo, D. (2000). Smoking cessation counseling with pregnant and postpartum women: A survey of community health center providers. *American Journal of Public Health, 90,* 78-84.

Sample Employment Contract

EMPLOYMENT AGREEMENT (the "Agreement") made as of May 1, 2004, by and between EMPLOYER, INC., a Maine corporation with its principal place of business in Portland, Maine ("EMPLOYER") and EMPLOYEE, an individual resident of Portland, Maine (the "Employee").

1. **Purpose and Employment**. The purpose of this Agreement is to define the relationship between EMPLOYER and Employee. EMPLOYER hereby employs Employee, and Employee hereby accepts employment by EMPLOYER, upon all of the terms and conditions of this Agreement.

2. **Duties**

   2.1 Employee shall serve EMPLOYER by providing women's health services to EMPLOYER's clients, and shall further perform such similar duties as may be assigned to Employee from time to time by EMPLOYER. EMPLOYER anticipates that it will schedule Employee to work approximately sixteen (16) hours per week, with additional hours added according to practice demands and both parties mutual consent.

   2.2 Employee shall (i) devote Employee's attention and best efforts to the duties hereunder, including the promotion of the success of the business of EMPLOYER, (ii) perform such duties in a reasonable, prompt, honest and faithful manner. Only by mutual consent will 1) Employee accept work as a NP for another entity and 2) EMPLOYER hire an additional NP. (iii) not participate actively in any other business during the term of Employee's employment under this Agreement without EMPLOYER's consent.

   2.3 Employee acknowledges that Employee owes full loyalty to EMPLOYER, and shall not engage in any activity or enter into any transaction that would constitute a conflict of interest with the duties and loyalties owed to EMPLOYER.

   2.4 EMPLOYER is employing Employee based on Employee's representations that she is a licensed and certified R.N., M.S. and F.N.P. Employee shall, upon EMPLOYER's request, provide proof of such professional certifications. At Employee's sole expense, Employee shall also take any and all such steps (including, without limitation, timely acquisition of continuing education units) as are necessary to maintain said professional license throughout the term of this Agreement (and any extensions thereto).

3. **Contract at Will**

   3.1 The term of Employee's employment under this Agreement will commence on May 1, 2004 (the "Commencement Date") and continue through April 30, 2005 (the "Initial Term"). Either party may terminate this contract by giving written notice of no less than sixty days to the other of a desire to terminate. This agreement will automatically extend for twelve (12) month periods commencing on the first anniversary of the Commencement Date and each subsequent anniversary thereof. Unless either party gives written notice to the other of a desire not to extend the term of this Agreement at least sixty (60) days before the end of the Initial Term or any extension, the Agreement will automatically be extended for successive additional twelve (12) month periods commencing on the first anniversary of the Commencement Date and each subsequent anniversary thereof.

   3.2 Employee's employment under this Agreement may be terminated prior to the end of the Initial Term or any extension thereof as provided below:

   (a) upon the death of Employee, this Agreement will automatically terminate, and the only obligation EMPLOYER will have under this Agreement will be to pay Employee's personal representative, administrator or executor Employee's unpaid base salary through the date of Employee's death;

(b) EMPLOYER may terminate Employee's employment hereunder at any time without notice for cause. Upon such termination for cause, the only obligation EMPLOYER will have under this Agreement will be to pay Employee's unpaid base salary through the date of termination. For purposes of this Agreement, "for cause" shall mean:

  (i) Employee's disability;

  (ii) Breach of conduct as defined in the employee policy manual;

  (iii) any other conduct by Employee generally recognized under applicable laws as cause for termination;

  (iv) a sale of all or substantially all of the assets of Company;

  (v) a staff reduction or reorganization resulting in the elimination or substantial redefinition of Employee's position with EMPLOYER or

  (vi) a termination or substantial curtailment of the business of EMPLOYER within the area or division in which Employee works.

For purposes of this Agreement, "disability" shall mean any physical or mental condition which prevents Employee, after EMPLOYER has made such accommodations as may be required by law, from performing Employee's full duties to EMPLOYER for any cumulative period of three (3) months during any six (6) month period.

3.3 Notwithstanding the above, before terminating the employment of Employee for any of causes (iii) through (vi) above, EMPLOYER shall give Employee ten (10) days' written notice and an opportunity to cure, except that if the nature of Employee's conduct is such that EMPLOYER may be materially harmed if it so postpones terminating Employee's employment, then EMPLOYER need not give Employee an opportunity to cure and may terminate Employee's employment immediately.

4. **Compensation**. Employee shall be compensated at the rate of $35 per hour, payable weekly or in accordance with Company's payroll policies. EMPLOYER shall withhold state and federal taxes to the extent required by applicable law. Hourly compensation shall be subject to review at 6 months and then annually thereafter.

5. **Employee Benefit Plans; Fringe Benefits**. Employee shall be entitled to benefits as per EMPLOYER stated policies that hold for any other EMPLOYER employee.

6. **Expenses**. If EMPLOYER requires Employee to incur any travel, entertainment or similar expenditures for the benefit of the Practice during the term hereof, it will reimburse Employee for such expenditures on the basis of vouchers submitted by Employee which have been approved by Employee's supervisor. Employee is responsible for all expenses of her professional liability insurance. During the term of this Agreement (plus extensions thereto), Employee shall maintain professional liability insurance coverage and with coverage equal to or greater that of the other Nurse Practitioner.

7. **Property of Company**. All records, files, client lists, or plans, developed or created by Employee during the term of this Agreement, individually or in conjunction with others, which may directly or indirectly relate to the practice of EMPLOYER or any of its affiliates shall be the property of EMPLOYER.

8. **Restrictive Covenants**.

8.1 Nondisclosure. Employee acknowledges, covenants and agrees that:

(a) During employment by EMPLOYER under this Agreement, Employee has and will come to have knowledge and information with respect to confidential plans, projects, practice methods, operations, techniques, clients, client lists, employees, financial condition, policies and accounts of EMPLOYER and its affiliates with respect to their practice ("Confidential Information"),

(b) During the term of Employee's employment and for one (1) year, Employee will not divulge, furnish or make accessible to anyone (other than in the regular course of Employee's performance of services for the benefit of EMPLOYER, its successors, assigns and affiliates) any knowledge or information with respect to any Confidential Information, and

(c) All organizational or administrative papers and records, including all memoranda, notes, plans, data, or other documents, and any and all copies thereof, whether made by Employee or not, reasonably related to EMPLOYER's practices are the sole and exclusive property of EMPLOYER. Employee shall not remove from the Practice's premises any such written information concerning the Practice's business.

8.2 Solicitation. Employee agrees that at all times during the term of employment under this Agreement and for a period of twelve (12) months after the termination of employment with EMPLOYER under this Agreement or otherwise, Employee will not, directly or indirectly, for or on behalf of any other practice solicit, divert, take away or accept the medical records of any of the clients of EMPLOYER that were served by EMPLOYER during the term of employment or any prospective clients of EMPLOYER that EMPLOYER actively served within one (1) year prior to the termination of this Agreement for the purpose of selling the services provided by EMPLOYER during the term hereof to any such client or prospective client. Employee further agrees that Employee will not, within the foregoing period of time, directly or indirectly, attempt or seek to cause any of the foregoing clients of EMPLOYER to refrain from seeking care from EMPLOYER.

8.3 Interference with Employees. Employee agrees that during employment under this Agreement and for a period of twelve (12) months after the termination of Employee's employment with EMPLOYER under this Agreement or otherwise, Employee will not, directly or indirectly, for or on behalf of any other practice request or induce any other employee of EMPLOYER or its affiliates to terminate employment of such persons with EMPLOYER or its affiliates.

8.4 Remedy for Breach. The parties recognize that the services to be rendered under this Agreement by Employee are special, unique, and of an extraordinary character, and that in the event of a breach of this Agreement by Employee or EMPLOYER, then either party shall be entitled to institute and prosecute proceedings in any court of competent jurisdiction, either in law or in equity, to obtain damages, or to enforce the specific performance of any terms, conditions, obligations and requirements of this Agreement, or to enjoin the party who breached the Agreement from continuing those actions which cause a breach of this Agreement, or to take any or all of the foregoing actions. Nothing herein contained shall be construed to prevent the pursuit of any other remedy, judicial or otherwise, in case of any breach of this Agreement by either party.

8.5 Effect of Termination. Expiration of the term of Employee's employment under this Agreement or termination of Employee's employment either by EMPLOYER or Employee shall in no way limit or restrict Employee's obligations under this Section 8 which shall remain in full force and effect for the remaining periods set forth in such Section.

9. **Paragraph Headings**. Paragraph headings contained in this Agreement are for convenience only and shall in no manner be construed as a part of this Agreement.

10. **Amendment**. This Agreement may be amended or modified only in writing signed by both parties.

11. **Counterparts**. This Agreement may be executed in two or more counterparts each of which shall be deemed to be an original but all of which together shall constitute one and the same instrument.

12. **Waiver**. The failure of either party hereto in any one or more incidences to insist upon the performance of any of the terms or conditions of this Agreement, or to exercise any rights or privileges conferred in this Agreement, or the waiver of any breach of any of the terms of this Agreement shall not be construed as waiving any such terms and the same shall continue to remain in full force and effect as if no such forbearance or waiver had occurred.

13. **Applicable Law**. This Agreement shall be construed according to the laws of the State of Maine.

14. **Severability**. In the event any term of this Agreement shall be held invalid or unenforceable by any court of competent jurisdiction, such holding shall not invalidate or render unenforceable any other term contained in this Agreement.

15. **Entire Agreement**. This Agreement embodies the entire understanding of the parties with respect to Employee's employment with EMPLOYER and incorporates any previous agreement, written or oral, relating to such employment.

16. **Assignment and Successors**.
    16.1 Employee's rights under this Agreement shall not be assignable by Employee.
    16.2 This Agreement may be assigned by EMPLOYER and shall inure to the benefit of and be binding upon EMPLOYER, its successors and assigns.

17. **Mediation**. If a dispute arises under this Agreement which the parties are unable to resolve through direct negotiations, the parties agree to engage jointly the services of a professional mediator and to participate in good faith in such mediation. If the dispute is not resolved as a result of such mediation within thirty (30) days after such mediation is commenced or such longer period to which the parties may agree, each party shall be free to pursue any legal or equitable action as it considers appropriate.
    IN WITNESS WHEREOF, EMPLOYER has hereunto caused its corporate name to be signed and sealed, and Employee has hereunto set her hand, all being done in duplicate originals, with one original being delivered to each party as of the day and year first above written.

EMPLOYER, INC.

By: _____
EMPLOYER

_____
Employee

Sample Collaborative Practice Agreement

It is the intent of this document to authorize the nurse practitioner(s) at the _____ clinic(s) to practice under these protocols without direct supervision, as specified in the Medical Practice Act, Texas Civil Statutes, Article 4495b, section 3.06(d)(5) and (6). This document sets forth guidelines for collaboration between the supervising physician(s) and the nurse practitioner(s).

Development, Revision and Review

The protocols are developed collaboratively by the nurse practitioners, delegating medical director, and supervising physicians. These protocols will be reviewed annually and revised as necessary.

Approval

The protocols will be approved annually on the initial approval date by the nurse practitioners, medical director, and supervising physicians. The *Statement of Approval* will be signed by all the above parties recognizing the collegial relationship between the parties and their intention to follow these protocols. Signature on the Statement of Approval implies approval of all the policies, protocols and procedures in this document. Nurse practitioners and physicians who join the staff mid-year, or who cover the practice also signify approval of the protocols. It is the task of the medical director to see that the written approval of all the above parties is obtained.

Setting

The nurse practitioners will operate under these protocols at the (Name of Institution) clinics listed below:

Clinic 1: (name and address)
Clinic 2: (name and address)

Supervision

The nurse practitioners are authorized to practice under the protocols established in this document without the direct (on-site) supervision or approval of the supervising physicians. Consultation with the supervising physicians or their designated back-up, is available at all times, either on-site or by telephone when consultation is needed for any reason.

Consultation

The nurse practitioners are responsible for providing health services to clients of the (name of clinic or agency). The nurse practitioners will provide health promotion, screening, safety instructions, management of acute episodic illness and stable chronic diseases. Referrals will be made, as needed to other health care providers. Physician consultation will be sought for all of the following situations and any others deemed appropriate. Whenever a physician is consulted, a notation to that effect, including the physician's name must be recorded in the patient's medical record. Consultation will occur:

- Whenever situations arise that go beyond the intent of the protocols or the competence, scope of practice, or experience of the nurse practitioners.
- Whenever the patient's condition fails to respond to the management plan within an appropriate time frame, based on the provider's clinical judgment.
- For any uncommon, unfamiliar, or unstable patient condition.
- For any patient condition which does not fit the commonly accepted diagnostic pattern for a disease/condition.
- For any unexplained physical examination or historical finding or abnormal diagnostic finding.
- Whenever a patient requests.
- For all emergency situations after initial stabilizing care has been initiated.

Medical Records

The nurse practitioners are responsible for the complete, legible documentation of all patient encounters using the SOAP format.

Education and Training

The nurse practitioners must possess a valid Texas license as a Registered Nurse and be recognized by the Texas Board of Nurse Examiners as a Nurse Practitioner.

Evaluation of Clinical Care

Evaluation of the nurse practitioners will be provided in the following ways:

A minimum of a monthly review by the supervising physicians of a minimum of 10% of patient charts.

A written record of the review is to be kept.

Annual evaluation by the supervising physicians based on written criteria.

Informal evaluation during consultations and case review.

Periodic chart review a part of chart audits by the Quality Assurance Committee.

Practice Guidelines

The nurse practitioners are authorized to diagnose and treat common medical conditions under the following current guidelines (including, but not limited to): Barker, LR, Burton, JR & Zieve, PD. (1999). *Principles of Ambulatory Medicine* 5th Ed., Williams & Wilkins or comparable current edition of medical references available on-site at the respective clinics.

OR

Other published, accepted sources of medical information, as agreed upon by the collaborating parties and/or identified below:

- OSHA guidelines
- CDC guidelines for immunizations
- Uphold, CR & Graham, MV (1998). *Clinical Guidelines in Family Practice*, 3rd Ed. Gainesville, FL: Barmarrae Books, Inc.

Drug Prescriptions

Nurse practitioners at this facility shall be authorized to prescribe dangerous drugs (excluding, controlled substances) as authorized by the Texas Board of Nurse Examiners (BNE) under Rule 222, Advanced Practice Nurses Limited Prescriptive Authority and the Texas Board of Medical Examiners (BME) under Rules 193.2-193.4 and 193.8, Delegation of Prescriptive Authority. Authority shall be delegated by the Medical Director of the Methodist Health Care Ministries and supervision of prescribing activity shall be conducted by the Medical Director and supervising physicians as indicated in the Rules. It is the responsibility of the nurse practitioners to obtain prescription ID numbers from the appropriate Board. The Medical Director shall inform the BME, in writing, of his intent to delegate prescriptive authority as required in the Rules. References for prescriptions will be the current Physician's Desk Reference and/or the Nurse Practitioner/Physician Monthly or Quarterly Prescribing Guide. Additionally, there may be limitations placed on prescriptions to an approved formulary for the MHCM.

Collaborating Parties: Statement of Approval

We, the undersigned, agree to the terms of this Collaborative Practice Agreement as set forth in this document.

_____ Medical Director

_____ Supervising Physician

_____ Supervising Physician

_____ Supervising Physician

_____ Nurse Practitioner

_____ Nurse Practitioner

_____ Nurse Practitioner

Approval Date _____

Renewal Date _____

Renewal Date _____

NOTE: This is an example of a broad collaborative practice agreement. Permission is given to download, copy or modify. Each state will have different board of nursing or public health code rules and regulations that will need to be identified in the wording.
Copyright: Judith C.D. Longworth, 1998, 2001

INDEX

A

AANA. *See* American Association of Nurse Anesthetists

AANM. *See* American Association of Nurse-Midwives

AANP. *See* American Academy of Nurse Practitioners

ABC Coding Systems for Third Party Billing, 731

Abortion, legalization of, 26

Academic Center of Evidence-Based Nursing, website of, 264

Accommodation in resolution of ethical conflict, 401

Accountability, 784
  patient, 424

Accreditation, 787-788
  APN, websites for, 796b, 841b
  collaborative practice and, 353

Acetaminophen overdose, consultation for, 244

ACNM. *See* American College of Nurse-Midwives

ACNP. *See* Acute care nurse practitioners

Active listening, indications for, 165

Activism, political
  by APN case manager, 652-653
  leadership in, 313, 321-323
  and regulatory process, 805-806

Activities of daily living, outcome indicator studies of, 904t

Acute care by APN case managers, 635-637

Acute care hospitals, comparative performance and benchmarking data resources for, 925t

Acute care nurse practitioners, 35-36, 475-514
  advanced degrees held by, 509
  versus blended role advanced practice nurses, 536
  in bone marrow transplantation service, 502
  case management by, 495
  certification of, 482
  challenges for, 507-509
  in collaborative practice, 494-495
  competencies of, 487-495
  core competencies of, 487
  in critical care, reimbursement for, 507
  in diagnosis/management of disease, 488, 489b-490b, 490-491
  diagnostic skills of, 496
  in diagnostic/interventional services, 502
  in direct clinical practice, 488
  education of, 503-504
  in ethical decision making, 495
  in heart failure services, 502-503
  history of, 477-478
  implementation examples, 500-503

Acute care nurse practitioners (*Continued*)
  individualization by, 487
  institutional employers of, 483-486
  job description of, 484b-485b
  Medicare coverage of, 505-507
  in orthopedic services, 503
  outcome studies of, 895-896
  physician collaboration with, 486, 499
  professional organizations of, 479-482
  profile of, 495-500
  in promoting health/preventing disease, 491, 493
  reimbursement for, 505
  relationships with physicians, 508
  roles of, 851
    versus other APNs and physician assistants, 497-499
  scope of employment of, 483-485
  scope of practice for, 478-487
  service-related scope of practice of, 486-487
  settings for, 495
  in specialty care settings, 496
  specialty competencies of, 488-495
  state regulation of, 482-483

Administrative Case Management Certification, 669, 671

Administrators, pressures on, 849, 849t

Admissions, inpatient, per 1000 covered lives, calculation of, 663

Advance directives, ethical dilemmas involving, 383, 405-406

Advanced Billing Concept, 169

Advanced diabetes managers, 693-695
  multidisciplinary approach of, 694

Advanced practice nurse case management
  billing methods in, 668
  business aspects of, 661
  competencies and care management strategies in, 660f
  indirect costs of, 667
  marketing of, 668
  organizational structures/cultures in, 661-662
  productivity/acuity of, 666-667
  shared accountability for utilization in, 662-666

Advanced practice nurse case managers, 5, 617-675
  in acute care complication management, 635-637
  versus blended role advanced practice nurses, 536
  certification/credentialing requirements for, 668-669, 670t, 671
  in chronic care management, 637
  in coaching/guidance, 646t, 648-649
  competencies of, 645-660
  in consultation/collaboration, 646t, 649

953